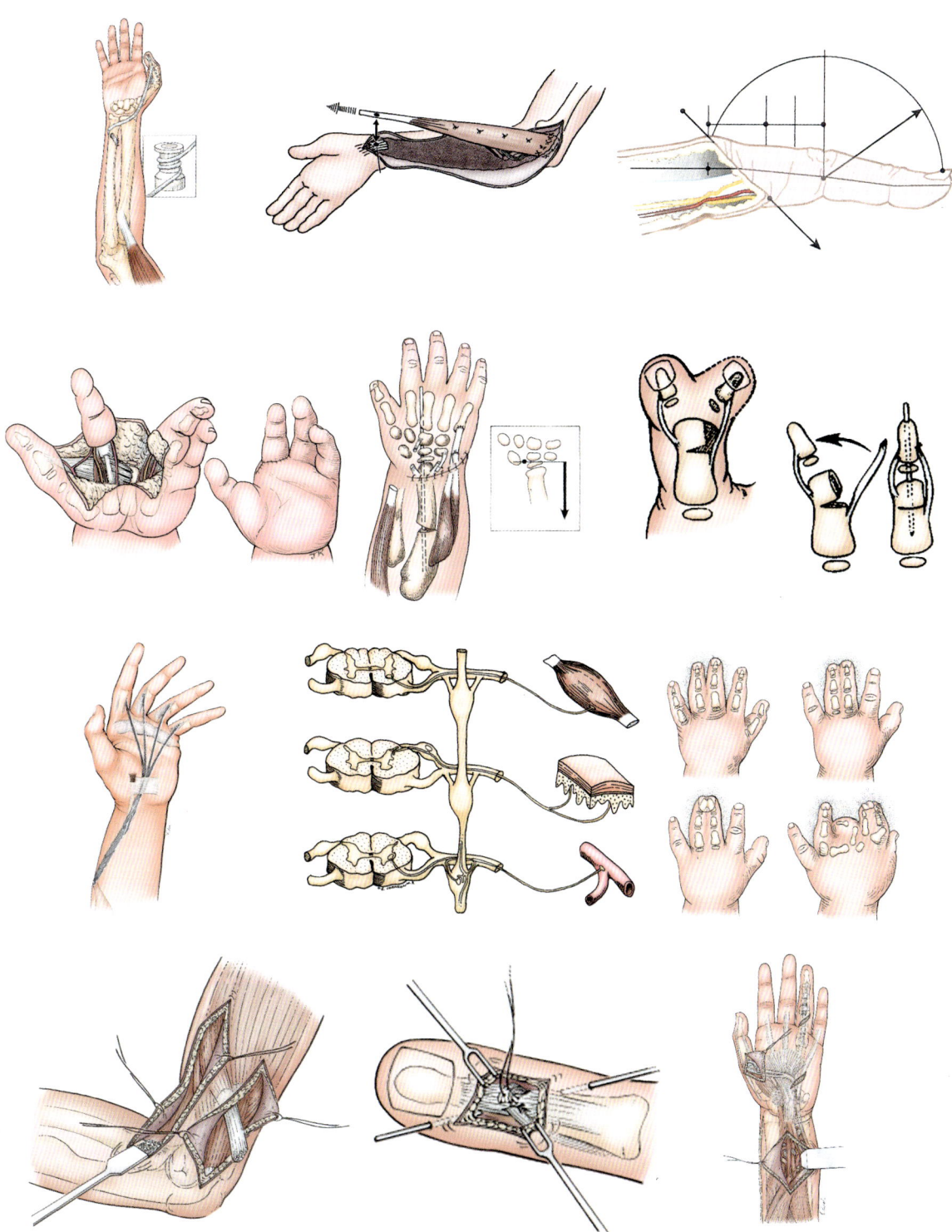

Plastic Surgery

Plastic Surgery

First Edition

Editor:
Joseph G. McCarthy, MD

Editors, Hand Surgery volumes:
James W. May, Jr., MD
J. William Littler, MD

Plastic Surgery

Second Edition

Editor
Stephen J. Mathes, MD
Professor of Surgery
Chief, Division of Plastic Surgery
University of California, San Francisco
School of Medicine
San Francisco, California

Editor, Hand Surgery Volumes
Vincent R. Hentz, MD
Professor of Surgery
Chief, Division of Plastic and Hand Surgery
Stanford University School of Medicine
Stanford, California

With illustrations by Kathy Hirsh and Scott Thorn Barrows, CMI, FAMI

Shireen L. Dunwoody, Editorial Coordinator

VOLUME *VIII*

THE HAND AND UPPER LIMB, PART 2

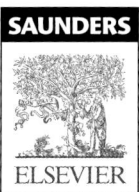

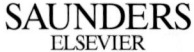

SAUNDERS
ELSEVIER

1600 John F. Kennedy Blvd.
Ste 1800
Philadelphia, PA 19103-2899

PLASTIC SURGERY, 2nd ed.

Volume I 0-7216-8812-8/978-0-7216-8812-1
Volume II 0-7216-8813-6/978-0-7216-8813-8
Volume III 0-7216-8814-4/978-0-7216-8814-5
Volume IV 0-7216-8815-2/978-0-7216-8815-2
Volume V 0-7216-8816-0/978-0-7216-8816-9
Volume VI 0-7216-8817-9/978-0-7216-8817-6
Volume VII 0-7216-8818-7/978-0-7216-8818-3
Volume VIII 0-7216-8819-5/978-0-7216-8819-0
8-Volume Set 0-7216-8811-X/978-0-7216-8811-4

Notice

Knowledge and best practice in this field are constantly changing. As new research and experience broaden our knowledge, changes in practice, treatment and drug therapy may become necessary or appropriate. Readers are advised to check the most current information provided (i) on procedures featured or (ii) by the manufacturer of each product to be administered, to verify the recommended dose or formula, the method and duration of administration, and contraindications. It is the responsibility of the practitioner, relying on his or her own experience and knowledge of the patient, to make diagnoses, to determine dosages and the best treatment for each individual patient, and to take all appropriate safety precautions. To the fullest extent of the law, neither the Publisher nor the Editors assume any liability for any injury and/or damage to persons or property arising out of or related to any use of the material contained in this book.

The Publisher

Previous edition copyrighted 1990.

Library of Congress Cataloging-in-Publication Data
Mathes, Stephen J.
    Plastic surgery / Stephen J. Mathes ; editor Vincent R. Hentz.—2nd ed.
      p. cm.
    ISBN 0–7216–8811–X
    1. Surgery, Plastic. I. Hentz, Vincent R.   II. Title.
RD118.M388 2006
617.9′5—dc21

2003041541

Acquisitions Editors: Sue Hodgson, Allan Ross, Joe Rusko, Judith Fletcher
Senior Developmental Editor: Ann Ruzycka Anderson
Publishing Services Manager: Tina Rebane
Senior Project Manager: Linda Van Pelt
Design Direction: Steven Stave
Cover Designer: Shireen Dunwoody

Printed in China

Last digit is the print number: 9 8 7 6 5 4 3 2 1

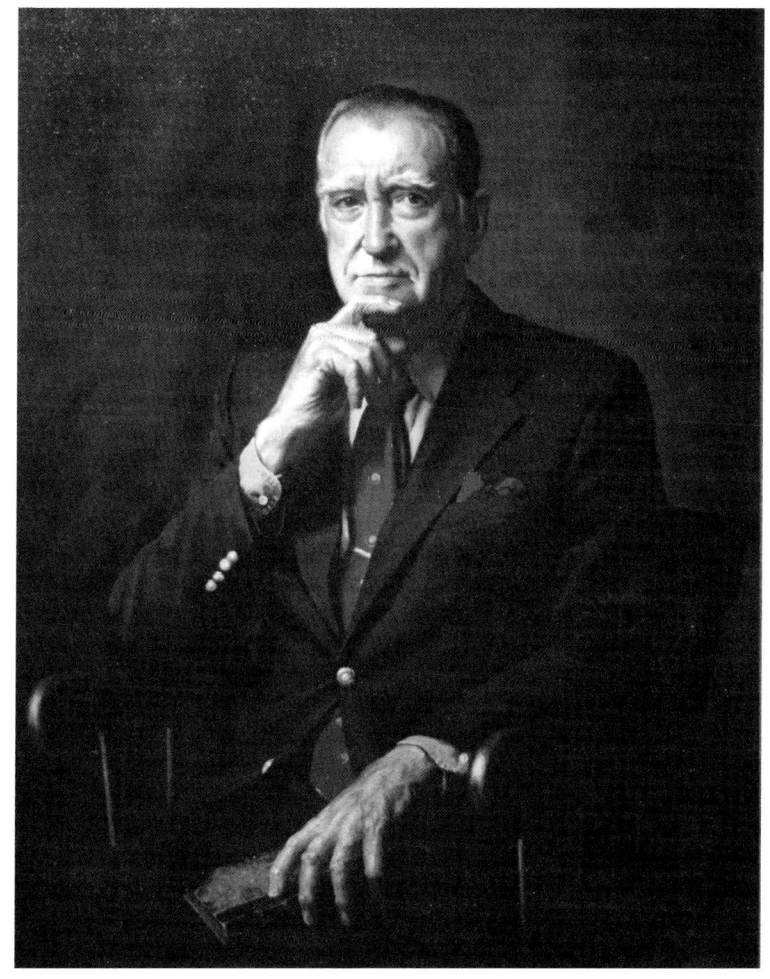

Portrait by Richard Whitney

J. William Littler, MD

Born: Manlius, New York, October 7, 1915; died: Providence, Rhode Island, February 27, 2005.

Volumes VII and VIII, the two hand volumes, are dedicated to Dr. J. William Littler. Innovator, educator, artist, master surgical craftsman, and Renaissance man, he lived and loved life to the fullest.

✦ CONTRIBUTORS

LOREN J. BORUD, MD
Instructor
Harvard Medical School
Attending Surgeon
Beth Israel–Deaconess Medical Center
Boston, Massachusetts

JOHN M. EGGLESTON III, MD
Assistant Professor of Hand Surgery
Department of Plastic and Reconstructive Surgery
Johns Hopkins University School of Medicine
Attending Surgeon
Johns Hopkins Hospital and Johns Hopkins Bayview
    Medical Center
Baltimore, Maryland

ALAIN GILBERT, MD
Associate Professor of Orthopedics
University of Saint-Antoine Paris Faculty of Medicine
Director
Institut de la Main
Paris, France

CAROLYN GORDON, OHT, CHT
Clinical Hand Therapist
Stanford University Hospitals and Clinics
Rehabilitation Services
Stanford, California

EDWARD J. HARVEY, MD, MSc
Assistant Professor of Surgery
McGill University Faculty of Medicine
Head of Hand and Microvascular Surgery
Chief, Orthopaedic Trauma
Medical Director
Bone/Fracture Metabolism
McGill University Health Center
Montreal, Quebec, Canada

VINCENT R. HENTZ, MD, FACS
Professor and Chief
Division of Plastic and Hand Surgery
Department of Surgery
Stanford University School of Medicine
Director, Robert A. Chase Hand and Upper Limb Center
Stanford University Hospital and Clinics
Stanford, California
Chief, Hand Surgery Center
Veterans Affairs Palo Alto Health Care System
Palo Alto, California

JAMES HOUSE, MD, MS
Professor Emeritus of Orthopaedic Surgery
University of Minnesota Medical School–Minneapolis
Minneapolis, Minnesota
Staff Physician
Gillette Childrens Specialtycare
St. Paul, Minnesota

NEIL F. JONES, MD, FRCS
Professor, Division of Plastic and Reconstructive Surgery
Professor, Department of Orthopaedic Surgery
David Geffen School of Medicine at the University of
    California, Los Angeles (UCLA)
Chief, Hand Surgery
UCLA Medical Center
Los Angeles, California

**KAYVAN T. KHIABINI, MD, MSc,
FRCS(C), FACS**
Assistant Professor of Surgery
Division of Plastic Surgery
University of Nevada School of Medicine
Head, Section of Hand and Microsurgery
University of Nevada Patient Care Center
Las Vegas, Nevada

AMY L. LADD, MD
Professor of Surgery
Department of Orthopaedic Surgery
Stanford University School of Medicine
Staff, Robert A. Chase Hand and Upper Limb Center
Stanford, California
Chief, Hand Clinic
Lucile Packard Children's Hospital at Stanford
Palo Alto, California

PREM LALWANI, OTR, CHT
Clinical Hand Therapist
Stanford University Hospitals and Clinics
Rehabilitation Services
Stanford, California

DONNA LASHGARI, OTR, CHT
Clinical Hand Therapist
Stanford University Hospitals and Clinics
Rehabilitation Services
Stanford, California

MAURICE LeBLANC, MSME, CP
Lecturer
Biomechanical Engineering Department
Stanford University School of Medicine
Stanford, California

L. SCOTT LEVIN, MD, FACS
Professor of Plastic and Orthopaedic Surgery
Duke University School of Medicine
Chief, Division of Plastic, Reconstructive, Maxillofacial
    and Oral Surgery
Duke University Medical Center
Durham, North Carolina

RALPH T. MANKTELOW, MD, FRCS(C)
Professor of Surgery
University of Toronto Faculty of Medicine
Staff Surgery
Division of Plastic Surgery
Toronto General Hospital
Toronto, Ontario, Canada

JENNIFER J. MARLER, MD
Assistant Professor of Surgery
Division of Plastic Surgery
University of Cincinnati College of Medicine
Pediatric Surgeon
Cincinnati Children's Hospital Medical Center
Cincinnati, Ohio

TIMOTHY R. McADAMS, MD
Assistant Professor of Surgery
Department of Orthopaedic Surgery
Stanford University School of Medicine
Staff
Robert A. Chase Hand and Upper Limb Center
Stanford University Hospital
Stanford, California

ANNIE DIDIER-JEAN PILLET, MD
Private Practice
Pillet Hand Prostheses, Ltd.
New York, New York

JEAN PILLET III, MD
Private Practice
Pillet Hand Prostheses, Ltd.
New York, New York

GERALD STARK, BSME, CP, FAAOP
Guest Lecturer
Northwestern University Prosthetic-Orthotic Center
Chicago, Illinois
Director of Education and Technical Support
Fillauer, Inc.
Chattanooga, Tennessee

JOSEPH UPTON III, MD
Associate Clinical Professor of Surgery
Harvard Medical School
Attending Surgeon
Children's Hospital, Beth Israel–Deaconess Medical
    Center, and Shriners Burns Hospital
Boston, Massachusetts

ANN VAN HEEST, MD
Associate Professor of Orthopaedic Surgery
University of Minnesota Medical School–Minneapolis
Minneapolis, Minnesota
Staff Physician
Shriners Hospital for Children—Twin Cities Unit
Minneapolis, Minnesota
Gillette Children's Specialtycare
St. Paul, Minnesota

RONALD M. ZUKER, MD, FRCS(C), FACS
Professor of Surgery
University of Toronto Faculty of Medicine
Staff Plastic Surgeon
The Hospital for Sick Children
Toronto, Ontario, Canada

✦ PREFACE

It is a great thing to start life with a small number of really good books which are your very own. Through the Magic Door (1908), Sir Arthur Conan Doyle

My meeting for lunch with Joseph McCarthy in Boston in 1998 during the annual meeting of the Society of Plastic Surgery was arranged to discuss the possibility of my becoming the editor of the new edition of *Plastic Surgery.* I was well aware of the responsibility of assuming this giant project. My admiration of the past editors, including Joseph McCarthy for the 1990 edition of *Plastic Surgery* and John Marquis Converse for the 1964 and 1977 editions of *Reconstructive Plastic Surgery,* was great since these texts in my estimation really defined our specialty of plastic surgery and provided the platform for future advances in treating congenital and acquired deformities. My memory of Converse's first edition started with my residency in plastic surgery on my first rotation at the private practice of William Schatten, John Hartley, and John Griffith in Atlanta, Georgia. There, in moments when I was not involved in patient care activities, I would enjoy reading the pages of clinical advice on all subjects related to plastic surgery in the five volumes of *Reconstructive Plastic Surgery.* Subsequently, in 1977, as a faculty member at Washington University, I was privileged to be able to purchase my own copy of the then six-volume edition of *Reconstructive Plastic Surgery,* again edited by Converse. This time, my reading of the exciting pages was less relaxed, since I was using the text as the reference in preparation for my plastic surgery board examinations.

By 1990, I was able to contribute a chapter to *Plastic Surgery,* edited by Joseph McCarthy, and I personally knew most of the contributors, having witnessed the evolution of many of the new advances and unique contributions contained within the then eight volumes. With this background, I was excited and honored to have been recommended as the next editor of this text, which has so well reflected the greatness of the specialty of plastic surgery. My meeting was punctuated by advice regarding the importance of the text and the selection of experts who would provide both guidance and stimulation to future readers on the many subjects important to physicians involved in plastic surgery. The complexity of orchestrating so many contributors in a timely fashion was also emphasized. I left this luncheon inspired to undertake this project, with the anticipation of capturing the best and most innovative surgeons as contributors to achieve an edition in keeping with the unique traditions of excellence of the past editions of *Plastic Surgery* and *Reconstructive Plastic Surgery.*

My first step was to find an academic hand surgeon to edit the two hand volumes. J. William Littler had served as the editor of the hand and upper extremity volume in Converse's two editions of *Reconstructive Plastic Surgery.* Littler was a master hand surgeon and one of the foremost innovators in hand surgery. McCarthy selected a unique combination of academic hand surgeons, James W. May and J. William Littler, to edit the two volumes dedicated to upper extremity and hand surgery in the 1990 edition of *Plastic Surgery.* With the many new techniques related to microvascular surgery, the space devoted to this important aspect of plastic surgery had been expanded into two volumes. Jim May, like Bill Littler, is a master hand surgeon, a gifted teacher, and an innovator in all aspects of plastic surgery and was able to include both his contributions and those of many other hand surgeons, who all took part in advancing this important discipline.

Fortunately, the decision regarding who should be the hand editor for this edition of *Plastic Surgery* was obvious. Vincent R. Hentz is a master hand surgeon and past president of the American Society of Surgery of the Hand. As an accomplished educator and chief of the division of plastic and hand surgery at Stanford, he is the ideal person to follow in the footsteps of Littler and May. In keeping with the many innovations and new techniques in upper extremity and hand surgery, this edition contains two volumes devoted to hand surgery. Of interest, we have shifted the editorial geography from the East Coast (New York City and Boston) to the West Coast (San Francisco and Palo Alto). Unfortunately, despite the improvement in weather characteristics of the western coastline of the United States, the commitment to continue the excellence of this text has kept the editors mostly indoors during the complex editing process necessary to complete these volumes.

The goal of this edition is to cover the scope of plastic surgery. The key was to select the best contributors to define the problems encountered in plastic surgery, to provide both the most current and the most successful solutions, and to deliver the challenge for future innovation in each area of plastic surgery. In this new edition, there are 219 chapters with 293 contributors. Each of the senior authors of the 219 chapters was carefully selected for his or her recognized expertise in the assigned subject of the chapter. Each author has personally contributed to the advancement in knowledge related to his or her area of expertise in our specialty.

The authors selected are inspirational leaders due to their many innovations toward improvement in the management of the plastic surgery patient. After the manuscripts were submitted, each chapter was carefully reviewed by the editors to ensure that all aspects of the authors' assigned topics were adequately covered and well illustrated so that the reader could readily incorporate the chapter content into the practice of plastic surgery.

In the eight volumes included in this edition, all subjects pertinent to the scope of plastic surgery are covered. Many new topics, 67 in all, have been developed or were enlarged from broader subjects and warranted a new individual chapter. Thirteen of these new chapter topics are included in Volume I: General Principles. The enlargement of the volume containing general principles reflects the continuing expansion of our specialty, the emphasis on experimental and clinical research, and the impact of research on the practice of plastic surgery. In the remaining volumes, devoted to specific clinical topics, two new types of chapter formats were added: 25 technique chapters and 7 secondary chapters. The technique chapters are added to complement the overview chapters and are designed to focus on particular techniques currently in use for a clinical problem. Likewise, the secondary chapters are again an extension of the overview chapters on particular subjects but focus on problems that persist despite the application of primary plastic surgery solutions. These secondary chapters are designed to demonstrate areas where operations may fail related to improper patient or technique selection or technique failures. They also discuss procedures to correct unsatisfactory outcomes following primary plastic surgery.

Volumes II through VII are divided into specific topographical areas of plastic surgery. Volume II: The Head and Neck (Part 1) is devoted to cosmetic procedures and contains six new topic chapters, seven new technique chapters, and three new secondary chapters. This volume now contains color illustrations, which will help the reader evaluate problems and results following cosmetic procedures. Many important subjects are expanded and introduced. For instance, there are now five chapters on the face lift, which provide the reader with the ability to compare techniques and focus on specific aspects of the procedure. Volume III: The Head and Neck (Part 2) is dedicated to reconstructive procedures and contains 10 new topics as well as the traditional subjects used in the previous edition. Volume IV: Pediatric Plastic Surgery contains five new topics and provides multispecialty approaches to children presenting with congenital facial anomalies. Volume V: Tumors of the Head, Neck, and Skin has seven new topics. Along with management principles of head and neck cancer, identification and treatment of melanoma and non-melanoma skin cancer have been added in new topic chapters. Volume VI: Trunk and Lower Extremity contains 34 added topics. For example, in the area of postmastectomy reconstruction, 12 new chapters have been added to provide specific diagnostic, management, and technical information on breast reconstruction issues. Similarly, four new chapter topics have been added on body contouring procedures. With emphasis on bariatric surgery and body contouring procedures, these chapters provide a complete array of information on techniques and outcomes. Volume VII: The Hand and Upper Limb (Part 1) contains introductory and general principles related to diagnosis and management of acquired disorders, both traumatic and nontraumatic. Volume VIII: The Hand and Upper Limb (Part 2) contains three parts: congenital anomalies, paralytic disorders, and rehabilitation. The two volumes on hand and upper extremity surgery contain an additional 22 chapters introducing new subjects to this edition of *Plastic Surgery*.

Education involves the process of observation as well as contact with teachers, mentors, colleagues, and students and the literature. Each component is essential to learning a specialty in medicine and maintaining competence in the specialty over the course of one's career. In plastic surgery, the abundance of master surgeons gives everyone the opportunity to observe excellence in technique, during residency and later through educational programs. Contact with teachers and colleagues must be maintained in order to keep abreast of the new innovations in medicine and to measure one's outcomes in the context of standard of care. Our professional society meetings and symposia, both locally and nationally, provide us with this opportunity. Contact with mentors and students is critical for innovation. The physician must seek out these sources of inspiration and stimulation to improve patient care. Collaboration with professionals is a unique opportunity to allow further growth in our specialty and is available in every medical environment. The literature allows the physician to see where we have been, where we are currently, and what the future holds. The physician can hold a piece of literature in the hand and review its message both in critical times, when patient management decisions must be made on a timely basis, and during leisure times, when a subject is studied and carefully measured against personal experience and knowledge acquired through professional contacts. It is hoped that this edition of *Plastic Surgery*, like its predecessors, can serve the purpose of literature in teaching. Its eight volumes contain more than 6800 pages of information carefully formulated by recognized experts in our specialty in plastic surgery. It is designed, as initially stated, to define the current knowledge of plastic surgery and to serve as a platform for future creativity to benefit the patient we see with congenital and acquired deformities.

Stephen J. Mathes, MD, 2005

✦ ACKNOWLEDGMENTS

So many talented and dedicated professionals are necessary to complete a text of this magnitude. It is impossible to really thank everyone adequately, since there are so many people behind the scenes who were silently working toward the completion of this project. However, I shall endeavor to acknowledge the people who provided scientific, technical, and emotional support to make this edition of *Plastic Surgery* possible.

My first contact with the publisher (Saunders, now Elsevier) started with my meeting with Allan Ross and Ann Ruzycka Anderson. Allan Ross, executive editor, was assigned to guide this text to publication. He is a dedicated publishing executive who was most supportive at the inception of this project. Ann Ruzycka Anderson, senior developmental editor, has been working in medical publishing for 20 years. This text was most fortunate to have Allan and Ann assigned as the guiding forces at the onset. Ann states that working on this text is "something exciting, worthwhile, and important" because she is helping to "produce the largest book in medical publishing history."

Because this book took 5 years to complete, there were changes in the personnel involved in the project. Joe Rusko, medical editor, assumed the responsibilities of guiding the development of the text, with Allan Ross taking on the role of consultant. Joe has great enthusiasm and provided great ideas for the format of this book and for associated advertising. During the past year, the project was turned over to the leadership of Sue Hodgson, currently the publishing director and general manager for Elsevier Ltd. With Sue living in London, the project took on a more international outlook, with Sue flying between London, Philadelphia, New York, and San Francisco to keep the project moving ahead to completion. Both Sue Hodgson and Allan Ross have a great deal of success in guiding complex publications to press. Sue has published highly successful books in dermatology, and now, it is hoped, she will be able to make the same claim for the field of plastic surgery. For sure, she can now lay claim to publishing the largest medical book in existence. Recently, Sue Hodgson summed up her role in the publishing industry as follows: "The opportunity to create new products to answer the market's educational needs and handling high-profile and demanding projects are what get me out of bed in the morning." All plastic surgeons who use this text are indebted to the perseverance and commitment of these publishing leaders: Allan Ross, Joe Rusko, and Sue Hodgson.

"The quality of a person's life is in direct proportion to their commitment to excellence, regardless of their chosen field of endeavor."

—Vince Lombardi

After the authors were selected for the 219 chapters, it was obvious that we needed someone special to serve as the editorial coordinator between the editors and the authors. Thanks to the advice of Allan Ross and Ann Ruzycka Anderson, Shireen Dunwoody was recommended for this position. Shireen is an accomplished computer programmer and musician and has served as a senior medical writer, media programmer/editor, and developmental editor since 1991. Among the high-profile medical texts on which she has worked are *Clinical Oncology* (Martin Abeloff et al., editors), *Surgery of the Liver and Biliary Tract* (Leslie Blumgart, editor), and *Fundamentals of Surgery* (John E. Niederhuber, editor). Shireen has worked closely with the editors and our assigned authors during every step of the process—obtaining the manuscripts (including a multitude of meetings and phone calls with authors), helping find artists when needed, confirming references, discovering historical information as related to the many subjects covered in *Plastic Surgery*, and coordinating all these data with the publishing staff in Philadelphia and New York. When asked to describe what this job was like, she described the process as follows: "At times, this project has been a struggle, but most of the time it has been a joy (kind of like raising eight children). On any given day, working on this project has given me a reason to (1) get up in the morning; (2) stay up all night; (3) despise the morning; (4) stay sober; (5) get drunk; (6) laugh; (7) cry; (8) live; (9) lie; (10) rejoice. Who could ask for anything more? It has certainly kept things interesting!" Shireen credits special members of the publishing staff for helping this immense project move ahead at a fairly steady pace. In Philadelphia, Linda Van Pelt, senior project manager, book production, and RoseMarie Klimowicz, freelance copyeditor, have been with this project since its inception. They have both dedicated vast amounts of blood, sweat, tears, and personal time. Ann Ruzycka Anderson has been dedicated to this project since the onset and has also worked closely with Shireen. Judy Fletcher, publishing director, provided the support needed for timely layouts and served as an advocate for this project even when layout or illustrations were changed to maintain the continuity and artistry of the chapters. Finally, Shireen acknowledges her two amazing assistants in Palm Springs, California, Donna Larson and Carla Parnell, who have helped her scan, copy, crop, sort, mail, and stay sane. Without the dedication and brilliance of Shireen Dunwoody in bringing out the best in the editors, publishers, authors, and artists, this text would not have the quality and completeness it now possesses.

My immediate family was always supportive of this project despite the time-consuming work associated with text preparation. I wish to acknowledge and thank my family for their exciting accomplishments, which are a source of pride and enjoyment: Mary, Norma, Paul, Leslie, Isabelle, Peter, David, Brian, Vasso, Zoe, Ned, Erin, Maggie, and Rick.

In any profession, the support and encouragement of one's colleagues are essential for productivity. I wish to thank the faculty in our division of plastic surgery for their specific contributions to the text and their active roles as outstanding teachers for our residents and students at the University of California in San Francisco. The faculty, both full time and clinical, include the following: Bernard Alpert, Jim Anthony, Ramin Behmand, Kyle Bickel, Greg Buncke, K. Ning Chang, Tancredi D'Amore, Keith Denkler, Issa Eschima, Robert Foster, Roger Friedenthal, Gilbert Gradinger, Ronald Gruber, William Hoffman, Clyde Ikeda, Gabriel Kind, Chen Lee, Pablo Leon, Mahesh Mankani, Robert Markeson, Mary McGrath, Sean Moloney, Douglas Ousterhout, John Owsley, Lorne Rosenfield, Vivian Ting, Bryant Toth, Philip Trabulsy, D. Miller Wise, and David Young.

During the time span in which this book was edited, a group of outstanding residents completed their plastic surgery residencies at UCSF. All these residents contributed to both the care of many of the patients included in the chapters written by our faculty and the development of concepts used in the chapters of this edition. Each resident listed has contributed to the advancement of our knowledge in plastic surgery: Delora Mount, Richard Grossman, Jeff Roth, Laura McMillan, Kenneth Bermudez, Marga Massey, Yngvar Hvistendahl, Duc Bui, Te Ning Chang, Hatem Abou-Sayed, Farzad Nahai, Hop Nguyen Le, Clara Lee, Scott Hansen, Jennifer Newman-Keagle, and Wesley Schooler. General surgery residents, research fellows, and students who participated in the project include Lee Alkureishi, Julie Lang, Edward Miranda, and Cristiane Ueno.

Without the dedication of our staff, the preparation of this text would not have been possible. Crystal Munoz served as our office manager during most of the preparation time. My patient coordinators, Marian Liebow and, later, Skye Ingham, are patient advocates and made the arrangements necessary to treat the patients discussed in our chapters. Our nurses, Janet Tanaka and, later, Ann Hutchinson, were essential to the overall care of patients presenting to our clinical practice. Our staff provides the support needed to allow the faculty to have the time necessary to participate in the creative activities expected in academic plastic surgery.

Plastic surgeons depend on visual assessment of problems; thus, illustrations are an essential part of our scientific literature. Numerous artists were involved in the chapters selected by the individual authors. However, two artists were available to all the contributors and provided outstanding art to accompany many of the chapters. Kathy Hirsh, located in Shanghai, China, and Scott Barrows, in Chicago, have worked diligently to provide accurate artistic interpretations of the surgical procedures recommended throughout this text.

"Mental toughness is many things. It is humility because it behooves all of us to remember that simplicity is the sign of greatness and meekness is the sign of true strength. Mental toughness is spartanism with qualities of sacrifice, self-denial, dedication. It is fearlessness, and it is love."

—Vince Lombardi

All the authors who contributed to these volumes exemplify mental toughness. To complete a chapter for a text is often considered an unappreciated task. However, thanks to the great reputation established by the prior editors of this comprehensive work, John M. Converse and Joseph G. McCarthy, and the previous editors of the hand volumes, William Littler and James May, the top plastic surgeons in their respective fields have given their time and efforts to maintain the excellence associated with past editions of this text. Thanks to these contributors, this book provides information at the forefront of innovation and current practice in the specialty of plastic surgery. The contributors and their families are thanked for their perseverance and sacrifice in the completion of these chapters and for their dedication to our specialty, plastic surgery.

SJM

✦ CONTENTS

✦ VOLUME II

The Head and Neck, Part 1

◆ VOLUME III

THE HEAD AND NECK, PART 2

✦ VOLUME IV

Pediatric Plastic Surgery

◆ VOLUME VII

The Hand and Upper Limb, Part 1

INTRODUCTION AND GENERAL PRINCIPLES 1

ACQUIRED DISORDERS—TRAUMATIC 151

♦ VOLUME VIII

The Hand and Upper Limb, Part 2

THE HAND AND UPPER LIMB: CONGENITAL ANOMALIES 1

PARALYTIC DISORDERS 451

REHABILITATION 555

The Hand and Upper Limb

Congenital Anomalies

Embryology of the Upper Limb

LOREN J. BORUD, MD ✦ JOSEPH UPTON III, MD

MORPHOLOGIC DEVELOPMENT
DEVELOPMENT OF SPECIFIC TISSUES
    Skeletal Development
    Arterial Development
    Neural Development
    Muscle Development
MOLECULAR BIOLOGY OF LIMB DEVELOPMENT
    Classic Model
    The Three Dimensions

MOLECULAR BASIS OF HUMAN UPPER EXTREMITY
DISORDERS
    Apert Syndrome
    Pfeiffer Syndrome
    Central Synpolydactyly
    Postaxial Polydactyly

Embryology, the study of the formation and development of organisms, is essentially the story of life. As such, it has been inextricably linked not only to science but also to theology, mythology, philosophy, and politics. Although there are records of primitive peoples, such as the Assyrians and ancient Egyptians, speculating about the reproduction of humans,[1] the most serious and long-lived theories in the Western world originated with Aristotle, who is credited with the first text on embryology, a five-volume compendium.[2] Other ancient Greek intellectuals shared his fascination and spent considerable effort postulating on the growth, development, and reproduction of the human organism. Since Aristotle's death in 322 BC, human reproduction and embryology have continued to be topics of great interest among philosophers, scientists, and political theorists—and even modern-day politicians and religious leaders. One of the more interesting and thorough discussions of historical theories of embryology can be found in Needham's excellent review.[3]

Aristotle's theory of spontaneous generation of organisms was widely held until as recently as 300 years ago (Fig. 201-1). In fact, it was not persuasively refuted until 1861, when Louis Pasteur proved that living organisms such as bacteria do not originate spontaneously but instead can be borne on other living organisms.[4] The modern era of embryology was ushered in by Wolpert in 1969 with his formulation of the "French flag problem."[5] Development, he argued, is contingent on pattern formation. How could cells be programmed to migrate, divide, and organize themselves into, for example, a red, white, and blue stripe pattern like the French flag (Color Plate 201-1)? This led to the study of the ways that positional information, specified by concentration gradients or biophysical forces, could direct cells to form the basic patterns that are the foundation of the growing organism.

Nowhere in the embryo is pattern formation better represented and studied than in the developing limb. Throughout the phylogenetic progression—from fish fins to chicken wings to human extremities—the developing limb is characterized by patterns of repeated motifs, regulated growth, and programmed segmentation. Historically, congenital limb deformities caused social ostracization, were associated with wives tales, and were occasionally documented by artists or anatomists (Fig. 201-2).

One century ago, our knowledge was founded on careful anatomic dissections of aborted products of conception, embryos, and deceased newborn children. Bardeen and Lewis's treatise is one of the most elegant on this subject (Figs. 201-3 to 201-5).[6,7] With the explosion of new technologies in cellular and molecular biology, computer science, DNA testing, and genetics, our understanding of limb development is profoundly more sophisticated than even a decade ago. Responsible pediatric hand surgeons must have a basic understanding of the process of limb development. This knowledge will allow surgeons to understand the spectrum of possible abnormal anatomic patterns, to identify other associated malformations or syndromes of importance to the child, to explain the defect, and to provide proper counseling to the new generation of Internet-savvy parents.

Text continued on p. 11

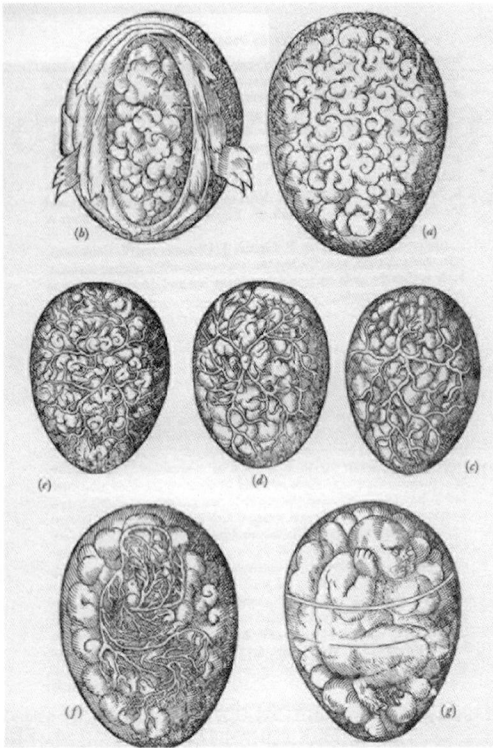

A

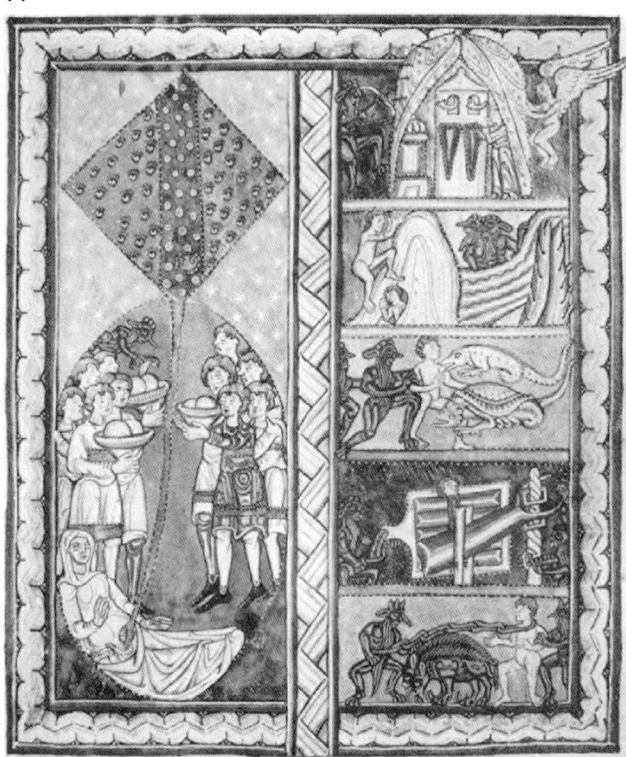

B

FIGURE 201-1. Historical theories of embryology. *A,* These images depict Aristotle's theory of conception, beginning with a mixture of "seeds" that develop and grow within the uterus.[77] *B,* In an early manuscript, *Liber Scivias,* St. Hildegard of Bingen in Rhineland describes her vision of the soul descending into the uterus of a pregnant woman containing what appears to be a complete human form.[78]

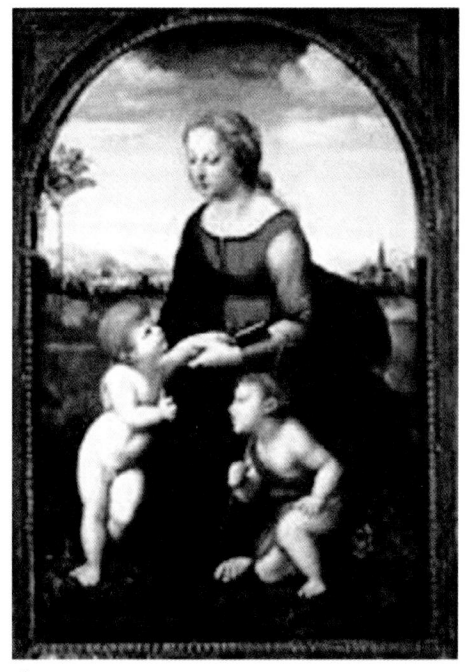
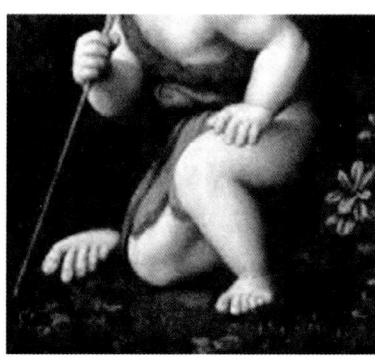

FIGURE 201–2. Depiction of limb deformities throughout history. *A* and *B,* Raphael's depiction of the infant John the Baptist in *La Belle Jardinière* (Paris, Musée National du Louvre) includes a sixth toe. (After Mimouni.[45])

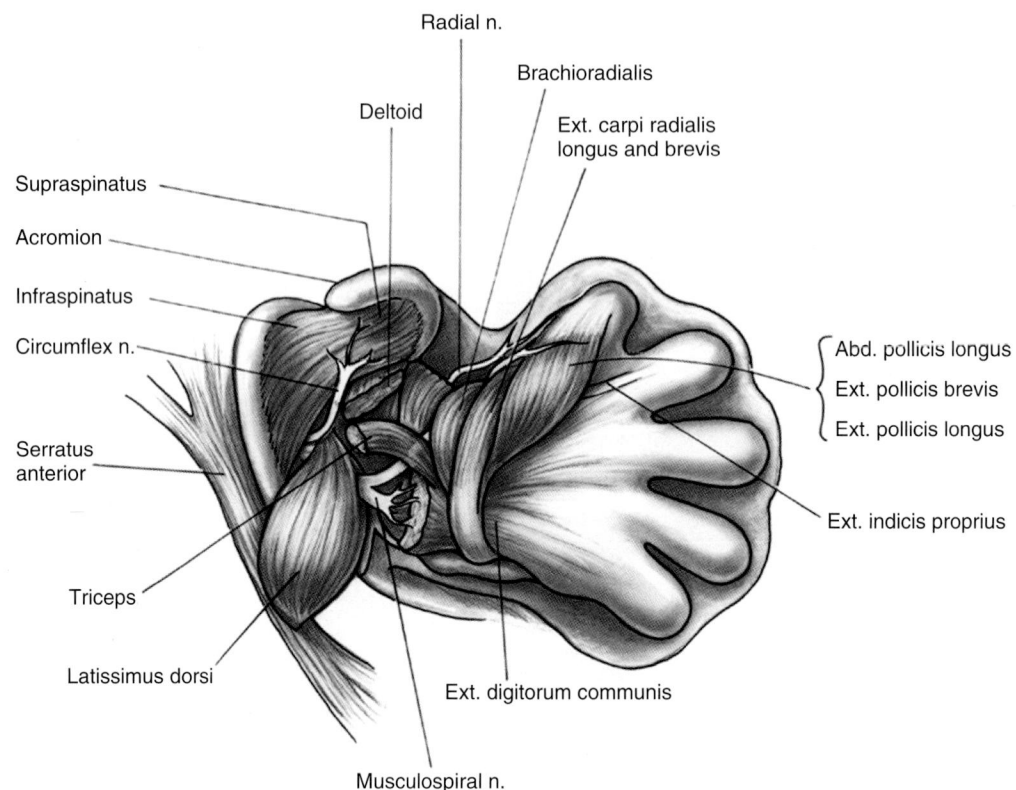

A *Window dissection*

FIGURE 201-3. Anatomic dissections, crown-rump length of 11.0 mm. *A,* This diagram represents development at 4 to 5 weeks of age. The dorsal view of the muscles to the limb shows the trapezius, latissimus dorsi, levator scapulae, and serratus anterior muscles at a more advanced stage of development. At the forearm level, small triceps and biceps muscle fibers are present, with extrinsic wrist extensors. The window dissection within the triceps demonstrates the radial nerve in its course to the outcropping muscles, extensor pollicis brevis and abductor pollicis longus of the thumb. The hand plate is well formed. *B,* Palmar (ventral) view of musculature and its relationship to the chest wall are demonstrated. The pectoralis major and minor muscles exist as a common mass that extends from the second and third ribs to the proximal portion of the humerus. It is not well differentiated into sternal or clavicular portions. The brachial plexus is well formed into lateral (dorsal) and medial (ventral) divisions, and these nerves are large in comparison with other structures. Trunks, cords, and major divisions are well formed. With distal progression, the flexor mass within the forearm is not as well differentiated, but superficial and deep layers are present (the median nerve lies between these two layers). The flexor carpi ulnaris has attached to the fifth metacarpal base (pisiform region). *C,* The arm skeleton consists of condensations of cartilage with greater degrees of differentiation in the more proximal portions. A poorly defined clavicle is attached to the scapula. The shaft of the humerus is surrounded by thick perichondrium. There is no evidence of joint cavitation at this stage, nor is there ossification. Radius and ulna are continuous with the humerus as well as the hand plate. Multiple centers of increased condensation correspond to eventual carpal bones. The scaphoid is in line with the radius and the lunate with the ulna. At this stage, the hand and carpus are not in ulnar deviation. (Redrawn from Bardeen and Lewis[6] and Lewis.[7] Drawings by J. Bittl.)

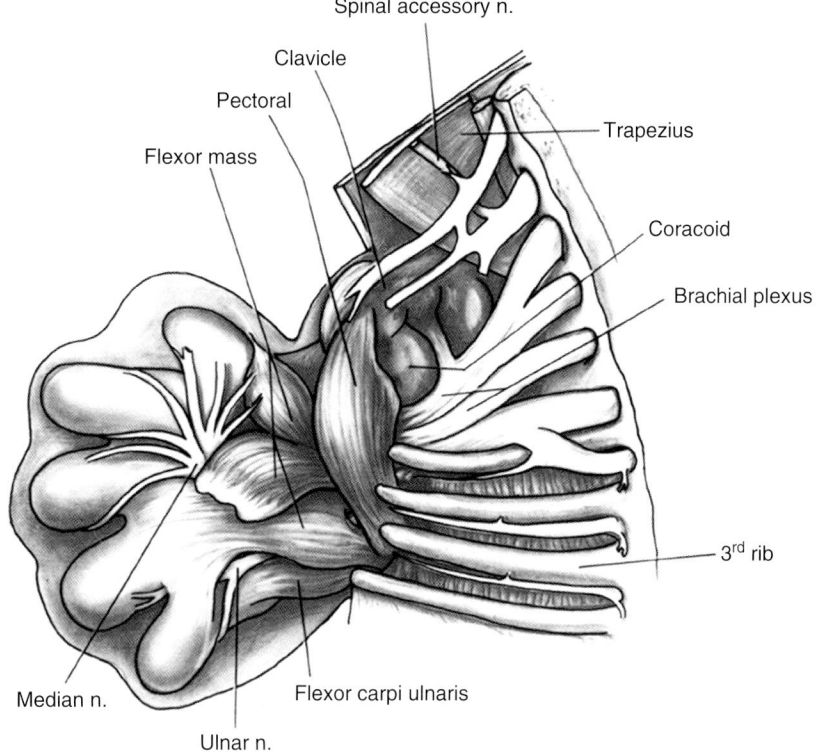

B *Pisiform region*

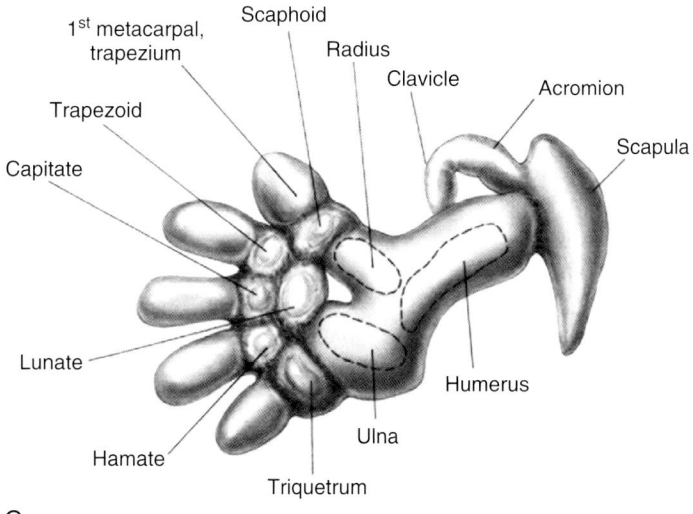

C

FIGURE 201-3, cont'd.

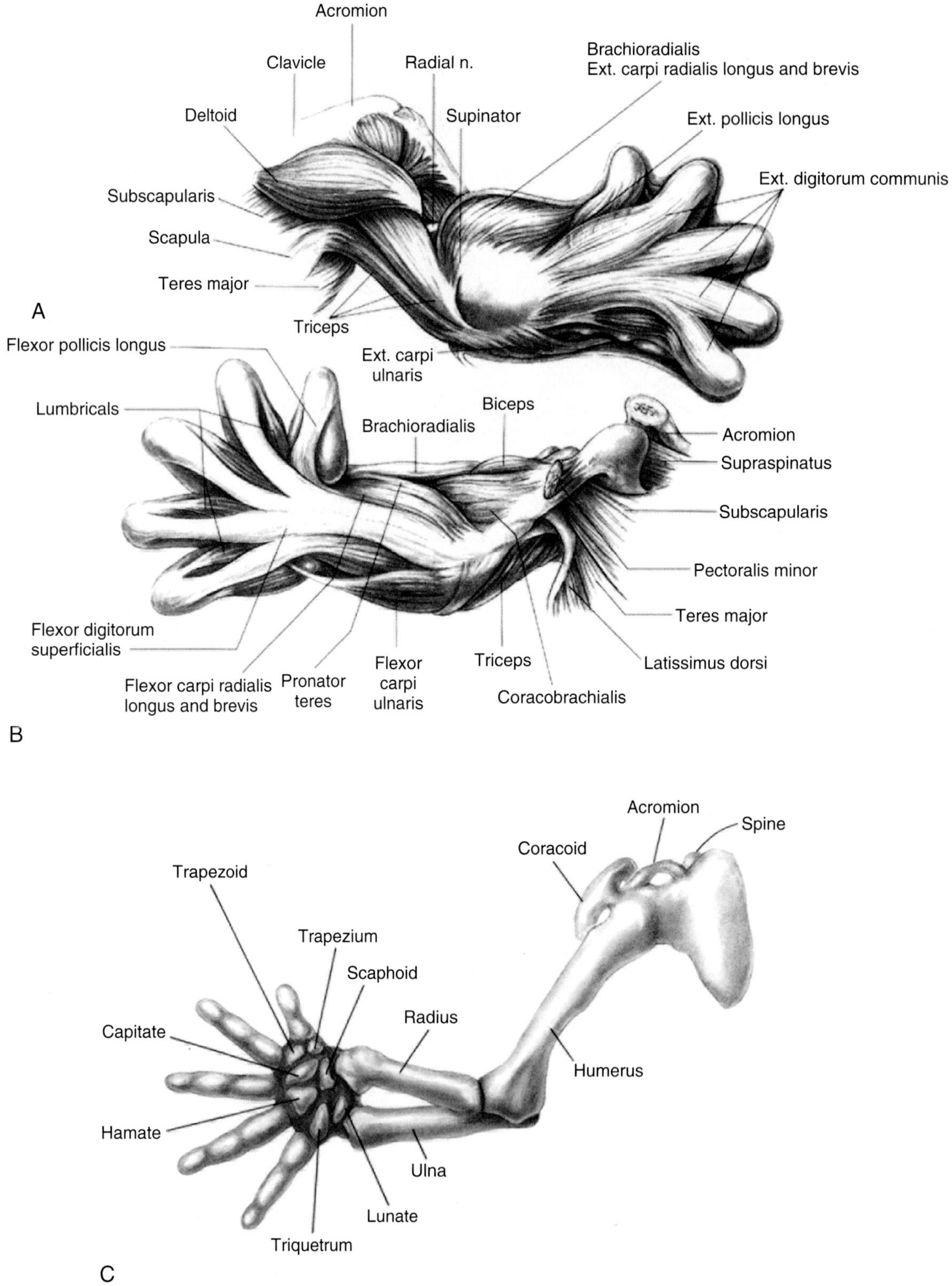

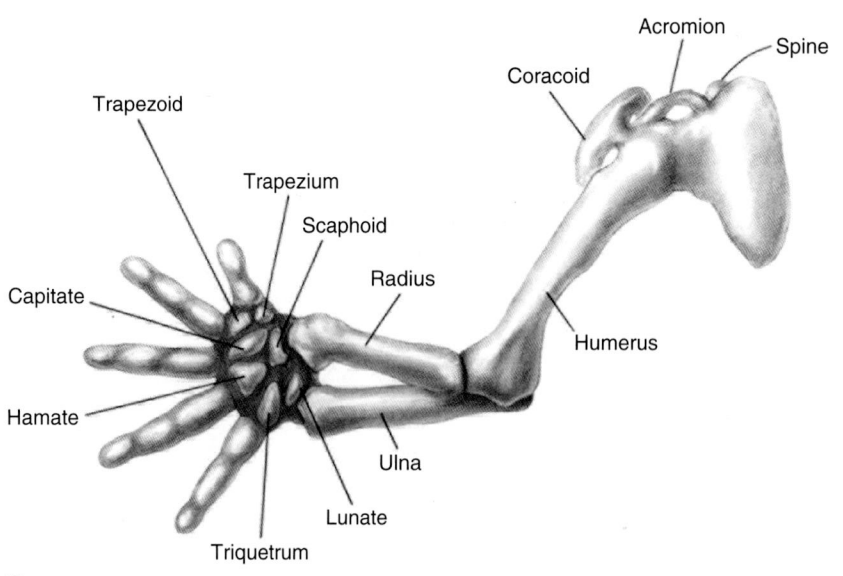

A

Acromion
Clavicle
Radial n.
Brachioradialis
Ext. carpi radialis longus and brevis
Deltoid
Supinator
Ext. pollicis longus
Subscapularis
Ext. digitorum communis
Scapula
Teres major
Triceps
Ext. carpi ulnaris

B

Flexor pollicis longus
Biceps
Acromion
Lumbricals
Brachioradialis
Supraspinatus
Subscapularis
Pectoralis minor
Teres major
Latissimus dorsi
Flexor digitorum superficialis
Flexor carpi radialis longus and brevis
Pronator teres
Flexor carpi ulnaris
Triceps
Coracobrachialis

C

Trapezoid
Acromion
Spine
Coracoid
Trapezium
Scaphoid
Capitate
Radius
Hamate
Humerus
Ulna
Lunate
Triquetrum

FIGURE 201-4. Anatomic dissections, crown-rump length of 16.0 mm. *A,* Dorsal view of the arm, forearm, and hand shows well-differentiated triceps and deltoid muscles. The subscapularis, teres major, and teres minor muscles are now in adult relationships. The triceps muscle has two distinct heads. The extrinsic extensor muscle groups are well differentiated and extend to the wrist and hand, but their development has not been as rapid as that of their antagonists on the flexor side.

FIGURE 201-4, cont'd. The brachioradialis still shares a common muscle origin with the two radial wrist extensors, over which pass the abductor pollicis longus, extensor pollicis brevis, and extensor pollicis longus. Common extensors to the digits are formed and are distinct from the extensor indicis proprius and extensor digiti quinti minimi proprius. *B,* Palmar (ventral) view of the same arm shows pectoralis insertion reflected to demonstrate insertions of teres major and latissimus dorsi muscles into the humerus. The triceps has three distinct origins at this stage, and the elongated triceps shows a long head extending to the coracoid process and a short head originating in common with the coracobrachialis muscle. The flexor muscles of the forearm are more advanced than the extensors and show separation into wrist flexors, superficial finger flexors, and deep finger flexors. The pronator teres muscle passes deep along the middle third of the radius. These muscle masses are broad and thin and extend to but not beyond the level of the carpal bones, where they connect to well-formed tendons. The lumbrical muscles have formed, but the other intrinsic muscles are still represented by less well differentiated masses of tissue adjacent to the metacarpals. *C,* The scapula, composed primarily of cartilage, has grown and has migrated posteriorly. The coracoid process of acromion is distinct. The humerus is longer and more slender than in the preceding stage and has broadened at either end, but there still is no joint cavity at either end. The radius and ulna are still continuous with the humerus and with each other over their proximal third of the forearm. Capsular structures are beginning to form over future joint cavities. The carpals are still a condensed mass with demarcations between future bones; the distal row is more easily distinguished. Metacarpals are beginning to form, with distal phalanges attached, and are represented by long, slender condensations of cartilage. There are no joint cavities. None of the metacarpal condensations come into contact with the radius. (Redrawn from Bardeen and Lewis[6] and Lewis.[7] Drawings by J. Bittl.)

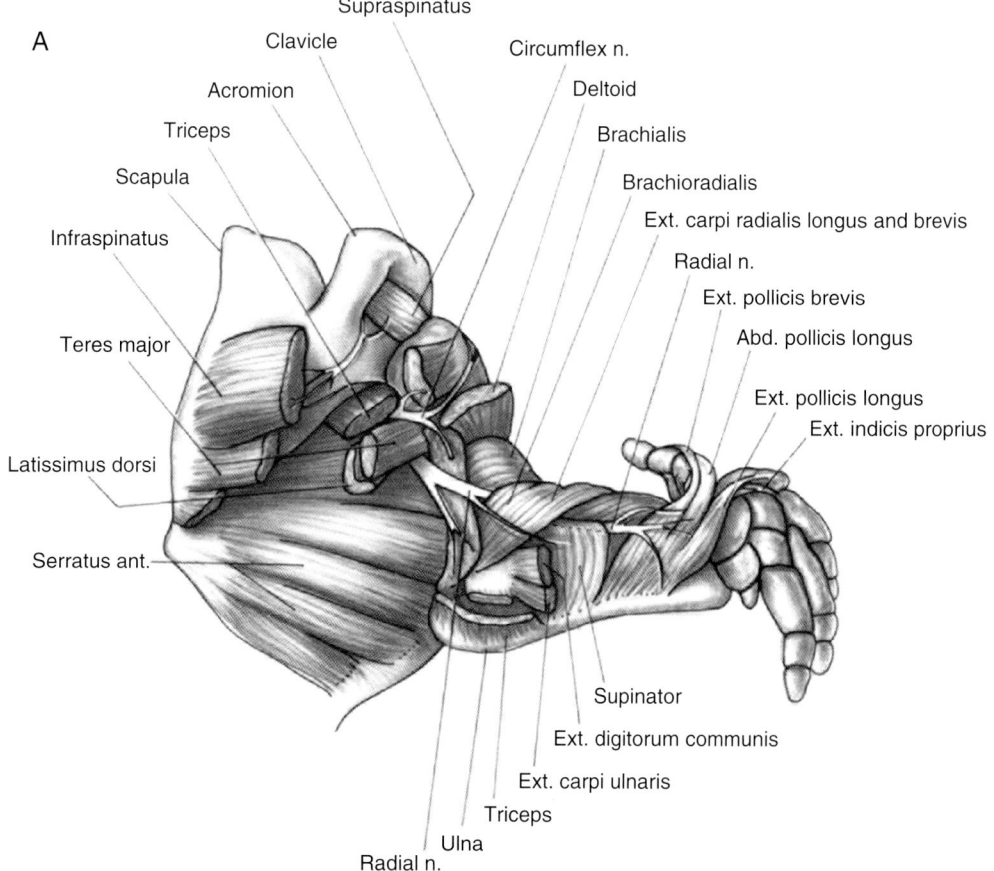

FIGURE 201-5. Anatomic dissections, crown-rump length of 20.0 mm at 7 weeks of age. *A,* In this dorsal dissection, many of the proximal limb muscles have been cut to show the distinct innervation around the shoulder. The deltoid, supraspinatus, infraspinatus, latissimus dorsi, serratus anterior, teres major, and teres minor are all well differentiated. The position of the radial nerve (musculospiral nerve) as it spirals around the humerus to innervate the wrist and finger extensors is demonstrated. The size of the peripheral nerves is still relatively great in comparison with other structures. The brachioradialis and extensor carpi radialis longus and brevis muscles are now distinct. The extensor carpi ulnaris has been cut away to show the supinator, through which passes the posterior interosseous nerve, a branch of the radial nerve. In the forearm, the abductor pollicis longus and extensor medius proprius now have distinguishable ulnar portions adjacent to the index extensor digitorum communis. A common extensor muscle mass (not shown) extends to the metacarpal level before tapering into four distinct tendons. *Continued*

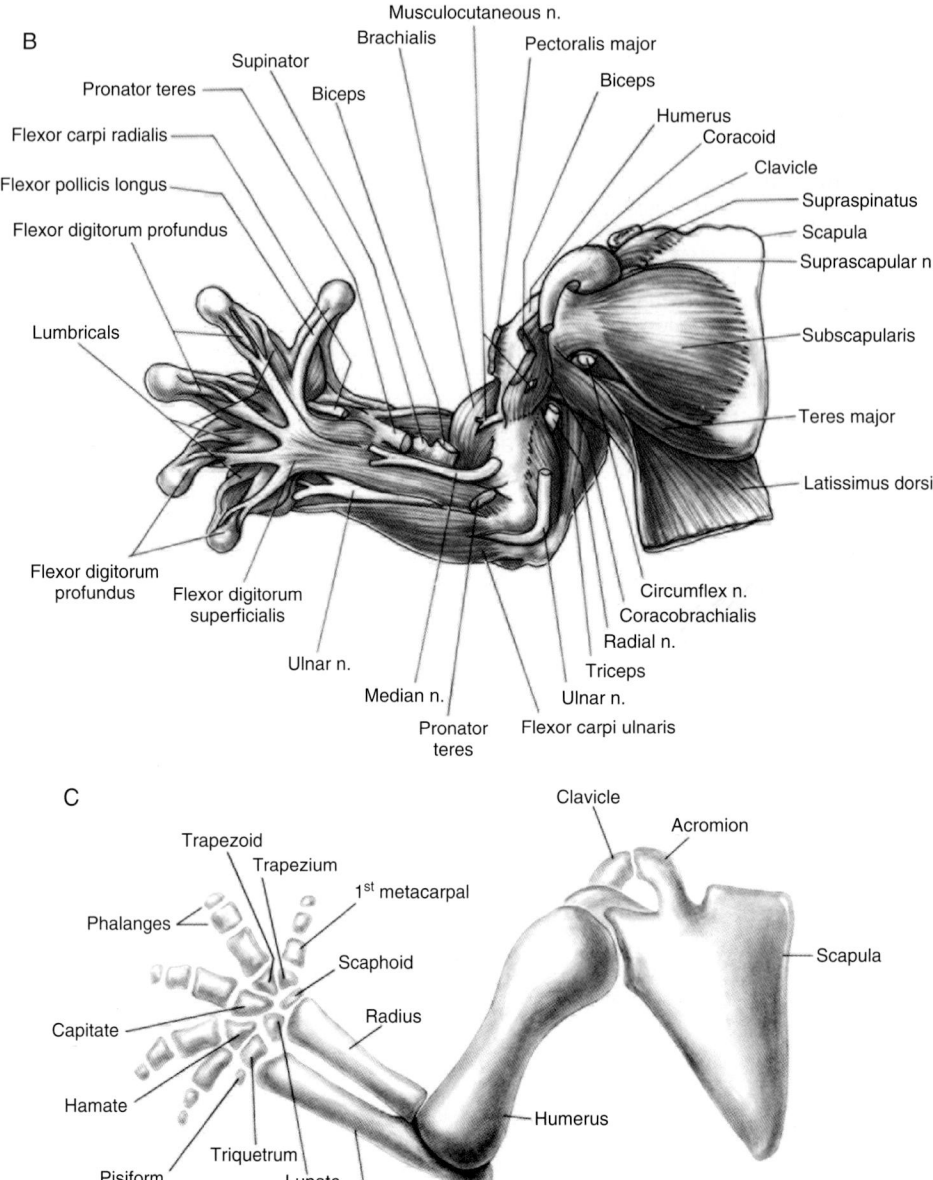

FIGURE 201-5, cont'd. *B,* On the palmar (ventral) surface of the same arm, portions of many superficial flexor muscles have been sectioned to show the relationship between the median and ulnar nerves. The broad latissimus dorsi muscle inserts onto the medial border of the humerus distal to the insertion of the subscapularis, which as a muscle group is still relatively large in comparison with the rest of the limb. The biceps muscle belly has been cut away to show its innervation, the musculocutaneous nerve, which also passes through the coracobrachialis muscle. The brachialis muscle has its origin along the humerus and is located deep in the biceps muscle. In the proximal forearm, the median nerve is shown where it passes between the deep and superficial (cut away) heads of the pronator teres muscle. The flexor digitorum superficialis muscle group is a large mass within the forearm tapering to tendons within the hand, which at this stage have split to allow the penetration of the flexor digitorum profundus. The well-formed lumbrical muscles extend to the radial side of their respective digits, where they condense with perichondrium. They are distinct from the palmar interosseous muscles. *C,* The skeletal representation shows that the scapula is larger and in a more posterior position than in the earlier stage. An acromioclavicular ligament has formed. The cartilaginous humerus is broader and thicker, and a coracohumeral ligament is present. There is still no glenohumeral joint. The radius and ulna are larger, and the olecranon, coracoid, and styloid processes are beginning to form as condensed tissue. No joints are present, and perichondrium between the two bones is still continuous. All carpal bones are still cartilaginous, and ligaments are beginning to form. The carpus has not yet begun to flex and deviate ulnarward. Five metacarpals are distinct, with the first on the preaxial side being the shortest. At the digital level, the front two rows of phalanges are evident. (Redrawn from Bardeen and Lewis[6] and Lewis.[7] Drawings by J. Bittl.)

MORPHOLOGIC DEVELOPMENT

The embryonic period refers to the time interval between fertilization and the completion of formation of the major structures. In humans, this period continues until the end of the eighth week after fertilization. Development of the limbs occurs primarily during the period of organogenesis, which extends from the fourth week to the eighth week of the embryonic period. During this phase, the developing embryo is most susceptible to the effects of teratogens. The fetal period—the remaining 7 months of gestation—is characterized by further growth and differentiation of the organ systems.

At about the fourth intrauterine week, the upper limb bud, also known as Wolff crest, forms on the ventrolateral side of the embryo.[8] The upper limb bud extends from the 8th to 12th myotome, corresponding to the C6-T2 vertebral level. In the fifth intrauterine week, the limb straightens and develops a depression, which becomes the axillary fossa. By day 37, the hand plate is present as a flat, paddle-like structure with small nubbins of nascent digits. Vessels enter the limb, initially supplying the ectodermal surface,

and nerve trunks soon follow.[9] Not long after, muscle groups appear around cartilage anlage, and joint interzones can be seen. By day 28, about when the mother realizes she is pregnant, the basic pattern formation in the upper limb is complete in the fetus, which measures about 3.0 cm long. The lower limb forms in parallel but lags behind by 2 to 3 days.

In 1949, Streeter[10] divided human upper limb development into 23 stages, from fertilization of the egg to penetration of the humerus by the nutrient artery. To avoid confusion, the morphologic changes in various tissues are discussed first, followed by a brief, systematic review of the molecular biology underlying these events (Table 201-1 and Fig. 201-6).

DEVELOPMENT OF SPECIFIC TISSUES

Skeletal Development

Bones develop first as cartilaginous precursors. These cartilage anlage are first seen in the embryo as clear, avascular areas known as condensations, which arise by recruitment of mesenchymal cells. In the fifth

TABLE 201-1 ◆ STAGES OF THE EMBRYOLOGIC DEVELOPMENT OF THE UPPER LIMB[10]

Streeter Stages of Human Embryonic Development			
Stage	Age (days)	C-R Length*	Events
1			Fertilization
2			Zygote divides
3			Early blastocyte
4	6		Implantation begins
5	9-10		Complete blastocyte implantation
6	11-15		Primary villi
7	16-20		Notochord appears
8	20-21		Neural plate develops
9	21-22		Neural groove develops
10	23	2.0-3.5	Embryo straight; heart begins to beat
11	24-25	2.5-4.5	Embryo curved
12	26-27	3.0-5.0	Arm buds appear
13	28-31	4.0-6.0	Arm buds are flipper-like
14	32	5.0-7.0	Forelimbs are paddle shaped
15	33-36	7.0-9.0	Hand plates form
16	37-40	8.0-11.0	Foot plates form
17	41-43	11.0-14.0	Finger rays appear
18	44-46	13.0-17.0	Notches between finger rays
19	47-48	16.0-18.0	Fingers begin to separate
20	49-51	18.0-22.0	Fingers separate and elongate
21	52-53	22.0-24.0	
22	54-55	23.0-28.0	Toes separate and elongate
23	56	27.0-31.0	Head rounded

*Crown-rump length in millimeters.

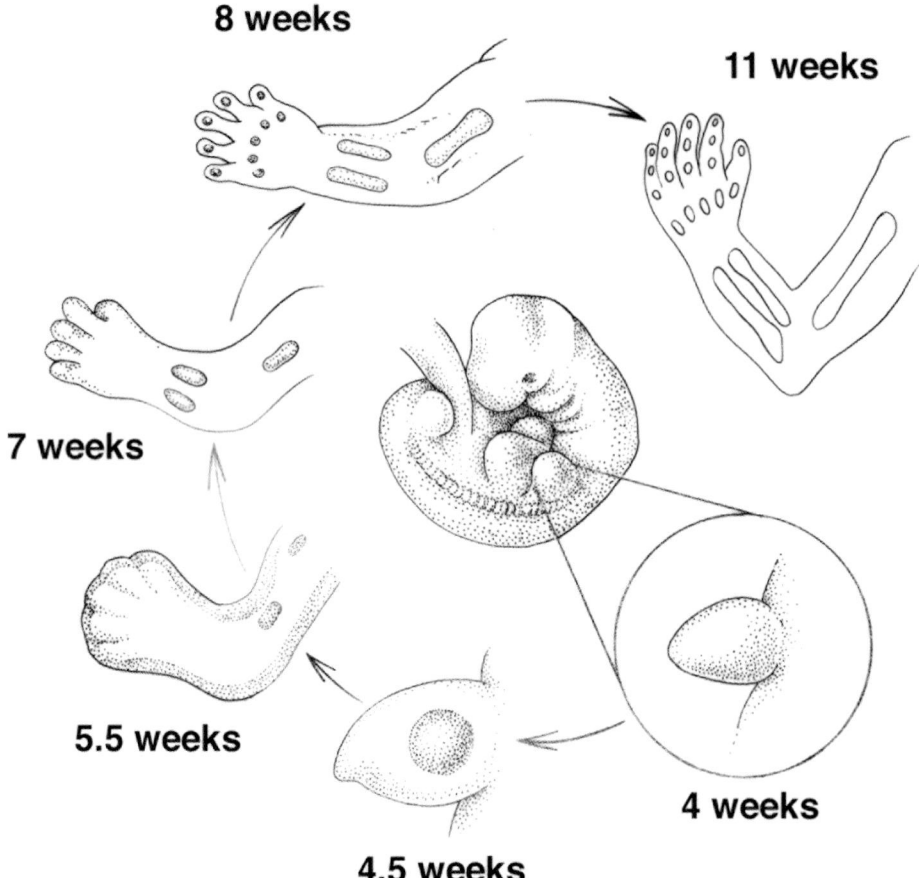

8 weeks

11 weeks

7 weeks

5.5 weeks

4 weeks

4.5 weeks

FIGURE 201-6. Timeline of development of the human upper limb. Stages of human upper extremity development are depicted. At 4 weeks, the limb bud is present. At 4.5 weeks, the distal flattened ectoderm known as the apical ectodermal ridge is seen. By 5.5 weeks, condensations representing the clavicle and humerus can be identified. At 7 weeks, the condensations representing the radius and ulna are visible and the digits have begun to separate. By 8 weeks, metacarpal and digital ossification centers are noted, with digital separation almost complete. By 11 weeks, digital separation is complete and all phalangeal ossification centers are present. (After England.[79] Illustration by J. Bittl.)

intrauterine week, chondrification begins as chondrocytes secrete an extracellular matrix. In contrast to the membranous bones of the craniofacial skeleton, which ossify by direct mineralization, the bones of the extremities ossify by a process known as endochondral ossification, in which cartilaginous precursors are gradually replaced by bone. The humerus first begins to ossify at the sixth week, followed by distal progression, skipping the carpal bones and proceeding to the distal phalanges.[11] Bone growth and remodeling continue throughout the prenatal and postnatal periods.

Whereas the humerus, radius, ulna, and phalanges ossify prenatally, the carpal bones and epiphyses do not. Therefore, the degree of ossification of the carpal bones and epiphyses is a useful determinant of skeletal maturity. In the congenitally deformed limb, ossification is typically delayed. Although the development

of the carpus is complex and beyond the scope of this text, the process can be briefly summarized. Only the trapezium, trapezoid, and capitate develop in their original form. The other carpal bones migrate and fuse in a complicated process that eventually results in two rows of carpals.[12] Components of the scaphoid and lunate form during the seventh week of intrauterine development but do not fuse to form their ultimate configuration until the fetus reaches a 50-mm crown-rump length (see Figs. 201-3 to 201-5).

Joint formation begins 6 weeks after fertilization through a process of cavitation. Mesenchymal cells in the future joint space lose their differentiation, creating a segmentation of the cartilaginous condensation (Fig. 201-7). The sides of this cavity form the joint capsules and ligaments. A synovial mesenchymal layer with blood vessels forms between the capsule and periosteum. By the seventh week, hypertrophic chondrocytes

Formation of interzone

Three-layered interzone

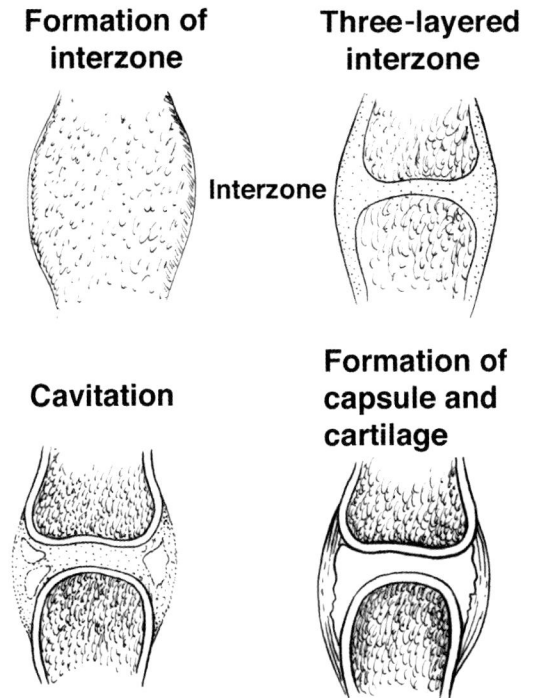

Interzone

Cavitation

Formation of capsule and cartilage

FIGURE 201-7. Formation of joints. Joints begin as a homogeneous swelling of the blastema known as an interzone. Soon the interzone displays three distinct layers. A cavity then forms within the central segment of the interzone, followed by the formation of articular cartilage, synovial tissue, and a joint capsule. (After Cihak.[19] Illustration by J. Bittl.)

form plates of cartilage at the proximal and distal sides of the cavity, which ultimately become articular cartilage.[13] In utero motion is then required for subsequent normal development of the joint, and embryos paralyzed before complete development of joints will have abnormal joints characterized by flat articular surfaces joined by fibrous tissue.[14,15]

Finally, at approximately day 38, the hand begins to take on its adult form, except for the soft tissue "webbing" between the digits. These interzones between the joints begin to recede through a process of programmed cell death known as apoptosis. As the interdigital mesoderm degenerates, the digits separate (see Fig. 201-9). Members of the bone morphogenetic protein family have been implicated in this process (see Fig. 201-6).[16]

Arterial Development

Much of our knowledge of the early development of the vascular and musculoskeletal systems in the human is based on careful work by anatomists at Charles University in Prague. In the late 1960s and early 1970s, Cihak and Mrazkova, among others, carefully sectioned tissue from a large number of aborted human embryos. The following discussion is largely based on their meticulous studies.[12,17-20]

By the third postovulatory week, the subclavian artery can be seen among a series of thin-walled vessels entering the developing limb bud. A marginal sinus (sinus marginalis) develops along the periphery of the limb bud and communicates with a discrete capillary complex, which gradually develops a venous drainage system emptying into a subclavian vein. The median artery is the first major branch off the brachial artery to the forearm and extends along the central axis of the limb (Fig. 201-8). According to the classic studies of Caplan and Koutroupas,[21] myogenic areas of the limb bud become vascular, and chondrogenic areas become clear and avascular. By the sixth week, the ulnar artery is apparent and branches from the brachial artery, progressing down the hand plate to form the deep palmar arch. The radial artery develops later and is more variable, progressing down the preaxial side of the limb. Eventually, the median and interosseous arteries decrease in size, and the median artery degenerates, providing only some blood supply to the median nerve.[20] The small vestige of the interosseous artery terminates in many small branches (rete system) in the carpus (Fig. 201-9).

The process of vascular development in the limb is poorly understood but results in remarkable anatomic variation.[22,23] Similar variation is noted in the development of both the muscles and tendons. It is well known that interruption of the developing blood supply results in malformations distal to the injury.[24,25] The molecular aberrations involved in vascular malformations are unknown.

Neural Development

Nerve growth proceeds in a fashion analogous to blood vessel growth, and the growth of sensory and motor nerves within the developing limb is a subject of great experimental and clinical interest. Unlike in lower vertebrates, in which there is an individual spinal nerve dedicated to control of each separate muscle, the human system is much more complex. In the human, all nerves to the limb traverse a cervicobrachial plexus, which is formed by the fourth week of intrauterine life (see Fig. 201-3).[6] However, we are still left to question how growing nerves are guided to their destinations.

Experimental work has yielded some clues about nerve development. In avian limbs, with removal of somatic mesoderm, a limb with no muscle will subsequently develop. Despite this, peripheral nerves develop normally, although they lack branches to the missing muscles. Therefore, it appears that muscle destinations are not the primary controls of nerve development.[26] Sensory nerves are derivatives of the neural

3.0–5.0 mm CR   **4.0–6.0 mm CR**

15.0 mm CR   **18.0 mm CR**

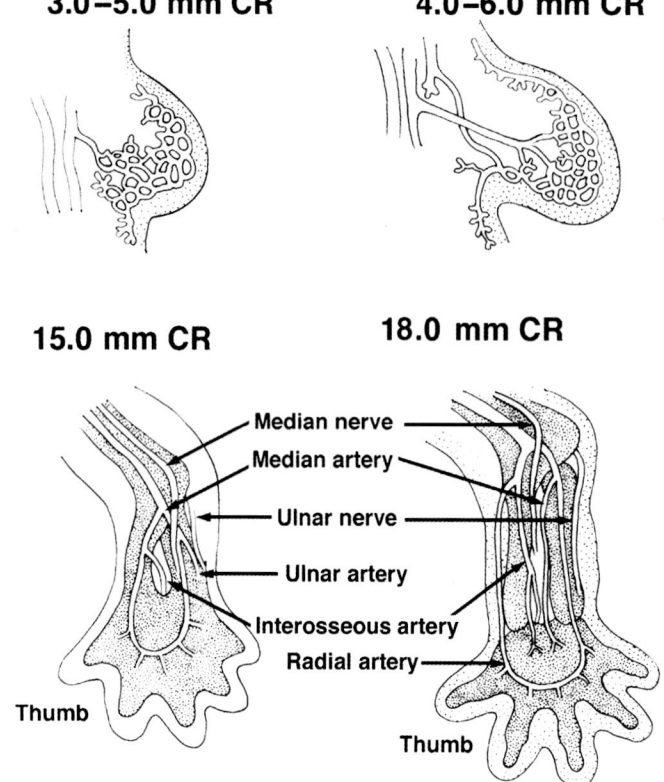

Median nerve

Median artery

Ulnar nerve

Ulnar artery

Interosseous artery

Radial artery

Thumb

Thumb

FIGURE 201-8. Vascular development. At a crown-rump (CR) length of 3.0 to 5.0 mm, the primary subclavian artery can be identified anastomosing with the digital capillary network. At a CR length of 4.0 to 6.0 mm, the primary subclavian vein provides venous egress from the limb bud. By the 15.0-mm CR stage, a vascular arcade has formed, dominated by the median artery, with an interosseous artery passing into the space between what will become the radius and ulna. The partially formed median nerve and the formation of the ulnar nerve and ulnar artery can also be seen at this stage. Finally, by the 18.0-mm CR stage (8 weeks), the median and interosseous arteries have been dwarfed as the new arcade of the radial and ulnar arteries takes on its adult role. The ulnar, median, and radial nerves have formed. (From Caplan A, Koutroupas S: The control of muscle and cartilage development in the chicklimb: the role of differential vascularization. J Embryol Exp Morphol 1973;29: 571. Reprinted with permission of The Company of Biologists, Ltd.)

Embryo at 4 weeks

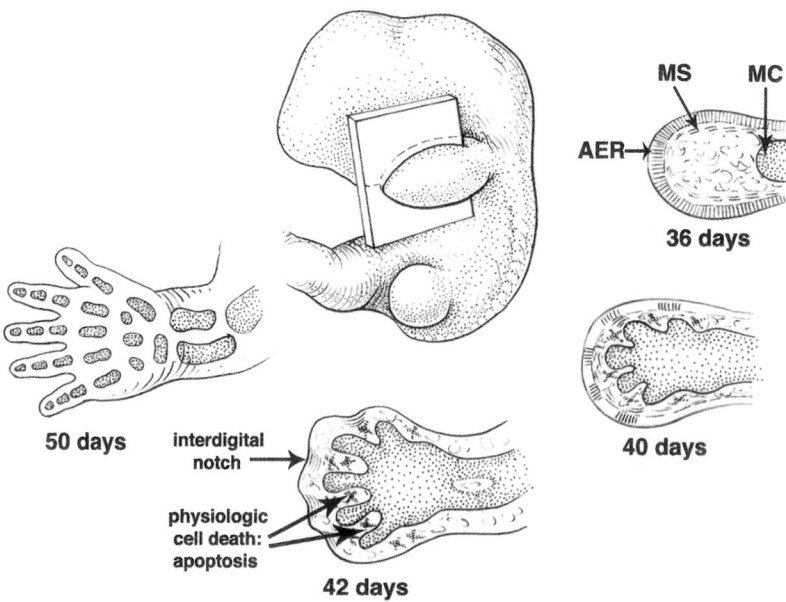

MS   MC

AER→

36 days

50 days   interdigital notch

40 days

physiologic cell death: apoptosis

42 days

FIGURE 201-9. Separation of the digits (clockwise, from center). At 4 weeks, the limb bud is formed. By 36 days, the bud has become paddle shaped and is composed of an apical ectodermal ridge (AER) and an underlying mesoderm. MS, marginal sinus; MC, mesenchymal condensation. By 40 days, the cartilaginous skeletal framework has begun to separate, and 2 days later, external ridging is present. By 7.5 weeks, the bone morphogenetic protein-mediated process of apoptosis results in complete digital separation. (From Yasuda M: Pathogenesis of pre-axial polydactyly of the hand in human embryos. J Embryol Exp Morphol 1975;33:745. Reprinted with permission of The Company of Biologists, Ltd.)

tube, whereas motor nerves are derivatives of the neural crest, and transplanted segments of spinal cord are able to sprout spinal nerves and join a nearby limb plexus.

On the basis of avian limb bud experiments, after the subclavian artery is well established, leading axons from the spinal nerve roots (C6-T1) sprout. Mixed motor and sensory nerves exit the plexus and enter the limb as a pioneer growth cone, which is soon surrounded by mesenchymal cells that form a perineural sheath. Once a dominant branch innervates a muscle, it is stretched distally with the growing limb and muscle. Although individual muscles in humans are supplied by complex interconnections of nerve routes through the brachial plexus, the anterior divisions generally supply the flexor muscle mass, and the posterior divisions generally supply the extensor muscle mass.

Muscle Development

Muscle development is a poorly understood process and parallels the development of the skeletal system of the limb. The somites divide into a sclerotome, which forms vertebral bodies and ribs; a dermatome, which forms skin and fascia; and a myotome, which forms segmented muscles. Myoblasts, which give rise to the limb musculature, either arise from limb bud mesenchyme or migrate into the limb from the somite.[27,28]

The dorsal muscle blastema gives origin to the extensor muscles, and the ventral muscle blastema gives origin to the flexor muscles. Parallel to skeletal development, the proximal muscles differentiate before distal muscles. By the eighth intrauterine week, all major muscle groups have formed.

There is evidence that muscle development is within the control of local factors and is not programmed by its somite origin or influenced by growing nerves.[29,30] Tendons develop separately from their muscle bellies and then fuse to form muscle-tendon units. In patients with abnormal development or absence of their normal bone of attachment, tendons will adhere to the nearest bone, tendon, or fascial layer, accounting for the many bizarre tendon insertions observed in congenital hand malformations. In patients with central clefts of the hand, for example, tendons often attach abnormally to phalanges on the adjacent digit, resulting in camptodactyly (see Fig. 201-9). If a tendon does not join its muscle belly, the tendon will degenerate.[31,32] In contrast, tendonless muscles can survive, but they do require innervation for growth.[30] This is clinically evident in the dissection of adactylous or monodactylous hands, in which tendons are present but fused in abnormal positions (Fig. 201-10).

In the forearm, the superficial muscles differentiate before the deeper muscles do. The blastemas of origin, differentiation, and migration of the extrinsic and intrinsic muscles of the hand are a fascinating

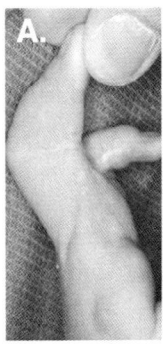
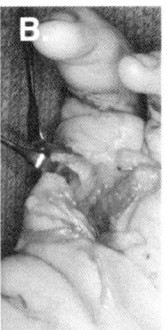
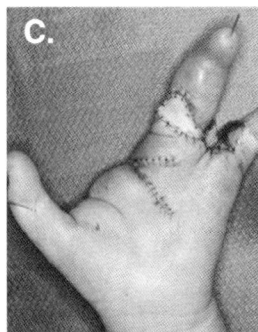
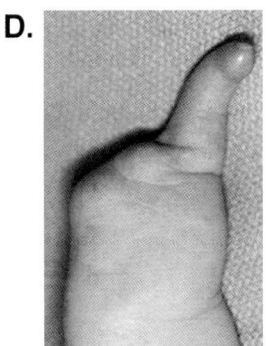
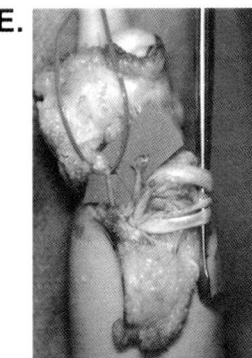

FIGURE 201-10. Abnormal fusion of tendons in monodactylous, adactylous, and cleft hands. *A,* Despite previous releases of the flexion contracture in this ring finger of a patient with a typical cleft hand, the deformity recurred with continued growth of the digit. *B,* Five extra flexor tendons (in addition to the ring superficial and deep flexor tendons) have been released. These tendons developed proximal to their normal distal insertions onto the index and long digits, which did not develop. *C,* A skin graft was used to resurface the skin defect. Sixteen years later (at the time of skeletal maturity), the contracture had not recurred. *D,* The gross appearance of a monodactylous hand in a child with the cleft hand–cleft foot syndrome. Thumbs were constructed by a toe to hand transfer with use of the only toe on either foot. *E,* At surgery, a complete fusion of the extrinsic flexor to the extensor tendon to each of the missing digits or thumb was identified. Only one was needed to motor the new thumb. Distal tendinous fusions are common in monodactylous and cleft hands.

subject well described by Cihak.[12,19] The intrinsic muscles arise from five embryonic muscle layers, which differentiate and fuse in a logical but complex fashion (Figs. 201-11 and 201-12).

MOLECULAR BIOLOGY OF LIMB DEVELOPMENT

Limb development has been studied in a wide variety of animal models, beginning with the silkworm. Zebra fish are known to regenerate their fins when they are severed, yielding a simple model for growth

and segmentation of bones. Insects, such as the cricket, and amphibians, such as the newt, are known to regenerate severed limbs and have become interesting models for researchers. Because the *Drosophila* fruit fly has a relatively simple and well-described genome, its limb development has been studied extensively.

Currently, the two primary animal models for limb development work are the chick and the mouse. Chicken eggs can easily be "windowed" for access to the embryo, permitting an endless variety of surgical manipulations, cell labeling experiments, and modification of gene expression. The mouse model is ideal

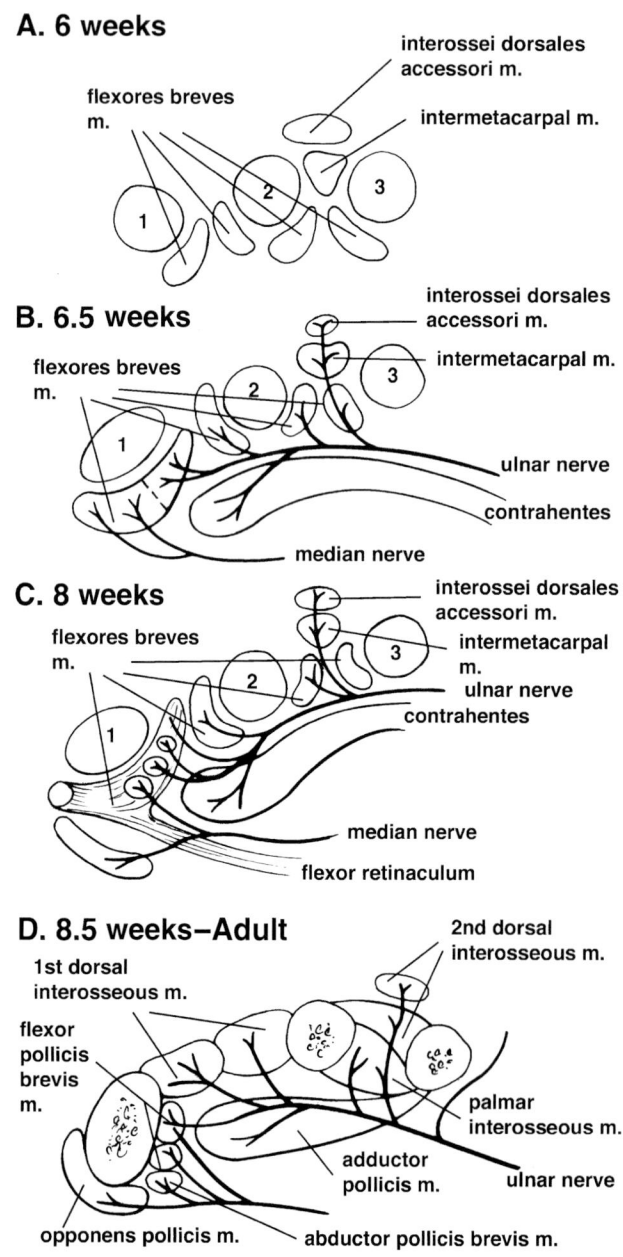

FIGURE 201-11. Intrinsic muscle development. The numbered segments represent the metacarpals. *A,* By week 6, three embryonic layers of intrinsic muscles are seen: interossei dorsales accessorii (IDA), intermetacarpals (IM), and flexores breves profundi (FBP). *B,* At 6.5 weeks, the more superficial ulnar-innervated fourth layer, or contrahentes, is present. Ulnar nerve branches innervate the IDA, the IM, and the FBP. The median nerve–innervated muscle group on the volar and most radial aspect of the thumb metacarpal is also noted. *C,* By 8 weeks, the innervation of these four muscle layers is developed. The median nerve has managed only to innervate the volar radial half of the thumb FBP. *D,* In the adult hand, the first dorsal interosseous is composed of the embryologic FBP layer. The second, third, and fourth interossei are composed of fused muscle groups of the FBP, the IDA, and the IM. The palmar interossei are derived from the FBP. The contrahentes layer has brought its ulnar innervation to all of the interossei from their volar sides. The ulnar nerve has innervated its contrahentes remnant—the broad adductor pollicis from its dorsal aspect—as well as the deep head of the flexor pollicis brevis. The median nerve has maintained its innervation of the volar radial half of the FBP, which has developed into the opponens, the abductor pollicis brevis, and the superficial head of the flexor pollicis brevis. (After Cihak.[19] Illustration by J. Bittl.)

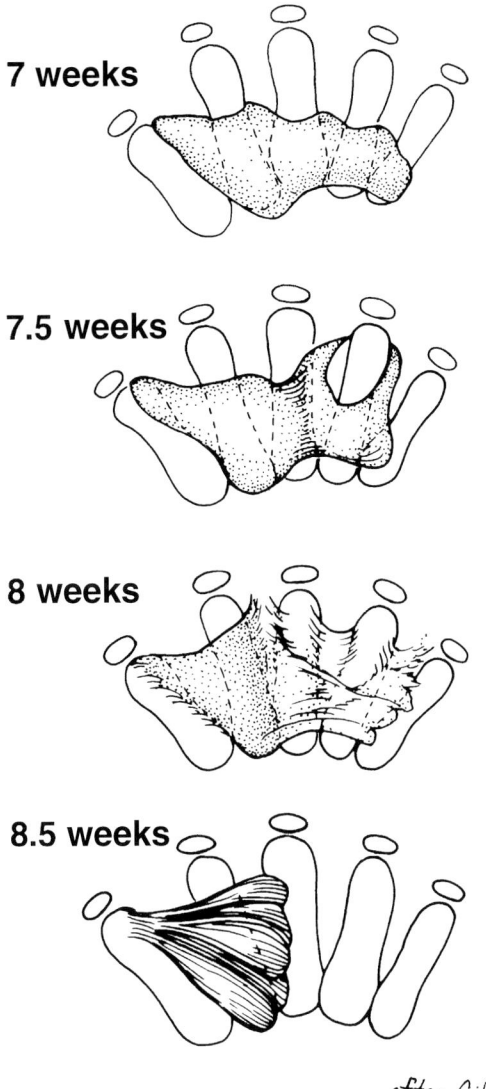

7 weeks

7.5 weeks

8 weeks

8.5 weeks

after Cihak

FIGURE 201-12. Adductor pollicis development. The development of the adductor pollicis muscle involves the formation of the contrahentes layer between the first and fifth metacarpal at 7 weeks of age. By 7.5 weeks, the layer is beginning to degenerate from the fourth and fifth metacarpals; by 8 weeks, there is a noticeable loss of muscle tissue; and by 8.5 weeks, the layer inserts only into the third metacarpal.

for performing and assessing specific genetic manipulations, and countless mutant mouse strains with limb malformations have been produced. Transgenic strains can be engineered to alter the expression of particular gene products. Alternatively, the loss of function of genes can be assessed by selectively inactivating them to produce knockout strains. Such mice are engineered to fail to produce a specific gene product. Various mating schemes to combine heterozygous or homozygous forms of such strains can be employed in ingen-

ious ways to further probe the effects of altered gene expression. A full description of these techniques is beyond the scope of this chapter.

Classic Model

On the basis of classic experiments by Summerbell,[33] Saunders,[34] and others, the so-called progress zone model of limb development has been proposed. Although recent work is likely to necessitate alterations and further refinements of this theory, the basic model is a widely accepted starting point for understanding limb development (Figs. 201-13 and 201-14). It holds that the duration of time that an individual cell spends in the progress zone determines its differentiation and ultimate position.

The limb bud is covered at its apex by a thick band of ectoderm known as the apical ectodermal ridge. Removal of the apical ectodermal ridge results in cessation of growth and limb truncation.[35] This truncation can be rescued by replacing the apical ectodermal ridge with a bead soaked in fibroblast growth factor (FGF) 4.[36] However, current research suggests that FGF-4 is not essential for limb development. There are now more than 24 known members of the FGF family, and there appears to be a complex interplay at the apical ectodermal ridge involving FGF-8, FGF-9, and FGF-17.

Initiation of limb bud formation is poorly understood. It appears that limb-forming potential is present, at the very least, along the entire length of the lateral mesoderm from the normal upper extremity position to the normal lower extremity position. Current work focuses on the gene products expressed very early in the limb bud, including FGF-10, snail, twist, Tbx-4, and Tbx-5.

The Three Dimensions

Limb development is a three-dimensional process, occurring in the anterior-posterior (or radial-ulnar) axis, the dorsal-ventral axis, and the proximal-distal axis. It will be most clear to consider these separately.

ANTERIOR-POSTERIOR AXIS

What accounts for the fundamental anterior-posterior polarity of the hand? Classic experiments by Saunders showed that transplantation of a small area of the posterior zone of the limb bud to the anterior limb zone results in mirror image duplication with posteriorization of the anterior hand plate (Fig. 201-15; see also Fig. 201-14). Because of the polarizing influence of this posterior limb bud tissue, it has become known as the zone of polarizing activity (ZPA). An early candidate for the active factor in the ZPA was retinoic acid because transplantation of a retinoic acid bead

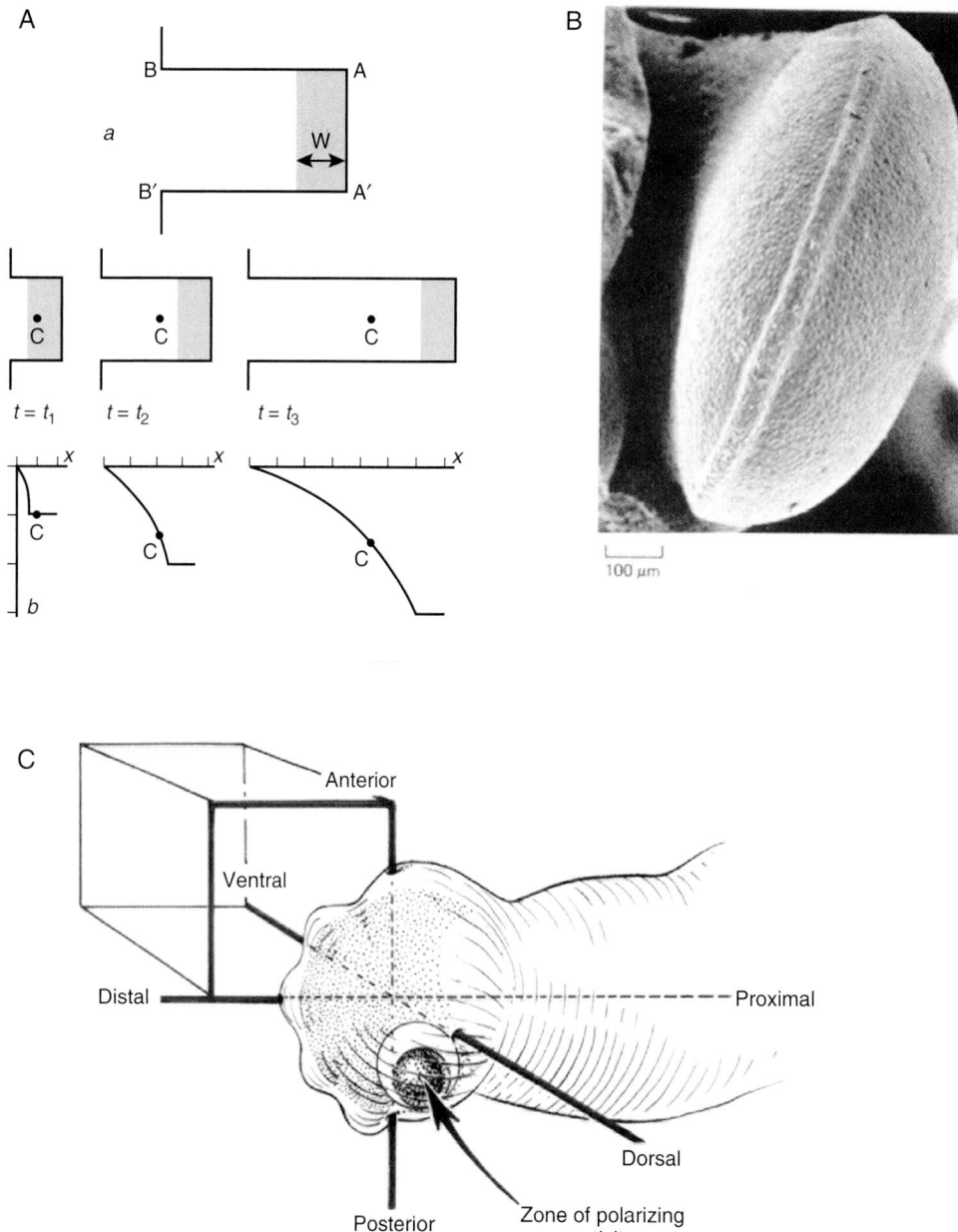

FIGURE 201-13. Progress zone model. *A,* This is the original illustration from the classic paper of Summerbell et al[35] in 1973. The authors, rather than postulating an external signal, proposed that cell differentiation and thus pattern formation along an axis may be a function of the time spent in the advancing distal progress zone. This represented a possible solution to the French flag problem. (Nature, v. 244, 1973. Reprinted by permission from Nature. Copyright 1973 Macmillan Magazines Limited. http://www.nature.com/nature.) *B,* This electron micrograph shows the apical ectodermal ridge in a developing chick embryo. *C,* This simplified schematic diagram describes the progress zone model. Maintenance of a hard ectodermal cap (the apical ectodermal ridge) covering the growing limb bud is necessary for development. Just beneath it lies the progress zone mesenchyme, which in part determines proximal-distal patterning. The zone of polarizing activity is mediated by Sonic hedgehog; it provides a posteriorizing (i.e., ulnarizing) influence and participates in radioulnar patterning. In truth, interaction between these various "layers" is exceedingly complex.

can duplicate the effect of ZPA transplantation. However, it has subsequently been shown that retinoic acid does not have a biologic role in the normally developing limb and that the ZPA activity is due to a secreted protein signal known as Sonic hedgehog (Shh).

Researchers now believe there is a complex positive feedback mechanism between Shh in the ZPA and FGF-4, FGF-9, and FGF-17 in the apical ectodermal ridge. The importance of Shh can be inferred from its phylogenetic conservation. Shh is present in settings as diverse as the regenerating zebra fish fin, the regenerating newt limb, and all higher vertebrates studied thus far.

DORSAL-VENTRAL AXIS

The early limb bud is divided into two distinct compartments, dorsal and ventral. Labeling studies have shown that no cells violate the dorsal-ventral border. The ectodermal covering of the limb bud appears to have some influence over the dorsal-ventral division because excision and rotation of the ectoderm results in reversal of the dorsal-ventral axis. Expression of the protein Engrailed (En-1) is strictly limited to the ventral compartment, and En-1 is thought to be under control of one or more of the bone morphogenetic proteins. Bone morphogenetic protein mediates its effect by

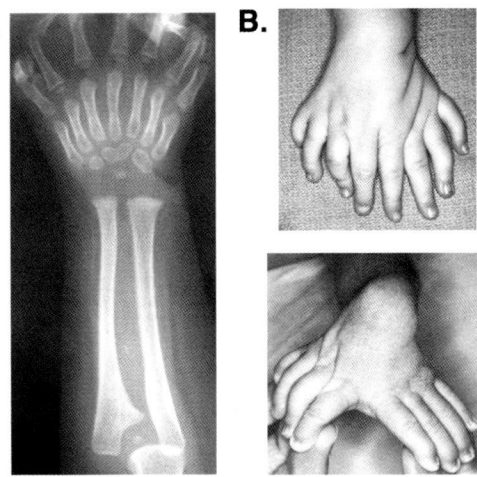

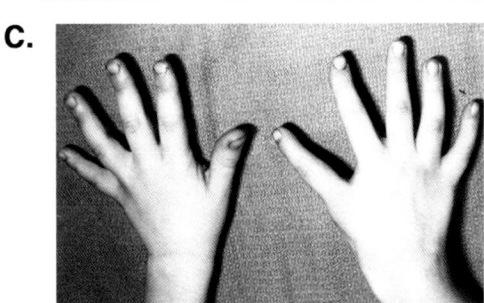

FIGURE 201-15. Mirror hand (ulnar dimelia). *A,* A clinical radiograph of a patient with a mirror hand and forearm, which contains two ulnae. These ulnae are not as anatomically symmetric as the digital and carpal skeleton. *B,* These eight digits are true mirror images of one another. *C,* This shows both hands after a rotation-recession osteotomy of the best accessory digit. These new thumbs are never completely normal. (Photographs courtesy of Vincent Hentz, MD.)

En-1, which suppresses Wnt-7a in the ventral compartment. Unopposed Wnt-7a activity presents a dorsalizing influence, possibly mediated by bmx-1. Knockout mice lacking Wnt-7a have a normal ventral compartment and a duplicated ventral compartment on the dorsal side.

PROXIMAL-DISTAL AXIS

Various factors arising from the apical ectodermal ridge are thought to signal proximal-distal patterning. A large gene superfamily, known as the homeobox or HOX genes, constitutes the most understood and perhaps most important determinant of proximal-distal patterning. In humans, there are four clusters of HOX genes labeled A, B, C, and D. In mice, analogous genes are represented in lowercase (e.g., *hoxa11*). HOX genes (Fig. 201-16) are expressed sequentially in a complex overlapping pattern within the developing limb and are numbered from proximal to distal. *HOX9* is expressed in the nascent humerus, *HOX11* in the forearm,

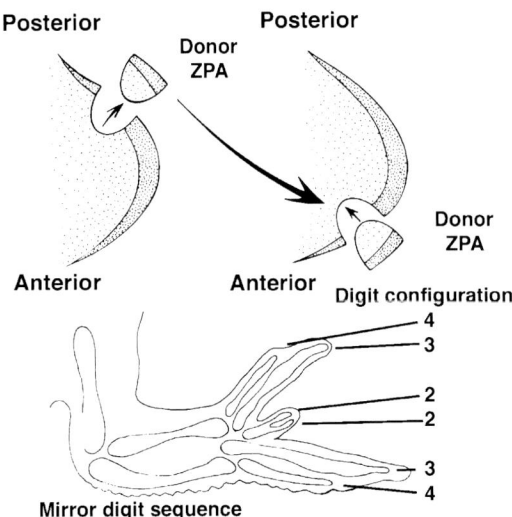

FIGURE 201-14. Mirror hand resulting from transplantation of the zone of polarizing activity (ZPA). A transplanted segment of ZPA is harvested from the posterior (ulnar) element of a donor limb bud. It is placed into the anterior segment (radial side) of another recipient limb bud with its normal posterior ZPA left untouched. The result is a posteriorizing influence mediated by Sonic hedgehog expression in the transplanted ZPA. The limb develops as a "mirror hand" (a mirror wing in the experimental case) with a 4, 3, 2, 2, 3, 4 digit configuration instead of the 1, 2, 3, 4 digit configuration of the normal wing. (After Saunders.[34] Illustration by J. Bittl.)

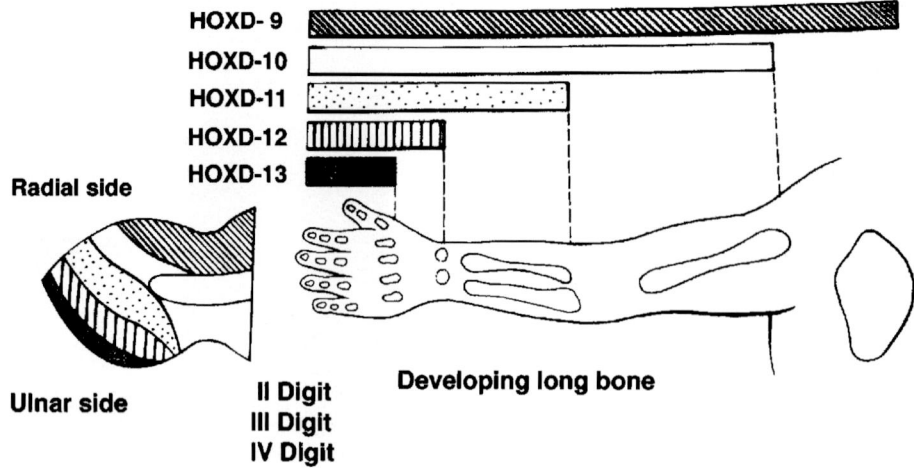

FIGURE 201-16. HOX genes control proximal-distal patterning. The homeobox family of HOX genes is expressed in complex overlapping patterns, which significantly influences proximal to distal patterning in the developing limb. (From Morgan B, Tabin C: Hox genes and growth: early and late roles in limb bud morphogenesis. Development [suppl] 1994;181. Reprinted with permission of The Company of Biologists, Ltd.)

HOX12 in the carpal region, and *HOX13* in the hand. There appears to be some redundancy built into the system because in mice, deletion of *hoxa11* or *hoxd11* has no apparent effect. However, loss of both *hoxa11* and *hoxd11* results in a mouse strain lacking the radius and ulna. The cascade of HOX expression is regulated in part by FGFs secreted by the apical ectodermal ridge and is influenced also through the Shh pathway.

The impact of human mutations in the HOX region has been recognized. For example, *HOXD13* is known to signal terminal digit formation, the most distal element in the limb. Mutations in *HOXD13* are associated with a complex synpolydactyly identified in a Portuguese family in the Boston area (Color Plate 201-2).[37]

MOLECULAR BASIS OF HUMAN UPPER EXTREMITY DISORDERS

By the standard molecular biology techniques of chromosome analysis, linkage analysis, and positional cloning, the genetic causes of several congenital hand disorders have been identified (Table 201-2). A closer examination of a few illustrative examples may be instructive.

Apert Syndrome

The Apert syndrome, or acrocephalosyndactyly, is characterized by midface retrusion, parrot beak nose, craniosynostosis, and mirror image complex syndactyly of the hands and feet. For unclear reasons, the severity of the craniofacial manifestations in an individual patient appears to be inversely proportional to the severity of the hand deformities.[38]

All Apert children who have been genetically analyzed display one of two point mutations in the gene encoding FGF receptor 2 *(FGFR2).*[39] Both the Ser252Trp and Pro253Arg mutations are located in the exon IIIA region of the *FGFR2* locus. Craniofacial and hand surgeons have long observed that patients with Apert syndrome experience inversely proportional deformity with respect to the cranial and hand involvement. The Ser252Trp mutation is now known to be associated with the "good hands, bad head" phenotype, and the Pro253Arg mutation is associated with the "bad hands, good head" phenotype.[40]

Pfeiffer Syndrome

The Pfeiffer syndrome, characterized by broad thumbs and halluces, has similarly been mapped to FGF receptor domains. Mutations in *FGFR1* (8p) are associated with a mild phenotype, whereas *FGFR2* (10q) mutations are associated with a more severe phenotype.[41]

Central Synpolydactyly

The first isolated human congenital hand disorder to be definitively mapped to a specific gene was a familial synpolydactyly.[37] A large, multigeneration family of Portuguese descent in the Boston area was noted to have an autosomal dominant severe synpolydactyly affecting the upper and lower extremities. Because of a phenotypic similarity with a particular mutant mouse strain, *HOXD13* (2q31) was postulated as a candidate gene. A polyA repeat sequence mutation was, in fact, identified in this region in affected individuals (Color Plate 201-3; see also Color Plate 201-2).[42]

TABLE 201-2 ✦ GENES THAT HAVE BEEN LOCALIZED OR IDENTIFIED FOR CONGENITAL HAND MALFORMATIONS

Disorder	Location	Gene	Reference
Preaxial polydactyly, type II and type III	7q36	?	Hootnick et al[24]
Preaxial polydactyly	7q36	?	Tsukurov et al[46] Heus et al[47]
Synpolydactyly (syndactyly type II)	2q31	HOXD13	Muragaki et al[37]
Split hand-split foot (SHSF)	7q21	?	Scherer et al[48]
SHSF 1, autosomal dominant			Crackower et al[49] Cobben et al[50] Nunes et al[51] Marinoni et al[52]
SHSF 2, X-linked	Xq26	DSS1?	Faiyaz ul Haque et al[53]
SHSF 3, autosomal dominant	10q24-25	?	Nunes et al[51] Gurrieri et al[54] Raas-Rothchild et al[55]
Split hand	6q21-23	?	Tsukahara et al[56]
Postaxial oligodactyly	6q21	?	Gurrieri et al[54]
Brachydactyly type C	12q24	?	Haws[57] Polymeropoulos et al[58]
Brachydactyly type D Hand, foot, genitalia		HOXD13 HOXA13	Del Campo et al[59] Mortlock and Innis[60]
Limb-mammary	3q27	?	van Bokhoven et al[61]
EEC	3q27	?	Celli et al[62]
Ulnar-mammary	12q23-24.1	TBX3	Bamshad et al[63]
Mirror hands, feet	4q13	?	Matsumoto et al[64]
Hand-heart	12q2	TBX5	Basson et al[65]
Holt-Oram		HOS1	Bonnet et al[66] Terrett et al[67] Li et al[68] Olsen et al[69]
Cephalopolysyndactyly (Greig syndrome)	7p13	?	Pettigrew et al[70] Brueton et al[71]
Acrocephalosyndactyly (Apert syndrome)	10q	FGFR2	Wilkie et al[39] Park et al[40] Slaney et al[72] Matsumoto et al[64]
Saethre-Chotzen	7p	?	Brueton et al[71]
Pfeiffer syndrome	8p 10q	FGFR1 FGFR2	Lajeune et al[73] Schell et al[74] Robin et al[75]
Trichorhinophalangeal (TRP1)	8q	?	Hamers et al[76]

Postaxial Polydactyly

Greig syndrome—or cephalopolysyndactyly syndrome—is characterized by craniofacial and limb abnormalities including postaxial polydactyly.[43] A series of patients with Greig syndrome was found to have point mutations in the *GLI3* gene. *GLI3*, or zinc finger gene, has also been implicated in postaxial polydactyly type A and Pallister-Hall syndrome. Recent work demonstrated that *GLI3* regulates Shh and is important in determining digit number and digit identity.[44]

REFERENCES

1. Zervos S: On Babylonian and Assyrian obstetrics and gynaecology. Arch Gesch Med 1912;6:401.
2. Aristotle: De Generatione Animalium. Oxford, Oxford Press, 1912.
3. Needham J: A History of Embryology. Cambridge, Cambridge University Press, 1959.
4. Pasteur L: Fermentations et generations dites spontanees. Oeuvres de Pasteur reunies par P. Vallery-Radot 1861;2:210.
5. Wolpert L: Positional information and the spatial pattern of cellular differentiation. J Theor Biol 1969;25:1.
6. Bardeen D, Lewis W: Development of the limbs, body wall, and back in man. Am J Anat 1901-1902;1:1-35.
7. Lewis W: The development of the arm in man. J Anat 1901-1902;1:146.
8. O'Rahilly R, Gardner E: The timing and sequence of events in the development of the limbs in the human embryo. Anat Embryol 1975;148:1-23.
9. Feinberg R, Saunders JW Jr: Effects of excising the apical ectodermal ridge in the development of the marginal vasculature in the wing bud of the chick. J Exp Zool 1982;219:345.
10. Streeter G: Developmental horizons in human embryos IV. A review of histogenesis of cartilage and bone. Contrib Embryol 1949;33:149-167.
11. Gray D, Gardner E, O'Rahilly R: The prenatal development of the skeleton and joints of the human hand. Am J Anat 1957;101:169-223.
12. Cihak R: Ontogenesis of the skeleton and intrinsic muscles of the human hand and foot. Ergebn Anat Entwicklungsgesch 1972;46:1.
13. Haines R: The development of joints. J Anat 1947;81:33-55.
14. Drachman D, Banker B: Arthrogryposis multiplex congenita. A case due to disease of the anterior horn cells. Arch Neurol 1961;5:77-93.
15. Drachman D, Sokoloff L: The role of movement in embryonic joint development. Dev Biol 1966;14:401-420.
16. Zou H, Niswander L: Requirement of BMP signaling in interdigital apoptosis and scale formation. Science 1996;272:738.
17. Cihak R: Connections of the abductor pollicis longus and brevis in the ontogenesis of the human hand. Folia Morphol (Praha) 1972;20:102-105.
18. Cihak R: Reduction of insertion of m. interosseous dorsalis accessorius in human ontogenesis. Folia Morphol (Praha) 1973;21:228-231.
19. Cihak R: Differentiation and rejoining of muscular layers in the embryonic human hand. Birth Defects 1977;13:97.
20. Mrazkova O: Ontogenesis of arterial trunks in the human forearm. Folia Morphol (Praha) 1973;21:193.
21. Caplan A, Koutroupas S: The control of muscle and cartilage development in the chicklimb: the role of differential vascularization. J Embryol Exp Morphol 1973;29:571.
22. Edwards E: Organization of the small arteries of the hand and digits. Am J Surg 1960;99:837-846.
23. Coleman S, Anson B: Arterial patterns in the hand. Surg Gynecol Obstet 1961;113:409-424.
24. Hootnick D, Levinsohn EM, Randall PA, Packard DS Jr: Vascular dysgenesis associated with skeletal dysplasia of the lower limb. J Bone Joint Surg Am 1980;62:1123-1129.
25. Zaleske D, Holmes L: Vascular patterns in the malformed hind limb of DH/+ mice. In Fallon J, Caplan A, eds: Limb Development and Regeneration, Part A. New York, Alan R. Liss, 1983:317-326.
26. Chevallier A, Kieny M, Mauger A: Limb somite relationship: effect of removal of somatic mesoderm in the wing musculature. J Embryol Exp Morphol 1978;43:263.
27. Zwilling E: Morphogenetic phases in development. Dev Biol Suppl 1968;2:184.
28. Newman S, ed: Lineage and pattern in the developing wing bud. In Ede D, Hinchcliffe JR, Balls M, eds: Vertebrate Limb and Somite Morphogenesis. Cambridge, Cambridge University Press, 1977.
29. Chevallier A, Kieny M, Mauger A: Limb-somite relationship: origin of limb musculature. J Embryol Exp Morphol 1977;41:245-258.
30. Jacob H, Christ B: On the formation of muscular pattern in the chick limb. In Merker H, Nau H, eds: Teratology of the Limbs. Berlin, Walter de Gruyter, 1980.
31. Kieny M, Chevallier A: Autonomy of tendon development in the embryonic chick wing. J Embryol Exp Morphol 1979;49:153-165.
32. Graham JM Jr, Stephens TD, Siebert JR, Smith DW: Determinants in the morphogenesis of muscle tendon insertions. J Pediatr 1982;101:825-831.
33. Summerbell P: The zone of polarizing activity: evidence for a role in normal chick limb morphogenesis. J Embryol Exp Morphol 1979;50:217-233.
34. Saunders J: The experimental analysis of chick limb bud development. In Ede D, Hinchcliffe JR, Balls M, eds: Vertebrate Limb and Somite Morphogenesis. Cambridge, Cambridge University Press, 1977.
35. Summerbell D, Lewis JH, Wolpert L: Positional information in chick-limb morphogenesis. Nature 1973;244:492.
36. Niswander L, Tickle C, Vogal A, et al: FGF-4 replaces the apical ectodermal ridge and directs outgrowth and patterning of the limb. Cell 1993;75:579.
37. Muragaki Y, Mundlos S, Upton J, Olsen BR: Altered growth and branching patterns in synpolydactyly caused by mutations in HOXD13. Science 1996;272:548.
38. Upton J: Classification and pathologic anatomy of limb anomalies (in the Apert syndrome). Clin Plast Surg 1991;18:321-355.
39. Wilkie A, Slaney SF, Oldridge M, et al: Apert syndrome results from localized mutations of FGFR2 and is allelic with Crouzon syndrome. Nat Genet 1995;9:165.
40. Park W, Theda C, Maestri NE, et al: Analysis of phenotypic features and FGFR2 mutations in the Apert syndrome. Am J Med Genet 1995;57:321.
41. Meyers G, Goldberg R, Daentl DL, et al: FGFR2 exon IIIa and IIIc mutations in Crouzon, Jackson-Weiss, and Pfeiffer syndromes: evidence for missense changes, insertions, and a deletion due to alternative RNA splicing. Am J Hum Genet 1996;58:491.
42. Askarsu A, Stoilov I, Yilmaz E, et al: Genomic structure of HOXD13 gene: a nine polyalanine duplication causes synpolydactyly in two unrelated families. Hum Mol Genet 1996;5:495.
43. Kalff-Suske M, Wild A, Topp J, et al: Point mutations throughout the Gli3 gene cause Greig cephalopolysyndactyly syndrome. Hum Mol Genet 1999;8:1769.
44. Litingtung Y, Dahn RD, Li Y, et al: Shh and Gli3 are dispensable for limb skeleton formation but regulate digit number and identity. Nature 2000;29:979.
45. Mimouni D, Mimouni M: Polydactyly reported by Raphael. Br Med J 2000;321:1622.

46. Tsukurov O, Boehmer A, Flynn J, et al: A complex bilateral poly-syndactyly disease locus maps to chromosome 7q36. Nat Genet 1994;6:282.

47. Heus D, Hing A, van Baren MJ, et al: A physical and transcriptional map of the preaxial polydactyly locus on chromosome 7q36. Genomics 1999;57:342.

48. Scherer S, Poorkaj P, Allen T, et al: Fine mapping of the autosomal dominant split hand/split foot locus on chromosome 7, band q21.3-22.1. Am J Hum Genet 1994;55:12.

49. Crackower M, Scherer SW, Rommens JM, et al: Characterization of the split hand/split foot malformation locus SHFM at 7q21.3-q22.1 and analysis of a candidate gene for its expression during limb development. Hum Mol Genet 1996;5:571.

50. Cobben J, Verheij JB, Eisma WH, et al: Bilateral split hand/foot malformation and inv(7)(p22q21.3). J Med Genet 1995;32:375.

51. Nunes M, Schutt G, Kapur RP, et al: A second autosomal split hand/split foot locus maps to chromosome 10q24-q25. Hum Mol Genet 1995;4:2165.

52. Marinoni J, Boyd E, Sherman S, Swartz C: Familial split hand/split foot bone deficiency does not segregate with markers linked to the SHSF1 locus in 7q21.3-q22.1. Hum Mol Genet 1994;3:1355-1357.

53. Faiyaz ul Haque M, Uhlhaas S, Knapp M, et al: Mapping of the gene for X-chromosomal split hand/split foot anomaly to Xq26-26.1. Hum Genet 1993;91:17.

54. Gurrieri F, Prinos P, Tackels D, et al: A split hand-split foot (SHFM3) gene is located at 10q24-25. Am J Med Genet 1996;62:427.

55. Raas-Rothchild A, Manouvrier S, Gonzales M, et al: Refined mapping of a gene for split hand-split foot malformation (SGSF3) on chromosome 10q25. J Med Genet 1996;33:996.

56. Tsukahara M, Yoneda J, Asuma R, et al: Interstitial deletion of 6q21-23 associated with split hands. Am J Med Genet 1997;69:268.

57. Haws D: Inherited brachydactyly and hypoplasia of the bones of the extremities. Ann Hum Genet 1963;26:201.

58. Polymeropoulos H, Ide SE, Magyari T, Francomano CA: Brachydactyly type C gene maps to human chromosome 12q24. Genomics 1996;38:45.

59. Del Campo M, Jones MA, Veraksa AN, et al: Monodactylous limbs and abnormal genitalia are associated with hemizygosity for the human 2q21 that includes the HOXD cluster. Am J Med Genet 1999;65:104.

60. Mortlock D, Innis JW: Mutation of HOXA13 in hand-foot-genital syndrome. Nat Genet 1997;15:179.

61. van Bokhoven H, Jung M, Smits AP, et al: Limb mammary syndrome: a new genetic disorder with mammary hypoplasia, ectrodactyly and other hand/foot anomalies maps to human chromosome 3q27. Am J Med Genet 1999;64:538.

62. Celli J, Duijf P, Hamel BS, et al: Heterozygous germline mutations in the p53 homolog p63 are the cause of the EEC syndrome. Cell 1999;15:143.

63. Bamshad M, Root S, Carey JC: Clinical analysis of a large kindred with the Pallister ulnar-mammary syndrome. Am J Med Genet 1996;65:325.

64. Matsumoto K, Urano K, Kubo Y, et al: Mutation of the fibroblast growth factor receptor 2 gene in Japanese patients with Apert syndrome. Plast Reconstr Surg 1998;101:307.

65. Basson C, Solomon SD, Weissman B, et al: Genetic heterogeneity of heart-hand syndrome. Circulation 1995;91:1326.

66. Bonnet D, Pelet A, Legeai-Mallet L, et al: A gene for Holt-Oram syndrome maps to the distal long arm of chromosome 12. Nat Genet 1994;6:405.

67. Terrett J, Newbury-Ecob R, Cross GS, et al: Holt-Oram syndrome is a genetically heterogeneous disease with one locus mapping to human chromosome 12q. Nat Genet 1994;6:401.

68. Li Q, Newbury-Ecob RA, Terrett JA, et al: Holt-Oram syndrome is caused by mutations in TBX, a member of the Brachyury (T) gene family. Nat Genet 1997;15:21.

69. Olsen E, Srivastava D: Molecular pathways controlling heart development. Science 1996;272:671.

70. Pettigrew A, Greenberg F, Caskey CT, Ledbetter DH: Greig syndrome associated with an interstitial deletion of 7p: confirmation of Greig syndrome to 7q13. Hum Genet 1991;87:452.

71. Brueton L, van Herwerden L, Chotai KA, Winter RM: The mapping of a gene for craniosynostosis: evidence for linkage of the Saethre-Chotzen syndrome to distal chromosome 7p. J Med Genet 1992;29:681.

72. Slaney S, Oldridge M, Hurst JA, et al: Differential effect of FGFR2 mutations on syndactyly and cleft palate in Apert's syndrome. Am J Med Genet 1996;58:923.

73. Lajeune E, Ma HW, Bonaventure J, et al: FGFR2 mutations in Pfeiffer syndrome. Nat Genet 1995;9:108.

74. Schell U, Hehr A, Feldman NH, et al: Mutations in the FGFR1 and FGFR2 cause familial and sporadic Pfeiffer syndrome. Hum Mol Genet 1995;4:323.

75. Robin N, Feldman GJ, Mitchell HF, et al: Linkage of Pfeiffer syndrome to chromosome 8 centromere and evidence for genetic heterogeneity. Hum Mol Genet 1994;3:2153.

76. Hamers A, Jongbloet P, Peeters G, et al: Severe mental retardation in a patient with tricho-rhino-phalangeal syndrome type I and 8q deletion. Eur J Pediatr 1990;149:618.

77. Rueff J: De Conceptu Generatione Hominis et iis quae circa haec potissimum consyderantur. Libri sex. Zurich, Froschorus, 1554.

78. Hildegard of Bingen S: Liber Scivias. Codex B. Wiesbaden, 1150.

79. England M: Color Atlas of Life Before Birth. London, Wolfe Publications, 1983.

80. Yasuda M: Pathogenesis of preaxial polydactyly of the hand in human embryos. J Embryol Exp Morphol 1975;33:745-756.

81. Izpisúa Belmonte J, Tickle C, Dolle P, et al: Expression of the homeobox Hox-4 and the specification of position in the chick limb bud. Nature 1991;350:1991.

82. Izpisúa Belmonte J, Duboule D: Homeobox genes and pattern formation in the vertebrate limb. Dev Biol 1992;152:26.

83. Morgan B, Tabin C: Hox genes and growth: early and late roles in limb bud morphogenesis. Dev Suppl 1994;181.

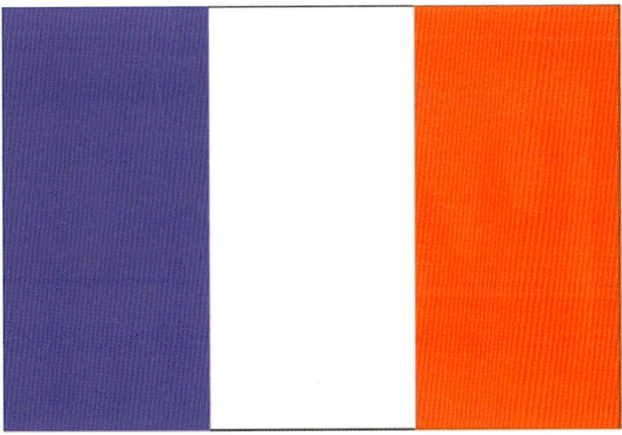

COLOR PLATE 201-1. The French flag problem. The modern era of embryology began in 1969, when Wolpert proposed the French flag problem. How do developing biologic systems create a pattern?

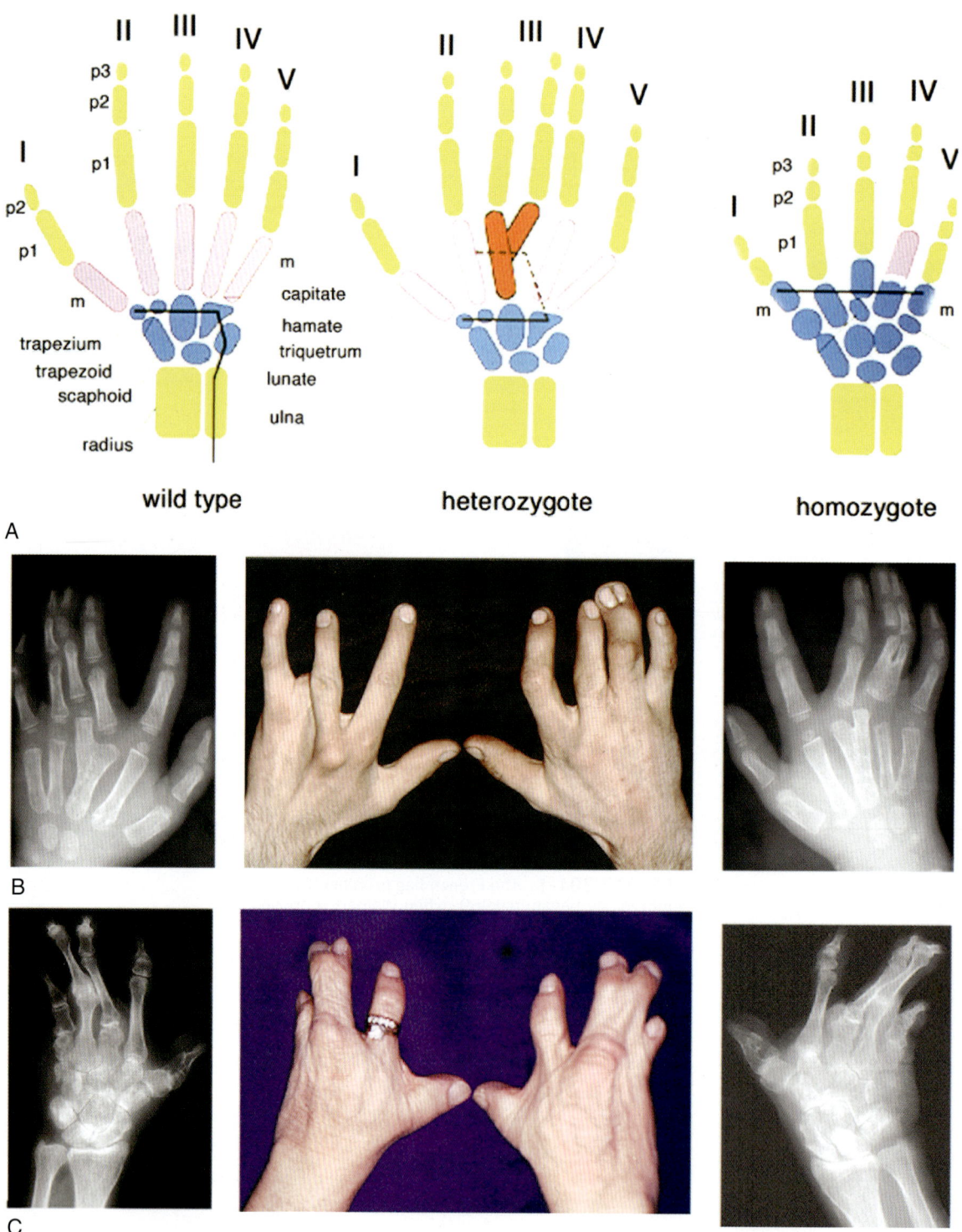

COLOR PLATE 201-2. Synpolydactyly clinical forms. *A,* The diagram of the hand skeleton of a normal (wild type) individual is compared with heterozygous and homozygous distal upper limbs in individuals with synpolydactyly. Carpal bones are in blue. The pisiform is not shown. Digits are represented by Roman numerals, phalanges by the letter *p,* and metacarpals by the letter *m.* In the heterozygote, metacarpal III is branched and gives rise to an extra distal digit. In the homozygote, the metacarpals are fully or partially replaced by carpal-like bones. Note the short p2 in all the digits. *B,* The clinical appearance and radiographs of a heterozygous individual. After a syndactyly release of the left hand, the ring digit was lost because of vascular compromise. This complication occurred in 1959. *C,* The mother of the individual shown in *B* was a homozygous individual. No surgical correction was ever performed, and she wore her ring on the left index digit. Her feet were equally deformed and constituted her major disability.

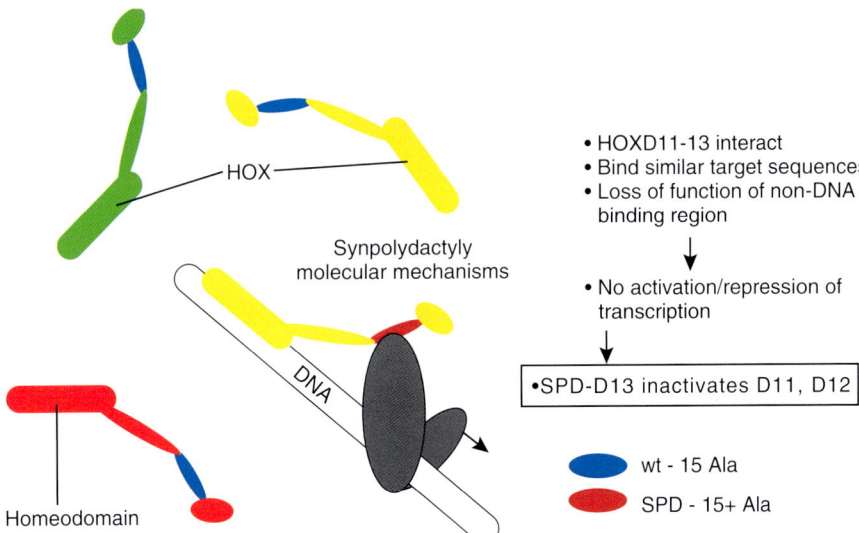

HOX

Synpolydactyly
molecular mechanisms

DNA

Homeodomain

- HOXD11-13 interact
- Bind similar target sequences
- Loss of function of non-DNA
  binding region

- No activation/repression of
  transcription

•SPD-D13 inactivates D11, D12

wt - 15 Ala

SPD - 15+ Ala

COLOR PLATE 201-3. Mechanism of mutation in synpolydactyly (SPD). The molecular mechanisms responsible for the development of synpolydactyly are unknown. One hypothesis is that the alanine stretch on the nonbinding portion of DNA creates a repression of transcription. (Courtesy of Stefan Mundlos, MD, and Bjorn Olsen, MD.)

Classification of Upper Limb Congenital Differences and General Principles of Management

JOSEPH UPTON III, MD

Hand surgery as a discipline has blossomed since the initial impetus it received from the organization of regional hand centers by Sterling Bunnell during World War II. During the past 50 years, the subject of congenital anomalies has remained a quiet backwater compared with the torrent of information in other subject areas, such as trauma, arthritis, tendon surgery, and microsurgery. Paradoxically, congenital hand deformity was one of the earliest topics to be pursued by medical academe and remains one of the most influenced by recent advances in surgical techniques and bioengineering technology.

Early references to limb anomalies are found in the Old Testament of the Bible; for example, Goliath was a member of a band of giants with polydactyly.[1] In 1634, Ambroise Paré documented monsters and pedigrees with limb malformations that he described as secondary to "bad thoughts or deeds," which could be damaging enough to terminate a pregnancy.

Further, the stigma of a congenital malformation has always been present in varied forms. In Biblical times, a six-fingered hand was so common in one Arabian tribe, the Hyabites, that a child with five digits was considered abnormal and subsequently sacrificed![2] Extra digits in England were considered a sign of royalty owing to the frequent appearance of polydactyly in the royal line since Mary Queen of Scots.[3] In the late 19th century, American art has shown evidence of untreated polydactyly (Fig. 202-1). As early as 1832, St. Hilaire[4] published a detailed classification of congenital deformities of the hand; soon after, Velpeau[5] (1847) and Vrolik[6] (1849) produced thoughtful treatises on the subject. Although most deformities of that time were unapproachable surgically, the treatment of syndactyly was hotly debated in 1892 when Felizet[7] proposed his classic techniques for separation of digits.

The embryology of the upper limb has been studied in great detail for more than 100 years; the interested reader is referred to the eloquent 40-page dissertation of Bardeen and Lewis.[8] Yet, despite this long history, the classification and treatment of congenital anomalies of the hand have only recently reached a high degree of definition and consensus, elevating the study of this branch of hand surgery to the level of its kindred subspecialties. During the 1960s, the thalidomide tragedy served to focus renewed attention on limb anomalies, providing a stimulus for basic research and development of new surgical solutions. Even today, with thalidomide babies entering their 40s and 50s, progress is still being made with regard to their treatment.

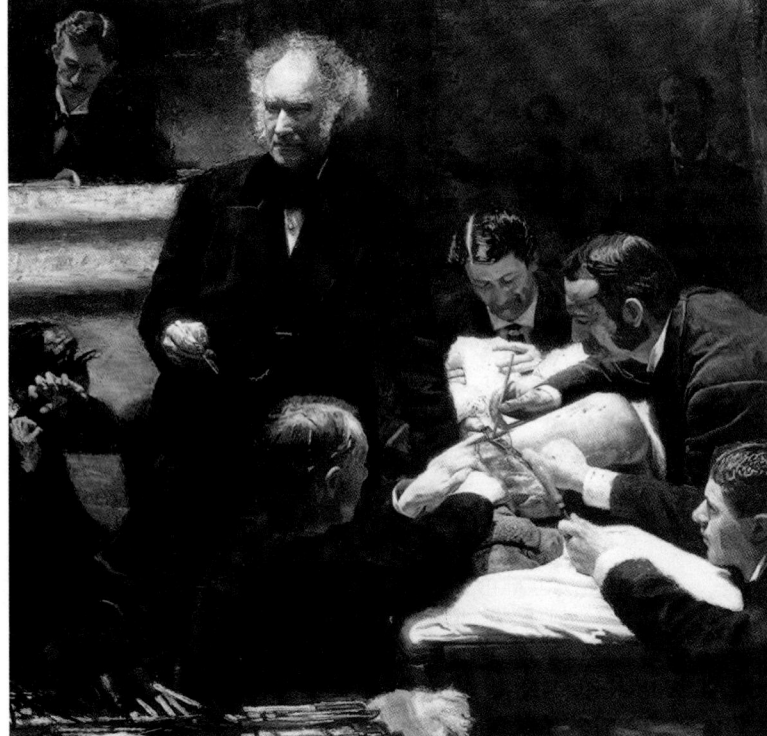

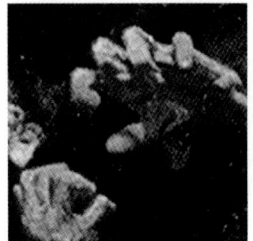 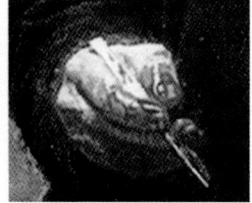 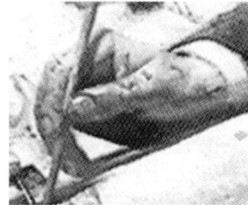

FIGURE 202-1. *The Gross Clinic.* Artist Thomas Eakins' most celebrated painting, which hangs in the Jefferson Medical College in Philadelphia, depicts Dr. Samuel D. Gross at work in his surgical clinic. It serves well to illustrate the nature of surgery and medical education in the late 1800s. Supremely confident and charismatic, Professor Gross is performing several tasks simultaneously—operating, setting an example, teaching. The light focuses on his head, revealing extreme concentration, and on his bloody hand, which holds the scalpel. Quite obviously, he and his first assistant are performing an operation. Modern viewers may be surprised to learn that the shaded figure who is witnessing this routine medical procedure is probably the patient's mother; during this era, it was not uncommon for one family member to remain at the bedside. The woman's face is shaded by her shawl and polydactylous left hand, and her suffering goes unnoticed by everyone in the room. All the participants in this work lived and worked in the Germantown section of Philadelphia in 1875 when this painting was made.[83] Interestingly, many of the family pedigrees studied throughout our discovery of the synpolydactyly gene were descended from German immigrants who initially lived in this region.[84] The mother's hand shows a type III ulnar polydactyly.

One cannot always transfer the principles of adult hand surgery to the treatment of congenitally deformed children. Quite obviously, surgery on the infantile hand is always restricted by the small size of the anatomic structures. The child is not merely a miniature adult, which presents many problems in both evaluation and treatment. For example, it is difficult to predict the psychological and functional responses to a deformed limb or to a proposed reconstruction because valid preoperative evaluation is difficult to obtain when a child is too young to articulate his or her needs precisely.[9]

Further complicating matters, the medical history is usually obtained from a parent, who may prove surprisingly uncertain of the manual dexterity and limitations of the child. Unfortunately, objective methods for sensory evaluation are few, and radiographic evaluation is of limited value because the infant hand is composed mostly of cartilage. Primary and secondary ossification centers appear at different ages in different bones of the upper limb, and knowledge of these is essential in planning treatment (Fig. 202-2). Surgical decisions and recommendations will be greatly influenced by careful observation of the development of hand function, hand-eye coordination, and growth.

Although the actual terrain of such surgery is often very small, particular care and time will be necessary to obtain a truly informed consent. The surgeon who examines and operates on a baby is actually treating an entire family. Parents may be devastated by guilt when an imperfection is identified in their otherwise normal child. Beginning with the initial consultation and continuing through every aspect of treatment, parents must be counseled honestly and informed clearly about potential benefits and complications. When a complex deformity exists, family members and patients should not be given unrealistic expectations about the anticipated functional result; every attempt

OSSIFICATION CENTERS

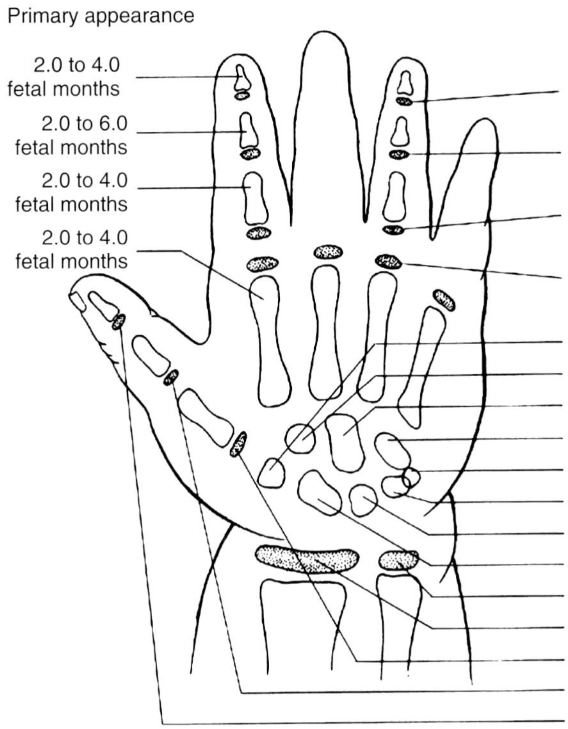

Primary appearance	Secondary appearance		Secondary fusion Boys/Girls (mean)	
2.0 to 4.0 fetal months	5.0 mo. to 2.0 yr.		13.1	11.2
2.0 to 6.0 fetal months	5.0 mo. to 2.0 yr.		16.0	12.7
2.0 to 4.0 fetal months	5.0 mo. to 2.0 yr.		14.5	12.9
2.0 to 4.0 fetal months	10.0 mo. to 2.0 yr.		14.4	13.1
	Trapezium	1.5 to 10.0 yr.	9.1	9.0
	Trapezoid	2.5 to 5.0 yr.	9.1	9.0
	Capitate	Birth to 6.0 mo.	15.0	13.1
	Hamate	Birth to 6.0 mo.	15.0	13.1
	Pisiform	6.5 to 16.5 yr.		
	Triquetrum	6.0 mo. to 4.0 yr.	12.7	11.1
	Lunate	6.0 mo. to 9.5 yr.	15.3	10.3
	Scaphoid	2.5 to 9.0 yr.	9.4	8.8
	4.0 to 9.0 yr.		10.3	9.9
	3.0 mo. to 1.5 yr.		16.3	15.8
	13.0 mo. to 4.0 yr.		12.6	12.0
			12.9	12.0
			13.6	12.0

FIGURE 202-2. Ossification centers. The time of appearance of primary and secondary ossification centers in the hand[85] and the average time of fusion of secondary centers for both boys and girls are outlined. There is great variation in these numbers among different ages and individuals. The time of appearance and of fusion can also be altered in the presence of a congenital anomaly.[49] The time for secondary fusion is given in years.

should be made to answer their questions with precision and sincerity. When there are multiple alternative methods of treatment, it is often wise to enlist the help of a knowledgeable colleague for a second opinion. Perhaps most important, if it is better for the patient, there is no disgrace in referring the child to a more experienced surgeon.[10] With these complex procedures, there can be little room for error.

DYSMORPHOLOGY APPROACH

Although some hand surgeons think geneticists are often speaking a foreign language, it is important to understand their terms, which are actually straightforward and simple. The 3.0% figure of babies born with some type of congenital malformation has not changed during the 100 years these statistics have been recorded. Only 0.7% of all babies born have multiple malformations; these often involve the upper limb.[11] A clear understanding of the alterations in morphogenesis is necessary in the evaluation of the malformation, the formulation of a treatment plan, and the counseling of parents.

Initial evaluation by the hand surgeon should consist of (1) a complete family history; (2) a thorough pregnancy history, including information about medical illnesses, medications, alcohol and substance abuse, onset and vigor of fetal movements, gestational timing, any indications of uterine irritability, delivery, and neonatal adaptations; and (3) postnatal growth and development. Minor and major abnormalities should all be recorded. Major anomalies are those that have serious medical and surgical implications and characteristically involve the renal, pulmonary, cardiovascular, or central nervous system. Hand anomalies are usually classified as minor. However, when three or more minor anomalies exist in a single patient, there is a 90% chance that a major anomaly will also be found.[12]

The term *congenital malformation syndrome* may be confusing because there are problems with all three components of the term. *Congenital* refers to something present at birth, but not all conditions, such as bone dysplasias and vascular malformations, are evident at birth. *Malformation* is used to define a gross structural anomaly and, according to some, should not be used for biochemical and nonstructural changes.[13] The anomalies that represent the breakdown of previously normal tissue could more accurately be identified as disruptions, and the anomalies that represent the normal response of tissue to unusual mechanical forces are termed deformations. Both of these stand in contrast to malformations, which denote a primary problem within the morphogenesis of the tissue. *Syndrome* is even more difficult to define but is generally used to describe a combination of anomalies in a patient (particularly if there is a familial tendency for this combination), a single known biochemical or chromosomal cause for this combination, or a developmental sequence that results in the combination. The distinction between a syndrome and the chance association of three or more anomalies can be an artificial one (Fig. 202-3).

Within the developing hand, there are two basic types of deformations: those in which the problem is due to an intrinsic abnormality within the tissues of the hand, such as gigantism associated with a vascular malformation; and those in which the deformation is caused by mechanical forces extrinsic to the fetus, such as the constriction ring in the amnionic band sequence. However, even with these two distinct categories, the interpretation of the patient's anomaly may not be simple (Fig. 202-4). Reference should be made to published stages of prenatal development for an estimate of the time at which the particular deficiency developed.[14] Multiple problems in morphogenesis may be explained in terms of a sequence, which is a single simple problem leading to a cascade of subsequent problems.

Developmentalists and geneticists have designated three types of sequences: malformation, deformation, and disruption (see Figs. 202-3 and 202-4).[14] In a *malformation sequence,* poor formation of tissue within the fetus initiates the chain of defects, which may range from minimal to severe. A good example is radial dysplasia, in which one may see anything from an isolated loss of thenar muscles to a complete absence of the radius with clubhand posturing. Another example is the multiple soft tissue and skeletal anomalies in the Apert syndrome. Recurrence rate for malformations is usually in the range of 1% to 5%.

In a *deformation sequence,* there is no intrinsic problem with the fetus or embryo, but abnormal external mechanical or structural forces cause secondary distortion or deformation. Leakage of amniotic fluid is a common cause for external deformation of the intact fetus in this sequence. In contrast to malformations, recurrence rate in this category is low, unless the cause is a persistent anatomic defect such as a bicornuate uterus. An example is forearm skin necrosis in cutis aplasia, which may be caused by prolonged labor or by a compression of the arm between the pelvis and uterine wall after breech presentation.

In a *disruption sequence,* the normal fetus or embryo is subject to tissue breakdown or injury, which may be vascular, infectious, mechanical, or metabolic in origin. The proximal limb deficiencies caused by thalidomide or alcohols are dramatic examples. Tethering or constriction of limb parts by amniotic bands in the constriction ring syndrome is one of the most common disruptions seen in the upper limb.

It is often important to recognize that not all of the patient's problems can be explained by a single initiating factor. As a general rule, when single or multiple anomalies exist in combination without any known unifying cause, the term *malformation association* is preferred by most diagnosticians. Similarly, when the anomalies appear to be the result of multiple defects

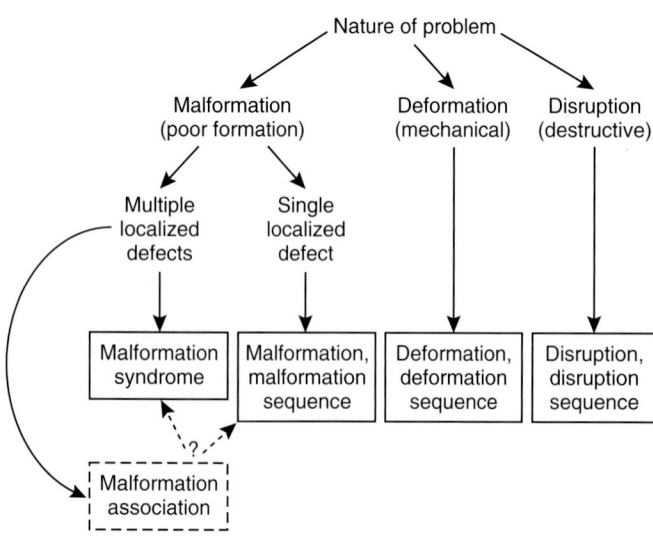

FIGURE 202-3. Dysmorphology. Most patients with more than one defect will be placed into one of these five categories by the developmentalists. The natural history of the malformation, the treatment options, the prognosis, and the possible outcomes may vary tremendously and depend greatly on the organ systems involved. When there are multiple structural defects that cannot be explained by a single initiating cause and its consequences, the term *malformation syndrome* is used. An accurate diagnosis of the 0.7% of babies born with multiple defects is important in terms of providing both a prognosis and a plan of management. (From Jones K: Smith's Recognizable Patterns of Human Malformation, vol 1, 4th ed. Philadelphia, WB Saunders, 1988:673.)

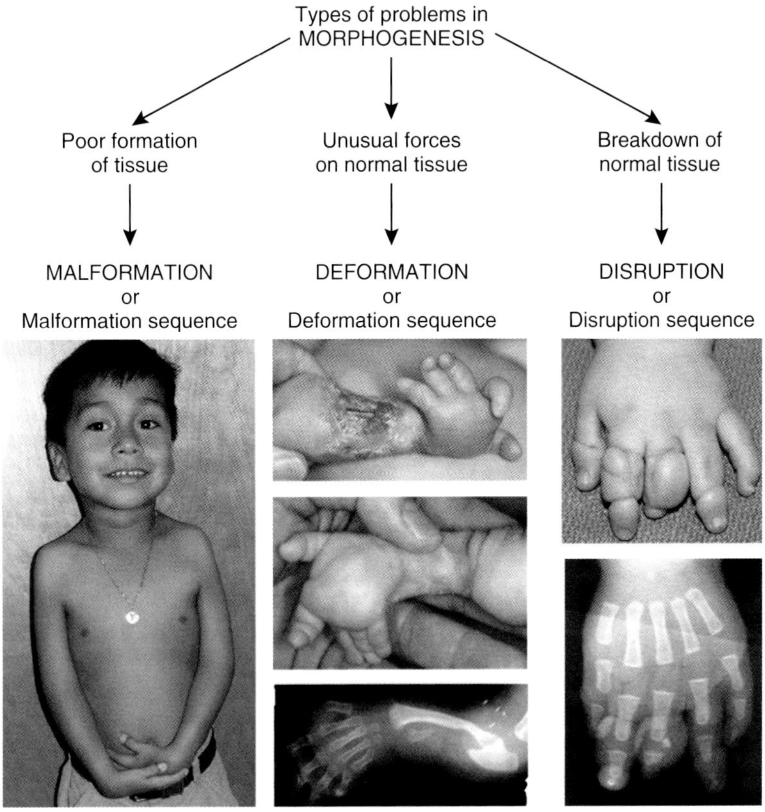

FIGURE 202-4. Dysmorphology. Three types of structural defects that can result in a chain of defects (a sequence) by the time of birth are demonstrated here. On the left is a child with multiple joint contractures associated with arthrogryposis, which is due to poor muscle formation. In the center is the forearm of a 4-week-old infant who sustained an in utero compression necrosis of soft tissue similar to a Volkmann ischemic injury. By 1 month of age, an impressive extension contracture had developed. On the right is the hand of a child with the constriction ring syndrome. This disruption was caused by the amniotic bands, which became entangled around the normally developing digits. (Modified from Graham J, Hanson JW, Darby BL, et al: Independent dysmorphology evaluations at birth and 4 years of age for children exposed to varying amounts of alcohol in utero. Pediatrics 1988;81:772-778.)

in one or more tissues, malformation syndrome is also used. Although the specific etiology of many syndromes is not known, some known causes include chromosomal abnormalities, mutant gene disorders, and teratogens such as thalidomide.

Geneticists employ important general principles and terms in their evaluation of multiple anomalies. The hand surgeon must understand these terms as they are used by geneticists, pediatricians, and other primary care physicians. *Nonspecificity* of an individual defect means that a single anomaly will not necessarily invoke a specific diagnosis. Instead, the surgeon may be forced to rely on the overall pattern of a collection of minor and major anomalies. For example, a defect such as clinodactyly or syndactyly may appear as part of many diagnostic categories, but considered alone, it will not lead to a specific diagnosis of a syndrome. *Variance* in the extent or expression of a defect is common among individuals—even within the same individual. *Pleiotropism,* another commonly used term, is synonymous with variance.[15] A good example is the Holt-Oram syndrome, in which hand manifestations may include absence of a thumb, hypoplastic thumb, or even a triphalangeal thumb, all defects involving the radial ray. Similarly, patients with absence of the radius and clubhand posturing in one limb may demonstrate only

hypothenar muscle absence on the other. The term *heterogeneity* is used often because many deformities with the same phenotype, such as simple syndactyly, or similar physical characteristics may have different etiologies. In the multiply deformed child, it is important to withhold a diagnosis (and its consequences) until there is a close resemblance between the overall pattern of anomalies seen in the patient and the syndrome under consideration.

Roughly half of cases with multiple anomalies fall into syndromes; the remaining have not been specifically labeled. In the absence of known genetic information, it is impossible to give accurate information about the potential risk for recurrence for future malformations. Temtamy and McKusick's work[1] is the only comprehensive treatise devoted to the genetics of hand malformations. Without very specific knowledge, the hand surgeon should not tell the parents that their child's condition is rare and will not occur in future children. In these situations, geneticists recommend telling parents that the lowest risk is 0% and the highest 25% with each pregnancy.[14]

Meanwhile, investigation of the genetic causes of upper limb anomalies is expanding at an exponential rate. Referral to a local birth defects service (if available) or a clinical geneticist may be particularly helpful for parents with multiply deformed children and advisable for the patients when they reach childbearing age. If uncertain about the possible association of upper limb anomalies with other malformations, one should refer to texts by Smith,[14] Jones,[16] and Temtamy and McKusick.[17]

SYNDROMES

The hand surgeon must not only recognize that a hand anomaly may have the likelihood of future occurrence within a given family or kindred but also consider that the deformity may be part of a syndrome. Identification of a syndrome may be difficult because not all of the cardinal features may be present and observations may be limited by the interest of the observer, but as Greenfield states, "a three-legged dog is still a dog."[18] With many syndromes, the upper limb surgeon is only peripherally involved, especially when the diagnosis has been made shortly after birth (Fig. 202-5). Major lifesaving cardiovascular, renal, or gastrointestinal procedures must often be performed before anything is indicated for the hand or upper limb. It is important for these patients to have periodic evaluations by a single surgeon and occupational therapist; they will then know the patient and accurately recognize important changes in function.

Syndrome diagnoses are difficult for the surgeon to make if he or she is not working with these children on a daily basis. Even though most are related to some chromosomal aberration (single gene, multiple gene, or sex linked), only 5% of all upper limb malformations occur as part of a well-recognized syndrome.[11] Over the years, geneticists have become fascinated with four particular hand anomalies: syndactyly, which is part of at least 38 different syndromes; clinodactyly,

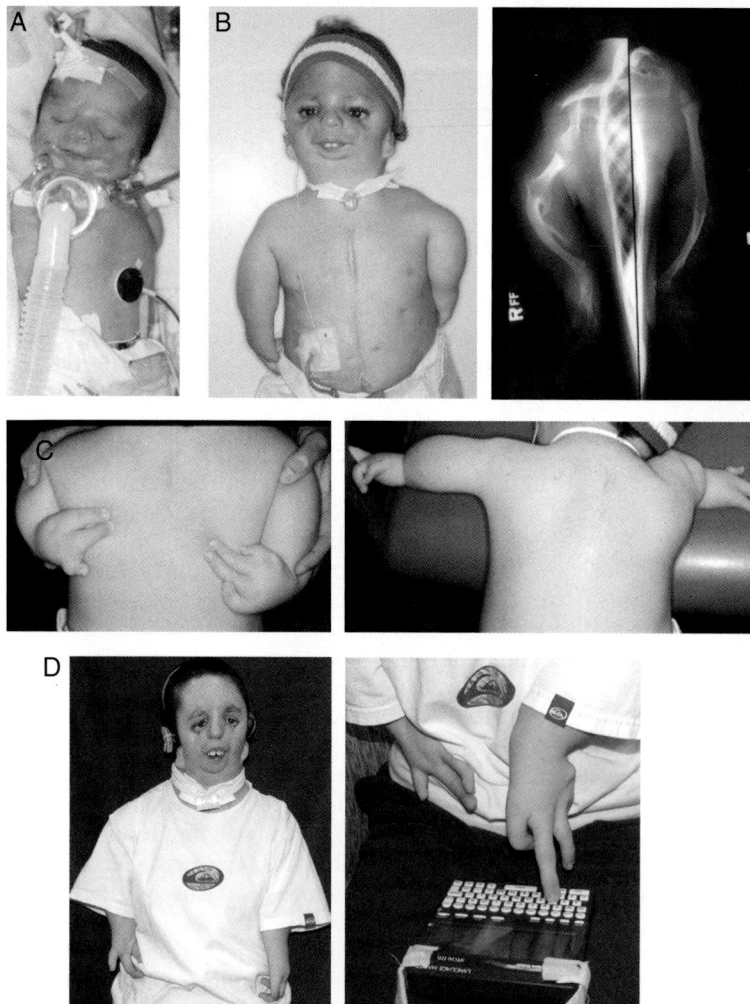

FIGURE 202-5. Malformation syndrome. *A,* This infant was born with severe craniofacial and limb abnormalities consistent with the diagnosis of Nager syndrome (acrofacial dysostosis). The facial abnormalities include mandibular and maxillary hypoplasia, severe micrognathia, cleft palate, abnormal external ears and microtia, atretic temporal bones, and severe conductive hearing loss.[19,87] The upper limbs are short with associated radial ray defects, including partial and complete absence of the thumb, hypoplasia of the radius and ulna, and radiohumeral synostosis. *B,* The boy's appearance at age 18 months. He has had multiple thoracic and abdominal surgeries for life-threatening conditions. A permanent tracheostomy is in place. The radiograph of his limbs shows bilateral humeroradial synostoses. As he grows, these upper limbs become relatively shorter because of the closure of growth plates at the elbow level. *C,* The behind-the-back posturing of these limbs is similar to that seen in patients with longitudinal ulnar failure of formation. *D,* As a teenager, his hand function with computers and digital games was remarkable. He has had no surgical correction in his hands but has had extensive surgery in other regions and is presently having his maxilla and mandible distracted anteriorly.

part of 56 syndromes; camptodactyly, part of 40 syndromes; and brachydactyly, part of 18 syndromes.[19] Many potential associations (with radial ray defects) will be made by the hand surgeon. These include Fanconi pancytopenia or syndrome, thrombocytopenia-absent radius (TAR) syndrome, Holt-Oram syndrome, and the VACTERL association (in which the hand anomaly may be the most obvious malformation in a patient with life-threatening hematologic, cardiac, genitourinary, or other musculoskeletal anomalies).

The often-fatal Fanconi anemia can now be diagnosed with a DEB (diepoxybutane) test[20,21] at the time of birth. During the past 25 years, we as hand surgeons were the first specialists to make this diagnosis in the cases of five children with small stature and varying degrees of radial dysplasia. One is referred to appropriate genetics textbooks for a full description of these syndromes.[14] Temtamy and McKusick's work[1] is the only one currently available that specifically deals with genetics of upper limb anomalies. An excellent review of the International Nomenclature of Constitutional Diseases of Bone and the Hand is contained in Poznanski's book[18] on the radiology of hand syndromes. The glossary of Flatt's books[3,22] contains a useful outline of common syndromes and eponyms involving the upper limb. The interested hand surgeon should also check the appropriate Web sites on the Internet to become up to date in this field, which is changing dramatically on a weekly basis.

HAND SURGEONS' APPROACH
Historical Perspective

During the past 100 years, attempts to establish a universal classification of congenital hand anomalies have been frustrated by the wide array of Greek and Latin terms used to describe similar deformities with the emphasis on different pathologic features. With no systematic approach, there has been confusion, duplication, and overlapping of terms, and some anomalies have seemed too bizarre to fit into any specific category at all. Isidore St. Hilaire[4] proposed probably the first classification in 1832, introducing terms such as phocomele (seal limb), hemimele (part of limb missing), and ectromele (complete absence). Since then, numerous authors have championed their own versions at regular intervals.[23,24] Not surprisingly, in the first comprehensive book devoted to the diagnosis and treatment of congenital hand anomalies, Kelikian wrote, "congenital anomalies of the hand do not lend themselves to a comprehensive classification."[24] This statement is as true today as it was more than 30 years ago.

In fact, there was so much confusion by the middle of the 20th century that the National Research Council adopted the Frantz and O'Rahilly[25] classification, which was based on skeletal appearance and still contained terms such as micromelia (partial limb) and amelia (missing limb). This system distinguished between a defect beyond which structures were absent (terminal defect) and a defect with the absence of parts between the proximal and terminal portions of the limb (intercalary defect). These terms were a reflection of the spectrum of skeletal reduction defects treated in prosthetic clinics. Ten years later, Frantz and O'Rahilly revised this system and added subcategories transverse and longitudinal to each category. In addition, a distinction was made between the preaxial or postaxial position of the limb for the intercalary defects.[25]

Many years later, this system was amended as the concept of central deficiencies was introduced.[26] Interestingly, a committee for the International Society for Prosthetics and Orthotics then simplified this approach and designated all conditions as either transverse or longitudinal deficiencies.[27] During this time, the hand surgeons realized that they did not have a good system of their own. For example, although there may be a missing "intercalary" defect within the upper limb, the remaining skeletal structures may not be normal. From this time to the present, the principal underlying difficulty in identification has been our limited understanding of embryogenesis.

International Classification

An ideal classification system should contain simple descriptive terms, permit easy recording of common conditions, but also allow full categorization of complex cases. While being specific, it should not be so detailed that its use becomes burdensome. Few of the flawed systems are likely to hold a surgeon's interest for long, nor have any of the myriad systems advanced the treatment of any specific anomaly. Nonetheless, until surgeons, pediatricians, embryologists, geneticists, and others who deal with these conditions use the same terms, communication and advances in treatment remain difficult, particularly when international boundaries are crossed. For example, the true incidence of a deformity and international comparisons are impossible to establish unless the classification is common to all.

Toward this end, in 1968, the American Society for Surgery of the Hand and the International Federation of Societies for Surgery of the Hand (IFSSH) adopted a classification proposed by committees within the IFSSH.[28-30] This system is based on grouping conditions according to the anatomic parts that have been primarily affected by certain embryonic failures (Table 202-1). The IFSSH system is basically a morphologic schema derived from a limited knowledge of embryologic failures. Blauth, Muller, and other German

TABLE 202-1 ✦ CLASSIFICATION OF CONGENITAL HAND DIFFERENCES (EXPANDED VERSION)

I. Failure of formation
  A. Transverse arrest
    a. Shoulder
      i. Shoulder level (amelia)
      ii. Clavicle
    b. Upper arm
      i. Upper arm level
        1. Long above elbow (AE)
        2. Short above elbow (AE)
    c. Elbow
      i. Elbow level
    d. Forearm
      i. Forearm level
        1. Long below elbow (BE)
        2. Short below elbow (BE)
    e. Wrist
      i. Wrist level (acheiria)
    f. Carpal
      i. Carpal level (no metacarpals present)
        1. Proximal carpal row
        2. Distal carpal row
    g. Metacarpal
      i. Metacarpal level (adactyly)
    h. Phalanx
      i. Phalangeal level
        1. Proximal phalangeal level
        2. Middle phalangeal level
        3. Distal phalangeal level
  B. Longitudinal arrest
    a. Radial ray (preaxial)
      i. Normal radius
        1. Thumb hypoplastic—functional
          a. Type I
          b. Type II
          c. Type III (floating thumb)
        2. Thumb hypoplastic—nonfunctional
          a. Type IV
        3. Thumb absent
      ii. Hypoplasia of the radius (complete but small)
        1. Thumb hypoplastic—functional
          a. Type I
          b. Type II
          c. Type III
        2. Thumb hypoplastic—nonfunctional
          a. Type IV (floating thumb)
        3. Thumb absent
          a. Type V
        4. Madelung deformity
        5. Other
      iii. Partial absence of the radius (distal end absent)
        1. Thumb hypoplastic—functional
          a. Type I
          b. Type II
          c. Type III
        2. Thumb hypoplastic—nonfunctional
          a. Type IV (floating thumb)
        3. Thumb absent
      iv. Complete absence of the radius
        1. Thumb hypoplastic—functional
          a. Type I
          b. Type II
          c. Type III
        2. Thumb hypoplastic—nonfunctional
          a. Type IV (floating thumb)
      v. Absent/hypoplastic thenar muscles
        vi. Absent/hypoplastic extensor muscles
        vii. Absent/hypoplastic flexor muscles
    b. Central ray(s) (cleft hand)
      i. Central ray deficiency
        1. Typical type (deficiency type)
          a. Metacarpal absent, digit hypoplastic
          b. Metacarpal present, digit hypoplastic or absent
          c. Metacarpal, digit absent
        2. Atypical type (symbrachydactyly)
          a. Triphalangeal type
          b. Diphalangeal type
          c. Monophalangeal type
          d. Aphalangeal type
          e. Ametacarpia type
          f. Acarpia type
          g. Forearm amputation type
    c. Ulnar ray (postaxial)
      i. Ulnar ray deficiency
        1. Normal ulna
          a. Metacarpals, digits hypoplastic
          b. Metacarpals hypoplastic, digits absent
          c. Metacarpals, digits absent
        2. Ulna hypoplastic (complete but small)
          a. Metacarpals, digits hypoplastic
          b. Metacarpals hypoplastic, digits absent
          c. Metacarpals, digits absent
        3. Partial absence of the ulna (distal end absent)
          a. Metacarpals, digits hypoplastic
          b. Metacarpals hypoplastic, digits absent
          c. Metacarpals, digits absent
        4. Complete absence of ulna
          a. Metacarpals, digits hypoplastic
          b. Metacarpals hypoplastic, digits absent
          c. Metacarpals, digits absent
        5. Defect of ulna with humeroradial synostosis
        6. Hypoplastic/absent hypothenar muscles
        7. Hypoplastic/absent extensor muscles
        8. Hypoplastic/absent flexor muscles
    d. Intersegmental (intercalated) type of longitudinal arrest
      i. Phocomelia
        1. Proximal type (hand to forearm to trunk)
        2. Distal type (hand to arm to trunk)
        3. Total type (hand to trunk)
      ii. Other
II. Failure of differentiation (separation) of parts
  A. Soft tissue involvement
    a. Disseminated
      i. Arthrogryposis
        1. Arthrogryposis multiplex congenita (upper and lower limb involvement)
        2. Distal type
          a. Severe (shoulder, elbow, hand)
          b. Moderate (forearm and hand)
          c. Mild (wrist and hand)
    b. Shoulder level
      i. Undescended shoulder

1. Sprengel shoulder
2. Other
  ii. Absence of thorax muscles (including Poland syndrome)
    1. Pectoralis major complete or partial absence
    2. Pectoralis major and minor absence
    3. Other
  c. Elbow and forearm level
    i. Aberrant muscle
      1. Aberrant extrinsic flexor muscles
      2. Aberrant extrinsic extensor muscles
      3. Aberrant intrinsic muscles of the hand
      4. Other
  d. Wrist and hand level
    i. Cutaneous syndactyly (simple complete or incomplete)
      1. Radial (1st interdigital web space)
      2. Central (2nd, 3rd interdigital web space)
      3. Ulnar (3rd interdigital web space)
      4. Combination of 1 ± 2 or 3
    ii. Congenital flexion contracture (camptodactyly)
      1. Fifth digit alone
      2. Multiple digits
      3. Syndromic types with multiple digits
      4. Others
    iii. Thumb-in-palm deformity
    iv. Deviated finger without skeletal deformity (laxity secondary to differentiation of muscle, ligament, or capsule)
      1. Radial-ulnar
        a. Isolated digit
        b. Congenital ulnar drift
          i. Freeman-Sheldon syndrome
          ii. Congenital ulnar drift "windblown hand"
          iii. Arthrogryposis
        c. Other
    v. Congenital trigger digit or thumb
    vi. Other
  e. Skin and appendages
    i. Pterygium (webbing) of axilla or elbow
    ii. Cutis aplasia congenita
    iii. Congenital clubbing of nails
    iv. Other nail deformities
    v. Other
B. Skeletal involvement
  a. Shoulder level
    i. Congenital humerus varus
    ii. Other
  b. Elbow level
    i. Elbow synostosis
      1. Humeroradial
      2. Humeroulnar
      3. Total
    ii. Elbow ankylosis (joint segmentation present)
  c. Forearm
    i. Proximal radioulnar synostosis
      1. Without radial head subluxation or dislocation
      2. With radial head dislocation
    ii. Distal radioulnar synostosis
  d. Wrist and hand

    i. Synostosis of carpal bones
      1. Lunate-triquetrum
      2. Capitate-hamate
      3. Scaphoid-lunate
      4. Others
    ii. Synostosis of metacarpal bones
      1. Ring-small
        a. Type I: proximal third
        b. Type II: up to one half
        c. Type III: total
      2. Others
    iii. Synostosis of phalanges (osseous syndactyly, complex syndactyly)
      1. Radial (1st-2nd rays)
      2. Central (2nd-3rd, 3rd-4th rays)
      3. Ulnar (4th-5th rays)
      4. Mitten hand
        a. Apert syndrome
        b. Others
    iv. Symphalangia
      1. Proximal interphalangeal joint
      2. Other
    v. Congenital deviation (clinodactyly)
      1. Idiopathic clinodactyly
        a. Fifth finger
        b. Thumb (including "delta" phalanx)
        c. Others
    vi. Hypersegmentation
      1. Triphalangeal thumb
        a. Type I: rudimentary extra phalanx
        b. Type II: short middle phalanx
        c. Type III: trapezoidal middle phalanx
        d. Type IV: long rectangular middle phalanx
        e. Type V: hypoplastic triphalangeal thumb (include five-fingered hand)
        f. Type VI: triphalangealism associated with thumb duplication
      2. Others
C. Congenital tumorous anomalies
  a. Vascular system
    i. Hemangioma
      1. Congenital hemangioma
        a. Rapidly involuting congenital hemangioma (RICHe)
        b. Noninvoluting congenital hemangioma (NICHe)
        c. Infantile
        d. Hemangiomatosis
      2. Pyogenic granuloma
      3. Kaposiform hemangioendothelioma
      4. Rare tumors
        a. Glomus tumor
        b. Giant cell angioblastoma
        c. Hemangiopericytoma
        d. Hemangioendothelioma
        e. Angiosarcoma
        f. Others
      5. Others
    ii. Malformation
      1. Telangiectasias
        a Cutis marmorata telangiectasia congenita (CMTC)
        b. Hereditary hemorrhagic telangiectasia

Continued

TABLE 202-1 ✦ CLASSIFICATION OF CONGENITAL HAND DIFFERENCES (EXPANDED VERSION)—cont'd

2. Capillary (CM)
   a. Port-wine stain
   b. Other
3. Venous (VM)
   a. Pure venous
   b. Glomovenous
   c. Blue rubber bleb nevus syndrome
   d. Others
4. Venolymphatic (VLM)
5. Lymphatic (LM)
   a. Pure lymphatic
   b. Lymphangiomatosis
6. Arterial (AM) with arteriovenous fistula (AVF)
   a. Type I: generalized aneurysmal
   b. Type II: confined to axial patterns
   c. Type III: diffuse
7. Combined (eponymous) slow-flow malformations
   a. Capillary lymphatic venous malformation (CLVM, Klippel-Trénaunay syndrome)
   b. Bannayan-Riley-Ruvalcaba syndrome
   c. Maffucci syndrome
8. Combined (eponymous) fast-flow malformations
   a. CAVM (Parkes Weber) syndrome
9. Others
   b. Neurologic
      i. Neurofibromatosis
      ii. Others
   c. Connective tissue
      i. Juvenile (aponeurotic) fibroma
      ii. Infantile digital fibroma
      iii. Others
   d. Skeletal (not including overgrowth syndromes)
      i. Osteochondromatosis (including multiple hereditary exostoses)
      ii. Enchondromatosis
      iii. Fibrous dysplasia
      iv. Epiphyseal abnormalities
         1. Arm and forearm
         2. Carpal
         3. Metacarpal and phalanges
   v. Other

III. Duplication
   A. Whole limb
   B. Humerus
   C. Radius
   D. Ulna
      a. Mirror hand (ulnar dimelia)
      b. Other
   E. Digit (include metacarpal level)
      a. Polydactyly
         i. Radial (1st ray)
            1. Type I: distal phalanx
            2. Type II: interphalangeal joint
            3. Type III: proximal phalanx
            4. Type IV: metacarpophalangeal joint
            5. Type V: metacarpal
            6. Type VI: carpometacarpal joint
            7. Triphalangeal thumb
            8. Special thumb
         ii. Central
         iii. Ulnar
            1. Type I: small soft tissue connection
            2. Type II: skeletal articulation
            3. Type III: entire ray

F. Epiphyseal (extra)
   a. 1st ray
   b. 2nd ray
   c. Others
IV. Overgrowth
   A. Whole limb
      a. Hemihypertrophy
      b. Associated with a vascular condition
         i. Klippel-Trénaunay (CLVM)
         ii. Parkes Weber (AVM with AVFs)
         iii. LM
      c. Other
   B. Partial limb
      a. Associated with vascular condition
      b. Other
   C. Hand (includes carpal, metacarpal, and digit levels)
      a. Macrodactyly
         i. Lipomatous
         ii. With neurofibromatosis
         iii. With bone or cartilage exostoses
         iv. Others
V. Undergrowth
   A. Whole limb
   B. Forearm and hand
   C. Hand alone
      a. Entire
      b. Partial
   D. Metacarpal
      a. Brachymetacarpia
         i. 5th ray
         ii. Other
      b. Other
   E. Phalangeal (digit)
      a. Brachysyndactyly
         i. With associated hypoplasia/aplasia of thorax muscles (Poland syndrome)
         ii. Without associated absence of thorax muscles
      b. Brachydactyly
         i. Defect of middle phalanx only (brachymesophalangia)
         ii. Defect of two or more phalanges
         iii. Defect of either proximal or distal phalanx
         iv. Other
VI. Constriction ring syndrome (amniotic band disruption sequence, Streeter dysplasia, others)
   A. Focal necrosis
      a. Constriction ring (partial or complete circumferential)
         i. With lymphedema
         ii. Without lymphedema
         iii. Multiple
      b. Acrosyndactyly
   B. Amputation ("intrauterine")
      a. Arm
      b. Forearm
      c. Wrist
      d. Metacarpal
      e. Digit
      f. Combination of c and d, d and e
      g. Other
VII. Generalized syndromes
   A. Apert
   B. Other craniosynostoses
   C. Holt-Oram

D. Thrombocytopenia-absent radius (TAR)
E. Fanconi anemia
F. Hemifacial microsomia (also craniofacial microsomia)
G. Nager

H. Trichorhinophalangeal
I. Cleft hand, cleft foot
J. Arthrogryposis multiplex congenita
K. Others

This is an expanded version of the classification adopted by the Congenital Committee of the International Federation of Societies for Surgery of the Hand, which included the American Society for Surgery of the Hand and the American Association for Hand Surgery. Clearly, one anomaly or group of congenital differences may be included in more than one category. Some malformations, such as tumorous conditions, may not be considered by some to be genuine upper limb anomalies.

Notation is as follows:
I. Main category
   A. Subcategory
      a. Level of deformity
         i. Diagnosis
            1. Subclassification
               a. Details

surgeons were the first to describe "teratologic progression" of a deformity from its least to most severe forms, and their system for thumb hypoplasia and aplasia is widely used today[31-33] because it is simple, practical, and helpful in clinical decision-making. Within this classification system, provisions for the continued use of widely accepted terms that are easily understood and cause no confusion have been made. They include -*melia* (limb), *cheir-* (hand), *-dactyly* (fingers), *-phalangia* (segments of fingers), *brachy-* (short), *syn-* (together), *poly-* (many), and *macro-* (large). All authors agree that it is beneficial to avoid confusion and to minimize the use of Latin and Greek derivatives in the description of these anomalies.

In the 10 years after its inception, this system was clinically tested by Flatt[34] and refined by Swanson and colleagues twice.[29,30] Each refinement offered further subdivisions of the major categories. Currently, there are seven major categories that cover the overwhelming majority of congenital hand differences. Failure of formation of parts (arrest of development) is divided into two sections, transverse and longitudinal. Longitudinal defects include all those that are not in the transverse category. Failure of differentiation (separation) of parts is divided into failure at shoulder, arm, forearm, and hand, which are in turn classified into carpal, metacarpal, and digital anomalies. The remaining groups include duplication, overgrowth (gigantism), undergrowth, constriction ring syndrome, and generalized skeletal anomalies. The author's expanded version of this classification system is shown in Table 202-1.[35] An excellent glossary of terms is provided in Flatt's textbooks,[3,22] and a comprehensive discussion of classifications is found in Kelikian's classic work.[24]

With our present state of knowledge, it is best to generalize that classifications "are only conveniences, and it is not possible to precisely classify all hand malformations."[22] Nevertheless, hand surgeons are compulsive individuals who are inevitably drawn to simple, anatomically distinct classifications. In spite of this fact, many malformations may still fit into two or more categories. A classic controversy persists in the distinction between hands with central syndactyly, central syndactyly with short digits (brachysyndactyly), central loss with hypoplastic digits (symbrachysyndactyly), and central loss with no digits.[36-41] Similarly, in the past, the clinical distinction was made between a typical cleft hand and an atypical cleft hand, which now is commonly labeled symbrachydactyly (Fig. 202-6). Each may represent "a morphologic classification in search of an embryologic explanation."[42] As the more experienced clinicians review their cases, they realize that some simply do not fit into any category (Fig. 202-7).[43]

All systems are relative and subject to change. Thirty years ago, vascular anomalies were loosely described as strawberries, salmon patches, and hemangiomas. Twenty years ago, a biologic system was proposed[44] and made the distinction between those lesions that involuted (hemangiomas) and those that did not (malformations). During the past 10 years, our knowledge has expanded exponentially; each major category has been significantly subdivided, and many exceptions have been identified, such as the noninvoluting congenital hemangioma. The relationships and distinctions between certain low-grade vascular tumors, such as hemangioendotheliomas, kaposiform hemangioendotheliomas, and mixed malformations, are often easily made and constantly challenge our present knowledge. Inevitably, these distinctions are likely to change as more scientific and clinical knowledge is gained.

Lumpers and Splitters

In light of our limited knowledge of genetics, molecular biology, and embryologic mechanisms of

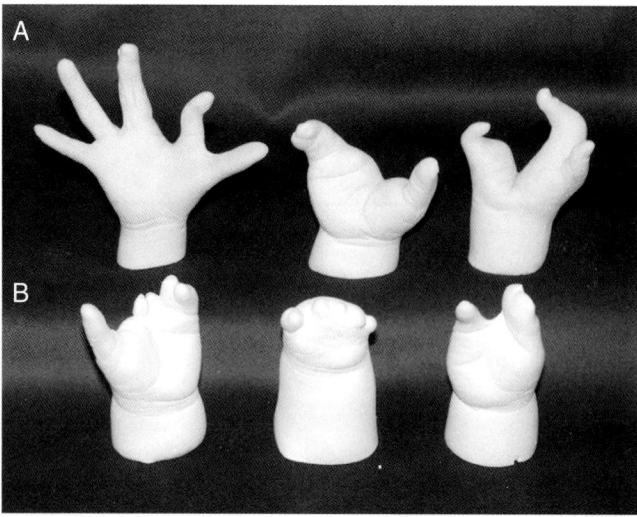

FIGURE 202-6. Classification, cleft hand controversy. Japanese and German surgeons and embryologists have pointed out that there are different types of central hand deficiencies. *A,* Three variations of a "typical cleft hand" are seen in right hands. On the left is a hypoplastic index between the thumb and long finger—from which it is separated by a shallow central cleft. The center is a complete absence of the index and long rays. On the right, a complete absence of the long and ring rays, with hypoplastic thumb and fifth digits, is seen. *B,* A characteristic "atypical cleft hand," now called symbrachydactyly, is shown on the left. This morphologic sequence represents mesenchymal damage to the hand plate with an intact or partially intact apical ectodermal ridge.[36] These surgeons would recommend that the hand in the center be called the same but be placed farther down the teratologic sequence. The mold on the right represents a right hand with thumb polydactyly and abnormal phalanges containing longitudinal epiphyseal brackets. The small hand contains only the border first and fifth metacarpals. At present, we have no classification for this hand.

malformations, a comprehensive classification will be frustrating for the strict constructionist. Many anomalies will continue to fit easily into two or more categories. Some current authors hypothesize that polydactyly, syndactyly, and the typical cleft hand may have a common teratologic mechanism on the basis of similarities of osseous fusions.[45,46] The two opposing trends in nosology must include traditional "lumpers" and "splitters." The lumpers try to find new things in common, an attempt that seems logical because it is easier to find similarities and variance (pleiotropism) within many syndromes. However, splitting a subclassification into smaller subcategories becomes necessary as genetic and biochemical heterogeneity becomes apparent. This is especially important when prognostication depends on specific biochemical or genetic factors. Splitting congenital hand deformities strictly on morphologic grounds, however, can be an exercise in futility. Hand surgeons work with a degree of precision that can breed a subclassification within every group of congenital upper limb differences. All of these, of course, are subject to change but satisfy objectives such as communication within the literature, formation of registries, and categorization of slides and digital images, among others. Ultimately, most of these systems still rely on the radiologic appearance of the limb.

RADIOLOGY

Radiologic measurements of the hand are the parameters most commonly used for evaluation of maturation, which includes the presence or absence of ossification centers, modeling characteristics, and presence or absence of epiphyseal closure (see Fig. 202-2). Although skeletal maturation and size may be related, they can develop independently. Variations exist in all 28 bones of the hand and wrist in terms of length, width, mineralization (density), relative size, and position. To be clinically useful, these features must be compared with normative tables that specifically define sex, race, and nutritional and social background of the group studied.[18]

The skeletal structures of the upper limb vary tremendously in size, shape (which can be determined not only by genetics but also immobility), temperature, physical forces, and other environmental or endocrine causes. For years, both primary and secondary ossification centers of bones of the hand and wrist have been used to assess age and skeletal maturation (see Fig. 202-2).

Skeletal Maturation

The simplest method for evaluating maturation to identify congenital defects is to look through the standards

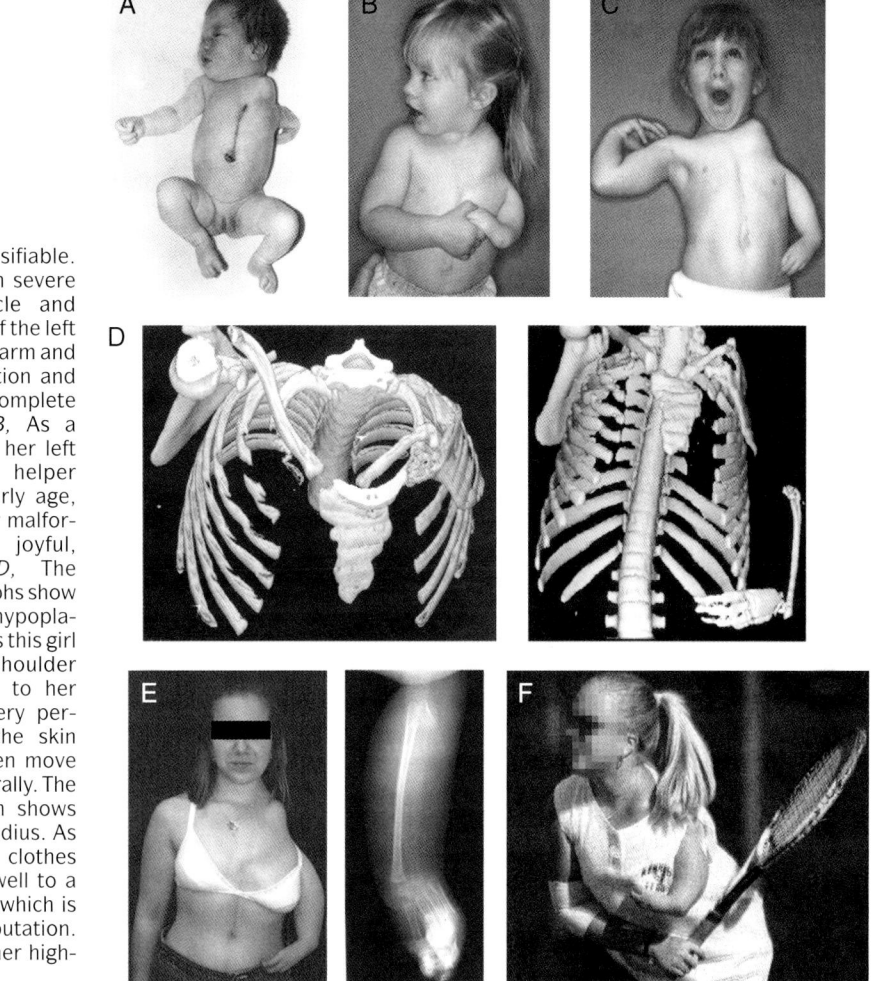

FIGURE 202-7. Unclassifiable. *A,* This child was born with severe hypoplasia of the clavicle and scapula and total absence of the left humerus. Her small left forearm and hand had good digital motion and sensation in spite of a complete absence of the radius. *B,* As a toddler, she began to use her left forearm and hand as a helper extremity. *C,* At a very early age, she learned to live with her malformation and developed a joyful, theatrical personality. *D,* The three-dimensional radiographs show the severe proximal limb hypoplasia and humeral absence. As this girl grew, the hypoplastic shoulder became positioned closer to her midline. *E,* The only surgery performed was to expand the skin lateral to the shoulder, then move the clavicle and scapula laterally. The radiograph of the forearm shows complete absence of the radius. As a teenager, she wore her clothes more easily and adapted well to a major shoulder deficiency, which is similar to a forequarter amputation. *F,* She has been a star on her high-school tennis team.

and find a radiograph that corresponds to the hand being studied[47] or to compare the onset of ossification centers.[48,49] When uncertain, comparison of individual maturation characteristics of each bone should be made.[50] Comparison of ossification centers in children with unilateral limb anomalies will often show delay on the affected side. No standards are available for common anomalies such as radial dysplasias, cleft hands, and hypoplastic hands.

OSSIFICATION CENTERS

The first indication of ossification within the fetal skeleton appears in the distal phalanges between 7 and 8 weeks, in the metacarpals and proximal phalanges by 10 weeks, and in the middle phalanges by 13 weeks. At birth, primary ossification centers have not appeared at the carpal level. However, during childhood and throughout adolescence, the appearance of primary and secondary ossification centers is routinely used

in the assessment of skeletal age, which should be clearly distinguished from chronologic age (see Fig. 202-2).

These measurements are of value if they are used consistently during a long period. Even in healthy youngsters, there are tremendous variations in the timing of the appearance of these centers between girls and boys, different races, different cultures, and different levels of nutrition. Therefore, evaluation of the ossification centers and skeletal age in hands with congenital differences is made difficult. With no standards available, we have relied on sequential films of both the abnormal and normal limbs for comparison. Although definitive studies have not been completed, our impression is that the relative differences measured at birth remain the same from birth through skeletal maturity with most conditions. The obvious exceptions are conditions that are associated with overgrowth, such as vascular malformations, macrodactylies, and syndromic gigantism like the Proteus syndrome, among other conditions.

GREULICH AND PYLE

One of the two most common methods of measuring skeletal maturation is the use of the Greulich and Pyle atlas,[47] in which maturation is correlated with radiographs of the left hand. The aim is for the observer to match his or her patient's radiograph to the appropriate image in the atlas. Maturity is defined as a specific skeletal age. The basis for this atlas is a series of radiographs of middle-class American children in Cleveland, Ohio, during the 1950s. The major disadvantage, of course, is that there may be a discrepancy between actual age and maturity. The advantage is that the system is quick and easy, and if it is used continually in a given child, it does give an accurate assessment of growth.

TANNER AND WHITEHOUSE

The Tanner and Whitehouse method[50] is based on the development of 19 individual bones that develop at the same rate within the hand. They include the carpal bones and the epiphyses of the distal radius and ulna. More complicated than the Greulich and Pyle system, these standards are obtained from radiographs of lower- and middle-class children in the United Kingdom during the 1950s. The first measurement records the finger bones, radius, and ulna; the second records the carpal bones; and the third is a combination of the two. The major advantage is that it does give a proper indication of maturity. However, the major problem, as with the Greulich and Pyle method, is one of racial variation.

RACIAL, GENDER, AND CLASS VARIATIONS

Racial variations have been well documented. For example, Japanese children mature at the same rate as those in the United Kingdom until 8 years of age, when they then progress much more rapidly. European children lag behind the equivalent youngsters in Africa, the Caribbean, and North America.[51] Disadvantaged, lower class, and poorly fed children tend to show a much slower maturation than the more affluent, upper-class children do. Girls tend to mature more rapidly than boys by 2 years, and poor environmental conditions are reported to slow maturation more in boys than in girls.

DYSHARMONIC MATURATION

Any anomaly in the maturation index of the normal population is termed dysharmonic. Variations, of course, occur within the different study populations, and it is difficult to compare results when different racial groups are under study. In addition, wide variations may exist between the right and left hands, between monozygotic twins, between siblings of a given pedigree, and between parents and their children. Delayed maturation is common in the affected hands and limbs of children with longitudinal or transverse deficiencies, some duplication, endocrine and metabolic disorders, and skeletal dysplasias. Advanced maturation is common after trauma, with some brachydactylies, and especially with fast-flow vascular malformations. The most enigmatic group includes the slow-flow venous and lymphatic anomalies, which may demonstrate both accelerated and delayed maturation in the same extremity. Unfortunately, there are no skeletal atlases for comparison of the numerous congenital differences.

Imaging Strategies

The hand surgeon presently has within his or her reach a potpourri of imaging techniques that can precisely define all of the soft tissue and skeletal structure of the upper extremity. Radiologists are no longer limited to an assessment of skeletal structures alone. Now, the attentive practitioner can define nerves, vessels, ligaments, tendons, and other connective tissue. The plain anteroposterior film of the hand or extremity set in comparison to the opposite side is the most important radiograph and is often all that is needed before an operation. For additional studies, the surgeon should collaborate with the pediatric radiologist.

Computed tomography is most useful for the evaluation of masses and any inflammatory processes involving bone. Its advantages over magnetic resonance imaging are the ability of computed tomography to obtain thinner slices, better resolution of bone detail, and three-dimensional reconstructions.[52] The ability of computed tomography to visualize skeletal structures from any plane can be particularly useful with complex limb malformations and their articulation with the shoulder or pelvis (see Fig. 202-7).

However, magnetic resonance imaging has an advantage over computed tomography in that magnetic resonance imaging can distinguish different tissues from one another. By contrasting the T1, T2, and other special sequences both with and without contrast enhancement, the clinician can obtain more specific information about the congenital malformation, particularly in the evaluation of tumors and vascular malformations.[53] Ultrasonography is rarely needed but is a cheap and quick method for distinguishing fast-flow vascular malformations from slower flow lesions.

The major indications for invasive angiography would be in the preoperative evaluation of patients with fast-flow vascular malformations with or without arteriovenous fistulas, complex central synpolydactylies, mirror hands, macrodactyly hands and limbs, hypoplastic hands before a distally based fasciocutaneous flap, and hands and feet before a microvascular transfer. Some surgeons feel comfortable with less expensive magnetic resonance angiography images, which visualize the same arterial circulation with much less detail. In most pediatric centers, these procedures have become safe and predictable and are performed by specialists with training in pediatric interventional radiology. At present, the use of multiple visualization techniques is confined primarily to the treatment of vascular anomalies.[53]

INCIDENCE

The frequency of congenital hand differences among various different populations is difficult to determine and is best expressed as the birth prevalence among live births.[54] Hand surgeons are more concerned with live birth prevalence and do not usually become involved with the details of genetic counseling. In one of the first studies by upper limb surgeons, Birch-Jensen[55] determined that congenital absence deformities occurred with a prevalence of 1:6438. Comparable ratios were reported as 1:1064 in Utah (United States)[56] and 1:2228 in England.[57] Flatt has pointed out that the major problem with most early studies is that they do not include the full spectrum of anomalies, particularly the most frequent—polydactyly. A well-performed and often cited study took place in British Columbia, reporting the prevalence of upper limb defects as 3.4:10,000 live births and 39.53:10,000 stillbirths.[58] This study underscores the high frequency of upper limb malformations. Perhaps the most pertinent data for the hand surgeon come from Flatt's clinic in Iowa, where polydactyly and syndactyly were the most common among 2758 diagnoses.[3] Twenty years ago, Lamb estimated the frequency of specific groups of malformations, including polydactyly, and gave an overall estimate of 18:10,000 malformations in 10.9:10,000 patients.[11] In general, this is thought to be a low estimate because many minor defects and large families with genetic conditions may not have been thoroughly screened. The data from 1673 diagnoses obtained from eight hand clinics have demonstrated a clinical experience similar to Flatt's.[11,41] Our experience at the Children's Hospital in Boston during the past 35 years is similar. Polydactyly (radial, central, and ulnar) and syndactyly as part of other individual diagnoses have been most frequently treated, but there has been a much higher percentage of vascular malformations, radial dysplasias, and overgrowth conditions because of our research interests with these problems.

Congenital anomalies of the hand and upper limb are not uncommon. Analysis of frequency data must be reviewed critically because of the tremendous variation in the genetic makeup of populations being studied, sampling, and inconsistencies in precise definitions.[17,24] The incidence of 1 in 4000 live births obtained by Birch-Jensen[55] in his classic study was low because he primarily considered congenital absence deformities in the Danish study population. A more realistic incidence of 1 in 626 live births was reported by Conway and Bowe,[59] who surveyed all of the births at the New York Hospital between 1932 and 1952. These and more recent frequency data studies cite camptodactyly, polydactyly (duplication), and syndactyly as the most common deformities in the upper limb.[3,11,60-62]

Flatt's systematic study[3] of limb anomalies in Iowa, conducted during a 15-year period, reflects the same relative incidence of individual anomalies evaluated and treated by the hand surgeons.[22] Geographic differences highlight the tremendous variation, for example, of polydactyly, which is two to three times more common in Asian countries and in certain well-studied regions within the United States where black and American Indian groups predominate (Tables 202-2 and 202-3).[62,63] Absence deformities, including constriction rings, occur much less frequently, with an incidence of 1 in 2000 to 3000 live births.[19] Between 2% and 4% of all children are born with a major or minor hand malformation, and approximately 0.7% have multiple anomalies. The relative incidence of individual anomalies varies with the population being studied. Table 202-3 summarizes frequency data for hand anomalies in four different clinic populations. These are consistent with other collaborative comparative studies.[11]

Minor anomalies cannot be fully evaluated by this method. For example, clinodactyly is probably not usually included on birth certificates, one of the sources of information for registries. On examination of 4322 infants with no major anomaly, Marden et al[64] found the incidence of clinodactyly to be 9.9 per 1000 live births, whereas in 90 babies with other major anomalies, the incidence was 122 per 1000 live births. In addition, some anomalies are evident on radiographic study only after a certain amount of maturation has occurred. Triquetrum-lunate synostosis (coalition), for example, cannot be clinically evaluated in youngsters. In a study of 7500 Africans, Garn et al[48] found the incidence to be 1.6 per 1000; in 11,663, the incidence was found to be 1 per 1000 during childhood.

The high associated coincidence of upper and lower limb anomalies is so common in many syndromes that they are almost always expected in entities such as the constriction ring syndrome. In the Apert syndrome (acrocephalosyndactyly), mirror image deformities of the feet are present. In the cleft hand-foot, ectrodactyly-ectodermal dysplasia-clefting (EEC), and Goltz

TABLE 202-2 ✦ RELATIVE FREQUENCY OF CONGENITAL UPPER LIMB ANOMALIES PER 1000 LIVE BIRTHS

	Incidence by Location				
Anomaly	Baltimore	Hungary	Sweden	Atlanta	Nebraska
Polydactyly	3.8			12.2	5.56
Whites	0.3			0.2	0.66
Blacks	3.5			12.0	4.9
Syndactyly	0.6		0.65	0.9	
Radial deficiency	0.03	0.09	0.08		
Ulnar deficiency	0.01	0.11	0.02		
Transverse deficiency	0.05	0.14	0.13	0.8	0.4
Camptodactyly (flexion deformity)	4.0				
Constriction ring	0.1	0.11			
Source study	Temtamy and McKusick[17]	Bod et al[60]	Kallen et al[61]	CDC[62]	CDC[62]

syndromes, the lower limbs are, almost by definition, abnormal.

EXAMINATION

The First Consultation

The birth of a baby is usually a greatly anticipated event, and when the child arises with an imperfection, many questions are asked by the parents, grandparents, family friends, and perhaps an entire neighborhood or city. The emotional response will often vary in relation to the extent of the malformation. The family of a child with a severe syndrome, such as the VACTERL association, will experience much more guilt, recrimination, and possibly blame toward care providers than the family of a child with ulnar polydactyly.

The pediatrician or obstetrician will often call about a referral. If at all possible, try to see the baby while he or she is still in the hospital, meet the family, and let them express their feelings and ask questions. Once they are reassured that treatment is possible and that there are specialists familiar with the specific malformation, much of their anxiety is often relieved. Plenty of time should be scheduled for the first consultation, which we purposely perform at the end of the day or on a weekend when there is not a waiting room full of patients to see. It is best to provide a detailed and factual explanation of the known etiology, genetics, natural history, and treatment options for the malformation. Pictures are better than words, actual molds are better than pictures, and referrals to patients who have been through the procedure are better than molds. Parents can also be introduced to Web sites and national and local parent support groups, which play an important role for families of patients with more extensive malformations. Pictures and radiographs of the child should be taken as soon as possible, and a detailed report

with answers to specific questions should be dictated. These are often helpful because most parents fail to absorb all of the information presented to them at the outset.

Every evaluation should include a thorough examination of the head and neck, trunk, genitalia, and lower extremities. Although the hand surgeon is a "regional specialist," he or she should be vigilant about identifying additional malformations that may easily be overlooked. More can be learned about the upper limb and hand by letting the baby play in the mother's lap, crawl and explore on a well-carpeted floor, or simply sort through a box of toys (Fig. 202-8). The elbow, shoulder, and thorax are often overlooked; however, they are essential to proper diagnosis and treatment because they support and position the hand in space. When treatment should be directed initially to the more proximal parts of the upper limb, a clear explanation should be provided.

The family should leave the consultation with a clear understanding of the treatment process and the options for reconstruction if needed at all. They will invariably return with specific questions about details. Although the parents know their child is "different," the patient will usually see his or her malformation as normal. Under ideal circumstances, the patient should be treated the same as siblings or other children, and care providers should avoid focusing undue attention on the curious anomaly.[65] The upper limb is an integral part of the child's exploration of the world during the first 3 years of life. When faced with difficulty while manipulating an object, most children naturally will use trial and error to find the "best way" to accomplish certain tasks. It is not unusual for a 9- to 10-month-old child, when left alone, to play with simple toy blocks for 30 to 60 minutes without interruption. Observing this unaided play can be a hand surgeon's most important diagnostic tool (see Fig. 202-8).

TABLE 202-3 ♦ RELATIVE FREQUENCY (PERCENTAGE) OF ANOMALIES SEEN IN FOUR HAND CLINICS

	Yokohama	Iowa	Hong Kong	Sapporo
Number of patients	227	1476	326	955
Failure of formation				
Transverse (arm, wrist, hand)	7.0	7.1	6.8	2.9
Radial ray	9.6	5.4	0.5	3.9
Ulnar ray		3.4		0.9
Central ray	5.8	3.9	2.5	3.2
Phocomelia (typical, atypical)	0.9	0.8		
Failure of differentiation				
Triphalangeal thumb		0.8		0.6
Clasped thumb		0.7	2.5	5.5
Trigger		2.3	6.3	21.0
Camptodactyly		6.9	2.0	7.2
Syndactyly	10.1	17.5	14.9	4.1
Proximal radioulnar		1.2	0.7	4.3
Synostosis		1.7		0.7
Madelung deformity	0.5	0.5	0.5	0.4
Symphalangism	1.3	5.6	1.8	1.3
Clinodactyly				
Duplication	28.6	14.3	39.9	18.4
Radial		6.4		16.3
Central		5.2		1.2
Ulnar		2.7		0.8
Ulnar dimelia		0.0		0.1
Overgrowth	1.3	0.8	0.5	0.5
Undergrowth				
Whole hand		0.8	2.0	
Brachydactyly	10.6	5.2		4.0
Brachysyndactyly	4.4			4.5
Ectrosyndactyly	7.5			
Hypoplastic thumb		3.6		
Constriction ring	1.3	5.3	4.5	4.8
Generalized skeletal anomaly			11.9	3.2
Poland syndrome		2.2		
Apert syndrome		2.1		
"Top four" anomalies in clinic	Duplication 28.6%	Syndactyly 17.5%	Duplication 39.9%	Trigger digit 21.0%
	Brachysyndactyly 10.6%	Duplication 14.3%	Syndactyly 14.9%	Duplication 18.4%
	Syndactyly 10.1%	Failure of formation, transverse 7.1%	Syndromes 11.9%	Camptodactyly 7.2%
	Radial ray defect 9.6%	Radial ray 5.4%	Failure of formation, transverse 6.8%	Clamped thumb 5.5%
Source study	Yamaguchi et al[91] (1973)	Flatt[63] (1980)	Leung et al[92] (1982)	Ogino et al[93] (1986)

Functional Development

MILESTONES WITHIN THE FIRST YEAR

The functional development of the hand from the in utero state through the first year of life follows a predictable sequence that has been studied in great detail by anthropologists,[66] occupational therapists,[67] psychologists,[68] neurologists,[69] and many others. From the first day of life, the hand is intricately involved in all aspects of development: motor control, social skills, language acquisition, and intelligence. There is well-defined proximal to distal or cephalad to caudad sequence of neurologic development, which is primarily controlled by the motor cortex and mediated through the brainstem.[70]

At birth, most of the baby's upper limb movements are reflexive, and a rudimentary grip using the digits is present. The thumb is held in a flexed and adducted clasped position within the palm but does extend when the baby is startled. Gradual maturation from reflexive to intentional conscious and unconscious movement patterns is dependent on a normal central and peripheral nervous system. Obviously, structural abnormalities in the congenitally different limb as well as neurologic malformations may significantly alter this developmental process. During the first few months of life, the visual and tactile (motor and sensory) systems develop independently of one another, and it is possible to have hand function without visual clues or monitoring.[67] During the latter part of the first year

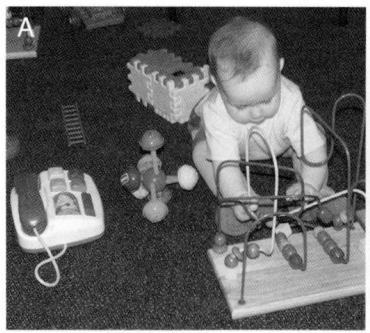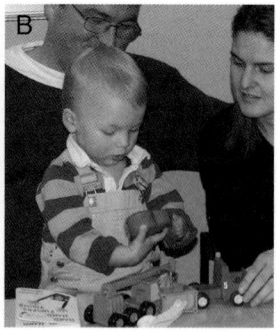

FIGURE 202-8. Examination. *A,* More information can be gleaned from watching the toddler play with safe toys than by trying to get him or her to cooperate with a hands-on approach. This 10-month-old child has good trunk and head control and is able to manipulate objects with both hands. By trial and error, she will find ways to use her hypoplastic left hand with no digits or thumb, revealing a great deal about her reconstructive needs. *B,* An uncooperative child will often play quietly when sitting in front of one or both parents. One toy may not hold his interest for very long, but multiple unfamiliar toys will. It is important to let the youngster know that he is in control during these sessions.

of life, more precise movements develop with hand-eye coordination. The child is able to manipulate small objects, hold objects, and—although still without discernible speech—effectively communicate with the hand. It is not surprising that toddlers can effectively use sign language long before they learn to speak.

In the normal child, prehension patterns develop within the first 15 months of life and are acquired by trial and error by the baby. The hand surgeon is referred to the work of Erhardt, who summarizes well the literature on this subject. The infant's grasp progresses from an ulnar power grip involving the ulnar three digits to a radial precision grip incorporating the thumb. This development can only occur when the child is able to bear weight on the upper limbs and raise her or his head. The grasping of a small dowel follows the same general pattern. The ability to grasp a pellet starts as a global, poorly controlled movement between the proximal portions of the hand and thumb. Gradually the thumb is able to grasp the pellet between more distal portions of the digits, usually the index, and by 10 months of age the child is able to hold the Cheerio between the tips of the thumb and index fingers. As wrist extension becomes stronger, greater precision movements are learned, and the distinction can be made between intrinsic movements within the hand and extrinsic movements of objects by the hand (Fig. 202-9).[71-73]

HAND DOMINANCE

Handedness or dominance is defined as the preference of a single hand to perform a motor task. Hand preference or dominance is usually not established within the first year of life and seems to correlate well with the development of a dynamic tripod pencil grasp between 4 and 6 years of age.[67] During the first year of life, the child uses trial and error to progress through stages of using both arms and both hands for individual tasks. As a rule, failure to develop dominance by 5 years of age is abnormal.[74,75] Once dominance is determined, the child can perform skillful activities with one hand alone. The incomplete development of handedness may result in "mirror movements" in the contralateral hand with voluntary motor activity of the performing hand. These can be seen with congenital anomalies, mostly neurologic, and are much more common in left-handed individuals.[76]

TIMING OF SURGERY

The optimal age for surgical correction of various deformities remains controversial. Ideally, one would like to perform all reconstruction within the first few months of life to provide the infant with everything possible for normal growth and development,[77] but this is impossible in our world today. Many physical and psychological factors will critically influence surgical judgment; agreement on the relative importance of these factors is not widespread, as some surgeons favor early (infancy) surgery, whereas others prefer later (childhood) correction.

Arguments that favor late correction of the congenitally malformed hands are many. Because the hand is larger, a more precise operation can be done on delicate structures. Difficulties with immobilization of skin-grafted regions, tenuous flaps, osteotomies, and ligament reconstructions are reduced. In addition, the infant may scar more readily than the older child, and precise incisional design may be more difficult in smaller hands. Developmental studies indicate that a primitive grasp mechanism functions early in infancy and that three-digit prehension with eye-hand coordination is not fully developed until 2 to 3 years of age.[78] Finally, the functional needs of the child can be evaluated more adequately, particularly in less severe deformities (Fig. 202-10).

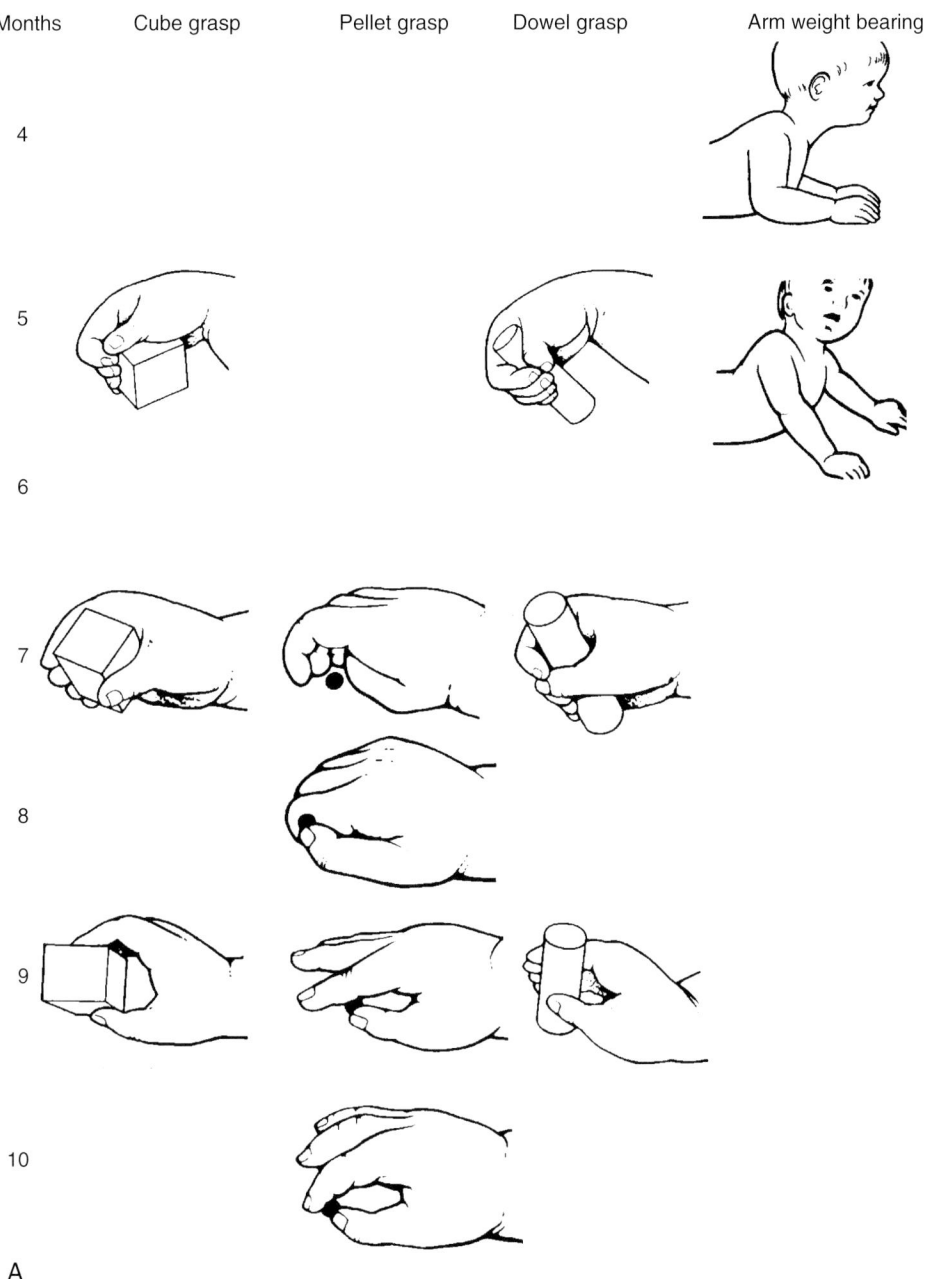

A

FIGURE 202-9. Pinch and prehension development. *A,* All the essential patterns of prehension develop within the first 15 months of life and follow a predictable progression. This summary of four specific functions is abstracted from Erhardt's Developmental Prehension Assessment (EDPA).[67,88,89] Various prehension patterns develop once the child can bear weight on the upper extremities. The cube grasp starts with the ulnar three digits, and by trial and error, the child moves the grasp in a more radial direction. At 9 months, the child is able to hold the cube between the thumb and index rays. Grasping of a small pellet starts between the dorsum of the thumb and the digits and moves to the side of the index finger by 8 months when the child is eating finger foods. Within the next 2 months, the child learns to separate the index from the rest of the hand and is able to hold the small pellet between the thumb and isolated index fingertip. Similar to the cube grasp, the dowel grasp follows an ulnar to radial progression within the hand and a palmar flexed to dorsiflexed wrist posture.   *Continued*

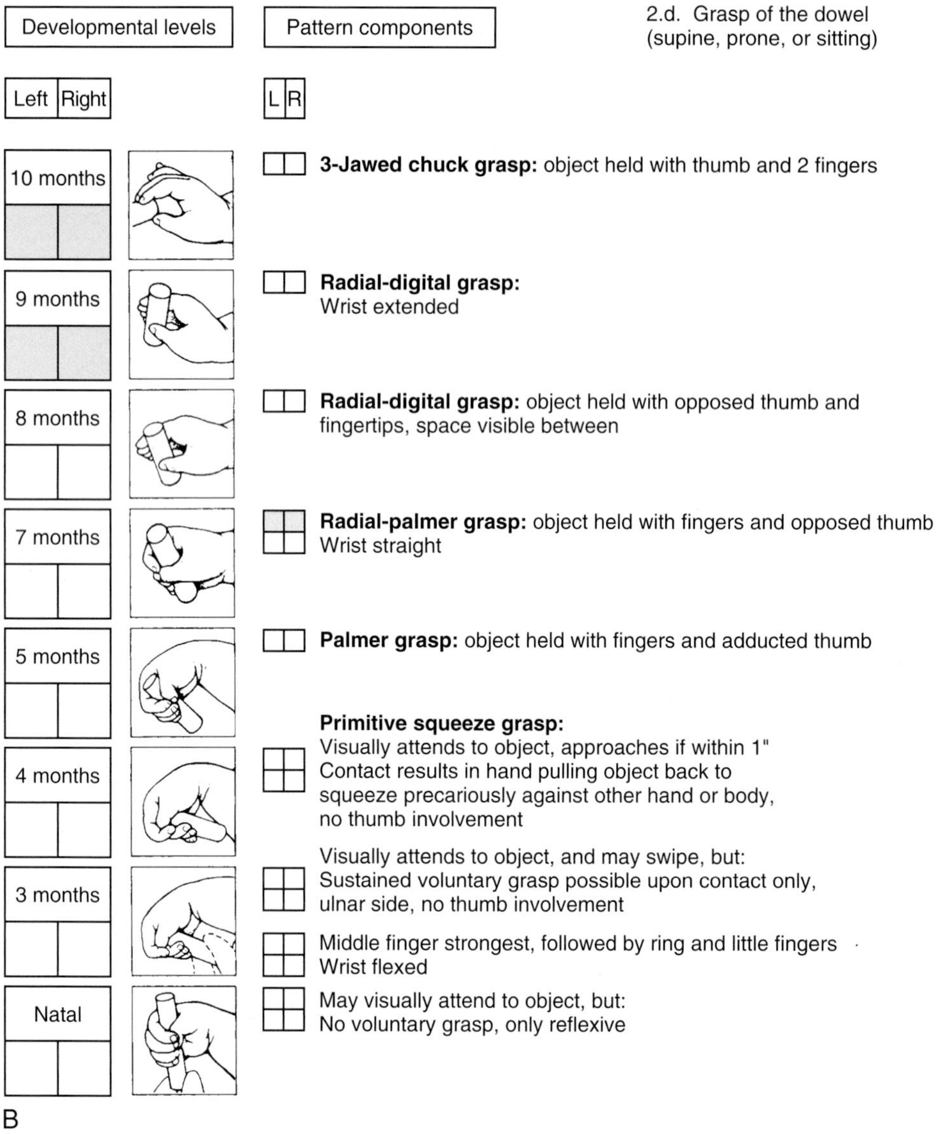

| Developmental levels | Pattern components | 2.d. Grasp of the dowel (supine, prone, or sitting) |

| Left | Right | | L | R | |

10 months — **3-Jawed chuck grasp:** object held with thumb and 2 fingers

9 months — **Radial-digital grasp:**
Wrist extended

8 months — **Radial-digital grasp:** object held with opposed thumb and fingertips, space visible between

7 months — **Radial-palmer grasp:** object held with fingers and opposed thumb
Wrist straight

5 months — **Palmer grasp:** object held with fingers and adducted thumb

Primitive squeeze grasp:
Visually attends to object, approaches if within 1"
Contact results in hand pulling object back to
squeeze precariously against other hand or body,
no thumb involvement

4 months

Visually attends to object, and may swipe, but:
Sustained voluntary grasp possible upon contact only,
ulnar side, no thumb involvement

3 months

Middle finger strongest, followed by ring and little fingers
Wrist flexed

Natal

May visually attend to object, but:
No voluntary grasp, only reflexive

B

FIGURE 202-9, cont'd. *B,* Example of age-related tasks from the EDPA. (Courtesy of Rhonda Erhardt, MS, OTR, FAOTA, Maplewood, MN.)

Many objective arguments favor early surgery, which is defined as that performed within the first 12 to 18 months of life. Tethering of adjacent structures, such as digits within a syndactyly, will result in irreversible angulation, rotation, and deviation of skeletal parts (Fig. 202-11). The infant or young child can begin to use the reconstructed part early in development and will develop fewer bad habits. Anatomic adaptation of the reconstructed part will occur with growth and the external forces placed on it. Examples include the broadening of the distal ulna after centralization of the radial clubhand[79] and intrinsic muscle hypertrophy and broadening of the metaphysis of the proximal phalanx of a pollicized index finger that has been moved into the metacarpal position.[80] Parental anxiety and potential psychological problems for the child are reduced with earlier surgery.[81] Functionless nubbins and the small floating thumb (pouce flottant) are best eliminated before the child or parents become psychologically attached. Many have stated that the congenitally malformed hand represents a static situation wherein changes occur only with growth or surgery. Early surgical release of tight deforming structures may unlock potential growth centers and lessen progressive deformity.[35]

The determination of the optimal time for correction of these varied hands is also guided in great part by the experience, knowledge, and special training of

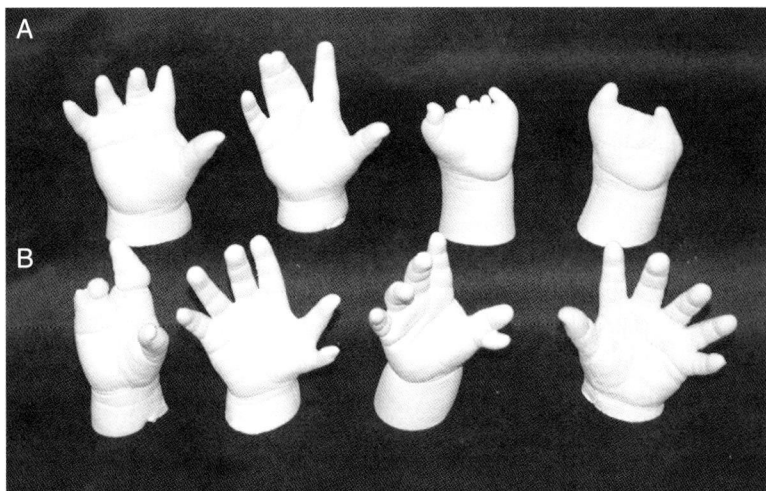

FIGURE 202-10. Timing. Most common congenital hand malformations are routinely corrected near the child's first birthday, when the hand is larger, making the procedure much easier. The operations required for these patients include the following: *A, left to right,* release of an incomplete simple syndactyly, release of a complete simple syndactyly, excision of hypoplastic nubbins and nonvascularized toe phalangeal transfer to thumb and fifth digits, and creation of a deeper web space with soft tissue flaps; *B, left to right,* excision and Z-plasty of a deep constriction ring, correction of a type VI radial polydactyly (Iowa classification) with first web space release, correction of a type IV radial polydactyly with thenar muscle transfers, and excision of a type III (Stelling classification) ulnar polydactyly.

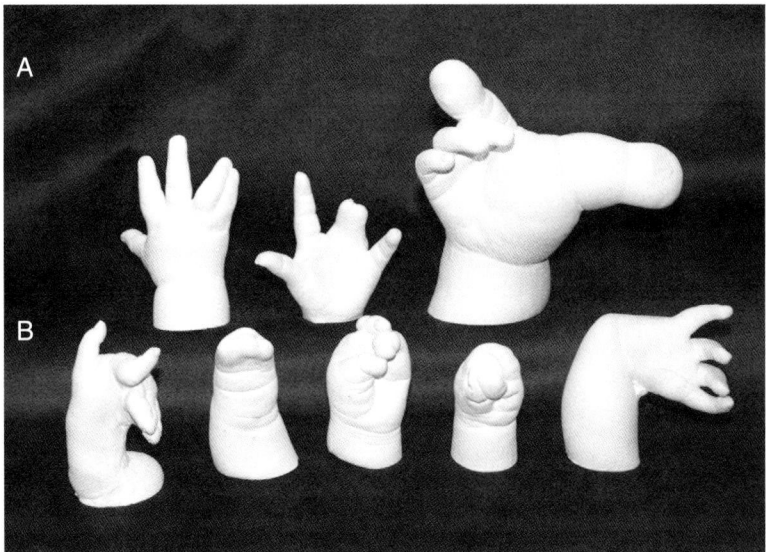

FIGURE 202-11. Timing. Many congenital hand malformations require a much earlier release because of massive overgrowth and displacement of adjacent structures, tethering of adjacent digits by tight scars, or distal skeletal coalitions. *A, left and center,* These hands demonstrate both dorsal buckling and lateral deviation at the proximal interphalangeal joint caused by the distal bone fusion within these complex syndactylies; *right,* the massive radial overgrowth of this 8-month-old hand has caused this child to neglect this limb. *B,* Relatively uncommon problems that require early surgical intervention include *(left to right)* a tight dorsal hand and wrist contracture in a child with cutis aplasia and loss of dorsal forearm and wrist soft tissue, the two-fingered "hoof" hand with interphalangeal flexion contracture, a tight acrosyndactyly in a patient with constriction ring syndrome, a tight type III Apert hand (Upton classification) with palmar skinfold maceration and infection, and the irreducible radial clubhand.

the surgeon.[77] Those who operate primarily on children and perform microsurgery on a regular basis will feel more confident with smaller structures and will achieve good results within the first year of a patient's life. Those who regularly reduce fractures, reconstruct ligaments, and perform osteotomies will be less tentative about early skeletal corrections. Those who work in rural regions or developing countries may need to wait and stage their procedures differently because of limited hospital facilities and equipment. The general condition of the patient and associated malformations will obviously influence the decision-making process. Correction of a congenital heart defect or gastrointestinal or genitourinary obstruction will obviously take precedence over a hand anomaly, which is not life-threatening. Severe mental retardation associated with impaired neurologic function may obviate any practical need for hand surgery. Some controversy will always exist with regard to which surgeons should perform congenital hand corrections. The complexity of the deformity and its correction should be directly proportional to the experience and skills of the surgeon (Fig. 202-12).

There seems no urgency to operate on most congenital hand anomalies until growth has been sufficient to allow exacting surgery. Early release of tethering structures, such as the radial clubhand, central polysyndactylies, complex syndactylies, transverse phalanges, and cleft hands, can safely be performed between 6 and 18 months (see Figs. 202-11 and 202-12). Other soft tissue releases of tight constriction rings and thumb-index web spaces can be done during the same period. Routine syndactyly release, polydactyly correction, and pollicizations are usually reserved for the second year of life (see Fig. 202-12). All major reconstructions should be completed by school age so that the deformity is less of a source of ridicule and so that maximum function can be achieved during the formative developmental period. Imbalance of major muscle-tendon units should be corrected early so that they will influence growth and proper skeletal alignment. Follow-up of all patients with complex deformity is mandatory until skeletal maturity is reached at the very least and preferably into adulthood.

On occasion, an adult presents for correction of a congenital anomaly to which he or she has adapted comfortably. The prime reason and primary motivation of such patients should be determined. Often, they have observed a functional correction in one of their children or have changed to an occupation that requires new functional demands. Just as frequently, however, the patient may be displacing anxieties to the obvious deformity and should be referred to a psychiatrist before any surgical recommendations are made.[82]

PRINCIPLES OF TREATMENT

It is well known that "the unique feature of the congenitally anomalous hand is that it represents a relatively static situation in which the only changes are caused either by surgery or growth. The former is slow and gradual and the latter is controllable."[22] The surgeon's general goal is to intervene at the most

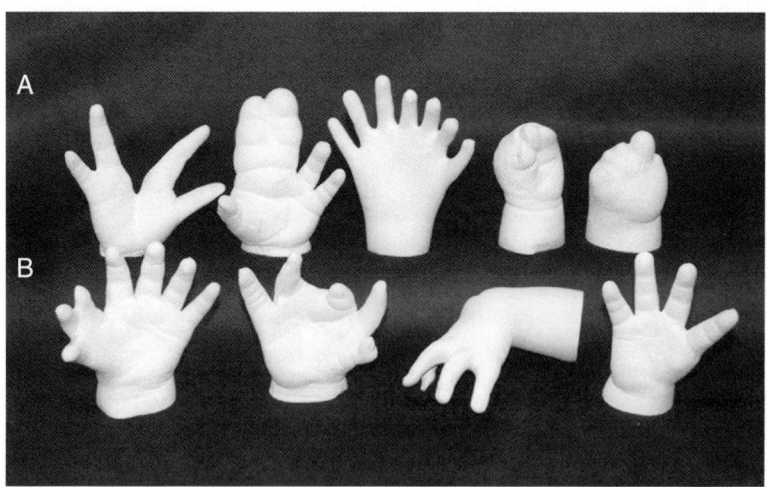

FIGURE 202-12. Timing. A wide variety of absent parts, extra parts, and overgrown or hypoplastic parts are seen in many hands. Each one requires special expertise from a surgeon. *A, left to right,* A typical cleft hand, which requires an index transposition; a massive macrodactyly in a newborn, which requires debulking and syndactyly release (or amputations); a mirror hand; a type II Apert hand; and a hypoplastic hand with no thumb before microvascular toe transfer. *B, left to right,* Additional complex malformations that can be difficult to correct: a triplicated thumb with deficient first web space; a complex cleft hand containing transverse phalanges, radial polydactyly, and fused metacarpals with deficient web spaces; a radial clubhand with stiff radial digits and flexion contractures; and a hand with thumb aplasia before index pollicization.

appropriate time to optimize potential function before disuse patterns, and even total neglect, begin to develop. Broad principles for treatment are

1. to provide the ability to place and control the upper limb and hand in space;
2. to provide good skin cover with intact sensation;
3. to maximize skeletal alignment and joint mobility;
4. to provide a volumetric grasp and precision pinch;
5. to provide the family a clear explanation of the malformation, the expected natural history, and options for reconstruction;
6. to maintain regular follow-up; and
7. to refer the child to a more experienced colleague when there is either doubt or controversy over treatment.

The treatment of congenital malformations of the upper limb will defy those who like routines and "standard operations" because every child and every hand are different. All combinations of deformity are possible with these hands, and the decision of what to do, when to do it, and how to operate is not always easy and may involve more than the existence of a simple syndactyly or polydactyly (see Figs. 202-11 and 202-12). Associated anomalies, syndromes, nutritional status, the child's health, and family all play a role.

During the past 20 years, potential problems with pediatric anesthesia and intensive care have been improved to the point that in most medical centers, it has become much safer to anesthetize babies and small children for relatively long times. Parents should be reassured that anesthesia in these babies is safe when it is delivered by a trained pediatric anesthesiologist.

In large pediatric centers where associated craniofacial, cardiac, gastrointestinal, and urologic malformations are treated, the life-threatening anomalies, of course, take precedence. In patients with multiple organ malformations, it is important to ensure and to make arrangements for appropriate intensive care stays in the immediate postoperative period. Apnea in the baby with Apert syndrome and arrhythmias in the child with Holt-Oram syndrome with radial dysplasia have frequently occurred in our patients and must be anticipated.

It is wise for the upper limb surgeon to be aggressive within the first 2 years of life and to perform the appropriate surgery and provide basic pinch and grasp by the time the youngster is ambulatory. By 12 months of age, children have fully integrated the use of their hands to express their needs and emotions, to manipulate the environment, and to communicate with others. Those with unilateral deformities will have adjusted to and compensated well for their unperceived loss, but it is still important to give their deformed hand or limbs maximal improvement. There is much greater urgency for those with bilateral absence of thumbs or hands. In these children, we have often completed toe to thumb transfers by 12 to 14 months of age.

As the surgeon observes these patients through adolescence and skeletal maturity, at times he or she is impressed by the unpredictable effect of the fourth dimension: growth. Corrected skeletal deformities involving abnormal growth plates, joint surfaces, synostoses, extra or anomalous phalanges, and hypoplastic arms or forearms can change rapidly from one year to another (Fig. 202-13). One of the most difficult problems for the surgeon who follows and recognizes these changes is when to intervene.

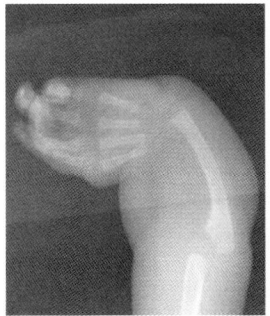 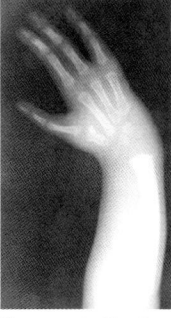 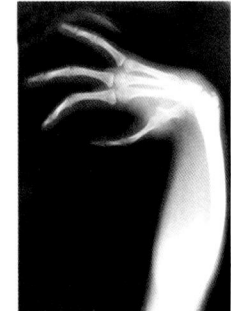

| Birth | Post-centralization, rotation-recession of index | 10 years later recontracted |

FIGURE 202-13. Secondary deformity with growth. At birth, this child with the VACTERL association presented with a radial clubhand and an apparent total absence of the radius. He was initially treated with stretching exercises and night splints. Centralization was completed well before his first birthday and pollicization of a relatively stiff index finger by his second. Note the broadening of the distal radius at this time. His hand function was good, and he was passively reduced to neutral position. Ten years later, he returned with a tight radial contracture, which was in part associated with a new fibrous anlage, which had formed between a hypoplastic proximal radius and the radial side of the carpus. His ulna is still growing.

In addition, the true extent of an anomaly is not evident on radiographs alone. Soft tissue, muscle, tendon, ligament, and capsular malformations are frequent in these patients and unless recognized will continue to affect growth and skeletal alignment. The complete excision of a fibrous anlage during a centralization of a radial clubhand or a complete excision of an intratendinous band causing the radial deviation (pollex abductus) in a hypoplastic or duplicated thumb is absolutely necessary to allow unrestricted potential growth.

Most hand surgeons recognize that the child's most noted period of growth is during the first 4 years of life and strive to complete all major reconstruction by the time the child enters school at the age of 5 to 6 years. The majority of subsequent problems occur between this age and late adolescence, when both boys and girls reach skeletal maturity (Fig. 202-14). Once these children enter junior high or high school, they have accepted and adapted to their limitations. They do not want to continue their yearly visits and commonly come in seeking correction of anomalies such

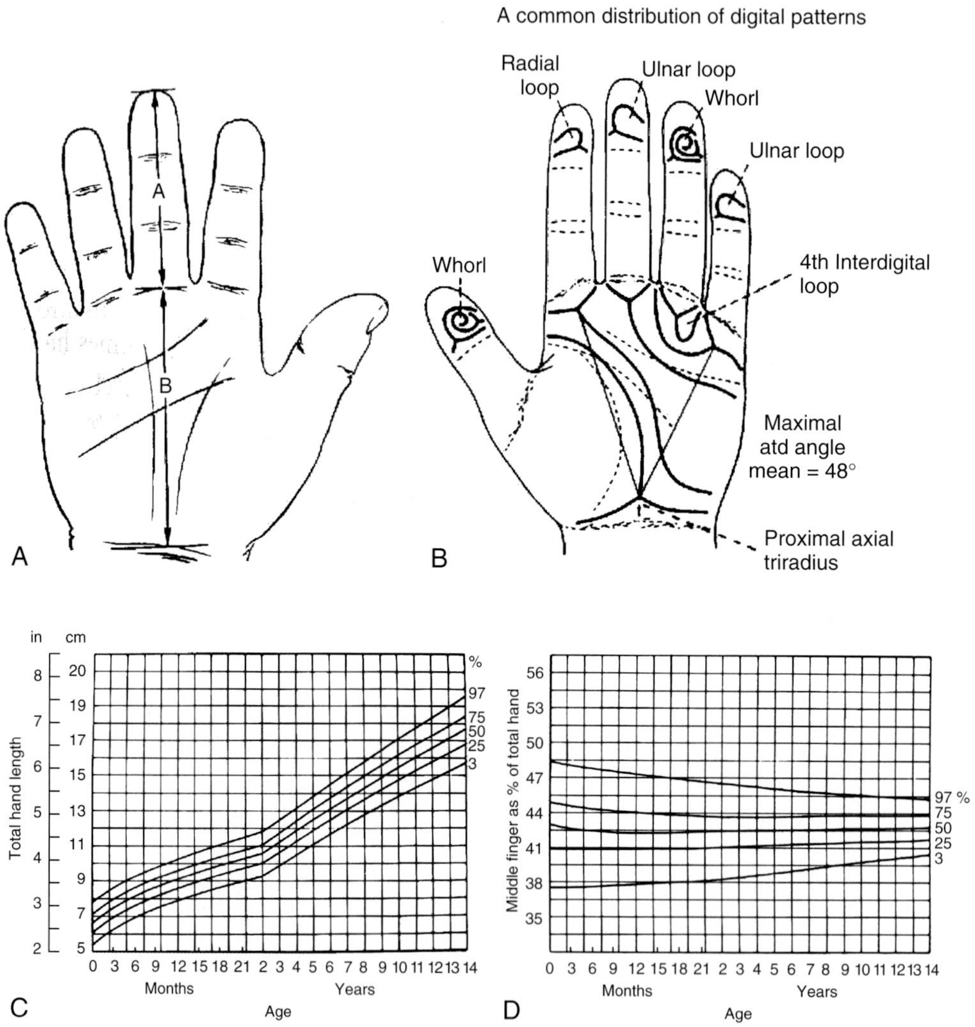

FIGURE 202-14. Hand size data. *A,* Hand measurements are made and recorded for the purposes of measuring growth. Two common measurements are (A) the length of the digit between the digital-palmar flexion crease and the fingertip and (B) the palm length between the distal wrist flexion crease and the digital-palmar flexion crease. *B,* Geneticists and pediatricians commonly describe digital dermatoglyphic patterns that are abnormal in many congenital differences of the hand. Radial and ulnar loops and whorls and the proximal triradius are most commonly described.[16] *C,* This graph shows the total hand length (A + B) as a function in time in American schoolchildren. *D,* The middle (third or long) finger length is graphed as a function of time in the same group.[90]

as the short forearm, the missing pectoral muscle, or the hypoplastic hand, which are all conspicuous and obvious to their peers. Simple procedures such as the release of a first web space or recurrent (web creep) syndactyly or osteotomy and lengthening of a short thumb can significantly improve appearance and function at these ages.

REFERENCES

1. Temtamy S, McKusick V: The Genetics of Hand Malformations. New York, Alan R. Liss, 1982.
2. Boinet E: Polydatylie et atavism. Rev Med (Paris) 1898;18:316-328.
3. Flatt A: The Care of Congenital Hand Anomalies. St. Louis, CV Mosby, 1977:131-140.
4. St. Hilaire I: Histoire generale et particuliere des anomalies de l'organisation chez l'homme et les animaux. Paris, JB Baillière, 1832:670-702.
5. Velpeau A: New Elements of Operative Surgery, vol I. Townsend PS, trans. New York, Samuel and Woods, 1847.
6. Vrolik W: Teratology. In Todd R, ed: Cyclopaedia of Anatomy and Physiology. London, Longman, Brown, Green, Longman, and Roberts, 1849.
7. Felizet G: Opération de la syndactylie congénitale (procédé autoplastique). Rev Orthop 1892;10:49.
8. Bardeen D, Lewis W: Development of the limbs, body wall, and back in man. Am J Anat 1901-1902;1:1.
9. Smith R, Lipke R: Treatment of congenital deformities of the hand and forearm. Parts 1 and 2. N Engl J Med 1979;300:344-349, 402-407.
10. Flatt A: The role of reconstructive surgery. In Flatt AE, ed: The Care of Congenital Hand Anomalies. St. Louis, Quality Medical Publishing, 1994:11-14.
11. Lamb D, Wynne-Davies R, Soto L: An estimate of the population frequency of congenital malformations of the upper limb. J Hand Surg Am 1982;7:557-562.
12. Holmes L: Congenital malformation. In Stark A, ed: Manual of Neonatal Care. Boston, Little, Brown, 1980:91-96.
13. Warkany J: Congenital Malformations (The Upper Extremities). Chicago, Year Book, 1971:967-968.
14. Smith D: Recognizable Patterns of Human Malformation. Philadelphia, WB Saunders, 1982:1-9.
15. McKusick V: On lumpers and splitters, or the morphology of genetic disease. Perspect Biol Med 1969;12:298-312.
16. Jones K: Smith's Recognizable Patterns of Human Malformation, vol 1, 4th ed. Philadelphia, WB Saunders, 1988:673.
17. Temtamy S, McKusick V: The Genetics of Hand Malformations. The National Foundation-March of Dimes. New York, Alan R. Liss, 1978. Birth Defects: Original Article Series; vol 14.
18. Poznanski A: The Hand in Radiologic Diagnosis, 2nd ed. Philadelphia, WB Saunders, 1984.
19. Goldberg M, Bartoshesky L: Congenital hand anomaly: etiology and associated malformations. Hand Clin 1985;1:405-415.
20. Auerbach AD, Rogatko A, Schroeder-Kurth TM: International Fanconi Anemia Registry: relation of clinical symptoms to diepoxybutane sensitivity. Blood 1989;73:391-396.
21. Alter BP: Fanconi's anemia. Current concepts. Am J Pediatr Hematol Oncol 1992;14:170-176.
22. Flatt A: Classification and incidence. In Flatt AE, ed: The Care of Congenital Hand Anomalies. St. Louis, Quality Medical Publishing, 1994:47-63.
23. Kelikian H, Doumanian A: Congenital anomalies of the hand. J Bone Joint Surg Am 1957;39:1002-1019, 1249-1266.
24. Kelikian H: Congenital Deformities of the Hand and Forearm. Philadelphia, WB Saunders, 1974:866-890.
25. Frantz C, O'Rahilly R: Congenital skeletal limb deficiencies. J Bone Joint Surg Am 1961;43:1202-1224.
26. Burtch R: Nomenclature for congenital skeletal limb deficiencies, a revision of the Frantz and O'Rahilly classification. Artif Limbs 1996;10:24-35.
27. Kay A: A proposed international terminology of the classification of congenital limb deficiencies. Orthot Prosthet 1974;28:33.
28. Swanson A, Barsky A, Entin M: Classification of limb malformations on the basis of embryological failures. Surg Clin North Am 1968;48:1169-1179.
29. Swanson A: A classification for congenital limb malformations. J Hand Surg Am 1976;1:8-22.
30. Swanson A, Swanson GD, Tada K: A classification for congenital limb malformation. J Hand Surg Am 1983;8:693-702.
31. Blauth W: The hypoplastic thumb [in German]. Arch Orthop Unfallchir 1967;62:225-246.
32. Blauth W, Gekeler J: Morphology and classification of symbrachydactylia [in German]. Handchirurgie 1971;3:123-128.
33. Blauth W, Schneider-Sickert F: Congenital Deformities of the Hand: An Atlas of Their Surgical Treatment. Berlin, Springer-Verlag, 1981:10-72.
34. Flatt A: A test of a classification of congenital anomalies of the upper extremity. Surg Clin North Am 1970;50:509-516.
35. Upton J, Burrows P: Congenital anomalies of the hand and forearm. In May JW Jr, Littler JW, eds: The Hand. Philadelphia, WB Saunders, 1990:5213-5398. McCarthy J, ed: Plastic Surgery; vol 8.
36. Miura T, Nakamura R, Horii E: The position of symbrachydactyly in the classification of congenital hand anomalies. J Hand Surg Br 1994;19:350-354.
37. Manske P, Halikis MN: Surgical classification of central deficiency according to the thumb web. J Hand Surg Am 1995;20:687-697.
38. Ogino T: Teratologic relationship between polydactyly, syndactyly, and cleft hand. J Hand Surg Br 1990;15:201-209.
39. Tada K, Yonenobu K, Swanson AB: Congenital central ray deficiency in the hand: a survey of 59 cases and subclassification. J Hand Surg Am 1981;6:434-441.
40. Tajima T: A brief review and a proposal for the classification of the congenital anomalies of the upper limb—my proposal for the classification of congenital upper limb anomalies. Hand Surg 1996;1:63-68.
41. Cheng J, Chow SK, Leung PC: Classification of 578 cases of congenital upper limb anomalies with the IFSSH system—a 10 years' experience. J Hand Surg Am 1987;12:1055-1060.
42. Kay S: Classification of congenital anomalies. In Gupta A, Kay SPJ, Scheker LR, eds: The Growing Hand. London, Mosby, 2000:125-136.
43. Buck-Gramcko D, Ogino T: Congenital malformations of the hand: non-classifiable cases. Hand Surg 1996;1:45-61.
44. Mulliken J, Glowacki J: Hemangiomas and vascular malformations in infants and children: a classification based on endothelial characteristics. Plast Reconstr Surg 1982;69:412-420.
45. Miura T: Syndactyly with split hand. Hand Suppl 1978;10:99-103.
46. Ogino T: Clinical and experimental study on the teratogenic mechanisms of cleft hand, polydactyly, and syndactyly. J Jpn Orthop Assoc 1979;53:535-543.
47. Greulich W, Pyle S: Radiologic Atlas of Skeletal Development of the Hand and Wrist, 2nd ed. Stanford, Calif, Stanford University Press, 1959.
48. Garn S, Frisancho AR, Poznanski AK, et al: Analysis of triquetral-lunate fusion. Am J Phys Anthropol 1971;34:431-433.
49. Stuart H, Idell S, Caornoni J, Reed RB: Onsets, completions and spans of ossification in the 29 bone-growth centers of the hand and wrist. Pediatrics 1962;29:237-249.
50. Tanner J, Whitehouse RH, Marshall WA, et al: Assessment of Skeletal Maturity and Prediction of Adult Height. London, Academic Press, 1975.

51. Hall C, Shaw DG: Normal radiologic variants and skeletal maturation. In Gupta A, Kay SPJ, Scheker LR, eds: The Growing Hand. London, Mosby, 2000:57-64.
52. Crass J, Miller C, Cohen AM: Radiological application of three-dimensional imaging systems. Semin Ultrasound CT MR 1992;13:94-101.
53. Upton J, Burrows P: Recent advances in the treatment of congenital vascular anomalies. In Saffar P, Amadio P, Fouchet G, eds: Current Practice in Hand Surgery. London, Martin Dunitz, 1998:125-131.
54. Larsen C: Demography and social impact. In Gupta A, Kay SPJ, Scheker LR, eds: The Growing Hand. London, Mosby, 2000:121-124.
55. Birch-Jensen A: Congenital Deformities of the Upper Extremities [thesis]. Copenhagen, Ejnar Munksgaard, 1949.
56. Woolf R, Broadbent T, Woolf G: Practical genetics of congenital hand abnormalities. In Littler JW, Cramer LM, Smith JW, eds: Symposium on Reconstructive Hand Surgery. St. Louis, CV Mosby, 1974:141-143.
57. Leck I: The incidence of limb deficiencies in recent years. In Swinyard CW, ed: Limb Development and Deformity: Problems of Evaluation and Rehabilitation. Springfield, Ill, Charles C Thomas, 1969:248-268.
58. Froster U, Baird PA: Upper limb deficiencies and associated malformations: a population-based study. Am J Med Genet 1992;44:767-781.
59. Conway H, Bowe J: Congenital deformities of the hands. Plast Reconstr Surg 1956;18:286-290.
60. Bod M, Dzeizal A, Lentz W: Incidence at birth of different types of limb reduction abnormalities in Hungary. Hum Genet 1983;65:27.
61. Kallen B, Rahmani TM, Winberg J: Infants with congenital limb reductions registered in the Swedish Registry of Congenital Malformations. Teratology 1984;29:73-85.
62. Centers for Disease Control: Congenital Malformations Surveillance Report. Atlanta, Ga, US Department of Health and Human Services, 1984.
63. Flatt A: Restoration of Function to Congenitally Deformed Hands. Final Report, 1980. National and Child Health Service Grant No. MC-R190356.
64. Marden P, Smith D, McDonald M: Congenital anomalies in the newborn infant, including minor variations: a study of 4412 babies by surface examination for anomalies and buccal smear for sex chromatin. J Pediatr 1964;64:357.
65. Walker B: A letter to my daughter. In Flatt AE, ed: The Care of Congenital Hand Anomalies. St. Louis, Quality Medical Publishing, 1994:3-5.
66. Goodall J: Tool-using primates and other vertebrates. In Lehrman DS, Hinde RA, Shaw E, eds: Advances in the Study of Behavior. New York, Academic Press, 1965:195-249.
67. Erhardt R: Developmental Hand Dysfunction: Theory, Assessment, and Treatment, 2nd ed. San Antonio, Therapy Skill Builders, 1994.
68. Paillard J: Basic neurophysiological structures of eye-hand coordination. In Bard C, Fleury M, Hay L, eds: Development of Eye-Hand Coordination Across the Life Span. Columbia, University of South Carolina Press, 1990:26-74.
69. Exner C: In-hand manipulation skills. In Case-Smith J, Pehoski C, eds: Development of Hand Skills in the Child. Bethesda, Md, The American Occupational Therapy Association, 1992:35-45.
70. Scherzer A, Tscharnuter I: Early Diagnosis and Therapy in Cerebral Palsy: A Primer on Infant Developmental Problems, 2nd ed. New York, Marcel Dekker, 1990.

71. Elliott J, Connolly KJ: A classification of manipulative hand movements. Dev Med Child Neurol 1984;26:283-296.
72. Napier J: The prehensile movements of the human hand. J Bone Joint Surg Br 1956;38:902-913.
73. Landsmeer J: Power and grip precision handling. Ann Rheum Dis 1962;21:164-170.
74. Crinella F, Beck FW, Robinson JW: Unilateral dominance is not related to neuropsychological integrity. Child Dev 1971;42:2033-2054.
75. Steffen H: Cerebral dominance: the development of handedness and speech. Acta Paedopsychiatr 1975;41:223-235.
76. Menkes J: Neurologic examination of the child and infant. In Menkes J, ed: Textbook of Child Neurology. Baltimore, Williams & Wilkins, 1995:1-28.
77. Eaton R: Hand problems in children; a timetable for management. Pediatr Clin North Am 1967;14:643-658.
78. McGraw M: The Neuromuscular Maturation of the Human Infant. New York, Hafner, 1943:93-101.
79. Zaricznyj B: Centralization of the ulna for congenital radial hemimelia. J Bone Joint Surg Am 1977;59:694-695.
80. Buck-Gramcko D: Congenital malformations of the hand: indications, operative treatment and results. Scand J Plast Reconstr Surg 1975;9:190-198.
81. Bradbury E: Psychology. In Gupta A, Kay SPJ, Scheker LR, eds: The Growing Hand. London, Mosby, 2000:21-24.
82. Upton J, Pap S: Congenital anomalies. In Goldwyn R, Cohen MN, eds: The Unfavorable Result in Plastic Surgery. Philadelphia, Lippincott Williams & Wilkins, 2001:693-710.
83. Berkowitz E: A History of the Institute of Medicine: To Improve Human Health. Washington, DC, National Academy Press, 1999.
84. Muragaki Y, Mundlos S, Upton J, Olsen BR: Altered growth and branching patterns in synpolydactyly caused by mutations in HOXD13. Science 1996;278:548-551.
85. Caffey J: Pediatric X-ray Diagnosis: A Textbook for Students and Practitioners of Pediatrics, Surgery, and Radiology, 7th ed. Chicago, Year Book, 1978.
86. Graham J, Hanson JW, Darby BL, et al: Independent dysmorphology evaluations at birth and 4 years of age for children exposed to varying amounts of alcohol in utero. Pediatrics 1988;81:772-778.
87. Lenz W: Forms and causes of human malformations. Acta Morphol Acad Sci Hung 1980;28:99-104.
88. Erhardt R: Erhardt Developmental Prehension Assessment (EDA). Tucson, Ariz, Therapy Skill Builders, 1989.
89. Erhardt R: Functional development of the hand. In Gupta A, Kay SPJ, Scheker LR, eds: The Growing Hand. London, Mosby, 2000:71-81.
90. Feingold M, Bossert HW: Normal values for selected physical parameters: an aid to syndrome delineation. Birth Defects Orig Artic Ser 1974;10(suppl 13), 1-16.
91. Yamaguchi S: Incidence of various congenital anomalies of the hand from 1961-1972. Proceedings of the Sixteenth Annual Meeting, Japanese Society of Surgery for the Hand, Fukuoka, 1973.
92. Leung P, Chan K, Cheng J: Congenital anomalies of the upper limb among the Chinese population in Hong Kong. J Hand Surg Am 1982;7:563.
93. Ogino T, Minami A, Fukuda K, Kato H: Congenital anomalies of the upper limb among the Japanese in Sapporo. J Hand Surg Br 1986;11:364-371.

Management of Transverse and Longitudinal Deficiencies (Failure of Formation)

JOSEPH UPTON III, MD

TRANSVERSE ABSENCES
    Upper Arm Level
    Intercalated "Phocomelia"
    Forearm Level
    Carpal and Metacarpal Level
    Phalangeal Level

LONGITUDINAL ABSENCES (FAILURE OF FORMATION)
    Classification
    Radial (Preaxial) Deficiencies
    Central Deficiencies (Typical Cleft Hand)
    Ulnar Deficiencies
    Symbrachydactyly (Atypical Cleft Hand)

TRANSVERSE ABSENCES

Upper Arm Level

CLINICAL PRESENTATION

Transverse absence at the upper arm level, also known as terminal transverse defect,[1] is rare, occurring in 1 in every 270,000 live births.[2] Aside from when they are seen in association with the constriction ring syndrome, these deformities are usually bilateral and have an autosomal recessive inheritance pattern with variable expression.[3] Children with transverse upper arm deformities become amazingly dexterous with their feet, although they are often embarrassed to use them in public settings. Other modes of prehension become important in later years when their hips, knees, and ankles become less flexible. The structure of the amputation stump is variable but usually bulbous and contains some useless rudimentary hand remnants. A deep dimple may be caused by attachment of these elements to whatever form of humerus is present. Remaining proximal parts of the limb are always hypoplastic, as is the chest wall musculature that attaches to the humerus.

TREATMENT

Surgical intervention is seldom necessary. However, this type of arm amputation has the highest incidence of distal bone overgrowth among transverse defects and sometimes necessitates surgery. Indications for treatment are covered in the section on intercalated phocomelia. In selected patients, prosthetic wear may be helpful but requires a considerable commitment on the part of the child and his or her family.

Intercalated "Phocomelia"

CLINICAL PRESENTATION

Phocomelia (seal limb) is characterized by an intercalated loss of upper arm and forearm elements.[1,4] It is distinguished from amelia (complete absence of the extremity at the shoulder level) by the presence of hand skeletal structures with at least one functional terminal element (Fig. 203-1). In most series, phocomelias are bilateral and account for only 0.8% of congenital limb deformities. Phocomelia became widespread in western Europe during the 1960s when the sedative thalidomide was taken by pregnant women who were between the 38th and 45th days of gestation.[5,6]

There are three basic types of phocomelia, which are distinguished by the features of the intermediate segment (Fig. 203-2). In the most severe type, called type I, arm and forearm skeletal elements are missing, and the hand attaches directly to the shoulder. In type II, a more moderate form, the upper arm segment, or humerus, is deficient, and the forearm-hand segment attaches directly to the shoulder. In type III, the mildest form, the forearm portion of the limb is absent, and the hand attaches to the humerus.[7,8] Arm, forearm, and hand segments are hypoplastic in the second and third types, and a longitudinal radial or ulnar deficiency is usually present[9] (see section

51

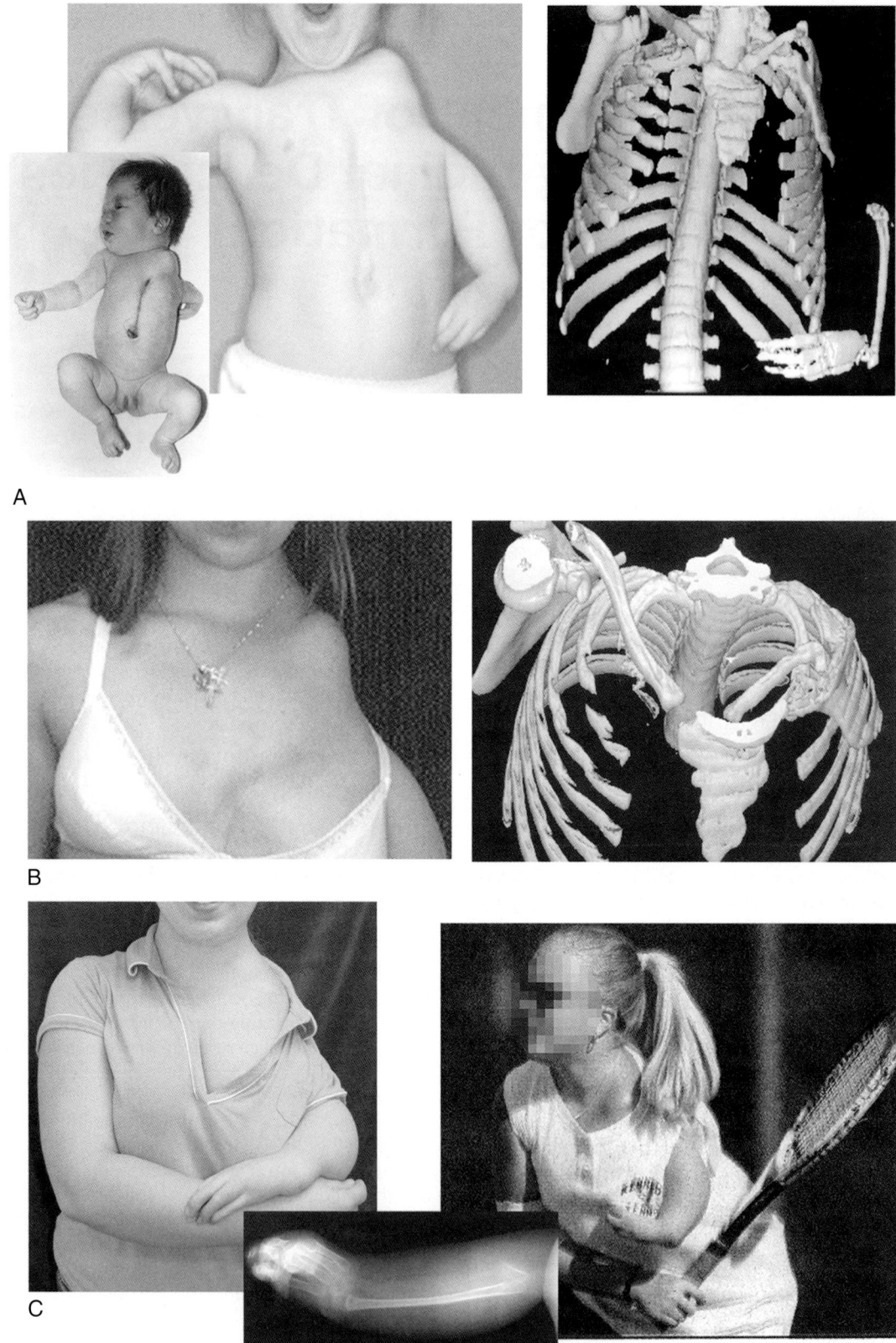

A

B

C

FIGURE 203-1. Radial dysplasia with intercalated deficiency. *A,* This child was born with a unilateral absence of the humerus, elbow joint, and radius. The forearm and hand emerged from the chest wall in a clubhand posture. The midline skin deficiency, or cutis aplasia, was not associated with any underlying chest wall or cardiac malformation. Three-dimensional skeletal reconstruction shows a hypoplastic scapula and clavicle, anteriorly positioned. *B,* Later in childhood, the scapula and clavicle were moved laterally and posteriorly so that she could wear clothes more easily. The preoperative position of the clavicle and scapula is contrasted with her normal right side. *C,* Like most children, she adapted well and developed many substitution patterns. No surgery was necessary on the left forearm and hand, which are used as helpers. She was a fierce competitor on her high-school tennis team.

---

entitled "Ulnar Deficiencies"). Digital function varies tremendously and is achieved primarily with intrinsic muscles. Although rarely normal, the strength and function of these digits are usually sufficient to manipulate shoulder or elbow locking mechanisms for control of myoelectric prostheses.

Half of the West German thalidomide patients studied presented with upper limb and lower limb deformities, and one fourth presented with upper limb involvement; more than 10% had congenital cardiac anomalies.[5,10-13] Syndromes in which phocomelia occurs include the Roberts syndrome, with four deficient limbs plus cleft lip or palate; the Holt-Oram syndrome, with congenital heart disease; and the adactyly-adontia syndrome, in which major proximal limb amputations may occur.[3]

TREATMENT

Phocomelia is generally managed without surgical intervention. Patients are more often referred to the prosthetist or mechanical engineer.[12,13] However, there are several indications for operative treatment. Digital function may occasionally be enhanced by web release, rotational osteotomy, or tendon transfer.[14] Associated radial or ulnar deviation of the hand may require centralization. These techniques are discussed in other sections (see Fig. 203-1). In addition, fitting of a prosthesis may be enhanced by lengthening of whatever humerus is present with or without bone grafts,[15]

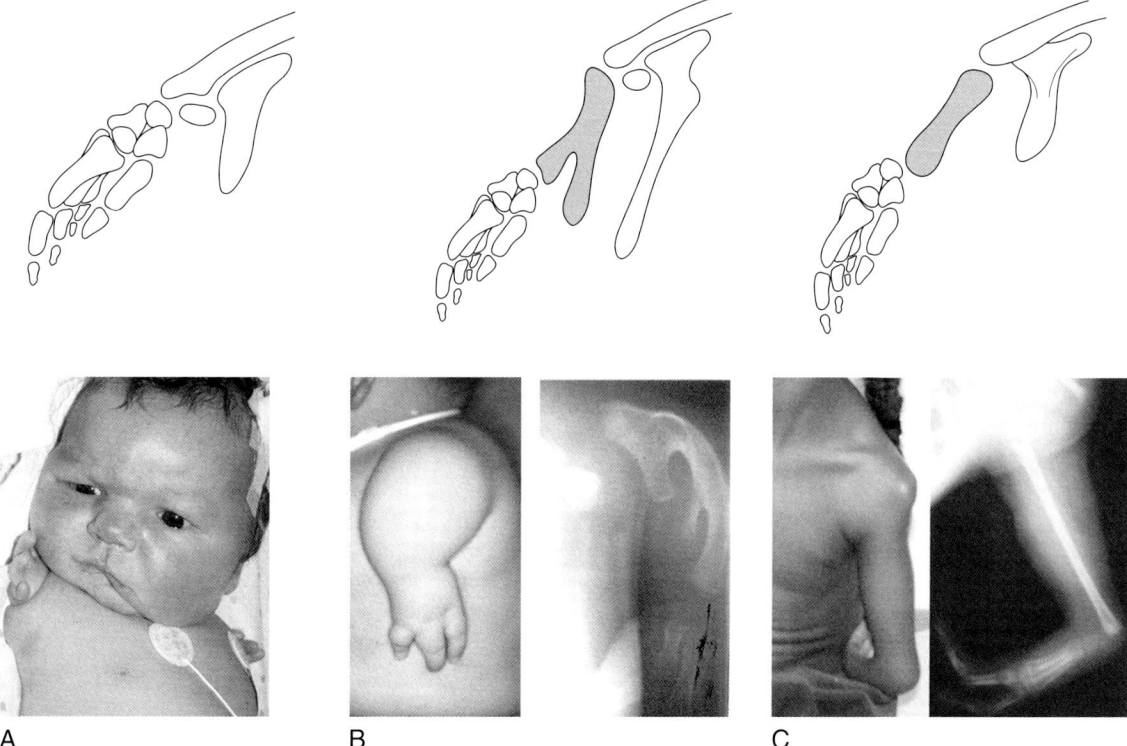

A   B   C

FIGURE 203-2. Phocomelia classification. *A,* In the most severe type of phocomelia, a small hand is attached to the clavicle and scapula. *B,* In the second type, there is an intercalated loss of the humerus and a small forearm with some type of fused radius and ulna that articulates with a small hand, in which there is a greater ulnar than radial deficiency. *C,* In the third type, the humerus is present and can be quite long, articulating with a hypoplastic hand that usually contains between one and three rays. Hand malformations are variable. (Illustration by Jean Biddl.)

removal of vestigial tags, mobilization of the clavicle,[5,6] and fibular transfer and fusion to the glenoid.

Amputation of hand remnants is rarely indicated, especially because the affected child can often use them to control a prosthetic terminal device. When a patient can reach his or her mouth with a phocomelic limb, fitting of a prosthesis is rarely indicated (Fig. 203-3).[16] In the rare circumstance that any surgical intervention is indicated, the objective is to gain a motor end organ with sensation that will achieve maximum function. Malformations can be corrected at an early age so function can be optimized; most patients will achieve some degree of upper extremity function.

If prosthetic wear is indicated, it is advisable to start at an early age to integrate the brain and functional development. The prosthesis, chosen from the wide variety of shoulder joints, elbow joints, and terminal devices available, must be individualized to the patient's age, size, opposite limb, and degree of adaptation. Shoulder motion may be used to trigger elbow and finger motion within prostheses. Newer myoelectric devices amplify impulses from muscle contraction to initiate prosthesis function.[12,17] These larger prostheses are readily accepted by patients and playmates as soon as curiosity is overcome (see Fig. 203-3). As long as prosthetic limbs are painless, functional, durable, and within the "gadget tolerance" of the patient and family, they are well tolerated. The principle of sensory feedback between a terminal device and an implanted electrode within a major nerve has been introduced, and although appealing, it is not clinically predictable at this time.[8]

Forearm Level

CLINICAL PRESENTATION

Transverse absence at the forearm level is more common than absence at the upper arm level, occurring once in 20,000 live births.[2] It is generally unilateral and most often involves the left arm. Overall, transverse upper arm absence occurs with a 3:2 female predominance by sex. However, sex distribution is equal when transverse upper arm absence is seen in conjunction with the constriction ring syndrome. Growth of the forearm portion of the limb is usually decreased, rarely exceeding a mature length of 10 cm.[18] Most malformations occur in the proximal third of the forearm. Vestigial bulbous remnants and deep dimples connecting skin to fibrous anlagen are often present in the ends of these stumps. Rarely are well-developed hand structures present. Subluxation of the proximal radioulnar joint and dislocation of the radial head are common, and elbow flexion of more than 100 degrees is usually present, with normal shoulder musculature. The cause of transverse upper arm deficits, which occur sporadically, is not known.

TREATMENT

Surgery is indicated in less than 10% of patients with transverse absence of the forearm. Stump revision in the form of excision of functionless nubbins, recontouring of bulbous skinfolds, and elimination of deep dimples facilitate initial fitting of a prosthesis but are not always necessary. Soft tissue deepening of the axillary web may facilitate fixation of the stump socket. In patients with transverse amputations at the elbow level, humeral overgrowth is common. Stump capping with autogenous cartilage may be useful to help prevent overgrowth.[18] Angulation osteotomies have been advocated in selected patients to provide a 20- to 45-degree flexion at the elbow.[18,19] On occasion, lengthening of a humeral stump with a sliding osteotomy or distraction lengthening may be indicated.[15] However, stump lengthening with bone grafts and tubed pedicle flaps produces an unpredictable amount of resorption, and vascularized bone transfers have not been attempted in these patients, primarily because it is easier to revise a prosthesis than to perform surgery.

One option for patients with bilateral amputations below the elbow or at the wrist is the Krukenberg procedure,[20] in which a prehensile pincer is formed by separating the radius and the ulna.[21-23] With pronation, the two forearm bones adduct, and an adult with a Krukenberg arm can hold objects weighing up to 10 kg. With supination, the two limbs of the pincer abduct as much as 45 degrees. The best candidates for this operation are those with bilateral absence of the hand, particularly in regions of the world where prostheses are not available, and blind patients, who require constant sensory feedback for use of the extremity. Clinical reports of the Krukenberg procedure include primarily adults with bilateral traumatic amputations in Southeast Asia and other countries where machete accidents are common. The report by Chan et al[23] describing eight procedures for unilateral congenital amputees who underwent the Krukenberg procedure indicates that there may be a place for this operation in the treatment of congenital defects, but most affected children do not have a long enough forearm stump for the procedure. Sighted children with unilateral deformities (and their parents) find the pincer functional but so unattractive and conspicuous that they reject its use in public. However, despite their appearance, these limbs are incredibly functional. The Krukenberg arm is also compatible with prosthetic wear if desired.

Early fitting of a prosthesis is the treatment of choice in patients with congenital absence of the forearm. Early fitting can avoid substitution patterns, and sensory stimulation at the stump-prosthesis interface will stimulate visual cues.[13,19,24] The timing of the initial fitting has changed dramatically in the past 10 years.[12]

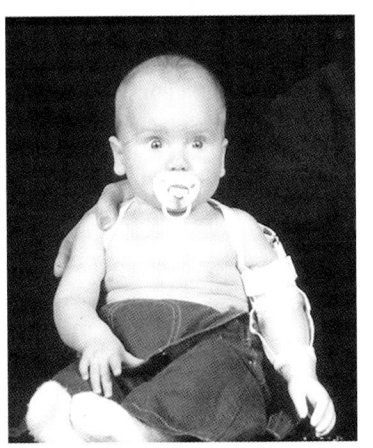
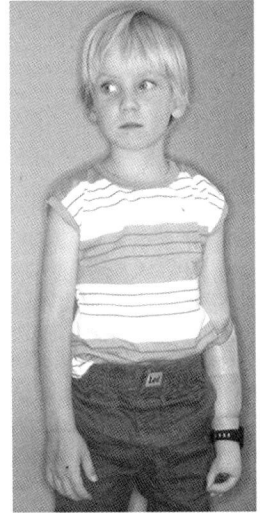

A

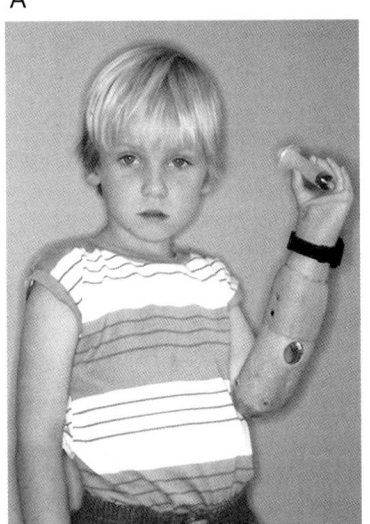
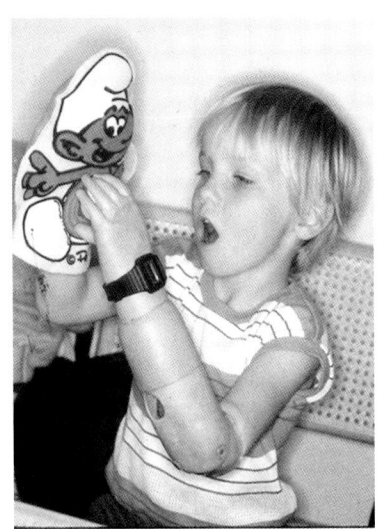

B

FIGURE 203-3. Early fit with myoelectric prosthesis. *A,* This boy with a unilateral congenital below-elbow amputation was observed from the time of birth. At 9 months of age, he was fitted with a static prosthesis with a terminal hand, which he used effectively during the first 3 years of life, after which he was fitted with a myoelectric device that he took to school and used for some bimanual functions. *B,* He used his hand for unilateral pinching and gripping maneuvers and for bimanual balancing tasks. On the playground, his prosthetic arm remained in his backpack. *C,* Although he managed to lose his prosthetic arm on occasion, it was always found, and repairs were necessary on a monthly basis. At age 25 years, he works as a computer programmer and no longer uses his myoelectric arm and hand.

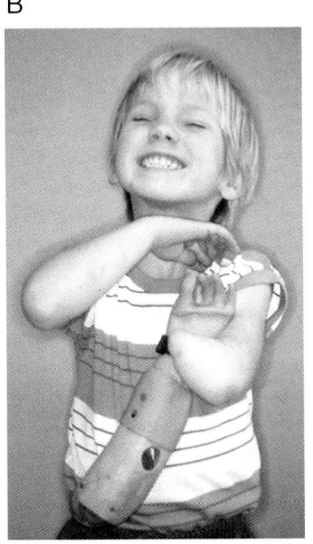
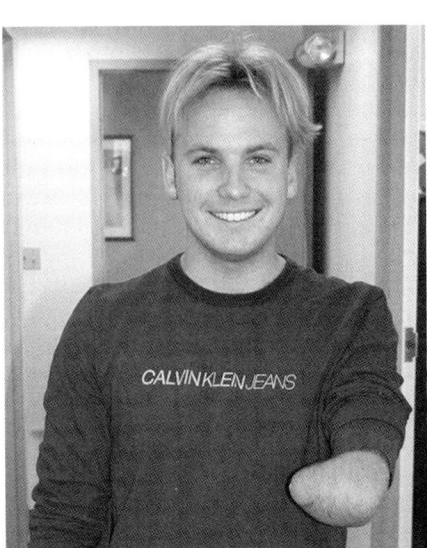

C

Most centers now recommend fitting below-elbow amputees with a smooth plastic mitten or paddle at 6 months of age so they can crawl, balance, and grasp with both extremities (see Fig. 203-3). At 18 to 24 months of age, a hook is added to the terminal device, and the child is taught to control it with a shoulder harness. More sophisticated myoelectric prostheses are now being introduced for children between 3 and 6 years of age.[25] Impulses from contracting muscles are amplified by skin electrodes to motor these devices, which provide a basic key pinch between thumb and index finger. The design and function of these prostheses have improved substantially in recent years.[26,27]

The child with unilateral arm or forearm amputation is an unpredictable user of a prosthesis, tending instead to use the deficient limb as a helper for support and hook activities. The normal limb, both of necessity and with development, becomes stronger, more dexterous, and adaptable. It is important to encourage use of a prosthesis, which may improve function, particularly bimanual function (see Fig. 203-3). Its continued use is ultimately determined by the patient, however, and not by an enthusiastic surgeon, therapist, or parent.

Continual retraining and refitting are necessary to ensure that the device becomes fully integrated into the child's activities of daily living and body image. Acceptance of the prosthesis is directly related to parental acceptance and participation in the prosthesis program.[28] The prosthetic goals should be restoration of optimal function, cosmetic effect, and comfort. Durability and adaptability are the most important features of a childhood prosthesis, and one of the greatest pitfalls has been to "over gadget" these devices in children, who provide the ultimate test for the most durable biomaterials.

Psychological concern about the limb absence deformity becomes a problem for most adolescents, who have adapted well, with or without a prosthesis. Counseling and open discussion with these children should be encouraged.

As a member of a prosthetic team, the surgeon must realize that the patient's acceptance of and willingness to wear a prosthesis may be difficult and unpredictable (see Fig. 203-3). These children should be fitted for prostheses only when necessary, and care should be taken not to make the patient's acceptance a focal point of family life.[24,29] Those working with such children are referred to the *Atlas of Limb Prosthetics* published by the American Academy of Orthopaedic Surgeons.

Carpal and Metacarpal Level

CLINICAL PRESENTATION

Transverse amputation of the hand at the wrist level (acheiria) or at the metacarpal level (adactyly) may be complete or incomplete. Congenital carpal and metacarpal amputations are usually unilateral and are not commonly associated with other malformations. They may present in a wide variety of clinical patterns, including true transverse absence, as part of a cleft hand, localized amputations within the constriction ring syndrome, and symbrachydactyly.[29,30] Strictly speaking, the presence of a hypoplastic nubbin with a small nail remnant in symbrachydactyly excludes this anomaly as a true transverse amputation (see section entitled "Symbrachydactyly"), and there are vestigial hypoplastic nubbins with or without miniature nail remnants. The dimpling or retraction of this tissue is indicative of extrinsic flexor and extensor tendons, which are usually abnormal but lie in normal position over the carpal and metacarpal portions of the hand and insert into the hypoplastic nubbins. These extrinsic flexor and extensor tendons may provide mobility of the radiocarpal joint. Grasping and pulling on the soft tissue nubbins will give the examiner some indication of the size of the skin envelope and the strength of the tendons. Radiographs are of limited predictive value early in life because the hypoplastic skeletal parts are not ossified.

TREATMENT

Vestigial nubbins without underlying skeletal elements or no functional potential should be excised early in life, before they become bizarre objects of curiosity and of psychological attachment for parent and child. Most authors agree that removal of the nubbins "removes the stigma of congenitalism" and establishes a more acceptable deformity that appears to be the result of trauma.[31,32] However, many patients polish these nails, do not feel self-conscious in public, and try to use them.

Treatment options for the carpal hand are difficult because the child adaptively uses the flexible wrist as a hook and manages to hold objects against the torso as a paddle. Fitting of a prosthesis may be not only unnecessary but also contraindicated because the prosthesis may interfere with normal sensory feedback between the sensate stump and the external environment.

When a mobile wrist is present, a palmar plate prosthesis may provide a post against which the child can grasp, pick up, and hold objects.[33] Many children develop two-point discrimination that is better than normal on both dorsal and palmar surfaces.[34] The size and length of the carpus can be increased by bone grafts beneath the soft tissue on the end of the extremity, which is often redundant. Distraction techniques and bone grafting at the carpal level to increase the amount of contact surface may be considered.

If metacarpal elements are present distal to the carpals, reconstructive possibilities increase substantially, essentially eliminating the need for a prosthesis. The goal should be to establish a "basic hand" that is more functional than a prosthesis; it contains a mobile ray on the radial side, a cleft, and a post or at least one additional mobile ray on the opposite side of the hand.[35] This is a realistic approach inasmuch as the first and fifth metacarpals are frequently present in this type of transverse deficiency (Fig. 203-4). The presence of a joint at the base of the thumb metacarpal, and of thenar intrinsic muscles, is the most critical factor in this reconstruction. Many surgeons believe that the unilateral deformity does not require reconstruction.[36]

The decision to perform any reconstruction requires careful evaluation, counseling, and planning. Every deformity is different, and there are many reconstructive possibilities. These should be carefully evaluated and discussed with parents, who should be urged to articulate their desires and questions. In few other areas of congenital hand surgery are the reconstructive options so great.

Web Deepening

Older methods of deepening the cleft to form a pincer mechanism between metacarpal remnants, or "phalangealization," will probably decrease in popularity as newer methods of distraction lengthening become available. Dorsal flaps are used to line the base of the commissure, and skin grafts are usually necessary.[14] The major problem with deepening webs to form a pincer between metacarpals is injury to intrinsic muscles, particularly the adductor pollicis muscle within the thumb-index web space, which may need to be detached and reattached more proximally on the metacarpal.

Metacarpal Transposition

Transfer of metacarpal remnants from the central portion of the hand to the border serves to lengthen an existing border ray or to deepen the central cleft. Consideration must be given to this procedure before any potentially useful hypoplastic metacarpals are discarded. The soft tissue may be lengthened by distraction techniques or with a combination of local flaps and grafts.[37]

Phalangeal Transfer

The transfer of a nonvascularized toe phalanx is effective for digital lengthening, given an adequate soft tissue envelope distal to the existing skeletal structures. (For indications and techniques of this procedure, see section "Symbrachydactyly.")

Metacarpal Distraction Lengthening

If sufficient metacarpal bone is present, satisfactory length can be achieved by the distraction method. The initial application of distraction lengthening was described by Codivilla[38] for use in the lower limb. Much later, Matev[39,40] applied it to the upper extremity for the correction of post-traumatic thumb deformities. Matev and others subsequently used distraction for treatment of congenital hand malformations.[41-44] The procedure is useful in clinical situations requiring increased length of a border ray or when an opposition post is necessary in a hand with no digits and a hypoplastic thumb. Most surgeons wait until the patient is 5 years of age to perform these staged procedures, although distraction can be undertaken earlier if enough bone stock is present to avoid damage to growth centers.

TECHNIQUE. Commercially available distraction devices consist of metal blocks that attach to a longitudinal screw mechanism on either side of the bone to be lengthened. Uniplanar devices are used for the hand. Turning the screw knobs 360 degrees will increase or decrease the interval distance 0.5 to 0.6 mm (see Fig. 203-4).

In the first stage of metacarpal distraction lengthening, the metacarpal osteotomy site is selected in the widest portion of the bone, sufficiently distant to the growth plate. Two or three small (0.28 or 0.35 mm) wires are passed transversely through the bone on either side of the planned osteotomy site. The holes within the metal blocks can be used as a drill guide. A dorsal skin incision is made, the extensor mechanism is retracted, the periosteum is *incised* transversely, and the osteotomy is completed. Direct observation of pin placement will prevent penetration of digital nerves or flexor tendons. The complete apparatus is assembled and stabilized with malleable struts connecting the block on either side of the hand or digit. In Matev's original work on the thumb,[40] the periosteum was not incised, and bone formation occurred by creeping substitution as the distractor was left on for several months. Owing to the unpredictable quality of this bone,[45-47] most surgeons prefer to insert a bone graft once satisfactory length has been achieved. The skin is closed and a protective splint is applied.

The lengthening is started several days later and proceeds at approximately 0.8 to 1.2 mm/day. Distraction is stopped temporarily if there is any sign of vascular compromise, skin irritation, or significant pain. In young children, the hand should be protected with a splint or bulky dressing. Parents can do the distraction at home by turning the screw knobs, which should all be marked with a reference point. At weekly intervals, the amount of distraction is measured radiographically. Most metacarpal distractions are completed within 4 to 5 weeks, at which point the child is admitted to the hospital for the second stage, a bone graft procedure.

Although autogenous donor sites from iliac crest or fibula are preferred, allografts[43] and demineralized

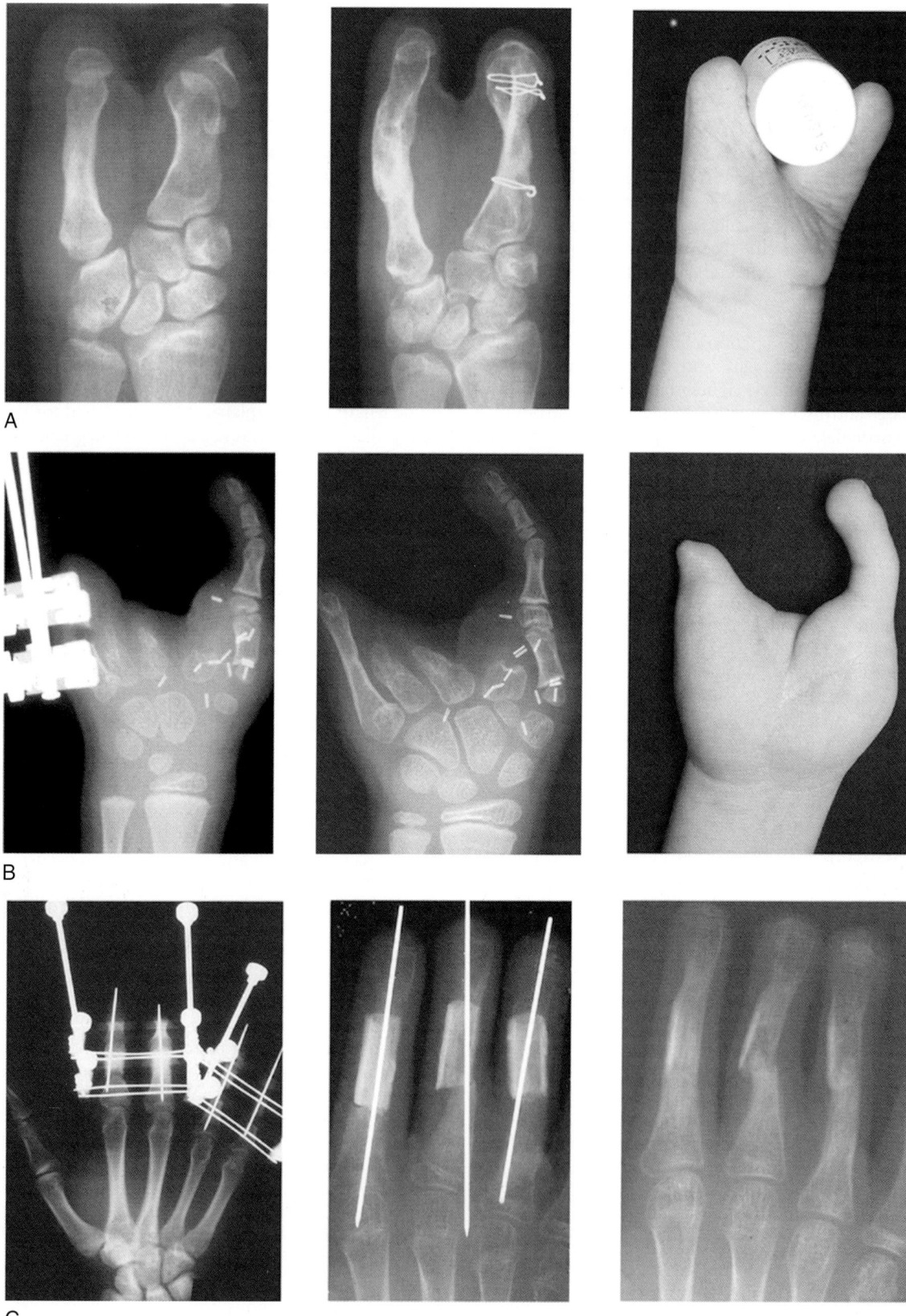

A

B

C

FIGURE 203-4. Distraction lengthening. *A,* The right hand of this patient with the constriction ring syndrome consisted of the first and fifth metacarpals with no functional phalanges. She had a congenital below-elbow amputation of her other upper limb. Thirty years ago, both metacarpals were lengthened with rudimentary devices and the gaps filled with autogenous bone grafts. After a web space was created, she maintained an excellent pinch and functioned effectively. Interosseous wires were used extensively before the development of plates and screws for the hand. *B,* The thumb in this child with symbrachydactyly was constructed with a second-toe microvascular transfer. The fifth metacarpal was lengthened 30 mm with slow distraction during 6 weeks. There was excellent regenerate bone during the 3-month period that the Kessler distractor, which was used extensively in the 1980s, was left in place, so autogenous bone grafting was not necessary. Now 22 years after reconstruction, the patient still maintains a strong thumb to fifth metacarpal pinch. *C,* Phalangeal distraction is less predictable than lengthening at the metacarpal level. Three digits in this child were simultaneously distracted at the middle phalangeal level. Because these gaps are not surrounded by well-vascularized muscle, the quality of the new bone formation is less than that of more proximal distractions. Demineralized bone grafts were used to fill the intercalated gaps. Note the malunion of the long finger; in the current era, miniplates and screws are used for internal fixation.

bone implants[48] have been useful (Fig. 203-4*C*). Nonfunctional skeletal segments within the hand may serve as bone graft donor sites, particularly at the metacarpal level in the cleft hand-foot and constriction ring syndromes and symbrachydactyly. Grafts are fixed with interosseous wires, miniplates and screws, or longitudinal K-wires. In selected patients, the lengthened segment may be transposed onto an adjacent ray.[36] In appropriate patients, adjacent metacarpals may also be inserted into the distracted segment as vascularized bone grafts. The transverse pins and apparatus are removed, and the extremity is immobilized in a cast.

Significant lengthening can be achieved within short periods. Usually only 30 to 40 mm of length is sufficient at the metacarpal level, but up to 80 mm has been reported. Intrinsic muscles cannot be rapidly stretched more than 75% of their resting length.[39,49] Skin and neurovascular bundles tolerate the 1.0- to 1.5-mm daily expansion well. In patients with previous surgery and scar formation adjacent to the bone to be distracted, especially in the first web space, the contracture should be released before distraction is performed.

COMPLICATIONS. Complications can occur early and late, and careful vigilance over these children is required. Active children will invariably bump and break a portion of the apparatus if the protective splints are not worn. Accordingly, an inventory of spare parts is necessary. Pin track irritation, skin blanching, a tight ridge between pins across the distraction site, and neurovascular compromise are best treated by stopping the distraction for a few days. Skin maceration can occur if the metal blocks of the apparatus are too close to adjacent skin surfaces. Possible late problems include contracture of joints distal to the distracted segment, intrinsic muscle fibrosis, and nonunion of the bone graft to the distal distracted segment. Infections are often related to soft tissue loss and skeletal extrusion associated with overly rapid distraction.

Bone Grafting

There is often an abundance of soft tissue beyond the hypoplastic metacarpal remnants. Insertion of autogenous bone grafts will transform the floppy palm or digital remnant into a rigid functional post with sensation. At a later date, this post can either be augmented with distraction methods or serve as the foundation for phalangeal reconstruction. Primary autogenous bone grafting to increase length at the digital level often results in significant graft resorption. On occasion, a local flap can be combined with a bone graft for functional border rays in the hypoplastic hand.[50,51]

Vascularized Toe to Hand Transfer

The most elaborate reconstruction for the missing digit is the toe to hand transfer. Like distraction methods, these techniques were initially developed for posttraumatic defects, and many surgeons have applied them to the hypoplastic hand with no digits or thumb (Fig. 203-5).[52-56] The prime indication is for the reconstruction of the thumb that has a carpometacarpal (CMC) joint but no phalangeal segments. (For technique and results of toe transfer, see Chapter 208.) The major disadvantages of toe transfers are the limitation of flexion arc and motion and the appearance. Gait alterations in the donor foot do not seem to be significant,[57] but some authors with extensive experience have raised doubts about functions such as running and walking on upwardly inclined surfaces.[58,59]

Transfer of the great or second toe is often more difficult in young children, and the function is less predictable than with a post-traumatic deformity because of the underdevelopment of necessary muscle-tendon units in the forearm. Typically, broad sheets of tendon attached to a common muscle mass are found in the dorsal and palmar forearm. Median and ulnar nerves are often so rudimentary that digital toe nerves must be joined to cutaneous branches at the carpal level.[54-56] The major exception to the rule is constriction ring syndrome and chorionic villus sampling-related defects, in which most of the normal anatomic structures are present and well differentiated in the

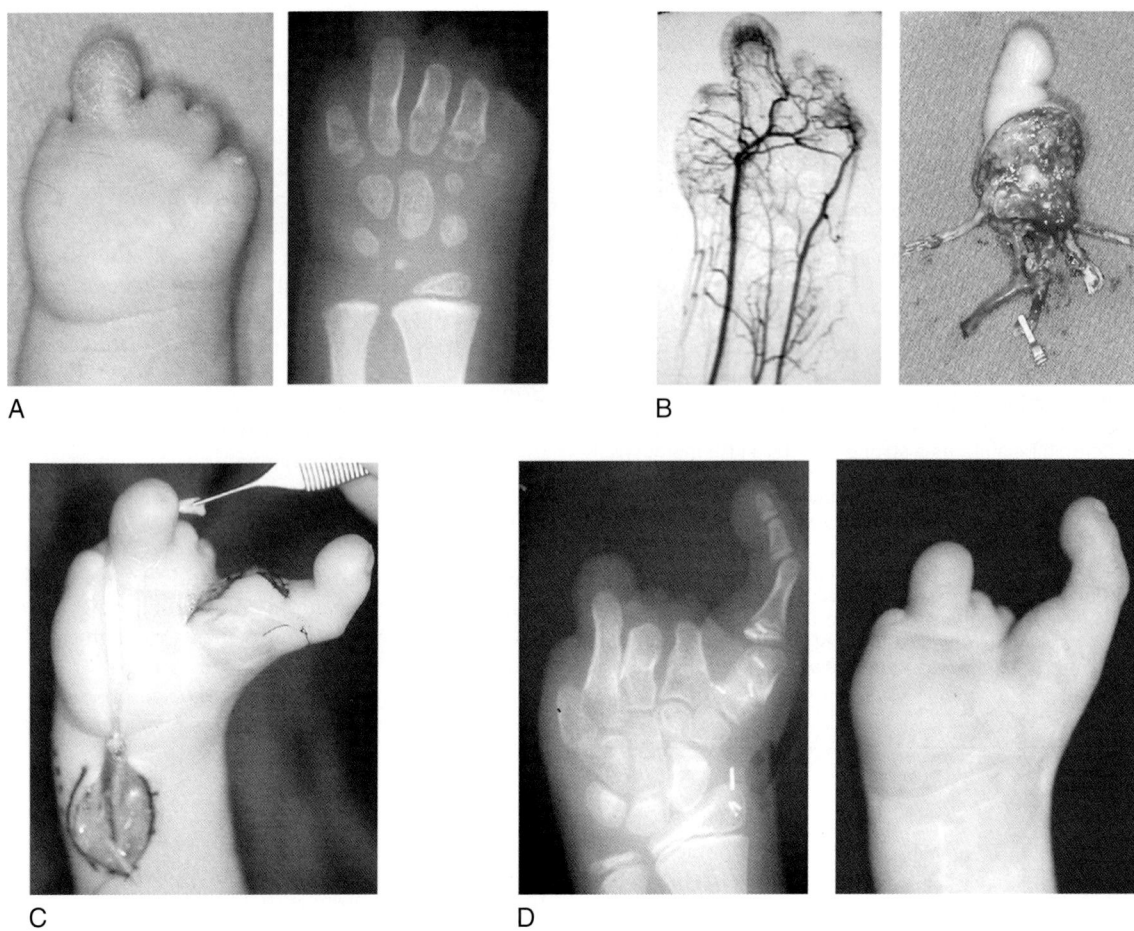

FIGURE 203-5. Second-toe to thumb transfer. *A,* The clinical appearance and radiograph of a right hand with transverse absence at the metacarpal level, which may also be classified as symbrachydactyly (aphalangia type), demonstrate an intact wrist and four metacarpals. There is no CMC joint on the radial side. *B,* All three vessels of the forearm are seen extending to the hand, with little direct communication between the radial and ulnar systems. The dissected ipsilateral second toe is in transit to the hand. *C,* A secondary adduction tendon transfer of the flexor carpi ulnaris plus palmaris longus graft to the "thoe" was necessary to strengthen pinch. Secondary procedures are commonly needed in these hands, which do not have normal extrinsic or intrinsic muscle-tendon units. *D,* The same hand is seen near skeletal maturity. Note the relative difference in growth between the ulnar metacarpal post and the transferred toe with three growth plates.

forearm until the level of constriction. The results of these transfers at the proximal phalangeal level can be very natural looking.

Phalangeal Level

CLINICAL PRESENTATION

At the digital level, amputations due to transverse arrest in development are less common than digital hypoplasia and are often classified as variants of the longitudinal deficiencies. Amputations of individual or multiple digits are most often seen in patients with the constriction ring syndrome or various types of brachydactyly, in which all fingers and the thumb may be involved, either alone or in combination, at any

phalangeal level. The hand or forearm is often hypoplastic.

In general, length and bulk are the presenting complaints, although abnormalities in alignment, mobility, and stability may also be present. Bulbous lymphedematous soft tissue masses may be present in the constriction ring syndrome (see Chapter 205). Anatomic structures present in a given patient with the constriction ring syndrome are best determined through a combination of radiographic and clinical evaluation. Terminal phalanges in this syndrome are characterized by a trumpet appearance, broad at the base and narrow at the tip. Extrinsic and intrinsic muscle-tendon units usually accompany a well-formed proximal phalanx. Anatomic structures proximal to the level of the transverse arrest are often normal, in contrast to the severely hypoplastic digit, in which proximal structures may be present but abnormal.

TREATMENT

Reconstruction is often beneficial and should be considered in the context of coexisting malformations of the hand. When the level of arrest is in the proximal half of the proximal phalangeal segment, nonvascularized phalangeal transfers or metacarpal distraction may be considered, especially if multiple digits and the thumb are abnormal (see "Symbrachydactyly"). Microvascular toe transfers may be a reasonable functional and aesthetic option but are often unacceptable to parents. In selected patients, complete and partial toe transfer may be indicated, although patients and parents tend to be less enthusiastic about such an operation in the setting of a congenital defect than with a post-traumatic deformity (see Fig. 203-5).[54,60] The functional gain achieved with excessive web deepening or phalangealization of the thumb is usually limited. Pollicization of a finger, partial ray ablation to establish a web space, or shifting of bone segments from one ray to another may be indicated. When the majority of the proximal phalanx is present, function is usually excellent and lengthening is rarely required.

Distraction methods have been used at this level with a lesser degree of predictability, particularly when hypoplastic phalanges are being manipulated. Although digital distraction restores length to the finger, it does not provide normal circumferential width or interphalangeal joint motion. Pin track infections and nonunion of the distal distracted fragment are the primary complications of digital distraction.

Partial or total finger prostheses are available commercially but are not consistently used by children, who prefer the shorter, sensate working surface of the native digit. Moreover, prostheses are also easily lost, damaged, and discolored by active children. However, Beasley[61] and Pillet[62,63] demonstrated that prostheses can be effectively worn by carefully selected children. Adolescents will wear them for social occasions. A partial hand prosthesis may be particularly advisable for the older child or adolescent with multiple digit amputations and a normal thumb.

LONGITUDINAL ABSENCES (FAILURE OF FORMATION)

Classification

Because there is no universally accepted system for subclassification of longitudinal upper extremity defects, for the sake of consistency, the same system as for the description of polydactyly is used, including the terms *radial, central,* and *ulnar.* In the past, the term *intercalated* was incorporated to describe losses at the shoulder or humeral levels, but it is not often presently used.

Longitudinal losses and absence include radial and ulnar dysplasias, which also involve the proximal portions of the limb. In addition, the typical cleft hand has been included as a longitudinal defect because it represents a failure of development of the central portion of the hand plate, but it is not associated with more proximal malformations. The presence of syndactyly of digits bordering the central cleft and the association of transverse and oblique bones within the hand may cause confusion with synpolydactyly,[64] which has been classified as a type of complex syndactyly primarily involving the long and ring rays of the hand.

Radial (Preaxial) Deficiencies

Radial deficiencies are those that are characterized by partial or complete absence of structures on the preaxial side of the limb. They range from minor abnormalities of the thenar muscles to complete absence of all preaxial structures as well as anomalies involving the upper arm and brachial plexus. They may be associated with postaxial deficits of varying severity.

PATHOGENESIS

The etiology of most radial deficiencies is unknown. Longitudinal radial deformities have been produced experimentally in chick embryos by Duraiswami,[65] who cauterized preaxial portions of the limb bud at critical periods of development, which correspond to the fourth through seventh postovulatory weeks in the human embryo.

Environmental factors such as drugs, radiation, nutrition, and viruses have been implicated in the pathogenesis of certain radial deficits. A well-known teratogen is the drug thalidomide. Used as a sedative in European countries during the 1950s and early 1960s, thalidomide came to be associated with short limbs (phocomelia) and radial ray defects when it was administered to pregnant women.[66,67] Other drugs responsible for radial ray deficiencies include aminopterin,[67] alcohol in excess,[68] phenobarbital,[69] and valproic acid.[70]

During the past 2 decades, Ogino, Kato, and Matsumura have demonstrated that administration of busulfan to WKAH/Hkm rats at critical periods of development, specifically E10-E11, causes limb deformities similar to the longitudinal deficiencies seen in humans.[71-74] The histologic study of affected limbs showed that the deformities were not due to localized damage to the limb bud and suggested that the cause of longitudinal defects is related to a deficiency of the mesenchymal cells below the apical ectodermal ridge.

INCIDENCE

The incidence of radial deficiencies has been estimated to range from 1 in 30,000 to 1 in 100,000 live births.[2,31,75-77] A more precise incidence is difficult to determine because of differences in classification systems and terminology. One explanation for the wide range is that many infants with this malformation die of other anomalies. The "clubhand" posture occurs bilaterally about as frequently as unilaterally. If one looks carefully in unilateral absence, some form of hypoplasia can usually be found in the opposite extremity.[78-80] In patients with bilateral absence, there is a 3:2 male-to-female ratio.[80,81] The severity of the hand abnormality may not be related to the amount of radial absence, which directly determines the degree of radial deviation and the extent of soft tissue deficiencies.[31,77,78,82-84]

ASSOCIATED MALFORMATIONS AND SYNDROMES

Associated anomalies are common, and many patients have recognizable malformation syndromes that can involve almost any organ system (Table 203-1). Although most do not have recognizable genetic causes, autosomal dominant genetic association has been recognized[77,78,84] in the context of well-recognized syndromes, such as thrombocytopenia-absent radius, Holt-Oram, craniofacial microsomia, and Fanconi anemia.[85,86] Because associated defects are particularly common, the limb anomaly should prompt investigation for associated anomalies, which are present in 40% of patients with unilateral absence and 77% of patients with bilateral absence. Possible defects include congenital heart disease (approximately 25%), pulmonary hypoplasia, and other anomalies of the genitourinary, gastrointestinal, hematologic, and musculoskeletal systems.[87-89] Only the anemias are not present at birth, typically becoming manifest later in childhood. Among associated anomalies, the Fanconi life-threatening pancytopenia[90,91] can now be recognized at birth with a DEB test,[92] which is performed in only a few centers worldwide because it involves a combustible gas, butane. All children with radial ray defects should be routinely screened with this blood test.

Syndromes most commonly associated with radial defects include the VACTERL association (vertebral anomalies, anal atresia, tracheoesophageal fistula, renal and limb abnormalities),[93] the Holt-Oram syndrome,[89,94] the ventriculoradial dysplasia syndrome,[95] the thrombocytopenia-absent radius syndrome,[96-98] and the Nager-acrofacial dysostosis syndrome (Fig. 203-6).[99] The cardiac defects most commonly seen are

TABLE 203-1 ✦ SKELETAL SYNDROMES ASSOCIATED WITH RADIAL DYSPLASIA*

Organ System	Condition or Syndrome
Skeletal	VACTERL association Klippel-Feil syndrome Costovertebral dysplasia or humeroradial synostosis (Keutel syndrome) Cervical rib–radial ray (Funston syndrome)
Hematologic	Thrombocytopenia–absent radius (TAR syndrome) Fanconi anemia Anemia–triphalangeal thumb (Aase-Smith syndrome)
Cutaneous	Cutaneous poikiloderma (Rothmund-Thomson syndrome)
Cardiac	VACTERL association Hand-heart syndrome (Holt-Oram syndrome) Ventriculoradial dysplasia
Renal	Renal–radial ray aplasia (Sofer syndrome)
Craniofacial	Acro-reno-ocular syndrome Eye-radial syndrome Radial ray–choanal atresia Lacrimo-auriculo-dento-digital (LADD) syndrome (Levy-Hollister syndrome) Oculo-auriculo-vertebral dysplasia (Goldenhar syndrome) Oro-cranio-digital syndrome (Juberg-Hayward syndrome) Acrofacial dysostosis (Nager syndrome) Micrognathia and limb anomalies (Hanhart syndrome) Craniofacial microsomia Roberts syndrome Mandibulofacial dysostosis (Treacher Collins syndrome)
Central nervous system–retardation	Cornelia de Lange syndrome Seckel syndrome

*Note: This list includes only common syndromes or those seen by the author during the past 30 years.

atrial septal defect and ventriculoseptal defects, but more severe anomalies, such as tetralogy of Fallot, aortic coarctation, transposition of the great vessels, and valvular anomalies, can also occur. There is no correlation between the extent of the respective radial ray and cardiac defects. Because of the high incidence of associated facial and cardiac malformations, many of these children are treated in conjunction with the craniofacial and cardiac programs in large children's hospitals. Owing to the frequent associations with other

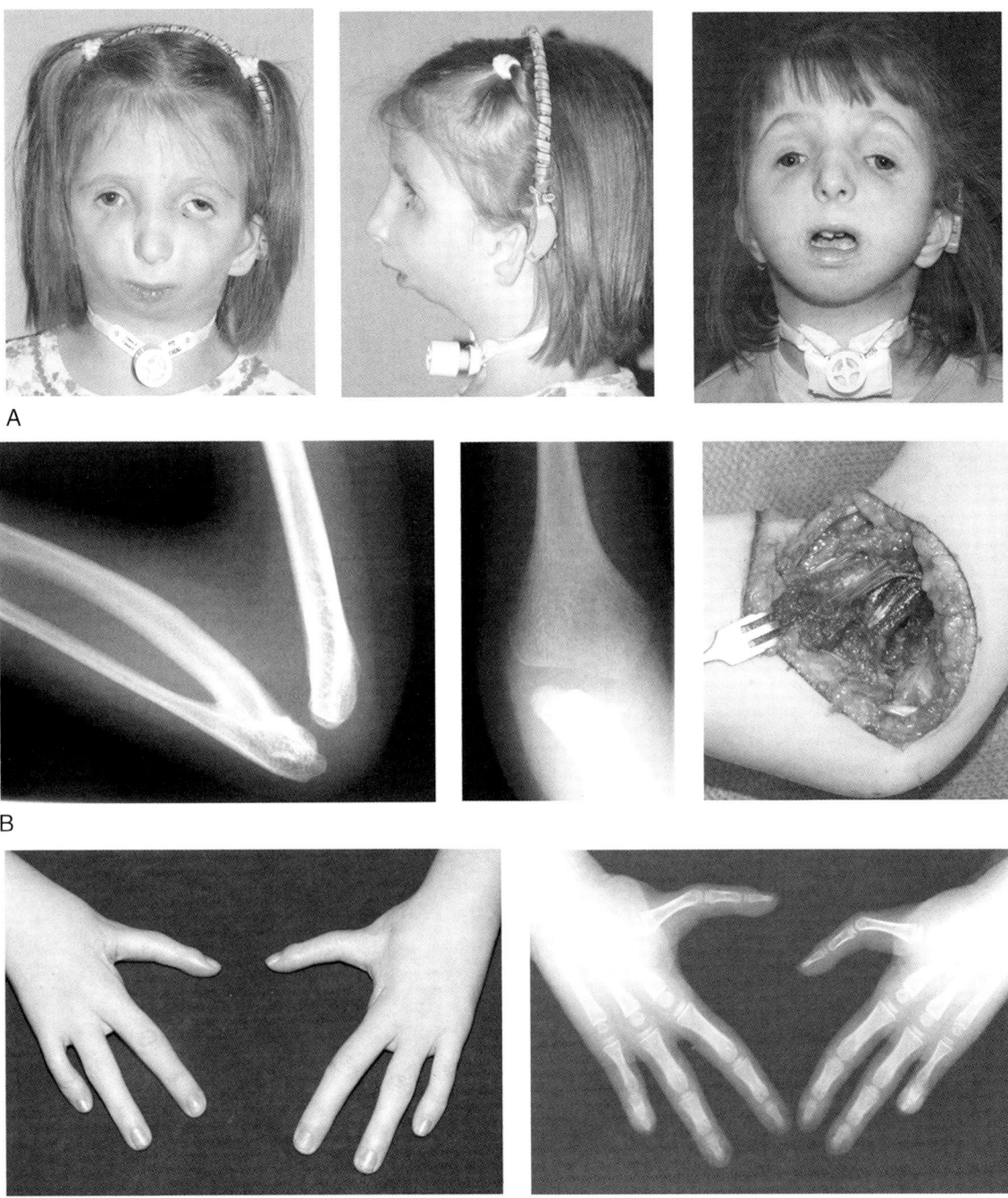

FIGURE 203-6. Radial dysplasia and facial malformations. *A,* This child with the Nager syndrome (acrofacial dysostosis) has had a tracheostomy since birth because of severe hypoplasia of the maxilla and mandible resulting in a marked upper airway restriction. She wears conductive hearing aids for severe hearing loss. On the right, she is seen 4 years later, after mandibular distraction lengthening by a process similar to that illustrated in Figure 203-4. *B,* Both of her radii were short and fused to the ulna just beyond the elbow joint, where total active motion did not exceed 90 degrees. The radioulnar synostosis was not treated, but elbow extension was improved with an anterior release followed by continuous passive motion therapy. *C,* Absent thumbs (type V) were treated with bilateral pollicization procedures.

anomalies, particularly facial and cardiac, patients with radial limb malformations should be evaluated by geneticists or other specialists as indicated.

CLASSIFICATION

Size of the radius is a practical criterion for classification of these deformities (Fig. 203-7).[79,100,101] Because of the hand and wrist deformities associated with radial dysplasia, this topic is covered in Chapter 208. Early correction or adjustment of arm, elbow, and wrist deformities must be carefully evaluated before any thumb construction is undertaken. Carpal abnormalities, particularly of the trapezium, scaphoid, and lunate, parallel the thumb, index, and long finger deficiencies.[80,82,83,102-106]

TYPE I: SHORT RADIUS. This variant is due to a growth deficiency of the proximal or the distal radial epiphysis. There is no radial bowing and little devia-

tion of the hand and wrist. The elbow is normal, and limb function is preserved. Support of the hand and wrist is adequate. No treatment is necessary for the forearm. Surgical procedures are confined to the hand, addressing the aplastic or hypoplastic thumb (see Chapter 208).

TYPE II: HYPOPLASTIC RADIUS. In this unusual variant, the radius is short due to abnormal growth of both the proximal and the distal epiphyses and presents as a radius "in miniature."[107] The hand is deviated and the ulna is thick, often bowed toward the radial side, although that deviation can be controlled with splinting, distraction, and bone grafting (see section on treatment of radial deficiencies). The thumb ray and its carpals are usually deficient.

TYPE III: PARTIAL ABSENCE OF THE RADIUS. Absence or hypoplasia of the middle and distal thirds of the radius is the most common radial deformity in

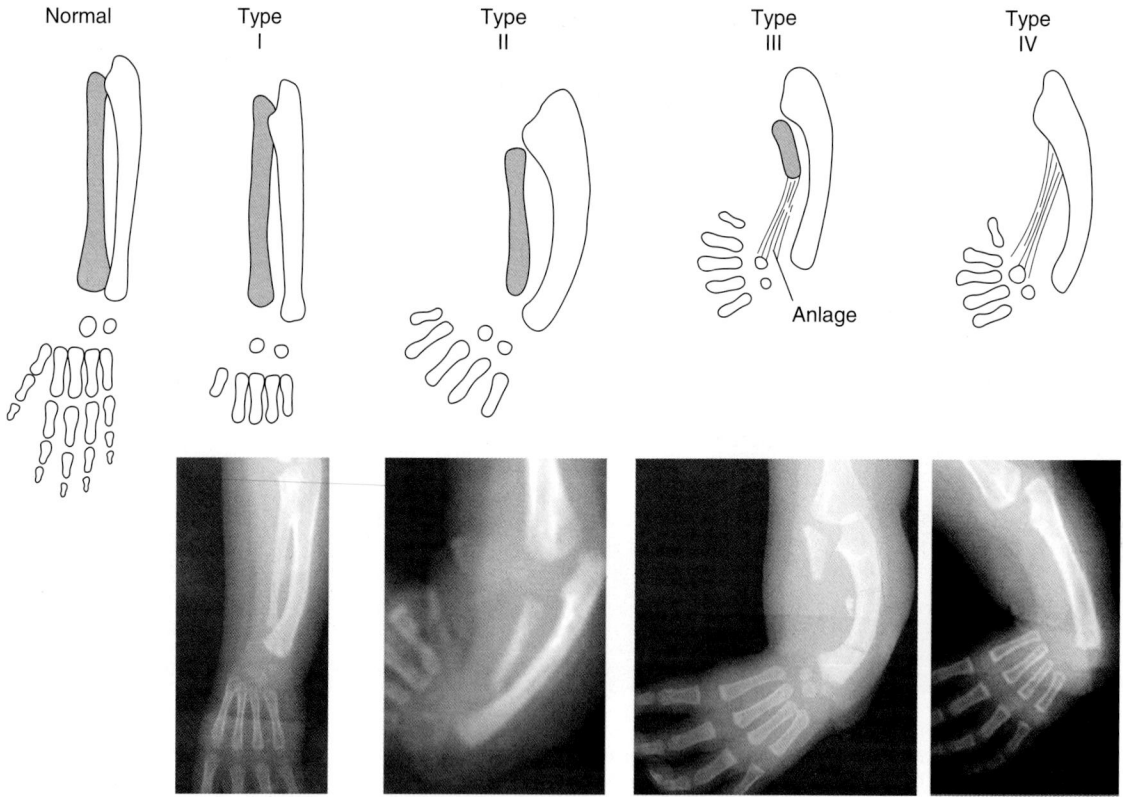

FIGURE 203-7. Classification of radial clubhand. The most commonly used classification system for radial forearm deficiencies has four categories. Type I: the radius is short but the elbow, wrist, and hand are normal. Type II (radius in miniature): the radius is short with proximal and distal epiphyses, the ulna may be slightly bowed, and the hand and wrist are radially deviated. Type III: the radius is partially absent, the ulna is bowed, and the hand and wrist are postured in radial deviation, pronation, and flexion. Type IV: the radius is completely absent, the ulna may be bowed, and the hand and wrist are in the same posture as in type III.[107] Although this system does not incorporate associated proximal limb deficiencies, there is a direct correlation between the severity of the forearm and hand deficiency and malformations of the elbow, humerus, shoulder, and, in many children, ipsilateral neck and chest wall. A moderate or marked amount of radial deviation may be present with types II, III, and IV. (Illustration by Jean Biddl.)

most reported series. The ulna is bowed, and deviation of the hand varies from moderate to extreme, depending on the length of the radius. The hand usually lies in a pronated, flexed, and radially deviated position. The thumb ray and carpals are usually deficient. The ulnar two digits are the most normal. A fibrous band or anlage is usually found in place of the deficient distal radius and contributes to bowing of the ulna. Abnormalities in muscles, tendons, nerves, and major arteries vary tremendously but usually correspond to the degree of skeletal deficiency. Blauth[108] and Heikel[100] observed that structures that are deficient but present tend to course radially at the distal end of the ulna. The radial nerve usually ends at the elbow, and the median nerve supplies the radial side of the existing hand. The median nerve is often thickened and may provide an unyielding obstacle to total passive correction of the wrist and hand. The ulnar nerve and artery are in their normal locations. In patients with severe deficiencies, preaxial flexor and extensor muscles and tendons are deficient; abnormalities of muscle, skeleton, nerves, and vessels may extend up to the shoulder level. The radial artery is usually absent.

The detailed descriptions of abnormal anatomy by Flatt[109] and others are recommended and should be reviewed before surgical intervention is undertaken.[82,88,110] Most patients with partial radial absence require some type of centralization procedure to improve hand function.

Type IV: Total Absence of the Radius. Total absence of the radius, the second most common presentation in the author's experience, demonstrates all the anatomic characteristics of the severe form of partial absence. The ulna is bowed and will never achieve its normal growth.[80,100] Elbow motion is restricted. The wrist is deviated and subluxed over the distal ulna. If it is left alone, a pseudarthrosis will develop with the distal ulna. The radial structures of the hand are deficient but not *all* may be severely deformed. The frequency of hand anomalies increases from the ulnar to the radial side. Index and long fingers rarely have normal range of motion and intrinsic tendons.[88] Aggressive soft tissue release with centralization or radialization is the most common form of treatment (Fig. 203-8).

James[102] proposed a classification system that incorporates abnormalities of the carpus and thumb with radial deficiencies, but not the more proximal humerus and glenohumeral joint.

CLINICAL PRESENTATION

Children with type I and type II deficiencies present with a shortened forearm and a mild clubhand posturing, which is usually passively correctable. The shoulder and elbow are functional, and the child can perform single and bimanual manipulative tasks with considerable adaptation. Digital sensation is normal. The thumb is present and in type II deficiencies may be stiff and severely hypoplastic. In such patients, grasp is good with the ulnar three digits, and many fine manipulative tasks may be accomplished with digital side-to-side pinching. Patients with bilateral radial involvement can still function remarkably well.

Children with type III and type IV deficiencies present with a severe clubhand posture, which may not be reducible. With complete or partial absence of the radius, the hand and carpus may be dislocated. The tight structures on the radial side of the wrist that prevent passive reduction include the median nerve, the flexor carpi radialis, and the fibrous anlage (scar band) present in place of the aplastic segment of the radius (Figs. 203-9 and 203-10). With severe deformities, the shoulder is dysplastic and flexor motion of the elbow is often missing. The elbow is extended and the hand is deviated radially at 90 degrees or more. The thumb is typically absent, but if present it may be severely hypoplastic and stiff. The one exception is the thrombocytopenia-absent radius syndrome,[111,112] in which the thumb is always present with varying degrees of function. The digital deformities and the intrinsic and extrinsic muscle and tendon abnormalities are more severe moving from ulnar to radial structures.[82] Tendon excursion and power also vary relative to the stability and the position of the wrist.[113,114]

TREATMENT

Treatment depends on the severity of the deformity, associated malformations, and functional deficits (Table 203-2).[88,115-120] Surgical correction often

---

TABLE 203-2 ◆ TREATMENT PRINCIPLES FOR RADIAL ABSENCE

Correct the "clubbed" position and place the hand and carpus in a normal position relative to the forearm,[80] which will stimulate optimal growth.[66]
Provide stability and preserve as much wrist motion as possible.[113,115]
Reposition the hand out of the "crotch" of the elbow into a more functional posture.[113]
Preserve length.[115,116]
Improve appearance.[117]

Options

Leave uncorrected
Passive stretching and splint immobilization indefinitely
Surgical centralization with tendon transpositions and capsular imbrication
Correction of radial bowing of the ulna
Distraction lengthening of the ulna
Elbow release and muscle transfer for flexion

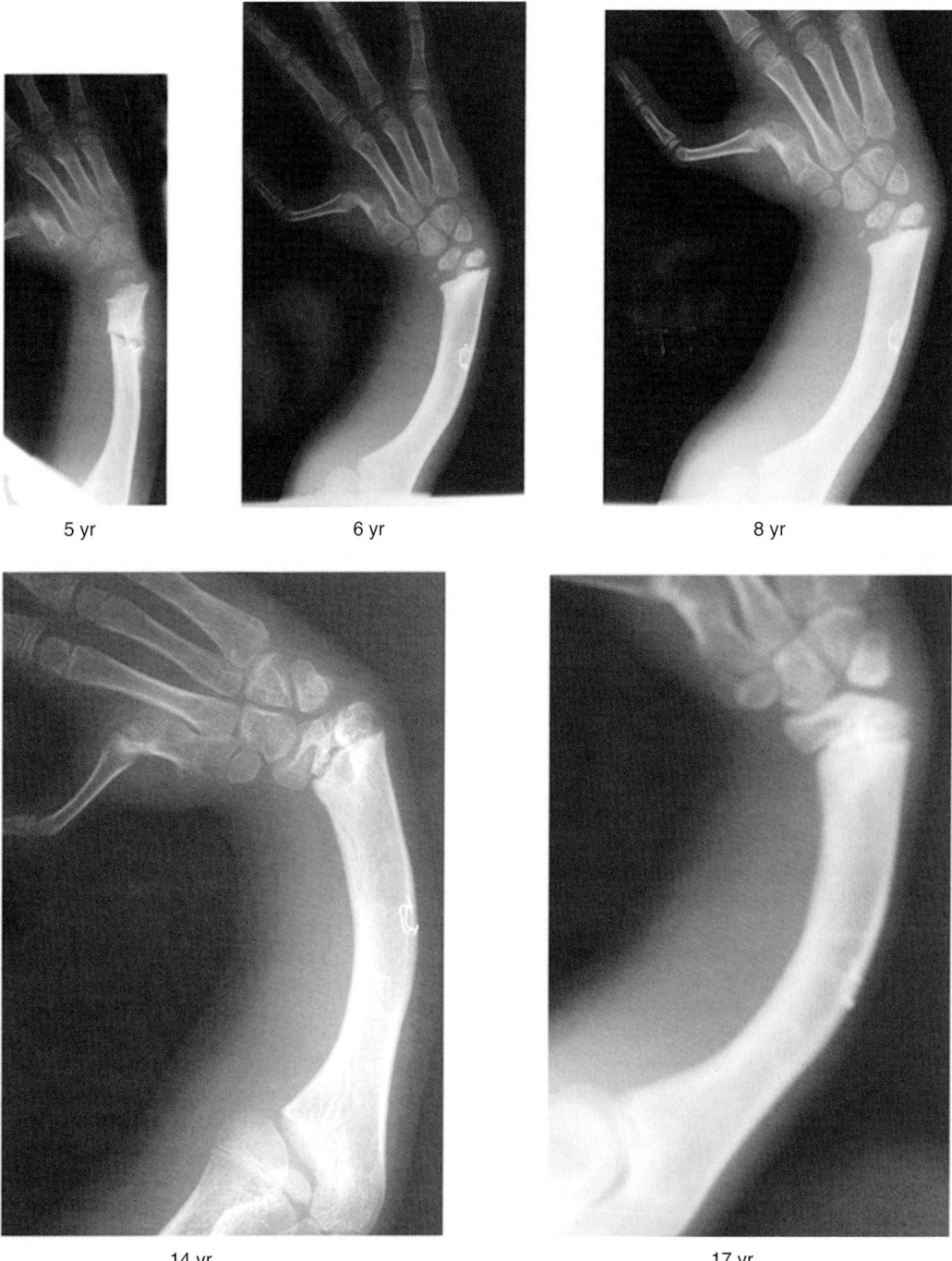

5 yr   6 yr   8 yr

14 yr   17 yr

FIGURE 203-8. Growth of the radial clubhand. Within the first year of life, this child, born with a complete agenesis of the radius, had a centralization of the hand and wrist over the distal ulna without carpal bone excisions. An index pollicization was completed on the same hand 1 year later. At the age of 5 years, 6 months, an osteotomy of the distal radius was performed to correct bowing and clubhand posturing. The interosseous wire that secures the closing wedge osteotomy can be used to document longitudinal growth of both proximal and distal portions of the ulna during a 12-year period. Note the persistent ulnar bowing that developed over time and the widening of the distal ulna, which looks more like a radius than an ulna at skeletal maturity. With time and growth, the hand has moved into more radial deviation with slight flexion. The muscle imbalance caused by the strong pull of the extrinsic flexors is responsible for the persistent distortion with growth. This marker demonstrates that the programmed growth at both ends of the radius has been deficient in comparison to the opposite, unaffected forearm, which was 16 cm longer at skeletal maturity.

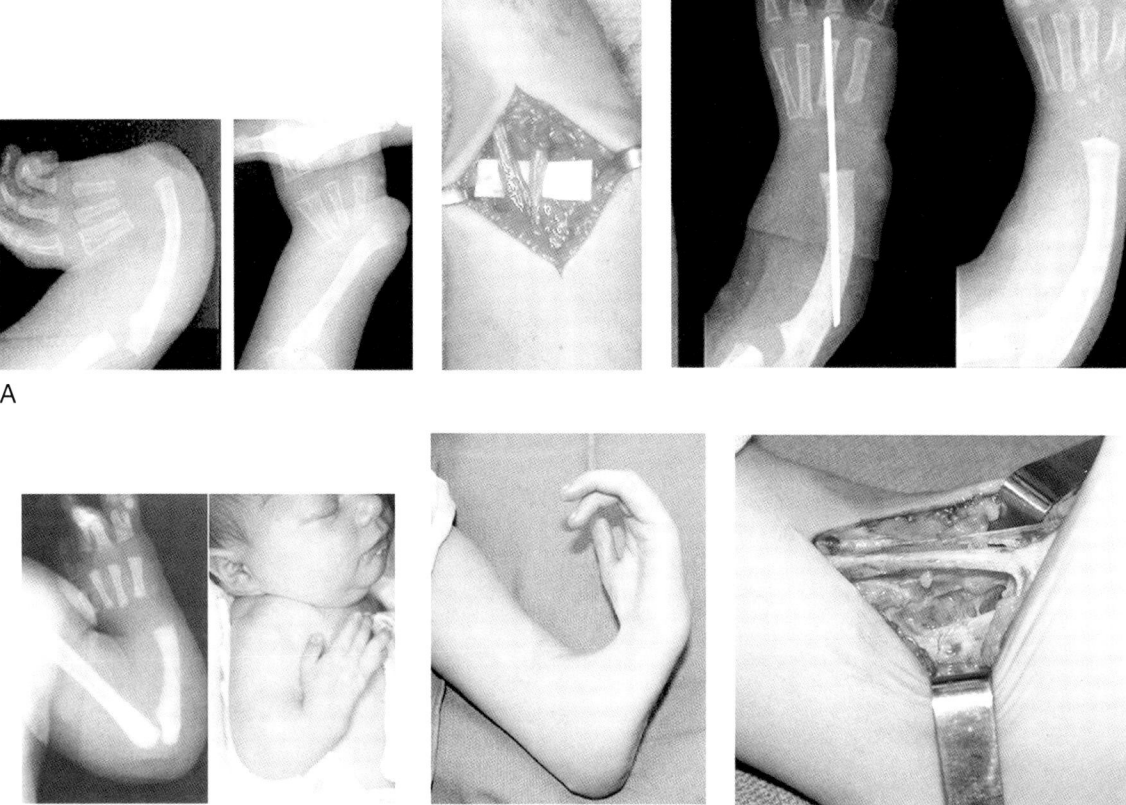

FIGURE 203-9. Centralization with anlage and radian nerve. *A,* This child born with complete absence of the radius (type IV) has an irreducible hand and carpus. Aggressive preoperative stretching and splinting were effective in correcting much of the deficit. At the time of centralization, the tightest structures were two portions of the median nerve seen in the radial position ("radian nerve"). The radiographs on the right show the position at the time of centralization and 1 year later. Note the early widening of the distal ulna, which has been stimulated by dynamic motion and compression forces at the radiocarpal joint. *B,* This child was diagnosed by ultrasound examination with a congenital absence of the radius. Although a segmented elbow joint was seen on radiography, she never gained any wrist motion and had a tight pterygium at the elbow level. At the time of Z-plasty and elbow manipulation later in childhood, a tight bowstringing median nerve was noted. All other tight soft tissue structures were released. Her hand function remains excellent.

presents the conflict between the need for cosmetic acceptance and the risk of functional loss. Until the last decade, some respected hand surgeons have seriously questioned the value of any surgery at all.[66,80,121] For select patients, no treatment may still be the best option. Type I patients with mild deformities, passively correctable wrists, and functional hands and thumbs may not require invasive therapy. Intervention also may not be indicated in babies with severe central nervous system retardation or life-threatening anomalies and a very short life span. Children with dysplastic shoulders, extended elbows with no flexor mechanism, and short arms and forearms should be carefully evaluated before any surgery because the native position of the hand, although abnormal, may be the most functional option for them. Adults with uncorrected radial clubhands, unfortunately, are rarely good candidates

for surgical intervention. Sadly, many are from rural areas where surgery for this anomaly was unavailable during their childhood—and ironically, many of them are parents of a child who has experienced a successful surgical outcome. However, these older patients do not benefit from later surgical intervention as much as young children do from procedures completed earlier in life. In addition, some may have psychiatric conditions triggered by a death, divorce, or other sudden life changes, which calls for a careful evaluation by an appropriately trained professional before surgery is undertaken.[122]

Timing

Ideally, all treatment starts in the newborn nursery with passive stretching and immobilization of the hand and carpus over the distal ulna. Surgical centraliza-

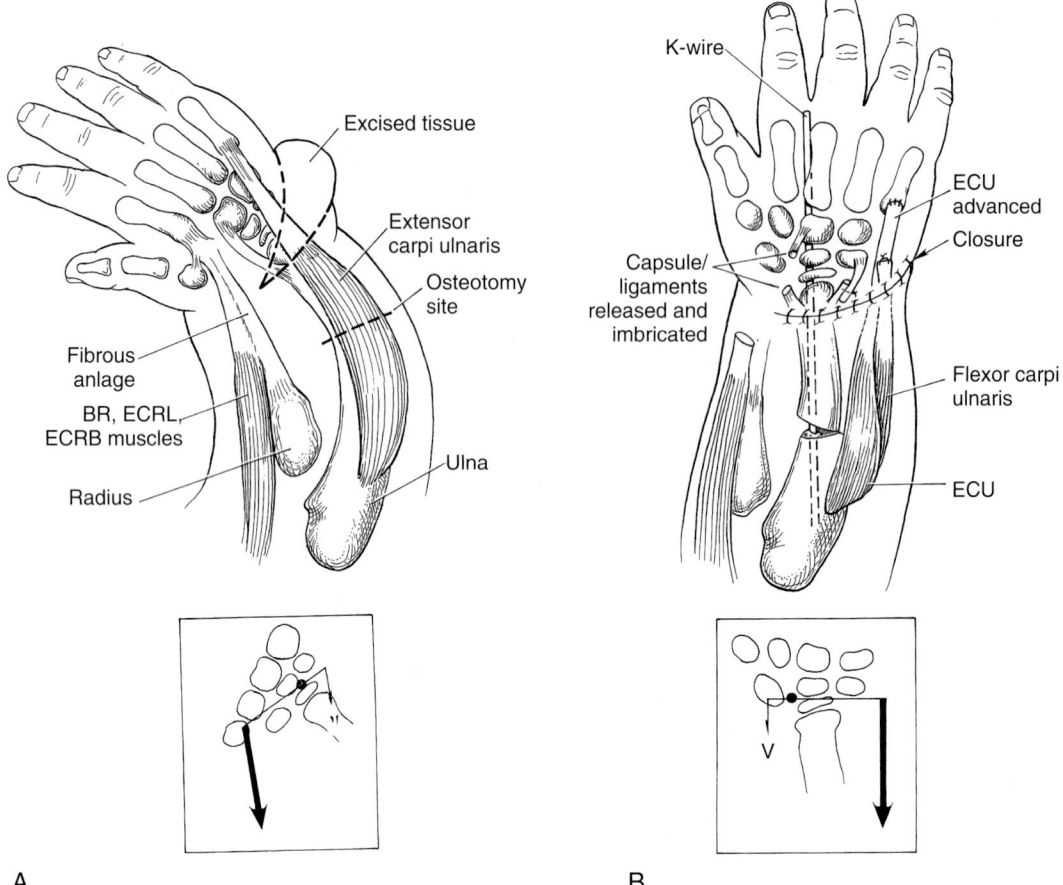

FIGURE 203-10. Centralization. *A,* Preoperative illustration of a type IV radial deficiency with clubbed hand and wrist posturing demonstrates the tight fibrous anlage or cord, which represents the radial wrist musculature that is not fully developed. With growth, ulnar bowing increases because of the inelastic quality of this cord. The preferred incision for centralization is outlined, and the osteotomy site for correction of the bowing is marked at the point of greatest bowing. The inset demonstrates the relative imbalance between the active flexor and extensor moment arms relative to the central axis of rotation of the wrist. *B,* During the centralization procedure, soft tissues released include the radial anlage (if present), dorsal muscle fascia, radial capsule, and ligaments. To rebalance the dynamic forces, the extensor carpi ulnaris is advanced and reinserted into the fifth metacarpal, and the flexor carpi ulnaris is transferred to the extensor carpi ulnaris to augment dorsiflexion and ulnar deviation of the wrist. When ulnar bowing is present, it is corrected with an opening wedge osteotomy held by the same intramedullary pin that holds the carpus and hand over the distal ulna. The inset illustrates the redistribution of forces with this exaggerated rebalancing. BR, brachioradialis muscle; ECRL, extensor carpi radialis longus muscle; ECRB, extensor carpi radialis brevis muscle; ECU, extensor carpi ulnaris muscle. (Illustration by Jean Biddl.)

tion should be completed between 6 and 12 months of life so the ambulatory child will have good wrist stability for both support and bimanual activities. Correction of deficient elbow flexion for those with more severe radial deficiencies must be considered within the first 2 years of life. Procedures for the hypoplastic or aplastic thumb should be completed by the time the child enters school at the age of 5 years.

Passive Stretching and Splinting

Reduction of the hand and carpus over the distal ulna with passive stretching is the cornerstone of initial treatment. This maneuver involves stretching of the hand and wrist out of the flexed and pronated position by application of axial traction. Serial casts or thin Aquaplast splints can aid in a remarkable correction if they are started early, but they should be considered of secondary importance to stretching and passive manipulation of the hand and wrist as well as of the elbow and shoulder in patients with type III and type IV deficiencies. If serial casts are used, they must extend proximal to the flexed elbow and be changed frequently. Passive splinting only helps maintain correction that has been achieved with stretching. In patients with the more severe type III and type IV deformities, preoperative distraction of the hand and carpus to the level of the distal ulna may facilitate centralization and obviate the need for carpectomy. Most experienced pediatric hand surgeons believe strongly that the most gains are achieved by the passive stretching by parents and therapists.

Some patients with clubbed hand posturing associated with type I or type II deformities will demonstrate excellent hand and thumb function in a splint. Although good candidates for surgical stabilization, they (or their parents) may elect treatment with an external splint indefinitely. Most of these children will come in as teenagers and request correction of the wrist and hand position.

Centralization and Radialization

Centralization can be delayed in passively correctable forearms, but it is usually completed within the first year of life and often by 6 months of age (see Figs. 203-9 and 203-10).

HISTORY. Centralization of the hand and wrist by replacement of the deficient radius with nonvascularized bone grafts, closing wedge osteotomies, or longitudinal splits of the ulna has a long and interesting history.[106,114,123-130] In Sayre's original centralization in 1893, an osteotomy was first made to correct the bowed ulna. Subsequently, the soft tissues were released and stretched with closed traction. Finally, during centralization, carpal bones were resected as needed to place the carpus over the shaved ulna.[128] Although these operations resulted in diminished growth and ultimate wrist fusion, many principles had been established: early stretching, correction of the bowed ulna, and avoidance of injury to intact nerves and tendons.

In the early years of centralization, various modified ulnar osteotomies were developed in an effort to provide a foundation for the wrist and hand. These involved multiple segmental osteotomies[124,128] or splitting of the ulna[130,131] and placement of the hand and wrist in between. Instead of disturbing the growth of the distal ulna, subsequent surgeons used the Y approach by inserting a fibular graft from the midshaft of the ulna to the radial side of the carpus.[106,114,123,129] In 1945, Starr proposed a three-stage approach: preoperative distraction to release soft tissues, ulnar osteotomy to correct bowing, and transfer of proximal fibula with intact epiphysis as a Y graft. However, it would take almost 50 years from Starr's innovation for someone to place a vascularized bone graft in this position.[132] Although many of the early transferred fibular grafts did not grow significantly,[114] centralization had become the procedure of choice by the 1970s.

Many modifications of centralization procedures have trimmed the distal end of the ulna without injuring the radius and have used partial carpectomies to receive the distal ulna, particularly when the hand and carpus could not be reduced over the distal ulna (Fig. 203-11).[67,80,105,133-136] Various modifications have emphasized the importance of soft tissue imbrication,[79] preservation of the ulnar growth plate,[80] preservation of motion with no carpal resection,[136] and tendon transfers.[79,80,134] Buck-Gramcko[115,137] also preserved motion and advocated "radialization" instead of centralization (Fig. 203-11C). His procedure places the hand and carpus ulnar to the distal ulna beneath the index metacarpal to produce a moderate overcorrection in position to decrease the chance of recurrent radial deviation. This forms a longer lever arm on the ulnar side and improves stability. At the same time, he transferred extrinsic motors to the dorsal and ulnar side of the wrist to counter the strong flexion and radial deviation caused by the extrinsic flexor forces (see Figs. 203-9 and 203-11).

Use of vascularized fibular grafts for centralization procedures has been promising to date, but it is still too soon to be assured of the long-term results. Such grafts are technically difficult because a separate pedicle to the proximal epiphysis of the fibula must be isolated and revascularized to ensure growth.[138,139] The new procedure by Vilkki,[132] in which the radius is replaced with a vascularized metatarsophalangeal joint with two intact growth plates, offers promising 10-year outcomes. There is no question that the technical advances of distraction lengthening and of microvascular transfer of vascularized bone or whole joint units have dramatically changed the treatment of difficult defects.

Arthrodesis of the wrist is usually reserved as a definitive posturing procedure after full growth has been achieved. The procedure should not be done in patients with bilateral deformities[80] or in patients with no elbow motion because of the resulting sacrifice of wrist motion.

TECHNIQUE. The goal of centralization is a stable wrist, centralized over the distal ulna with its motion preserved. Preoperative distraction may be employed for wrists that cannot be corrected passively (Figs. 203-12 and 203-13; see also Figs. 203-9 to 203-11).[117,140-142] The operation is performed under general anesthesia and with pneumatic tourniquet. A transverse incision is made over the distal ulna and carpus with an S-shaped extension into the dorsal and radial aspects of the forearm as needed. This extension is rarely necessary for visualization of the entire forearm. The flexor carpi ulnaris tendon and dorsal sensory branches of the ulnar nerve are identified and retracted. The extensor retinaculum is incised in an ulnar to radial direction after all extensor tendons, particularly the fourth dorsal compartment, have been identified. In most patients, the radial extrinsic flexors and extensors have

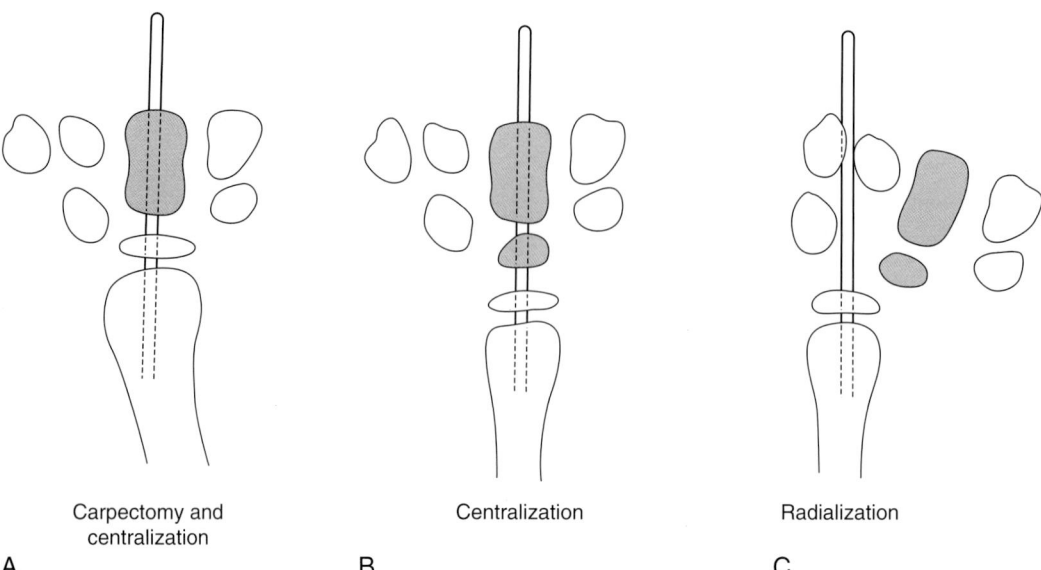

A   Carpectomy and
      centralization

B   Centralization

C   Radialization

FIGURE 203-11. Centralization and radialization. *A,* Initial procedures for centralization of a tight radial clubhand included judicious resection of carpals, usually the hypoplastic scaphoid and lunate, to make room for the ulnar head, which was carefully placed in this notch with its blood supply undamaged.[127,162] *B,* Subsequent modifications involved aggressive stretching and, in some cases, distraction lengthening to avoid carpal resections and to preserve motion.[117,118,136] The stippled capitate and lunate remained intact. *C,* A major modification in this technique was introduced by Buck-Gramcko,[159] who "radialized" the procedure by placing the ulna under the radial side of the wrist to counter the tendency of these hands to deviate again because of the strong flexion-pronation dynamic forces. (Illustration by Jean Biddl.)

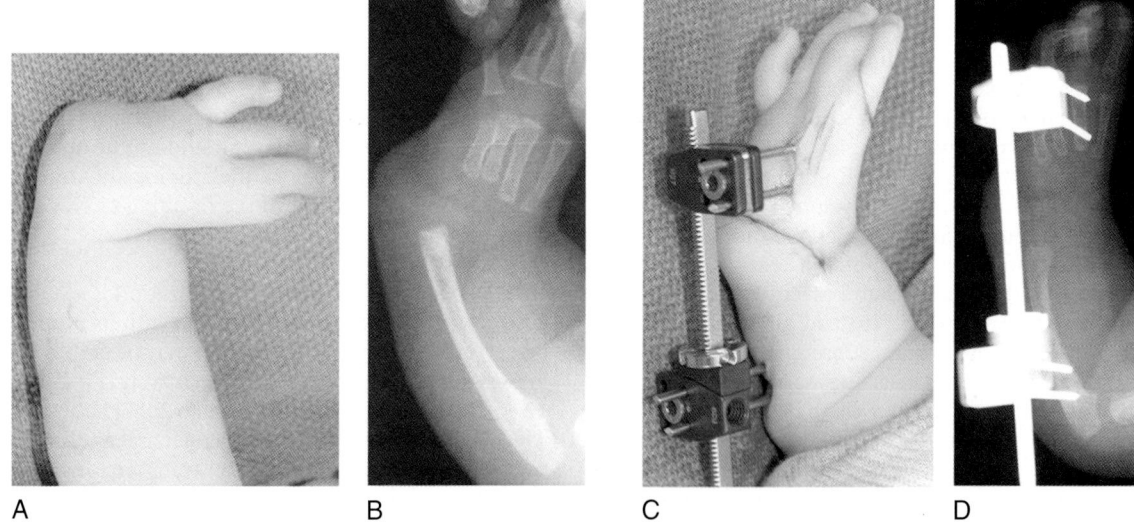

A   B   C   D

FIGURE 203-12. Preoperative distraction and radial dysplasia. *A to D,* Distraction lengthening has been useful in patients with partial or complete radial agenesis. At birth, the left hand and carpus of this child are dislocated relative to the distal ulna. Type IV arms are the most difficult to treat. The radiograph on the left is taken with maximal longitudinal traction on the hand after 6 weeks of aggressive stretching and splinting by the family and occupational therapists. In a separate surgical procedure before radialization, the tight radial soft tissues were released and a distraction apparatus was applied. Within 3 weeks, enough length was achieved to permit easy repositioning of the hand and wrist over the distal ulna.

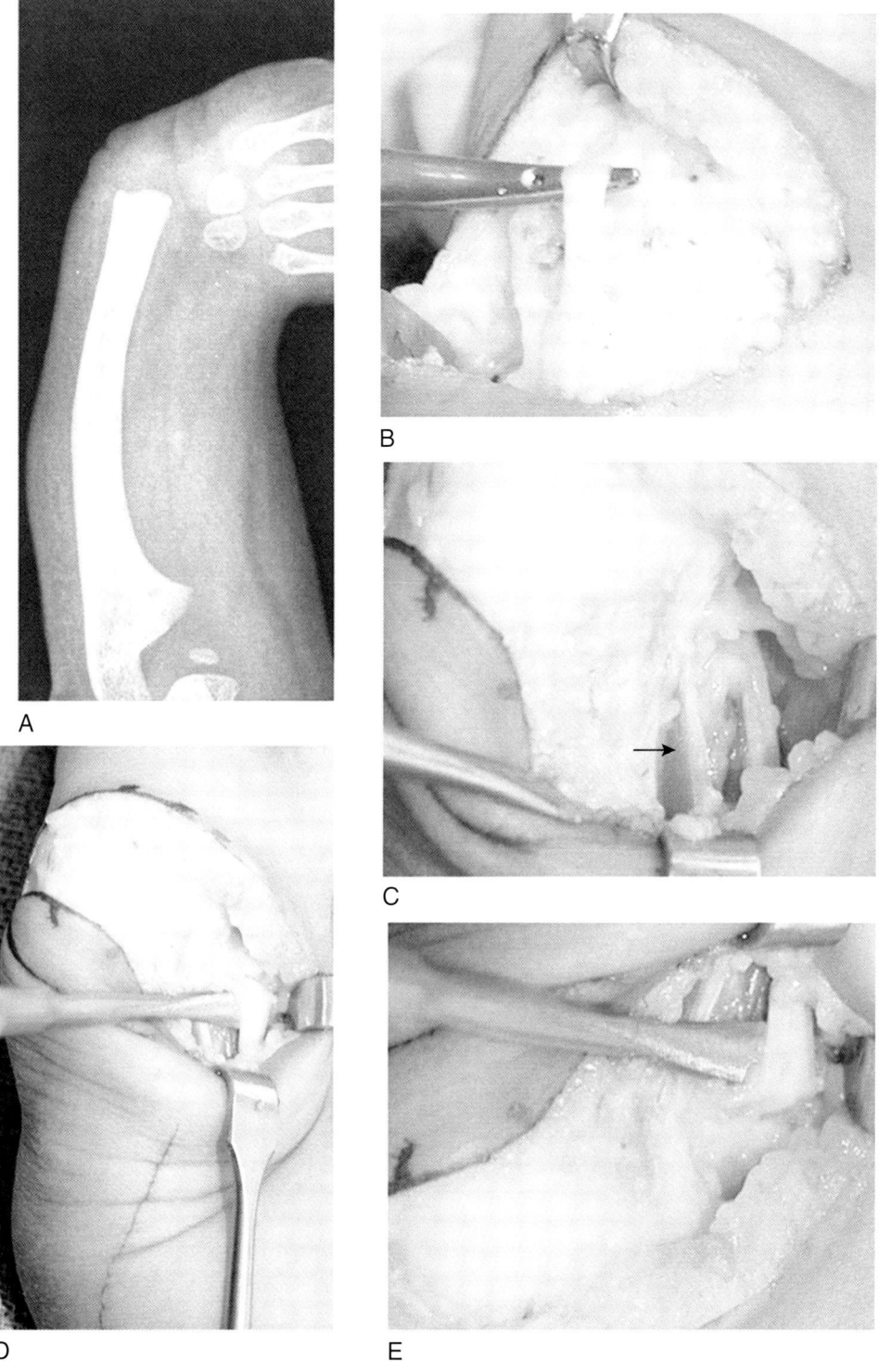

FIGURE 203-13. Centralization technique. *A,* A preoperative radiograph shows a radial clubbed hand and complete absence of the radius. *B,* The extensor carpi ulnaris is mobilized and isolated in the sixth dorsal compartment. *C,* With good retraction, easy exposure to the tight structures on the radial side of the wrist and forearm is gained through this dorsal incision. The arrow shows the radial muscle bellies after release of fibrous bands, muscle fascia, and fibrous anlage (if present). *D,* A nerve in this area is usually surrounded by fat and must be identified because it may be mistaken for a tendon. *E,* A closer view demonstrates the median nerve, which needs to be mobilized proximally. *Continued*

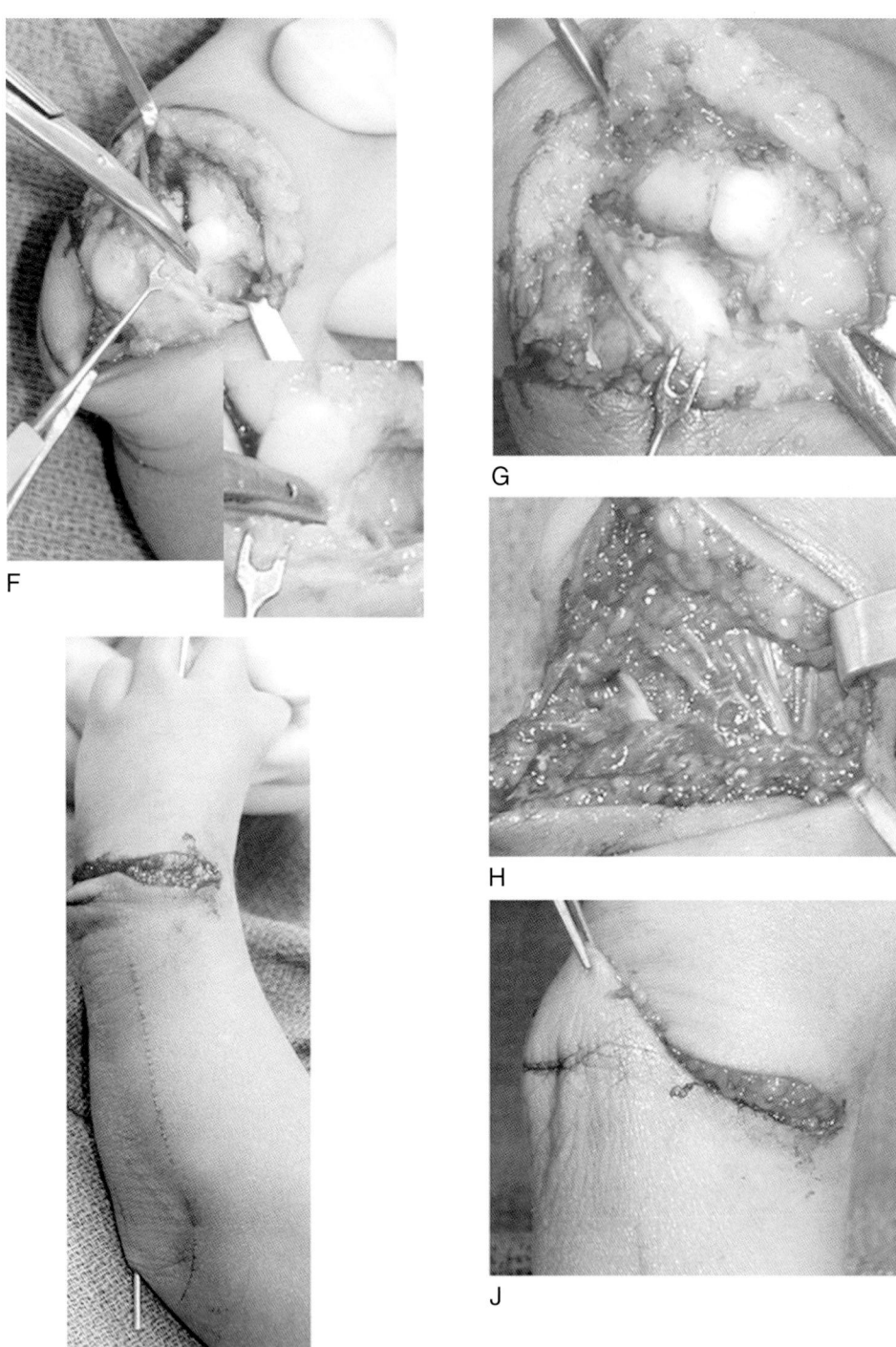

FIGURE 203-13, cont'd. *F,* The dorsal capsule is released as the small and fragile extensor tendons are carefully retracted. The inset shows the palmar and most radial capsule and ligaments, which are often the tightest of all the restricting soft tissue structures. Release often allows easy reduction of the hand and wrist over the distal ulna. *G,* Minimal shaving of the new articular surfaces may be necessary to achieve optimal contour. *H,* The extensor tendons in compartments 4 through 6 are seen after imbrication of the dorsal capsular structures. *I,* The hand and wrist are now in a well-centralized position. *J,* Excess skin may be trimmed and the incision closed with a careful subcuticular technique to avoid stitch marks. A bilobed flap may be used to transfer this excess tissue to the more deficient radial surface of the wrist.

a common muscle mass and need to be detached from the radial carpal bones. On occasion, separate tendons with metacarpal insertions are present. The distal ulna is exposed, and the interval between it and the carpus bones is located. The dorsal capsule and the second palmar joint capsule are incised transversely to mobilize the distal ulna, and the ulnar collateral ligament is preserved as a distally based capsular flap (see Figs. 203-9 to 203-13).

Fibrotic and contracted muscle or scar on the radial side may require release for mobilization of the carpus and hand. The tight muscle fascia within the entire forearm may require release. Although this can generally be accomplished through the dorsal incision, an additional incision over the forearm may be necessary for adequate visualization. A Z-plasty may be used for closure if length is needed.[79] Care should be taken to identify tendons, the median nerve, and medium-sized arteries before any structures are incised. If present, a tight fibrocartilaginous anlage should be excised; this is usually found in partial and complete radial absence deformities (types III and IV). Often what is called a type IV forearm with bowing is actually a type III deformity with a cartilaginous ulna connected to tight radial fibrous structures, which must be released. With mobilization of the joint capsule, the periosteum and blood supply to the growth plate of the distal ulna must not be injured. The median nerve, often in a radial position ("radian" nerve), becomes the most restrictive structure for mobilization of the radial side of the wrist. The hand is now ready for repositioning over the distal ulna.

CENTRALIZATION. In performing centralization (see Fig. 203-11),[80,107,127,136] the distal radius is exposed and shaved slightly to flatten its surface.[79,136] A Kirschner wire is then predrilled into the distal ulnar articular surface and passed down its shaft. A separate wire is then passed retrograde through the lunate and capitate and into the base of the third metacarpal. Lamb[80] chooses to prepare a notch for reception of the distal ulna with partial or complete excision of the lunate. The blood supply and soft tissues around the distal ulna are kept intact. The capitate and the metacarpal are then centered directly over the distal ulna, and the second pin is advanced in a retrograde fashion down the ulnar shaft. The hand and carpus are in neutral position between dorsiflexion and palmar flexion. Opening or closing wedge osteotomies may be performed to correct radial bowing of more than 30 degrees. Healing of these osteotomies is better if they are done in the distal third of the ulna. Radiographs are then obtained intraoperatively to confirm position.

RADIALIZATION. After aggressive mobilization of the hand and carpus with preservation of the ulnar

collateral ligament, in radialization (Fig. 203-14; see also Fig. 203-9),[143] the distal ulna is predrilled. The distal Kirschner wire is passed through the radial carpal bones and obliquely through the base of the second (index) metacarpal. After the articular surface of the ulna has been shaved to match the radial side of the carpus, the hand is positioned in an ulnar direction with the second (index) metacarpal and trapezium centered directly over the distal ulna. Wedge osteotomies may be incorporated within the distal third of the ulna to correct bowing.

In both centralization and radialization, the capsular structures are trimmed, and tight closure is performed with nonabsorbable sutures. Dynamic rebalancing is achieved by imbrication or advancement of the extensor carpi ulnaris, transfer of the flexor carpi ulnaris to become an extensor, and lengthening or tenotomy of well-formed radial tendons, if present. The flexor carpi radialis, extensor carpi radialis longus and brevis, and brachioradialis, often indistinguishable from one another, are transferred as a mass dorsally into the extensor carpi ulnaris insertion to become dorsiflexors and ulnar deviators.[143] Bora et al[144] have advocated use of some superficial flexors for the same purpose. Before transfers are made absolute, the muscle and tendon to be moved must be identified, as extrinsic flexors and extensors are often undifferentiated from one another. The dorsal retinaculum is then transposed between the extensor tendons and wrist capsule to prevent adhesions. Excess skin on the ulnar side of the hand is excised during closure with preservation of the dorsal sensory branch of the ulnar nerve. A well-padded long-arm cast extending well above the flexed elbow is applied. Active stretching of the fingers is initiated in the early postoperative period. The Kirschner wire is left in place for at least 8 weeks. After it is removed, active motion of the wrist is initiated.[79] Use of night splints that leave the fingers and elbows free is recommended until skeletal maturity has been reached.

The relative merits of centralization and radialization have been debated, but investigators seem to agree that radialization must be performed early in life to be effective and that centralization is an effective procedure in older children and adults. Ultimately, long-term follow-up studies will be necessary to determine the relative benefits and drawbacks of these two strategies.

Preoperative Distraction

In patients with severe "clubhand," even the most diligent stretching and splinting will not advance the hand and carpus to adequate length for a tension-free centralization or radialization. Distraction lengthening is an excellent technique and will reliably enable repositioning of the hand and wrist over the distal ulna much more easily (see Fig. 203-12).[141,142,145]

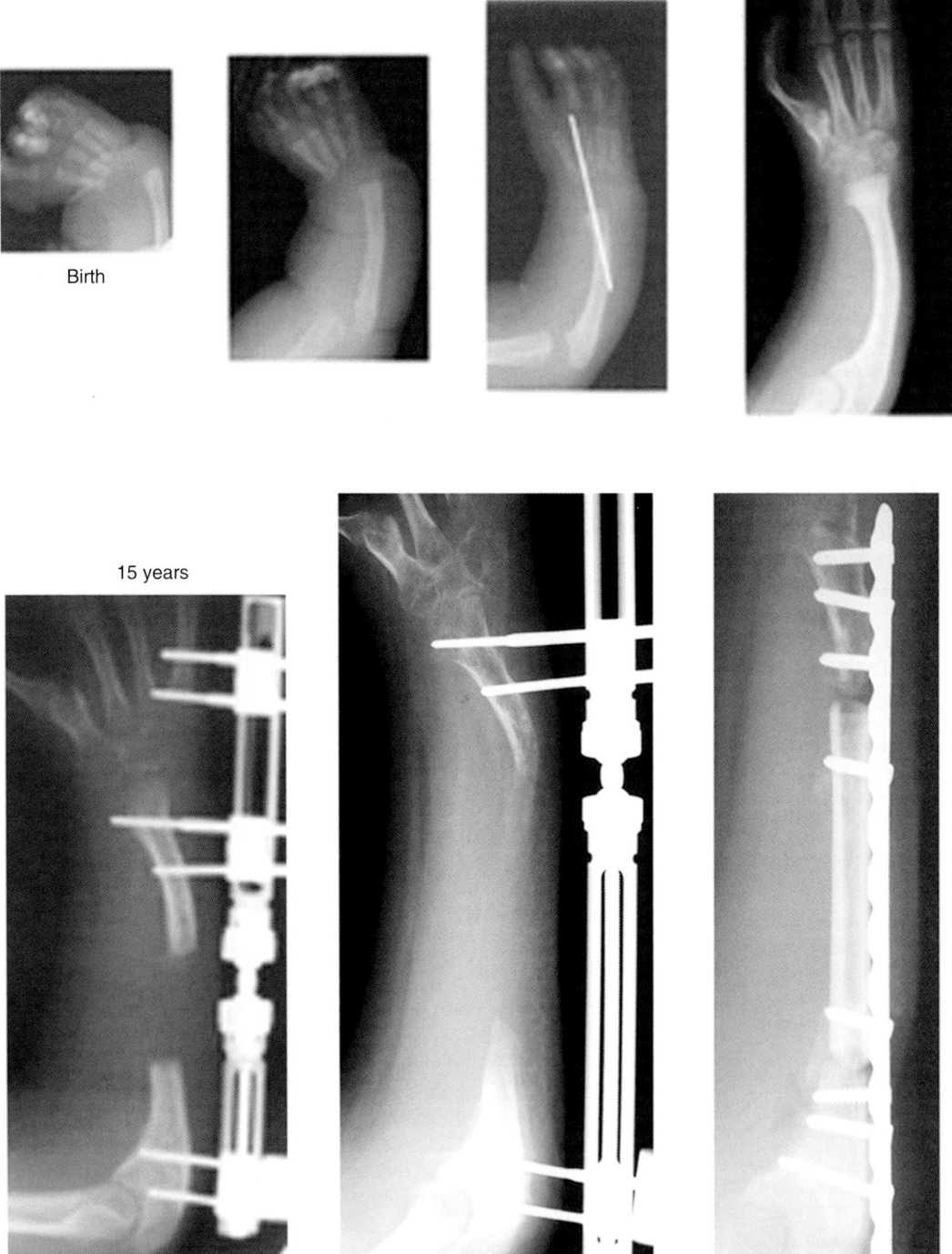

Birth

15 years

FIGURE 203-14. Radialization followed by distraction lengthening. *Above,* Serial radiographs of a child with a type IV radial deficiency demonstrate the characteristic pattern of development. After an aggressive stretching program, radialization without carpal resection was performed at 4 months of age. After 5 weeks, the longitudinal pin was removed and active motion started. Pollicization was completed at the age of 18 months. Radialization and the tendon rebalancing prevented recurrent radial deviation with growth, and the distal ulna widened so much that it resembled a radius more than an ulna. *Below,* As a teenager, he requested distraction lengthening of his short forearm. Distraction with a uniplanar device produced a 95-mm gap during 12 weeks. The intercalated gap was then filled with a demineralized cadaveric bone graft secured with a plate and screws. Of note, with slow distraction, his forearm flexors and extensors were not weakened.

Distraction is routinely accomplished as a separate procedure 3 to 4 weeks before radialization. Within the first few months of life, the soft tissues are supple and stretch easily. At the time of placement of the distraction apparatus, a dorsal incision is made and the tight structures on the radial side of the wrist and forearm are released. The fibrous anlage, if present, is excised, and fasciotomies are completed as needed over the forearm musculature. Many different distraction devices are available as necessary. The preferred device enables the anchoring of pins in the most stable skeletal elements, both proximal and distal to the gap, to be lengthened (see Figs. 203-12 and 203-14).

Muscle and Tendon Transfers

Reorientation of the skeletal structure alone is usually insufficient to achieve dynamic stability of the wrist. Tendon and muscle transfers are often preferred as components of the centralization or radialization procedure with different motors, depending on the severity of the forearm (and arm) deficiency. The extensor carpi ulnaris is most commonly used because it is always present and strong.[67,115,118,127,146] After skeletal realignment, the extensor carpi ulnaris is readvanced and sutured to the dorsal base of the fifth metacarpal to improve dorsiflexion and ulnar deviation of the centralized wrist and hand (see Fig. 203-10). The flexor carpi ulnaris can be transferred dorsally to augment this transfer.[115] The radial wrist flexor may be used if an adequate muscle-tendon unit is present.[80,147] This transfer is not possible in most type III and type IV deficiencies, in which these musculotendinous units are fibrotic and have no passive excursion, if they are present at all. The ring and long finger flexor digitorum superficialis muscles may be transferred either primarily or secondarily[134,144] to decrease flexor power and to augment dorsiflexion of the wrist. Some surgeons have advanced the abductor digiti minimi from the pisiform to the ulna to improve ulnar deviation.[67,134] The major problem with this simple transfer is excessive stretch of the neurovascular bundle supplying the hypothenar muscles.

With severe type IV and some type III deficiencies, elbow flexion may be weak or absent. Because elbow motion can severely affect the functional outcome of a centralization or radialization procedure, it is often beneficial to provide flexion to the elbow with a muscle transfer. Simple release of the posterior capsule and triceps tendon will allow elbow flexion by gravity.[148,149] Of the three available muscle transfers—triceps, pectoralis major, and latissimus dorsi—the most physiologic has proved to be the pectoralis transfer of the sternocostal portion of the pectoralis major muscle.[150] This transfer should be performed during the first 3 years of life once passive flexion of the joint reaches 90 degrees (Fig. 203-15).

Straightening of Ulnar Bowing

The ulna can be straightened with a single or multiple closing wedge osteotomies at the time of centralization.[7,67,80,85,118,121,151] It is generally recommended that the ulna be straightened before placement of the wrist and carpus, although these osteotomies can be performed later.[113,152] With either approach, the length of the forearm is not increased (see Fig. 203-9).[153] The short forearm can be lengthened with distraction later in life (Fig. 203-16; see also Fig. 203-14) and should not be lengthened at the time of centralization. It is preferable to perform an opening wedge osteotomy of the ulna at the point where the intramedullary pin breaks the posterior cortical surface of the ulna during the centralization-radialization procedure. A small separate incision is made to guide the pin into the proximal portion of the ulna.

Ulnar Lengthening

During the past 2 decades, distraction, by a variety of external fixation approaches, has been used to lengthen the ulna in type II, type III, and type IV forearms as a secondary procedure.[154,155] Distraction is also used to stretch the hand and carpus out to the length of the distal ulna before centralization or radialization in the most severe radial clubbed hands.[43,85,142,145] Ulnar lengthening is an effective procedure and can be repeated several times without significant morbidity, but it should not be performed at the time of centralization (see Figs. 203-14 and 203-16). The complications in young children are proportional to the duration of time the external fixation apparatus is left in place. Most patients and their families prefer to go through this process only once. Thus, it is preferable to wait until the adolescent growth spurt to perform the definitive lengthening procedure. Many external fixation apparatuses have been used for this process.[85,140,142,145,156]

Microvascular Transfer

Large intercalated gaps (more than 2 to 3 inches) formed during distraction lengthening are best filled with vascularized bone transfers and internal fixation. As discussed earlier, the fibula has been the most versatile donor. Smaller gaps do not require vascularized bone.

Vilkki[132] has stabilized the severe radial clubhand with a two-stage reconstruction: (1) distraction of the hand and wrist, followed by (2) vascularized transfer of the metatarsophalangeal joint of a second toe between the ulna and the radial side of the wrist and hand (Fig. 203-17). The growth of the toe ray parallels that of the distal ulna. Outcomes at 5 years have been encouraging; children undergoing this procedure have maintained their motion and have not experienced redeviation.

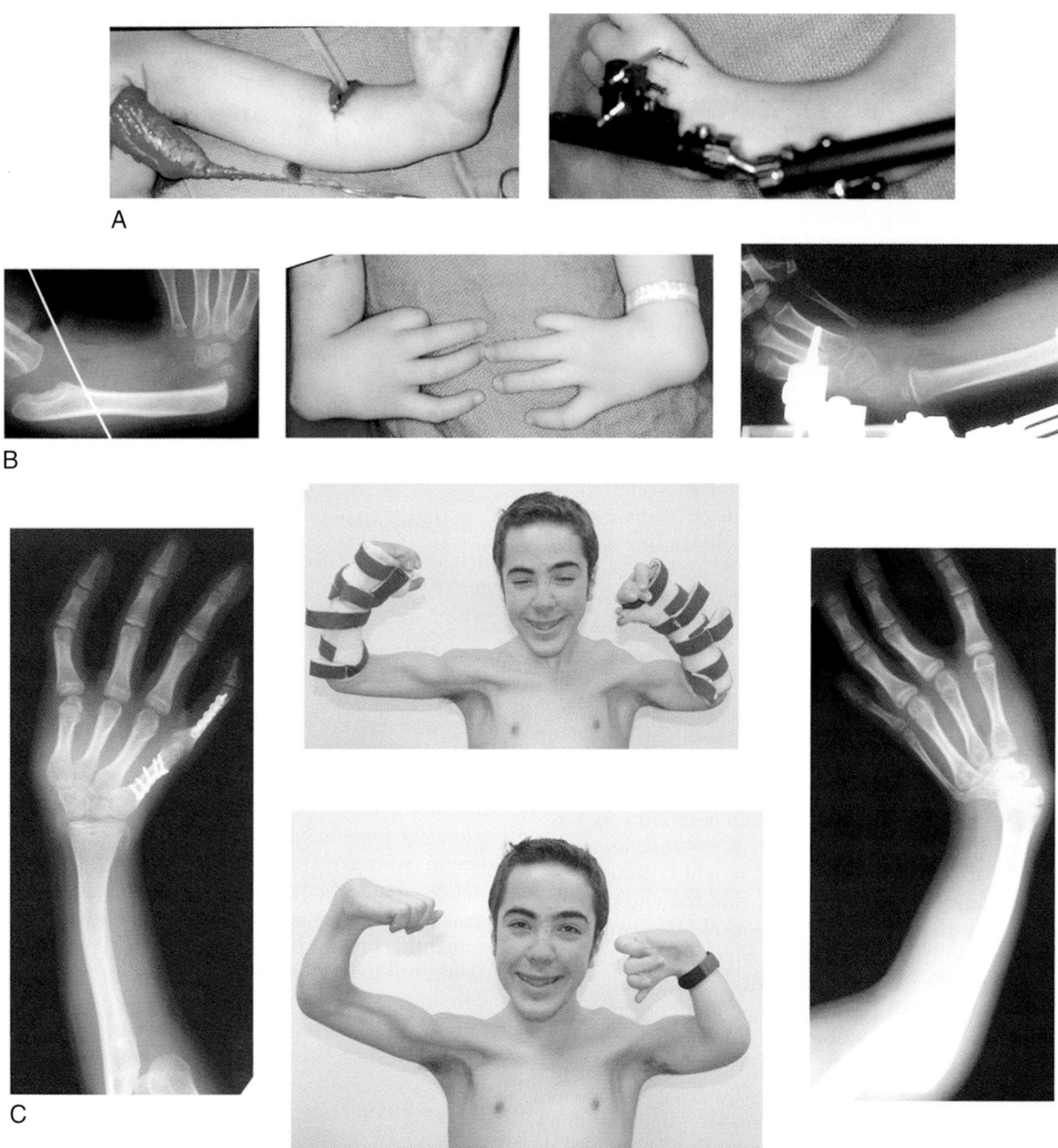

FIGURE 203-15. Pectoralis muscle transfer for elbow flexion. *A,* This child with bilateral type IV radial deficiencies presented late at 5 years of age with severe clubbed hand posturing, lack of elbow flexion, and severely limited function. No surgical correction had been attempted. Before the position of the wrists and hands in these short arms and forearms could be determined, elbow flexion was restored in a two-stage procedure: (1) posterior release and triceps lengthening, followed by (2) transfer of the sternocostal portion of the pectoralis major muscle. *B,* Once powerful flexion was established on both sides, the hand and wrist position was corrected with another two-stage procedure: (1) distraction, followed by (2) centralization at 7 years of age. The distractions were slow and difficult, and the wrist was kept in slight radial deviation because of the short forearms. *C,* The flexed and immobile index rays were repositioned with a combination of MP arthrodeses and metacarpal rotation-recession osteotomies.[32] Over the years, he had gradually built up both the bulk and strength of the transferred muscles.

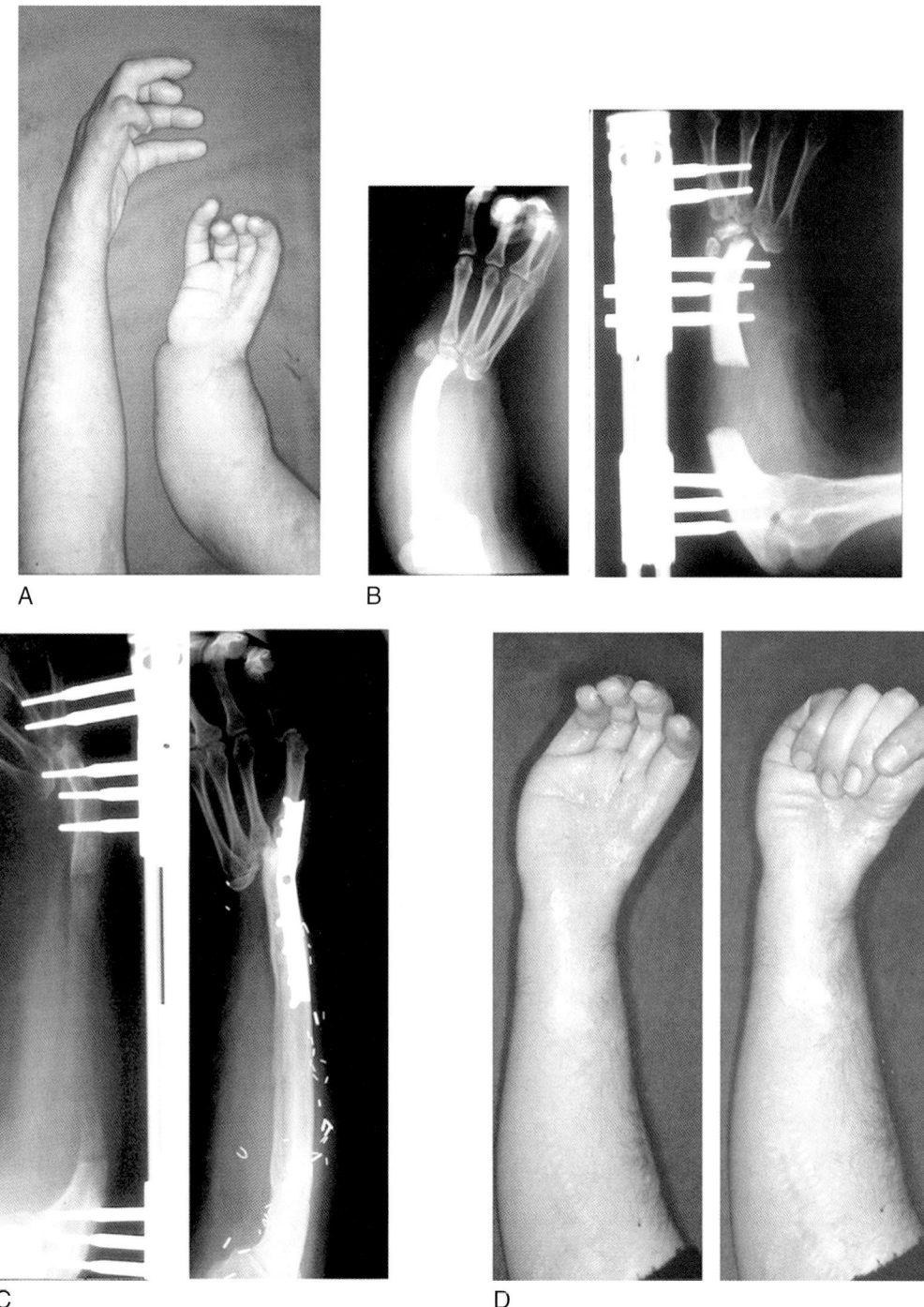

FIGURE 203-16. Ulnar distraction lengthening. *A,* This adult man presented with bilateral radial deficiencies, which consisted of a normal forearm and type IIIA flexed and immobile thumb on the left and a short forearm, complete radial absence, and type V (absence) thumb deficiency on the right. The length discrepancy was marked, and his primary objective was increased length. *B,* The preoperative radiograph shows a short ulna and a centralized wrist, which was accomplished many years earlier with carpectomies. The hand is also held with the apparatus to prevent flexion and radial deviation with gradual lengthening. *C,* During an 8-month period, a 178-mm gap (7 inches) was produced and filled with a vascularized fibular transfer. *D,* Despite the extent of this lengthening, his forearm flexors and extensors were maintained with daily exercising and nighttime splinting.

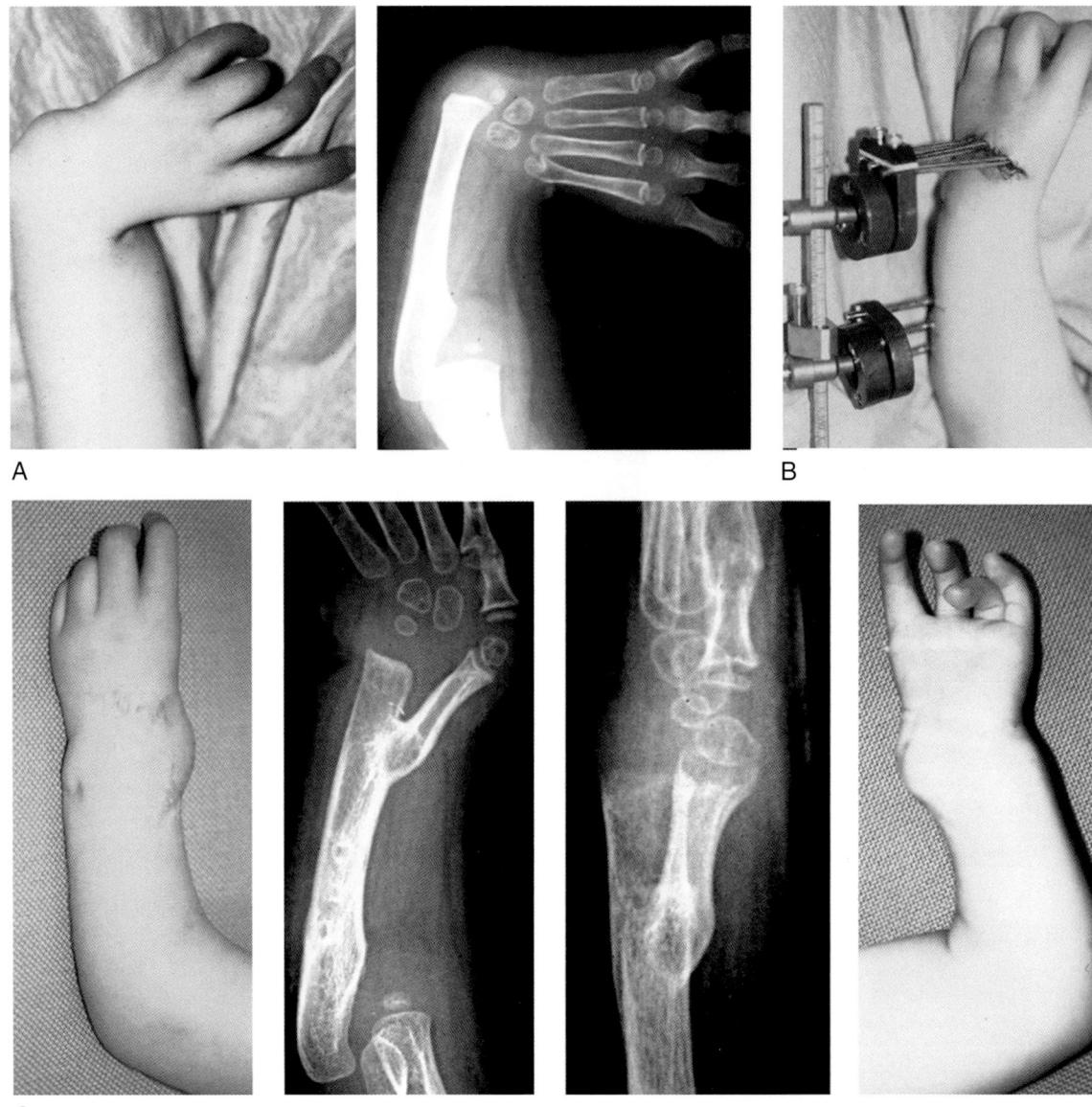

A

B

C

FIGURE 203-17. Vilkki procedure.[132] *A,* The clinical appearance and radiograph of a 4-year-old child with congenital absence of the radius and severe clubbed hand posturing. *B,* In the first-stage procedure, the hand and wrist were advanced beyond the level of the distal ulna. *C,* The second ray of one foot with an intact MP joint and dorsal vascularized tissue was transferred to the hand, with the metatarsal fused to the radial cortex of the distal ulna and the toe proximal phalanx placed beneath the index metacarpal. Five years postoperatively, both position and motion were maintained, and the growth of the toe ray paralleled that of the radius. (Courtesy of Simo Vilkki, MD.)

COMPLICATIONS

Recurrence of deformity is a common long-term problem after centralization procedures, short of an arthrodesis (Fig. 203-18).[157] In a study group of 15 surgeons who had collectively performed more than 700 procedures for radial clubhand, it was determined that severe deformities recur after soft tissue procedures. This problem may be due to poor pin fixation,

inadequate tendon balance, tight soft tissues, pin fractures, or progressive bowing of the ulna with growth. Ulnar bowing with growth can result from damage to one side of the ulnar epiphysis, excessive pull of radial muscles, or internal growth deficiency within the ulna. Patients who do not wear night splints or perform the prescribed exercises will achieve poor correction. However, the major cause of recurrence is growth and the predominant imbalance between the stronger

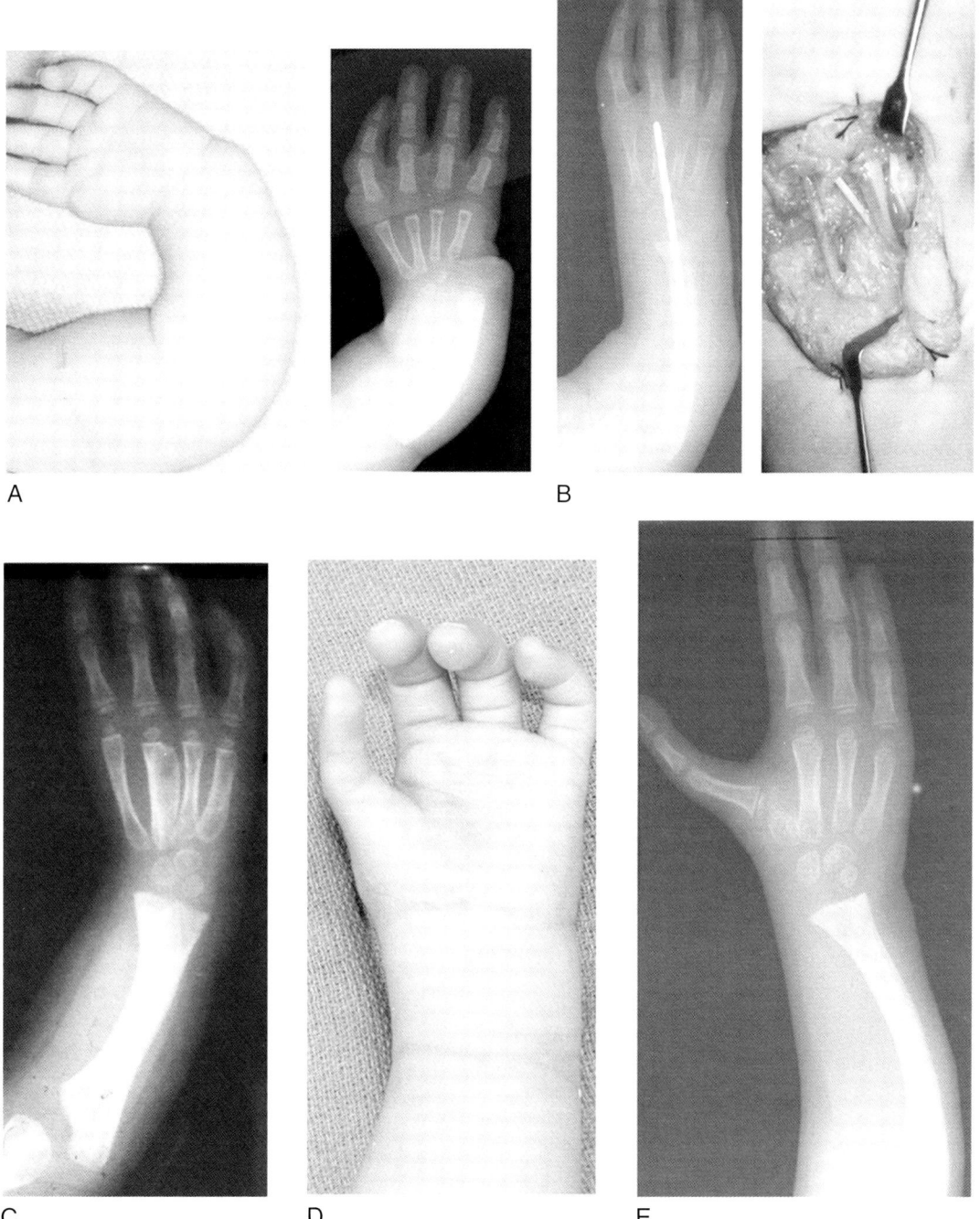

A   B

C   D   E

FIGURE 203-18. Outcome of centralization and pollicization. *A,* This child with a type IV radial deficiency was treated with a stretching and night splinting program 29 years ago. *B,* A standard centralization was performed at 5 months of age. The large pin was removed 6 months later. The extensor muscle-tendon units are seen in their centralized position. *C,* With wrist motion and dynamic compression, the distal ulna rapidly widened. Note the hypertrophy of the long metacarpal caused by the Steinmann pin. *D,* An index pollicization was performed at the age of 2 years. Because the preoperative motion of this digit was diminished in all three joints, the position of the new thumb is in less abduction than normal. His postoperative motion was also diminished. *E,* Within a year, the third metacarpals remodeled. The left hand remained in a centralized position. On the opposite upper limb, his radius was normal, and a type IIIA hypoplastic thumb reconstruction was performed. In college, he excelled in athletics as a midfielder on the varsity lacrosse team.

flexor forces of the forearm muscles. Repeated centralization with correction of deforming forces is indicated when recurrence affects function.

OUTCOMES

The natural history of untreated limbs has been well documented by Heikel[100] and later by his student Vilkki[132] in Finland (see Fig. 203-8). Most authors agree that the appearance of the extremity is improved with surgery, but outcomes of surgery for radial anomalies vary according to the severity of the malformation. There are few quantitative outcome measurements of this diverse group of patients. Radial deviation is one functional and aesthetic measure that can be assessed reliably. Lamb[80] reported an improvement of radial deviation from 78 degrees preoperatively to 22 degrees postoperatively. Manske[102,146] has emphasized that the position and stability of the wrist and hand are most important and has further defined the proper hand-forearm angle and the hand-forearm position. Radiographic assessment of a series of 29 limbs was subjected to a "survivorship analysis," and it was demonstrated that the recurrence rate of radial deviation and the need for revision were decreased when the ulna was straight and the hand and carpus were in an ulnar position relative to the distal ulna.[158] Ulnar osteotomy was found to be beneficial for correction of the bowed ulna. The major problem with this type of outcome analysis, which has become popular for total joint assessment, is the definition of failure, which is considered a revisionary procedure. This study and others have supported the concept of radialization.[159] Recurrence of radial deviation is common with growth in children with severe type III and type IV deficiencies, especially those in whom pre-radialization or modified centralization distraction was used. In these patients, the unstable platform provided by the distal ulna, which has not widened, and the strong flexor forces conspire to persistently pull the hand into a flexed and radially deviated posture (Fig. 203-19).

Wrist motion and digital function are also important outcome measures after centralization and radialization procedures. Wrist motion is in the range of 30 to 40 degrees in most patients with type III and type IV defects. With functional use and growth, the distal ulna broadens and becomes less bowed if it supports a well-balanced hand and wrist. The most predictable results are obtained in young patients (younger than 3 years) with ulnar bowing of less than 30 degrees and no significant preoperative soft tissue tightness. After radialization, wrist motion is reported to range between 40 and 90 degrees of flexion.[115] Although it is difficult to quantify digital function with radialization and centralization other than by assessment of motion, one report shows that digital function is improved to 27% of normal. Moreover, there is a pre-dictable improvement of grip strength from the ulnar three digits of the hand with centralization and stabilization of the wrist and hand.[80,115,160] Lamb has emphasized that improvement in motion, stability, and appearance are particularly dramatic in patients with bilateral deformities, although some surgeons discourage surgical centralization in children with bilateral malformations, relying instead on the adaptive capacities of each individual child.[161,162]

The potential loss of ulnar length after centralization has been debated. A detailed study of untreated patients in Iceland[100,163] demonstrated a marked deficiency of ulnar growth with both moderate and severe deficiencies. Hippe[164] reported a decreased growth of the distal ulna after centralization. Others think that with careful surgery performed before 8 years of age, ulnar growth is not disturbed.[80,144] As experience with distraction techniques increases, potential loss of ulnar length should no longer be an issue.

Central Deficiencies (Typical Cleft Hand)

Central deficiency comprises a range of deformities in which the central portion of the hand is missing. These are congenital hand malformations, characterized by a bizarre and remarkable function. The nosologies and classifications used are perhaps as confusing as any category of congenital hand differences. Communication within the hand literature is complicated by the potpourri of terms that have been used to describe these unusual hands, including ectrodactyly,[165] the offensive lobster claw hand[143] and crab claw hand,[166] median hypoplasia,[167] split hand complex,[168] split hand-foot complex,[169] syndactyly-cleft hand complex,[170,171] and typical and atypical cleft hand.[172,173] In current literature and practice, cleft hand is the most widely accepted term. A clear distinction has been made between the typical cleft hand and symbrachydactyly (Table 203-3). Although the morphologic appearance of different anomalies is often similar, the pathogenesis may be different.

CLASSIFICATION

A typical or true cleft hand has a V-shaped central cleft, is often associated with syndactyly or other deformities of digits adjacent to the cleft, and may be unilateral or bilateral. In Sandzen's early classification,[174] typical cleft hands constituted categories I and III. Category II hands, according to Sandzen's system, are those with symbrachydactyly. In contrast to typical cleft hands, those with symbrachysyndactyly have a U-shaped cleft, are unilateral and sporadic, and often have rudimentary nubbins in the place of digits. Much confusion was perpetuated by a German classification[175] that divided these hands into three groups: cleft with

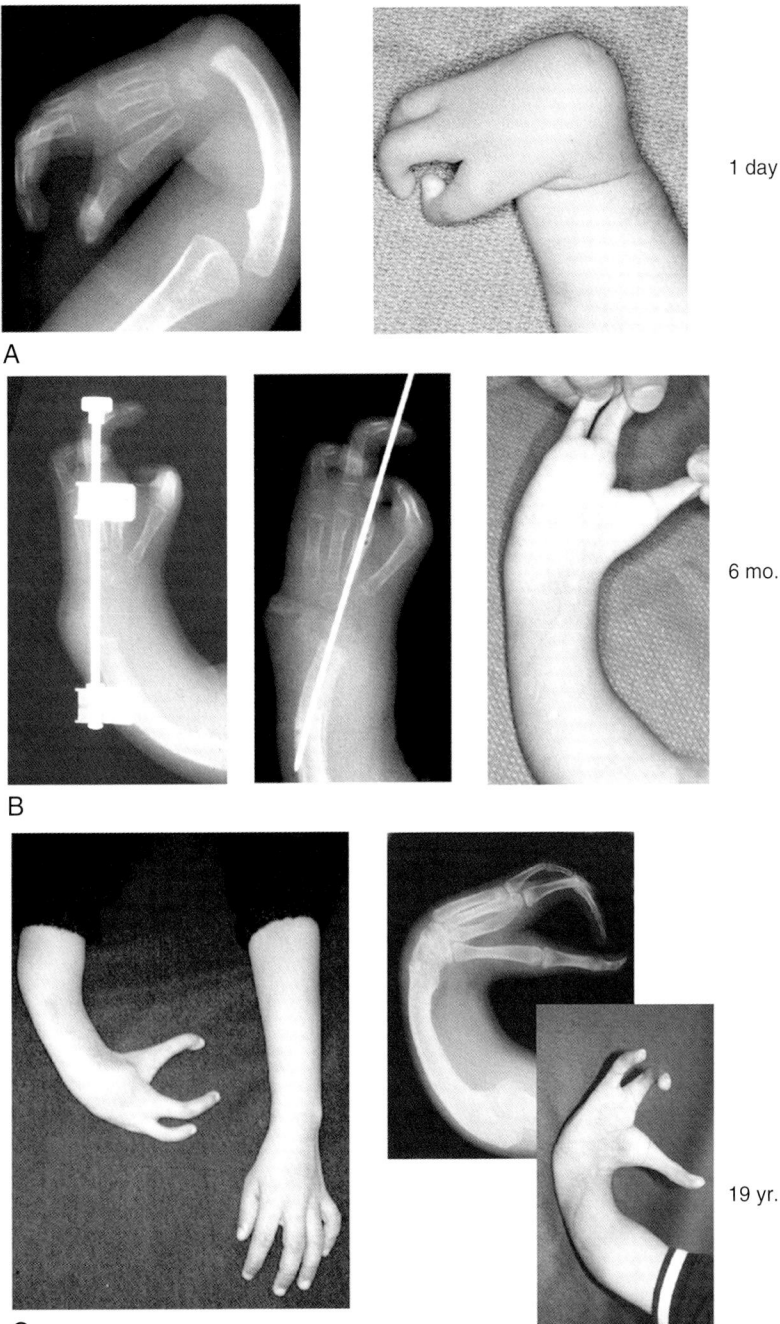

FIGURE 203-19. Outcomes of severe type IV deficiency. *A,* This child with the VACTERL association was born with multiple life-threatening malformations of the pulmonary, gastrointestinal, and genitourinary systems. *B,* At 1 day of age, a distractor was placed on the affected forearm and hand. Three weeks later, the pins were removed and a centralization was performed. The correction was held with night splints and stretching as he grew. *C,* No further surgery was recommended on the three-digit hand, which he learned to use effectively. There was marked length discrepancy between the forearms. The position of the hand is seen when he is about to enter college. The type IIIA left thumb was constructed with a first web space release, abductor digiti minimi transfer (Huber transfer), and collateral ligament constructions on both sides of the MP joint. He has become an accomplished violinist who uses the right hand for his bow.

TABLE 203-3 ✦ COMPARISON OF TYPICAL AND ATYPICAL CLEFT HAND

Characteristic	Symbrachydactyly	Typical Cleft
Origin	Sporadic, unknown	Positive hereditary
Hand involved	Unilateral	Often bilateral
Feet involved	No	Usually bilateral
Shape of defect	U shaped	V shaped
Depth of cleft	Shallow	Deep, metacarpal
Rays involved	Usually all digits	Few
Thumb involved	Rarely	Usually
Chest wall involved	Often involved	No
Lip, palate involved	No	Frequently cleft
Bones in digits	Short, hypoplastic small nails	Larger, transverse phalanges

aplasia, cleft with synostosis, and cleft with aplasia and synostosis. During the next 2 decades, a number of refined classifications and subclassifications were developed. The most detailed was proposed by Ogino,[64] who included the association of a cleft, syndactyly, and polydactyly. The fusion of osseous elements is graded according to the level of fusion: S-0, no fusion; S-1, distal phalanx; S-2, middle phalanx; S-3, proximal phalanx; and S-4, metacarpal. Similarly, the degree of polydactyly is designated by level: P-0, none; P-1, distal phalanx; P-2, middle phalanx; P-3, proximal phalanx; and P-4, metacarpal. Although it is possible to have a minimal cleft without any skeletal abnormalities,[176] the most common forms involve varying degree of hypoplasia or absence of the third (long) digit, with or without both polydactyly and syndactyly on either side of the cleft. Clefting between the ring and fifth rays is much less common[177,178] and in this author's experience is primarily seen in the ectodermal dysplasia syndromes.

Manske[179] has proposed a morphologic classification based on the condition of the first web space (Table 203-4). Manske's system accounts for the fact that in more extensive clefts, the central deficit may actually merge with the first web space or involve the thumb, which typically appears as a hand with no radial structures and, in patients with extreme defects, as a hand with no radial digits including the thumb (Fig. 203-20). This system is clinically relevant because it directly relates to both function and the indications for surgery. This system has been modified by subdivision of class V into type A, partial radial structure suppression, and type B, which designates complete suppression of the radial ray.

INCIDENCE

The incidence of typical cleft hand probably ranges somewhere between 1 in 100,000 and 4 in 100,000 live births.[180-183] Typical cleft hand is the fifth most common type of congenital hand difference in a large registry from Japan.[171] Prevalence data are difficult to interpret

because symbrachydactylies may have been included in some analyses and because of the variable phenotypic expression of this condition.[184]

When presenting as bilateral hand and foot clefts, the condition is typically inherited in an autosomal dominant pattern. The genetic defect responsible in patients with bilateral defects has a variable expressivity and penetrance such that morphologic features of the malformation may vary from one hand to the other and between affected individuals within the same pedigree. Syndromes with cleft hands include ectrodactyly-ectodermal dysplasia-clefting (EEC), unusual forms of ectodermal dysplasia (Goltz syndrome),[185] and rare syndromes in which cleft hands are associated with deafness and ocular abnormalities.

PATHOGENESIS

As the relationship between the apical ectodermal ridge and the underlying mesoderm was demonstrated by embryologists, several theories concerning cleft hand

TABLE 203-4 ✦ MANSKE'S CLASSIFICATION OF THE CLEFT HAND

Type	Description	Characteristics
I	Normal web	Normal first web space
IIA	Mildly narrowed	Mildly narrowed first web space
IIB	Severely narrowed	Severely narrowed first web space
III	Syndactylized	No web, thumb-index syndactyly
IV	Merged web space	Index suppressed, first web space merged with cleft
V	Absent	Thumb and web suppressed, ulnar rays only remain

From Manske P, Halikis MN: Surgical classification of central deficiency according to the thumb web. J Hand Surg Am 1995;20:687-697. Copyright 1995, with permission from The American Academy of Dermatology, Inc.

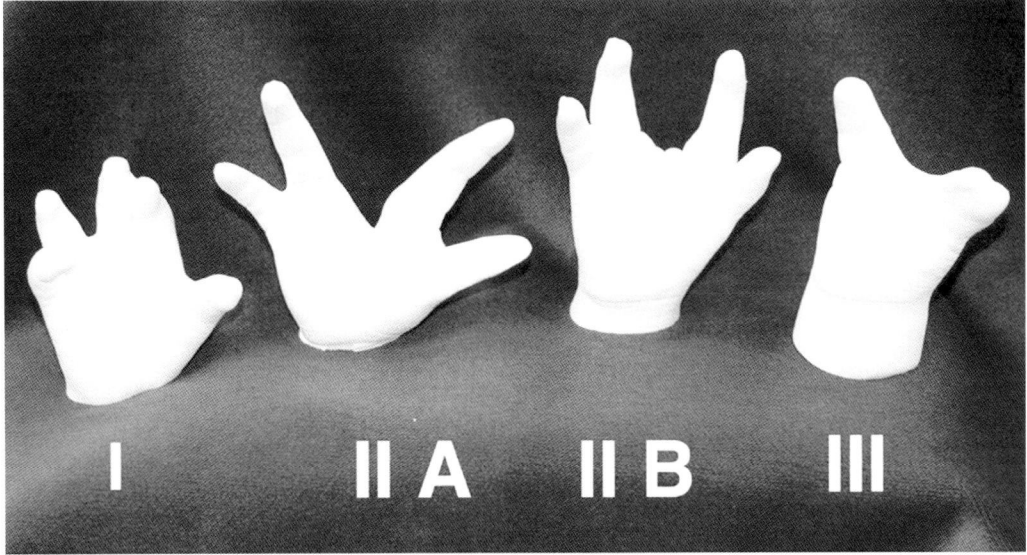

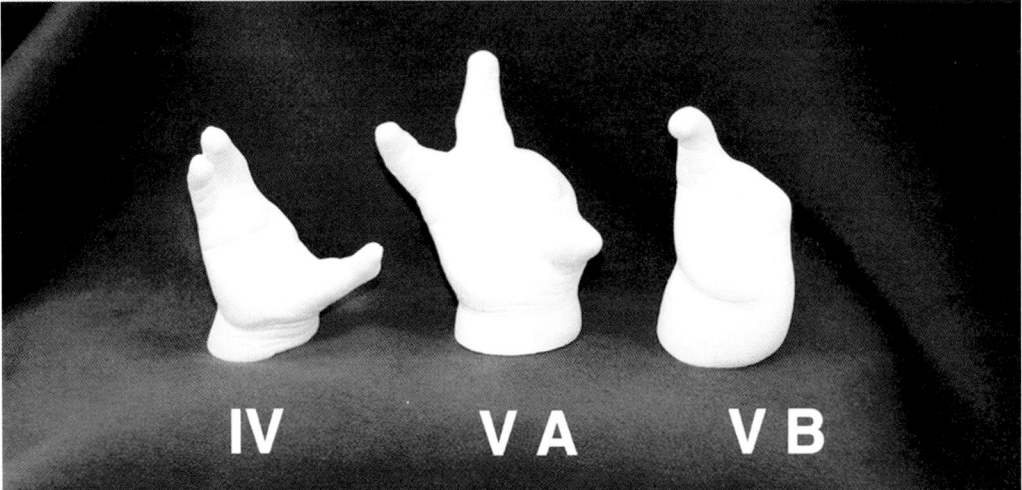

FIGURE 203-20. Classification of the typical cleft hand. In type I deformities, the first web space is narrowed. Type II malformations are classified as mildly (A) or moderately (B) narrowed. In type III varieties, the thumb and index ray are joined in a simple complete or incomplete syndactyly. In the type IV hand, the index ray is suppressed and the first web space is merged with the cleft. There are varying degrees of thumb suppression in type V, which is designated partial (A) and complete (B). In type V B hands, only the fifth digit remains on a one-digit hand.

were advanced. Müller[186] proposed that the typical cleft hand is caused by a central defect in the apical ectodermal ridge, which fails to develop, and that symbrachydactyly is caused by a primary mesenchymal disturbance in bone formation. Maisels' centripetal suppression theory of the developing hand, widely quoted during the past 3 decades, describes a cycle of suppression starting within the central portion of the hand plate.[184] The mildest form is a simple central soft tissue cleft with no skeletal deformity. In moderate forms, the radial rays are suppressed; and in the most severe forms, the ulnar rays are suppressed, which leads

to total suppression and an adactylic hand. Suppression progresses in a radial to ulnar direction. In patients with more extreme defects, a monodactylic hand with only a fifth ray (including digit) may result. In contrast, the severe forms of symbrachydactyly or atypical cleft hand present with the thumb as the last remaining digit. In the light of our limited knowledge of the mechanisms of these malformations, Maisels' system is consistent with the clinical findings.

The potential role of teratogens in the development of cleft hand has been elegantly explored by Ogino,[187-189] who administered busulfan at various points in embryonic fetal development in mice, producing the whole spectrum of cleft hand defects seen in humans, including syndactyly and polydactyly. Others have suggested that central polydactyly leads to central cleft formation and a progressive syndactyly of adjacent rays[178,190-192] as a result of damage to the apical ectodermal ridge causing a lack of differentiation (syndactyly), an exaggerated differentiation (polydactyly, transverse bones), or a defective differentiation (cleft hand) of the underlying mesoderm.[175]

GENETICS

Although cleft hands occasionally occur in isolation, the majority of patients present with cleft hands and feet, a combination that has been designated split hand and split foot (SH/SF) complex.[193,194] The transmission of this defect shows strong autosomal inheritance with variable penetrance, with phenotypic abnormalities in more than two thirds of affected probands. Ianakiev and collaborators[194a] demonstrated that an abnormality in the chromosome 3q.27 region is important in the development of the central portion of the apical ectodermal ridge, and patients with these deficiencies present with SH/SF syndromes such as the Cornelia de Lange syndrome, orodigital complex, Wildervanck syndrome (otodigital complex), Russell-Silver syndrome, EEC syndrome, and Goltz syndrome (ectodermal dysplasia).[195] Other genetic loci have been implicated in the development of cleft hand as well: SHFM1 on 7q21[196]; SHFM2, an X-linked locus on Xq26[197]; and SHFM3 on 10q24-25.[198,199] Limb-mammary syndrome includes hand-foot anomalies to 3q27.[200]

ASSOCIATED MALFORMATIONS

A multitude of congenital anomalies involving almost all organ systems has been associated with cleft hand. The most common associated anomalies are lower limb defects, and the severity of the foot malformation is often commensurate with that of the hand. Common lower limb anomalies include short femurs, tibial defects, and cleft feet. Associated upper limb malformations include short humerus, synostoses of the elbow and proximal forearm, and absent ulna. Common syndromic associations include Cornelia de Lange, Russell-Silver, EEC, and a wide variety of oro-oculo-oto syndromes. It is essential that babies with cleft hand undergo comprehensive evaluation by a geneticist and other subspecialists as indicated.

ABNORMAL ANATOMY AND CLINICAL PRESENTATION

Cleft hand defects may involve one or both upper limbs. Most defects are unilateral,[201] but when they are bilateral, the feet are typically involved as well and the patient fits a recognized syndrome. The classic type of typical cleft has a V-shaped defect of variable depth within the central portion of the hand. Transverse tubular bones may be present at the depth of the cleft,[202,203] and partial or complete simple syndactyly is often present adjacent to the cleft (Fig. 203-21; see Tables 203-3 and 203-4). In severe forms, syndactyly between the thumb-index or ring-small interdigital spaces may be present, and the central (long) ray is absent (see Figs. 203-20 and 203-21). Alternatively, a third metacarpal may be split and fused to the adjacent second and fourth metacarpals. A more complete form may include a complete absence of the second and third rays. The digits, including metacarpals, adjacent to the cleft are often long and wider than the normal digits.[204] A fusion between rays at either the metacarpal or phalangeal level with formation of a large "superdigit" is common.[205] The hand is not hypoplastic, but the thumb may be hypoplastic in association with a complete syndactyly with the index finger. Digital symphalangism at the phalangeal level may occur. Early radiographs often appear to have well-segmented joints, which rapidly close later in childhood. Attempts to release these cartilaginous bars surgically have been unsuccessful. Digital range of motion is often deficient, particularly in fingers adjacent to the cleft.

Soft tissue abnormalities parallel the skeletal malformations. The level of the simple syndactyly is variable. Most problematic for treatment is complete simple syndactyly between the thumb and index rays, which always includes a thick fibrous band within the soft tissue fusion. With absence of a metacarpal, the extrinsic flexor and extensor tendons form a tendon loop at the base of the cleft. This occurs most commonly in the Manske type V defect when the radial rays are suppressed (Fig. 203-22). With partial skeletal absence, they often attach to the adjacent digits and cause a camptodactyly of the proximal interphalangeal (PIP) joint. These flexion contractures are the result of excessive pull from the flexor side. Many abnormal fusions and distal insertions of the extrinsic flexors and extensors can be expected adjacent to the cleft (Figs. 203-23 and 203-24).[175,206,207] Angiography shows normal digital arteries within rays that have a full complement of skeletal elements.[208] Intrinsic muscle deficiencies also parallel the skeletal defects. The degree of development of the adductor pollicis muscle, critical for pinching maneuvers, is variable (Fig. 203-25). When the third metacarpal is normal, the adductor pollicis is normal. A full complement of median-innervated thenar muscles and ulnar-innervated hypothenar muscles is usually found when the first and fifth rays of the hand are normal. With digital absence and partial metacarpal hypoplasia, the interosseous muscles within the cleft will attach

Text continued on p. 92

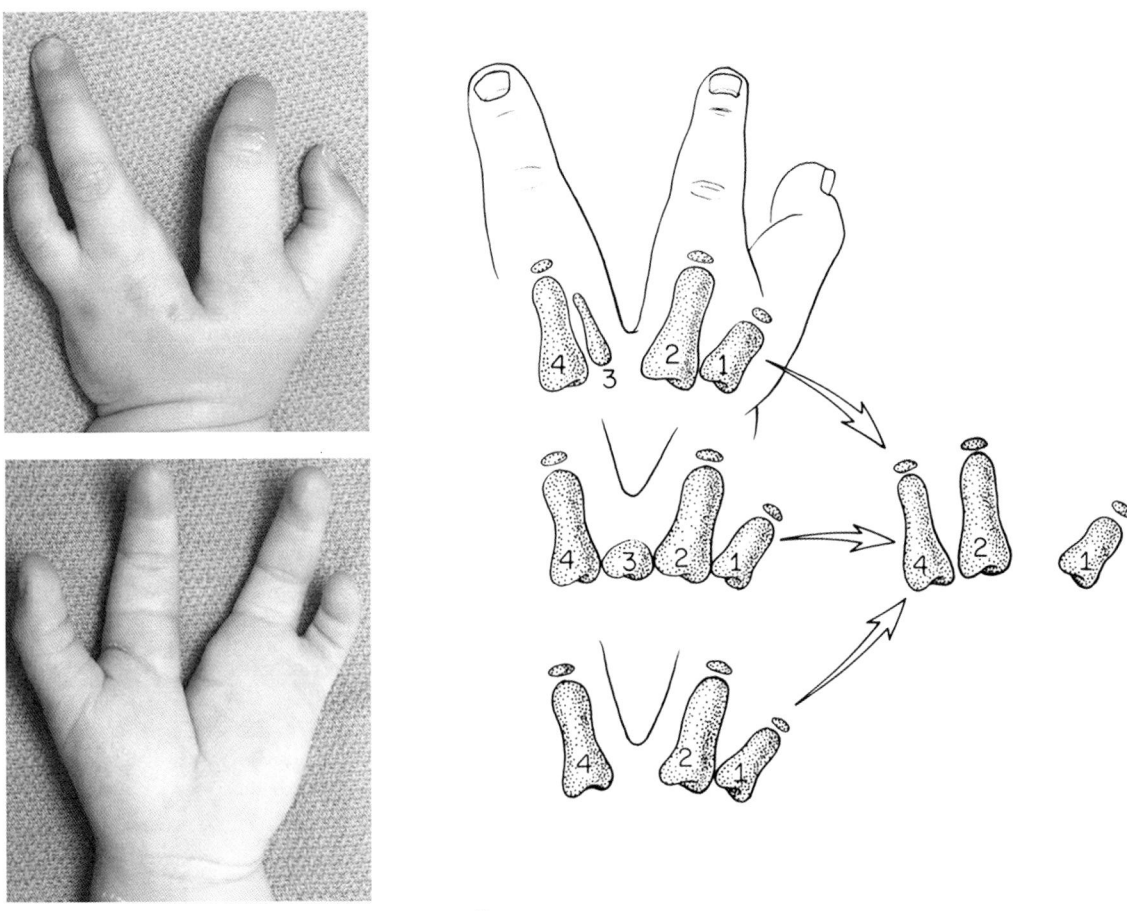

A   B

FIGURE 203-21. Depth of cleft. *A,* Appearance of a typical cleft hand with a deep central cleft. *B,* With deeper clefts, the long metacarpal may be slim and hypoplastic *(top),* very short *(central),* or completely absent *(below).* Index metacarpal transposition is best accomplished at the CMC joint level, where shortening and trimming of the joint surfaces will ensure a precision fit. Whatever adductor pollicis muscle is attached to the small long metacarpal should be saved. 1, thumb metacarpal; 2, index metacarpal; 3, long metacarpal; 4, ring metacarpal. (Illustration by Jean Biddl.)

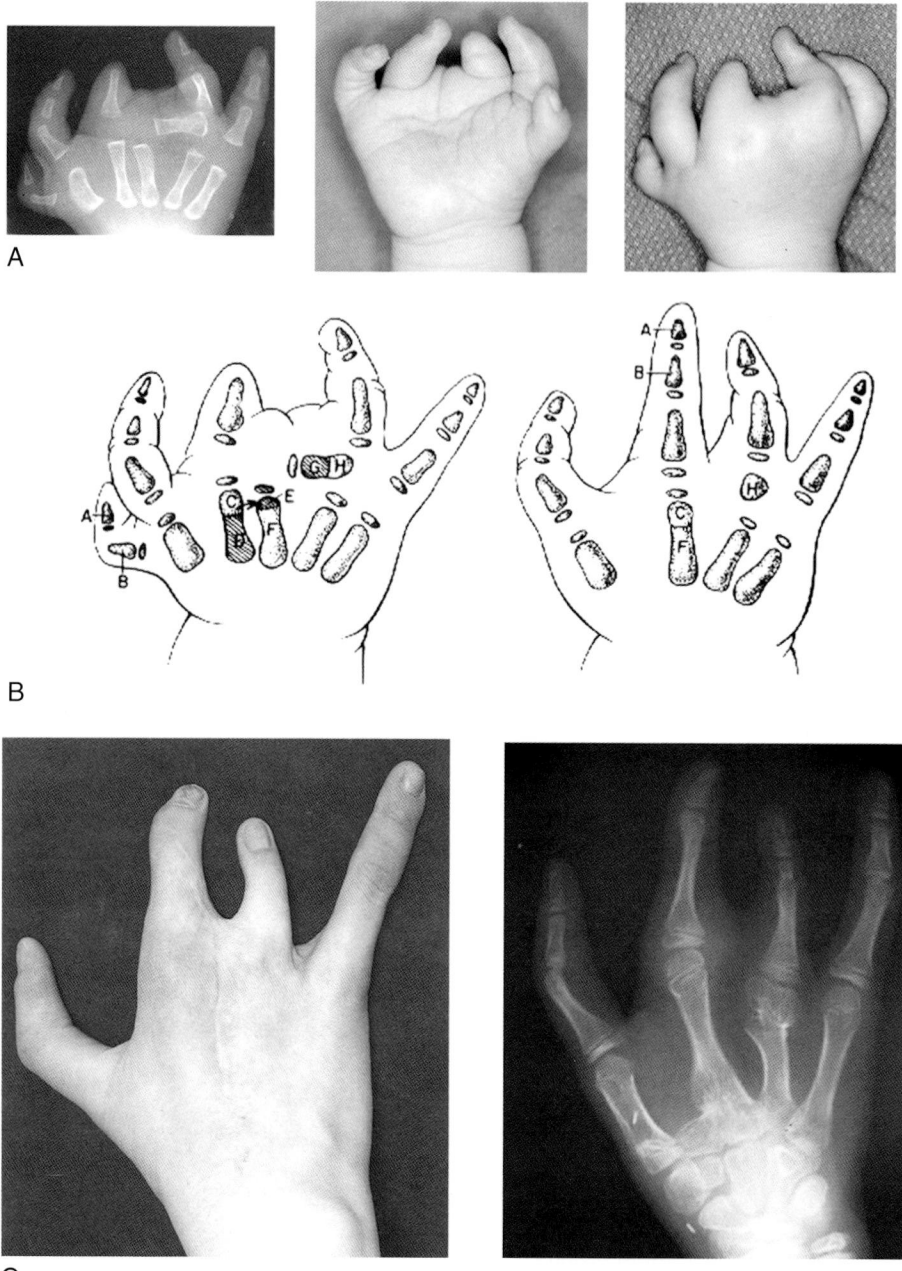

FIGURE 203-22. Cleft with tubular bones and thumb duplication. *A,* This child with the EEC syndrome has bilateral cleft hands and feet and an associated cleft palate like her mother and older brother. Her right hand contained a thumb duplication at the metacarpal level (type V, German classification), a triphalangeal ulnar thumb, a short thumb-index web space, an index finger missing two phalanges, a central cleft with intact long metacarpal, a transverse phalanx articulating with the ring MP joint, and a short ring digit. *B,* The first stage of her reconstruction consisted of transposition of the index ray (C) on top of the long metacarpal after excision of the index metacarpal base (D) and distal long metacarpal (E). A portion of the transverse phalanx was removed (G), but the segment articulating with the joint space was left intact. Six months later, the second-stage procedure consisted of widening of the thumb-index web space with local flaps and transfer of the radial thumb on top of the index finger as a free tissue transfer. The long triphalangeal thumb was not altered because of her excellent function. *C,* The clinical appearance and radiograph 16 years later. No web deepening has been requested. She excelled in high school as a Merit Scholar and has won numerous regional piano competitions. Identical malformations were reconstructed on both hands. (Illustration by Jean Biddl.)

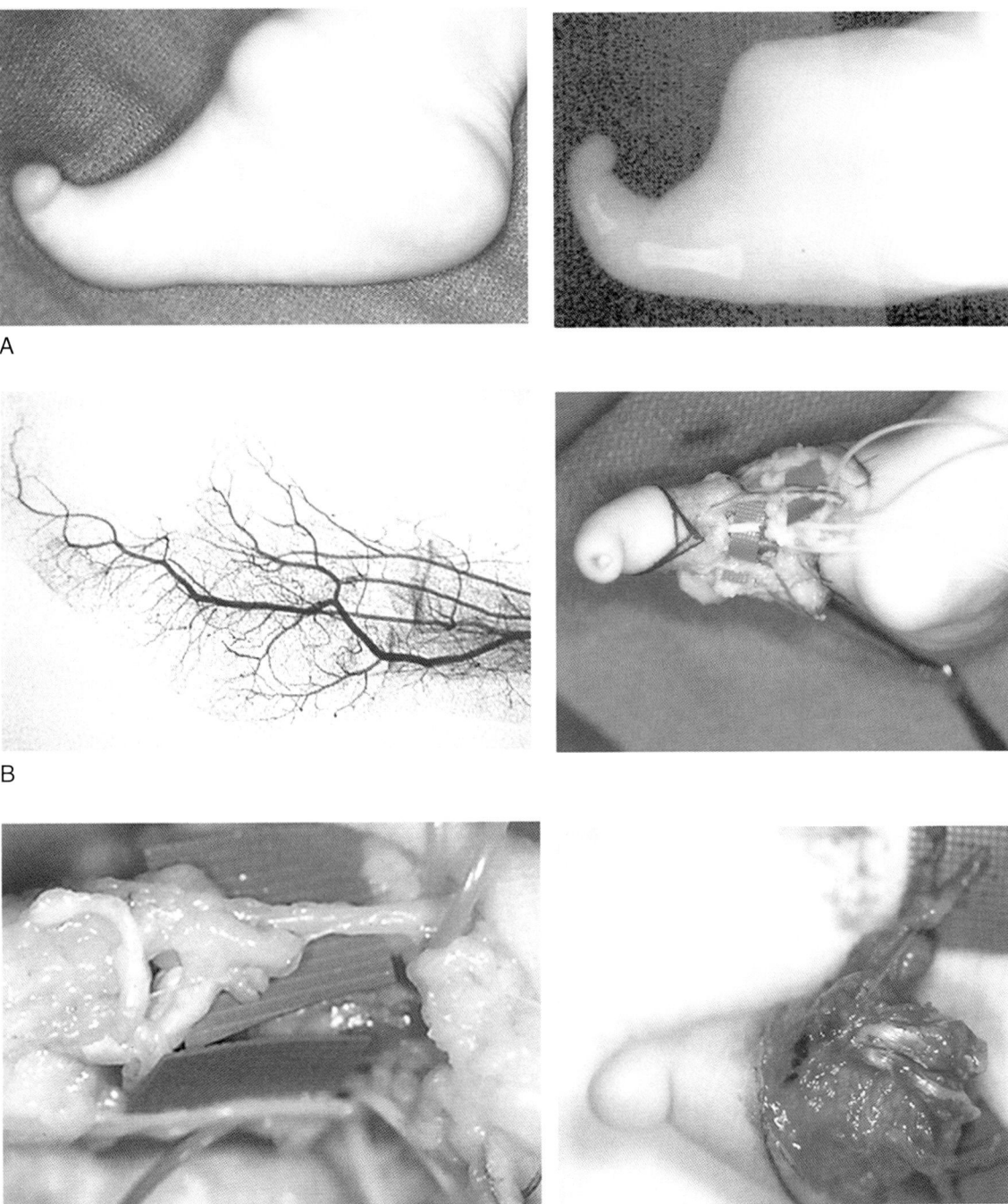

FIGURE 203-23. Single-digit (type V B) hand reconstruction. *A,* The potential foot donor site in this patient with the cleft hand-foot syndrome has small but present phalangeal components and a hypoplastic nail. *B,* An angiogram shows only one persistent branch of the lateral plantar artery to this toe. The artery, nerve, and veins, all anomalous structures, are identified. The flexor mechanism is an intrinsic muscle-tendon unit that deviates the toe medially. *C,* A close-up view of the neurovascular structures shows the medial location of the single artery, vein, and plantar nerve supplying this toe. On the right, the dissected toe with short pedicles is in transit.   *Continued*

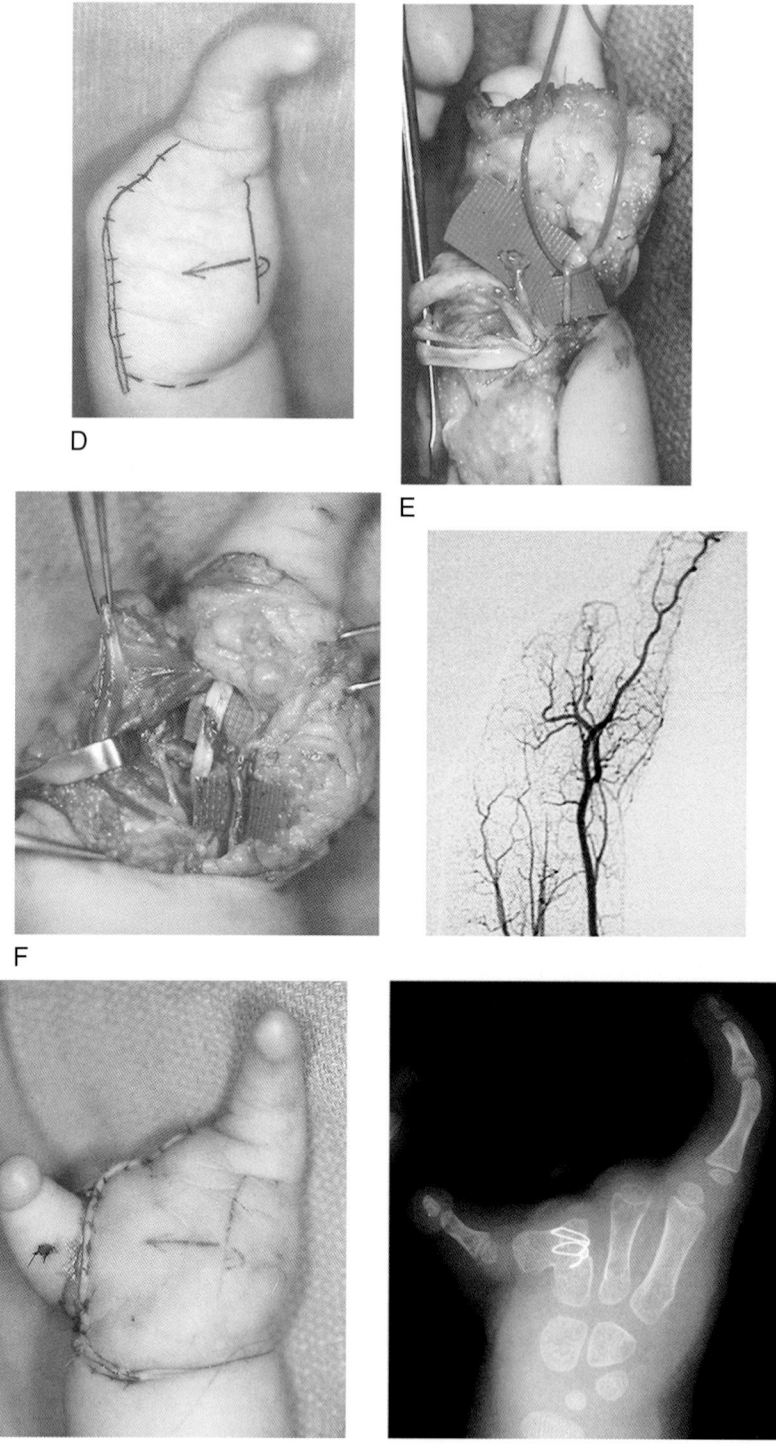

FIGURE 203-23, cont'd. *D,* The incisions in the recipient site are outlined. *E,* The extrinsic flexor and extensor tendons to the missing thumb, index finger, and ring finger are joined as a single tendon distal to the metacarpals. *F,* The anatomy of the ulnar artery, with its branch to the palmar arch, corresponds with the preoperative angiogram. A single deep flexor tendon is present. A sensory nerve to the missing digits is seen near the retractor. *G,* The new "thoe" has been transferred to the radial side of the hand and secured with bone to bone fixation. The tendon with the greatest passive excursion was joined to the thoe flexors and extensors.

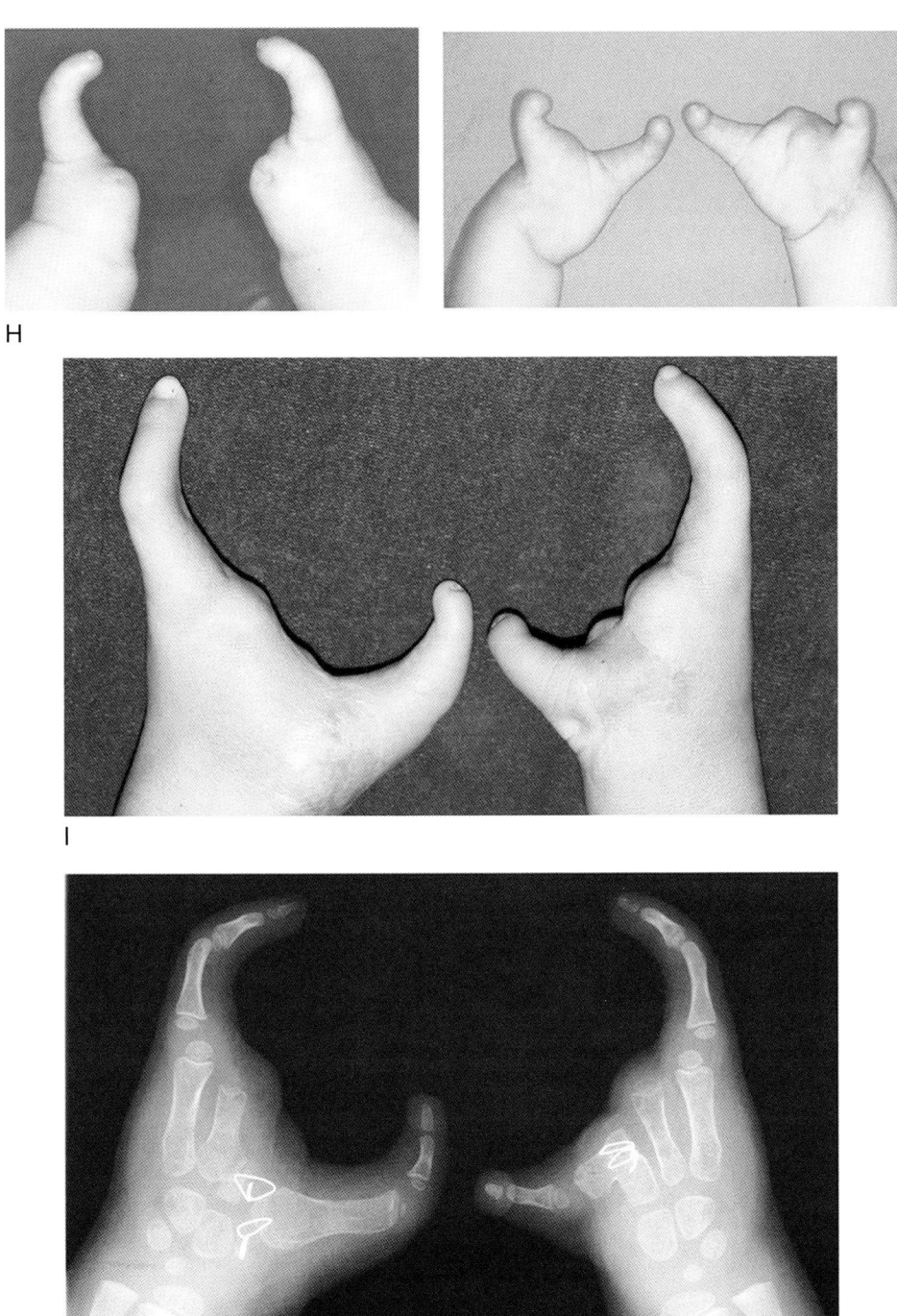

FIGURE 203-23, cont'd. *H,* Both hands are depicted, once at age 6 months before transfers and again at age 14 months after two independent toe transfers. *I,* Three years later, her adaptive hand function has been amazing. *J,* A postoperative radiograph demonstrates that the entire metatarsal was transferred with the thoe to the left hand and left on the foot with the right hand transfer. Transfer of at least a part of the metatarsal, which adds both increased stability and length, is recommended. There was no difference in the foot donor site's function.

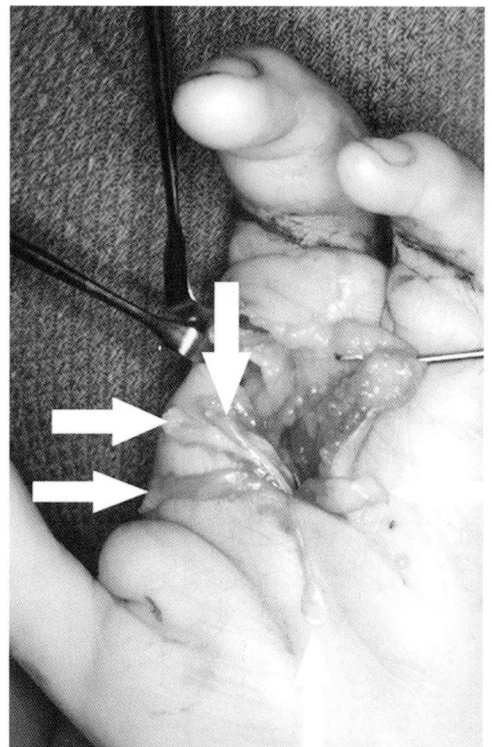

A

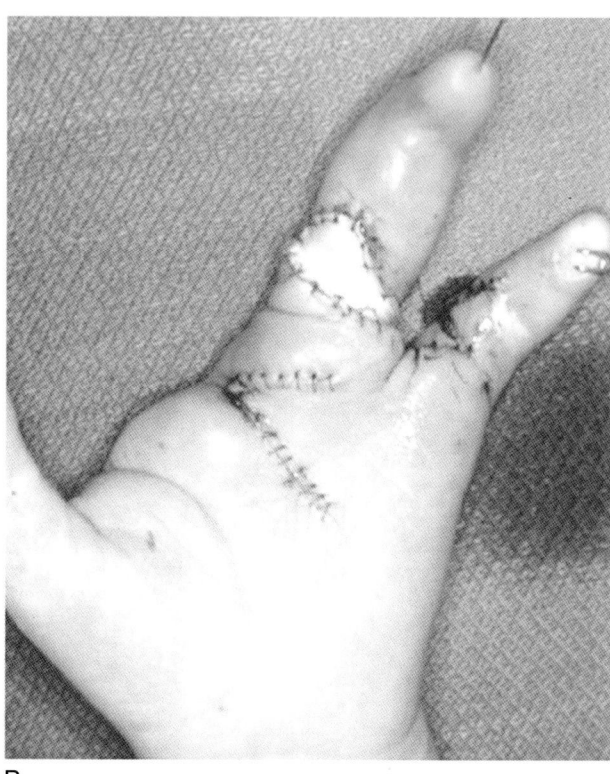

B

FIGURE 203-24. Digital flexion contractures. *A,* Extrinsic flexor (and extensor) tendons will attach to skeletal struc-tures bordering the cleft. The arrows indicate five flexor tendons attached to the proximal phalanx of the ring digit, causing an imbalance and contracture at the PIP joint. *B,* After multiple tenotomies and joint release, skin grafting or other tissue replacement is often necessary. An incomplete syndactyly in the ring to small finger web space has also been separated and closed with a commissure flap and skin grafts. The zigzag incision in the palm was used to facili-tate clarification of the expected abnormal anatomy.

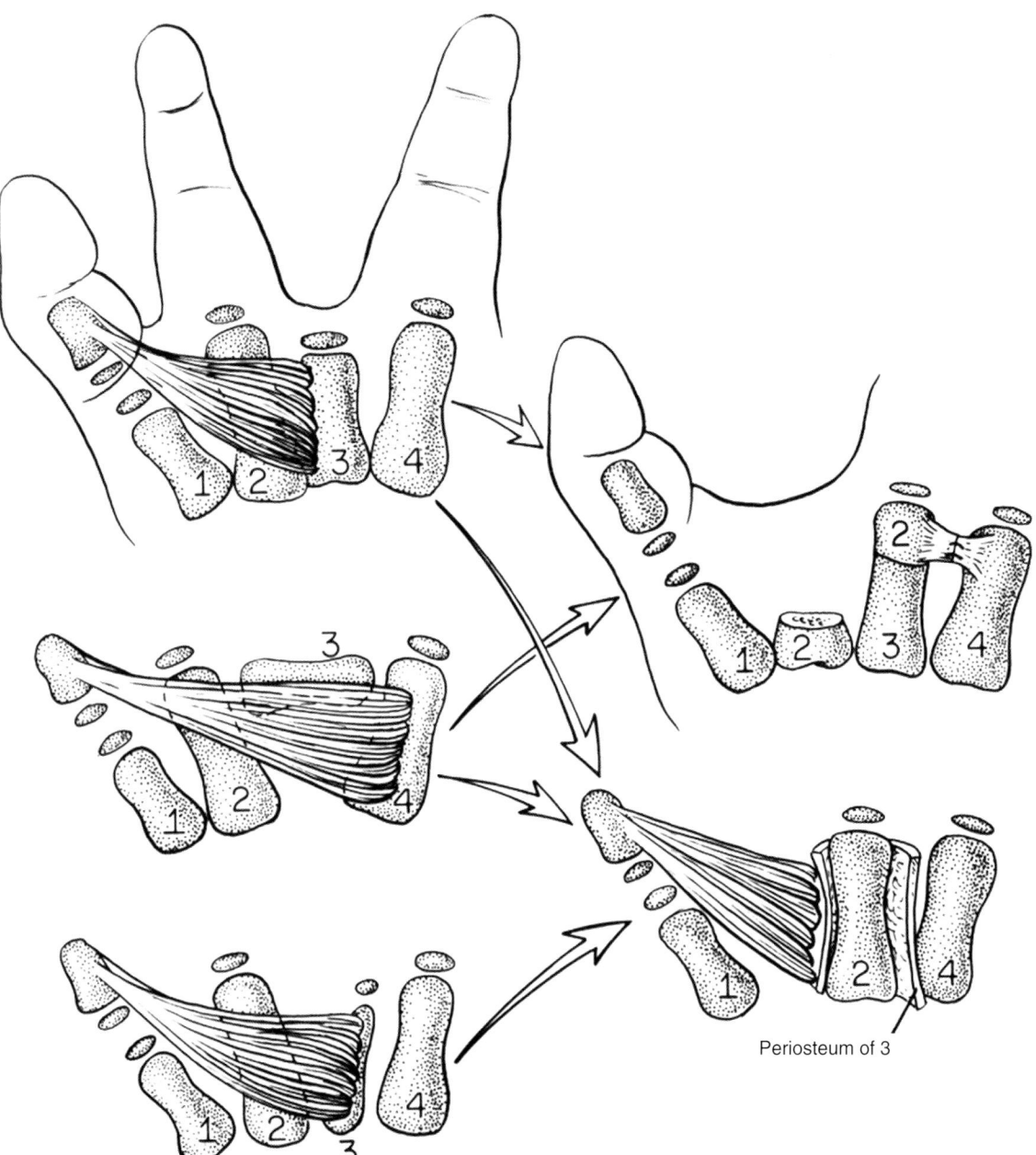

FIGURE 203-25. Adductor pollicis muscle variations. *Left,* A strong adductor muscle should be saved because a weak pinch is a predominant feature of the cleft hand. Three common variations of cleft hands are shown on the left: a hypoplastic metacarpal with a strong muscle and no distal digit; a transverse phalanx with the adductor inserting into the next ulnar bone; and a severely hypoplastic metacarpal with a muscle deficiency. *Right,* Two alternatives for treatment of these hands are (1) transposition of the distal index metacarpal on top of the existing long metacarpal and (2) subperiosteal removal of a hypoplastic long metacarpal and transposition of the index metacarpal into the periosteal sleeve. The transverse phalanges seen in the left center are excised completely, including removal of all periosteum, which would otherwise produce bone as the child grows. 1, thumb metacarpal; 2, index metacarpal; 3, long metacarpal; 4, ring metacarpal. (Illustration by Jean Biddl.)

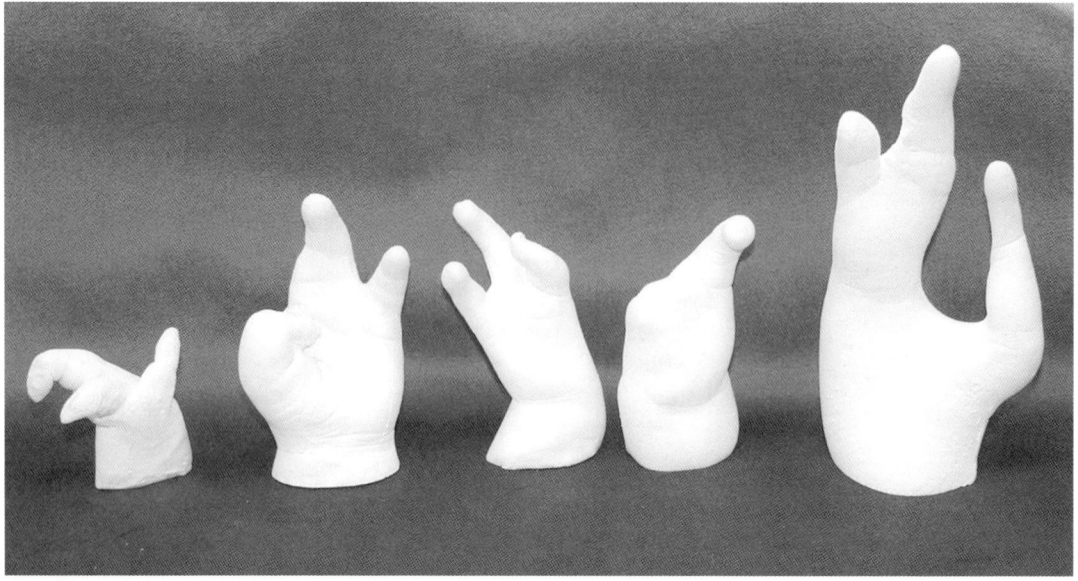

FIGURE 203-26. "Functional triumph, aesthetic disaster." Photographs of hand molds are from children with typical cleft hand malformations. The remarkable function of each hand has verified Adrian Flatt's commonly quoted observation that these hands are functional triumphs and aesthetic disasters.[109] It is interesting that the parents of four of these five patients recognized their child's adaptability and elected to have no surgery. The toe transfer in the one-fingered hand is depicted in Figure 203-23.

distally into either the phalangeal bases or the extensor expansion.

Although hand function is usually satisfactory, the cosmetic appearance of the hand is conspicuously poor, forming what Flatt[109] has referred to as a functional triumph and social disaster. Despite the remarkable capacity for adaptation observed in many children, hand function is often severely impaired. Grasp is usually achieved either within the central cleft or between the thumb and fifth finger. In most hands, simple pinch or grasp is blocked by the index ray, which is positioned in a functional "no man's land" between the thumb and the cleft (Fig. 203-26). The primary goal of treatment in these hands is to transpose the index ray into a position where it does not interfere with thumb pinching and gripping. Abnormal rotation of the ulnar digits (usually in supination), hypoplasia of the thumb, flexion contractures of the PIP joints, or diminished interphalangeal joint motion may contribute to functional limitation. Wrist motion and anatomy are usually normal.

INDICATIONS FOR TREATMENT

The indications for and timing of surgery for cleft hand are debatable. Facial clefts in syndromic patients are more conspicuous and require early surgical correction. However, parents often wait to consider hand surgery and are impressed by their child's adaptive abilities. Interestingly, functional problems with the hands often bother young patients more than appearance

does. If one parent with the same deformities has experienced previous complications, he or she is often reluctant to subject his or her child to the possibility of similar adverse outcomes.[209]

The major indications for surgery are severe flexion contracture of one or more digits, malpositioned index ray that interferes with function, tight syndactyly involving the thumb, absent thumb, and major functional limitations of the child. Deformities such as joint contractures and web space limitation may become marked with growth. Most patients have functional problems with their feet long before they recognize major problems with their hands. The treatment of the foot, not discussed in this chapter, is important and must parallel that of the hand.

It is preferable to operate before 1 year of age and plan to complete reconstruction by the time the child enters school at 5 to 6 years of age. Skeletal and soft tissue corrections are performed simultaneously.

TREATMENT

Almost all children with cleft hands will benefit from surgical reconstruction (Table 203-5). With the exception of individuals with adactylic or monodactylic hands, all patients with a cleft hand have an intact basic hand consisting of a mobile preaxial ray, an intervening cleft or web space, and a mobile digit or post on the postaxial portion of the hand. Because sensation is intact, these hands can be used effectively, and functional difficulties are proportional to the extent of the

TABLE 203-5 ✦ COMPONENTS OF A TYPICAL CLEFT HAND RECONSTRUCTION

Preservation and formation of a mobile, unscarred, stable thumb
An index ray transposed to the ulnar side of the cleft
An adequate first web space
Interdigital web spaces lined with normal flaps, not scar tissue
Index metacarpals not excessively long or rotated
Reconstructed transverse metacarpal head ligaments
Preservation of all intact adductor pollicis intrinsic muscles

---

malformation. There is such variation in the morphologic features of cleft hands that no standard treatment exists. Operations must be tailored to the individual patient's needs and functional difficulties. Not all procedures designed to improve appearance will improve function.[210]

Many surgical approaches to the cleft hand have been used during the past 40 years,[115,174,179,211-216] among which the Snow-Littler method has been most popular. The preferred approach incorporates and refines important components of most of these procedures.[202,217]

Incisions

Keep it simple! The widely used methods described by Snow (Fig. 203-27),[215] Miura,[212] and others include designs of small, randomly based flaps of dorsal or palmar skin that may die and ultimately result in contracture of the first web space or metacarpophalangeal (MP) joint flexion contracture.[214] It is preferable to use a simple circumferential incision around the index ray to be transposed, straight-line incisions within the cleft, and extensions to the thumb (Fig. 203-28). The raised dorsal and palmar flaps then provide a clear exposure of the entire metacarpal portion of the hand, including intrinsic muscles, common neurovascular structures, extrinsic tendons, and skeletal structures, all of which can then be precisely repositioned if necessary. The index-long commissure is lined with a small flap based on the radial side of the ring ray with a 45-degree dorsal to palmar inclination.

Index Ray Position and Length

The index ray is often on the radial side of the cleft in a functional "no man's land" and must be transposed adjacent to the next complete ray of the hand (usually the ring ray). Severely hypoplastic nonfunctional digits are best ablated, but this recommendation may be unpopular with parents. In patients with a deep central cleft, the index metacarpal is often much longer than the adjacent ring metacarpal and should be short-

ened appropriately. At the time of transposition, the digit should be positioned with appropriate pronation to allow good pulp to pulp contact during key pinch.

Intermetacarpal Ligament Reconstruction

Elaborate tendon graft fixations at the MP joint level have been described,[216] but these may compromise potential tendon gliding and motion at the MP joint. When present, the transverse metacarpal ligaments are sutured with the metacarpal heads as close together as possible (Fig. 203-29). A second alternative is a large circumferential suture around the two adjacent metacarpals.

Adductor Pollicis and Long Metacarpal

All adductor intrinsic muscles are preserved. Preoperatively, the location and size of the third metacarpal correlate well with the presence and size of this important pinch muscle. The incision described before provides excellent visualization not only of this muscle but also of the arterial anatomy on the radial side of the hand. A decision must be made about the third metacarpal. If a normal metacarpal is present, the muscle is left intact and the index digit is transposed to the distal third metacarpal (see Figs. 203-22, 203-25, and 203-29). If the metacarpal is hypoplastic, the muscle is left attached to the periosteal sleeve and the index metacarpal is positioned within this sleeve. Any recession or partial myotomy of the adductor pollicis muscle will result in a predictable weakening of pinch strength.

In some cleft hands with transversely oriented abnormal phalanges, all or some of the adductor pollicis muscle may originate from the ring metacarpal. The author has never seen an origin from the fifth metacarpal. Transverse tubular bones at the metacarpal level must be removed before index ray transposition (see Fig. 203-22). It is occasionally necessary to save a portion of these abnormal skeletal structures to provide stability for the ring finger MP joint.

The first dorsal interosseous muscle will often have a bipennate origin from the thumb and index metacarpals and must be completely released from the first metacarpal before transposition (see Fig. 203-29).

A metacarpal osteotomy is used only when a good third (long) metacarpal and intact adductor pollicis muscle are present. The transverse cut is made at the distal diaphyseal level (see Fig. 203-29). When the metacarpal sleeve technique is employed, it is preferable to disarticulate the index at the CMC joint, adjust the height of the new index metacarpal with cartilage trimming, and position the metacarpal base into the long metacarpal CMC joint. No motion is present as this remains the "fixed unit" of the hand skeleton.[218] The method of internal fixation should not restrict MP joint motion.

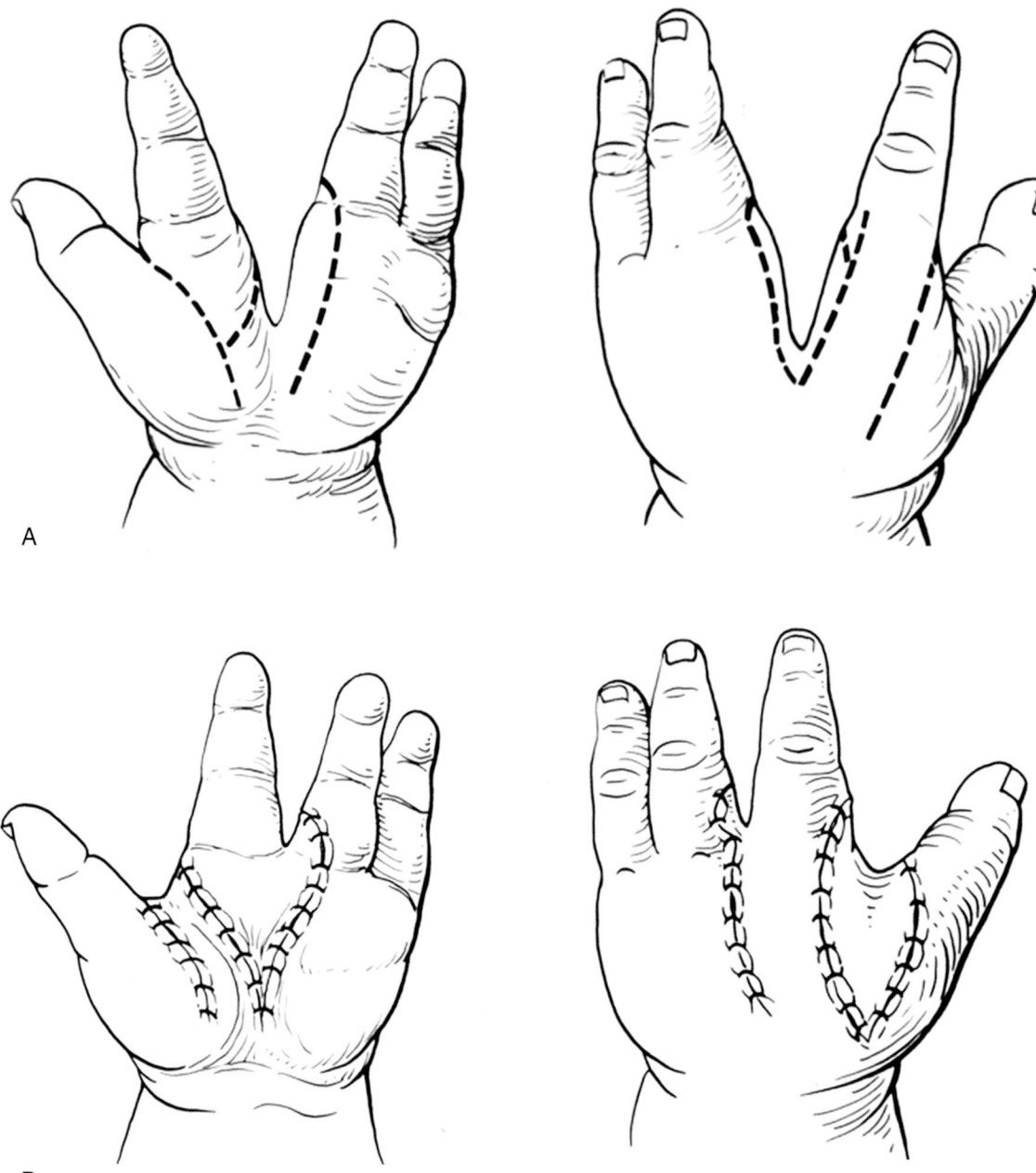

FIGURE 203-27.   Snow-Littler incisions.[215] *A,* The incisions for this technique show a narrow dorsal skin bridge over the dorsal and palmar surfaces of the index metacarpal and the base of the cleft. The palmar-based flap is raised before the index ray is transposed into a more ulnar position. *B,* Skin closure after index transposition is outlined. Necrosis of the distal portion of the palmar flap, which now forms the first web space, is a potential problem. (Illustration by Jean Biddl.)

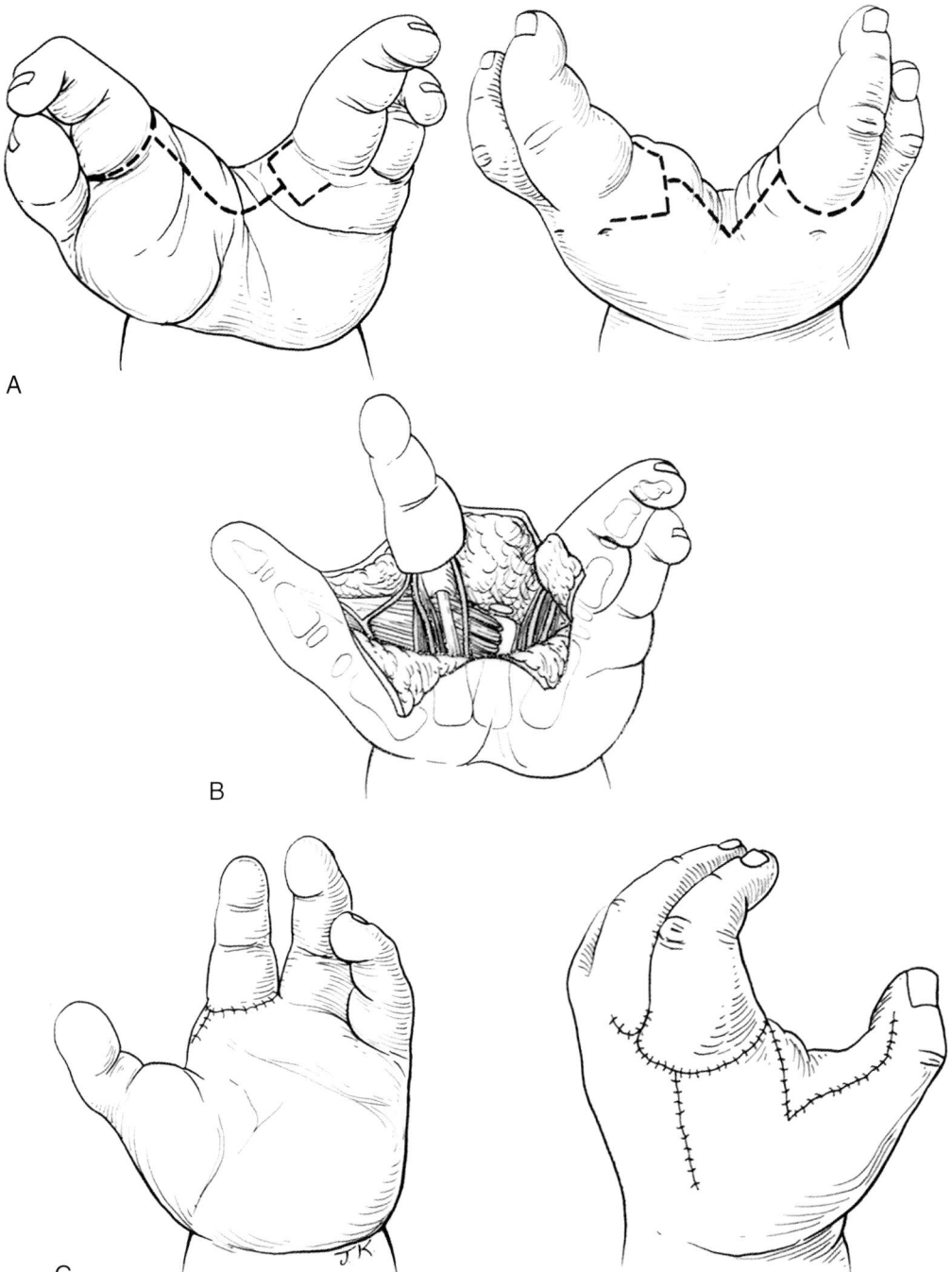

FIGURE 203-28. Modified cleft hand incisions. *A,* Incision outlines on dorsal and palmar surfaces of the hand show a commissure flap on the radial side of the ring digit and equal division of tissue within the depth of the central cleft. All glabrous tissue remains palmar, and nonglabrous (hair-bearing) tissue remains dorsal. The major difference from the Snow-Littler incision is that the author's incision does not depend on a dorsally based flap to line the first web space. *B,* After flap elevation, there is wide exposure of all important neurovascular structures, the adductor pollicis, the first dorsal interosseous muscles, and all skeletal structures. There is easy access to all anatomy down to the CMC joint level. This incision is the hand equivalent of the coronal incision used by the craniofacial surgeon. Complete exposure of all important structures is afforded by a direct incision. *C,* After transposition of the index ray, both flaps are moved into the first web space. Z-plasties or other transposition flaps can be used for improvement of contour.

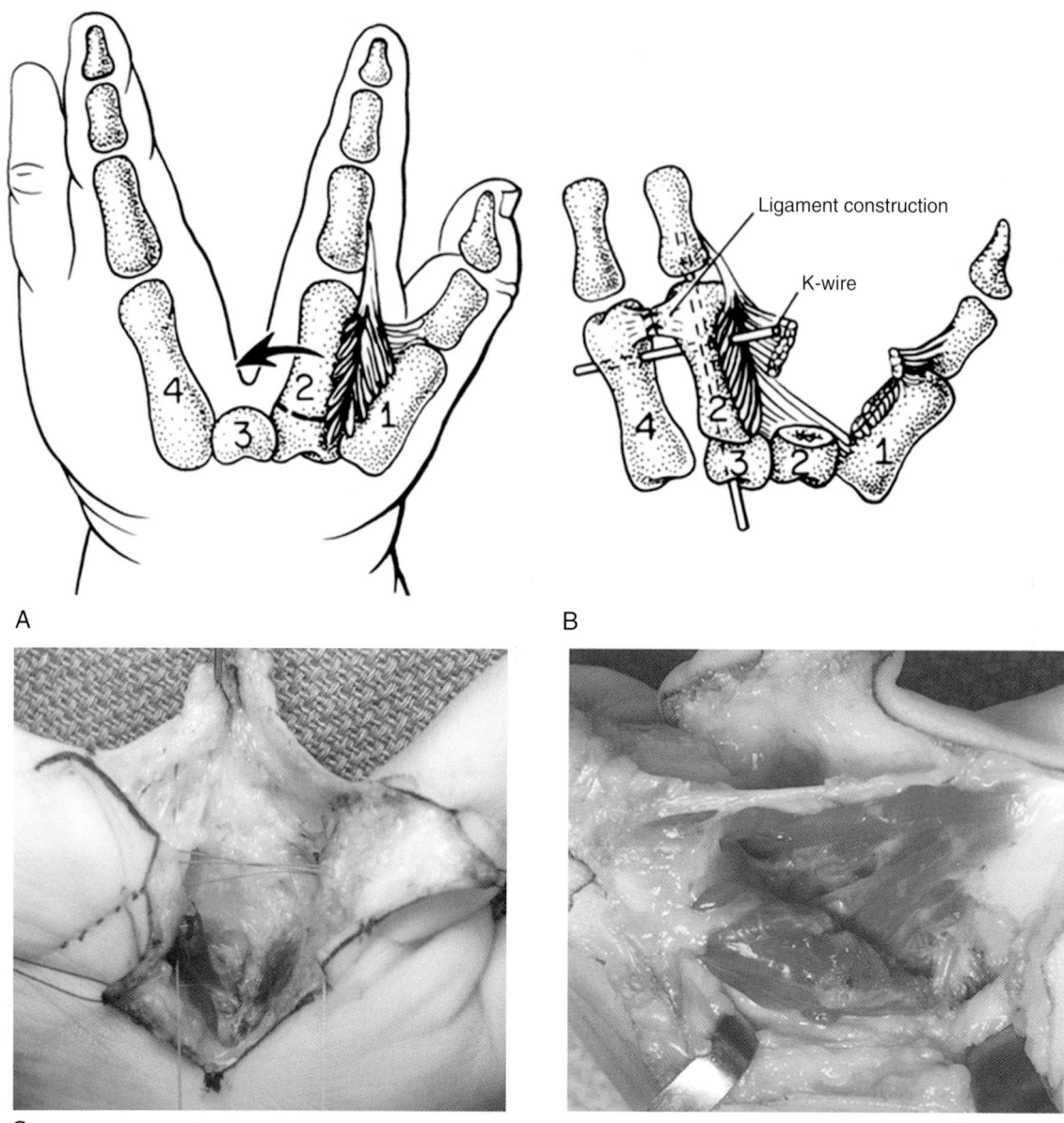

FIGURE 203-29. Intermetacarpal suture and first dorsal interosseous muscle release. *A,* A deep central cleft is present with a tight first web space. An osteotomy is made at the base of the index metacarpal before transposition into the long position. The most limiting structure will be the thumb metacarpal origin of the first dorsal interosseous muscle, which must be released at a deep enough level to allow complete movement of the index ray. Interosseous wire fixation is helpful. *B,* The transverse metacarpal ligament is constructed with a substantial nonabsorbable suture or, alternatively, with a tendon graft. *C,* The first dorsal interosseous muscle has been released from the thumb metacarpal on the right. The adductor pollicis muscle remains intact. 1, thumb metacarpal; 2, index metacarpal; 3, long metacarpal; 4, ring metacarpal. (Illustration by Jean Biddl.)

Digital Flexion Contractures

Tight PIP joint flexion contractures are often seen in the digits adjacent to central clefts of the hand because of the imbalance caused by the attachment of multiple intrinsic muscles and extrinsic tendons that developed in the palm but had no distal digit to join. After complete detachment of these structures, the secondarily contracted volar plate and accessory collateral ligaments may require release before the PIP joint can be fully extended. Glabrous skin grafts are often needed (see Fig. 203-24).

First Web Space (Thumb to Index)

After skeletal transposition and fixation, tendon release, intrinsic muscle release, or repositioning and intermetacarpal ligament fixation, wound closure can be performed. The new commissure flap is first sutured to the ulnar side of the index ray, which is now in the long position. With the index finger in extension, the flaps are repositioned around it under no tension. A skin deficiency may exist in patients with a deep cleft and should be covered with a full-thickness glabrous skin graft. An interosseous wire between the first two metacarpals will hold the thumb in maximum palmar abduction. In this position, the skin flaps are draped without tension on both sides of the index ray. In most patients, they are sutured around both sides of the index ray, and enough tissue is present within the web for formation of a well-contoured first web space (Fig. 203-30; see also Fig. 203-28). At this point, Z-plasties or other preferred local rotational or transposition flaps can be incorporated to provide the best contour to the web space and to break up a straight line. The most appropriate time to make these decisions is after the skeletal transposition has been completed. In most instances, these modifications are not obvious before musculoskeletal reconstruction. Subcuticular suture techniques are used for all dorsal incisions, and glabrous

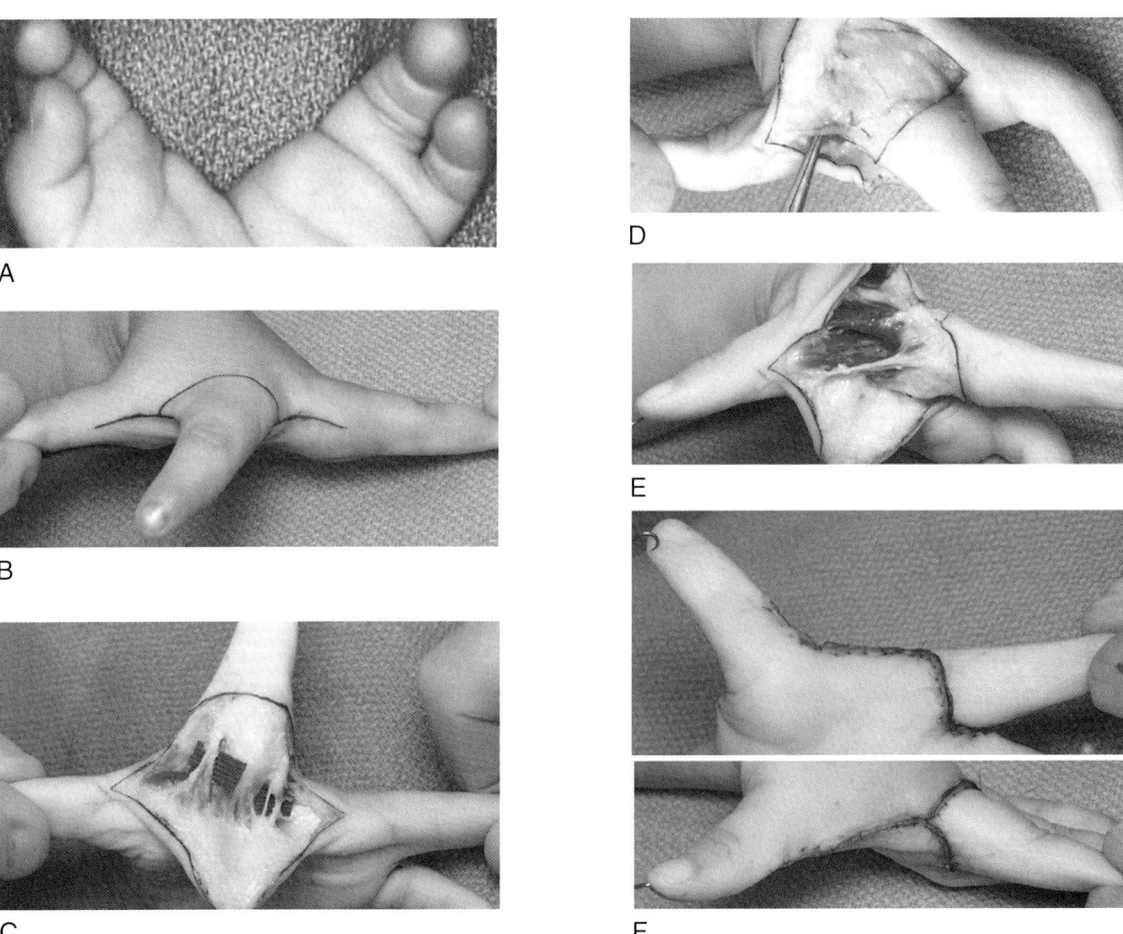

FIGURE 203-30. Simple correction of the cleft hand. *A,* This central cleft exists at the level of the long ray. The index ray is radial to the cleft, and a small thumb-index web space is present. *B,* The incision extends between the thumb and ring finger, around the index finger. *C,* After incision and retraction of the palmar flap, the fascia is released and all neurovascular structures are identified. *D,* Beneath the dorsal flap is the omnipresent fibrous band between the thumb and index metacarpals. The tightest and thickest part of the band is usually parallel to the leading edge of the adductor pollicis muscle. *E,* The thenar intrinsic muscles are easily identified, and all fascial investments are appropriately released down to the CMC joint if necessary. *F,* After index transposition, the dorsal and palmar flaps are closed to construct a new thumb-index web space. Z-plasties are easily incorporated at this stage if necessary. (Illustration by Jean Biddl.)

surfaces are closed externally with fast-absorbing 6-0 mild chromic sutures.

Full-thickness skin grafts from a non-hair-bearing donor region are used to cover exposed portions of the index ray (occasionally palmar) and thumb. Syndactyly release with grafts can also be performed between the ring and small digits.

The contact pulp prehension surfaces on the ulnar side of the distal thumb phalanx and the radial side of the index finger should be surfaced with local skin. Incisions should be appropriately designed. The hypothenar donor site is ideal for harvesting of dorsal, palmar (glabrous), or combined full-thickness skin grafts. If more skin is needed, the groin is preferred as a donor site.

Thumb Duplications and Other Variations

In complex forms of typical cleft hands with a relatively shallow central cleft and extra transversely oriented phalanges, thumb duplications with or without a triphalangeal thumb may be present. In these hands, the more deficient radial duplicate partner may be used as a free tissue transfer to augment the distal portion of a deficient finger, usually located on the index or long ray (Fig. 203-31). Preoperative angiography is mandatory. Triphalangeal thumbs often do not require shortening as the additional length increases thumb-index span. It is best to assess the patient's functional status before sacrificing a mobile thumb joint or length.

Monodactylic Hand

A monodactylic hand is usually associated with a cleft hand-foot presentation and consists of an intact fifth ray with a metacarpal and phalanges on the ulnar side of the hand. A hypoplastic radial metacarpal is usually present (see Fig. 203-23). The goal of reconstruction is to design a hand consisting of a mobile radial digit, a web space, and at least one digit or a post on the ulnar side of the hand (Table 203-6). Three treatment options are available for monodactylic hands: no intervention, great-toe transfer, and distraction of the radial metacarpal. Transfer of the hypoplastic distal portion of the great (medial) toe is the treatment of choice.[219-222] Despite arguments to save all metatarsal length, func-

tional thumbs may be constructed when the metatarsophalangeal joint has been transferred intact and solidly fixed to bone on the radial side of the hand (see Fig. 203-23). Gait function is not significantly altered. In monodactylic hands, excellent extrinsic flexor and extensor motors have been found in the depth of the cleft as a single, well-differentiated tendon. If the capability to perform a microvascular toe transfer is not available, the other options are reasonable. Even without treatment, children with monodactylic hands demonstrate remarkable functional adaptability.

Traditional methods of osteoplastic reconstruction with tubed pedicle or local flaps to cover nonvascularized corticocancellous bone grafts are no longer used. When a skeletal distraction technique has been chosen, a uniplanar device is all that is necessary. The distraction is performed in two stages, (1) distraction and (2) bone graft and internal fixation. Leaving an external apparatus attached to a young child's hand while waiting months for adequate bone regenerate to form is not necessary and will predictably lead to pin track-related complications. When the desired length has been obtained, it is best to remove the pins, adjust proper rotation and angulation, and then insert a bone graft into the intercalated distraction gap.

OUTCOMES

Regardless of reconstructive treatment, cleft hands are never normal. The conclusions reported in this chapter are based on personal operative and nonoperative experience with 108 typical cleft hands, which have been evaluated at follow-up ranging from 1 to 27 years (Fig. 203-32).[202] Because these hands are individually unique, general impressions are recorded here. Early in my experience, the Snow-Littler incisions and intrinsic releases were used in eight hands. Partial flap necrosis and a limited first web space prompted incisional modifications. When these children were observed into adolescence, persistent radial angulation at the MP joint and long index metacarpal became obvious. Nine patients, who were initially seen well after their primary correction, required extensive surgery for salvage of complex problems, including an array of transverse tubular bones, shared joints, side-to-side fusions at the metacarpal or phalangeal level, and contracted index digit next to a functionless thumb (see Fig. 203-22). In these children and teenagers, a stable and mobile thumb was constructed with a good first web space. The transposed index and released ring fingers were stiff at the interphalangeal joint level, and the fifth digit was the most functional element of the hand. Grip strength averaged 15% of normal, and key pinch between the thumb and fifth digit was 25% of normal. Overall, function of these hands in all activities of daily living was markedly

---

TABLE 203-6 ✦ COMPONENTS OF A RECONSTRUCTED MONODACTYLIC HAND

A mobile thumb on the radial side
Skeletal stability of the thumb
A web space lined with full-thickness skin flaps
Adequate space between the two digits
Rotation of the two digits in opposition for pinch and grasp

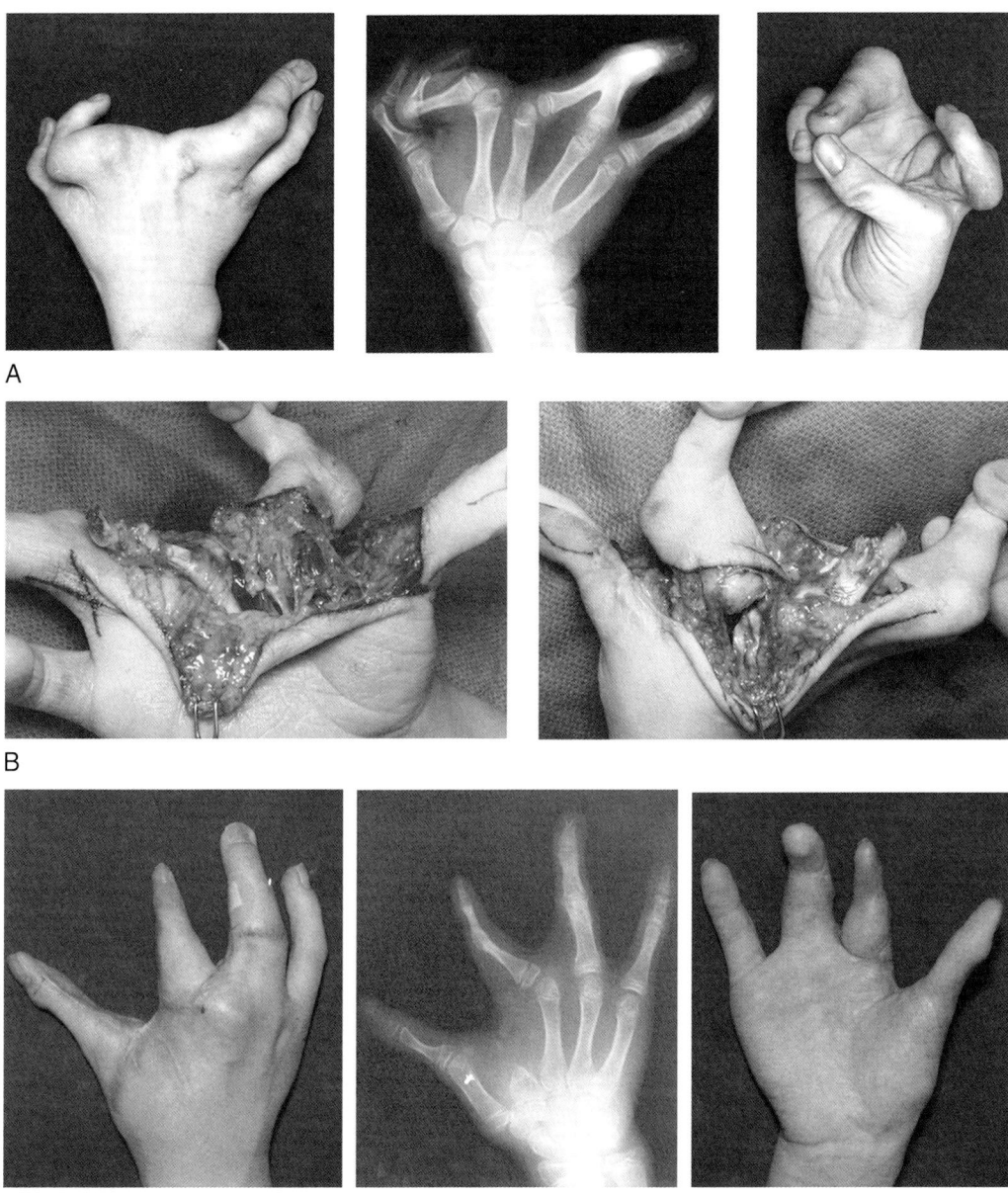

FIGURE 203-31. Complex secondary cleft hand reconstruction. *A,* This photograph shows the hand of a patient with the EEC syndrome who had bilateral hand and foot clefts and wide bilateral cleft lip and palate. The patient presented 6 years after thumb-index syndactyly release elsewhere. The ring finger is a "superdigit" containing the long and ring digits joined at the proximal phalangeal level, where there is a fixed 90-degree flexion contracture. There is no first web space, the thumb is flail at the MP joint, and the index is severely contracted. The mother strongly desired preservation of the index ray and construction of a pinch and grip to this hand, which was not used. In fact, the patient concealed it most of the time. *B,* A complex reconstruction was performed in three stages, with excision of skin grafts on the thumb, tendon graft stabilization of the thumb MP joint, transposition of the index ray on top of the long metacarpal after excision of the distal long metacarpal with its proximal phalanx, release of the ring flexion contracture and osteotomy of the proximal phalanx, realignment of the ring flexor and extensor tendons, chondrodesis of the index distal interphalangeal joint, and dorsal flap advancement to line the first web space. All structures involved in this difficult secondary reconstruction are easily approached through this incision. *C,* The clinical appearance and radiographs of the hand after reconstruction. This boy now has a stable pinch between the thumb and all three digits and has developed a strong grip between the thumb and ulnar two digits. The index finger is in good position and does not interfere with pinch or grip functions. The released ring PIP joint is in better position for pinch and grip with the thumb.

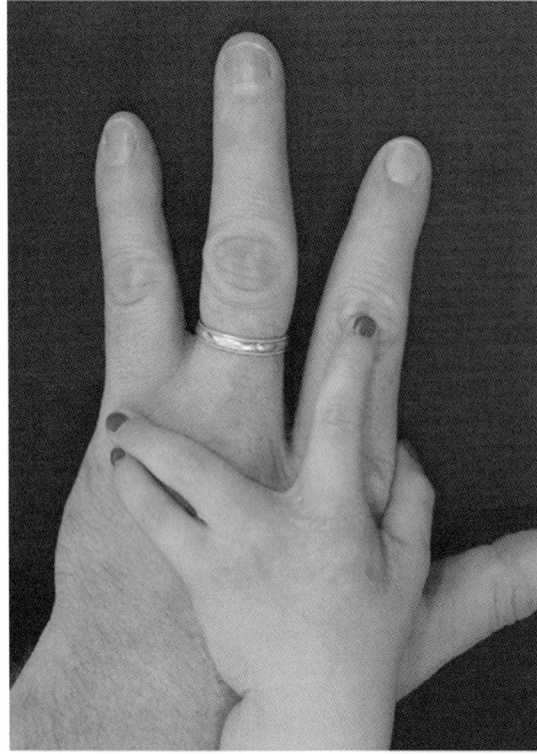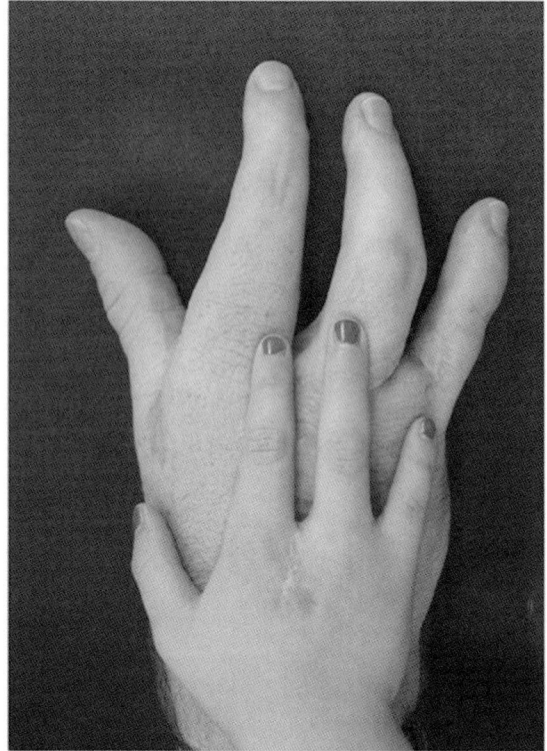

A

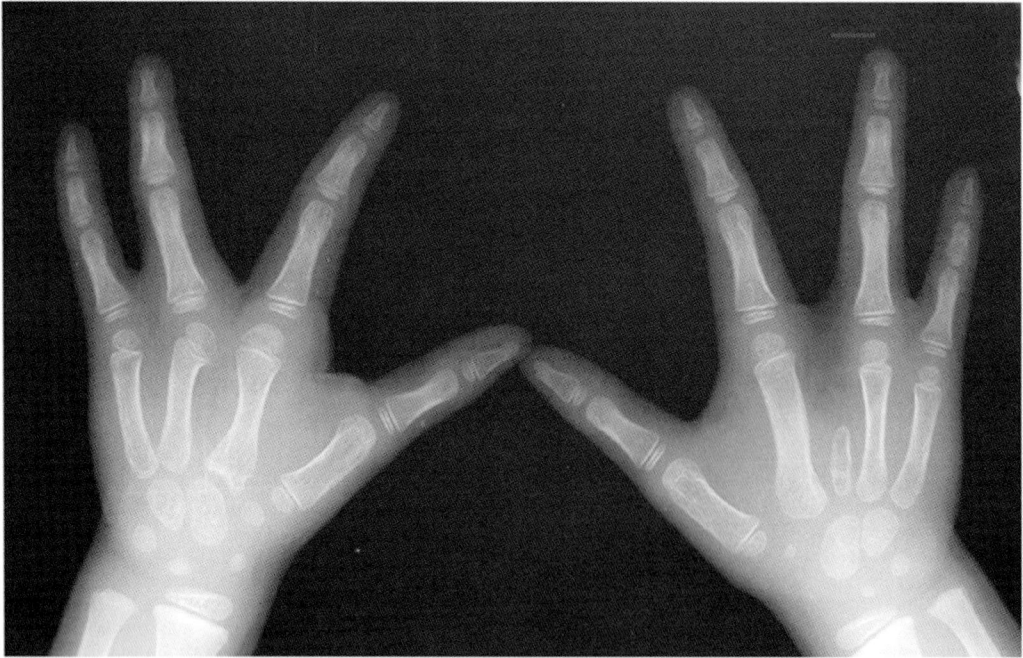

B

FIGURE 203-32. Typical outcome. *A,* The uncorrected hands of a 4-year-old child shown with the hands of her father, who underwent correction 28 years earlier. The initial central cleft was asymmetric in both patients. *B,* The radiograph of the daughter's left hand shows the typical increased length, radial deviation, and slight supination of the index ray, which was transposed at the CMC level. This was corrected with a secondary metacarpal osteotomy and might have been avoided with a greater release of the first dorsal interosseous muscles from the thumb metacarpal and more extensive shortening of the index metacarpal at the time of initial transposition. Note that the small third metacarpal on the left hand was not excised.

improved. All nine of these patients felt much less conspicuous about their hands.

In 82 hands treated with modified incisions (see Fig. 203-28), there were no flap losses. Visualization was excellent for dissection of the intrinsic muscles and index ray transposition at the CMC joint level. Secondary procedures have been performed in 15 hands, including excision of hypertrophic scars (5 hands), Z-plasties and other modifications of the first web space (9 hands), osteotomy of the index metacarpal (2 hands), tendon transfer of the extensor carpi radialis longus plus tendon graft to restore index abduction (2 hands), correction of MP or PIP joint flexion contractures (2 hands), tendon transfer to strengthen adductor pollicis function (2 hands), and arthrodesis for correction of joint instability or malposition (4 hands). Excessive pronation of the transposed index digit has not been a problem with pinch, which has been weak in all patients (see Fig. 203-32).

TREATMENT OF THE FOOT

In children with bilateral upper and lower limb involvement, the treatment of the foot must parallel that of the hand. The same general principles of treatment apply, and most patients adapt to their foot deficiencies remarkably well. Although the hand surgeon may not be involved with the foot surgery, her or his opinion will be sought by the parents. Foot deformities are classified into six groups[223] on the basis of skeletal anatomy. In types I and II, all metatarsals are present; in type VI, only the fibular ray is intact with phalangeal segments. Transverse bones, polydactyly, syndactyly, and marked deviation occur within the intermediate groups as the central rays are suppressed before the medial (tibial) ray.

Surgery is rarely necessary but may improve function. These patients are likely to complain more about their feet than their hands because of the weight-bearing function of the lower extremities. Excision of anomalous bones, osteotomies for correction of major deviation, and partial cleft closure will often release symptomatic pressure points and facilitate shoe wear.

Ulnar Deficiencies

CLASSIFICATION

The manifestations of ulnar failure of formation are so diverse, with numerous combinations of deformities at all skeletal levels, that a universal classification system is impossible. Nevertheless, many systems have been proposed for classification of these anomalies.[224-229] Bayne's system[118] combines features of many different systems and is most useful clinically (Fig. 203-33).

In type I deformities, the distal ulnar epiphysis is present but deficient. There is minimal shortening or clinical deviation of the hand. The proximal ulna, elbow, and shoulder are normal. In type II deformity, the most common type, the distal or middle third of the ulna is deficient. A fibrous anlage is present, and there may be bowing of the radius. In two thirds of patients, an inert cartilage block, which is radiopaque within the first year of life, is present and may contribute to progressive radial head migration. The radial head may be dislocated, and the distal radial epiphysis may be slanted in an ulnar direction. The proximal ulna is present and articulates with the humerus. The hand and wrist may be deviated and may exhibit deformities unrelated to the severity of the forearm abnormality. Some postaxial hand deficiency is invariably present. In type III deficiencies, the ulna is completely absent, there is no ulnar anlage, deviation of the hand is minimal, and the radius may be straight but is often bowed. The elbow is unstable, and the radial head is dislocated. Two clinical subtypes of type III deformity exist, including those with (1) severe elbow flexion contractures, "pterygium cubitale," and (2) progressive radial head dislocation. Severe hand deformities are present. In type IV deficiencies, there is a radiohumeral synostosis with shortening of the entire limb. The ulna is usually completely absent but may be represented by a small olecranon fused to the humerus. The hand and forearm are usually supinated away from the body and held in a posterior posture, sometimes referred to as "hand behind back" or "hand on flank" position. A fibrous ulnar anlage is usually present with severe radial bowing, and hand anomalies are always present.[118,224,230,231]

Patients with ulnar clubhand posturing due to a congenital pseudarthrosis of the ulna associated with neurofibromatosis are not included in this group.

INCIDENCE

Ulnar deficiencies are uncommon, and almost all are sporadic. Birch-Jensen[180] reported an incidence of 1 in 100,000 live births, and most authors find one ulnar absence for every 5 to 10 radial deficiencies.[229,232,233]

Between 25% and 50% of affected patients have associated defects, which are usually musculoskeletal, including femoral focal deficiency, fibular defects, scoliosis, clubfeet, and congenital dislocation of the hip. In contrast to radial defects, ulnar deficiencies are rarely associated with abnormalities in the hematopoietic, gastrointestinal, genitourinary, and cardiopulmonary systems. Only 25% of patients have contralateral upper extremity defects.[226,227,229,230,234,235]

ETIOLOGY

There is no clear understanding of the pathogenesis of ulnar failure of formation other than the work of Ogino.[72,187] Although the etiology of ulnar deficiency

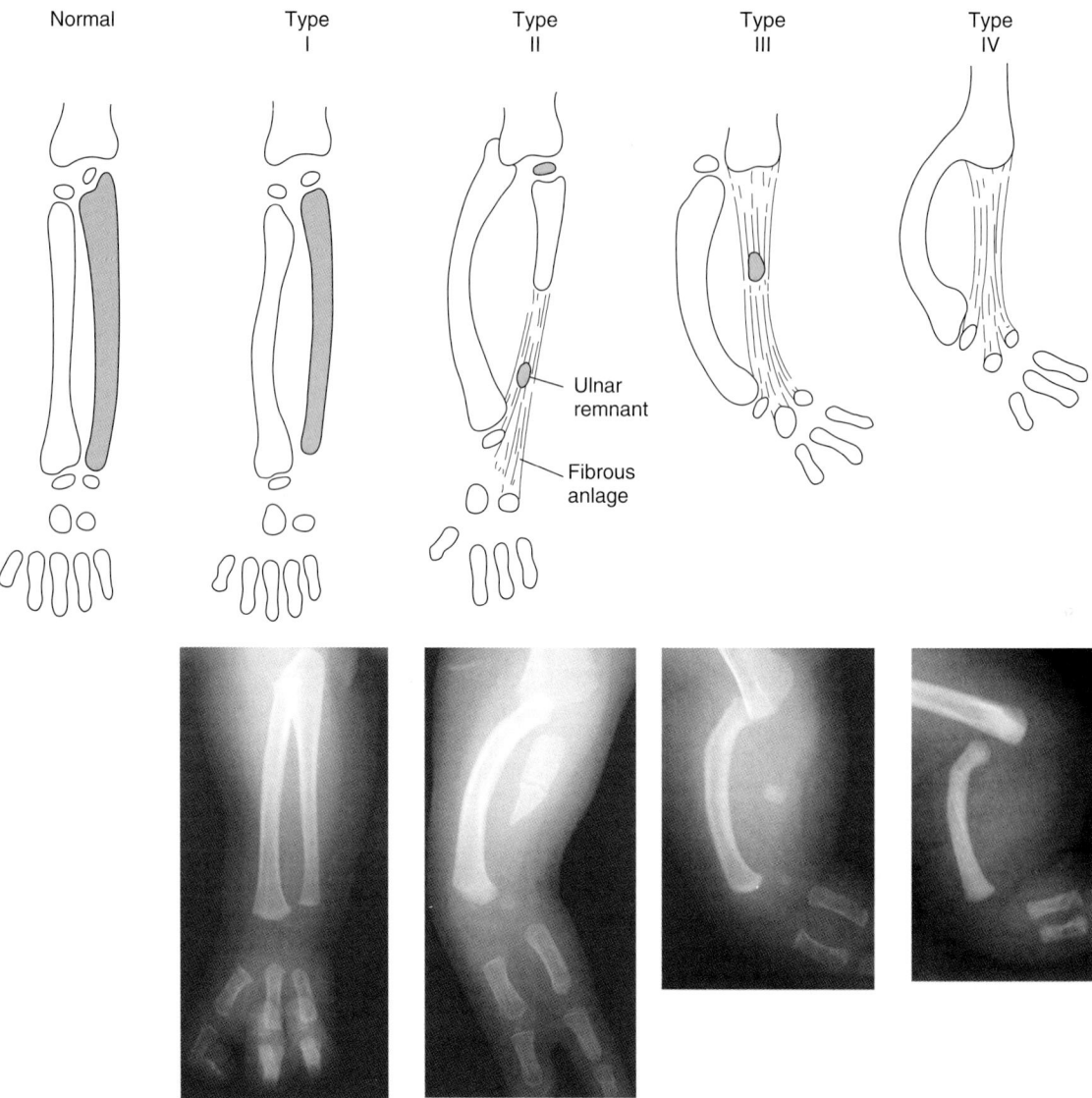

FIGURE 203-33. Classification of ulnar failure of formation. The four categories of ulnar failure of formation (ulnar clubbed hand) are contrasted to a normal hand and arm. In all cases, the forearm is shorter than normal. Associated hand deformities are variable. In type I, the ulna is present but short. In type II, which is the most common type, the proximal one or two thirds of the ulna is present and there may be bowing of the radius. There is bowing with or without radial head dislocation in type III and type IV deformities. The "hand behind back" or "hand on flank" posture is commonly seen in the type IV defects, which are characterized by humeroradial synostosis and total absence of the ulna. (Illustration by Jean Biddl.)

is unknown, and no teratogenic associations have been identified, familial inheritance has been described.[169] Although most instances occur with autosomal dominant inheritance, they may also occur with syndromes that demonstrate great variation in mendelian inheritance patterns.[169,231]

Ulnar defects may be found in patients with several malformation syndromes, including orofacial malformations, Cornelia de Lange syndrome, femur-fibula-ulna syndrome, and ulnar-mammary syn-

drome.[194] The ulnar-mammary syndrome is interesting because it presents with a wide variety of ulnar defects of the arm-forearm-hand, hypoplasia of mammary glands, and underdeveloped external genitalia. In humans, the *TBX3* gene is important in limb, mammary gland epithelial, genital tubercle, and uterine development,[236] and mice lacking the *tbx3* gene show forelimb and hindlimb deficiencies similar to those seen in humans with the ulnar-mammary syndrome.[237]

CLINICAL PRESENTATION

Ulnar deformities predominantly involve the hand, wrist, forearm, and elbow. In a review of major reported series, Johnson[231] found that only 11% of individuals with ulnar deficiencies have a normal complement of digits, syndactyly is present in more than one third of patients, and metacarpals are usually absent proximal to missing digits.

Hand

To a great extent, hand anomalies determine functional status in this condition (Fig. 203-34). Interestingly, the extent of the hand anomaly does not always correspond to the severity of wrist, forearm, or upper arm deficiencies. A full complement of digits is present in 9% to 11% of patients,[230,234] and four digits are present in 12% of patients. A reduced number of digits is common, and the ring and fifth rays are most frequently deficient. More than 50% of patients have a radial-sided thumb deficiency, ranging from complete absence to hypoplasia to duplication.[230,233,238] All digits including the thumb ray are often in the same plane. Extra phalanges with longitudinal bracketed epiphyses are often found within the soft tissue syndactyly, and there is often a terminal phalangeal fusion. Many of the one-, two-, three-, and four-fingered hands are positioned on top of an intact radius-ulna and are reported under the ulnar failure of formation category. Some authors have designated them "special thumbs" or unclassifiable malformations. All of the affected hands are hypoplastic (see Fig. 203-34). Various combinations of tendon and neurovascular anomalies may be present.

Wrist

At the wrist level, carpal bones are frequently missing, and ossification centers appear delayed, in descending frequency, in the pisiform, hamate, triquetrum, capitate, and trapezoid.[101,227,234] In 25% of patients, carpal bones fail to differentiate, manifesting as coalitions that articulate well with the radius (see Fig. 203-34).[7] In contrast to radial ray defects, in which deformity is common, only 30% of patients demonstrate any ulnar deviation, and most of these have an ulnar slant to the radial articular surface. The degree of ulnar deviation is less than 30 degrees in most patients.[223] In a minority of patients, the deviation is severe, measuring more than 30 degrees and significantly affecting growth and formation.[231,233,234,239-241] Total active motion of the wrist averages 70 degrees of normal and is not severely affected by radial head dislocation or bowing. There has been disagreement about the cause of ulnar deviation. Some believe it is secondary to an intrinsic mesenchymal defect during development,[233] whereas others hold that the bowing is secondary to the tethering effect of the fibrous anlage, which has been compared with a fiberglass fishing pole that will bend but not lengthen.[231,234,242]

Forearm

Abnormalities of the forearm are variable. Type II deformities are present in almost two thirds of patients. In patients with type II defects, there is partial hypoplasia of the forearm, and although a distal ulnar epiphysis does appear, growth is delayed. Whereas some patients demonstrate "catch-up" growth, the forearm grows proportionately with the rest of the limb in most patients.[231,234,242] There is variable bowing of the radius and ulnar deviation of the hand. Anomalies of tendons, muscles, and neurovascular structures are related to the degree of the deformity and are best documented by Stoffel.[110,231,234,242]

The existence of an anlage in type II and type III deformities has aroused considerable interest.[243] Some surgeons believe that as the patient grows, this "fibrous cord" acts as a tether on the distal radius and contributes to bowing of the radius, dislocation of the radial head (which is often present at birth), and ulnar slant of the distal radius (Figs. 203-35 and 203-36), and they recommend excision of the cord early in life to prevent these developments.[227,228,232] Others maintain that severe ulnar deviation occurs so infrequently that routine resection of the anlage is warranted only for patients showing progressive deviation with growth.[226,231,233] Absence of extrinsic flexor and extensor muscles within the forearm parallels the degree of the deformity. Although the ulnar artery is often absent, the ulnar nerve is usually present in type II defects, lying directly beneath the fibrous anlage.

Although growth does occur and provides adequate support for the wrist and hand, in both minimal and moderate deformities, the distal radial epiphysis is present but demonstrates delayed growth in 60% of patients. The radius is almost always short. In severe deformities, there does not appear to be a correlation between the ulnar tilt of the distal radius and the degree of radial bowing.

Elbow

Although the hand is usually stable at the wrist, the elbow is frequently unstable or fused. In type I limbs, the joint configuration is almost normal, but elbow abnormalities occur in all patients presenting with severe defects. A radial head dislocation is usually present at birth and may or may not improve with growth but frequently affects motion. These patients may have functional but limited pronation and especially supination. A humeroradial synostosis is present in the most severe deficiencies. In these patients, the humerus is hypoplastic, and the hand and forearm are usually not positioned optimally, lying in a supinated position in the posterior axillary line

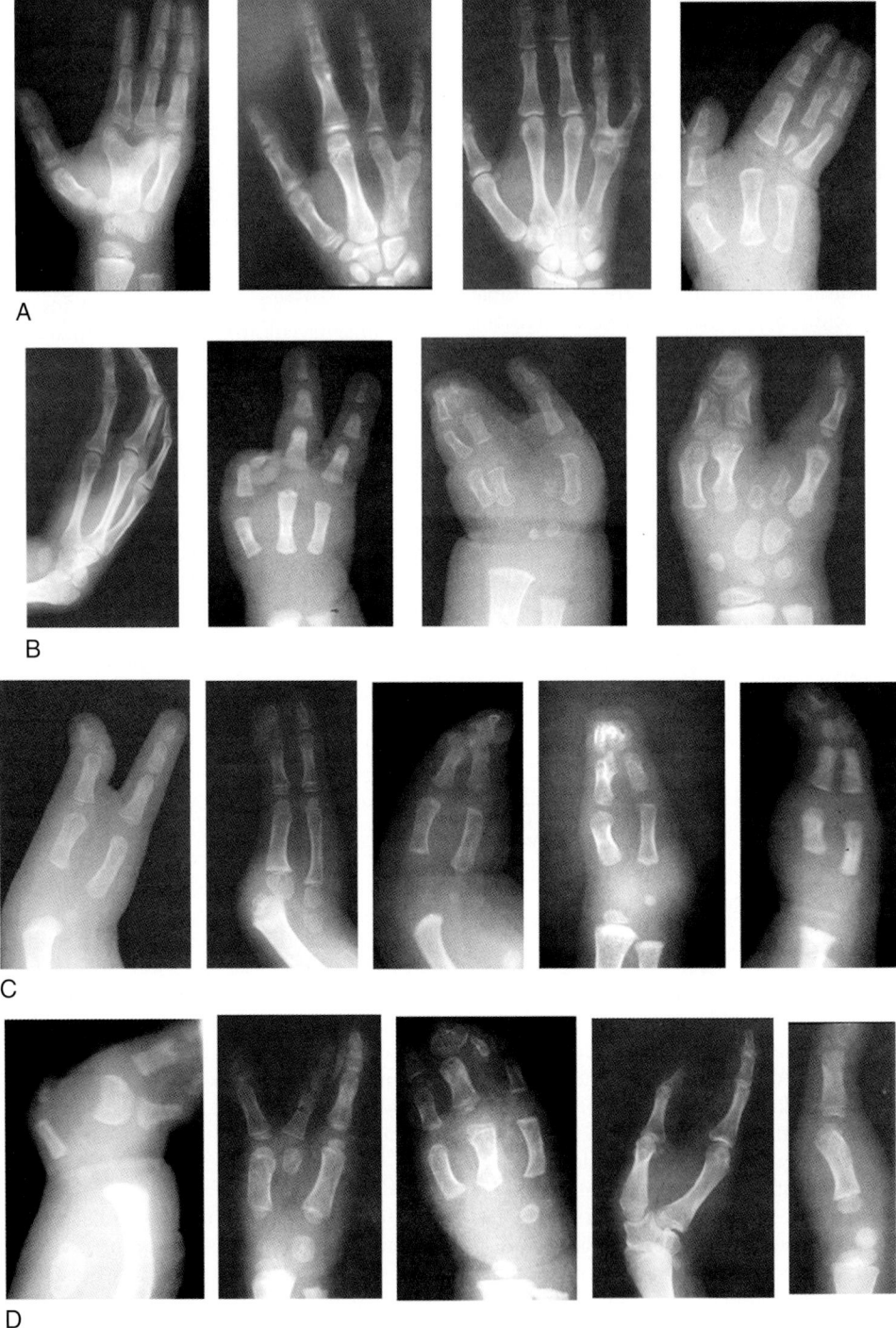

A

B

C

D

FIGURE 203-34. Spectrum of hand malformations in patients with ulnar deficiencies. Patients with ulnar failure of formation have a wide variety of hand malformations, which do not necessarily correlate in severity with the forearm deformities. *A,* In four- and five-fingered hands, the thumb is free and many variations of metacarpal fusion are seen. There may also be a central set of phalanges without metacarpal articulation. *B,* In three-fingered hands, the thumb may be free or joined to the index ray in a simple or complex syndactyly. The most common variation, shown in the second panel, contains a thumb and two rays, all separated from one another. *C,* In two-fingered hands, the digits are joined in a complete syndactyly. These are associated with all types of ulnar deficiency but most often with type III and type IV. *D,* Other forms of one-, two-, and three-fingered hands with and without evidence of skeletal fusions may be encountered.

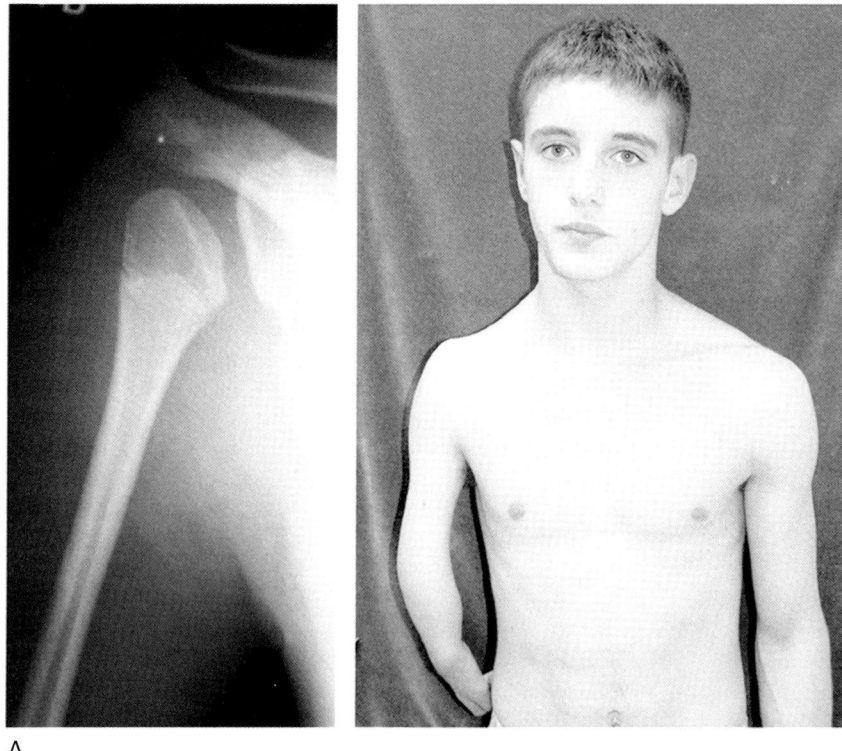

A

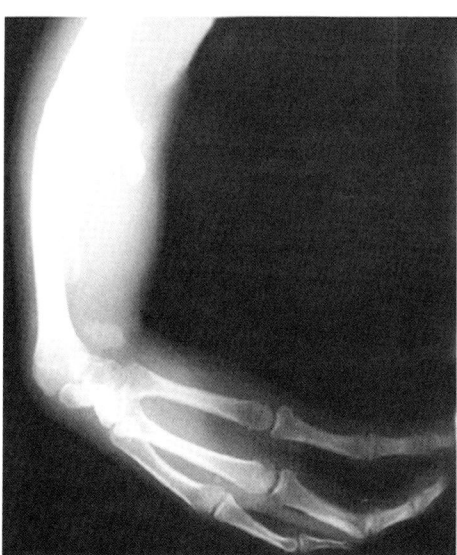

B

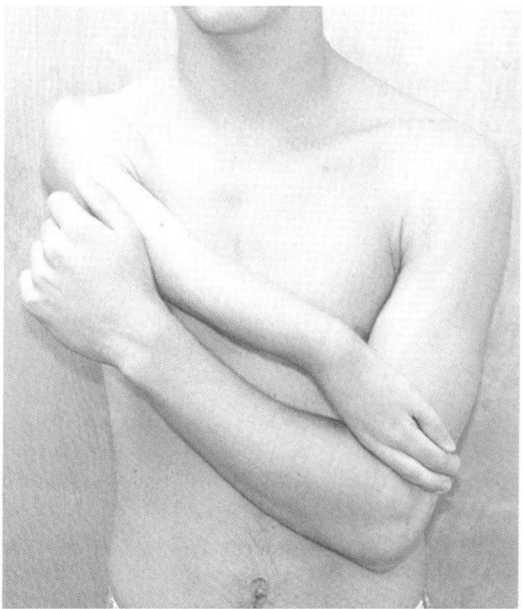

FIGURE 203-35. Shoulder and forearm in type IV ulnar deformities. *A,* Frequently overlooked is the ipsilateral shoulder hypoplasia in these patients. Both the glenoid and humeral head are deficient. *B,* The humeroradial synostosis is always associated with a marked shortening of the forearm. The only surgery performed on this boy was on his hand. As a teenager, he will have lengthenings at both arm and forearm levels.

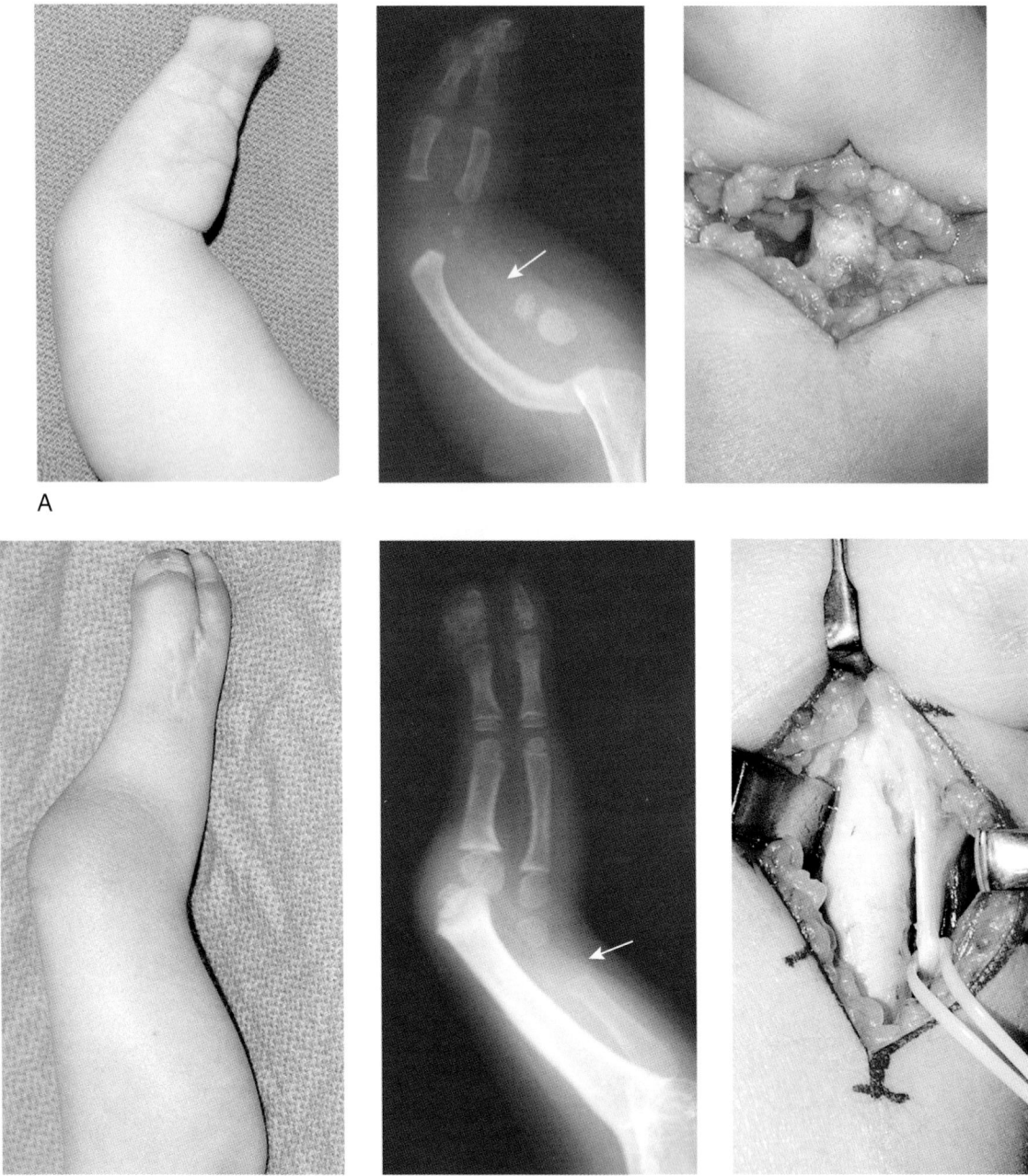

FIGURE 203-36. Forearm bowing and anlage. *A,* The arrow indicates the position of the fibrous anlage in this child with a two-fingered hand and type III ulnar deficiency. The histologic examination of this fibrous cord often shows cartilage, which represents primordial bone. *B,* Another two-fingered hand in a child with a type II ulnar deficiency is shown. The loop is encircling the anlage, which was composed entirely of cartilage.

(Fig. 203-37). These children with bilateral deformities are unable to reach their mouths.

Upper Arm and Shoulder

Despite an extensive body of literature concerning ulnar deficiencies, the arm and shoulder are rarely mentioned in surgical series. The author's experience is similar to that of Buck-Gramcko, who observed that shoulder strength and mobility are usually normal when the only malformations are in the distal portion of the extremity. The shoulder is never completely normal when there are deficiencies at the forearm, elbow, and arm levels. Deficiencies of the muscles and hypoplasia of both the glenoid fossa and humerus are common (see Fig. 203-35), but synostosis at the glenohumeral joint is rare.

Despite significant anatomic deformities, patients with ulnar deficits function well. "The deformed limb is much more useful than its anatomical condition would lead one to expect."[241] Grip is significantly reduced and prehension difficult, especially in children with limited numbers of digits.[231,244] Functional testing by Flatt,[109] Johnson,[231] and Blair[244] demonstrated that the hand deformity provides the greatest functional limitation and that patients with ulnar deficiencies generally adapt to and use these limbs much better than expected.

TREATMENT

Conservative

Infants with ulnar deviation should receive manipulation or splinting as early as possible to achieve passive correction. Splints should be worn continuously during the first year of life and at night thereafter in an effort to achieve maximum correction early. Conservative treatment is of no benefit and is contraindicated in children who are having functional difficulty.

Hand

Surgical treatment in patients with ulnar deficiencies is primarily limited to the hand. In our experience, approximately 90% of all procedures performed on these children were distal to the wrist.[118,230,233-245] Hand deformities vary, and absence of rays on the ulnar side is common. Complete syndactylies between the thumb-index and index-long webs should be released early to avoid discrepant growth. A rotational osteotomy at the metacarpal level is often necessary for opposition of mobile digits that are present (Fig. 203-38). These operations are frequently delayed until the thenar muscles have had a chance to develop and rotate the thumb ray into palmar abduction after an adequate first web space has been established. For the two-digit hand or hand with no thumb, a formal pollicization of the radial digit is recommended. Osteotomies of both metacarpals in the two-digit hand

are often necessary to form a pulp to pulp pinch of opposing digits. A rotational flap with a modified Z-plasty may be helpful.[233] However, it is preferable to use a dorsal advancement-rotation flap.[116] Short metacarpals with functional digits are easily lengthened with distraction techniques and bone grafts.

Wrist and Forearm

Some surgeons recommend resection of the fibrous anlage early in life for patients with severe radial bowing, ulnar slant to the radial articular surface, and radial head dislocation, before growth accentuates these deformities (Fig. 203-39; see also Fig. 203-36).[227] Resection of the cord should start as far distally as possible in type II and type III deformities, and care must be taken to avoid injury to the ulnar nerve, which is directly beneath the fibrous anlage, and to the posterior interosseous nerve in the proximal forearm. At the same time, the forearm can be straightened with an opening wedge osteotomy and bone graft (see Fig. 203-39).

Early resection of the anlage remains controversial, and many surgeons prefer to wait because the natural history of more severe deformities indicates that radial bowing may improve spontaneously, the ulnar tilt of the epiphysis is rarely extensive, the radial head dislocation is not progressive, and the functional results without anlage resection are usually excellent.[231,233,234] Most authors agree that resection of the fibrous anlage improves ulnar deviation and should be considered for angulation greater than 30% that occurs during a period of 6 months. It is preferable to excise the anlage in severe type II and most type III and type IV deformities and to correct excessive angulation of the short, bowed radius with osteotomy and bone graft.

The formation of a one-bone forearm by fusing the proximal ulna to the distal radius has been recommended for type III and type IV deformities.[226,243] Advantages of this approach include increased forearm length, removal of the obstruction to full extension caused by the radial head, stable forearm, and better appearance. These gains come at the expense of pronation and some supination (see Fig. 203-39). Distal distraction of the radius before radioulnar synostosis facilitates fusion. Other useful forearm procedures in fully grown patients include complete wedge osteotomies for correction of excessive bowing and derotational osteotomies for correction of excessive pronation or supination. Resection of the dislocated radial head is seldom performed and must be combined with construction of a one-bone forearm.[118] This procedure is reserved for patients with a demonstrable decrease in elbow motion and greater proximal migration of the radial head.[246]

Distraction devices can be used to maximize potential length lost by overriding of the proximal radius,

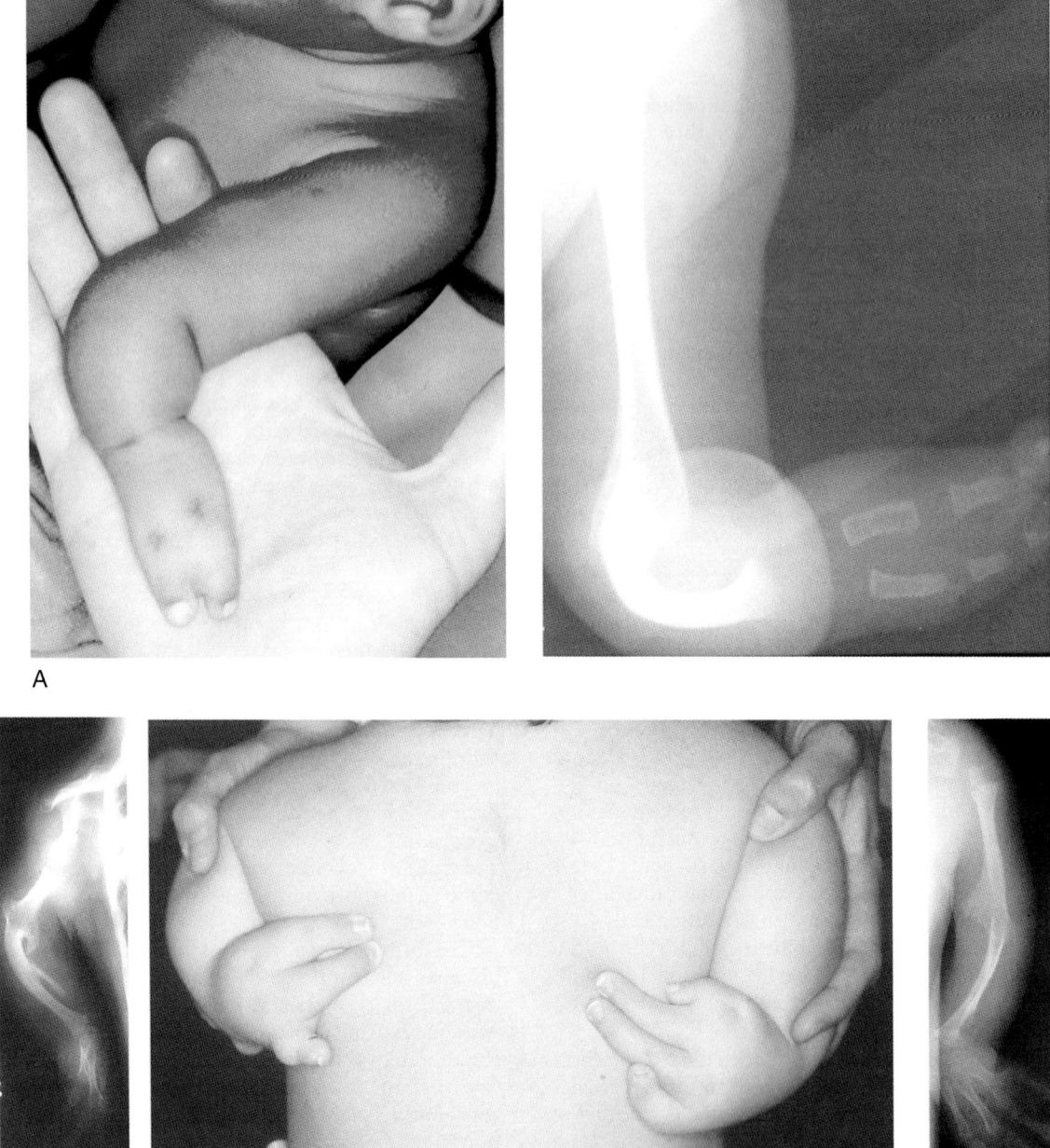

FIGURE 203-37. Humeroradial synostosis and hand behind back. *A*, The "hand behind back" position of both hands in this patient is due to the marked angulation and supination of the radius distal to the site of synostosis. *B*, The same hand posture is seen in this child with the Nager syndrome. Note the asymmetric ulnar deficiency, with type IV on the left and type III on the right.

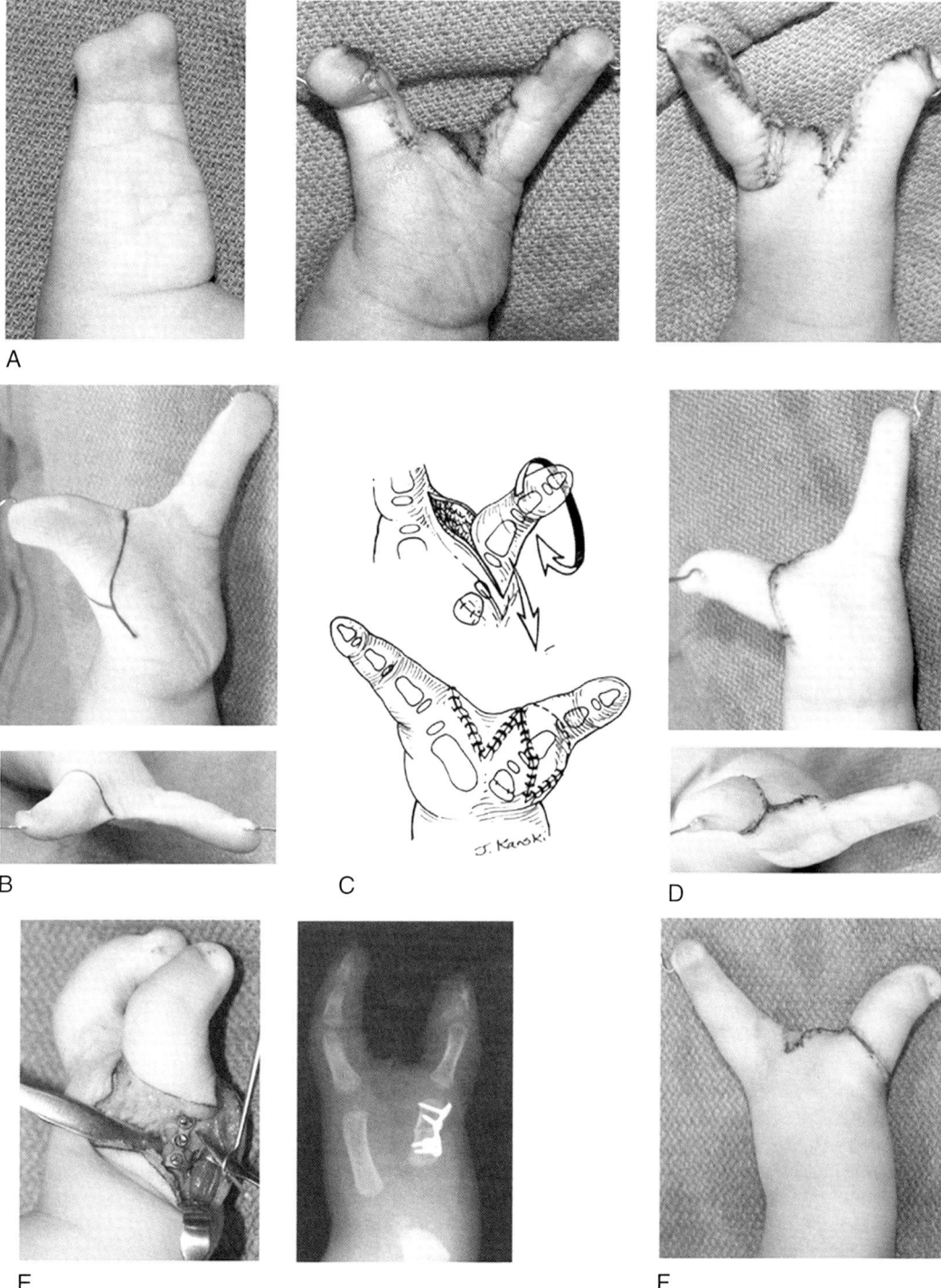

FIGURE 203-38. Two-fingered hand. *A,* The first procedure in this child with a two-fingered hand was a simple syndactyly release in which all available soft tissue was placed within the commissure. Skin grafts and distal closures were also used. No osteotomies were performed during this stage. *B,* The incisions for a rotation-recession osteotomy of the thumb are marked 2 years later. The degree of rotation was determined by the degree of development of the thenar intrinsic muscles and the corresponding pronation of the first ray after syndactyly release. *C,* An illustration of the procedure shows a Y-V advancement of the thumb and a Z-plasty within the expanded first web space. *D,* The appearance of the hand after closure. *E,* Miniplate and screw fixation was used for fixation after osteotomy. *F,* The web space has been widened and adjusted to ensure the optimal position for opposition of the two digits for pinch.

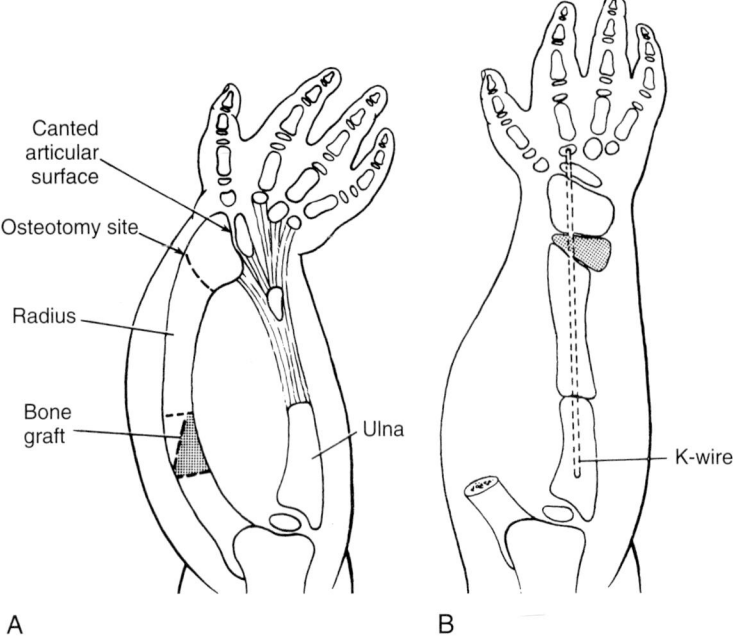

FIGURE 203-39. Creation of one-bone forearm. *A,* This illustration shows a type II deformity with significant bowing. The fibrous anlage and canted articular surface of the distal radius are demonstrated. A cartilage block that does not grow cannot be seen on routine radiographs but is typically present. The planned osteotomy sites within the radius are marked. A portion of the proximal radius will be used as a graft after opening wedge osteotomy in the distal third of the radius. *B,* A one-bone forearm has been constructed by transposing the radius onto the proximal ulna. A bone graft has been used to correct the ulnar angulation. The current approach is to gain additional length with distraction of the radius and hand after excision of the anlage (if present). (Illustration by Jean Biddl.)

especially in the construction of a one-bone forearm.[242] Patients with type II, type III, and type IV deformities have extremely good function. Although range of motion at the elbow and strength of the wrist and grip are markedly reduced, these youngsters, including those with bilateral deformities, manage well.

Elbow

Surgery on the upper arm and forearm frequently precedes refinement procedures on the hand. Derotational osteotomy of the humerus is necessary in most patients with type IV deformities if the hand is to be of functional value. Osteotomy is most effectively performed at the humeroradial synostosis, with direct observation of the abnormal neurovascular structures to avoid kinking and entrapment. The goal of the procedure is to place the hand in front of the body and in midforearm rotation with approximately 60 degrees of elbow flexion. Removal of a segment of bone often releases tension on neurovascular structures.

Arthroplasty of congenital elbow synostoses in patients with ulnar deficiencies does not produce predictable stability or motion, and total joint replacement with alloplastic materials has not been reported. Vilkki[163] has used a vascularized metatarsophalangeal joint from the foot for elbow mobilization. Patients with fixed elbow contractures of more than 90 degrees are often better treated with amputation to facilitate prosthetic supplementation. Children with elbow contractures secondary to skin deficiencies respond well to preoperative expansion.[247]

Symbrachydactyly (Atypical Cleft Hand)

Symbrachydactyly (*sym,* together; *brachy,* short; *dactyl,* digit) literally refers to a hand with short, webbed digits. As several investigators have demonstrated, a wide spectrum exists within this broad definition,[186,204,248-250] and these hands do not represent a terminal failure of formation.

POLAND SYNDROME

The most notable instance of symbrachydactyly was described originally in the *Guy's Hospital Reports* in 1841.[251,252] Alfred Poland, then a student dissector within the department of anatomy, described the chest wall and limb anomalies of a deceased street person, George Elt. This report contained detailed drawings of the axillary and chest wall anomalies and demonstrated the absence of the sternal head of the pectoralis major muscle and a portion of the serratus anterior muscle. The hand was described as hypoplastic with short webbed digits but was not illustrated. One hundred years later, Patrick Clarkson, the senior hand surgeon in Guy's Hospital, noted the hand in the archives of the hospital's museum and described it in detail.[253] Thus, the eponym Poland syndrome was established.[253-257] Poland syndrome has come to denote a variety of phenotypic features to specialists, and its use in the literature has been inconsistent. To the upper extremity surgeon, Poland syndrome consists of two primary components, an absent sternocostal portion of the pectoralis major muscle and a hypoplastic hand with short webbed digits. Within this group of patients, a wide spectrum of hand malformations exists, from a hand with central short digits to a hand with no digits at all. Similarly, these patients may also have a wide variety of additional ipsilateral chest wall skeletal and soft tissue abnormalities (see Chapter 204).

The severity of the brachysyndactyly in patients with Poland syndrome has been classified as mild, moderate, and severe.[258] All of these patients have triphalangeal digits, with most variation in the middle phalanx. Most of the clinical features seen in this syndrome occur at stage 19 of embryonic life[259]; these include splitting of the pectoralis muscle mass into sternal and clavicular portions, early separation of the digits, and chondrification of the middle phalanges. The radiologic features of these middle phalanges vary, but the more hypoplastic forms show a central sclerotic nidus characteristic of vascular compromise. The cause of these abnormal changes has been proposed to be a vascular arrest[258,260,261] at this critical stage. A more extensive vascular arrest involving the hand plate would account for more severe absence deformities within the teratologic spectrum seen in symbrachydactyly.

INCIDENCE

There are few published reports estimating the incidence of symbrachydactyly. A house-to-house survey from Brazil revealed an incidence of 4 to 5 per 10,000 live births.[262] Only half of the affected individuals in that study had pectoral muscle abnormalities,[256] with a reported incidence of 1 in 20,000 to 30,000 live births. Yamauchi, who used a much broader definition of symbrachydactyly,[29,263] estimated close to 1 in 10,000 live births.

Given the broad morphologic spectrum of types, overlapping terminology, and wide differences in both reporting and analysis of data, one cannot reach a more specific conclusion about the prevalence of this condition. A more accurate estimate of incidence is difficult to determine.

CLASSIFICATION

The original classification by Pol[264] separated patients with digital reduction and syndactyly into two groups according to the presence or absence of pectoral defects. His system was further refined to the system presently used that recognizes a definite reduction sequence of skeletal parts.[186,249,265,266] According to the current system, the reduction initially affects the central three (index, long, and ring) rays of the hand and gradually progresses to a total absence of digits and finally to a total absence of the thumb. The term *symbrachydactyly* is appropriate if the absent digits are represented by small rudimentary nubbins. Hands with

TABLE 203-7 ✦ FOUR BASIC TYPES OF SYMBRACHYDACTYLY

The *short-finger type,* characterized by the presence of a thumb and four short coalesced stiff digits, which may have one or more missing phalanges within these digits

The *oligodactylic* or *"atypical cleft hand" type,* characterized by a central aplasia of digits, with thumb and fifth digit present

The *monodactylic type,* characterized by the presence of a thumb and four associated digital remnants

The *peromelic type,* characterized by a complete absence of all digits at the metacarpal level.

Modified from Blauth W, Gekeler J: Zur Morphologie und Klassifikation der Symbrachydaktylie. Handchirurgie 1971;3:123-128.

symbrachydactyly were originally divided into four basic types (Fig. 203-40 and Table 203-7).[249]

Yamauchi and Tanabu expanded this system into seven categories based on the radiologic pattern of skeletal reduction,[29,263] which is useful for clinical analysis and decision-making (Fig. 203-41 and Table 203-8).

ETIOLOGY

The cause of symbrachydactyly is unknown. Because almost all symbrachydactylies are unilateral malformations, many investigators doubt that there is a genetic cause or predisposition. Some authors have

TABLE 203-8 ✦ SYMBRACHYDACTYLY TYPES BASED ON RADIOLOGIC PATTERN OF SKELETAL REDUCTION

The *triphalangia type,* characterized by a hand with no missing bones, even though many phalanges (usually the middle phalanx) may be short

The *biphalangia type,* characterized by one or more missing phalanges in one or more digits

The *monophalangia type,* characterized by the presence of a thumb and one or more digits containing only one phalanx

The *aphalangia type,* characterized by the presence of a thumb and digital nubbins with no phalanges

The *ametacarpia type,* characterized by absence of the thumb and digits and absence of one or more metacarpals

The *acarpia type,* characterized by the absence of all digits and thumb and one or more carpal bones

The *forearm amputation type,* characterized by absence of the distal portion of the forearm with small rudimentary nubbins on the amputation stump

From Yamauchi Y, Tanabu S: Symbrachydactyly. In Buck-Gramcko E, ed: Congenital Malformations of the Hand and Forearm. London, Churchill Livingstone, 1998:149.

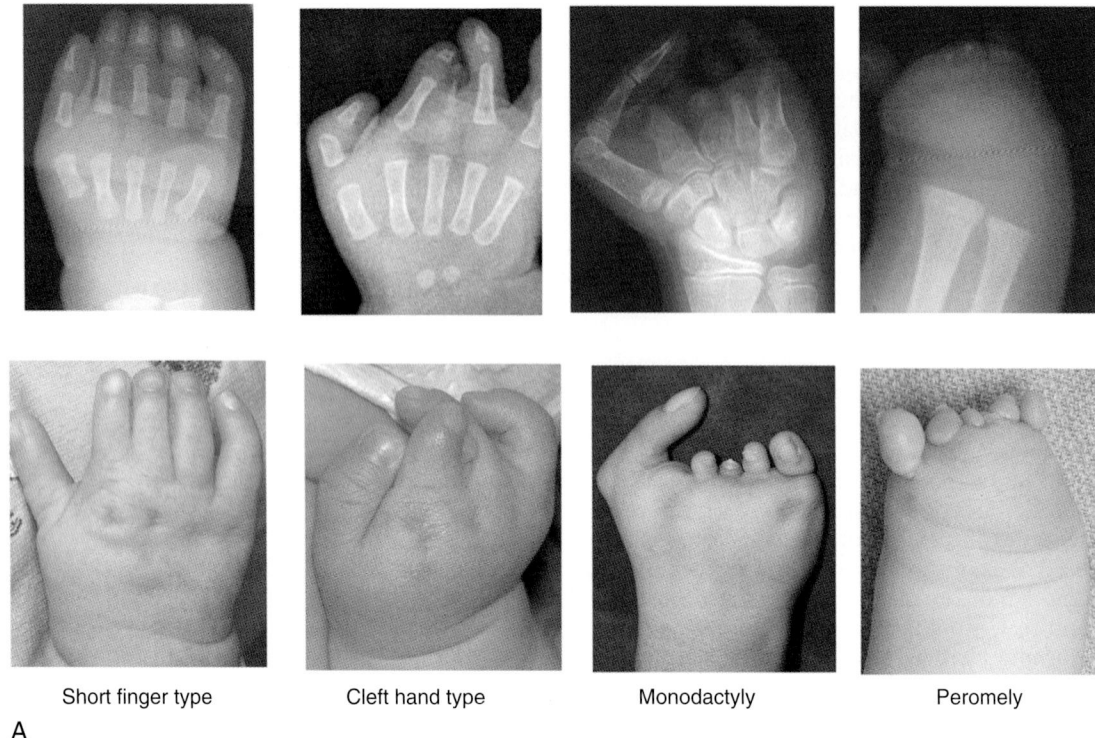

Short finger type   Cleft hand type   Monodactyly   Peromely

A

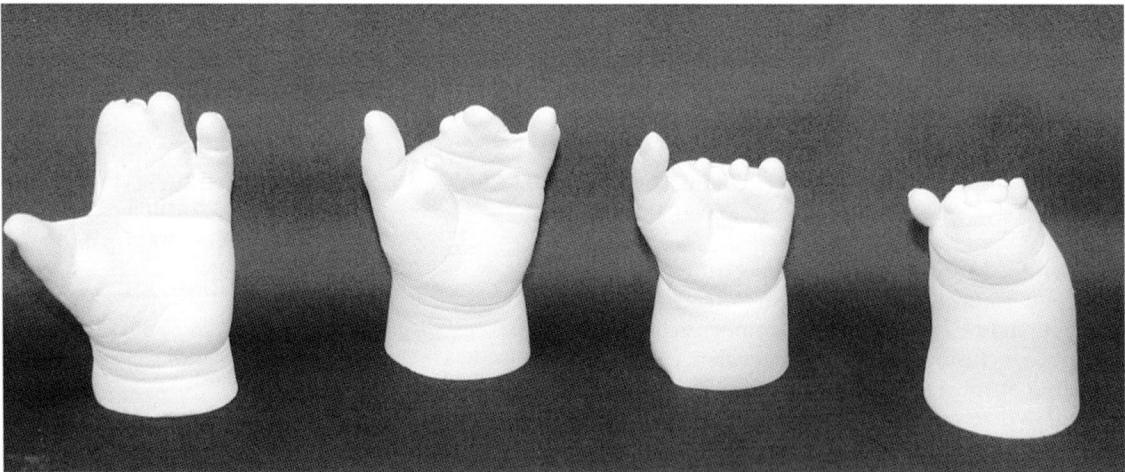

B

FIGURE 203-40. Symbrachydactyly classification. *A,* The original classification of symbrachydactyly was divided into four specific types, which are illustrated by these clinical pictures and radiographs. *B,* Clinical molds demonstrate the four types.

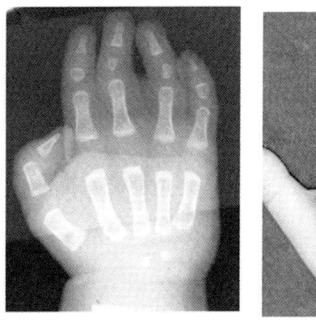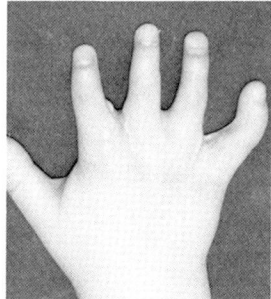

Triphalangia

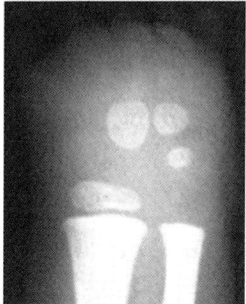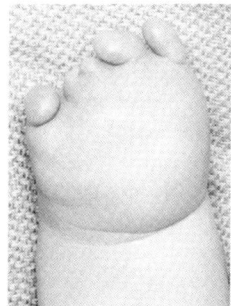

Ametacarpia

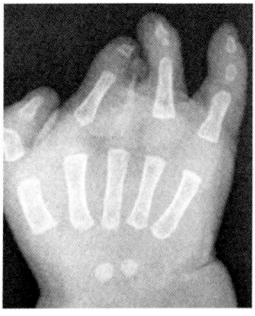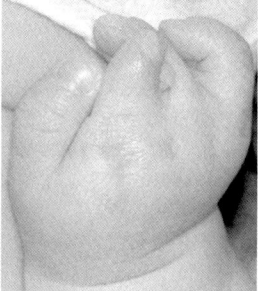

Biphalangia

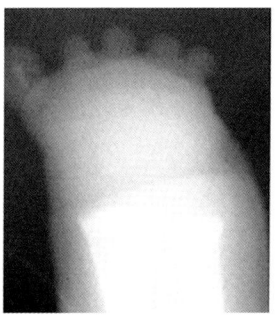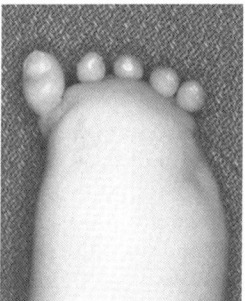

Acarpia

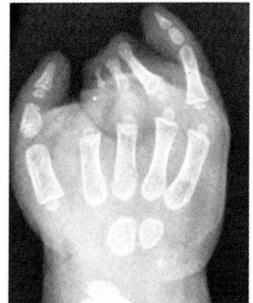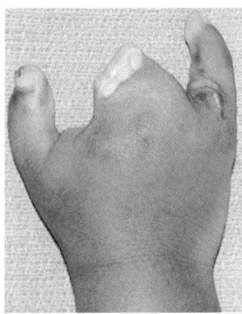

Monophalangia

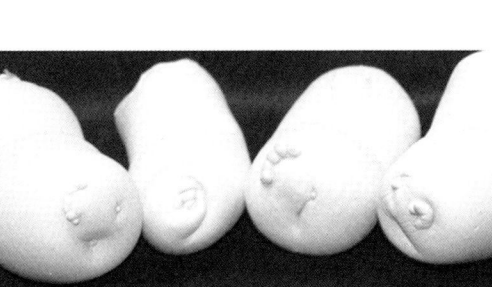

Forearm amputation

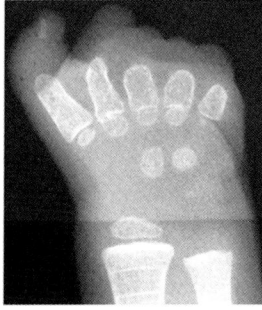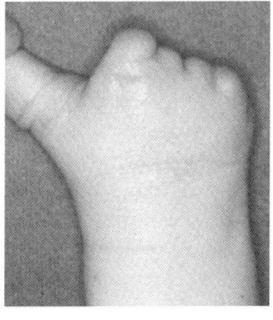

Aphalangia

FIGURE 203-41. Expanded symbrachydactyly classification. An expanded and clinically more useful classification incorporates the number of skeletal parts remaining at skeletal levels. The most common and clinically challenging varieties are at the monophalangeal and aphalangeal levels. Most of the acarpia and forearm level types are referred to the prosthetist. The characteristic diminutive hand nubbins are shown on these molds.

reported the occurrence of hand malformations other than symbrachydactyly in other members of the proband. Although many extrinsic causes are mentioned in the literature, there is no proven link to medication, radiation, trauma, infection, foods, or toxins. Imagawa[248] reported symbrachydactyly in the offspring of rats given 5-fluorouracil early in pregnancy. Several investigators have hypothesized that symbrachydactyly may be caused by necrosis of mesenchymal cells within the hand plate around Carnegie stage 17 to 20, during which time the cartilaginous anlage of skeletal structures is formed. According to this hypothesis, the syndactyly is due to the effect of this mesodermal aberration on the apical ectodermal ridge. By administering busulfan to pregnant rats, Ogino[72,189,267] produced central clefts, osseous syndactyly, and symbrachydactyly and has speculated that the defects are caused by a failure of induction of the digital rays within the hand plate. With respect to the Poland syndrome, no connection has been made between the hand deformities and the chest wall malformations, which are seen primarily in association with short-finger hand malformations.

Several investigators observed an association between the Poland syndrome and an ipsilateral hypoplasia of the subclavian artery,[261,265,268] primarily in children with coexisting congenital heart defects. This observation gave rise to the subclavian artery disruption sequence theory, which proposes that the constellation of malformations is the result of a vascular insult during the sixth week of gestation[258,265,269]; this is the embryonic stage when distinct subclavian and vertebral arteries branch off of the aorta, the pectoralis muscle develops, and digital separation occurs. Abnormalities of these developing vessels and vascular malformations of the ipsilateral hemithorax provided additional support for this theory.[260] The variability of the malformations is presumably related to the severity of the restriction of blood flow in utero. However, in an effort to reach some conformity concerning a confusing group of malformations, Müller,[186] Blauth,[249,250] Falliner,[270] and Buck-Gramcko[266] have suggested that there is a spectrum of maldevelopment extending from an intact hand with short middle phalanges (brachymesophalangia) and syndactyly to a hand with a thumb and no digits (oligodactyly or atypical cleft hand type) and finally to a hand with no thumb or digital rays (peromelic type).

It is proposed that the deficiency spectrum is due to progressive mesodermal deficiency, with insufficient skeletal framework to support the overlying soft tissues. Left unsupported, the digits do not differentiate and grow, instead forming small rudimentary nubbins with small nail appendages.[72,271] This process may affect all or only some digits and consistently involves digits, in descending order, as follows: index, long, ring, fifth, thumb.[137,248,249,255,267,271-273]

The sequence of deficiency seen in the middle phalanx is interesting and corresponds with our general understanding of embryology. Abnormalities of the middle phalanx are constant features in the more complete Poland hands with three phalanges (four-finger type or triphalangeal type). An ischemic insult to the digit probably occurs during embryonic stage 19, which corresponds to postovulatory day 47,[259] at which time chondrification of the middle phalanx occurs. The proximal and distal phalanges chondrify at stages 18 and 20, respectively. The normal sequence of development of the tubular bones in the hand progresses from condensation of mesenchyme to chondrification and then ossification.[274] The initial chondrification starts in the midportion of the bone and then spreads in a circular fashion, first proximally and then distally. The shapes seen in these smaller-than-normal middle phalanges (brachymesophalangia) progress from complete absence or aplasia to a small nidus,[258] a round or circular phalanx, a triangular or delta-shaped phalanx, and finally a larger or truncated phalanx. The epiphyses of these middle phalanges are abnormal and have great similarity to those seen in conditions with abnormal chondrification, such as the Goltz syndrome.

Why is the distal phalanx present in these symbrachydactylies? The distal phalanges chondrify during embryonic stage 20. However, only the proximal two thirds of this bone will ossify through chondrification; the distal portion develops through intramembranous ossification. This may explain the presence of diminutive distal phalanges in the hypoplastic nubbins when other phalanges are absent from these digits.

CLINICAL PRESENTATION

The presentation of patients with symbrachydactyly is highly variable, and no two hands are alike. In all types, the entire hand is hypoplastic relative to the normal contralateral hand. Although patients with bilateral deformities have been described,[250,272,275] they are rare. In the author's experience with 270 symbrachydactyly patients, only three have had bilateral involvement. Within this group are six sets of monozygotic twins, one of whom has a unilateral symbrachydactyly.

In the short-finger type, all extrinsic and intrinsic muscles are intact. The triphalangeal variety is characterized by a normal thumb and fifth ray with the central three digits usually joined by an incomplete simple syndactyly. There is no skeletal coalition. The middle phalanx is the most hypoplastic, and there is moderate shortening of the proximal phalanx. The most frequently hypoplastic digit is the index, followed by the long and ring fingers (Fig. 203-42).

In the biphalangeal type, the index and long digits are also the most commonly affected. The middle

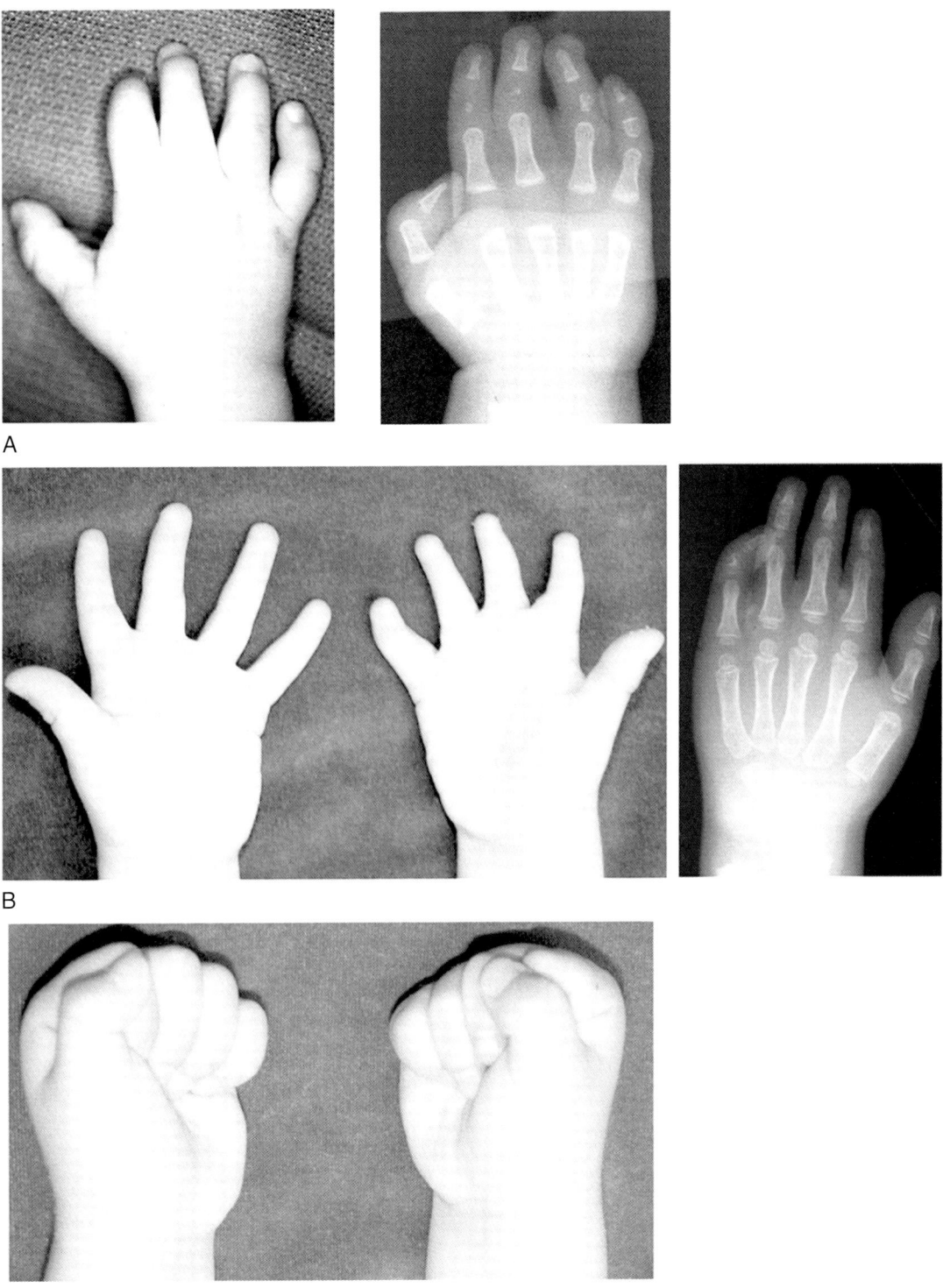

FIGURE 203-42. Symbrachydactyly, short-finger type. *A,* The typical short-finger type has the normal number of digits with the normal complement of phalanges joined by a simple, incomplete syndactyly. *B,* After routine syndactyly releases, the shortness of the digits can be appreciated. The middle phalangeal segments are the most deficient, and there is usually radial clinodactyly of the fifth digit. *C,* With flexion of all digits, there is full motion of the PIP joints and either little or no motion at the distal joint level, which translates into a diminished grip power.

phalanx is absent in one or more digits. Often during the first few years of life, only the proximal phalanx is visible. A distal phalanx eventually appears. When the cutaneous syndactyly to the long finger is released, instability between these two phalanges is inevitable. During digital separation, there may be a coalescence between the superficial and deep flexor tendons as well as an adhesion of flexor tendons to surrounding soft tissue structures.[272] The thumb is smaller than normal with two phalanges and a stable MP joint. When the third (long) metacarpal is present, the important adductor pollicis muscle is intact. A typical variation of this type is a hand with intact thumb and fifth rays and coalesced index to fifth rays containing one, two, two, and three phalanges, respectively (Fig. 203-43).

In the monophalangeal type, the single remaining phalanx is usually larger than a distal phalanx alone and possesses a rudimentary nail, which may represent a merging of the proximal and distal phalangeal elements. At the carpal level, the extrinsic flexor tendons are bundled within a common sheet. The border rays, thumb, and index finger are hypoplastic and often do not have extrinsic flexor or extensor muscle-tendon units. The absence of an interphalangeal thumb flexion crease is indicative of an absent flexor pollicis longus. Thenar and hypothenar muscles are usually present, but intrinsic muscles of median and ulnar nerve innervation are hypoplastic or absent in the central portion of the hand. The MP joint of the hypoplastic fifth digit is characteristically unstable and will require surgery to stabilize a strong thumb to fifth digit pinch (Fig. 203-44).

In the aphalangeal type, the degree of deficiency is greatest in the index ray, followed by the long and ring rays. The thumb and fifth rays are hypoplastic, and both may lack extrinsic flexors and extensors. The extent of intrinsic muscle deficiency is proportional to the skeletal deficiency. If the fifth finger has either one or two phalanges, the MP joint is unstable and pulled toward the thumb by the remnants of the central three digits. After soft tissue release, it is often difficult to stabilize this joint (Fig. 203-45).

TREATMENT

Syndactyly

The digital syndactyly in these hands is always cutaneous and the usual principles should be observed (Table 203-9; see Fig. 203-42). Excessive deepening of the triphalangeal (short-finger) type may form an abnormal-appearing hand with no functional improvement. Both sides of a hypoplastic digit should not be released simultaneously. Rudimentary digits should be excised through a single straight incision, which can then be lengthened with one or more Z-plasties to improve the contour of the intradigital cleft. There is no standard type of cutaneous syndactyly

TABLE 203-9 ◆ COMPONENTS OF A SYMBRACHYDACTYLY (ATYPICAL CLEFT HAND) RECONSTRUCTION

Excision of rudimentary nubbins
Formation or preservation of a mobile, unscarred thumb with stable joints
Formation or preservation of a broad first web space
Maintenance of a thumb and at least one digit with sensation
Formation or preservation of an intact fifth ray with metacarpophalangeal joint motion and stability
Separation of digital syndactylies
Preservation of digital proximal interphalangeal joint motion in triphalangeal digits and metacarpophalangeal joint motion in biphalangeal digits

release, and the surgeon should use the method with which she or he is most comfortable.

In some triphalangeal and biphalangeal types, the first web space may be tight. In such patients, one has the option of excising the index ray or augmenting the web space with a local or distant fasciocutaneous flap. With greater central digit (index, long, and ring) deficiencies, there is usually more than enough tissue available to widen the web space between functional digits sufficiently (see Fig. 203-45).

Functional priority is always given to the first web space in the less severe types of symbrachydactyly, especially for patients with the Poland syndrome. Splinting and stretching of these small hands are usually ineffective but should be pursued with cooperative families. When enough tissue is available for a four-flap Z-plasty, this technique is preferred (Fig. 203-46). Techniques that involve multiple transposition flaps or a dorsal rotation flap plus a skin graft[276] form either excessive scar tissue or a conspicuous dorsal skin graft. For severe deficiencies, it is preferable to use either free or locally pedicled fasciocutaneous flaps[56,217] or skin expansion techniques.[56,217,247] Careful attention should be given to the size of the metacarpals, especially the third, and a functioning adductor pollicis muscle, which, if it is present, is the most important muscle in these small hands.

In biphalangeal and monophalangeal hands that involve two or more of the central digits, cutaneous webbing and digital dissections should be avoided if transfer of one or more toes is planned later in childhood. During the past 30 years, some of the prime candidates for double or triple toe transfers have been patients with symbrachydactyly or constriction ring syndrome, in whom the proximal phalanges and MP joint within the central portion of the hand are intact (see Fig. 203-43). When placed on top of an intact

Text continued on p. 121

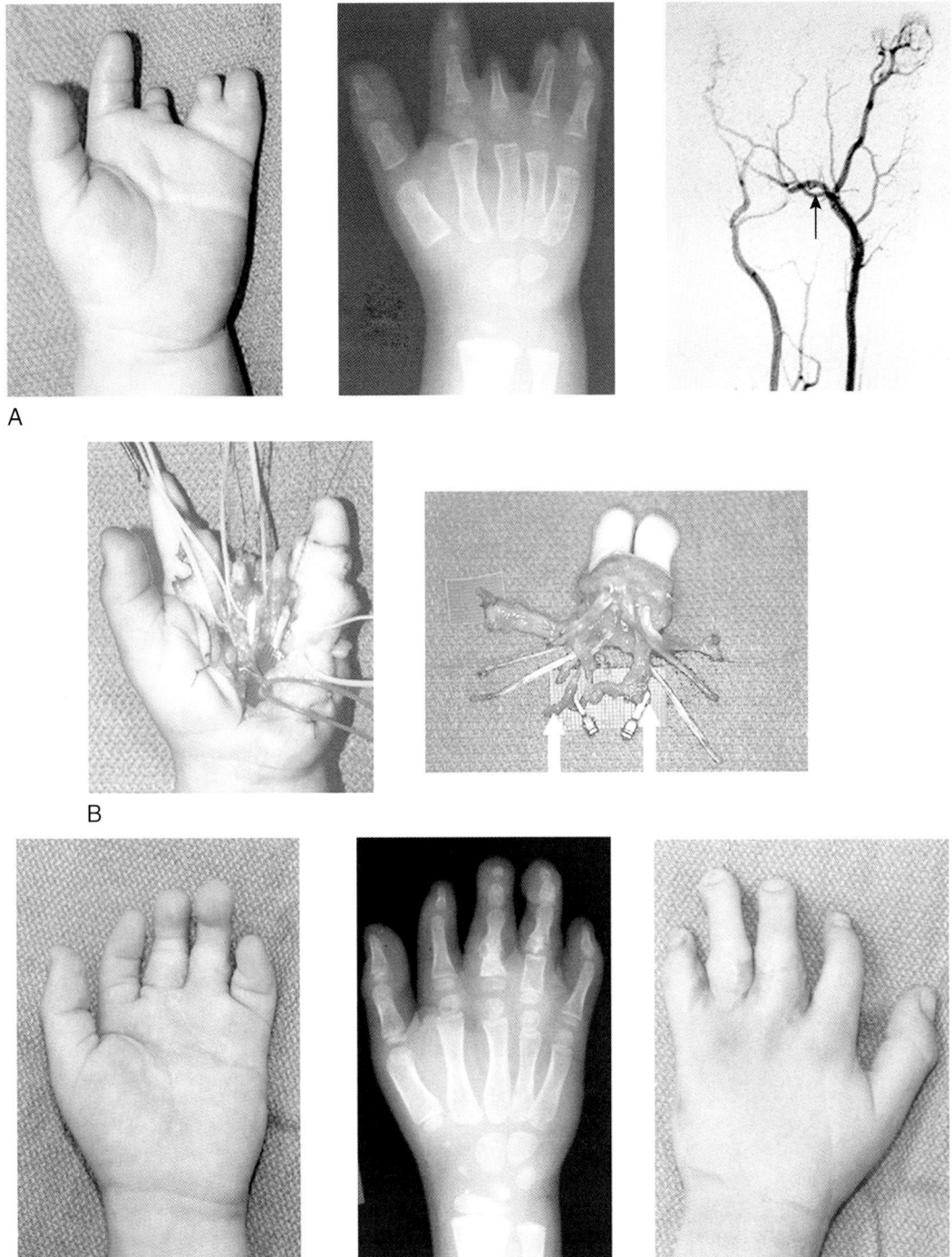

FIGURE 203-43. Symbrachydactyly, biphalangeal type. *A*, The photograph, radiograph, and angiogram of a patient with deficient central digits show a normal thumb, normal metacarpals, and MP joints with intact proximal phalanges. The arrow marks the midportion of the palmar arch, into which the double toe transfer will be spliced. The index phalanges are large compared with other hands of the biphalangeal type. *B*, Dissection of the midpalmar region of the hand shows the neurovascular structures and the dissected and prepared double second-third toe in transit. *C*, Several months after transfer, a routine syndactyly release was performed. The clinical appearance and radiograph are seen 18 months after transfer. Two-point discrimination is 4.0 mm on both sides of the transferred digits. Metacarpophalangeal joint motion is normal and interphalangeal joint motion is 50% of normal.

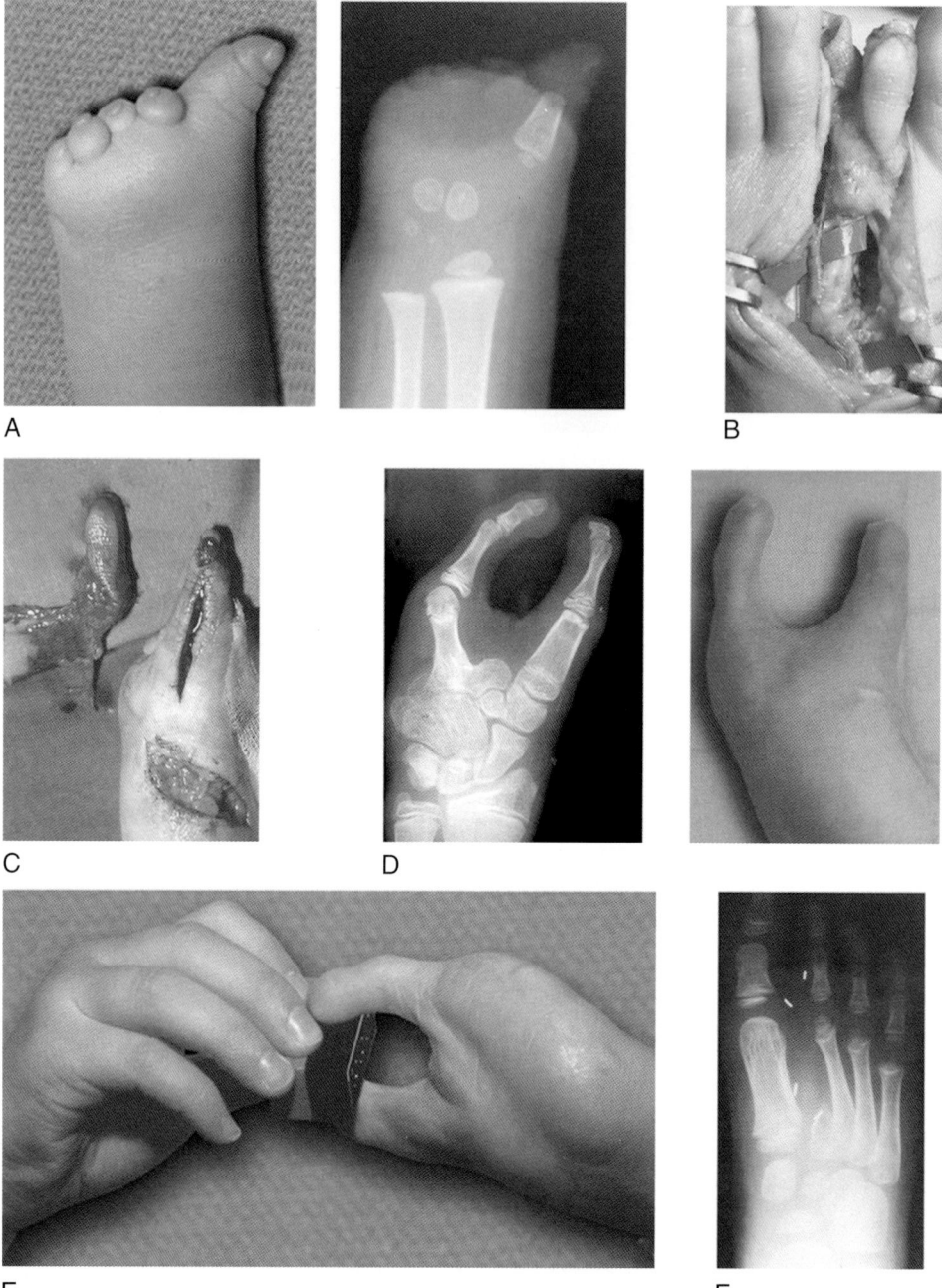

FIGURE 203-44. Symbrachydactyly, monophalangeal type. *A,* The photograph and radiograph show a symbrachydactyly hand with no proximal phalanx and one metacarpal. Only the distal portion of the distal phalanx is present. (This is the portion of the bone that ossifies by intramembranous ossification rather than by chondrification.) *B,* The reconstruction consisted of a second-toe transfer from each foot to the radial and ulnar sides of the hand. The transfer to the thumb position included the proximal and middle phalanges with an intact PIP joint and some dorsal skin. The metatarsal has been elevated here to facilitate dissection of the dominant plantar vessels to the toe. An entire second ray of the opposite foot was transferred to the ulnar side of the hypoplastic hand. *C,* A separate proximal incision was made at the base of the thumb for isolation of a recipient dorsal vein for the transfer to the radial side of the hand. *D,* A postoperative radiograph many years later, when the patient was approaching skeletal maturity, shows the partial toe transfer to the thumb articulating at the MP joint and a complete second-toe or second-ray transfer on the ulnar side of the hand. *E,* The patient developed two-point discrimination of 4.0 mm in both transferred digits and an excellent pinching mechanism. *F,* There were no donor site problems. Shoe wear and gait were unaffected. (Courtesy of Guy Foucher, MD.)

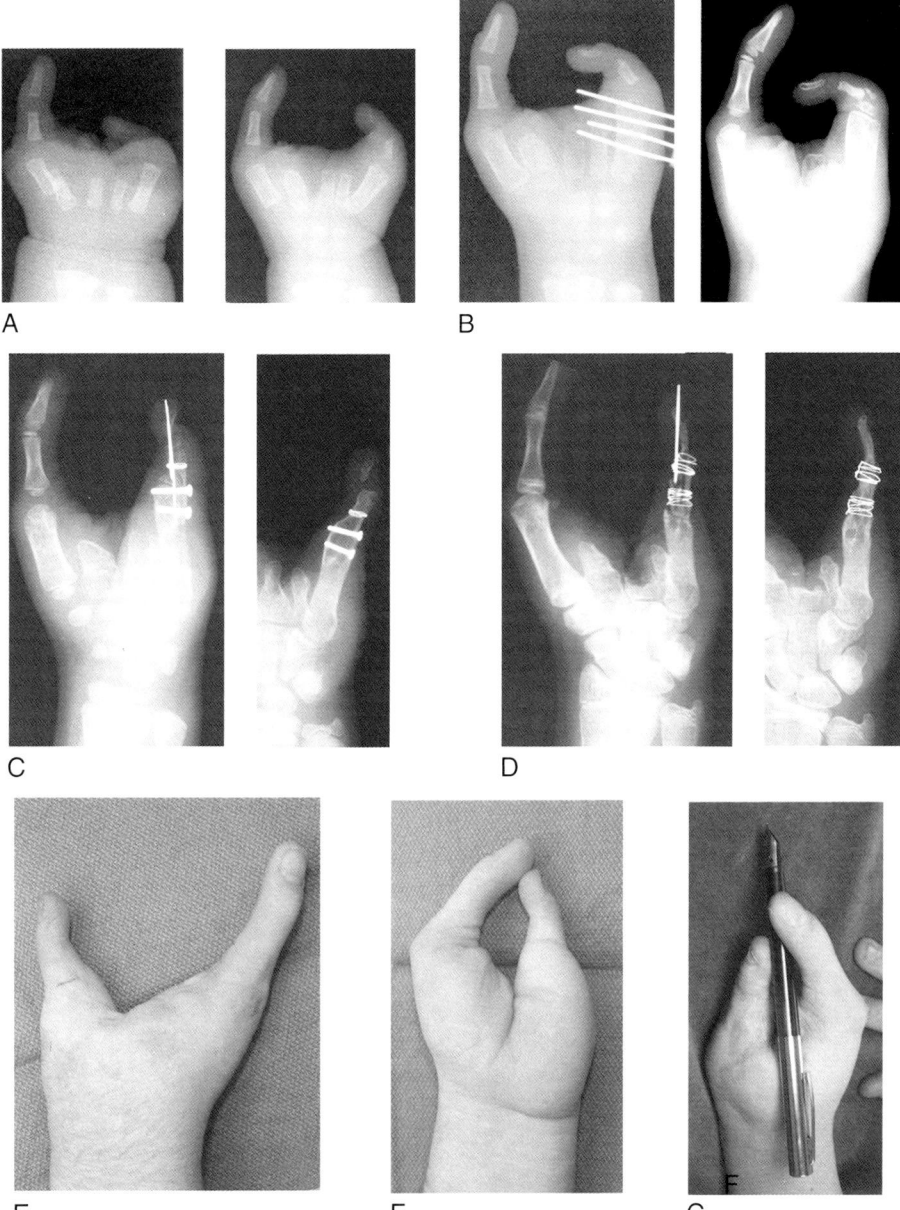

FIGURE 203-45. Symbrachydactyly, biphalangeal type. *A,* This child was born with unilateral symbrachydactyly, with a strong biphalangeal thumb and a floppy fifth digit that contained only a distal portion of the distal phalanx. The hypoplastic nubbins representing the index, long, and ring digits were excised within the first 3 months of life. Additional Z-plasties were performed to gain maximum breadth and depth of the web space. *B,* At 10 months of age, the floppy fifth digit was stabilized with a nonvascularized phalangeal transfer harvested from the right fourth toe. *C,* At age 3 years, the fifth metacarpal was lengthened to provide a longer ulnar post and a better pinching mechanism. The fifth digit still remained in a flexed position, but he used this hand well. *D,* A few years later, poor growth was noted in the toe phalanx, which had become unstable at the MP joint level. *E,* By 10 years of age, the unstable toe phalanx was fused to the tip of the metacarpal and augmented with a corticocancellous bone graft. A nonunion developed between the bone graft and the existing distal phalanx, which was severely hypoplastic. *F,* This region was lengthened and regrafted a year later. Note that the lengths of the fifth ray and the thumb are almost equal. *G,* At 20 years of age, he continues to use this constructed post for both grip and pinching functions. The thumb has grown and is much longer. He has fractured the fifth digit twice and has achieved primary bone healing on both occasions. He perceives little limitation with this, his nondominant hand.

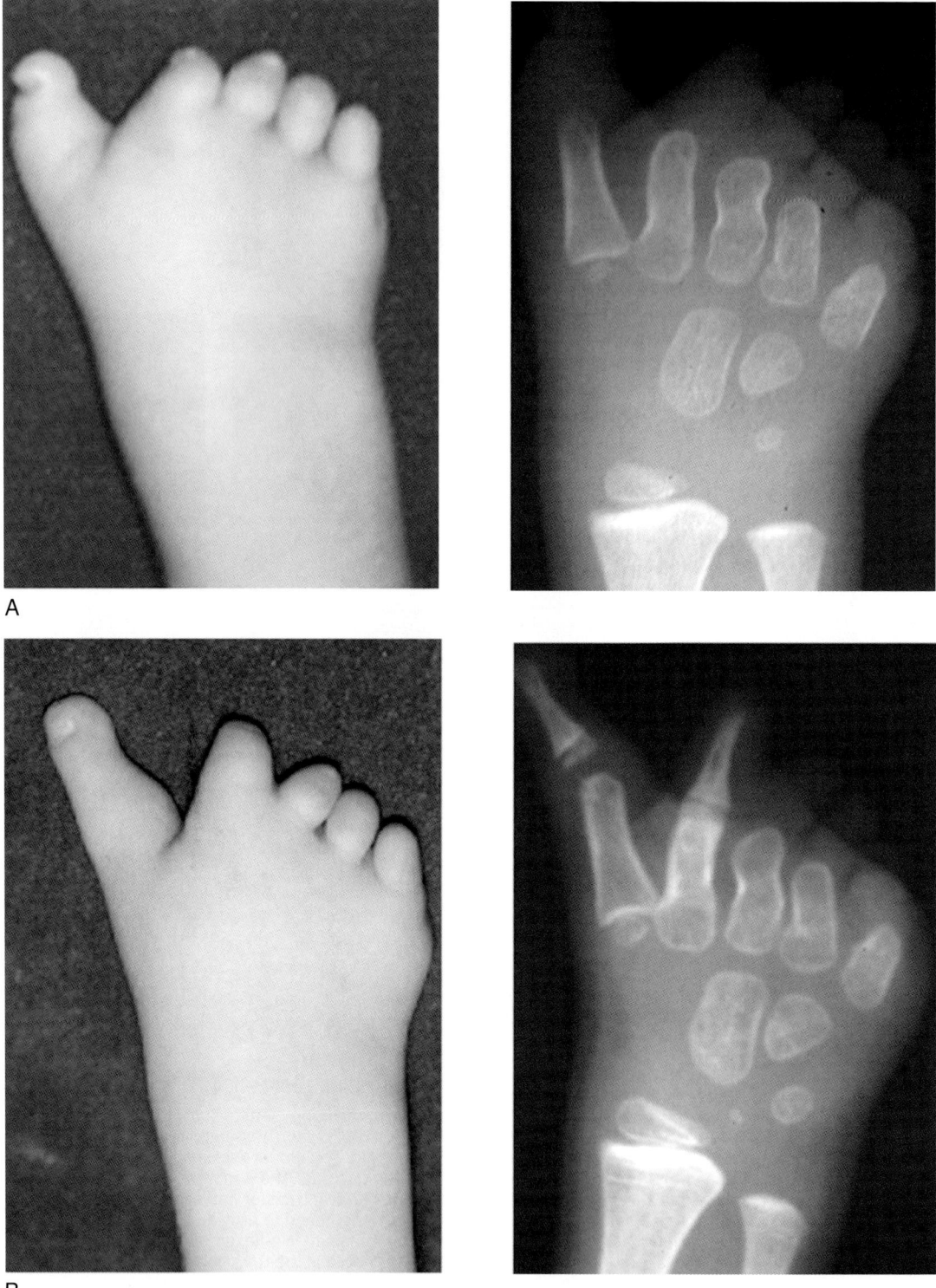

A

B

FIGURE 203-46. Symbrachydactyly, aphalangeal type. *A,* This boy with an aphalangeal symbrachydactyly has good soft tissue nubbins, large enough to support the framework of a bone, representing all five digits and no first web space. *B,* One year after nonvascularized toe phalangeal transfers to the thumb and index metacarpals, plus a four-flap Z-plasty, a basic pinch has been constructed. The transferred phalanges have continued to grow.

proximal phalanx, these toes, termed tingers, actually look and function more like fingers than toes.

The tight pterygium, or web, in the anterior axillary line in patients with pectoralis muscle anomalies is easily released with a Z-plasty transposition flap. The tight cord within the web is usually a fibrous band or anlage of the sternal portion of the muscle and should be excised. Neurovascular structures are usually not involved.

Hypoplastic Nubbins

Hypoplastic nubbins are digital remnants with no functional potential and are best ablated early in life. The retraction of these nubbins with wrist or thumb motion is due to very small extrinsic flexor and extensor tendons, which connect to forearm muscles. If they are left in place beyond the age of 1 year, children and parents may become psychologically attached to these parts, which may later become a source of embarrassment. However, functionally, there is nothing wrong with leaving them intact. Many girls are proud of their nails and take delight in polishing them meticulously.

Hypoplastic Digits

In the triphalangeal type, both proximal and distal interphalangeal joints are intact. Attempts to lengthen these digits are not advised because the extensor mechanism becomes adherent to the bone regenerate, and distal motion and function are severely compromised. In the biphalangeal type, preference should be placed on preservation of MP motion with PIP joint stability. In monophalangeal and aphalangeal hands with adequate soft tissue in the digital remnants, nonvascularized toe phalangeal transfers may be effective (Figs. 203-47 and 203-48).[117,277-279] Monophalangeal digits in the index position are generally not very functional and are best removed to improve the web space. In these patients, the bone segment removed may be effectively used as a graft elsewhere in the hand (Fig. 203-49; see also Fig. 203-48).

Technique of Nonvascularized Toe Transfer. The nonvascularized transfer of the proximal phalangeal segments of toes may be useful to fill floppy soft tissue masses that have attached extrinsic tendons. The presence of these muscle-tendon units can be seen by deep retraction of distal skin dimples at the end of amputation stumps. When phalanges are used to fill redundant soft tissue nubbins distal to hypoplastic metacarpals, remarkable improvement in function can be achieved, particularly with the thumb. Prerequisites are that the child be younger than 1 year, have normal neuromuscular control of the limb and hand, and have a suitable phalanx on the foot for transfer. Although extrinsic tendons are preferred, transferred toe phalanges can also be attached to

the soft tissue structures surrounding the metacarpal head.

The technique preferred by most surgeons involves removal of the third- and fourth-toe proximal phalanges through dorsal incisions, which use the MP extension creases (see Fig. 203-47). Other surgeons prefer the second-toe phalanx because of its size. It is preferable to save the second toe if there is a remote possibility that it may be used for a microvascular transfer. The soft tissue envelope of the digital remnant is opened and dissected, and its maximum length is measured. If the pocket is large enough, a transfer can be done.

The foot incisions are made along the sides of the toes and the dorsal extension creases. Dorsal veins and nerves are retracted and the extensor mechanism is raised from one side, exposing the distal portion of the proximal phalanx. The toe PIP joint is disarticulated, and the proximal phalanx is easily raised once the flexor sheath has been incised. At the MP joint level, the collateral ligaments, capsule, and volar (palmar) plate may be retained with periosteum and attached to the phalanx.

The recipient metacarpal head is exposed through a dorsal incision. A dorsal transverse incision is preferred when more than one phalanx is transferred; individual incisions may be made along each nubbin (see Fig. 203-47). Flexor and extensor tendons may be fused together over the metacarpal head (see Fig. 203-23E). With retraction of the distal digital nubbin, these small tendons are seen to attach to a cartilaginous nubbin supporting the nail matrix. These are all detached, and the collateral ligaments and volar plate are exposed. The articular cartilage may be shaved on opposing surfaces if no pseudojoint function is desired. Flexor and extensor tendons are then attached to the transferred phalanx. On occasion, these tendons attach to a nonossified cartilaginous bone. In such patients, the phalanx is placed on top of this cartilaginous bone. These patients achieve the best functional outcome because they have an intact MP joint. Internal fixation of the phalanx may result in premature closure of the central portion of the transferred physis,[279] and stabilization can be maintained with extraosseous pins (see Fig. 203-47). It is easier to place a pin through the phalanx, set the bone into the soft tissue pocket, and then advance the pin into the metacarpal.

The foot is closed with absorbable 6-0 chromic sutures after the flexor and extensor tendons are coapted with a single mattress suture. The donor toe will predictably retract and will be less stable than its neighbors, but gait will not be altered. This issue is of prime importance to parents and must be explained thoroughly.[57] The donor site graft may be filled with a free corticocancellous iliac crest graft obtained from the anterior portion of the ilium.[55] The plug is harvested percutaneously by a dowel technique and

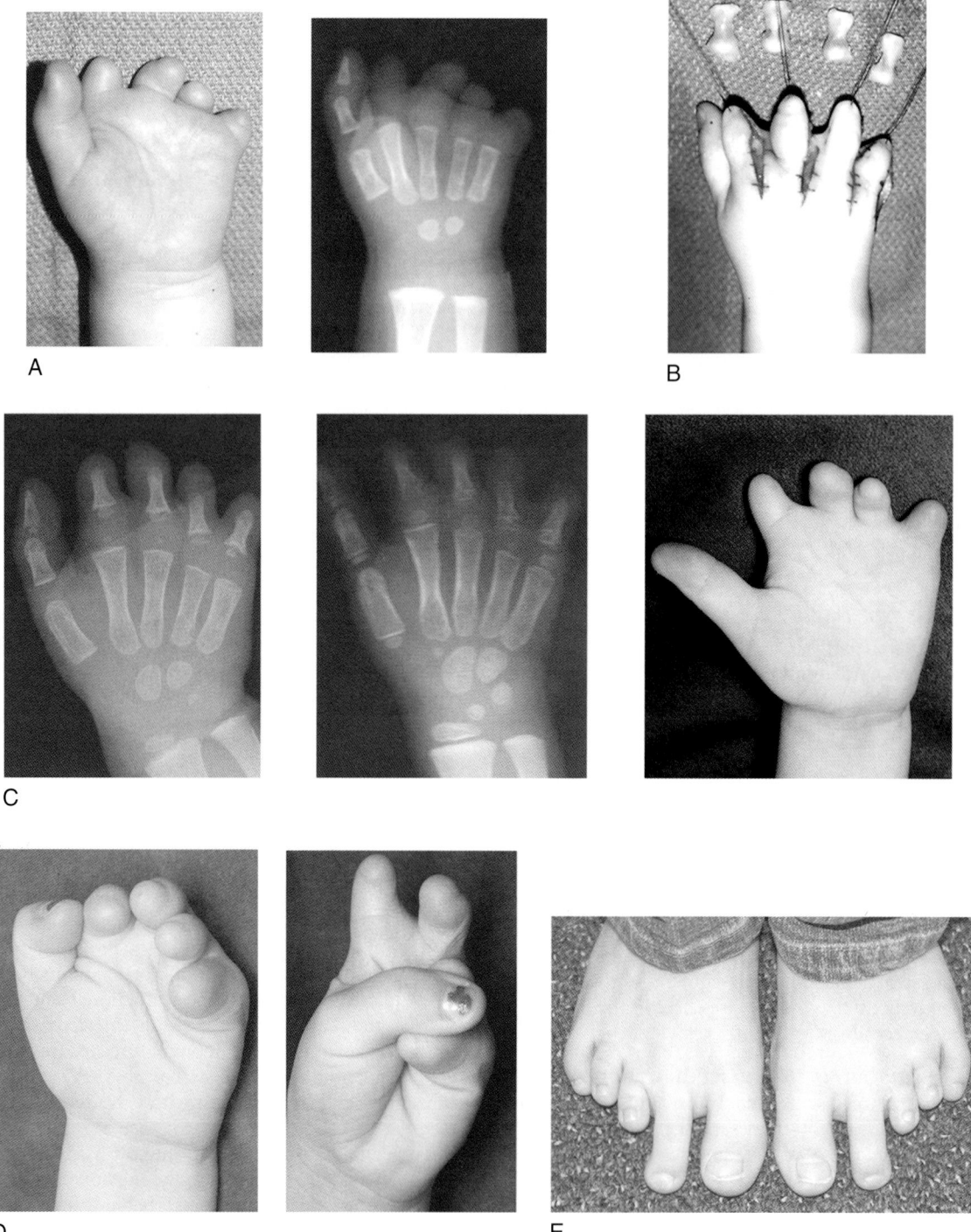

FIGURE 203-47. Nonvascularized toe phalangeal transfers. *A,* This 1-year-old child has a good thumb, four intact metacarpals, and good retraction of the abundant soft tissue nubbins, indicating the presence of extrinsic flexor and extensor tendons. *B,* Four toe proximal phalanges harvested from the third and fourth toes on either foot were used to fill these nubbins and were placed on top of small cartilaginous proximal phalanges to which the tendons attached. A single dorsal incision would be used today. *C,* Radiographs 1 and 2 years postoperatively demonstrate that the phalanges have maintained good position and have continued to grow. *D,* With time and growth, the MP joint motion of all four digits has continued to improve. The patient has developed a strong thumb to index finger key pinch and an effective thumb to fifth finger gripping mechanism. *E,* The donor feet are seen at 15 years of age.

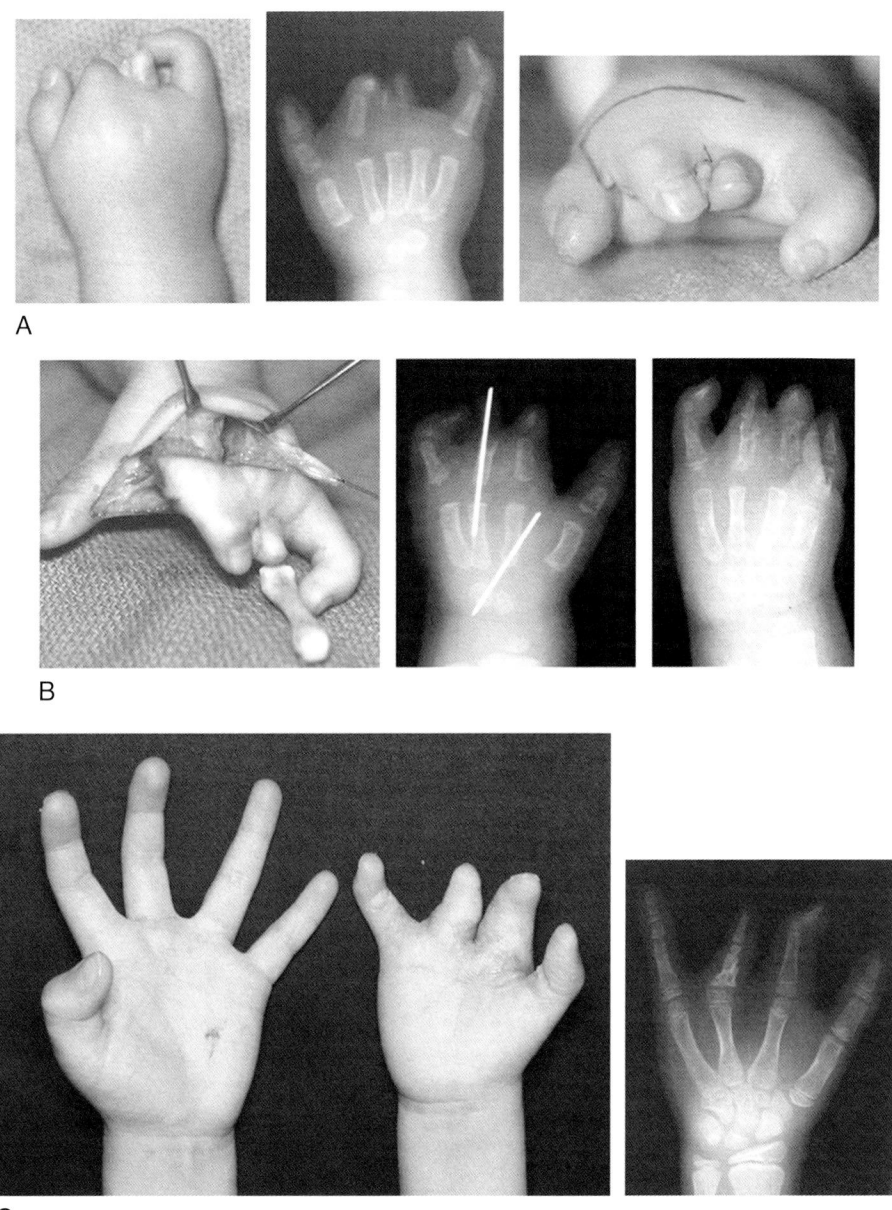

FIGURE 203-48. Symbrachydactyly, nonvascularized toe transfers. *A,* The clinical appearance and radiograph of a unilateral hand deformity, which primarily affects the central three digits. The index ray contains an intact MP joint and is tethered side-by-side to the long and ring digits by tight fibrous bands. The radial clinodactyly of the fifth finger is caused by the small, delta-shaped middle phalanx. The first web space is tight. Although hypoplastic, the border thumb and fifth rays are intact and functional. Three previous hand consultants recommended partial resection of the three central rays. *B,* The construction of a more functional hand consisted of resection of the long ray, transposition of the index ray into the long position at the CMC level, and placement of the long metacarpal between the ring metacarpal and distal phalanx as a nonvascular free bone graft. During the first 2 years postoperatively, there was resorption, but remineralization did occur with some shortening. At the same time, a V-Y lengthening of the first web space was achieved and provided excellent exposure for the free bone graft to the ring finger. *C,* The hand and radiograph are seen 5 years later. The webbing between the index and ring digits has been deepened, and both digits have good MP joint motion. Neither digit obstructs thumb to fifth finger pinch and grasp, and the index is effective with the thumb. The growth of the free transferred phalanx to the ring finger lags behind that of the other three native proximal phalanges.

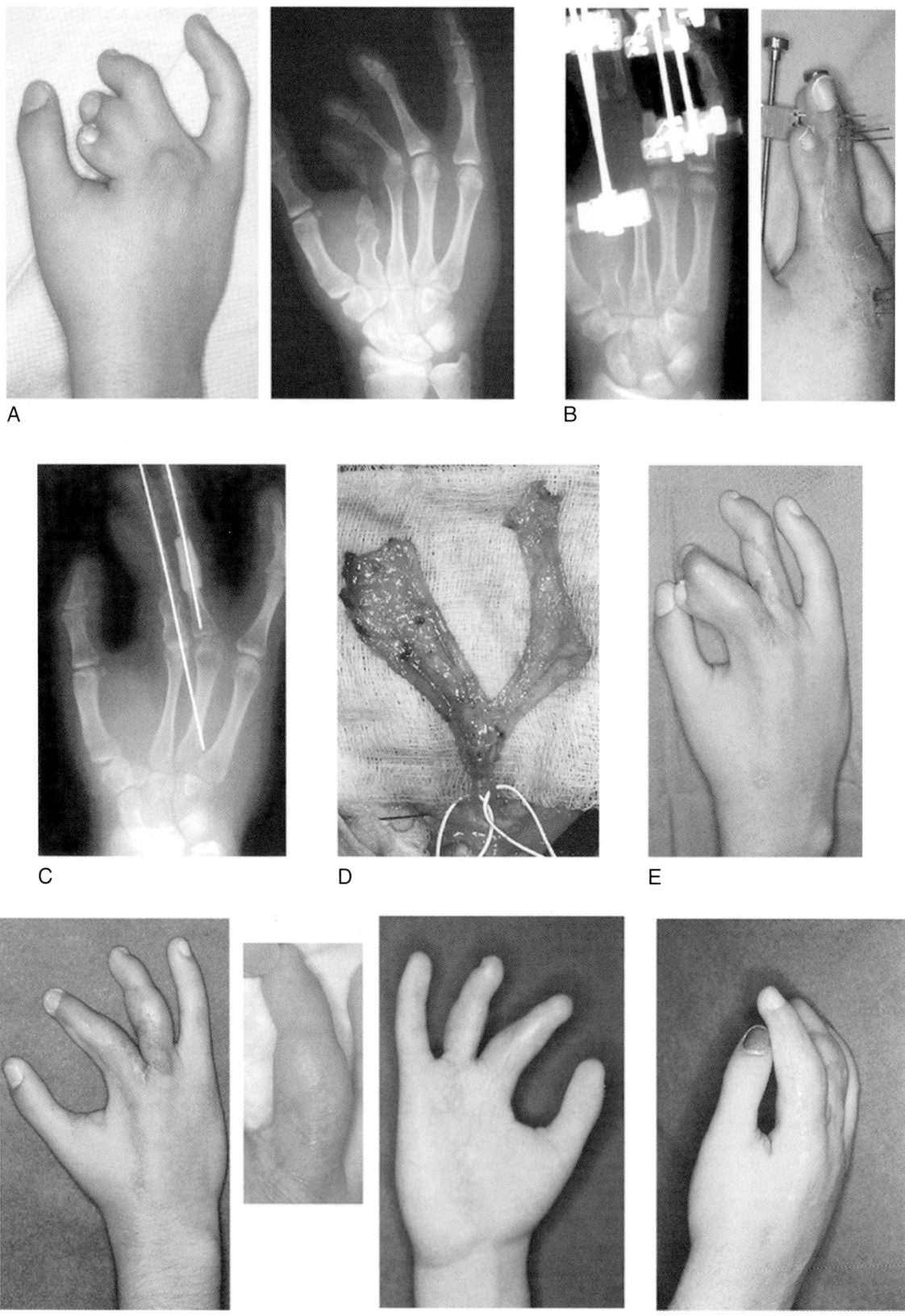

FIGURE 203-49. Symbrachydactyly, distraction lengthening and free tissue transfer. *A,* This girl with a unilateral right hand congenital symbrachydactyly presented, with her parents, at the age of 15 years with the objective of improved appearance and function. She had become adept at hiding her conspicuous hand and covered it with a prosthetic glove in public. The radiograph shows that the index was much more hypoplastic than the deficient long and ring rays. *B,* The first-stage procedure consisted of distraction lengthening of the long finger at the MP joint and of the ring finger through the proximal phalanx. *C,* When the desired length was achieved, the gap in the long ray was filled by the metacarpal and proximal phalanx of the index ray, and that in the ring digit with a demineralized bone graft. The patient did not wish to have an autogenous iliac crest graft. The syndactyly is intact. *D,* At the time of separation of the long and ring digits, a split temporoparietal fascial flap was wrapped around each digit to increase the circumference to the normal proportions of a digit. The usual dorsal and palmar commissure flaps and full-thickness skin grafts were used. *E,* The distal index finger remnant was removed a few months later. *F,* The appearance of the hand was greatly improved and enthusiastically accepted by the patient, now 30 years of age. The MP joints of the two constructed digits were intentionally placed in enough extension to prevent them from hindering any pinch or grasp between the thumb and fifth digit. She has a strong thumb to index pinch, no longer hides her hand, and is the mother of several children. Most important, she uses this hand.

---

contains 4 to 5 mm of cartilaginous apophysis and 10 mm of corticocancellous bone. The graft is held in place with an interosseous wire for 4 to 6 weeks postoperatively. All grafts have remained visible on radiographs for at least 1 year after transfer. The long-term outcomes are not available.

OUTCOMES. The reported success of toe phalangeal transfer varies from normal growth in 159 phalanges transferred without periosteum[280] to 90% growth in 20 of 27 phalanges transferred with intact periosteum and collateral ligaments that were then attached to skeletal elements.[87] Most authors agree that considerable resorption occurs when the toe segment is transferred as a free-floating segment within a soft tissue tube and when patients are older than 12 months at the time of transfer. Even if the epiphysis remains open and growth occurs, the maximal length gained is not great owing to the natural size disproportion of toe and finger phalanges.[277,278,281] Buck-Gramcko[277] reported that at least one third of toe phalanges transferred after 1 year of age show some resorption on radiographs. It has been suggested that free, nonvascularized phalangeal transfers both stimulate adjacent bone growth and are incorporated more effectively when they are attached to bone or used as interpositional grafts.[279] Some of our best results have been transferred phalanges placed between a metacarpal

head and distal phalanx for floppy thumbs or digits. Growth of transferred phalanges is similar to that of native toes and is not as predictable as growth after vascularized "thoe" or "tinger" transfers. In the future, phalangeal transfers will be performed in conjunction with skeletal distraction methods.

Thumb

There are basic principles for thumb construction (see Chapter 208). Two techniques used extensively in patients with symbrachydactyly are microvascular toe transfer and nonvascularized toe phalangeal transfer.

With few exceptions, in patients with the short-finger type, the thumb is hypoplastic despite being the most intact portion of the hand. The skeletal elements may be reduced to variable degree, but a metacarpal bone and an intact CMC joint are usually present. Interphalangeal flexion is usually diminished or absent. The long flexor is replaced by an abnormal intrinsic thumb flexor. Most functional motion is at the MP joint through the activity of normal thumb intrinsic muscles and an abnormal long flexor, if present.

In the triphalangeal and biphalangeal types, median-innervated thenar intrinsic muscles are present, and well-segmented stable joints are present at all three (CMC, MP, and IP) levels. Absolute priority should be given to the thumb. It is often best to do nothing. In the more deficient monophalangeal type, the extrinsic flexor and, less often, the extensor mechanism are abnormal. The intrinsic muscles flex the MP joint. Flexor tendon grafts intended to restore interphalangeal flexion and power must be joined to adequate forearm motors with a good excursion, usually a wrist flexor. Staged flexor reconstructions are necessary with the absence of a flexor pulley mechanism. Lack of thumb palmar abduction may be restored with either a hypothenar muscle transfer or an available extensor tendon lengthened by a tendon graft. The timing of these operations is critical, and it is often best to wait until the youngster is old enough to cooperate with postoperative therapy, usually beyond 2 to 3 years of age.

On occasion, the aphalangeal type may have a metacarpal with a distal phalanx and a good soft tissue tube. These flail thumbs can effectively be stabilized with a nonvascularized toe phalangeal transfer between the metacarpal and distal phalanx. If they are transferred with intact periosteum and collateral ligaments intact within the first 12 to 18 months of life, these phalanges are likely to revascularize and grow.[277] Although a microvascular toe transfer is preferred, many parents in the United States balk at a complicated procedure,[34] although it seems to be performed more frequently in the United Kingdom[55,56,59] and Asian countries (see the later section on microvascular toe transplantation in the discussion of the monodactylic or adactylic hand).

Fifth Digit

The ulnar digit in a patient with symbrachydactyly will often have an unstable MP joint and radial clinodactyly caused by its asymmetric proximal phalanx. This constitutes the major functional problem with monodactylic or oligodactylic hands. The flexor tendons are strong and the extensors are present but unbalanced. Stabilization of the MP joint with chondrodesis, bone grafts, or transfers of nonvascularized toe phalanges has been performed with varying degrees of success. Distraction lengthening[45,144,282] and metacarpal rotational osteotomies have been useful for the proper positioning of this digit. When it is positioned as a stable post with or without MP joint motion, the ulnar ray functions well for both hook and balancing maneuvers and grasping with the thumb (see Fig. 203-45).

Tendon Transfers

In the more severe types of symbrachydactyly, thumb and digital motion may be poor after the formation of a basic hand. Extrinsic flexors and extensors and intrinsic muscles are absent or severely hypoplastic. Tendon transfers may be useful for gaining digital motion if motors are available. Wrist flexors and extensors, or hypothenar muscles, are suitable if they are available, but digital flexors and extensors generally are not because they are poorly differentiated from one another in the distal forearm and hand, where they fuse as a common tendon mass at the level of the carpal tunnel. The surgeon should be cautious before transferring a tendon to improve thumb or fifth finger flexion or adduction of the two-fingered hand.

Monodactylic or Adactylic Hand

The options for treatment of the monodactylic or adactylic type of symbrachydactyly are the same as those outlined in the cleft hand portion of the chapter. A floppy thumb that possesses an intact metacarpal may occasionally be treated with a nonvascularized toe phalangeal transfer, especially in patients with either the Möbius or Poland syndrome. A better method for transfer of a second toe is by microvascular techniques (see Fig. 203-23).[51,54,56,59,132,219,283-285] Although motion may be limited because of underdeveloped forearm muscles, the adaptive functional gain with hooking, balancing, and probing may be remarkable, especially in children with bilateral absence of hands. Accurate assessment of the postoperative outcome of these procedures requires several years of follow-up.

In patients with a stable digit and an additional metacarpal, distraction lengthening of this metacarpal is an option if microvascular toe transfer is declined. If a thumb metacarpal is present with a mobile CMC joint, one may elect to distract and lengthen the thumb as a mobile post and shift the toe to the ulnar side of the adactylic hand. When there is a stiff first ray, toe transfer to this ray is recommended. Every hand must be considered individually because no two are the same.

TOE TRANSPLANTATION (MICROVASCULAR). The concept of transplantation of an intact composite toe to the hand is not new. Nicoladoni[286] completed a pedicled transfer to the thumb before the turn of the last century. Fifty years later, others duplicated these efforts and in their reports emphasized the difficulties of keeping the patients' hands attached to their feet in awkward positions.[287] The first clinical toe transfers for traumatic defects[288] opened the door to use of this technique in congenital differences.[289] The more severe forms of symbrachydactyly constitute one of the most frequent indications for single or multiple toe transfers.[263]

The clinical appearance of the hand is not necessarily an indication of the anomalous anatomy of the forearm, wrist, and palm of the hand. Tendon grafts, nerve grafts, and venous conduits for arterial reconstruction are frequently needed as a bridge across hypoplastic or aplastic structures within the palm. Toe transfers may also be performed with similar frequency for thumb and digital reconstruction. There is a difference in the expected anatomy between the longitudinal and transverse types of malformations. Most toe transfers are performed for transverse deficiencies in which neurovascular and musculotendinous structures are present to some degree in the palm. In contrast, many of these structures are absent in longitudinal deficiencies and must be transferred from an adjacent ray to motor and to innervate a toe transfer.[56,132] The hand anatomy proximal to transverse absences associated with the constriction ring syndrome is predictably normal.

Extensive preoperative preparation with patients (if older) and parents is mandatory. Parents must be guided through the decision-making process with a careful, realistic description of the surgery, expected results, and potential complications, including those involving the donor site.[56,290,291] Hand molds, videotapes of patients, pictures, and interactions with other patients and their families are useful. There is no absolutely right or wrong decision. The parents should be reassured that their child will adapt and function well, even those children with adactylies. A percentage of expected functional or aesthetic gain after surgery cannot be given. If parents are reluctant, it is often best to wait to undertake intervention; these parents are often those who would prefer that the child make his or her own decision later in childhood. In the author's 29-year experience with toe transfers, seven children have requested toe transfers when they were old enough to understand the procedure. All had severe deficiencies, one with adactyly and five with thumb and digit amputations associated with the constriction ring syndrome. Kay[56,59] provides a nice discussion and illustration of the hands most suitable for toe transfers. The only situation in which the author strongly advocated this surgery is that of the child with bilateral adactylies with no thumbs.

Which toe should be transferred? In published series, the second toe is most frequently transferred.[132,219,283,289,292-294] However, this toe should not always be transferred to the thumb position. For example, if a normal thumb is present on the opposite hand, a modified toe transfer is preferred.[295] When it is placed next to a normally existing digit, the transferred toe should resemble that digit as much as possible. If the appearance of the transferred toe will be conspicuous, it may be advisable not to perform the procedure.[296] In most symbrachydactyly hands, digits are small and narrow, so second and third toes are usually acceptable (see Figs. 203-43 and 203-44). Exceptions include patients with the constriction ring syndrome, in which there are often few or no toes available for transfer. Donor site cosmesis is important. The loss of the second ray on the foot results in a minimal cosmetic or functional problem, particularly if toes have been harvested from both feet. Although many eschew second-third or second-third-fourth toe monobloc harvest,[56] it may be used in patients with constriction ring syndrome to design a basic hand containing a mobile thumb, a good first web space, and one or two digits on the opposite side.

Technical difficulties that may be encountered in patients with symbrachydactyly include the paucity of arterial vessels within the hand; a predominance of the plantar vessels in the foot; other anomalous anatomy of the foot; the lack of sensory nerves within the palm of the hand; the attachment of the flexor tendons to a common aponeurosis within the palm; and the small size of the nerves, tendons, and vessels.

Technique of Second-Toe Transplantation.
The second toe or ray of the foot is the most frequently used donor site for toe transfers for congenital hand differences. The procedure in children follows a standard progression of steps with a few exceptions. Before surgery, the indications for the transfer with emphasis on donor site morbidity, immediate postoperative care, postoperative rehabilitation, potential problems with growth, and expected functional and cosmetic outcomes should be discussed in detail with the patients and their families.[56] This process may be slow, but the family should not be rushed, and all of their queries should be answered carefully. Children older than 5 to 6 years should be involved in the decision-making process—after all, it is their toe that is being autotransplanted.

Timing. The precise timing for toe transfer to the hand in children is not known but is most practically governed by the surgeon's experience and ability, the size of the hand and foot, the facility within which the surgery is to be performed, and finally the absence of more important cardiac, gastrointestinal, pulmonary, and hematologic anomalies. It is not clear that earlier surgery (before the age of 5 to 6 years) makes much difference in terms of adaptability and cerebral cortical plasticity. It may be advisable to transfer a toe to establish a thumb at 1 year of age in a child with no thumbs or digits on either hand, but it is preferable to wait to pursue elective thoe and tinger transfers between 2 and 4 years of age. In years past, surgery was delayed until 7 to 10 years of age, and these children adapted to and used their new hands remarkably well.

Anesthesia. A thorough preoperative evaluation with the family is essential before any prolonged anesthetic. An epidural catheter is placed in older children to alleviate postoperative donor site pain. Upper limb pain and possible vascular spasm may also be curtailed with a brachial block. Preoperative visits to the operating suite and intensive care unit will help familiarize these children and their parents with the ordeal they are about to endure. During the actual anesthetic, care is taken to carefully calculate fluid losses, not to overhydrate children, and to keep them relatively light during the long anesthetic.

Toe Harvest. Preoperative planning is the key to any microsurgical procedure. The foot should be examined with a Doppler probe, and if any doubt exists about the presence of the first dorsal metatarsal artery or its pedicle length, an angiogram should be obtained. It is not advisable to perform magnetic resonance angiography because of the lack of specific detail. Before any incision is made, the operation should be performed mentally much like the oral surgeon calculates her or his osteotomies with molds mounted on an articulator.

The skin incision on the toe is invariably a V-shaped flap that should fit nicely into the hand. With the tourniquet at the midhumeral level, incisions are first made on either side of the second toe and then extended down the dorsum of the foot to the level of the base of the second metatarsal. Flaps are reflected, the large dorsal veins are followed back to their coalescence into a single vein, and dorsal sensory nerves are identified and marked (Fig. 203-50).

The arterial anatomy is then identified with a direct approach into the first web space.[295] In the majority of feet, the plantar vessels constitute the dominant arterial conduit to the toe. If a large first dorsal metatarsal artery is present, simple ligation of the plantar system is all that is needed. Pedicle length is crucial, and every millimeter can be determined from the preoperative planning. Instead of dissecting down through the interosseous musculature of the foot, it is preferable to make a dorsal wedge osteotomy at the base of the second metatarsal, simply elevate the second metatarsal

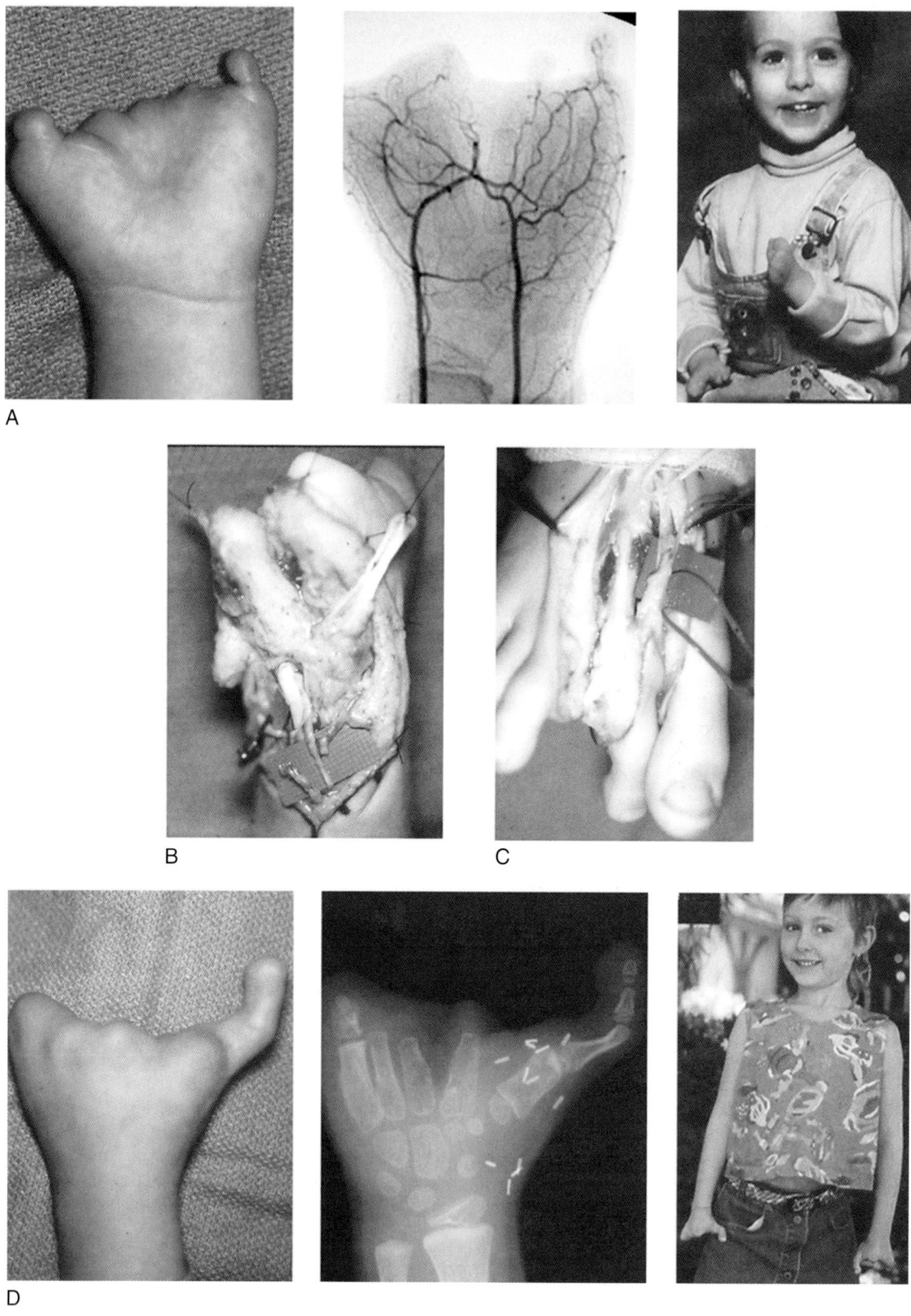

FIGURE 203-50. Second-toe to hand transfer. The microvascular transfer of the second toe to the thumb position is the most commonly performed toe to hand transfer in those with congenital hand differences. The procedure follows a standard series of steps: preoperative evaluation, recipient site dissection, donor site dissection, transfer, tendon repair, muscle realignment, vascular anastomoses, nerve repair, closure, and finally postoperative care and rehabilitation. *A,* This child with a bilateral combined symbrachydactyly and transverse absence of all digits and thumbs on both hands presented more than 20 years ago. Chorionic villus sampling had been performed on the mother during the first trimester. A preoperative angiogram, which was routinely performed in the 1980s, showed intact radial and ulnar arteries draining into an intact palmar arch. The arterial anatomy appears normal at the metacarpal level. In these patients, similar to those with the constriction ring syndrome, the proximal anatomy is normal. *B,* The dissection of the recipient site involves isolation of extrinsic flexor and extensor tendons and identification and partial mobilization of thumb intrinsic muscles (all of which were present and normal). The radial artery, two venae comitantes, and the large cephalic vein have been prepared as recipient vessels at the level of the wrist. *C,* The second toe is isolated on either the first dorsal metatarsal artery or a plantar artery. Both vessels have been dissected and tagged through a direct approach on either side of the second toe. The veins have been followed to a large common draining vein on the dorsal surface of the foot. Once isolated as a vascular island, the toe is ready for transfer. *D,* The second-toe transfer has been placed on top of the first metacarpal and secured with a chondrodesis. Excellent interphalangeal joint motion was achieved. After transfer of both second toes to become thoes, she developed such an effective pinch and grasp between the thoe and the mobile fifth ray that she did not wish to have any lengthening or additional toe transfer for elongation of the fifth ray of the hand.

(see Fig. 203-44*B*), and visualize the arterial system back to the plantar arch. A 15- to 20-mm arterial pedicle is formed by this simple maneuver.[292] With upward reflection of the bone, an atraumatic dissection to the level of the plantar arch is possible.

Once the vascular and neural anatomy has been defined and isolated with loops, the intrinsic muscles are detached from their extensor origins and the extrinsic flexor and extensor tendons sharply transected at the proximal metatarsal level. Note: if the flexor pollicis longus is isolated and transected behind the medial malleolus, it will not always "pull through" easily into the distal foot because of intratendinous connections proximal to the tarsal tunnel. The same is true for the flexor profundus to the second toe. The extensor digitorum brevis tendons are always easy to isolate but are rarely incorporated into the reconstruction.

The joint capsule and collateral ligaments are then transected, and the toe is isolated as a vascular island. The soft tissue structures on the lateral side of the second toe are usually the last to be separated.

The medial and lateral plantar nerves are easily identified by their proximity to arterial structures, the presence of pacinian corpuscles, and their association with adipose tissue. They are usually dissected and isolated with the arterial anatomy.

The tinger has now been isolated as a vascular island on the most prominent artery (usually the plantar) and a large dorsal vein and is ready for transfer.

Skeletal Fixation. Fixation is usually achieved in the simplest way possible. Every consideration is given to avoidance of potential injury to the growing epiphysis. Small longitudinal interosseous wires are preferred for longitudinal alignment accompanied by sutures for correction of rotation. Early motion is possible with this combination. When the transfer involves a joint articulation, the hyaline cartilage lining both joint surfaces is minimally shaved to conformity, and the collateral ligaments and volar plate are repaired. These joints may function remarkably well. The use of crossed interosseous wires should be avoided because they may cause pin track–related problems.

Tendon and Muscle Repair. Both extensor tendons (extensor digitorum communis and extensor indicis proprius) are repaired when recipient donor tendons are available. The extensors are secured under some tension similar to index pollicization into the thumb position. The flexor digitorum communis of the toe is repaired second. In those with congenital differences, especially the symbrachydactyly category, the excursion of the extrinsic digital and toe extensors may be compromised. In children with monodactyly in the cleft hand-foot syndrome, the extrinsic flexor and extensor tendons are joined as a perfect tendon at the distal metacarpal level. Although all intrinsic tendons available may be routinely repaired, an appreciable effect with lumbrical reconstitution may not be observed. However, when thenar muscles are present at the base of the thumb, transfer into the second toe can result in an excellent palmar abduction or adduction of the thoe. These anatomic considerations are seen primarily in the constriction ring syndrome and defects of hands related to chorionic villus sampling.

Vascular Anastomoses. Whereas some authors repair only one artery and one vein,[56] it is preferable to anastomose at least two arteries and either one large vein or two smaller veins. Often, the major artery is the plantar vessel to the second toe. Although the arteries may be smaller than those of adult "replant" patients, they are clean and free of any vascular disease. Beware of toe transfers in children with collagen vascular diagnoses (the author's only failure with 70 pediatric toe transfers occurred in a teenager with undiagnosed homocystinuria). Vein grafts are rarely needed. Anastomoses are routinely irrigated with a heparin-saline (5000 units heparin + 500 mL normal saline) solution and doused with papaverine before clamp release. Spasm in these young patients is most

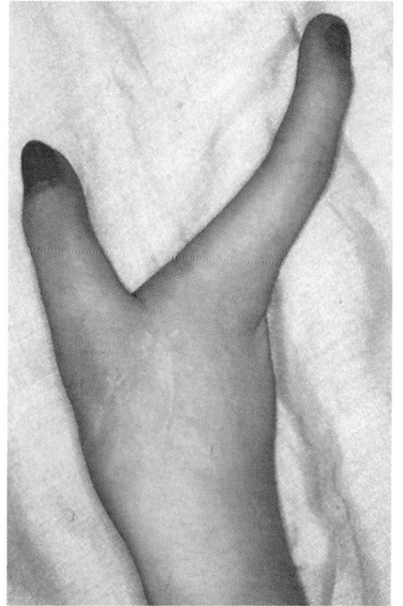
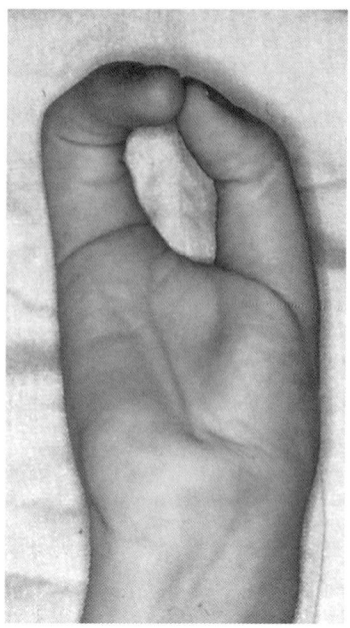

A

B

FIGURE 203-51. Prosthetic wear. *A,* This patient was born with a two-digit hand with a narrow web space. At 2 years of age, a modified pollicization of the radial digit was performed with a rotation-recession osteotomy at the metacarpal level and a V-Y lengthening of the web space (see Fig. 203-38C). Functional use and appearance were excellent at the age of 21 years. *B,* In public or at formal social functions, she still preferred to keep her hand hidden within a prosthetic hand or glove.

likely to be secondary to a rough donor or recipient site dissection than an intrinsic property of pediatric vessels. The vein repair is performed after the artery and often involves a long venous pedicle draining into one large vein, which is joined to a recipient vein at the level of the wrist.

Nerve Repair. The neural repairs are performed last and are routinely sealed with a fibrin glue preparation. When volar digital nerves are available (constriction ring syndrome, split hand-foot syndrome, chorionic villus sampling), direct nerve junctures are preferred. When no digital nerves (symbrachydactyly) or abnormal digital nerves (macrodactyly) are present, one should perform nerve junctures to normal dorsal sensory nerves.

Skin Closure. The skin is closed with absorbable sutures under no tension. Open areas including those containing vascular anastomoses are resurfaced with thick split-thickness skin grafts. If there is a consideration of closure under tension and graft, the graft is always performed. The transferred thoe is monitored with both a Doppler probe over the vessels and a pulse oximeter placed on the transferred part. At the time of discharge, the limb is immobilized with a long-arm cast extending proximal to the elbow flexed 90 degrees.

Prosthetic Wear

Although the major goal of hand surgery is to improve the function of the limb and hand, the appearance of these small hands is also important. The notion that cosmesis is important only to female patients is fallacious; parents and patients of both genders place equal importance on the appearance.[59,61,63] The appearance of the hand is not a trivial issue to these patients, who often understand the importance of function and reconstructive surgeries. Some patients are willing to have multiple staged reconstructions to achieve a better-looking hand without a major difference in function. Others will prefer to wear a hand prosthesis over their reconstructed and more functional hand during appropriate social events (Fig. 203-51). Others will often discard their prostheses after struggling with them in public view.[209] Single-digit or thumb prostheses worn with a ring at the base of the digit seem to be the most consistently worn in the author's practice.

Although some children will wear a prosthetic digit or thumb or hand consistently, most will not unless there is some type of sensory feedback. Those in grade school will also manage to lose or damage these expensive accessories, which then require replacement. Requests for prostheses may often come from older children and adolescents with either total or subtotal hand absence or an incomplete loss of the thumb. Patients with functional restorations may also wear a prosthesis for selected social occasions.

REFERENCES

1. Frantz C, O'Rahilly R: Congenital skeletal limb deficiencies. J Bone Joint Surg Am 1961;43:1202.
2. Birch-Jensen A: Congenital Deformities of the Upper Extremities. Odense, Denmark, Andelsbogtrykkeriet, 1949:15-36.
3. Temtamy S, McKusick V: The Genetics of Hand Malformations. New York, Alan R. Liss, 1978:73-181.
4. Smith R, Lipke R: Treatment of congenital deformities of the hand and forearm (two parts). N Engl J Med 1979;300:344-349, 402-407.
5. Taussig H: A study of the German outbreak of phocomelia: a thalidomide syndrome. JAMA 1962;180:1106-1114.
6. Sulamaa M, Ryoppy S: Early treatment of congenital bone defects of the extremities: aftermath of thalidomide disaster. Lancet 1964;Jan 18:130-132.
7. Swanson A: Phocomelia and congenital limb malformation: reconstruction and prosthetic replacement. Am J Surg 1965;109:294-299.
8. Clippinger F, Avery R, Titus B: A sensory feedback system for an upper-limb amputation prosthesis. Bull Prosthet Res 1974;Fall:247-258.
9. Kay HW, Day HJ, Henkel HL, et al: The proposed international terminology of the classification of congenital limb deficiencies. Dev Med Child Neurol Suppl 1975;34:1-12.
10. Stephens T: Proposed mechanisms of action in thalidomide embryopathy. Teratology 1988;38:229-239.
11. Fletcher I: Review of the treatment of thalidomide children with limb deficiencies in Great Britain. Clin Orthop 1980;148:18-25.
12. Hooper G: Phocomelia. In Gupta A, Kay SPJ, Scheker LR, eds: The Growing Hand: Diagnosis and Management of the Upper Extremity in Children. London, Churchill Livingstone, 2000:143.
13. Aitkin G, Frantz C: Management of the child amputee. Instr Lect Am Acad Orthop Surg 1960;17:246.
14. Kelikian H: Congenital Deformities of the Hand and Forearm. Philadelphia, WB Saunders, 1974:780-824.
15. Dick H, Tietjen R: Humeral lengthening for septic neonatal growth arrest: case report. J Bone Joint Surg Am 1978;60:1138-1139.
16. Posner M: Upper limb prostheses. In Bora FJ, ed: The Pediatric Upper Extremity. Philadelphia, WB Saunders, 1985:400.
17. Kadfors R, Taylor C: On the feasibility of myoelectric control of multifunctional orthoses. Scand J Rehabil Med 1973;5:134.
18. Marquardt E: The multiple limb-deficient child. In The American Academy of Orthopaedic Surgeons: Atlas of Limb Prosthetics: Surgical and Prosthetic Principles. St. Louis, CV Mosby, 1981:595.
19. Pellicore R, Lambert C: Congenital limb deficiencies: upper limb deficiencies. In The American Academy of Orthopaedic Surgeons: Atlas of Limb Prosthetics: Surgical and Prosthetic Principles. St. Louis, CV Mosby, 1981:518.
20. Krukenberg H: Über plastiche Umwertung von Amputationsstumpfen. Stuttgart, Ferdinand Enke, 1917.
21. Sung R: Experience with the Krukenberg plastic operation. Chin Med J 1957;7:212.
22. Nathan P, Trung N: The Krukenberg operation: a modified technique avoiding skin grafts. J Hand Surg Am 1977;2:127-130.
23. Chan KM, Ma GF, Cheng JC, Leung PC: The Krukenberg procedure: a method of treatment for unilateral anomalies of the upper limb in Chinese children. J Hand Surg Am 1984;9:548-551.
24. Murray J, Shore B, Trefler P: Prostheses for children with unilateral congenital absence of the hand. J Bone Joint Surg Am 1972;54:1658-1664.
25. Marquardt E: The Heidelberg pneumatic arm prosthesis. J Bone Joint Surg Br 1965;47:425-434.

26. Lamb D: Prosthetics in the upper extremity. J Hand Surg Am 1983;8(pt 2):774-777.

27. Lamb D, Law H: Upper Limb Deficiencies in Children: Prosthetic, Orthotic, and Surgical Management. Boston, Little, Brown, 1987:127.

28. Laboriel M, Setoguchi Y: Research in juvenile prosthetics. In The American Academy of Orthopaedic Surgeons: Atlas of Limb Prosthetics: Surgical and Prosthetic Principles. St. Louis, CV Mosby, 1981:642.

29. Yamauchi Y, Tanabu S: Symbrachydactyly. In Buck-Gramcko E, ed: Congenital Malformations of the Hand and Forearm. London, Churchill Livingstone, 1998:149.

30. Lister G: The Hand: Diagnosis and Indications. New York, Churchill Livingstone, 1984:312.

31. Flatt A: The Care of Congenital Hand Anomalies. St. Louis, CV Mosby, 1977:286.

32. Hentz V, Littler J: The surgical management of congenital hand anomalies. In Converse JM, ed: Plastic and Reconstructive Surgery. Philadelphia, WB Saunders, 1977:3306-3349.

33. Lamb D, Kuczynski K: The Practice of Hand Surgery. Edinburgh, Blackwell, 1981.

34. Lister G: Toes to the hand. In Flatt A, ed: The Care of Congenital Hand Anomalies. St. Louis, Quality Medical Publishers, 1994:180.

35. Entin M: Reconstruction of congenital anomalies of the upper extremities. J Bone Joint Surg Am 1959;41:681-701.

36. Dobyns J, et al: Congenital hand deformities. In Green DP, ed: Operative Hand Surgery. London, Churchill Livingstone, 1982:277.

37. Buck-Gramcko D: Hand surgery in congenital malformations. In Jackson I, ed: Recent Advances in Plastic Surgery. London, Churchill Livingstone, 1981:115-129.

38. Codivilla A: On the means of lengthening in the lower limbs, the muscles and tissues which are shortened through deformity. Am J Orthop Surg 1905;2:353-369.

39. Matev I: The distraction method in reconstructive surgery of the hand. In Tubiana R, ed: The Hand. Philadelphia, WB Saunders, 1985:535-549.

40. Matev I: Gradual elongation of the first metacarpal as a method of thumb reconstruction. In Stack H, Bolton H, eds: Proceedings of the Second Hand Club, 1956-1967. London, Royal College of Surgeons, 1975:431.

41. Kessler I, Baruch A, Hecht O: Experience with distraction lengthening of digital rays in congenital anomalies. J Hand Surg Am 1977;2:394-401.

42. Cowen N: Shortened digits can be stretched to normal length with new technique [interview with BJ Montgomery]. JAMA 1978;240:89.

43. Smith R, Gumley G: Metacarpal distraction lengthening. Clin Hand Surg 1985;1:417-429.

44. Upton J, Clarke H: Allongement progressif des membres. In Gilbert A, Buck-Gramcko D, Lister G, eds: Les malformations congenitales du membre supérieur. Paris, Expansion Scientifique Française, 1991:117-129.

45. Ulitskyi G, Malygin G: Roentgenological dynamics of reparative regeneration in lengthening of metacarpals by the distraction method. Acta Chir Plast 1973;15:82-92.

46. Mulliken J, Curtis R: Thumb lengthening by metacarpal distraction. J Trauma 1980;20:250-255.

47. Seitz WH Jr: Distraction treatment of the hand. In Buck-Gramcko D, ed: Congenital Malformations of the Hand and Forearm. London, Churchill Livingstone, 1998:119-128.

48. Upton J, Boyajian M, Mulliken JB, Glowacki J: The use of demineralized xenogenic bone implants to correct phalangeal defects: a case report. J Hand Surg Am 1984;9:388-391.

49. Seitz W: Distraction treatment of the hand. In Buck-Gramcko D, ed: Congenital Malformations of the Hand and Forearm. London, Churchill Livingstone, 1998:119-130.

50. Reid D: The Gillies thumb lengthening operation. Hand 1980;12:123-129.

51. Lister G: The Hand: Diagnosis and Indications, 2nd ed. New York, Churchill Livingstone, 1984:324.

52. O'Brien BM, Black MJ, Morrison WA, MacLeod AM: Microvascular great toe transfer for congenital absence of the thumb. Hand 1978;10:113-124.

53. May J, Smith R, Peimer C: Toe-to-hand free tissue transfer for thumb reconstruction with multiple digit aplasia. Plast Reconstr Surg 1981;67:205-213.

54. Gilbert A: Toe transfers for congenital hand defects. J Hand Surg Am 1982;7:118-124.

55. Kay S, Wiberg M, Bellew M, Webb F: Toe to hand transfer in children. Part 2. Functional and psychological aspects. J Hand Surg Br 1996;21:735-745.

56. Kay S: Microvascular toe transfer in children. Part A. Congenital defect. In Gupta A, Kay SPJ, Scheker LR, eds: The Growing Hand. London, Churchill Livingstone, 2000:987-999.

57. Lipton H, May JJ, Simon S: Preoperative and postoperative gait analyses of patients undergoing great toe-to-thumb transfer. J Hand Surg Am 1987;12:66-69.

58. Leung P: Problems in toe to hand transfer. Ann Acad Med Singapore 1982;12(suppl):377-381.

59. Kay S, Wiberg M: Toe to hand transfer in children. Part 1. Technical aspects. J Hand Surg Br 1996;21:723-734.

60. Tonkin MA, Nanchahal J, Kwa S: Ulnar-sided cleft hand. J Hand Surg Am 2002;27:493-497.

61. Beasley R: Cosmetic considerations in surgery of the hand. Surg Clin North Am 1971;51:471-477.

62. Pillet J: Esthetic hand prostheses. J Hand Surg Am 1983;8(pt 2):778-781.

63. Pillet J: Esthetic prostheses. In Gupta A, Kay SPJ, Scheker L, eds: The Child's Hand. London, Churchill Livingstone, 2000:1079-1090.

64. Ogino T: Cleft hand. Hand Clin 1990;6:661-671.

65. Duraiswami P: Experimental causation of congenital skeletal defects and its significance in orthopedic surgery. J Bone Joint Surg Br 1952;34:646-698.

66. Kelikian H: Cleft hand. In Kelikian H, ed: Congenital Deformities of the Hand and Forearm. Philadelphia, WB Saunders, 1974:467-495.

67. Goldberg M, Meyn M: The radial club hand. Orthop Clin North Am 1976;7:341-349.

68. Pauli R, Feldman PF: Major limb malformations following intrauterine exposure to ethanol: two additional cases and literature review. Teratology 1986;33:273-280.

69. Lindhout D, Stewart PS, Reuss A, et al: Prenatal ultrasound in antiepileptic drug exposure. Teratology 1988;37:473-474.

70. Verloes A, Frikiche A, Gremillet C, et al: Proximal phocomelia and radial ray aplasia in fetal valproic syndrome. Eur J Pediatr 1990;149:266-267.

71. Ogino T: Clinical and experimental study on the teratogenic mechanisms of cleft hand, polydactyly, and syndactyly. J Jpn Orthop Assoc 1979;53:535-543.

72. Ogino T: Teratogenic mechanisms of longitudinal deficiency and cleft hand. Handchir Mikrochir Plast Chir 2004;36:108-116.

73. Kato H, Ogino T, Minami A, Ohshio E: Experimental study of radial ray deficiency. J Hand Surg Br 1990;15:470-476.

74. Matsumura T: Congenital hand malformations—local disturbance in the limb bud and longitudinal deficiency: an experimental study on the pathogenesis. Nippon Seikeigeka Gakkai Zasshi 1994;68:234-249.

75. Bod M, Czeizel A, Lenz W: Incidence at birth of different types of limb reduction abnormalities in Hungary 1975-1977. Hum Genet 1983;65:27-33.

76. Kallen B, Rahmani TM, Winberg J: Infants with congenital limb reduction registered in the Swedish Register of Congenital Malformations. Teratology 1984;29:73-85.

77. Wynne-Davies R, Lamb DW: Congenital upper limb anomalies: an etiologic grouping of clinical, genetic, and epidemiological data from 387 patients with "absence" defects, constriction bands, polydactylies, and syndactylies. J Hand Surg Am 1985;10:958-964.

78. Forbes G: A case of congenital club hand with a review of the etiology of the condition. Anat Rec 1938;71:181-199.

79. Bayne L, Klug W: Long-term review of the surgical treatment of radial deficiencies. J Hand Surg Am 1987;12:169-179.

80. Lamb D: Radial club hand: a continuing study of sixty-eight patients with one hundred and seventeen club hands. J Bone Joint Surg Am 1977;59:1-13.

81. Urban M., Osterman AL: Management of radial dysplasia. Hand Clin 1990;6:589-605.

82. Skerik S, Flatt A: The anatomy of congenital radial dysplasia. Clin Orthop 1969;66:125-143.

83. Lourie G, Lins RE: Radial longitudinal deficiency: a review and update. Hand Clin 1998;14:85-99.

84. Goldenberg R: Congenital bilateral complete absence of the radius in identical twins. J Bone Joint Surg Am 1948;30:1001-1003.

85. Upton J: Congenital anomalies of the hand and forearm. In May JW Jr, Littler JW, eds: The Hand. Philadelphia, WB Saunders, 1990:5213-5398. McCarthy JG, ed: Plastic Surgery; vol 8.

86. Cox H, Viljoen D, Versfield G, et al: Radial ray defects and associated anomalies. Clin Genet 1989;35:322-330.

87. Goldberg M, Bartoshesky L: Congenital hand anomaly: etiology and associated malformations. Hand Clin 1985;1:405-415.

88. D'Arcangelo M, Gupta A, Scheker LR: The growing hand. In Gupta A, Kay SPJ, Scheker LR, eds: The Growing Hand. London, Churchill Livingstone, 2000:147-170.

89. Lin A, Perloff J: Upper limb malformations associated with congenital heart disease. Am J Cardiol 1985;55:1576-1583.

90. Fanconi G: Familial constitutional panmyelocytopathy. Fanconi's anemia (F.A.) I. Clinical aspects. Semin Hematol 1967;4:233-240.

91. Gmyrek D, Syllm-Rapoport I: Zur Fanconi Anämie. Analyse von 129 beschriebenen Fallen. Z Kinderheilkd 1964;91:297-337.

92. Auerbach A, Sagi M, Adler B: Fanconi anemia: prenatal diagnosis in 30 fetuses at risk. Pediatrics 1985;76:794-800.

93. Quan L, Smith D: The VATER association: vertebral defects, anal atresia, T-E fistula with esophageal atresia, radial and renal dysplasia: a spectrum of associated defects. J Pediatr 1973;82:104-107.

94. Holt M, Oram S: Familial heart disease with skeletal malformations. Br Heart J 1960;22:236-242.

95. Carroll R, Louis D: Anomalies associated with radial dysplasia. J Pediatr 1974;84:409-411.

96. Hall J: Thrombocytopenia with absent radius (TAR) syndrome. J Med Genet 1987;24:79-83.

97. Hays R, Bartoshesky L, Feingold M: New features of thrombocytopenia and absent radius syndrome. Birth Defects Orig Artic Ser 1982;18:115-121.

98. Dell PC, Sheppard JE: Thrombocytopenia, absent radius syndrome: report of two siblings and a review of the hematologic and genetic features. Clin Orthop 1982;162:129-134.

99. Smith D: Recognizable Patterns of Human Malformation: Genetic, Embryologic and Clinical Aspects, 3rd ed. Philadelphia, WB Saunders, 1982:236.

100. Heikel H: Aplasia and hypoplasia of the radius: studies of 64 cases of epiphyseal transplantation in rabbits with the mutated defect. Acta Orthop Scand Suppl 1959;39:1-55.

101. O'Rahilly R: Morphological patterns in limb deficiencies and duplications. Am J Anat 1951;89:135-194.

102. James M, McCarroll HR Jr, Manske PR: The spectrum of radial longitudinal deficiency: a modified classification. J Hand Surg Am 1999;24:1145-1155.

103. Kato K: Congenital absence of the radius with review of the literature and report of three cases. J Bone Joint Surg 1924;6:589-626.

104. Imamura T, Miura T: The carpal bones in congenital hand anomalies: a radiographic study in patients older than ten years. J Hand Surg Am 1988;13:650-656.

105. O'Rahilly R: An analysis of cases of radial hemimelia. Arch Pathol Lab Med 1947;44:28-33.

106. Riordan D: Congenital absence of the radius. J Bone Joint Surg Am 1955;37:1129-1140.

107. Bayne L: Radial club hand. In Green DP, ed: Operative Hand Surgery. New York, Churchill Livingstone, 1982:219-233.

108. Blauth W: Zur Morphologie und Therapie der radialen Klumphand. Arch Orthop Unfallchir 1969;65:97-123.

109. Flatt A: The Care of Congenital Hand Anomalies. St. Louis, CV Mosby, 1977:99-117, 228-248.

110. Stoffel A, Stempel E: Anatomische Studien über die Klumphand. Stuttgart, Enke, 1909.

111. Temtamy S, McKusick V: The Genetics of Hand Malformations. The National Foundation-March of Dimes. New York, Alan R. Liss, 1978. Birth Defects: Original Article Series; vol 14.

112. Hedberg V, Lipton JM: Thrombocytopenia with absent radii. Am J Pediatr 1988;10:51-64.

113. Manske P, McCarroll HR: Radial club hand. In Buck-Gramcko D, ed: Congenital Malformations of the Hand and Forearm. London, Churchill Livingstone, 1998:433-447.

114. Riordan D: Congenital absence of the radius: a fifteen year follow-up. J Bone Joint Surg Am 1963;45:1783.

115. Buck-Gramcko D: Radialization as a new treatment for radial club hand. J Hand Surg Am 1985;10:964-968.

116. Buck-Gramcko D: Syndactyly between the thumb and index finger. In Buck-Gramcko D, ed: Congenital Malformations of the Hand and Forearm. London, Churchill Livingstone, 1998:141-147.

117. Upton J: Congenital anomalies of the hand and forearm. In May JW Jr, Littler JW, eds: The Hand. Philadelphia, WB Saunders, 1990:5213-5398. McCarthy JG, ed: Plastic Surgery; vol 8.

118. Bayne L: Ulna club hand (ulnar deficiencies). In Green DP, ed: Operative Hand Surgery. New York, Churchill Livingstone, 1982:245-256.

119. Dobyns J, Wood VE, Bayne LG: Congenital hand deformities. In Green DP, ed: Operative Hand Surgery. New York, Churchill Livingstone, 1993:288-303.

120. Flatt A: The Care of Congenital Hand Anomalies. St. Louis, Quality Medical Publishers, 1984.

121. Define D: Treatments of congenital radial club hand. Clin Orthop 1970;73:153-159.

122. Upton J, Pap S: Congenital anomalies. In Goldwyn R, Cohen MN, eds: The Unfavorable Result in Plastic Surgery. Philadelphia, Lippincott Williams & Wilkins, 2001:693-710.

123. Albee F: Formation of the radius congenitally absent: condition seven years after implantation of bone graft. Ann Surg 1928;87:105-110.

124. Hoffa A: Lehrbuch der orthopädischen Chirurgie, 4th ed. Stuttgart, Ferdinand Enke, 1902:557.

125. Gocht T: Ätiologie, Pathogenese und Therapie der Deformitäten im Allgemeinen. In Hoffa A, ed: Orthopädische Chirurgie. Stuttgart, Enke Verlag, 1925.

126. Gardemin H: Zur frühoperation der angeborenen Radiusaplasie. Langenbecks Arch Klin Chir 1964;306:183-185.

127. Lidge R: Congenital radial deficient club hand. J Bone Joint Surg Am 1969;51:1041-1043.

128. Sayre R: A contribution to the study of the club hand. Trans Am Orthop Assoc 1893;6:208-216.

129. Starr D: Congenital absence of the radius: a method of surgical correction. J Bone Joint Surg 1945;27:572-577.

130. Romano C: Grave, mano torta congenita. Raddrizzamento merce osteoectomia segmentaria trapezoidale del cubito e tenotomia del musculo grande palmare. Arch Ortop 1894;11:80-93.

131. Antonelli I: Su un caso di mancanza congenita bilaterale de radio. Gazz Med Ital Torino 1904;55:501-505, 519.

132. Vilkki S: Advances in microsurgical reconstruction of the congenitally adactylous hand. Clin Orthop 1995;314:44-58.

133. Blauth W: Die operative Behandlung der angeborenen Fehlbildungen der Hand. Verh Dtsch Ges Orthop Traumat 1969;3:386-402.

134. Bora FJ, Nicholson J, Cheema H: Radial meromelia, the deformity and its treatment. J Bone Joint Surg Am 1970;52:966-979.

135. DeLorme T: Treatment of congenital absence of the radius by transepiphyseal fixation. J Bone Joint Surg Am 1969;51:117-129.

136. Watson H, Beebe R, Cruz N: A centralization procedure for radial club hand. J Hand Surg Am 1984;9:541-547.

137. Buchler U: Symbrachydactyly. In Gupta A, Kay SPJ, Scheker LR, eds: The Growing Hand: Diagnosis and Management of the Upper Extremity in Children. London, Churchill Livingstone, 2000:213.

138. Weiland AJ, Daniel RK, Riley LH Jr: Application of the free vascularized bone graft in the treatment of malignant or aggressive bone tumors. Johns Hopkins Med J 1977;140:85-96.

139. Tsai T, Ludwig L, Tonkin M: Free vascularized epiphyseal transfer. In Urbaniak J, ed: Microsurgery for Major Limb Reconstruction. St. Louis, CV Mosby, 1987:318-324.

140. Smith AA, Greene TL: Preliminary soft tissue distraction in congenital forearm deficiency. J Hand Surg Am 1995;20:420-424.

141. Tonkin M, Nanchahal J: An approach to the management of radial longitudinal deficiency. Ann Acad Med Singapore 1995;24(suppl):101-107.

142. Nanchahal J, Tonkin MA: Preoperative distraction lengthening for radial longitudinal deficiency. J Hand Surg Br 1996;21:103-107.

143. Buck-Gramcko D: Cleft hands: classification and treatment. Hand Clin 1985;1:467-473.

144. Bora FW Jr, Osterman AL, Kaneda RR, Esterhai J: The radial club hand deformity. J Bone Joint Surg Am 1981;63:741-745.

145. Kessler I: Centralization of the radial club hand by gradual distraction. J Hand Surg Br 1989;14:37-42.

146. Manske P, McCarroll H, Swanson K: Centralization of the radial club hand: an ulnar surgical approach. J Hand Surg Am 1981;6:423-433.

147. Snyder M, Bora FJ: Leczenie wrodzonej reki koslawe. Chir Narz Ruchu Ortop Pol 1984;49:47-50.

148. Bunnell S: Restoring flexion to the paralytic elbow. J Bone Joint Surg Am 1951;33:566-571.

149. Menelaus M: Radial club hand with absence of the bicep muscle treated by centralization of the ulna and triceps transfer: report of two cases. J Bone Joint Surg Br 1976;58:488-491.

150. Clark J: Reconstruction of biceps brachii by pectoralis muscle transplantation. Br J Surg 1946;34:180-181.

151. Buck-Gramcko D: Congenital disorders: radial and ulnar club hand. In Berger RA, Weiss A-PC, eds: Hand Surgery. Philadelphia, Lippincott Williams & Wilkins, 2002:1453-1464.

152. Manske P, McCarroll HR Jr: Abductor digiti quinti minimi opponensplasty in congenital radial dysplasia. J Hand Surg 1978;3:552-559.

153. Glossop N, Flatt AE: Opening versus closing wedge osteotomy of the curved ulna in radial clubhand. J Hand Surg Am 1995;20:133-143.

154. Dick HM, Petzoldt RL, Bowers WR, Rennie WR: Lengthening of the ulna in radial agenesis: a preliminary report. J Hand Surg Am 1977;2:175-178.

155. Paley D: Distraction treatment of the forearm. In Buck-Gramcko D, ed: Congenital Malformations of the Hand and Forearm. London, Churchill Livingstone, 1998:73-118.

156. Pickford M, Scheker LR: Distraction lengthening of the ulna in radial club hand using the Ilizarov technique. J Hand Surg Br 1998;23:186-191.

157. CHASG (Congenital Hand Anomaly Study Group): Discussion of radial dysplasia recurrence; Fouchet G, ed. Strasbourg, France, 1999.

158. Geck M, Dorey F, Lawrence JF, Johnson MK: Congenital radius deficiency: radiographic outcome and survivorship analysis. J Hand Surg Am 1999;24:1132-1144.

159. Buck-Gramcko D, Lamb D, Tonkin MA, Valenti P: Radialization has certainly improved the treatment of radial club hand [debate]. European Congress of Hand Surgery, Paris, 1996.

160. Paradini AJ: Radial dysplasia. Clin Orthop 1968;57:153-177.

161. Frankel M, Goldner JL, Stelling FH: Radial club hand: is centralization necessary? A rational surgical approach. J Bone Joint Surg Am 1971;53:1026.

162. Lamb D: The treatment of radial club hand: absent radius, aplasia of the radius, hypoplasia of the radius, radial paraxial hemimelia. Hand 1972;4:22-30.

163. Vilkki S: Vascularized joint transfer for radial club hand. Techniques Hand Upper Extremity Surg 1998;2:126-137.

164. Hippe P, Blauth W: Erfahrungen mit Klumphandoperationen. Z Orthop 1979;117:863-872.

165. Warkany J: Syndromes. Am J Dis Child 1971;121:365.

166. Hartsinck J: Beschryving van Guiana of de Wilde Kust in Zuid-America, vol 2. Amsterdam, Gerrit Tielenburg, 1770:811-812.

167. Wood V: The cleft hand (central deficiencies). In Green DP, ed: Operative Hand Surgery. New York, Churchill Livingstone, 1982:233-245.

168. Kelikian H: Congenital Deformities of the Hand and Forearm. Philadelphia, WB Saunders, 1974:902-938.

169. Temtamy S, McKusick V: The Genetics of Hand Malformations. New York, Alan R. Liss, 1978.

170. Tada K, Yonenobu K, Swanson A: Congenital central ray deficiency in the hand—a survey of 59 cases and subclassification. J Hand Surg Am 1981;6:434-441.

171. Tsuge K, Ishil S, Ueba Y, et al: Report of the Japanese Society for Surgery of the Hand, Committee on Congenital Malformation of the Hand. Orthop Surg (Jpn) 1980;31:1959-1603.

172. Barsky A: Cleft hand: classification, incidence and treatment. Review of the literature and report of nineteen cases. J Bone Joint Surg Am 1964;46:1707-1720.

173. Lange M: Grundsatzliches über die Beurteilung der Entstehung und Bewertung atypischer Hand und Fußmißbildungen, Ges 3 1st Congress Konigsberg Pr. Z Orthop Suppl 1937;66:80-87.

174. Sandzen SJ: Classification and functional management of congenital central defect of the hand. Hand Clin 1985;1:483-498.

175. Blauth W, Falliner A: Zur Morphologie und Klassifikation von Spalthanden. Handchir Mikrochir Plast Chir 1986;18:161-195.

176. Ogino T, Kato H: Cleft hand without absence of a finger. Handchirurgie 1988;20:184-188.

177. Miura T: Congenital absence of the fourth metacarpal bone (congenital dysplasia of the ring finger). J Hand Surg Am 1988;13:93-96.

178. Watari S, Tsuge K: A classification of cleft hands based on clinical findings. Plast Reconstr Surg 1979;64:381-389.

179. Manske P, Halikis MN: Surgical classification of central deficiency according to the thumb web. J Hand Surg Am 1995;20:687-697.

180. Birch-Jensen A: Congenital Deformities of the Upper Extremity. Copenhagen, Munksgaard, 1949.

181. Calzolari E, Manservigi D, Garani GP, et al: Limb reduction defects in Emilia Romagna, Italy: epidemiological and genetic study in 173,109 consecutive births. J Med Genet 1990;27:353-357.

182. Froster-Iskenius U, Baird PA: Limb reduction defects in over one million consecutive live births. Teratology 1989;39:127-135.

183. Rogala E, Wynne-Davies R, Littlejohn A, Gormley J: Congenital limb anomalies: frequency and aetiological factors. J Med Genet 1974;11:221-233.

184. Maisels D: Lobster claw deformities of the hands and feet. Br J Plast Surg 1970;23:269-282.

185. Bixler D, Bennett SJ, Christian JC: The ectrodactyly-ectodermal dysplasia-clefting (EEC) syndrome. Clin Genet 1971;3:43-51.

186. Müller W: Die angeborenen Fehlbildungen der menschlichen Hand. Leipzig, Thieme, 1937.

187. Ogino T: A clinical and experimental study on the teratogenic mechanism of cleft hand, polydactyly and syndactyly. J Jpn Orthop Assoc 1979;53:535-543.

188. Ogino T: Teratologic relationship between polydactyly, syndactyly and cleft hand. J Hand Surg Br 1990;15:201-209.

189. Ogino T, Ischii S, Minami M, et al: Congenital anomalies of the hand. The Asian perspective. Clin Orthop 1996;323:12-21.

190. Miura T: Syndactyly and split hand. Hand 1976;8:125-130.

191. Tsuge K, Watari S: New surgical procedures for correction of club hand. J Hand Surg Br 1985;10:90-94.

192. Miura T, Nakamura R, Suzuki M, Watanabe K: Cleft hand, syndactyly and hypoplastic thumb. J Hand Surg Br 1992;17:365-370.

193. Zguricas J, Bakker WF, Heus H, et al: Genetics of limb development and congenital hand malformations. Plast Reconstr Surg 1998;101:1126-1135.

194. Schwabe G, Mundlos S: Genetics of congenital hand anomalies. Handchir Mikrochir Plast Chir 2004;36:85-97.

194a. Ianakiev P, Kilpatrick MW, Toudjarska I, et al: Split-hand/split-foot malformation is caused by mutations in the p63 gene on 3q27. Am J Hum Genet 2000;67:59-66.

195. Buss P: Cleft hand/foot: clinical and developmental aspects [review]. J Med Genet 1994;31:726-730.

196. Scherer SW, Allen T, Kim J, et al: Fine mapping of the autosomal dominant split hand/split foot locus on chromosome 7, band q21.3-22.1. Am J Hum Genet 1994;2:12-20.

197. Faiyaz ul Haque M, Uhlhass S, Knapp M, et al: Mapping of the gene for X-chromosomal split hand/split foot anomaly to Xq26-26.1. Hum Genet 1993;1:17-19.

198. Nunes M, Schutt G, Kapur RP, et al: A second autosomal split hand/split foot locus maps to chromosome 10q24-q25. Hum Mol Genet 1995;4:2165-2170.

199. Gurrieri F, Prinos P, Tackels D, et al: A split hand/split foot (SHFM3) gene is located at 10q24-q25. Am J Med Genet 1996;62:427-436.

200. Von Bokhoven H, Jung M, Smits AP, et al: Limb mammary syndrome (LMS): a new genetic disorder with mammary hypoplasia, ectrodactyly, and other hand/foot anomalies maps to human chromosome 3q27. Am J Hum Genet 1999;64:538-546.

201. Czeizel A, Vitez M, Kodaj L, Lenz W: An epidemiological study of isolated split hand/foot in Hungary, 1975-1984. J Med Genet 1993;30:593-596.

202. Upton J: Simplicity and the treatment of the typical cleft hand. Handchir Mikrochir Plast Chir 2004;36:152-160.

203. Wood V: The treatment of crossbones of the hand. Handchir Mikrochir Plast Chir 2004;36:161-165.

204. Miura T, Suzuki M: Clinical differences between typical and atypical cleft hand. J Hand Surg Br 1984;9:98-102.

205. Wood V: Superdigit. Hand Clin 1990;6:673-684.

206. Egawa T, Horiki A, Senrui H, Tada K: Charakteristische anatomische Befunde der Spalthand—ihre Bedeutung und Klassifikation. Handchirurgie 1978;10:3-8.

207. Otto A: Monstrorum Sexcentorum Descriptio Anatomica. Vratislaviae, Hirt, 1841.

208. Ueba Y, Nishjioma N, Hamanishi C, et al: Angiography in the treatment for congenital anomalies of the hand. J Jpn Soc Surg Hand 1984;1:269-272.

209. Walker B: A letter to my daughter. In Flatt A, ed: The Care of Congenital Hand Anomalies, 2nd ed. St. Louis, Quality Medical Publishers, 1994:3.

210. Flatt A: The Care of Congenital Hand Anomalies, 2nd ed. St. Louis, Quality Medical Publishers, 1994.

211. Flatt A: Cleft hand and central defects. In Flatt A, ed: The Care of Congenital Hand Anomalies. St. Louis, Quality Medical Publishers, 1977:265.

212. Miura T, Komada T: Simple method for reconstruction of the cleft hand with an adducted thumb. Plast Reconstr Surg 1979;64:65-67.

213. Nutt J, Flatt A: Congenital central hand deficit. Hand Surg 1981;6:48-60.

214. Rider MA, Tonkin MA, Wood VE: An experience of the Snow-Littler procedure. J Hand Surg Br 2000;25:376-381.

215. Snow J, Littler J: Surgical treatment of the cleft hand. Transactions of the 4th International Congress of Plastic and Reconstructive Surgeons, Rome 1967. Amsterdam, Excerpta Medica, 1969:888-893.

216. Ueba Y: Plastic surgery for the cleft hand. J Hand Surg Am 1981;6:557-560.

217. Upton J, Havlik RJ, Coombs CJ: Use of forearm flaps for the severely contracted first web space in children with congenital malformations. J Hand Surg Am 1996;21:470-477.

218. Littler J: Principles of reconstructive surgery of the hand. In Converse JM, ed: Plastic and Reconstructive Surgery. Philadelphia, WB Saunders, 1977:3103-3153.

219. Eaton C, Lister GD: Toe transfer for congenital hand defects. Microsurgery 1991;12:186-195.

220. Shvedovchenko I: Toe-to-hand transfers in children. Ann Plast Surg 1993;31:251-254.

221. Berger A, Reichert B: Heterotopic finger transfer in ulnar ray deficiency associated with contralateral postaxial polydactyly. J Reconstr Microsurg 1993;9:27-32.

222. Upton J: Discussion: Heterotopic transfer of ulnar ray from hand and foot and foot to hand. J Reconstr Microsurg 1993;9:109-110.

223. Blauth W, Borisch NC: Proposals for a new classification based on roentgenological morphology. Clin Orthop 1990;258:41-48.

224. Dobyns J, Wood VE, Bayne LG: Congenital hand deformities. In Green D, ed: Operative Hand Surgery. New York, Churchill Livingstone, 1993:251-548.

225. Kümmel W: Die Mißbildungen der Extremitäten durch Defekt, Verwachsung und Überzahl. Cassel, Fischer, 1895.

226. Miller J, Wenner S, Kruger L: Ulnar deficiency. J Hand Surg Am 1986;11:822-829.

227. Ogden J, Watson H, Bohne W: Ulnar dysmelia. J Bone Joint Surg Am 1976;58:467-475.

228. Riordan D, Mills E, Alldredge R: Congenital absence of the ulna. Proceedings of the American Society for Surgery of the Hand. J Bone Joint Surg Am 1961;43:614.

229. Swanson A, Tada K, Yonenobu K: Ulnar ray deficiency: its various manifestations. J Hand Surg Am 1984;9:658-664.

230. Carroll R: Congenital absence of the ulna. In Buck-Gramcko D, ed: Congenital Malformations of the Hand and Forearm. London, Churchill Livingstone, 1998:449-461.

231. Johnson J, Omer G: Congenital ulnar deficiency. Natural history and therapeutic implications. Hand Clin 1985;1:499-510.

232. Carroll R, Bowers W: Congenital deficiency of the ulna. J Hand Surg Am 1977;2:169-174.

233. Broudy A, Smith R: Deformities of the hand and wrist with ulnar deficiency. J Hand Surg Am 1979;4:304-315.

234. Buck-Gramcko D: Ulnar deficiency. In Tubiana R, Gilbert A: Tendon, Nerve, and Other Disorders. London, Martin Dunitz, 2004:439-455.

235. Temtamy S, McKusick V: Ulnar defects. In Temtamy S, McKusick V, eds: The Genetics of Hand Malformations. Birth Defects: Original Article Series; vol 14. New York, Alan R. Liss, 1978:48-51, 149-157.

236. Bambshad M, Lin RC, Wastkins WC, et al: Mutations in human TBX3 alter limb, apocrine and genital development in ulnar-mammary syndrome. Nat Genet 1997;16:311-315.

237. Davenport T, Jerome-Majewska LA, Papaioannou VE: Mammary gland, limb and yolk sac defects in mice lacking Tbx3, the gene mutated in human ulnar mammary syndrome. Development 2003;130:2263 2273.

238. Cole R, Manske PR: Classification of ulnar deficiency according to the thumb and first web. J Hand Surg Am 1997;22;479-488.

239. Marcus N, Omer GJ: Carpal deviation in congenital ulnar deficiency. J Bone Joint Surg Am 1984;66:1003.

240. Riordan D: Congenital absence of the ulna. In Lovell W, Winter R, eds: Pediatric Orthopaedics. Philadelphia, WB Saunders, 1978:714-719.

241. Southwood A: Partial absence of the ulna and associated structures. J Anat 1926-27;61:346-351.

242. Mulligan P: The elbow in the "ulnar club" hand. In Gupta A, Kay SPJ, Scheker LR, eds: The Growing Hand. London, Churchill Livingstone, 2000:197-202.

243. Straub L: Congenital absence of the ulna. Am J Surg 1965;109:300-305.

244. Blair W, Shurr D, Buckwalter J: Functional status of ulnar deficiency. J Pediatr Orthop 1983;3:37-40.

245. Watson H, Bohne W: The role of the fibrous band in ulnar deficient extremities. Proceedings of American Society for Surgery of the Hand. J Bone Joint Surg Am 1971;53:816.

246. Tachdjian M: Pediatric Orthopedics. Philadelphia, WB Saunders, 1972:232-247.

247. Coombs CJ, Mutimer KL: Tissue expansion for the treatment of complete syndactyly of the first web. J Hand Surg Am 1994;19:968-972.

248. Imagawa S: Symbrachydactyly: review of 50 cases and definition. Hiroshima J Med Sci 1980;29:105-115.

249. Blauth W, Gekeler J: Zur Morphologie und Klassifikation der Symbrachydaktylie. Handchirurgie 1971;3:123-128.

250. Blauth W, Gekeler J: Symbrachydaktylien. Beitrag zur Morphologie, Klassifikation und Therapie. Handchirurgie 1973;5:121-171.

251. Poland A: Deficiency of the pectoral muscles. Guys Hosp Rep 1841;6:191-193.

252. Clarkson P: Poland's syndactyly. Guys Hosp Rep 1962;111:335-346.

253. Glicenstein J, Pennecot G-F, Duhamel B: Le syndrome de Poland 17 nouvelles observations. Ann Chir Plast Esthet 1974;19:47-54.

254. Ireland D, Takayama N, Flatt A: Poland's syndrome. A review of forty-three cases. J Bone Joint Surg Am 1976;58:52-58.

255. Mace J, Kaplan JM, Schanberger JE, Gotlin RW: Poland's syndrome. Report of seven cases and review of the literature. Clin Pediatr 1972;11:98-102.

256. Sugiura Y: Poland's syndrome: clinico-roentgenographic study of 45 cases. Cong Anom 1976;16:17-28.

257. Ravitch M: Poland's syndrome—a study of an eponym. Plast Reconstr Surg 1977;59:508-512.

258. Al-Quattan M: Classification of hand anomalies in Poland's syndrome. Br J Plast Surg 2001;54:132-136.

259. Zaleskie D: Development of the upper limb. Hand Clin 1985;1:383-390.

260. Beer G, Kompatscher P, Hergan K: Poland's syndrome and vascular malformations. Br J Plast Surg 1996;49:482-484.

261. Bouwes-Bavinck J, Weaver D: Subclavian artery supply disruption sequence: hypothesis of a vascular etiology for Poland, Klippel-Feil, and Mobius anomalies. Am J Med Genet 1986;23:903-918.

262. Freire-Maia N, Azevedo JBC: Reduction deformities, twinning and mortality in Brazilian whites and negroes. Acta Genet Med Gemellol 1977;26:133-140.

263. Yamauchi Y, Nakamura S, Ando T, et al: On symbrachydaktylie. Seikeigeka 1975;26:1437-1440.

264. Pol R: "Brachydaktylie"—"Klinodaktylie"—Hyperphalangie und ihre Grundlagen: Form und Entstehung der meist unter dem Bild der Brachydaktylie auftretenden Varietaten, Anomalien und Mißbildungen der Hand und des Fußes. Virchows Arch Pathol Anat 1921;229:388-530.

265. DeSmet L, Fabray G: Characteristics of patients with symbrachydactyly. J Pediatr Orthop 1998;2:158-161.

266. Buck-Gramcko D: Symbrachydactylie. Classification et traitement chirurgical. In Gilbert A, Lister G, Buck-Gramcko D, eds: Les malformations congenitales du membre supérieur. Paris, Expansion Scientifique Française, 1991.

267. Ogino T, Ischii S, Minami M, et al: Studies on clinical features and roentgenograms of symbrachydactylies of human hands. Nippon Seikeigeka Gakkai Zasshi 1978;52:1753-1760.

268. Bouvet J, Maroteaux P, Briadr-Guillemot M: Le syndrome de Poland. Etudes clinique et genetique—considerations physiopathologiques. Nouv Presse Med 1976;5:185-190.

269. Bavinck J, Weaver DD: Subclavian artery supply disruption sequence: hypothesis of a vascular etiology of Poland, Klippel-Feil, Mobius anomalies. Am J Genet 1996;23:903-918.

270. Falliner A: Isolierte Symbrachydaktylie des Fusses. Z Orthop 1988;126:125-126.

271. Ogino T, Minami A, Kato H: Symbrachydactylie. Etude clinique et radiologique. In Gilbert A, Lister G, Buck-Gramcko D, eds: Les malformations congenitales du membre supérieur. Paris, Expansion Scientifique Française, 1991.

272. Senrui H: Clinical findings and treatment of symbrachydactyly. Seikeigeka Mook 1984;35:274-290.

273. Tanubu S: Clinical and roentgenological study of the hands in symbrachydactyly, constriction bone syndrome and cleft hand. Nippon Seikeigeka Gakkai Zasshi 1985;59:167-182.

274. Beatty E: Upper limb tissue differentiation in the human embryo. Hand Clin 1985;1:391-403.

275. Buck-Gramcko D: Classification and traitement chirurgical. In Gilbert A, Lister G, Buck-Gramcko D, eds: Les malformations congenitales du membre supérieur. Paris, Expansion Scientifique Française, 1991.

276. Friedman R, Wood VE: The dorsal transposition flap for congenital contractures of the first web space: a 20-year experience. J Hand Surg Am 1997;22:664-670.

277. Buck-Gramcko D: The role of nonvascularized toe phalanx transplantation. Hand Clin 1990;6:643-659.

278. Radocka R, Netscher D, Kleinert HE: Toe phalangeal grafts in congenital hand anomalies. J Hand Surg Am 1993;18:833-841.

279. Rank B: Long-term results in epiphyseal transplants in congenital deformities of the hand. Plast Reconstr Surg 1978;61:321-329.

280. Carroll R, Green DP: Reconstruction of the hypoplastic digits using toe phalanges. J Bone Joint Surg Am 1975;57:727.

281. Kleinert H, Brotherston M, Mesa-Betancourt F: Free toe phalangeal transfers in congenital hand anomalies. In Gupta A, Kay SPJ, Scheker LR, eds: The Growing Hand. London, Churchill Livingstone, 2000:1045-1048.

282. Hulsbergen-Kruger S, Preisser P, Partecke BD: Ilizarov distraction-lengthening in congenital anomalies of the upper limb. J Hand Surg Br 1988;23:192-195.

283. Foucher G: Toe transplantation in congenital malformations of the hand [in French]. Bull Acad Natl Med 1997;181:1737-1744.

284. Gilbert A: Congenital absence of the thumb and digits. J Hand Surg Br 1989;14:6-15.

285. Yamauchi Y, Fujimaki A, Yanaghiharam Y, et al: A free toe transfer for congenital unilateral monodactylia: a case report. Seikeigeka 1980;31:1594-1596.

286. Nicoladoni C: Daumenplastik. Wien Klin Wochenschr 1897;10:663-665.
287. Freeman B: Reconstruction of thumb by toe transfer. Plast Reconstr Surg 1956;17:393-398.
288. Cobbett J: Free digital transfer. Report of a case of transfer of a great toe to replace an amputated thumb. J Bone Joint Surg Br 1969;51:677-679.
289. Gilbert A, Morrison WSA, Tubiana R, et al: Transfert sur la main d'un iambeau libre sensible. Chirugie 1975;101:691-694.
290. Bradbury E, Kay SP, Tighe C, Hewison J: Decision-making by parents and children in paediatric hand surgery. Br J Plast Surg 1994;47:324-330.
291. Rylance G: Making decisions with children. BMJ 1996;312:794.
292. Foucher G, Moss AL: Microvascular second toe transfer: a statistical analysis of 55 transfers. Br J Plast Surg 1991;44:87-90.
293. Lister G: Microsurgical transfer of the second toe for congenital deficiency of the thumb. Plast Reconstr Surg 1988;82:658-665.
294. Wilson R, Yates APB: Paediatric microvascular surgery: anesthetic experience of 27 toe transfers. Paediatr Anaesth 1993;3:209-215.
295. Upton J: Direct visualization of arterial anatomy during toe harvest dissections: clinical and radiological correlations. Plast Reconstr Surg 1995;102:1988-1992.
296. Upton J, Littler JW: Discussion of microvascular thumb reconstruction with toe transfer: selection of techniques. Plast Reconstr Surg 1994;93:352-357.

Management of Disorders of Separation—Syndactyly

JOSEPH UPTON III, MD

For the pediatric hand surgeon, syndactyly remains one of the two most common congenital differences of the upper limb seen across cultures (see "Incidence"). Although interdigital webbing usually presents as an isolated anomaly, it is also frequently seen in association with other soft tissue and skeletal anomalies of the hand and malformations of other organ systems as part of a syndrome.[1,2] The main focus of the following discussion is diagnosis and treatment of syndactyly in the hands. Other anomalies, such as constriction ring, hypoplastic thumb, and vascular malformations, are discussed in specific chapters elsewhere in this volume.

CLASSIFICATION

Level

Syndactyly (Greek *syn*, together, and *daktylos*, digit) is first classified as either *complete* or *incomplete*, depending on the degree of webbing along the length of the digit (Fig. 204-1). A complete syndactyly extends to the tip of the terminal phalanx of the involved digit or thumb. An incomplete syndactyly may end anywhere between the level of the normal commissure and the fingertip but does not extend to the most distal point of the finger.

Soft Tissue and Skeletal Anatomy

In a *simple* syndactyly, the interdigital connection consists of only skin and abnormal fibrous connections; in a *complex* syndactyly, abnormal osseous or cartilaginous unions are present between adjacent fingers (Fig. 204-2). These interconnecting bands may have their origin both dorsal to and palmar to the neurovascular bundles along the sides of the digits. Growth deformities and joint abnormalities will occur as these fingers grow disproportionately while they are fused at or near the tip. Dorsal buckling or lateral angulation of the proximal interphalangeal joint of a long finger fused at the tip of a ring finger will, for example, progress unless the distal fusion is released.

Complexity of Skeletal Structures

A *complex* syndactyly contains abnormal osseous or cartilaginous skeletal unions between adjacent fingers plus or minus the thumb. The useful term *complicated* syndactyly is reserved for those patients with more

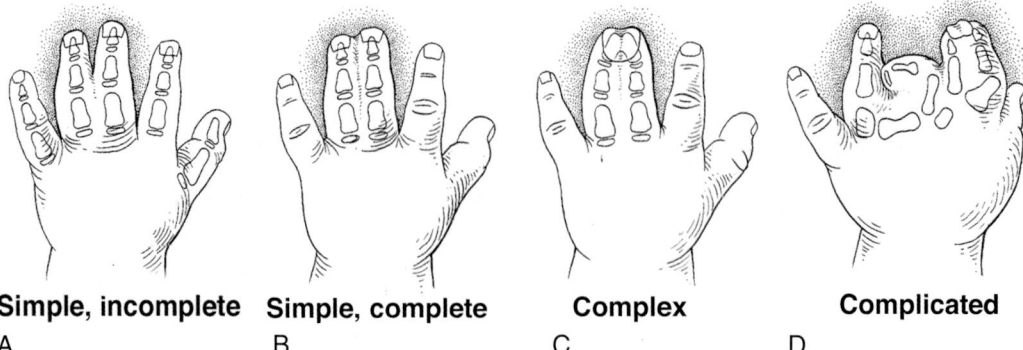

Simple, incomplete   Simple, complete   Complex   Complicated

A   B   C   D

FIGURE 204-1. Syndactyly classification. *A,* A simple, incomplete syndactyly involves soft tissue only and does not extend to the tip of the terminal phalanx. *B,* A simple, complete form extends to the tip of the involved digits. *C,* Skeletal union, usually at the distal phalangeal level, is present in complex varieties. Here, distal bone fusion will result in progressive proximal buckling or angulation owing to discrepant growth of the digits. *D,* In complicated forms, bone union, duplications, abnormal phalangeal segments (triangular [delta], trapezoidal, and others), and a bizarre disorganization of normal skeletal ray alignment are common.

than simple side-to-side bone fusions.[3-6] Examples include the Apert syndrome, central polysyndactyly, and typical cleft hand, in which an array of abnormal bones, joints, tendons, muscles, and nerves may be present. The degree of abnormality of skeletal elements within a web space is often a good indicator of other abnormal anatomic relationships involving soft tissues.

Thumb-Index Web Space (First Interdigital Web Space)

There are no specific practical classifications for this unique web space. Most surgeons have used the system of either incomplete versus complete or simple versus complex versus complicated. Complex and

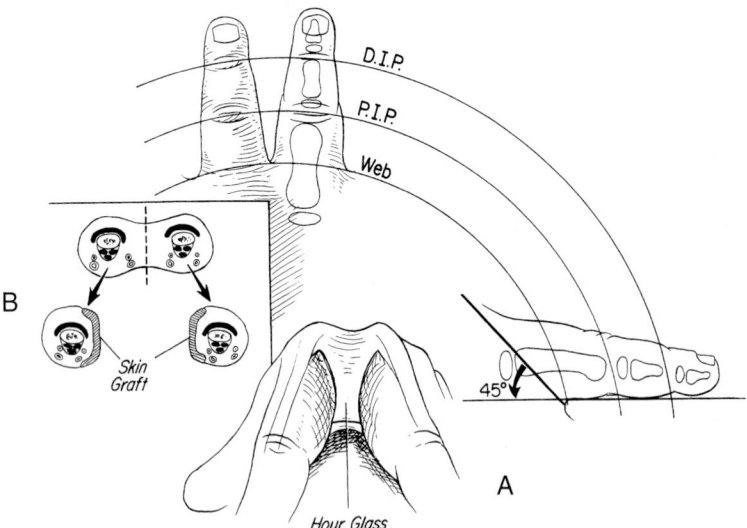

FIGURE 204-2. Interdigital anatomy. *A,* The normal anatomy of an interdigital web space demonstrates an hourglass configuration of non-hair-bearing skin that subtends at 45 degrees dorsal to palmar angulation. The base of the web commissure in the normal hand is located at the midportion of the proximal phalanx on the lateral view. In a 12-month-old child, this flap measures 16 to 18 mm in length and 8 to 9 mm in maximum width. The transverse width of the second and fourth web spaces is greater than that of the central (third) web space. *B,* A relative deficiency of skin always exists in most webbed digits, particularly at the base of the commissure adjacent to the borders of the commissure flaps. With a full release, additional skin is necessary to cover the raw area formed. In simple syndactylies, many authors have advocated aggressive defatting to avoid the use of skin grafts.[9,69,210,211] DIP, distal interphalangeal joint; PIP, proximal interphalangeal joint; Web, proximal level of web space.

complicated unions between the thumb and its adjacent digit are unusual, primarily seen in the Apert syndrome or in thumb duplications in the two- or three-digit hand.

INCIDENCE

The true incidence of syndactyly varies from one part of the world to another, but some type of interdigital webbing is seen in approximately 1 of every 2000 live births.[7-9] Half of the patients have bilateral defects, and boys are more often affected. Familial syndactyly is seen in 15% to 40% of most reported series. These patients usually represent some of the more complex and complicated forms of synpolydactyly. All different types of genetic inheritance patterns have been documented with syndactyly, the most common being sporadic with incomplete penetrance.[10] In families with the disorder, the dominant genes show a reduced penetrance and variable expression, meaning that there is little consistency from one generation to another.[8] The third (long-ring) interdigital web space in the hand and the second interdigital web space in the foot are the most commonly affected areas. The highest degree of penetrance within syndactyly pedigrees is seen within those families with synpolydactyly.[11]

The first (thumb-index) interdigital web space in the hand is the least frequently affected because the thumb separates from the rest of the hand at a much earlier embryonic stage. The incidence of ray involvement varies from one series to another but is generally as follows: first interdigital web space, 5%; second interdigital web space, 15%; third interdigital web space, 50%; and fourth interdigital web space, 30%.[6,11,12]

ETIOLOGY

Because of the varied presentations of interdigital webbing with or without osseous coalitions or other abnormalities, there are no well-accepted causes of syndactyly formation. Between the fifth and sixth weeks of gestation, interactions between the apical ectodermal ridge and the underlying mesenchymal tissue within the hand plate result in a distal to proximal cleft formation between each of the rays of the hand. By a process of "programmed cell death" or apoptosis, the soft tissue between the longitudinal cartilaginous rays of the hand disappears as separate digits and a thumb appear. In the constriction ring syndrome, the distal tissues of the digit are often rejoined by the constricting amniotic bands encircling them. This results in an inflammatory reaction, and the subsequent common scar often binds adjacent digits together. Just proximal to this common scar are dorsal to palmar epithelium-lined sinuses, which represent the presence of a commissure that had formed or was forming at the time of the band formation.

SYNDROMIC ASSOCIATIONS

Associated anomalies are common and occur in conjunction with defects in all other organ systems. Syndactyly is part of at least 28 syndromes, of which the most common are Poland, Apert (acrocephalosyndactyly), constriction ring, and multiple facial syndromes. Syndactyly is often one of the most treatable defects in the multiply deformed child.[1,2,7,13] The specific components of each syndrome can be obtained from commonly referenced textbooks.

Poland Syndrome

CLINICAL PRESENTATION

Poland syndrome is a common syndactyly-related syndrome. It typically consists of the absence of the sternocostal portion of the pectoralis major muscles; hypoplasia of the hand and, to a lesser degree, of the forearm and upper arm; simple complete or incomplete syndactyly; and short fingers (brachysymphalangism) (Fig. 204-3).[14-21] The cause of the condition is unknown, and there is no inheritance pattern or predisposition. There also are no commonly associated anomalies.[19,22] Because these limb anomalies can be seen with some associated head and neck malformations, some researchers believe they fall along a disruption sequence involving the brachiocephalic arterial system.[22-24] Disruption sequences in the distal portion of this system would present as the Poland syndrome. Disruption sequences in the more proximal portion of this arterial system would present with findings consistent with the Möbius syndrome[25] (bilateral seventh, fourth, and other cranial nerve palsies), the Klippel-Feil syndrome (cervical soft tissue, neurologic, and skeletal malformations), or the Pierre Robin syndrome[26] (cleft palate, severe retrognathia). On occasion, portions of several syndromes may coexist.[25] It is not uncommon for the hand surgeon to work with a craniofacial team while treating a child with one or more cranial nerve problems, a neck malformation, and an ipsilateral upper limb malformation that will fall somewhere within the teratologic sequence of symbrachydactyly (Fig. 204-4).

Children with the Poland syndrome present with a wide variety of hand malformations. The central digits (index, long, and ring fingers) are more commonly affected than the thumb and fifth rays, but a whole spectrum of variations of symbrachydactyly has been seen in the author's series of 190 children with this syndrome. Their hands follow a "teratologic sequence" previously described by a number of German authors.[27-30] The first web space is invariably restricted, and all degrees of skeletal hypoplasia are present within the digits, which are joined by simple syndactylies. In the most severe form of Poland syndrome, hypoplastic thumb and fifth fingers are present,

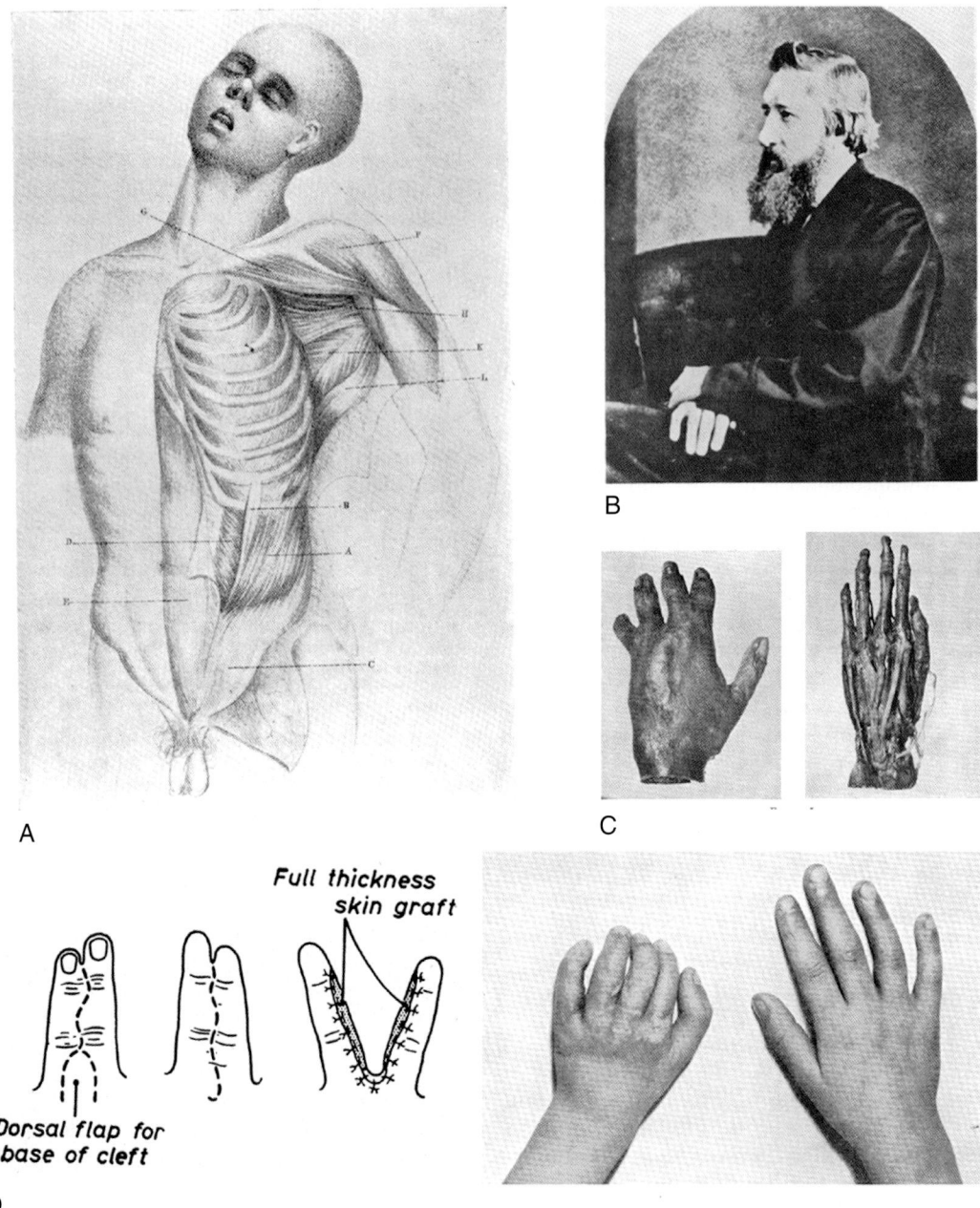

FIGURE 204-3. The Poland syndrome. *A,* The illustration in Poland's original article[20] showed the absence of the pectoralis major muscle but did not show the hand. *B,* Alfred Poland. *C,* Years later, Patrick Clarkson found the hand, shown dissected here with and without the skin envelope, in the museum archives.[16] *D,* Clarkson's preferred method of syndactyly correction used a large dorsal flap to form the commissure and full-thickness grafts to line the sidewalls. The postoperative result on the left shows that no skeletal correction had been done. (Reproduced from Clarkson P: Poland's syndactyly. Guys Hosp Rep 1962;111:335-346.)

and the remaining digits are represented by hypoplastic nubbins. The ipsilateral pectoralis major muscle deficit may also be associated with absence or hypoplasia of the serratus anterior, latissimus dorsi, and deltoid muscles; breast hypoplasia (33% of girls)[31,32]; rib cage deficiencies; scoliosis; and, rarely, dextrocardia.[33] The most common presentation involves the absence of the sternocostal portion of the muscle with or without all degrees of breast hypoplasia.

Associated chest wall, skeletal, and soft tissue deformities often require treatment, particularly in the adolescent girl with a hypoplastic breast. Restoration of

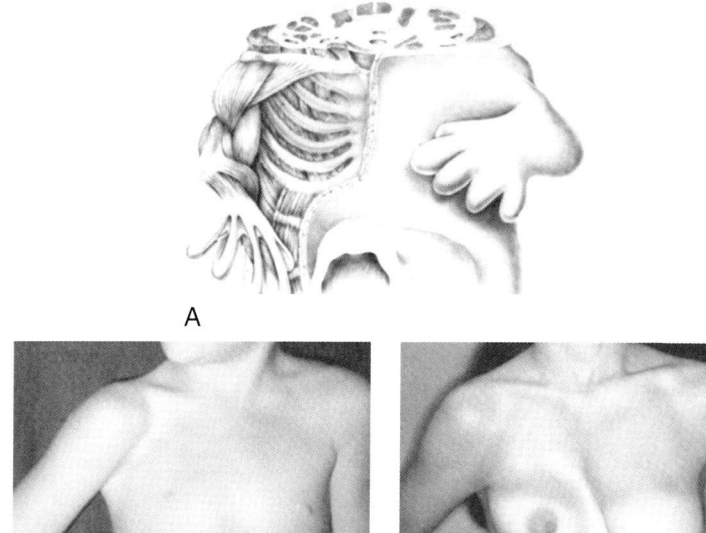

A

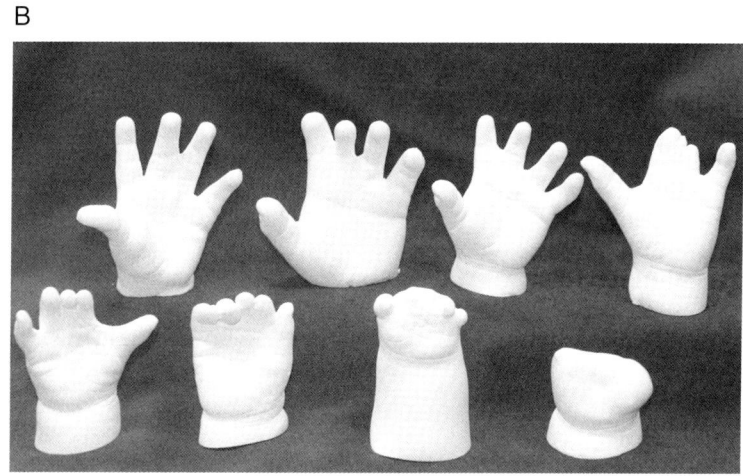

B

C

FIGURE 204-4. Poland variations. *A,* A schematic of the developing embryo shows the absence of the sternocostal portion of the pectoralis major muscle. The clavicular portion is often intact in these children. The degree of soft tissue and skeletal hypoplasia in the ipsilateral upper limb decreases from distal to proximal. *B,* A young girl with absence of the entire portion of the pectoralis muscle is shown at the age of 4 years and at the age of 37 years after two pregnancies. No breast surgery has been done. The relative growth of the breast buds cannot be accurately predicted before puberty. *C,* A wide variation of symbrachydactyly in these patients extends from *(upper left)* minimal skeletal hypoplasias with simple incomplete webbing involving the central three digits to *(lower left)* severe skeletal shortness and complete syndactyly to *(lower central)* the mitten hand with diminutive digits and finally to *(lower right)* aplasia of all digits including the thumb.

contour to ipsilateral chest wall deformities is seldom required. Although respiratory function is rarely compromised, some of these children may have severe pectus carinatum or pectus excavatum sternal deformities coupled with multiple rib hypoplasias or aplasias. Correction of these contour irregularities is not functional. Construction of the absent breast or augmentation of the hypoplastic breast in girls and restoration of pectoralis contour with latissimus transfers in boys invariably result in a dramatic improvement of self-image as these youngsters pass through adolescence and become young adults. Alloplastic materials rarely remain in place for a lifetime, and in the past 20 years, local latissimus dorsi muscle pedicle transfers and custom-made silicone implants have gained popularity.[15,32]

EPONYM

The designation Poland syndrome will mean many things to different medical and surgical specialists and represents the classic example of an eponym gone awry.[14] The original description by Alfred Poland in the *Guy's Hospital Reports*[20] was of a street person, George Elt, who had both ipsilateral chest wall and hand malformations. The major subject of the short paper was of the chest wall, well illustrated by one of Poland's colleagues, with only a short paragraph devoted to the hand "with short webbed fingers." A century later, the hospital hand specialist, Patrick Clarkson, found the hand, preserved in a jar, in the basement of the hospital's well-known museum. He then wrote a frequently referenced paper that outlined the

TABLE 204-1 ◆ CHARACTERISTICS OF
POLAND SYNDROME[16-33]

Unilateral shortened digits, mostly the central three
  digits
Syndactyly of the shortened digits, usually simple
  incomplete or complete
Hypoplasia of the hand and to a much lesser degree of
  the forearm and arm
Absent or hypoplastic sternocostal head of the
  pectoralis major muscle
Other reports have also associated this condition with
  unilateral:
  Absence of pectoralis muscle
  Absence or hypoplasia of the breast
  Contracture of the anterior axillary fold
  Absence or hypoplasia of the serratus anterior,
    latissimus dorsi, or deltoid muscles on the
    ipsilateral side
Rib deficiencies and pectus deformities
Dextrocardia

four characteristics of the syndrome. This list has subsequently been expanded to include additional associated anomalies (Table 204-1).[16] One may readily see
how this syndromic designation means dextrocardia
to the cardiac surgeon, unilateral breast hypoplasia to

the plastic surgeon, brachysyndactyly to the hand
surgeon, or rib absence combined with a pectus deformity of the sternum to the pediatric surgeon.

Apert Syndrome

CLINICAL PRESENTATION

The Apert syndrome, which affects all races, is the most
common of six acrocephalosyndactyly syndromes
seen by the hand surgeon. It has an autosomal dominant inheritance pattern and an incidence higher than
1 in 100,000 live births.[34] Geneticists have identified
and confirmed two chromosome loci in these children.[35,36] The author has observed that clinically, the
more frequent serine substitution at the FGFR-2
receptor represents the "good hands and bad head"
malformation; the less frequently observed proline substitution is more indicative of the "bad hands (type
III) and good head" combination.

The physical findings are striking. Facial features
consist of a wide variety of skull deformities due to
premature closure of the basal portions of the coronal
and, frequently, the lambdoid sutures. The orbits are
shallow, with exorbitism, and the forehead is deeply
furrowed (Fig. 204-5). There is a failure of forward
growth of the maxilla, with a parrot-beaked nose, a

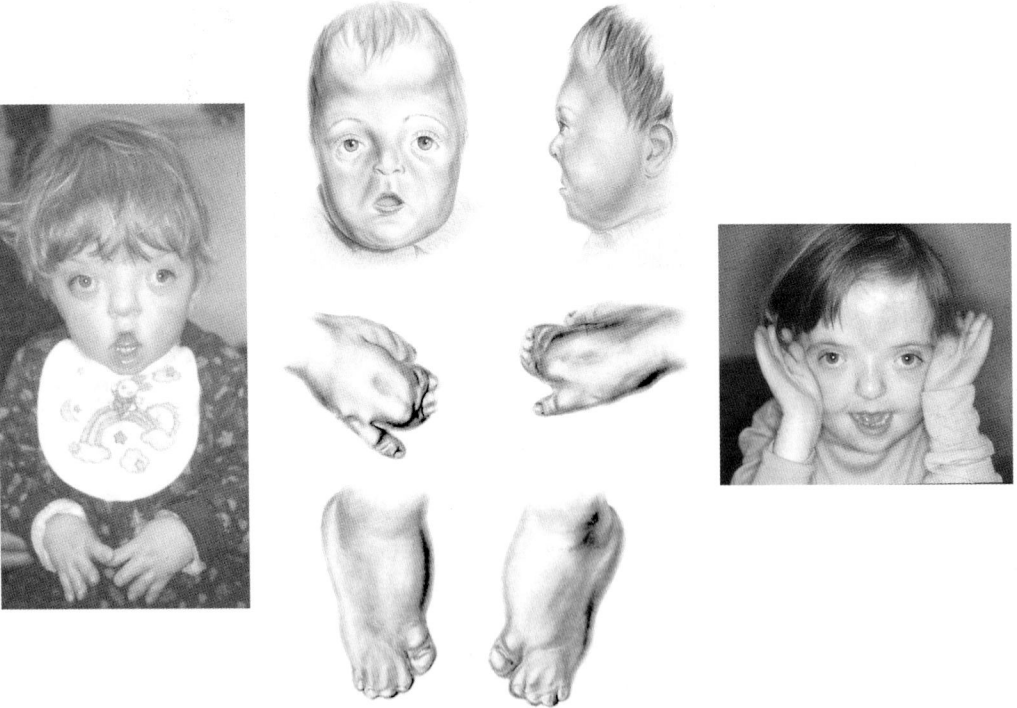

FIGURE 204-5. The Apert syndrome (acrocephalosyndactyly). The characteristic facial deformities seen
in the Apert child include brachycephaly, prominent supraorbital ridge, midface retrusion, exophthalmos,
and parrot beak nose. Respiratory difficulties including sleep apnea are frequent in these children. Bilateral mirror image (enantiomorphic) malformations of the hands and feet are always present. The severity
of these deformities may vary. The children are seen on either side after their digital separations. Both
were born with mild (type I) hand and foot deformities and severe cranial malformations.

high-arched palate, and crowding of maxillary teeth and tongue, which can frequently cause upper airway difficulty.

There are no commonly associated malformations, aside from those of the musculoskeletal and central nervous systems. Although mental retardation is *not* part of this syndrome, at least one third of affected children are delayed to the point that they require special assistance in school, but most are normal if intracranial pressure problems are aggressively treated in infancy. Historically, many of these individuals have been institutionalized, and their intellectual potentials never developed.[6] However, aggressive treatment of the craniostenosis and associated hydrocephalus has all but eliminated many of the central nervous system-related problems.

Symmetric complex and complicated syndactylies of both hands and feet are present.[37] There is usually skeletal dysplasia of the glenohumeral joint and occasionally of the elbow joint, which limits proximal limb function.[38] Three basic types of hand patterns are seen: the flat, spade-like hand; the constricted, cupped, mitten hand; and the tightly coalesced "hoof" or "rosebud" hand (Fig. 204-6 and Table 204-2). For ease of

clinical decision-making, these have been conveniently grouped into three types. Further refinements of this system have been described.[39-45] Common to all are a short, radially deviated thumb with an abnormal, delta-shaped proximal phalanx; a complex side-to-side fusion involving phalanges of the index, long, and ring fingers; symphalangism within the four digits; and a simple syndactyly involving the fourth web space. Fewer than half of these patients have syndactyly of the first web space.[6,46,47]

In types I and II, the syndactyly within the first web space is simple with all degrees of phalangeal hypoplasia involving the thumb. Conjoined nails are indicative of underlying distal phalangeal fusion. Longitudinal ridges represent distal phalanges with some separation, and the absence of ridges is indicative of a common coalesced distal phalanx. Only the type III hands contain a solid side-to-side distal phalangeal fusion, and in these hands, the sharply angulated conjoined nail may cause severe maceration of the glabrous pulp skin and frequent paronychial infections. These are the only Apert thumbs that may not have severe radial clinodactyly, and in many hands, the thumb terminal phalanx is deficient. Often, the

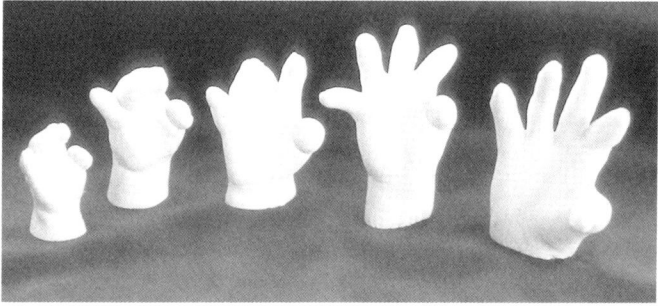

A

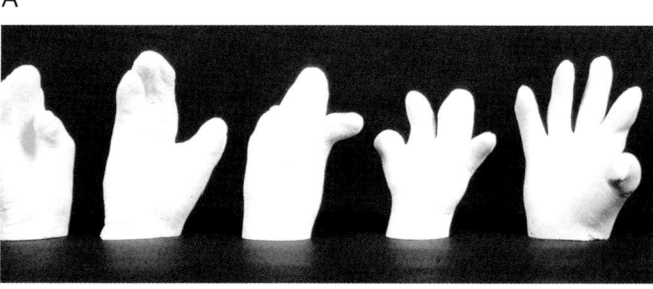

B

FIGURE 204-6. Syndactyly in the Apert hand. *A,* The molds of the right hand in an Apert child show the sequential digital separations between the ages of 6 months *(left)* and 7 years *(right)*. After separations, the border index and fifth digits often splay out in a sunburst fashion. Both were corrected with closing wedge osteotomies. The radial clinodactyly of the thumb was corrected with an opening wedge osteotomy and bone graft at 7 years of age. We now correct these much earlier, between the ages of 4 and 6 years. *B,* These patients may have between one and four digits. Most have four. Type III hands often have an insufficient index skeleton for a useable digit and consequently are best treated with ray resection.

TABLE 204-2 ✦ COMMON FEATURES OF THE APERT HAND

Characteristic	Type I	Type II	Type III*
Skin maceration	−	−	+
Short deviated thumb	+	+	+/−
Complex syndactyly, index-long-ring	+/−	+	+
Symphalangism	+	+	+
Simple syndactyly, fourth interdigital web space	+	+	+
Duplication, fifth ray (phalangeal level)	−	+	+

*Type III hands are characterized by paronychial infections, straight thumbs, synonychia without longitudinal ridging, coalesced distal phalanges, and a higher incidence of elbow problems.

thumb distal phalanx with overlying nail plate is barely visible beneath swollen folds on the radial side of the hoof configuration.[48]

The central three digits in the type I and type II hands have some degree of distal phalangeal fusions, which may not be obvious on radiographs obtained during the first year or two of life. Interzones between phalanges and longitudinal lucent areas parallel to the distal phalanges represent cartilaginous bridges. Bone coalescence is typically not seen within the ring-small simple syndactyly, which may be either complete or incomplete. The distal interphalangeal joint of the fifth finger is the most normal interphalangeal joint within all three types of Apert hands. In less than 15% of these children, an incomplete fifth finger duplication at the phalangeal level may be present and will result in a marked ulnar deviation and diminution of motion.[6,49]

There is a marked increase in the complexity of type III hands due to the fact that the distal portion of all five rays in the hand may be fused.[6,43,45] Folds of overlapping skin on the dorsal surfaces may partially obscure the nail plate of the thumb. Although separate phalangeal segments may be demarcated by longitudinal ridges, a smooth nail representative of a cloven hoof may be indicative of side-to-side fusions of multiple phalanges. Metacarpophalangeal joints lie directly beneath the dorsal dimples in all these hands and are always present for all rays. The character of the dorsal buckling or lateral splaying of the phalanges depends on the character of the distal skeletal fusions and subsequent designation of clinical types.

Acrosyndactyly

CLINICAL PRESENTATION

Acrosyndactyly denotes fused digits (Greek *daktylos*, digit; *syn*, formed or together; *acro*, peak) and is generally considered part of the constriction ring syndrome (see Chapter 205). Within these hands, there is always a proximal dorsal to palmar epithelium-lined space or sinus (see Fig. 205-23). Dissections by Losch and Duncker[50] and extensive studies by Patterson[51] and

Torpin and Faulkner[52] indicate that some type of disruption sequence initiated by an ischemic insult occurs after the digits have been separated and that the resulting scar tissue draws adjacent soft tissue and bone together. Patterson[51] has also noted the possibility that there is a more fundamental tissue problem because of the high number of associated anomalies, including facial clefts, congenital heart defects, and clubbed feet. Frequently, upper and lower limbs are involved. The author's experience with 225 patients with the constriction ring syndrome has an associated anomaly rate of 13%. It is possible that a combination of malformations, disruption, and deformation sequences may be involved in this syndrome.[53]

Walsh[54] and others[6,55] have documented a wide range of hand presentations and categorized them as mild, moderate, and severe, depending on skeletal structure alone (Fig. 204-7). A more detailed and refined classification has not been developed because it would not change clinical decision-making. Incomplete simple syndactylies may be a component in all three varieties. The two hands in any given patient never have identical mirror image deformities, commonly seen in congenital differences of genetic origin. In patients with mild deformities, three phalanges with two segmental joints are present with well-formed proximal clefts. In moderately involved hands, there are two phalanges and a single interphalangeal joint. In severe deformities, only hypoplastic nubbins with small phalanges are present. Of the 68 patients described by Walsh,[54] the presentation was mild in 4 patients, moderate in 44 patients, and severe in 20 patients. The author's experience with a much larger number of patients is similar. There is no standard pattern of involvement in a single hand or in opposite limbs of the same child.[6,54,56]

A characteristic pattern of syndactyly is present in all of these unique hands. Large and small epithelium-lined spaces or sinuses are present, denoting web commissures that are more distal than the normal commissure location.[57] Congenital transverse amputation of one or more digits is common, and soft tissue at and distal to the level of digital coalescence is always

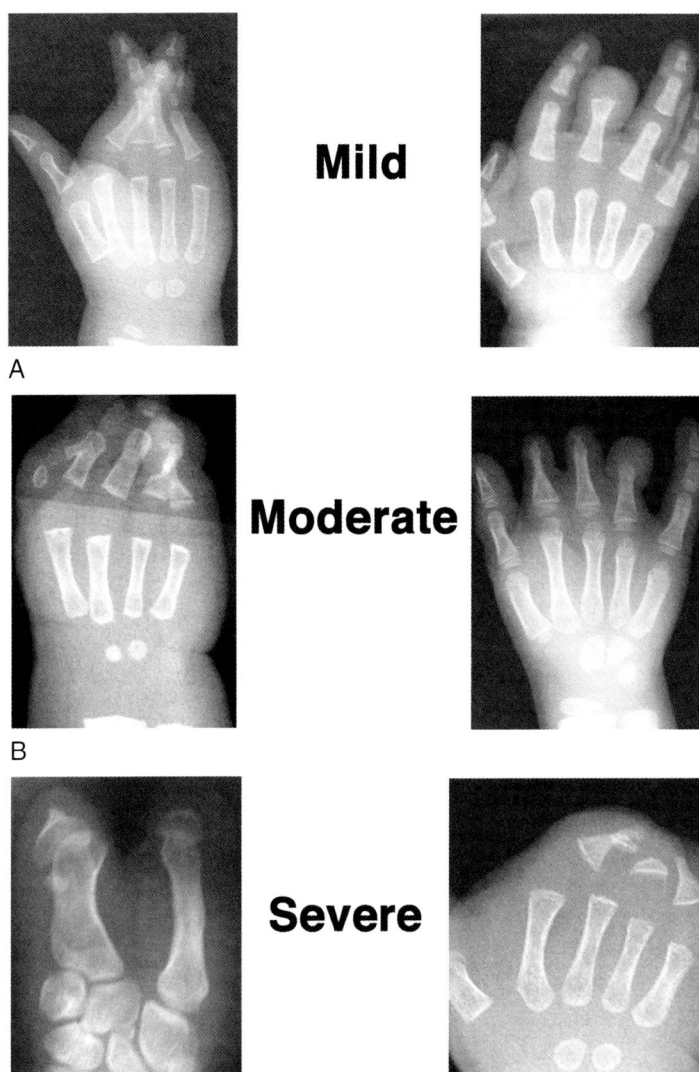

FIGURE 204-7. Syndactyly of the constriction ring syndrome. The severity of both skeletal and soft tissue involvement of constriction ring syndrome hands with syndactyly correlates well with the difficulty of reconstruction. A simple system has been used for the digits. The thumb deficiencies are described in Chapter 205. Simple syndactyly may be a component of any constriction ring syndrome hand. *A,* In patients with mild deformities, the metacarpals of all five rays are present, and most of the digits contain two or more phalanges and intact proximal interphalangeal and distal interphalangeal joints. The syndactyly is usually incomplete. The coalesced soft tissue and skeletal parts are joined by scar tissue. *B,* In moderate hands, the proximal phalanges are all present with small but present middle phalanges and at least one intact proximal interphalangeal joint. Dorsal to palmar epithelialized sinuses are often present adjacent to these phalangeal stumps. *C,* In patients with the most severe defects, no normal phalanges are present, and metacarpals may often be deficient. The digits are often functionless nubbins with or without proximal phalangeal remnants.

deficient. Digits are short, and osseous involvement is different from that in other forms of syndactyly. Extra skeletal parts are never found, and fusion is between common scars in a side-to-side or on-top position (see Fig. 204-7).

Other Syndromic Associations

Patients with either the Freeman-Sheldon (whistling face) syndrome or some form of arthrogryposis may present with a simple incomplete syndactyly of the second through fourth interdigital web spaces and a tight adducted thumb associated with a deficient first web space.[6,58-60] In both, flexion and ulnar deviation of the wrist and one or multiple proximal interphalangeal joint flexion contractures may require

correction. The interdigital webbing is simple and almost by definition does not contain extra skeletal elements. In contrast, hands within the typical cleft hand category may have complex and complicated syndactylies between the involved digits, but the syndactyly between the thumb and nomad index digit are simple and usually complete (Fig. 204-8). Complex and complicated syndactylies are also found in synpolydactyly and are addressed in detail in Chapter 206. In these hands, the degree of complexity is related to the level of duplications along the central ray.

Syndactyly is present in several other conditions that are not adequately described in all available surgical textbooks. These include the very hypoplastic hand containing a thumb on the radial side joined by a simple syndactyly to either one or two digits, an

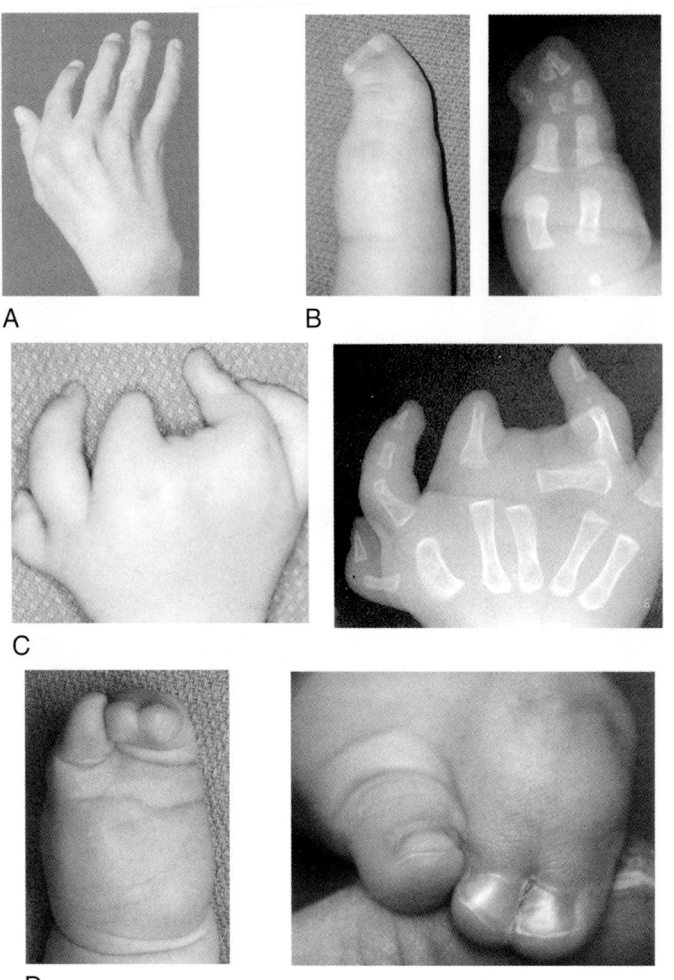

A

B

C

D

FIGURE 204-8. Additional syndactyly syndromes. *A,* The hand of a child with either arthrogryposis or the Freeman-Sheldon syndrome (whistling face syndrome) will often have simple incomplete interdigital webbing combined with ulnar drift of all digits and a tight adducted thumb with a deficient first web space. *B,* Those patients with two-digit hands often present with a complete syndactyly. The conjoined nail here with longitudinal ridges indicates that there are at least three distal phalangeal components. Two are part of a distal thumb polydactyly hidden within the syndactyly. *C,* Simple, simple complete, or complex syndactylies are often seen in the digits of the typical cleft hand. The digits involved are usually adjacent to the central cleft. *D,* This three-digit hand contains an incomplete syndactyly between the thumb and index rays and a complete webbing between the index and long digits.

abnormal thumb duplication joined to one or two other digits, and the small mitten hand with soft tissue webbing between a very small thumb and digits. Correction of the digits is identical to the usual procedures described, but liberation of a mobile thumb often requires the transfer of full-thickness tissue into the first web space. In both types, the extrinsic flexors, and sometimes the extrinsic extensor tendons, arise from the same forearm muscle.

ABNORMAL ANATOMY

Almost all permutations and combinations of abnormal soft tissue and skeletal anatomy can be present in syndactyly. A determination of abnormal can be made only after consideration of normal interdigital relationships (Color Plate 204-1). Skin is invariably deficient, especially in the region of the normal commissure. This can easily be demonstrated to curious parents by measuring the circumference of two digits

held together and comparing it with the sum of the circumferences of the individual digits.[4,6,61] Although infrequently webbed, the thumb-index web space is usually deficient in the hypoplastic hand, where webbing of the digits is commonly present.

Broad or short fascial interconnections are present in all webbed digits and extend across the interdigital space at the level of the proximal and middle phalanges in the midaxial line. These bands do not have names but may incorporate Cleland ligament palmar to the neurovascular bundle and Grayson ligament dorsal to the vessels on either digit. The configuration of the bands varies, and with careful dissection, the bands are picked up at the level of the distal interphalangeal joint during a retrograde separation. When the bands are seen in the first web space, they may appear to be above the adductor pollicis muscle, connecting the first and second metacarpals.[62] Adequate release of this fascia is often the single most important step in a first web release.[63] The transverse metacarpal ligaments, retinacular sheaths, investing fascia of intrinsic muscles, and palmar aponeurosis may be hypertrophied and tight in the small hypoplastic hand or Apert hand and may block normal growth and mobility. These tight, unyielding fascial interconnections are some of the most statically deforming structures as these patients grow.[5,6]

Bones and joints may present bizarre and erratic configurations. Central duplications within the web (polysyndactylies) often demonstrate interconnections of phalanges and metacarpals articulating with one another at any level. On occasion, alignment of skeletal elements into digital rays is impossible. Transversely oriented phalanges in the proximal portions of digits and symphalangism are encountered in the complex central problems as well as in the typical cleft hand deformities. Similar sharing of abnormal structures is seen in the typical cleft hand. Joints in patients with syndactyly may be incompletely developed, angulated, ankylosed, or even fused in a wide range of variations. What appears to be a well-segmented joint with no motion at birth may rapidly fuse to form a symphalangism, typically seen in digits of those with the Poland syndrome. Phalanges may be crooked, broad, short, long, or fused. These abnormal patterns occur with the highest incidence in the hereditary forms of syndactyly. The thumb proximal phalanx may often present as a triangular (delta) or trapezoidal instead of a rectangular bone, placing the distal portion of the thumb in radial or ulnar (uncommon) deviation. The middle phalanx of the fifth finger, the last to ossify in the hand, is abnormal, forming the familiar radial deviation known as clinodactyly.[7,13] This is so frequently seen in congenital hand differences that it is not specific for a given diagnosis. Missing or hypoplastic phalanges or metacarpals are as common as duplicated skeletal structures and are often accompanied by tendon, nerve, and ligament deficiencies.

Digital nerves and arteries often have a wide variety of branching patterns within a web space.[64-67] Distal branching is most common for both. An artery may loop around a digital nerve to form an arterial loop, and vice versa for the neural loop. Nerves can easily be teased apart under the microscope, but arterial loops present a much more complex problem if they represent the primary or only arterial conduit to a digit or thumb. In complex and complicated syndactylies, there are often incomplete or missing neurovascular structures on one or both sides of a digital ray. Flexor and extensor tendons may have similar distal branching patterns and interconnections within a web. Distal insertions may be abnormal in complex and complicated syndactylies. Often, the radiographic appearance of the skeletal structures and degree of hypoplasia are good indicators of associated tendon, nerve, arterial, or ligament abnormalities. The precise configuration must be individualized for each patient; few broad generalizations can be made. The most anomalous and bizarre neurovascular configurations are predictably seen in those with either central synpolydactyly or the complex and complicated typical cleft hands.

TREATMENT

Timing

Timing of surgical correction varies with the complexity of the deformity and the web space involved. Although there is no consensus, most hand surgeons agree that complicated and complex webbing involving adjacent digits with different growth potential warrants early release by 1 year of age (see Chapter 202). Patterns of prehensile function are established by 24 months, which should be the upper age limit for correction.[68] There has been interest in correction within the first 2 weeks of life in infants with an abundance of mobile skin and less complex deformities.[69,70] In any event, restoration of maximum functional potential and liberation of all digits should be completed by school age (Fig. 204-9).

An increasing body of knowledge in the field of neurophysiology has supported the hypothesis that there are ongoing changes in the cortical representation of the somatosensory portion of the cerebral cortex and that these changes are greatly influenced by input from the hand. The reorganization of the cortex of owl monkeys after digital syndactylization showed a complete loss of individual digit representation after the procedure.[71,72] These studies have been expanded by others following additional types of peripheral nerve manipulation.

It is preferable not to routinely release simple syndactylies in newborns, who are often born with large amounts of redundant skin, which obviates the need for skin grafts. In a limited number of patients,[6,69,70] the results may be dramatic (Fig. 204-10), and about half of these children needed minor revisions later in childhood. Complete webbing involving the important first (thumb-index) and fourth (ring-small) web spaces is best released by 6 to 12 months of age. For progression of skeletal deformities to be avoided in patients with complex syndactylies, which may not be corrected with growth once they are established, it is often necessary to perform surgery before 1 year of age. The urgency for correction increases with greater discrepancy between the webbed digits; thus, one should not wait as long with the thumb-index web space as with the middle-ring web space.

In general, the majority of simple and complex syndactylies are corrected between 12 and 24 months of age. Whenever possible, bilateral procedures should be performed on patients with deformities in both hands.[5,9,28,73-81] This is best completed in nonambulatory children who are younger than 12 to 14 months

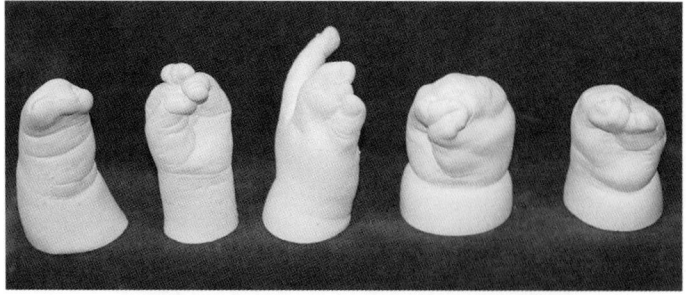

Thumb involved

A

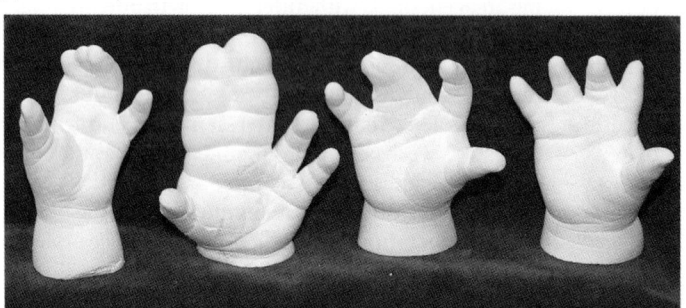

Digital deformities

B

FIGURE 204-9. Indications for early syndactyly release. *A,* Clinical situations for early separation of syndactyly involving the first web space include the three-fingered hand, acrosyndactyly (constriction ring syndrome), the Apert hand, and the mitten hand, among others. The border rays (thumb and fifth digit) should be liberated first. *B,* Situations that include isolated or combined digital syndactylies, illustrated here with a synpolydactyly, macrodactyly, synpolydactyly, and Poland symbrachydactyly *(right)*, are not urgent.

because by 2 or 3 years of age, the toddlers are more active and much more difficult to manage. In the older child, bilateral procedures should be avoided.[6,9] During the past 3 decades, there has been a definite trend to operate earlier and to perform bilateral procedures in babies before they begin to ambulate. The dictum "release by 5 years of age and revise as teenagers"[7] is no longer followed.

Alterations in this timetable are, of course, dictated by associated anomalies, size of the hand, medical problems of higher priority, and concerns about anesthesia exposures. Several authors of long-term review series cite a higher incidence for complications and resultant contractures with early surgery and recommend delay of initial procedures.[7,12,77,82-87] Although infants and children of any age can be safely anesthetized during a long operation, elective syndactyly releases may often need to be postponed in the multiply deformed child with cardiopulmonary, hematologic, central neurologic, or severe musculoskeletal problems. It is important to emphasize to the families that syndactyly releases, although delicate procedures, do not involve prolonged hospitalizations including intensive care unit stays, which may be necessary with correction of possible craniofacial, gastrointestinal, cardiovascular, pulmonary, urologic, or other malformations. This said, treatment of hand and

upper limb anomalies is all too often relegated to a secondary status by members of the treatment team and neglected until other major malformations have been corrected. In the child with multiple malformations and a normal neurologic system, maximal early treatment of the upper limb malformations definitely helps these children reach their developmental milestones at more appropriate ages.

In some patients, however, the correction of major skeletal deformities and digital separations are preferably completed before major craniofacial procedures in those with limb and facial malformations.[44,88] For example, one should try to complete all necessary digital and thumb separations in children with the Apert syndrome before they are scheduled for forehead or midfacial advancements or staged distraction procedures.

Historical Development

The history of the surgical correction of syndactyly is fascinating, and refinements made during the past 200 years have established many important principles (Fig. 204-11).[6,89] Clearly, the first and only goal was to separate coalesced digits. The evolution of described techniques has progressed through four overlapping periods—simple separation and epithelialization, use

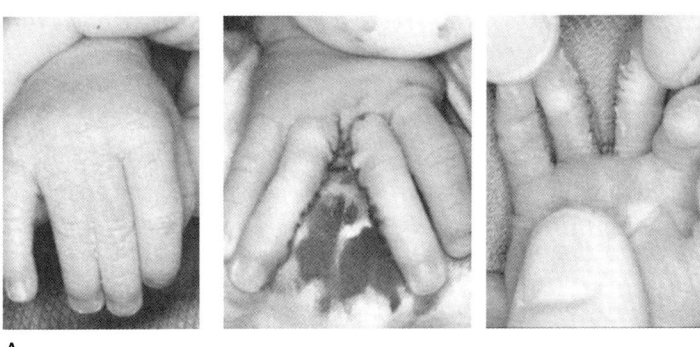

A

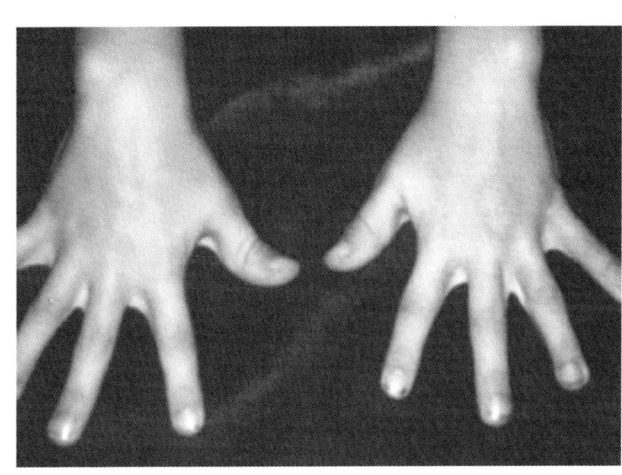

B

FIGURE 204-10. Syndactyly release in the newborn. Most syndactylies without digital buckling or deviation are now released at 1 year of age. An opportunity does exist in newborn babies, whose skin is often loose and redundant.[69] *A,* In this newborn, a simple incomplete syndactyly was present in the third interdigital web space. At 1 week of age, dorsal and palmar flaps[103] have been used to form the commissure, and the sidewall flaps are closed primarily during a procedure performed under local anesthesia with the baby properly sedated. *B,* With subsequent growth, the tightness at the base of the commissure was easily corrected with simple Z-plasties performed at 10 years of age on an outpatient basis. No further surgery was necessary.

of skin grafts, use of interdigitating sidewall flaps, and use of local island flaps—to the use of distant pedicled and free flaps.

The well-known early surgical operations date to the early 19th century, when lead beads, glass setons, rubber tubes, and ligatures were used to form epithelium-lined commissures and to separate the webbing segmentally.[90-104] Often, large raw surfaces were left to heal secondarily, resulting in contractures that accentuated growth deformities.[96,105]

The subsequent introduction of the use of skin grafts significantly decreased the contracture rate.[91,102] With improved knowledge of local and regional anatomy, almost every conceivable flap and graft design has been used for syndactyly separation. Constricting palmar scars are minimized with the use of zigzag incisions.[106,107] Historically, raw edges were left to epithelialize,[91,98,104,108] and tremendous contractures developed in many children; however, ingenious patterns of incision have been developed through the decades to avoid this specific problem. The most problematic region after release is still the palmar edge of the commissure; several helpful modifications have been made here either to overcorrect the commissure depth or to interdigitate flaps to break up a straight-line scar.[3,27,28,46,109-111]

As knowledge of the blood supply of the hand has improved, almost every conceivable local and regional flap has been introduced for the correction of congenital webbing.[3,4,7,57,77,87,111-144] Local island flaps based on subcutaneous tissue planes were next introduced. Many local pedicled flaps transferred as an island have been described after the dorsal metacarpal arterial system was described in detail.[145-151] During the past decade, there have been a number of reports that advocated flap closure without skin grafts. Reversed vascular island flaps based on the radial side of the first interdigital web space, practically the thumb-index web space, were essentially the same for the first 150 years (Fig. 204-12).

Obviously, during the past 4 decades, all combinations of local advancement and rotational flaps were described for release of the first web space, and many were ultimately incorporated in the treatment of congenital differences. The single Z-plasty and combinations of these transposition flaps have been described. One procedure, the four-flap Z-plasty, has become the "gold standard" for the release of mild and moderate first web space deformities.

Those interested in the history of this procedure have noted that surgeons characteristically have

Text continued on p. 159

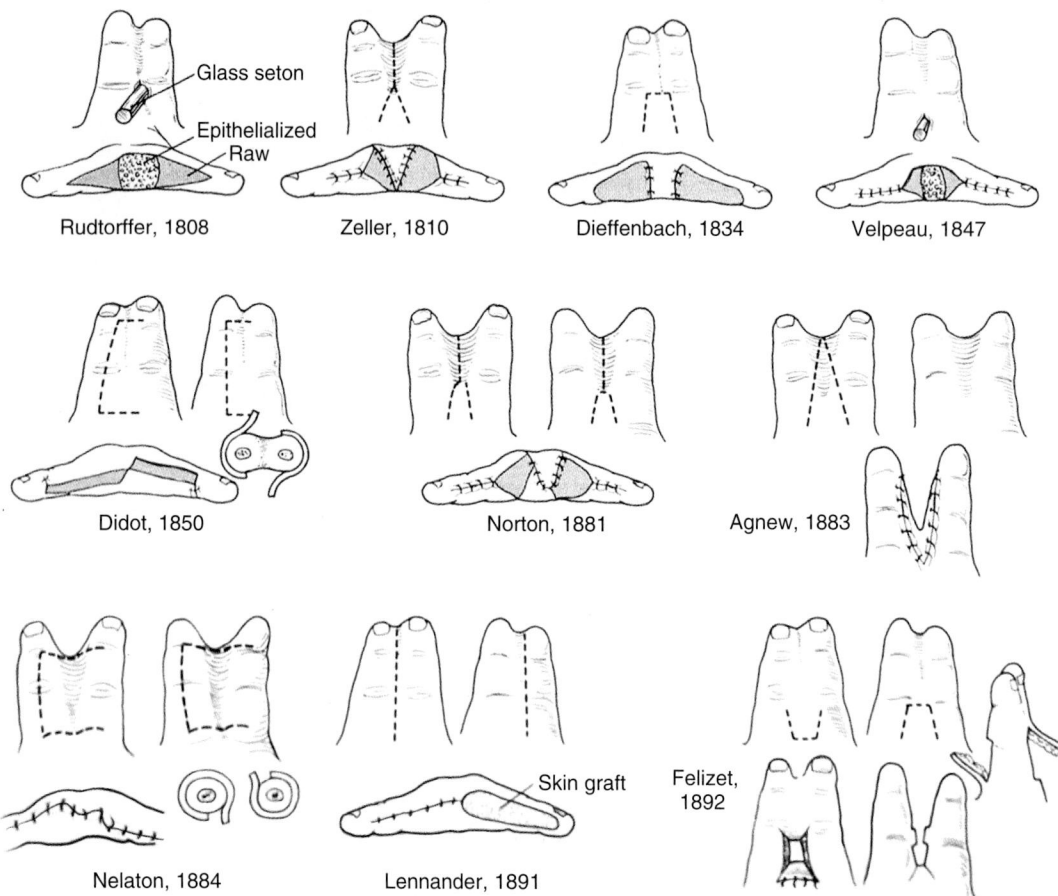

FIGURE 204-11. Historical methods of interdigital syndactyly release. The evolution of methods for correction of interdigital webbing has varied tremendously. Although early attempts at simple division were probably made before the 19th century, the literature documents methods beginning at the turn of the century. Earlier methods included the use of glass rods, setons, and other foreign bodies, which formed epithelialized tracks serving as the commissure base. One of the first to use skin grafts was Lennander.[102] Although primary closure of many of these incisions along the sides of the digits seems impractical, review of the original source articles indicates that many of these patients had simple incomplete syndactylies with wide interdigital webbing. The raw areas are indicated by dense stippling, epithelialized areas by pebbling, and skin-grafted areas by fine stippling. More recently, skin has been transposed into the commissure region from the dorsal surfaces with incisions that are extensions of previous techniques.

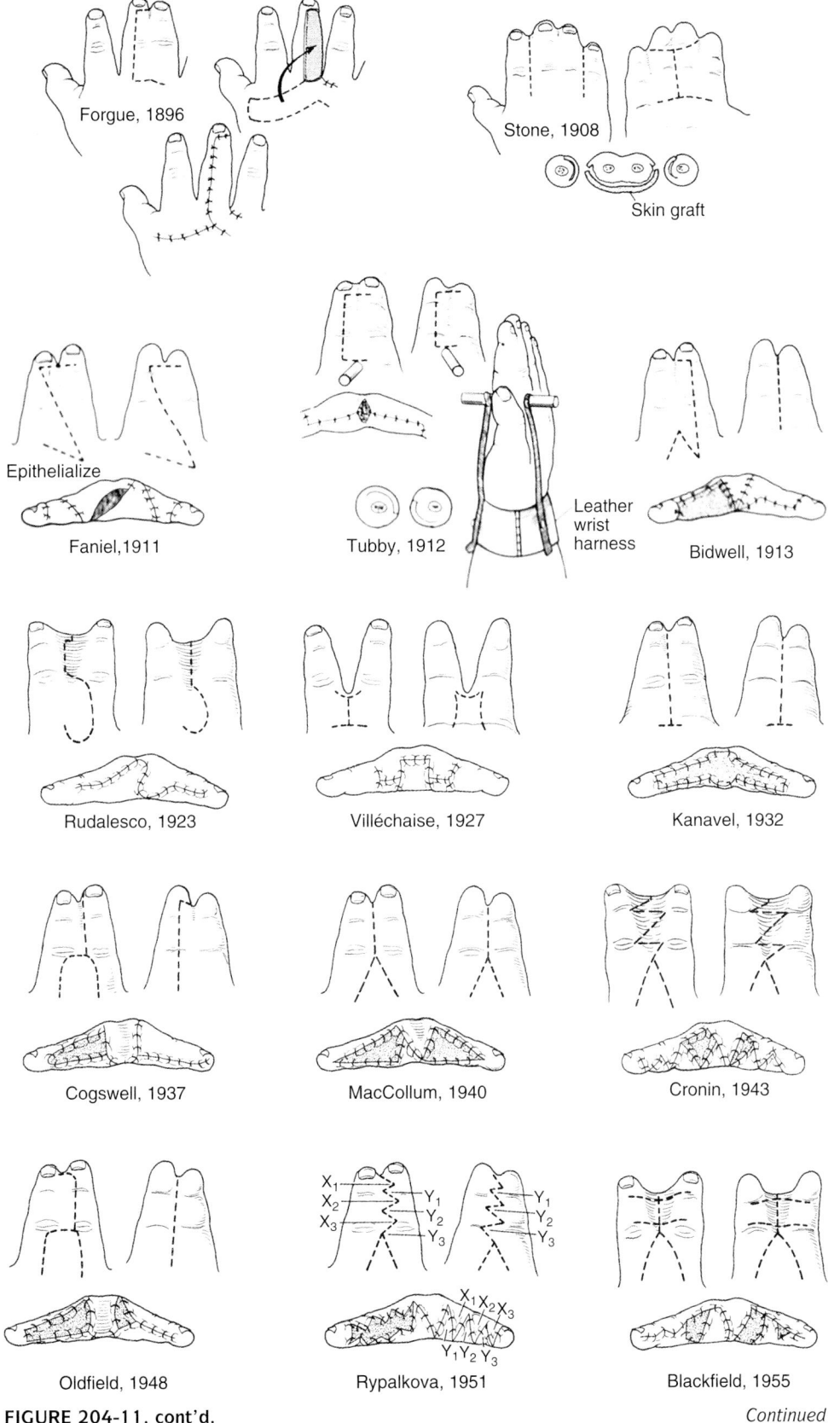

Forgue, 1896

Stone, 1908

Skin graft

Epithelialize

Faniel, 1911

Tubby, 1912

Leather wrist harness

Bidwell, 1913

Rudalesco, 1923

Villéchaise, 1927

Kanavel, 1932

Cogswell, 1937

MacCollum, 1940

Cronin, 1943

Oldfield, 1948

Rypalkova, 1951

Blackfield, 1955

FIGURE 204-11, cont'd.

Continued

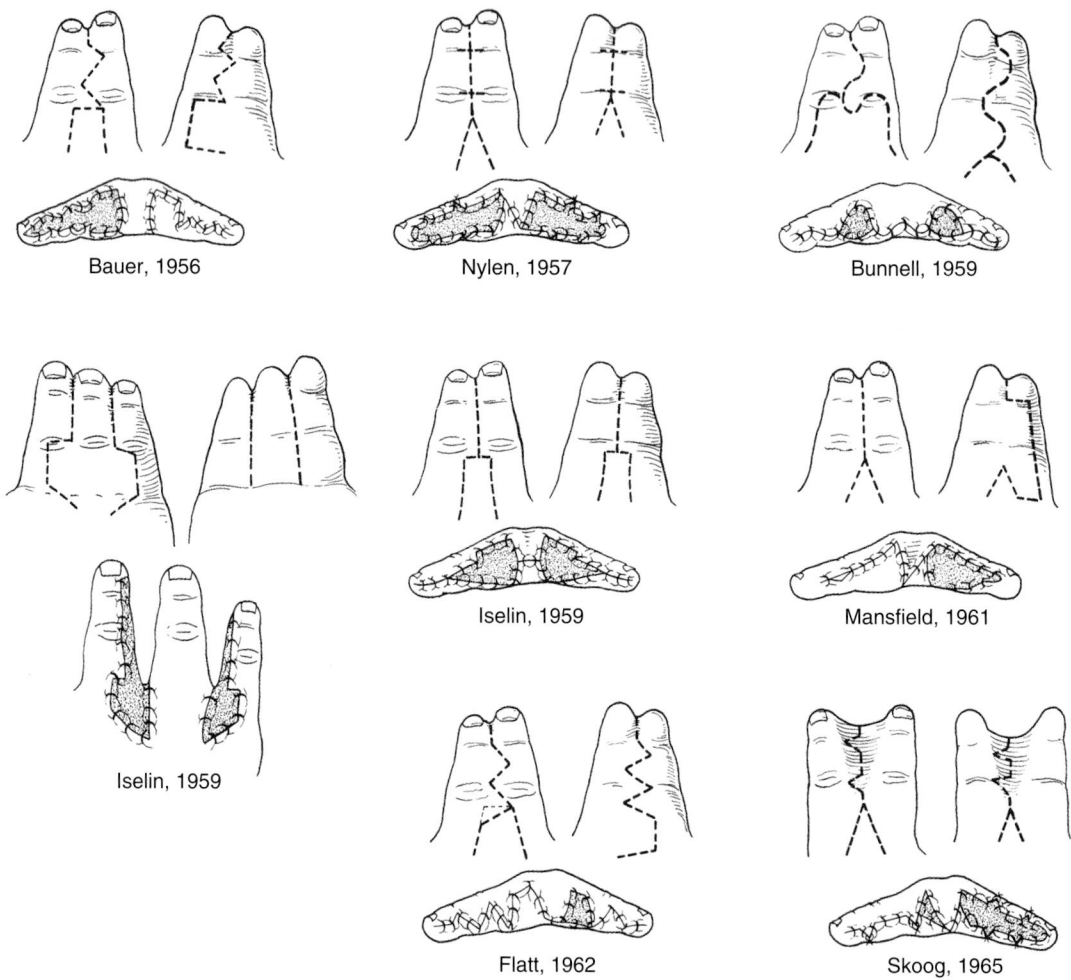

Bauer, 1956

Nylen, 1957

Bunnell, 1959

Iselin, 1959

Iselin, 1959

Mansfield, 1961

Flatt, 1962

Skoog, 1965

FIGURE 204-11, cont'd.

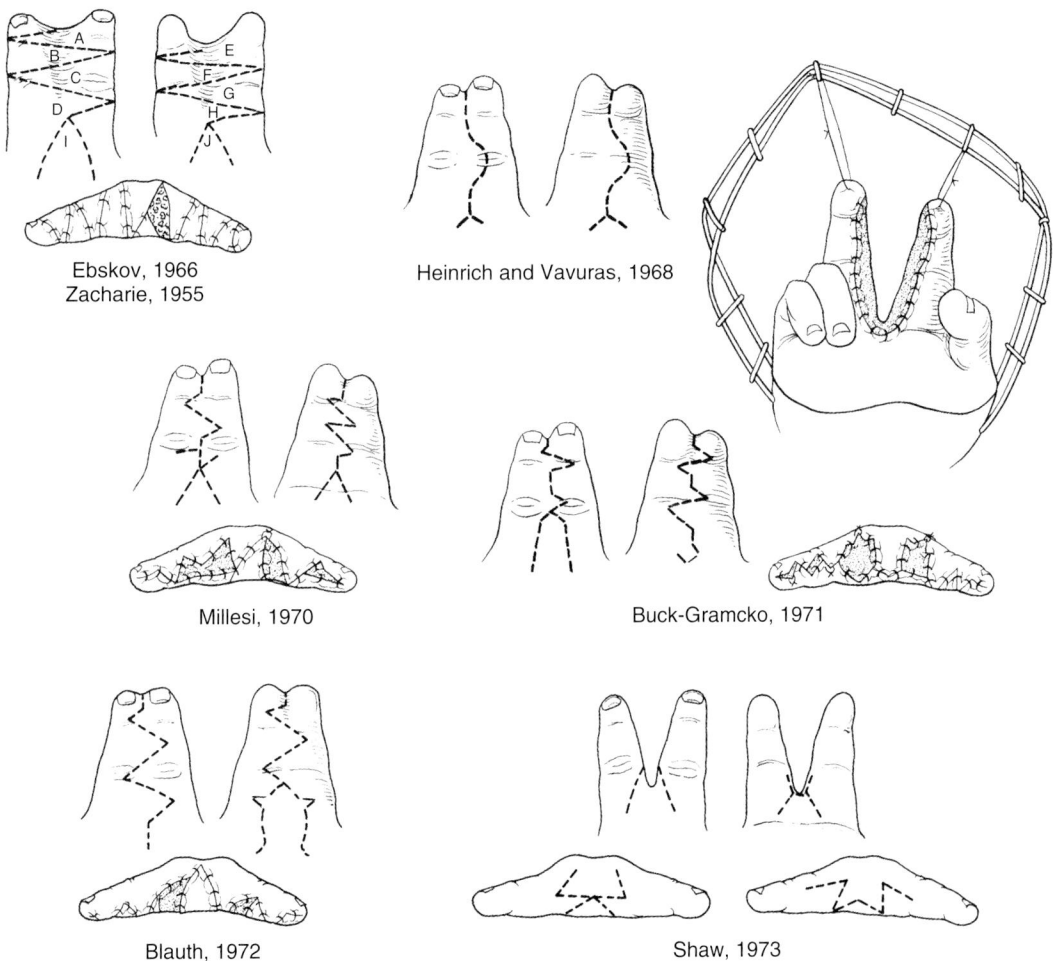

Ebskov, 1966
Zacharie, 1955

Heinrich and Vavuras, 1968

Millesi, 1970

Buck-Gramcko, 1971

Blauth, 1972

Shaw, 1973

FIGURE 204-11, cont'd.

Continued

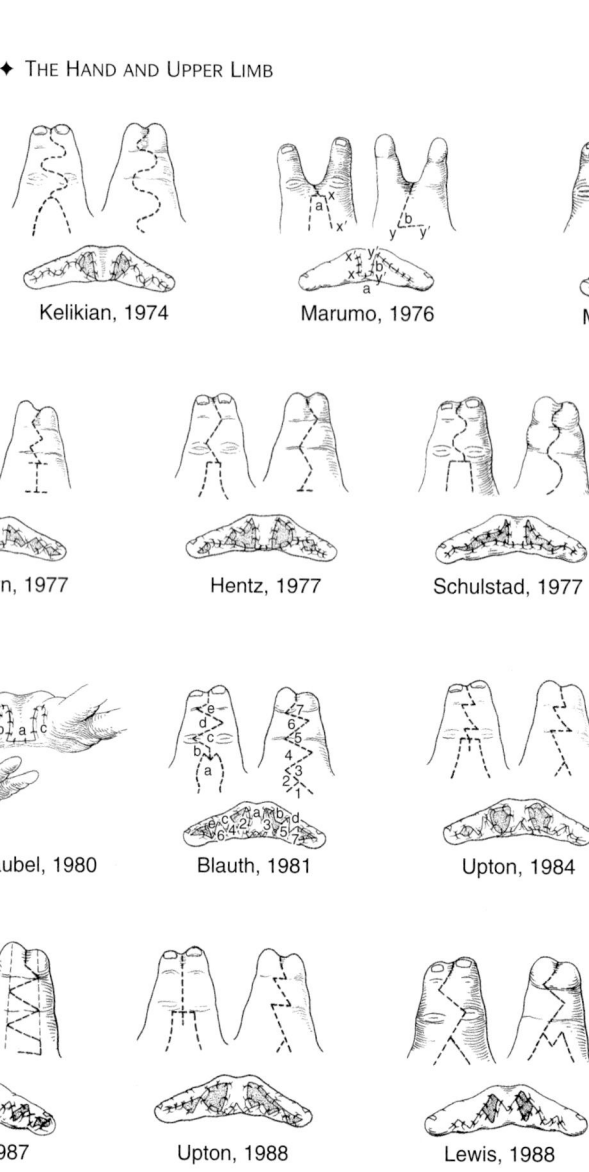

Kelikian, 1974

Marumo, 1976

Marumo, 1976

Brown, 1977

Hentz, 1977

Schulstad, 1977

Littler, 1978

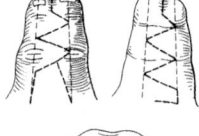
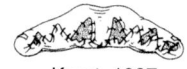

Schneider, Vaubel, 1980

Blauth, 1981

Upton, 1984

Gilbert, 1986

Keret, 1987

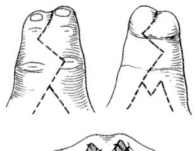

Upton, 1988

Lewis, 1988

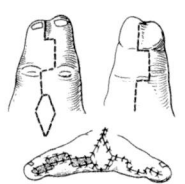

Colville, 1989

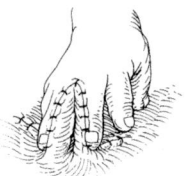

Zuker, 1990

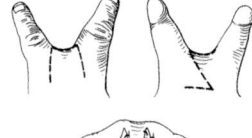

Ostrowski, 1991

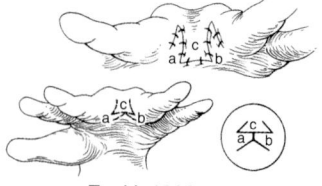

Ezaki, 1993

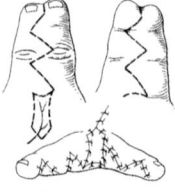

Sherif, 1998

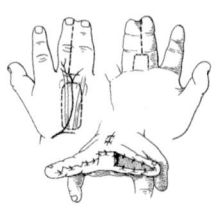

Segura-Castillo, 2002

FIGURE 204-11, cont'd.

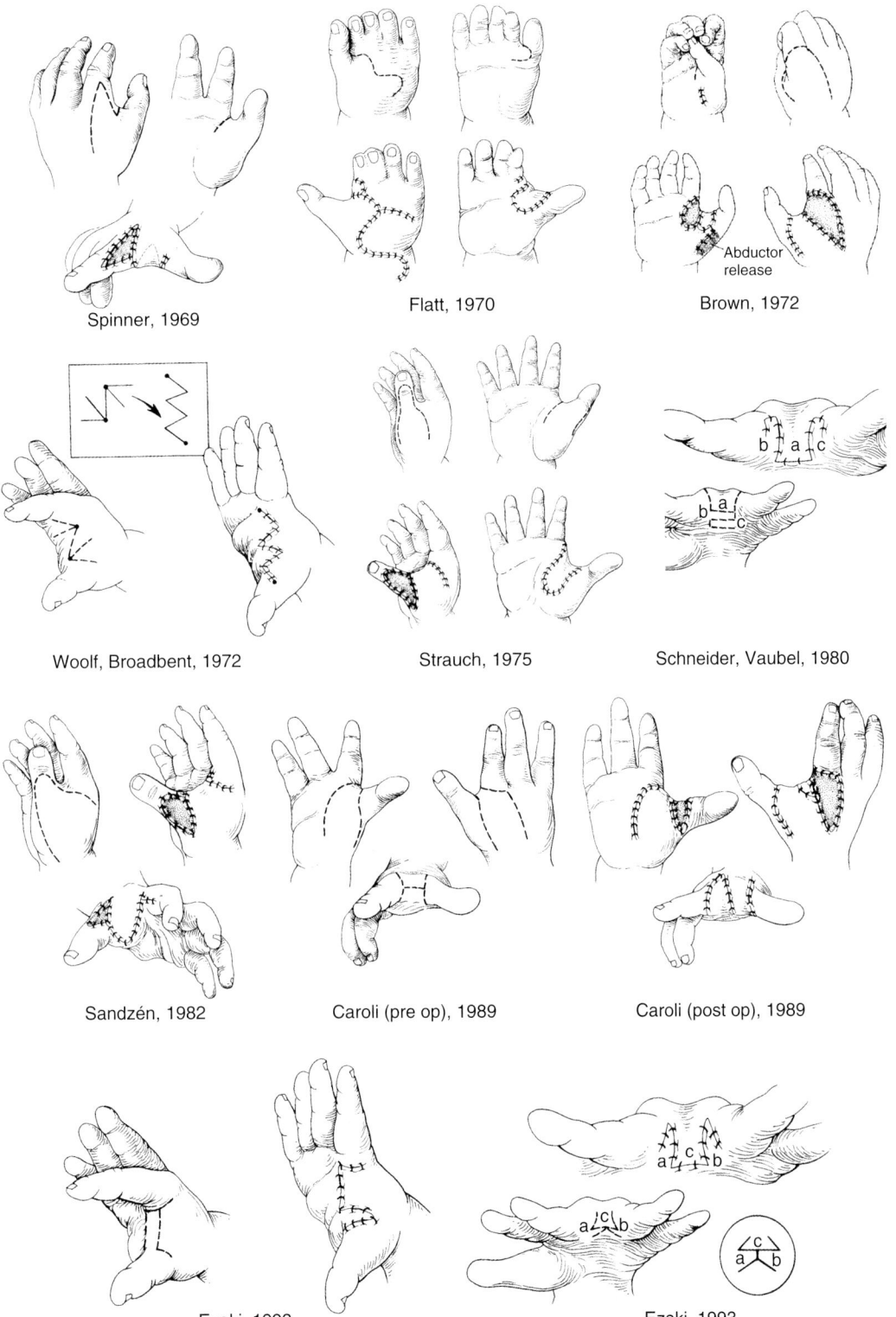

Spinner, 1969

Flatt, 1970

Brown, 1972

Woolf, Broadbent, 1972

Strauch, 1975

Schneider, Vaubel, 1980

Sandzén, 1982

Caroli (pre op), 1989

Caroli (post op), 1989

Ezaki, 1993

Ezaki, 1993

FIGURE 204-12. Historical methods of first web space release. Many of the previous methods have been applied to the release of the much broader thumb-index web space, which has different anatomic proportions. The evolution here parallels that of the interdigital spaces up until the past 20 years, during which time pedicled vascular island and free tissue transfers have been introduced. Of all methods available, the four-flap Z-plasty has remained the most predictable and commonly used for minimal and moderate deficiencies.

Continued

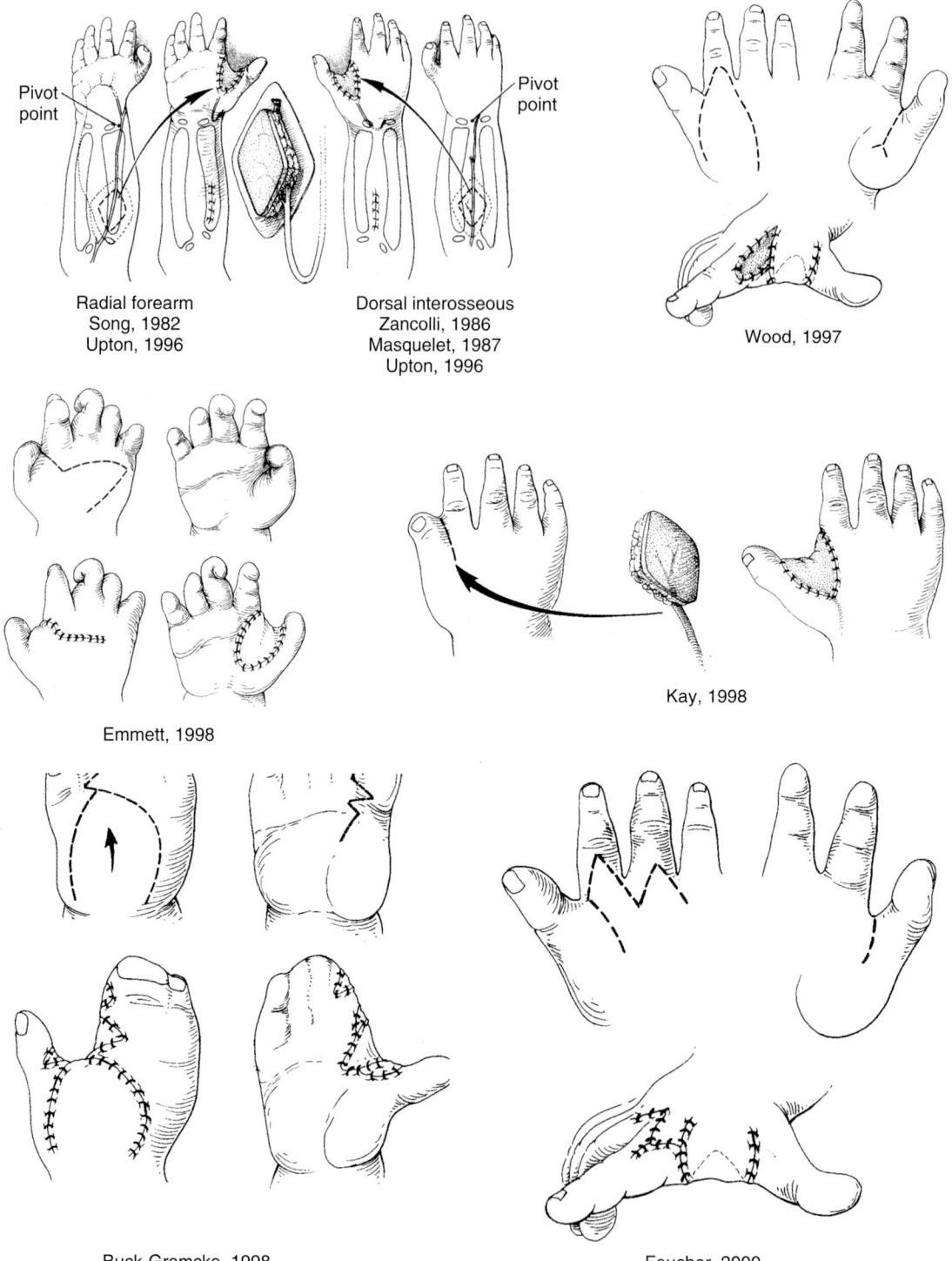

Pivot point

Radial forearm
Song, 1982
Upton, 1996

Dorsal interosseous
Zancolli, 1986
Masquelet, 1987
Upton, 1996

Pivot point

Wood, 1997

Emmett, 1998

Kay, 1998

Buck-Gramcko, 1998

Foucher, 2000

FIGURE 204-12, cont'd. For severe deficiencies, full-thickness tissue must be either added or advanced and re-advanced into this critical region.

"reinvented the wheel" by describing "new" and innovative procedures that had been both introduced and refined decades earlier.

Principles

Syndactyly separation is a "simple problem and should not be made more complicated."[4] The anatomy of the four normal interdigital web spaces has not changed with time and has been well described and illustrated.[4,152] It is important that each surgeon learn to execute his or her preferred technique well for given indications. Principles for the separation of all forms of syndactyly have become established during the past 7 decades (Table 204-3).[6,153,154]

Of course, good surgeons understand that principles and rules are made to be broken. In the Apert hand, for example, areas along the distal phalanges are left open to epithelialize, straight-line incisions are used, longitudinal epiphyseal brackets are excised early in life, and, at times, full-thickness grafts are not used.[44,45,155] These hands require exceptional surgical approaches for the best results to be achieved. Of all the principles listed in Table 204-3, the one that probably has the most impact on a favorable outcome is adequate postoperative immobilization, the one most surgeons take for granted (see "Outcomes").

Technique

THUMB TO INDEX (FIRST) WEB RELEASE

The first web space has the configuration of a diamond-shaped tetrahedron,[4] which has a large

tissue requirement for both glabrous (palmar) and nonglabrous dorsal skin. Complete syndactyly of this web space occurs in less than 10% of all patients, but this region is frequently deficient in the congenitally deformed hand, limiting abduction and independent motion of the thumb.[9,48,78,156,157] The thenar muscles are often deficient; their reconstruction is covered in Chapter 208. A well-executed first web space release, with liberation of an otherwise immobile thumb, is the single most functional operation performed by the pediatric hand surgeon working with congenital differences.

Correction of the thumb-index deficiency varies with the severity of the contracture. Although more comprehensive systems for evaluation have been described,[158] first web space deficiencies may be evaluated as mild, moderate, and severe. This characterization has the most direct impact on surgical treatment.

Mild

For small defects, many variations of Z-plasty transposition flaps have been described. Although single Z-plasty with two larger flaps is often sufficient to provide an adequate release within the first web space, it is preferable to use the four-flap Z-plasty because it provides excellent length and contour within the depth of the web space (Fig. 204-13).[159,160] In a similar procedure, a complex central V-Y, lateral Z-plasty approach may also accomplish the same result and may be more useful within the interdigital web space.[161,162] Techniques for providing dynamic muscle balance for palmar abduction (opposition) after soft tissue release are covered in other sections.

Moderate

With more restriction, the thumb is webbed by a simple incomplete or complete syndactyly, and palmar abduction and grasping ability are severely restricted. Tissue must be brought into the released web space, and all varieties of V-Y flaps, dorsal transposition flaps,[148,163,164] and dorsal rotation[165-168] or rotation-advancement flaps[48,156,157,169-173] with and without skin grafts have been described.

Orthopedic surgeons like to use local rotation flaps from the dorsal surface of the index metacarpal or proximal phalanx.[169,173-177] Plastic surgeons usually eschew this technique, which leaves a conspicuous skin graft on a visible surface.[178] Instead, they prefer to place these grafts on the lateral surfaces of the thumb or index finger because most of these patients come back as teenagers asking to have the graft removed.

Whenever possible, it is preferable to use variations of the advancement of dorsal skin into the defect. The mobility of the dorsal nonglabrous skin of the hand allows repeated advancement of this tissue. The base of this flap is broad, and all proximal soft tissue attachments to the flap are carefully preserved. A zigzag

---

TABLE 204-3 ✦ PRINCIPLES FOR THE SEPARATION OF ALL FORMS OF SYNDACTYLY

Use of full-thickness tissue for commissure reconstruction
Placement of the commissure at a dorsal to palmar 45-degree angle at the level of the midportion of the proximal phalanx in a normal-sized digit (see Color Plate 204-1 and Fig. 204-13)
Use of zigzag incisions on the palmar surfaces (Fig. 204-13)
Equal distribution of full-thickness skin grafts to cover raw areas
Meticulous surgical technique
Operation on one side of a digit at a time
Emphasis on construction of normal nails and nail folds
Earlier correction of skeletal deformities when there is no danger of injuring growth centers (see Fig. 204-9)
Adequate postoperative immobilization, which in our patients is in a well-padded long-arm cast[6,153]
Use of postoperative stents at night to maintain web configuration[6,154]

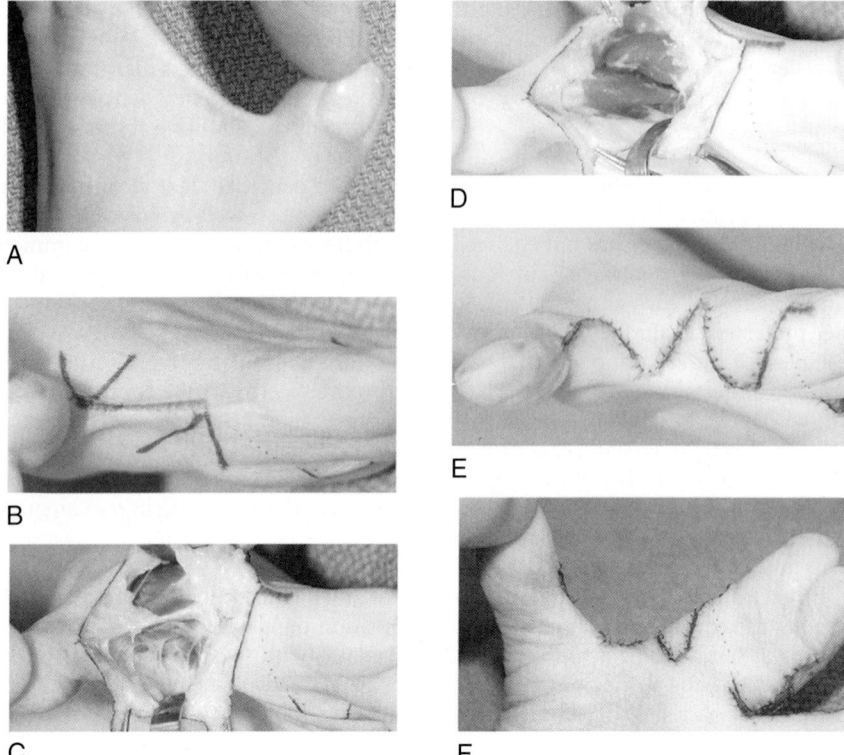

FIGURE 204-13. First web release with four-flap Z-plasty (technique). *A,* A simple incomplete syndactyly severely restricts the mobility of the thumb in this child with brachysyndactyly. *B,* Incisions for a four-flap Z-plasty are outlined. *C,* After flap incision and retraction, the investing fascia of the intrinsic muscles is hypertrophied. The thickest portion is the most distal between the two layers of muscle. *D,* After complete fascial excision, the first dorsal interosseous muscle (above) and adductor pollicis muscle are seen. There is a remarkable improvement of thumb abduction from the index ray. *E,* The flaps have been transposed and closed with 6-0 chromic sutures. *F,* The new first web contour has a gentle curve extending from the metacarpophalangeal joint of the thumb and index rays.

configuration of the incisions within the depth of the commissure will reduce the chance of secondary contracture.

Skin grafts are best placed along the lateral border of the thumb or index finger and not directly across the web space. Tissue expansion can be used with limited effectiveness and requires a cooperative family and patient.[179,180] A temporary pin is used to hold the thumb metacarpal in maximal abduction.

Severe

In the simple complete and complex first web spaces—such as those seen in the Apert hand, the typical cleft hand, some symbrachydactylies, the unilateral mitten hand, and the occasional radial clubhand—the entire diamond-shaped tetrahedron must be brought into the web. The release and excision of the fibrous band or bands between the thenar intrinsic muscles often includes a release of the carpometacarpal joint. Distal bifurcations of the common artery to the ulnar side of the thumb and the radial side of the index finger are often present. One must be ligated, usually that to the index if there is a normal vessel to the opposite side of this digit within the second interdigital web space.

A combination of local rotation-advancement flaps with or without skin grafts is preferred primarily because these flaps can be readvanced with subsequent operations.[157,181] Distal tubed pedicled flaps[7,111,182] are no longer used because they are too cumbersome. Distally based radial forearm flaps are an excellent source of regional tissue based on the radial artery system[181,183] or the dorsal interosseous vessels (Fig. 204-14),[59,181,184] but they have two disadvantages. First, they leave a forearm scar, and second, they are difficult to perform in a 6-month to 2-year-old child because of the large layer of adipose tissue.

Free flaps from groin, opposite forearm, or lateral arm donor sites constitute another option for the confident microsurgeon (Fig. 204-15).[185,186] A pin or external fixator must be used to hold the thumb in maximal abduction postoperatively. Skin expansion

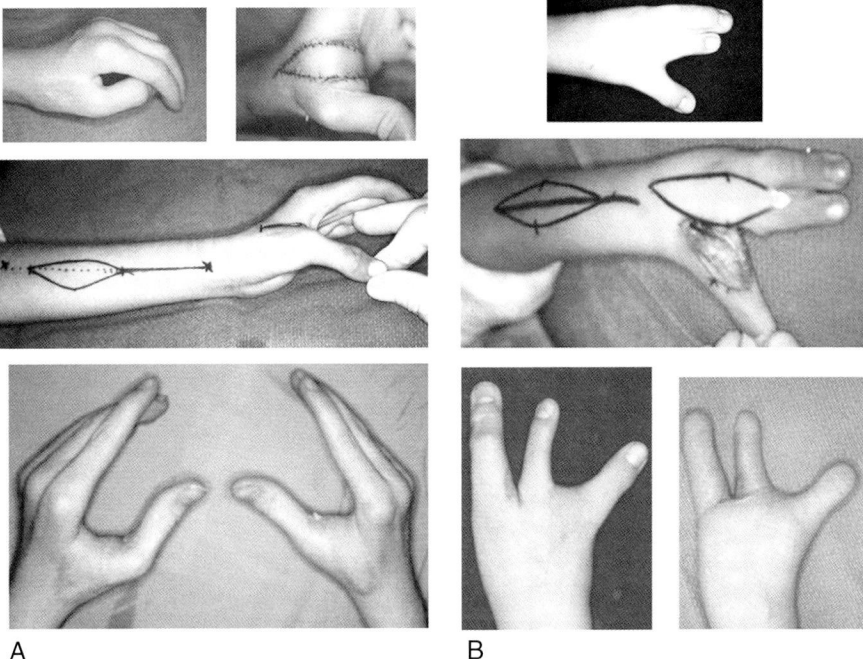

A   B

FIGURE 204-14. First web release with forearm flap (technique). *A,* The left hand in this child with arthrogryposis had been previously released twice with rapid contracture recurrence due to the extensive soft tissue deficiency. A distally based radial forearm flap is outlined in the middle third of the forearm. The postoperative picture of both hands illustrates the marked improvement in both thumb position and posture. *B,* The thumb in this three-digit hand lies in the same plane as the digits with a small first web space. The outline and template of a distally based dorsal interosseous flap are seen after a full release has been completed. The addition of tissue within the web space and a tendon transfer for palmar abduction have permitted the thumb much more independence and mobility.

has the same results in these hands as it does in the less restricted web spaces.[6,179,187] Finally, ray resection of the index finger is an excellent option and is preferred when the epiphysis of the proximal phalanx is abnormal or when three additional functional digits are present on the same hand.

RELEASE OF COMPLETE, SIMPLE SYNDACTYLY (SECOND, THIRD, AND FOURTH INTERDIGITAL WEB SPACES)

A syndactyly release is a simple but meticulous operation that should not be made more complicated than necessary. An almost inexhaustible number of techniques continue to be described (Fig. 204-16), most of which adhere to the principles outlined. No single method is perfect for every patient. It is important that the surgeon be comfortable with one or two methods and use them consistently. During the past 10 years, the author has used more straight-line dorsal incisions for aesthetic reasons and prefers either a large dorsal rectangular flap or a combination of dorsal and palmar triangular flaps for the commissure (see Fig. 204-11).

ANESTHESIA. General anesthesia is preferred. After routine preparation and draping, incisions are planned with the pediatric tourniquet deflated.

MARKING. The dorsal and palmar levels of the cleft are marked, and a large dorsal, slightly truncated rectangular flap is outlined. Dorsal skin dimples in chubby hands denote the metacarpophalangeal joint level. Measurements of adjacent web spaces and of the opposite hand are often useful. The normal web space has a palmar inclination of 40 to 45 degrees and an "hourglass" configuration (Fig. 204-17; see also Color Plate 204-1 and Figs. 204-11 and 204-16). The size of the dorsal flap varies; it is often 18 mm long and 9 mm wide in the normal 12-month-old child and extends almost to the proximal interphalangeal joint extension crease. The palmar flap inset is marked so that there is always slight 1-mm overcorrection. The inset for the third web space extends more distally than that for the second and fourth interdigital web spaces. Distal zigzag incisions are measured so that mirror images are formed on the two sides of each finger.

Sharp, acute angles are preferable to gentle, obtuse angles, which often become straight with growth.

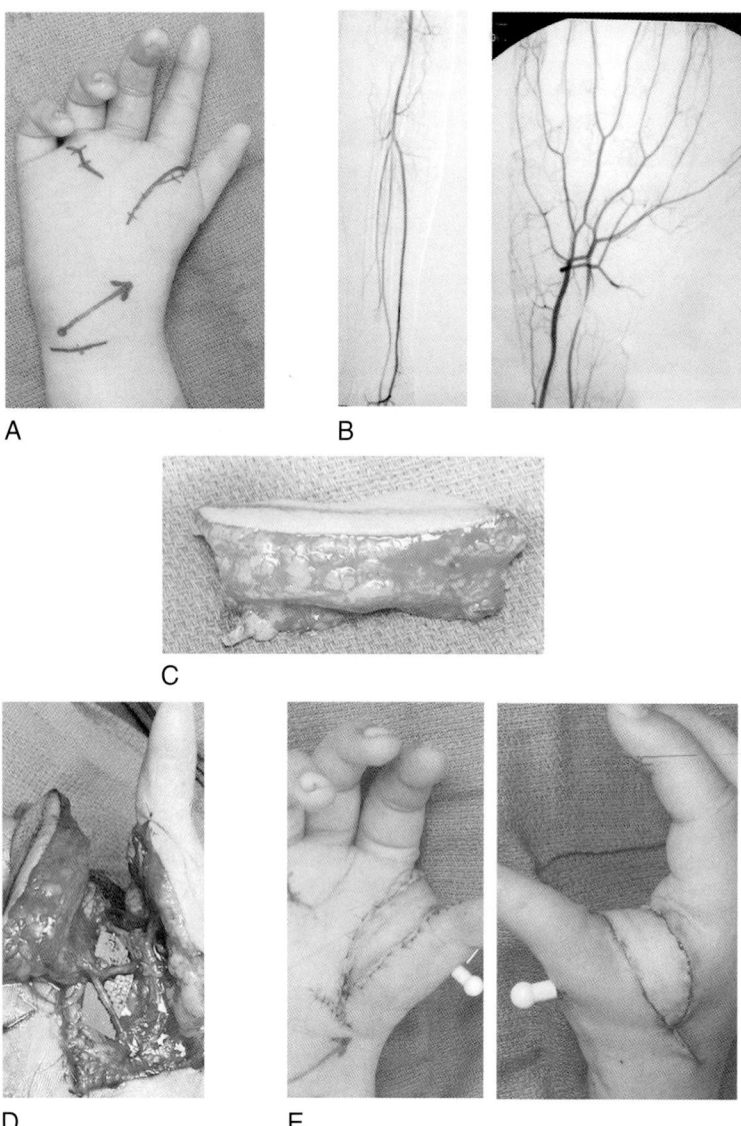

FIGURE 204-15. First web space release with free flap. *A,* The clinical appearance and markings of a patient with bilateral radial dysplasia and a type IIIA hand in which the carpometacarpal joint is intact. The first web space is deficient, and there are no functional median-innervated thenar intrinsic muscles. *B,* The preoperative angiograms of the forearm and hand show that there is no radial artery to the hand, which is supplied primarily by the ulnar system. The blockage in the prominent interosseous system negated possible use of a distally based forearm flap. *C,* A precise amount of full-thickness tissue was harvested from the opposite forearm, where the donor site was closed primarily. *D,* Two arterial anastomoses were performed: one to the radial side of the palmar arch and a second to the index radial digital artery, which required transection during the web release. Dorsal veins were used for the venous recipient vessels. *E,* A C wire to hold the web space apart was placed before flap inset and left in place for 4 weeks postoperatively. The ring flexor digitorum superficialis tendon transfer to the abductor pollicis aponeurosis was performed simultaneously to improve palmar abduction (opposition) of the thumb. Collateral ligament reconstruction at the metacarpophalangeal joint level was not necessary.

Marked reference points along the sides of the digits,[61] bent dental wires,[114] or 25-gauge needles passed through the webbing may help align this precision marking (see Figs. 204-11 and 204-16).[188] The flaps are equally distributed between the two digits. Techniques designed to totally resurface one side of the release with flap tissue and the other with a skin graft[9,116] often yield inconsistent results. When there is not enough distal skin to cover both sides of the release, a straight-line dorsal incision is recommended to minimize the visible skin graft deformity.

A number of techniques have been used to facilitate the markings for coordination of the dorsal and palmar surfaces. Simple marking on the sides of the digits,[9,189] making chevrons,[190] bending paper clips,[107]

and placing a needle between the interdigital webbing[6] are among the most common.

DISSECTION. After limb exsanguination and tourniquet inflation, the web is released, beginning distally and progressing proximally. A knife or small osteotome is often sufficient to release distal bone or cartilaginous coalitions beneath conjoined nails. Oscillating saws are necessary with large skeletal fusions in older children. Palmar pulp can often be defatted[9] and advanced dorsally to form a new paronychial fold. In some instances, a portion of the lateral nail matrix and underlying bone may provide enough space for advancement. Composite grafts from the lateral portion of the great toe[191,192] or the medial arch of the foot[193]

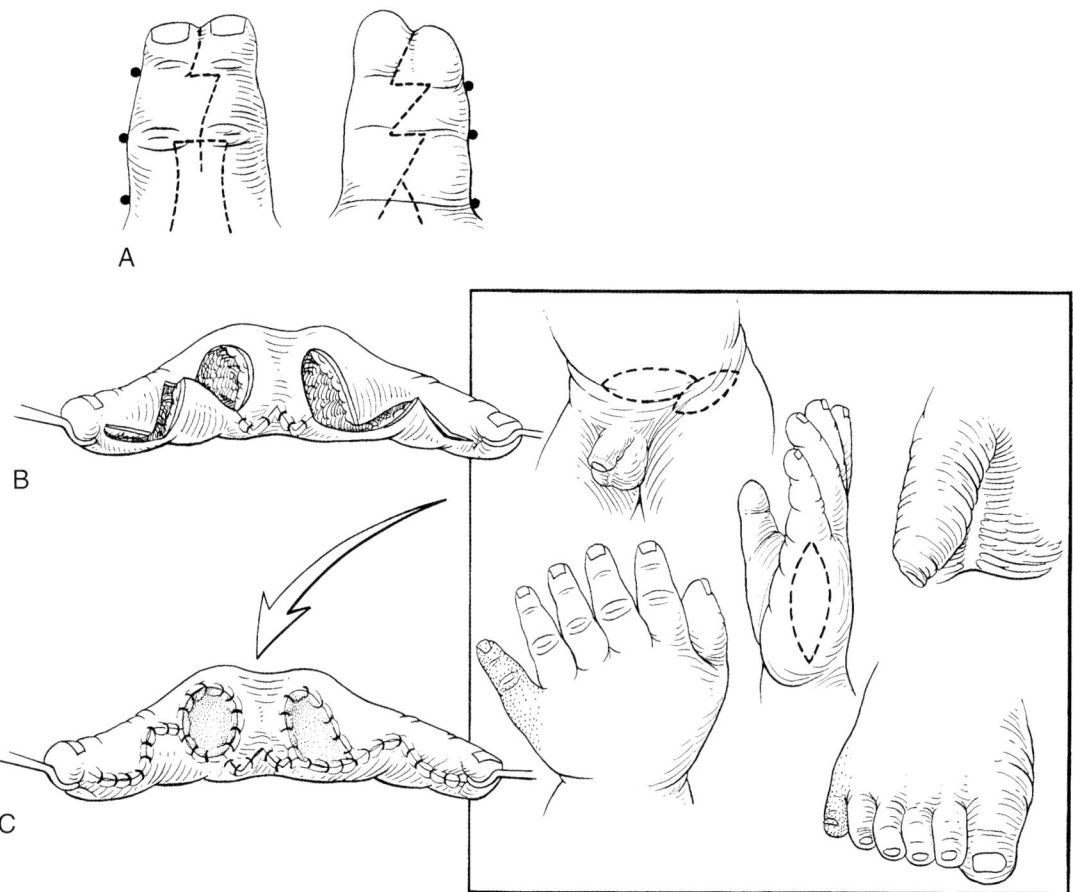

FIGURE 204-16. Principles of interdigital release and donor sites. *A,* One technique uses dorsal and palmar markings for zigzag incisions to minimize straight-line scar contractures with growth. A large dorsal hourglass flap is used to line the depth of the commissure. Reference points made on the side of the digit are helpful in obtaining correct alignment in the distal half of the digit, where enough tissue is available to obviate the use of skin grafts after flap interdigitation. *B,* After the flaps have been sutured within the commissure and along the distal sides of the digit, templates of the raw areas are made for skin grafts, which may be obtained from a variety of sources. *Inset:* "Like tissues" from a similar part, such as an extra finger or toe or the hypothenar region of the hand, are preferred but usually not available. The inguinal crease is most commonly used, and the lower abdominal flexion crease is used when large amounts of skin are required during sequential release of multiple web spaces in the same patient, such as the Apert child. Foreskin preputial grafts are described at periodic intervals but are not preferred because of their frequent infection and dark pigmentation. *C,* After tourniquet release, the full-thickness skin grafts are meticulously applied. The ensuing dressing and immobilization are imperative for a complete take of the graft.

may also provide a smooth, rounded fold (Figs. 204-18 and 204-19).[191] For complex syndactylies with a conjoined nail, some authors have advocated separation of the nail and application of a thenar flap as a preliminary procedure to web separation[194,195]; however, this procedure is not routinely performed.

With the distal portion of the digits held in maximal abduction by hooks, a spreading scissor dissection is used to identify neurovascular structures, and the interdigital separation is continued along the midline toward the proximal interphalangeal joint. The fascial interconnecting fibers between Cleland and Grayson ligaments on either digit are incised and

preferably excised if they are thick and fibrous (see Fig. 204-16). Magnification is essential in the dissection of this tissue from the underlying neurovascular structures on either side of the web. The dorsal flap is next raised with careful preservation of large dorsal veins. Nerves are identified and can easily be teased proximally if a distal bifurcation is found. The arborization of the common digital artery to the adjacent sides of the web space will often be the structure that limits the depth of the commissure release. At least one digital artery per digit should be preserved. If an artery is injured or cut in a digit with known absence of an artery on the opposite side,

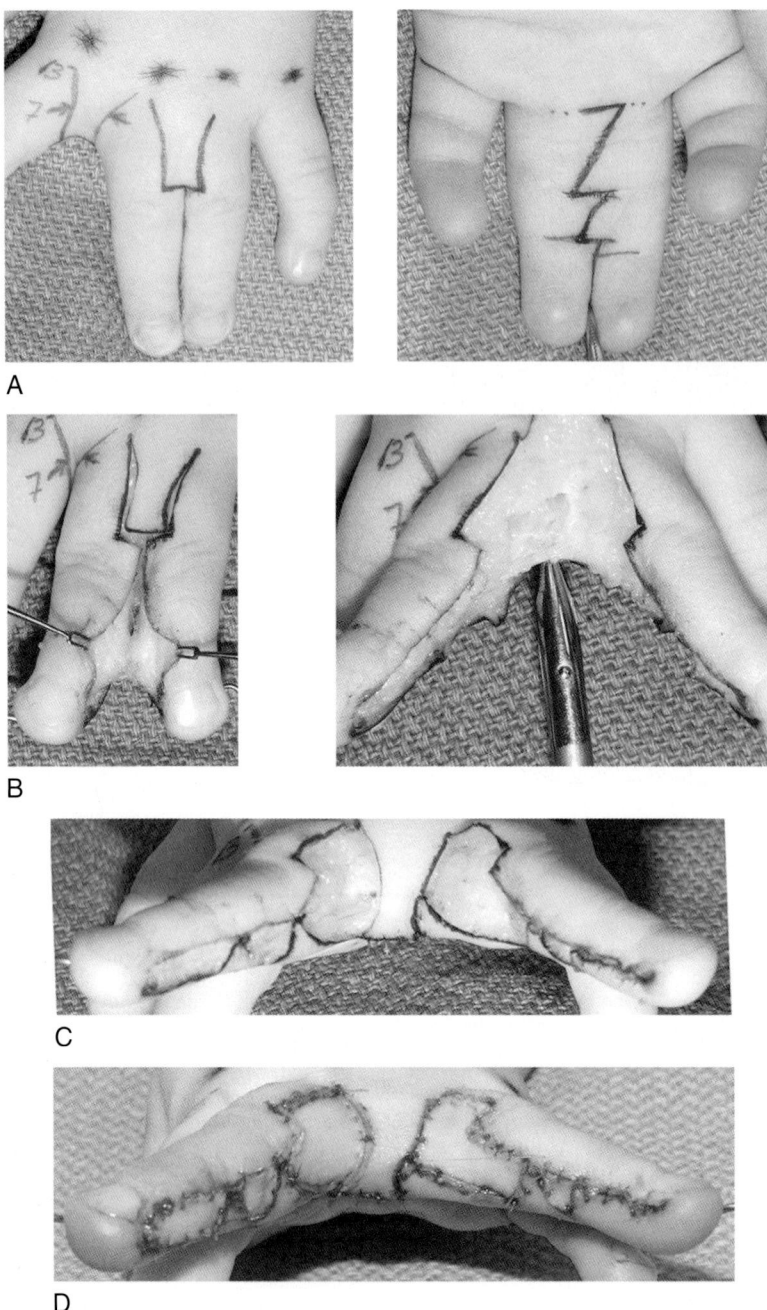

FIGURE 204-17. Release of interdigital web space. *A,* The dorsal and palmar markings show a large dorsal flap to line the commissure; the transverse components of the zigzag palmar incisions lie in the normal existing interphalangeal flexion creases. The length and width are 13 mm and 7 mm in this 11-month-old child. *B,* Thick interdigital fibrous bands may originate both dorsal and palmar to the neurovascular structures. They must be completely excised. *C,* The new commissure has been formed and the side flap sutured under no tension. Excessive defatting invites tight closures. *D,* The open areas have been covered with full-thickness skin grafts that are secured with absorbable sutures.

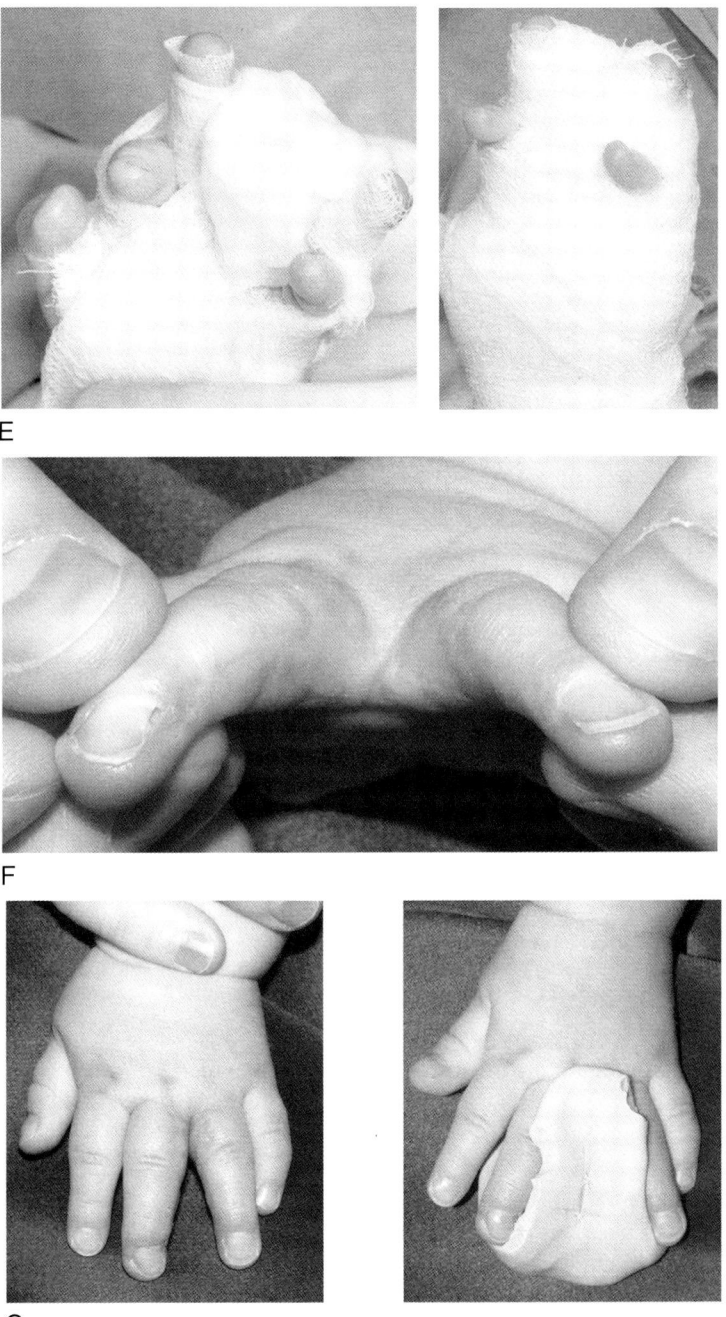

FIGURE 204-17, cont'd. *E,* A dressing with interdigital moist cotton is carefully applied before the extremity is immobilized with a long-arm cast. *F,* The flaps and grafts are seen 6 weeks later. *G,* For 6 to 8 weeks after cast removal, an interdigital stent secured with Coban is worn at night to maintain early correction and to keep the hand out of the baby's mouth.

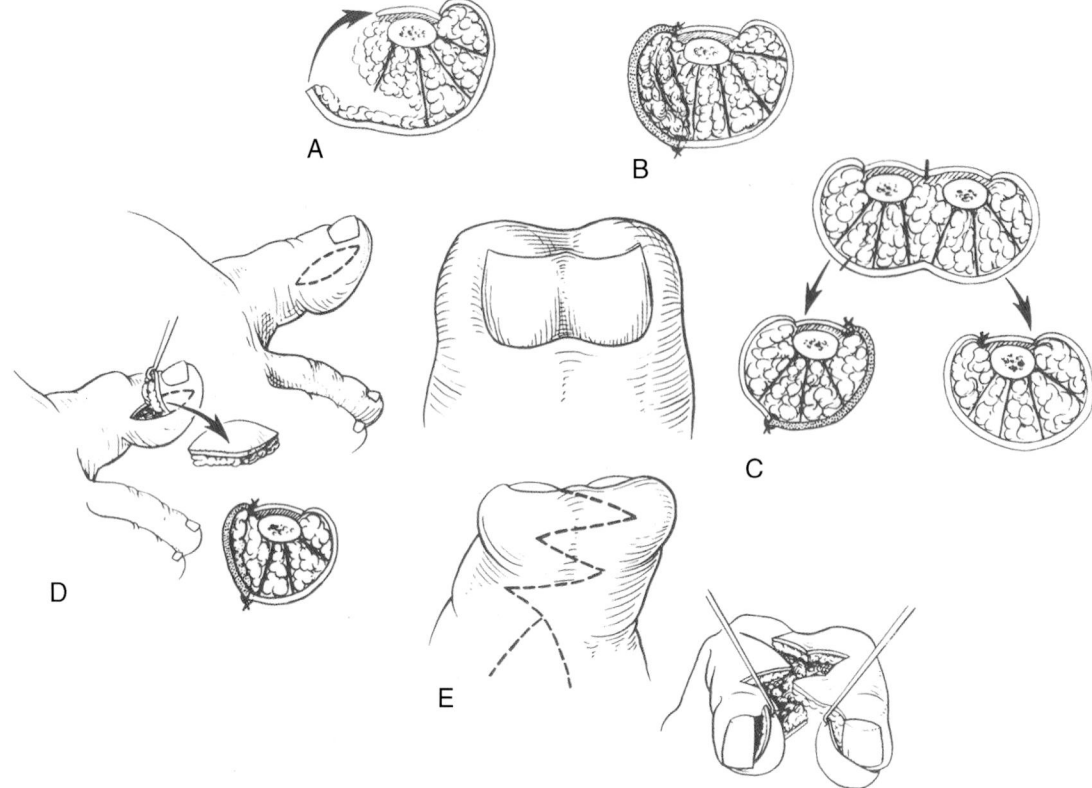

FIGURE 204-18. Nail folds. Paronychial and eponychial folds are one of the most difficult portions of the digit to construct. Many methods exist, but few are perfect. *A,* The lateral skin can be undermined and simply advanced with minor deficiencies. *B,* Full-thickness skin grafts may be used. Glabrous donor skin is preferred. *C,* After release, one side can be covered with skin and the other resurfaced with a graft. In these patients, there is never enough skin to cover both sides. *D,* Composite skin and pulp grafts from the lateral side of the great toe are effective.[192] *E,* Distal triangular flap from either side of the fingertip provides excellent paronychial fold coverage in complex syndactyly, such as the Apert hand.[197] (From Upton J: Congenital anomalies. In Jurkiewicz M, Krizek T, Mathes S, Ariyan S: Plastic Surgery Principles and Practice. St. Louis, Mosby, 1990:529-604.)

revascularization by use of the operating microscope is recommended.

SKELETAL CORRECTION. The transverse metacarpal ligament is identified and incised if greater metacarpal mobility is desired, as in the hypoplastic hand or Apert hand. Abnormal osseous structures may require rearrangement at this point, but most surgeons prefer to delay definitive osteotomies for skeletal correction until the patient is older. Damage to growth centers and periosteum must be avoided. However, duplicated skeletal parts should be excised, collateral ligaments reattached, and intrinsic muscles appropriately reattached or completely excised during correction of complex and complicated syndactylies, particularly within the central portions of the hand.

FLAP INSET. The dorsal flap is rotated into the depth of the release, and the palmar flap is interdigitated and secured with 5-0 or 6-0 absorbable sutures tied under no tension. In hands without significant skeletal abnormalities, the bifurcation of the common digital nerve often marks the normal depth of the web space. The distal flaps along the sides of the digits are closed with 6-0 chromic sutures. Excessive defatting[196] to gain mobilization and to close these flaps is not generally recommended but may be helpful along the borders.[185] Exact templates are made of all areas to be grafted. The tourniquet is released, flap circulation is checked, and bleeding is controlled with the bipolar cautery.

SKIN GRAFTS. A pressure dressing is applied while full-thickness skin grafts are harvested from the lower abdominal flexion crease or the inguinal crease, well lateral to the future hair-bearing escutcheon (see Fig. 204-16, *inset*). The donor site is closed with buried absorbable sutures and external Steri-Strips or skin adhesives. The skin grafts are defatted and sutured into position with 6-0 chromic sutures.

DRESSING. The dressing is all important! Grafts and incisions are covered with one layer of a medicated gauze, followed by a compressible synthetic foam or moistened cotton placed as a stent within the

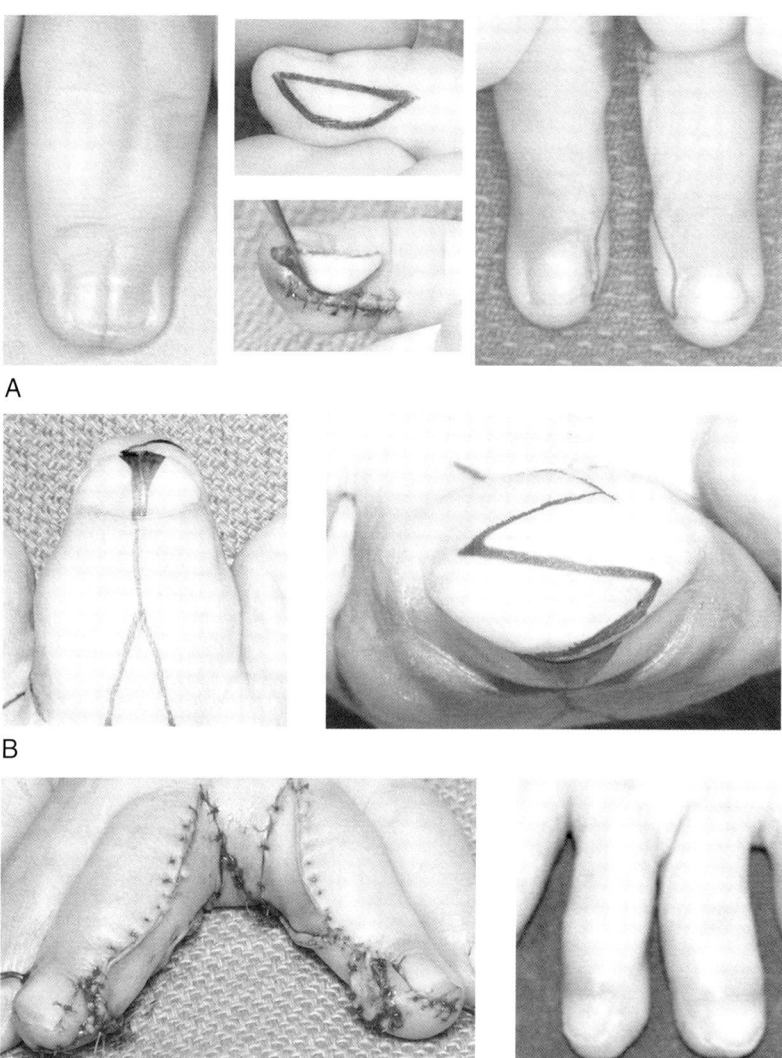

FIGURE 204-19. Composite nail fold grafts. *A,* After release of this complete simple syndactyly, the large open areas were covered with skin and pulp composite grafts harvested from the lateral border of each great toe. The grafts have grown well and are seen 6 years later. *B,* The markings for release of the central two digits in this Apert patient show planned excisions of nail plate and matrix and triangular pulp flaps, which will provide paronychial fold construction. *C,* The triangular flaps have been placed along the ulnar border of the long finger and radial side of the ring finger. Two years later, the relationship between these paronychial folds and the eponychial folds has been maintained.

interdigital web space. The fingers are positioned in abduction to avoid any kinking of the commissure flaps. Next, a bulky fluff dressing is applied and secured with a circumferential Kling wrap. The extremity is then immobilized with a well-padded long-arm cast or splint extending well above the flexed elbow.

The forearm of a 2-year-old child is bulky in its midportion and tapers distally, so casts easily slip off unless elbow flexion is maintained. Because of larger amounts of subcutaneous fat, breast-fed children younger than 1 year can be the most difficult to fit. The thumb or at least one other finger is left exposed distally to act as a monitor of hand position within the cast. A stockinette-sling is then passed around the cast and tied behind the child's back. The other end can also be tied to a line strapped above the child's bed for elevation at night.

Proper dressings and immobilization of an active child's arm are the most important factors in obtaining a satisfactory skin graft take. The cast is left in place for 2 to 3 weeks, depending on the amount of bone or soft tissue reconstruction performed (see Fig. 204-16). The parents are instructed to call if the exposed digit or thumb disappears into the cast. Excessive perspiration during the summer months and problem grafts or flaps, such as in the Apert child or in any child with hyperhidrosis, may require earlier inspection. Cast removal is usually most efficiently accomplished in the ambulatory surgery room under sedation or light general anesthesia for the uncooperative child or equally anxious parent. When healing has been incomplete and small areas of scar are present at the base of the commissure, small splints and molded inserts are made for the child to wear at night.

FINGERTIPS AND CONJOINED NAILS

In simple or complex complete syndactylies, the soft tissue deficiencies include the pulp at the distal phalangeal level, and a variety of techniques can be useful (see Figs. 204-18 and 204-19).[6] Reconstruction of paronychial and eponychial folds is one of the most challenging aspects of syndactyly surgery. The popular transposition flaps[194,197-201] require delicate incision and elevation but are the best technique for constructing paronychial folds. Nail matrices and underlying bone should be trimmed to normal proportions. Local fat and fascial tissue should then be advanced over the exposed distal interphalangeal joint or distal phalangeal bone after the proper amount of skeletal and nail trimming has been completed.

SKIN GRAFT DONOR SITES

The ideal is to replace the exact "tissue in kind"[202] from an amputated extra part. Glabrous skin is available along the hypothenar eminence of the hand or the instep of the foot, which as a donor site can be quite painful. Preputial grafts obtained from simultaneous circumcision have had periodic enthusiasts[203] but are no longer used by us because of initial infections or long-term hyperpigmentation.[6,204] Full-thickness grafts from the inguinal flexion crease must be harvested lateral to the future escutcheon and will result in a distracted scar. In contrast, grafts taken from the side of the buttock in most children will result in a wide scar with growth. A Pfannenstiel incision in the lower abdominal flexion crease provides a large amount of tissue in those with much larger graft requirements, as in the correction of bilateral mitten hands. When this incision is reused for subsequent graft harvests, the grafts should all be taken from the superior (cephalad) flap. Full-thickness grafts harvested with several millimeters of fat and areolar tissue will contract less and provide better contour for a missing pulp surface (see Fig. 204-17).[192] In some conditions, small areas after web release are left open to epithelialize spontaneously.[6,44,45,205,206] Historically, many authors have advocated the use of split-thickness skin grafts,[41,83,85] but most surgeons prefer full-thickness grafts, which are not associated with as much secondary scar contracture and deformity.[6,207] The ulnar side of the hand, hypothenar eminence, wrist,[6,207-209] antecubital flexion crease, and plantar surface of the foot[193] have also been used.

Donor sites are closed in layers with absorbable suture material. The last layer is a running intradermal or subcuticular stitch. The epidermal closure is reinforced with Steri-Strips placed along the same axis of the incision. Those placed perpendicular to the incision often cause blistering when they are applied with some tension. Some surgeons have advocated the use of split-thickness skin grafts because of the low incidence of web creep with symphalangism typically seen in the central three digits.[41] Defatting has been advocated by some[9,196] to avoid the use of skin grafts in selected patients.[210]

Tissue expansion before syndactyly release in difficult hands that require multiple interdigital separations, such as the Apert hand and mitten hand, has been reported in relatively small series of patients.[179,187,188,211-214] Both inflatable balloons and spring-loaded interdigital devices have been used. The author's experience with a large Apert population is similar to that of others[212]; namely, the additional procedures and complications in active babies and young children did not justify a continued use of these techniques.

TWO- AND THREE-DIGIT HAND

In the two- or three-digit hand, moderate to severe hypoplasia of skeletal and soft tissue structures is often found. The most radial digit invariably represents the thumb, and the design of a broad first web space is crucial to function of these diminutive hands. It is recommended that one use the same technique as outlined for simple syndactyly release but always line the depth of the commissure with a large full-thickness flap. Multiple interdigitating flaps and skin grafts are avoided. It is often necessary later to rotate and recess one of these digits (usually the radial) with an osteotomy to gain a more effective pinching mechanism. These maneuvers are best accomplished by a Y-V principle with incisions through unscarred tissue (Fig. 204-20). In these patients, use of a temporary threaded pin or a permanent bone block is recommended to secure the position of the metacarpals.

OUTCOMES

Release of First Interdigital Web Space

The best and most predictable results are obtained in the more moderate forms of syndactyly. The most critical single factor is the recognition and release of the fascial bands between and investing the intrinsic musculature within the web space. These bands do not expand with growth and are often responsible for web creep more than an overlying skin graft or surgical scar is. Local flap coverage is always sufficient, and the four-flap Z-plasty technique[159] provides the best contour of the web, which should extend from the metacarpophalangeal joint of the thumb and index finger, but many other techniques have been described. The single isolated large Z-plasty correction often results in a deep depression within the web space and a disruption of the normal contour.

For more moderate and severe contractures, additional tissue must be introduced into the first web

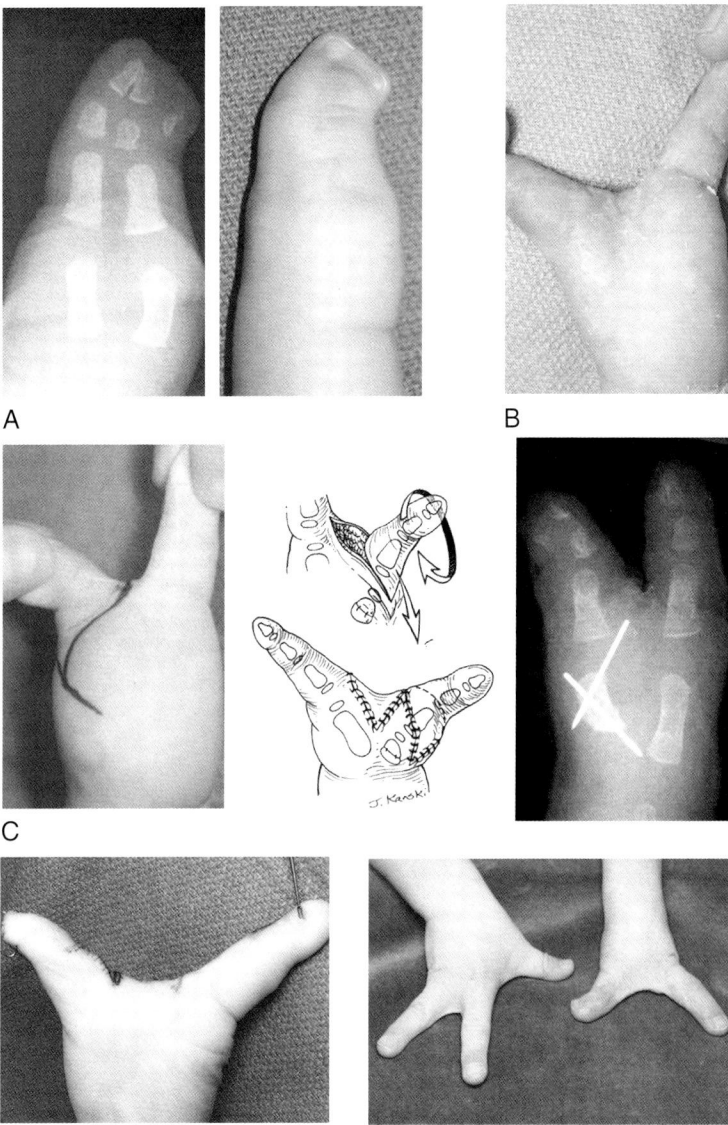

FIGURE 204-20. Syndactyly and special thumb. *A,* The clinical appearance and radiograph of a unilateral left hand malformation are shown. The radial ray has two distal phalanges; the radial partner is smaller and the ulnar phalanx is joined to the index ray. *B,* A large dorsal flap and zigzag incisions were used for the soft tissue separation. *C,* Six months later, a rotation-recession osteotomy of the thumb ray was performed at the metacarpal level through a Y-V incision. *D,* The original dorsal flap could be readvanced to further widen the web space between the thumb and index finger. *E,* Five years later, the broad web space seen here from the dorsal view is maintained on the left hand.

space. Skin grafts on either side of the release will contract, and the web space will get smaller with growth. A good strategy in small hands, such as the Apert hand, is to advance a single dorsal flap into the first web space and subsequently readvance the same flap when future procedures are performed on the hand. Multiple small flaps within this critical region simply translate into a tight scar with time and growth.

Release of Second Through Fourth Interdigital Web Spaces

The problems reported after simple and complex syndactyly release constitute a wide range. Although the problem can be secondary to simple scar contracture, it may represent the discrepancy between the growth of the tissues of the hand and the growth of the scar. Distal migration of the commissure, or web creep, is the most common, reported to occur in between 3% and 40% of large series[*] (Fig. 204-21). If one were able to observe these patients with simple syndactylies through skeletal maturity into their early 20s, the incidence of secondary contractures requiring Z-plasties or other revisions would be low. The author's

---

[*]References 12, 57, 61, 73, 76, 78-80, 82, 85, 86, 89, 110, 204, 157, 207, 215-226.

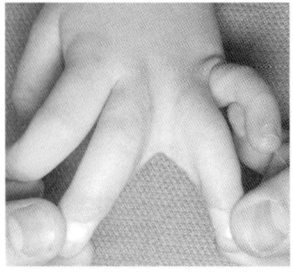
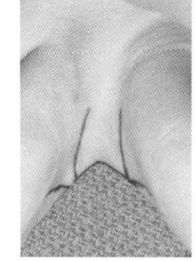
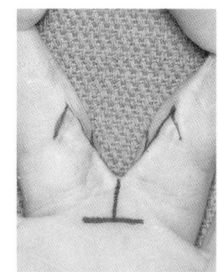
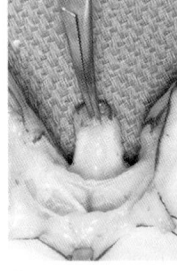
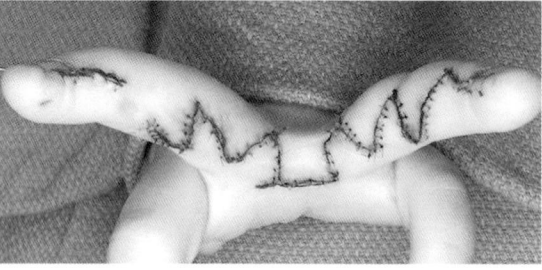

A

B

FIGURE 204-21. Recurrent syndactyly "web creep." *A,* Web creep or distal advancement of the interdigital commissure occurs in at least 15% of most published series. Scar tissue at the base of these commissures does not stretch as readily as the rest of the tissues with growth. The incisions have been marked out. Scar tissue and residual bands along the sides of these digits must be excised. The dorsal flap has been raised and readvanced. The bifurcation of the common digital artery is the normal level of the commissure base. Note the secondary paronychial fold revisions. *B,* The scar contractures in this child have caused a combined deviation and rotational deformity that will affect joint configuration with growth.

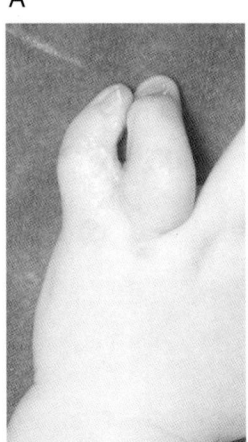
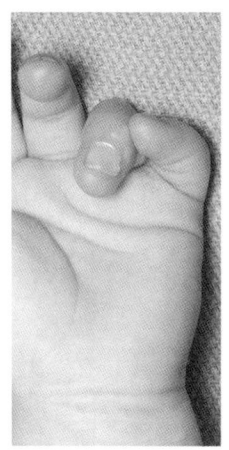
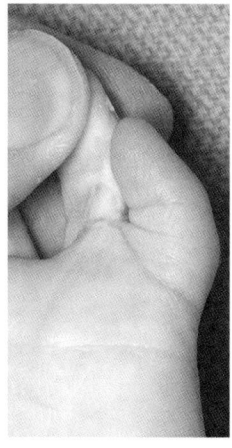

experience with more than 925 patients requiring more than 3000 web releases indicates that the need for secondary surgery is related to the complexity of the original syndactyly more than to any other single factor. Secondary soft tissue surgery was performed in 9% of patients observed for at least 15 years and in virtually all of the Apert patients observed at least 10 years after their original web releases had been completed.

TREATMENT OF SPECIFIC SYNDACTYLY SYNDROMES

Apert Syndrome

CLASSIFICATION

These hands have been broadly classified into three basic types, defined by varying degrees of soft tissue and skeletal abnormalities. Although several refinements to this system have been proposed, treatment decisions correlate well with the three-type system (Fig. 204-22 and Table 204-4).[6,37,39-42,155,227] Three-dimensional imaging is often helpful in the evaluation of complex type II and type III hands.[228]

PRINCIPLES FOR TREATMENT

The Apert hand is unique, often falling well outside the general rules for treatment of other malformations. Therefore, there are many additional principles that may be applied in the treatment of specific patients. For example, because of the symphalangism and the lack of interphalangeal motion of the central three digits, straight-line incisions can be safely used along the sides of the fingers (Table 204-5).[37,44,155,177,185,200,229-232]

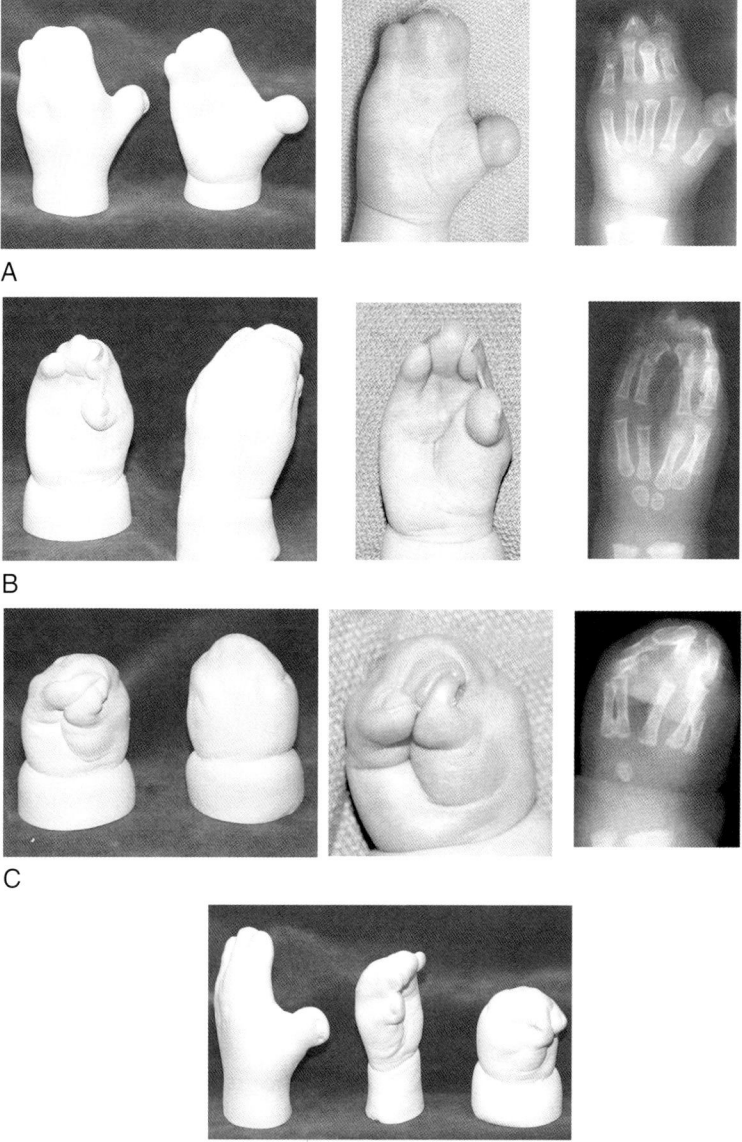

FIGURE 204-22. Classification of the Apert hand. *A,* In a type I Apert hand ("obstetrician's hand"), the plane of the digits is flat, the thumb is free, the index-long-ring digits are joined in a complex syndactyly, and the fifth digit is joined in a simple syndactyly. The distal joint of the fifth digit is mobile, and there may or may not be an ulnar duplication. The thumb has a radial clinodactyly (hitchhiker thumb). *B,* In a type II Apert hand ("cup hand"), the thumb is joined in a simple syndactyly, the transverse arch of the hand is cupped, and there is splaying apart of the digits at the metacarpophalangeal joint level. The syndactyly joining the fifth digit is usually simple. The radial clinodactyly of the thumb persists. *C,* In a type III Apert hand ("rosebud hand" or "hoof hand"), there is a tight skeletal union of all digits, which often results in severe maceration of the skinfolds on the glabrous surfaces. Nails often become ingrown and infected. The thumb phalanges are often small and can underlap the central three digits. Thumb radial clinodactyly may not be present. *D,* The presence or absence of thumb independence is appreciated in these molds of types I, II, and III hands.

TABLE 204-4 ✦ APERT HAND: GUIDELINES FOR TREATMENT

Procedure	Type I	Type II	Type III
Nail infections and maceration			Neonates
Release of border rays	4-12 months	4-12 months	4-12 months
Readvance dorsal flap or other first web space correction		1-4 years	1-4 years
Index ray resection with initial thumb release		4-12 months	4-6 months
Thumb radial clinodactyly correction	4-6 years	4-6 years	Often not necessary
Metacarpal synostosis correction	4-6 years	4-6 years	4-6 years
Revisions: metacarpal transposition, nail matrix excisions, graft excisions, osteotomies, ostectomies, carpometacarpal joint arthroplasties, Z-plasties, web space revisions	7-15 years	7-15 years	7-15 years
Tissue expansion (experimental)		1-2 years	1-2 years

TABLE 204-5 ✦ ADDITIONAL PRINCIPLES FOR TREATMENT OF THE APERT HAND

Straight-line incisions can be safely used along the sides of the fingers.

Separation of the thumb and fifth ray may be done first.

Separation of both hands may be done simultaneously before the age of 12 months.[37,185,229,230]

Treatment and resolution of nail fold infections and maceration-related problems may be done before skeletal separations.

Triangular flaps may be used for paronychial fold construction.[44,155,177,200,231,232]

Distal open areas are allowed to epithelialize.

Dorsal flaps are readvanced into the first web space with repeated procedures.

The thumb is lengthened at the phalangeal level.

Digits and thumb are debulked to approach normal width and circumference.

Release of the ring to fifth metacarpal synostosis is performed to allow pinch and grip with the thumb.

The lower abdominal Pfannenstiel incision is incorporated for skin graft harvest.

A ray resection of the index ray may be performed with very small dysplastic phalanges.

There should be little hesitation in performance of skeletal and soft tissue revisions later in childhood or adolescence.

SYNDACTYLY RELEASE (FIRST WEB SPACE)

Type I hands rarely need an additional first web release, but the addition of full-thickness flaps to form a good web is the key to a functional hand. It is preferable to use a modification of Buck-Gramcko's dorsal advancement flap, which can be readvanced with successive operations. Free groin flaps[186] and pedicled groin or lower abdominal flaps[182] have been effectively used. Intermetacarpal fascial bands are often prominent between the hypertrophied adductor pollicis and first dorsal interosseous muscles. In the most deformed type III hands, the phalanges and nails may be very small, and local available flap tissue may be marginal. In these children, the initial use of grafts on the side of the web release, followed by successive dorsal flap readvancements, is particularly effective. The eventual lengthening of the phalangeal portion of the thumb between the ages of 3 and 5 years will significantly enhance the first web space (Table 204-6).

SYNDACTYLY RELEASE OF INTERDIGITAL WEB SPACES

There is no optimal release for any type of complex syndactyly. The best outcomes with minimal secondary problems will occur if the surgeon adheres to the basic principles previously outlined. Because both dorsal and palmar soft tissues are at a minimum, it is important to outline equitable distribution to line three potential commissures (Fig. 204-23). It is preferable to use dorsal and palmar side-by-side flaps to line the commissure. Recurrent syndactyly, or web creep, often occurs in the second interdigital web space because of the presence of a pseudoepiphysis at the base of the index metacarpal, which results in a long index ray. This commissure may be lined with a dorsal hourglass flap that can easily be readvanced at the time of secondary revision. However, some surgeons prefer to line the commissures with pedicle flaps,[182] and others prefer to separate the distal skeletal unions of the central three digits in stages.[48,198]

In type III hands, the most crucial decision concerns the fate of the index ray. If the second ray is sacrificed, this extra tissue can be used to line a much broader first web space for the one-thumb and three-digit ("Mickey Mouse") hand. In type I and type II hands, the second interdigital web space is lined by a dorsal rectangular flap, which is easily readvanced in hands with web creep secondary to the abnormally long index metacarpal. This is caused by an extra growth plate at its base. Zigzag incisions are not necessary, and these digits grow well despite the presence of longitudinal incisions.

SECONDARY REVISIONS

It is unrealistic to think that maximal functional and aesthetic outcomes will be achieved once the digital and thumb separations have been completed before 2 years of age. As these small hands grow, the grafts and some incisions do not expand commensurately with the other tissues of the hand. In addition, the skeletal parts have asymmetric configurations and abnormal growth plates at both the phalangeal and

TABLE 204-6 ✦ TIMETABLE FOR TREATMENT OF THE APERT HAND

Age	Procedure
1-6 months	Incision and drainage of macerations and nail bed infections; thumb-index web space release; conversion of type III to type I hands
6-18 months	Digital separations; joint releases
4-6 years	Thumb clinodactyly releases; excision of metacarpal synostosis; skin graft excisions; nail bed revisions
7 years-adolescence	Digital osteotomies, ostectomies, graft excisions, web revisions, metacarpal arthroplasties, soft tissue debulking, and carpometacarpal joint arthroplasties

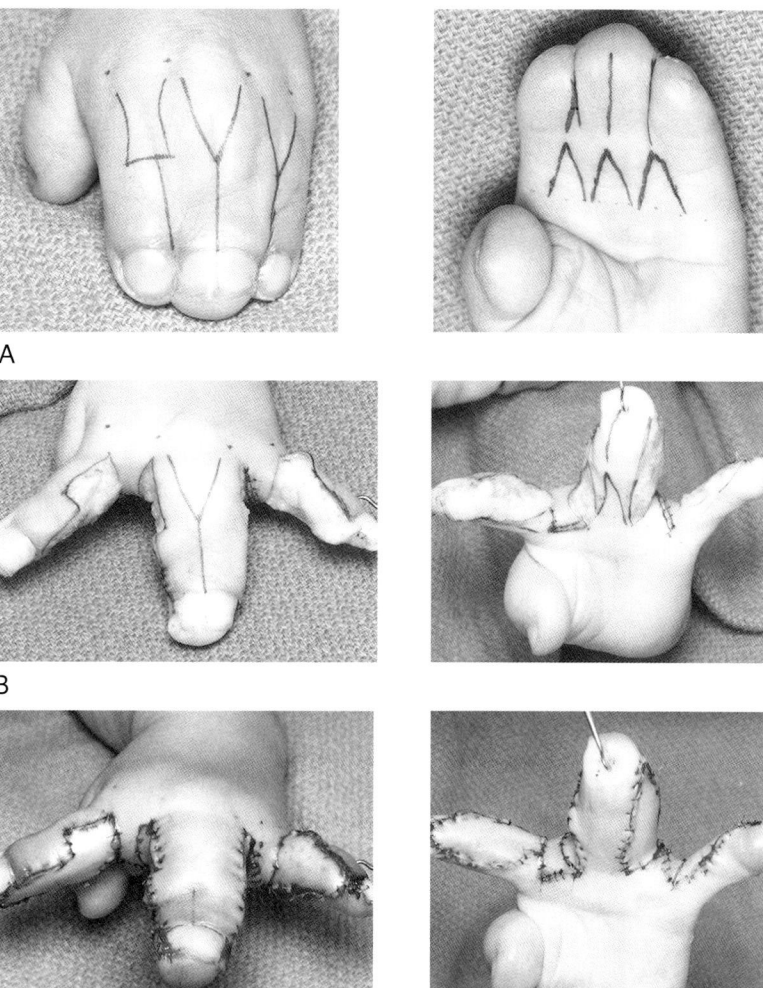

FIGURE 204-23. Interdigital release in an Apert hand. *A,* The outline of incisions on a type I Apert hand is made before any surgery has been done. Dorsal and palmar triangular flaps are usually sufficient. A dorsal hourglass flap for the index-long web space is often chosen because of the tendency for web creep, which is caused by the greater growth of the index metacarpal, which often has an extra proximal pseudoepiphysis. Straight-line palmar incisions are safe because of the symphalangism of the proximal and middle phalanges. *B,* The digits have been separated and the commissure flaps inset. Both techniques provide an excellent broad commissure. *C,* Full-thickness skin grafts are used to cover the raw areas.

metacarpal levels. Growth in many patients only accentuates the original deformity, especially of the thumb. Radial clinodactyly of the thumb is best corrected before the age of 4 to 5 years. The most critical factor in the decision to operate is the size of the proximal phalanx with its longitudinal epiphyseal bracket along the radial border, which prevents proximal to distal elongation on that side of the bone. It is preferable to perform an opening wedge osteotomy through the proximal phalanx and to fill this gap with bone from the synostosis, if it is present, between the fourth and fifth metacarpals (Fig. 204-24).

Whenever subsequent surgery is performed on these hands, it is beneficial to do as much as possible within reasonable tourniquet times. This includes, among others, correction of skeletal angulation, rotation, or excess breadth; excision of pigmented skin grafts; deepening of web spaces (first through fourth

if necessary); carpometacarpal joint arthroplasty; excision of deformed nail plates and matrices; and reconstruction of paronychial and eponychial folds (Fig. 204-25).

OUTCOMES

In shaking the hand of an adult Apert patient, it is obvious that this hand is not normal (Fig. 204-26).[43-45,185,232] The first web space is short, as are the digits, which do not bend. In essence, the Apert hand almost slips out of the grasp of a normal hand. Imagine what it feels like for the patient! The thumb is short, but thanks to the hypertrophied intrinsic muscles, pinch strength is well within normal ranges for adult men and women. Volumetric grasp strength averages 30% of normal values because of the lack of interphalangeal motion of the index, long, and ring fingers

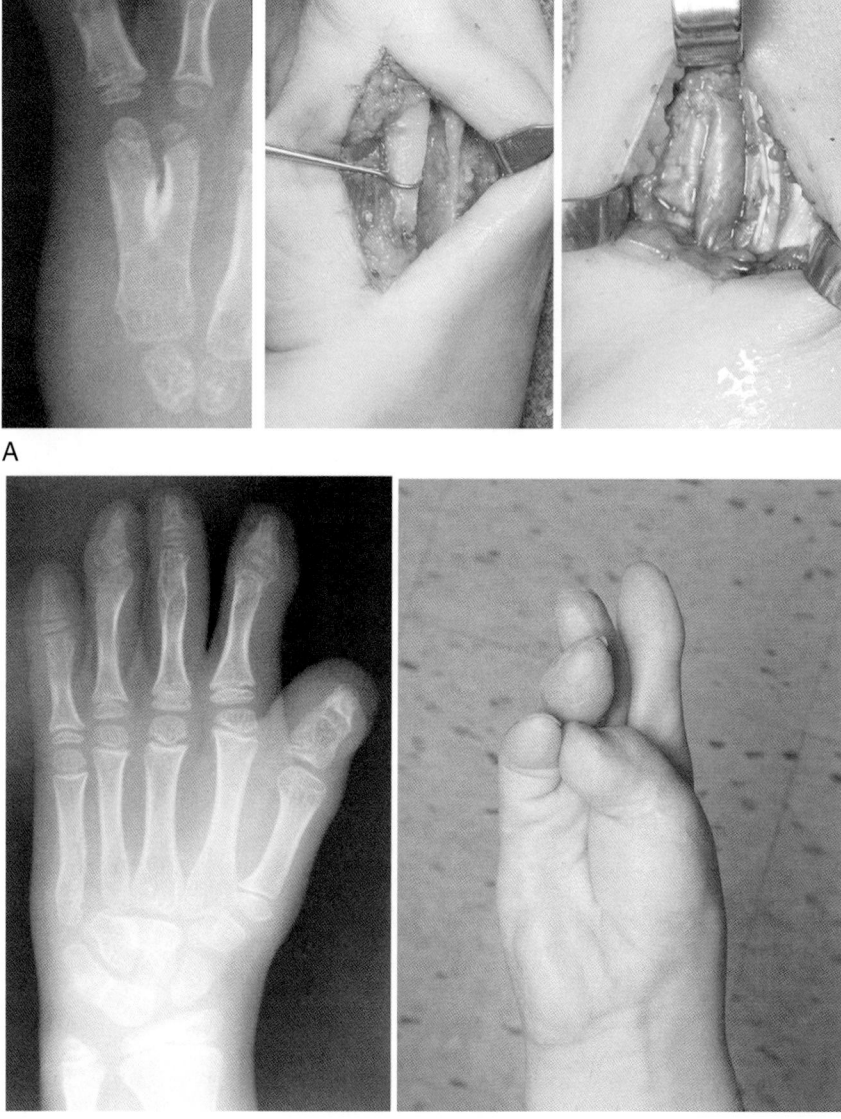

FIGURE 204-24. Apert metacarpal synostosis correction. *A,* A synostosis between the ring and fifth metacarpals is present in the majority of Apert patients and severely limits the mobility of the fifth ray. The radiograph on the left shows the synostosis before resection. A complete resection of the synostosis and periosteum is done. Hydrated cadaveric fascia lata has been interposed and wrapped around the fifth metacarpal to prevent repeated fusion across the site of resection. The presence of the dorsal ulnar capsule and collateral ligament at the carpometacarpal joint will prevent subluxation of the fifth metacarpal. *B,* Eleven years later, the site of resection has remained open, and, since the initial surgery, the patient has developed a functional thumb to fifth finger pinch and grasp.

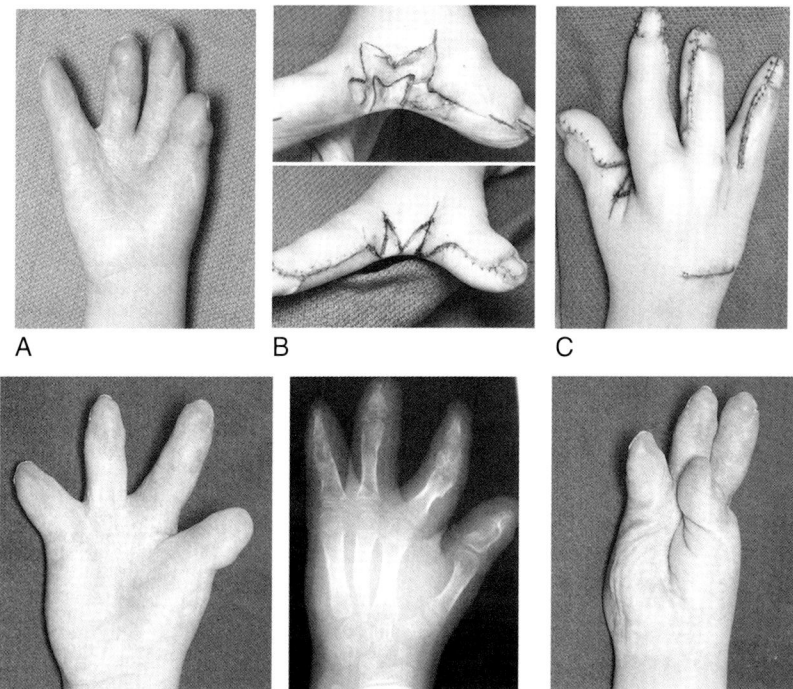

FIGURE 204-25. Apert hand secondary surgery. *A,* After early digital and thumb separations, this teenager presents with broad digits and thumb, a tight first web space, and multiple ugly overlapping nails. The fifth finger cannot oppose the mobile thumb. Secondary correction will definitely improve the function and appearance of these hands. *B,* The hyperpigmented skin grafts on the ulnar side of the thumb and radial surface of the long finger (index ray resection has been performed) have been excised, excess bone has been trimmed, and the dorsal skin is advanced and closed in the midaxial line. Thumb nail plate, matrix, and underlying bone have been trimmed, and a pulp flap is advanced to form a paronychial fold. Previous commissure flaps have been undermined and readvanced as a Y-V closure to further widen the first web space. *C,* The metacarpal synostosis has been excised and the gap filled with fascia. The hand is seen after nine separate revisions have been completed. *D,* The slight improvement of the digit and thumb size, position, and mobility has been major to the patient. After release of the synostosis, the most complete digit of the hand, the fifth finger, is now able to function in concert with the thumb.

and distal interphalangeal motion of the fifth finger. The presence of a mobile fifth ray at the metacarpal level is a tremendous asset because it allows both a thumb to fifth finger pinch and grasp (Fig. 204-27; see also Fig. 204-22).[188] On the whole, these patients adapt well and compensate at an early age, continuing to use the thumb to fifth finger grasp effectively throughout their adult lives.

Outcomes of the type III Apert hand fall into a separate category. The thumbs are always short in these "hoof" hands, and the first web spaces are frequently insufficient. In some children, proximal and distal phalanges may not ossify within the first year of life, although they will ultimately. Radial clinodactyly of the first ray is frequently not present. The digits are generally short, and the fifth ray may deviate in an ulnar direction because of duplication at the phalangeal level (see Fig. 204-22). Release of the metacarpal synostosis will enhance the thumb to fifth ray pinch and grasp

and is one of the most important functional improvements made in these patients.

Poland Syndrome

TREATMENT

Because these hands fall along a broad teratologic spectrum, treatment must be carefully individualized to both the hand and the patient. Those patients with well-formed digits and thumb are best treated with digital separations and the formation of as large a first web space as possible. Those with digital nubbins in the central rays are best treated with augmentation of the border rays with nonvascularized phalangeal transfers. Finally, those with no digits or thumbs are good candidates for toe to thumb transfers. Many permutations and combinations are available. Details for methods other than web releases are included in the section on symbrachydactyly in Chapter 208. These

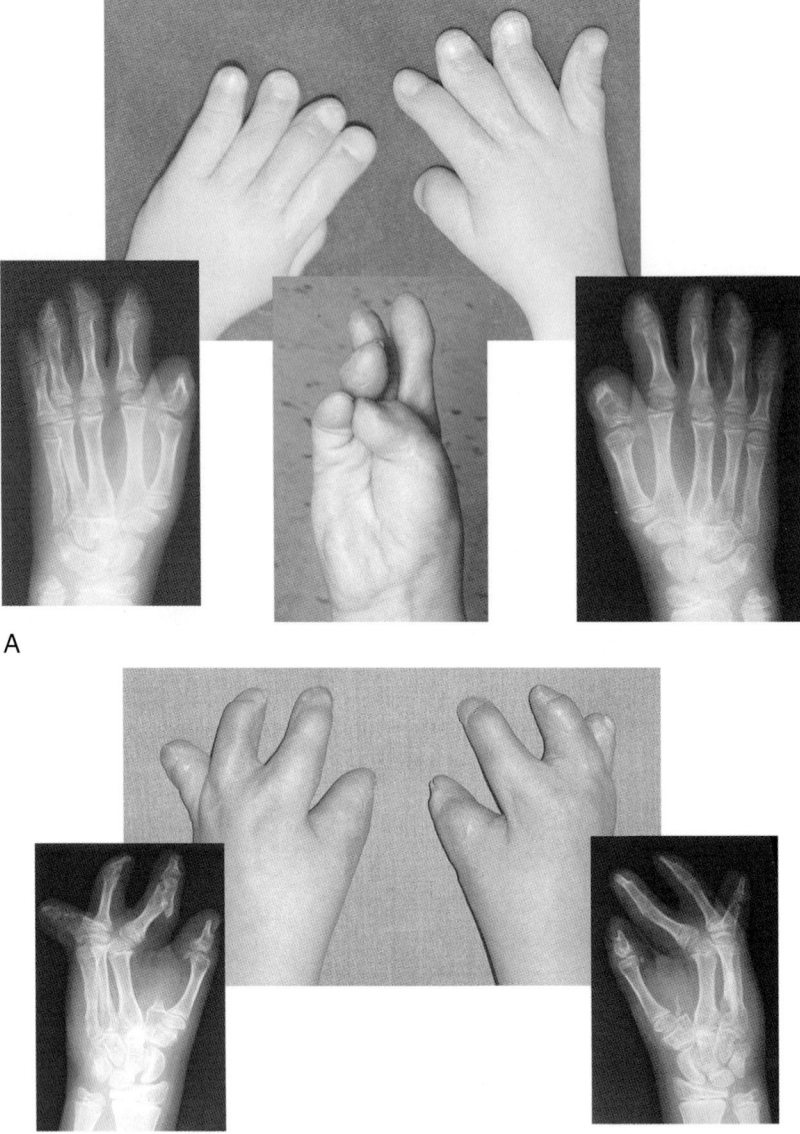

FIGURE 204-26. Apert hand outcomes. *A,* A representative example of type I Apert hands is shown 10 years after digital separations. Individual nail folds are present. The digits are straight and separated by good commissures. Digital motion is present only at the metacarpophalangeal joints and distal interphalangeal joint of the fifth finger. The thumb is short and broad with motion at the metacarpophalangeal joint. *B,* A teenage boy born with severe type III hands is seen after many surgeries. The first web spaces were formed with only an index ray resection. The thumb is broad and short. There was no radial clinodactyly. No lengthening has been performed. Both fifth digits deviate ulnarly because of the abnormal growth plate associated with an ulnar duplication at the phalangeal level. Metacarpophalangeal joint motion is limited. Hand function in this patient is severely compromised, in contrast to that in the type I patient.

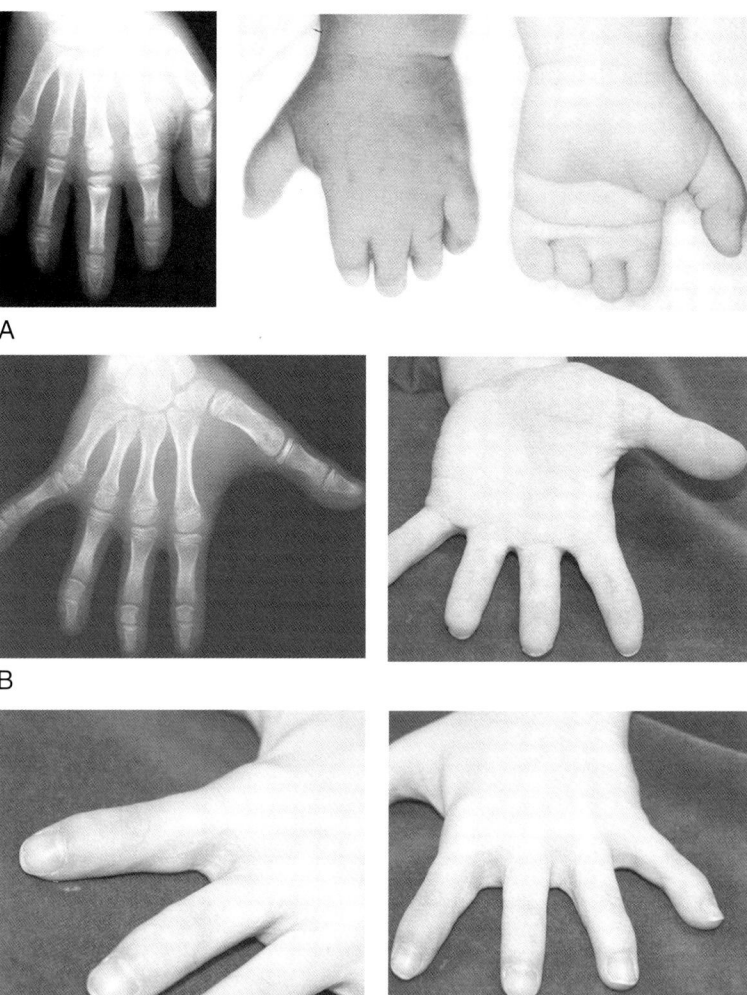

FIGURE 204-27. Poland symbrachydactyly hand. *A,* The clinical appearance and radiograph before digital separations for symbrachydactyly are shown. Very small middle phalangeal segments are seen. Flexion creases within the digits are indicative of clinical motion. Routine separations were completed in two stages. Dorsal hourglass flaps lined the commissures, and full-thickness skin grafts were placed along the sidewalls. *B,* At age 13 years, the middle phalanges are more visible and all epiphyses are open. There is no web creep, and the palmar level of the commissures has been well maintained. *C,* On closer inspection, the grafts are well contoured with a slight increase in pigmentation. Full digital abduction and adduction of the digits are made possible by the full-thickness lining of the commissures.

are truthfully the most difficult category of all congenital differences to treat. Parents often seek multiple consultations from a large number of experienced surgeons, all of whom may recommend a different course of reconstruction.

SYNDACTYLY RELEASE

There are no significant differences in the technique of syndactyly release for brachysyndactyly. The same principles come into play without significant alteration and are often coordinated with standard constriction ring correction (see Fig. 204-16).[56] Many surgeons like to exaggerate the depth of the web release in those with short digits.

OUTCOMES

Because these deformities are unilateral, function and appearance can always be contrasted with the con-

tralateral normal hand. Many have emphasized that the functional loss is much greater than in those nonsyndromic hands with syndactyly releases alone, indicating that there are additional soft tissue and skeletal anomalies contributing to the functional loss.[224] The experience of the author does not support this conclusion. Grip, pinch, and precision intrinsic muscle function are related to the degree of hypoplasia of the thumb and digits in these hands. There is no reason to think there is a difference in the outcomes after syndactyly release between these patients and other patients with simple syndactyly.

Acrosyndactyly

CLASSIFICATION

There is no system specifically described for the constriction ring syndrome (see Chapter 205). Terms such as the standard mild, moderate, and severe may be used as designations for the first web and incomplete and complete for the other interdigital web spaces. There are no mirror image deformities in this syndrome because each hand (and foot) is unique. There are no skeletal coalitions, but the tapered skeletal parts at the site of acrosyndactylies are joined only by a common scar. The bone stock at the site of congenital loss (ampu-

tation) or at the tip of an acrosyndactyly is typically tapered.

SYNDACTYLY RELEASE

The same techniques and principles are used in these hands as in those discussed previously (Fig. 204-28). In those with multiple transverse amputations, there

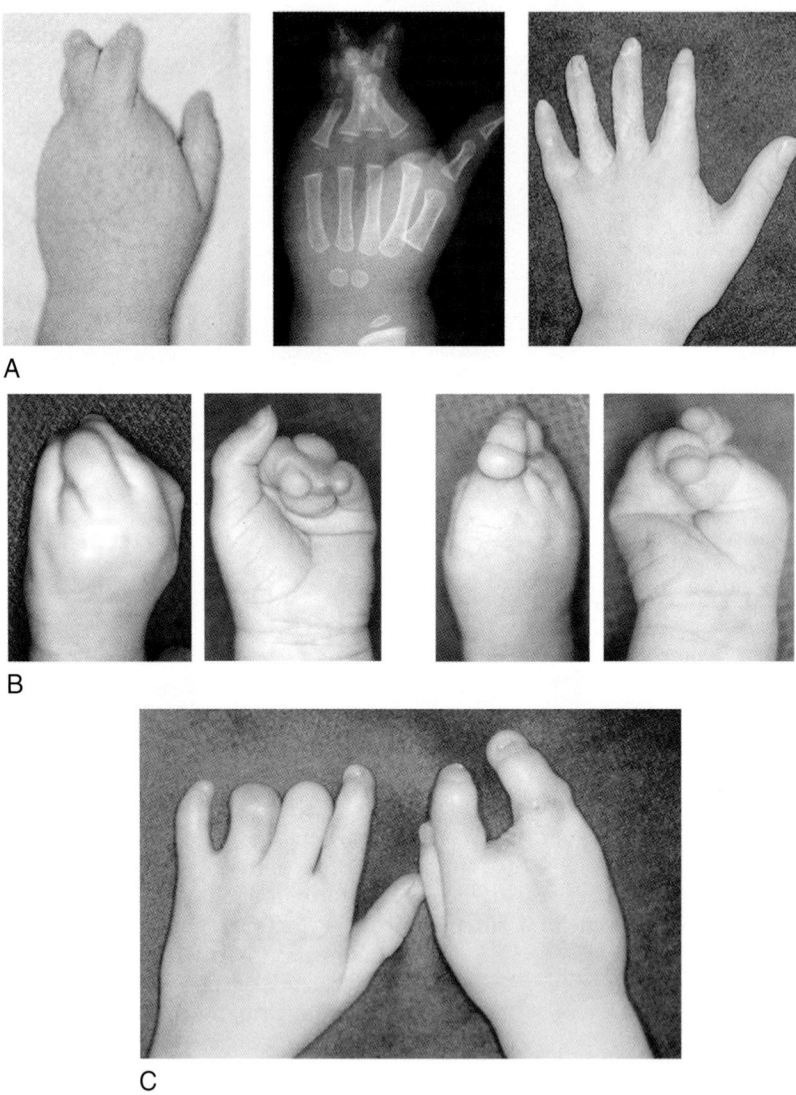

FIGURE 204-28. Acrosyndactyly. *A,* This child had acrosyndactyly composed of overlapping digits that were released one digit at a time. All available skin was used for commissures and the sidewall grafted. Ten years later, these digits have a satisfactory appearance but are short, thin, and stiff. *B,* The right and left hands of a child with severe acrosyndactyly are seen shortly after birth. It is difficult to discern which distal nubbins match respective proximal phalanges. *C,* The digits have been released and those phalanges with nails positioned on the tips. The commissure level is at the bifurcation of the common digital arteries. The tip of a digit with congenital amputation proximal to the nail is often bulbous, and the saved nail is often abnormal in appearance. Despite these limitations, both hands are extremely functional.

is a tendency to overcorrect and deepen the web to the level of the metacarpophalangeal joint. This can often be unsightly and does not provide a functional advantage. It is important to have all the webs at the same level. The epidermal lining of the dorsal to palmar sinuses can often be used for coverage of raw surfaces but does not have much usefulness because of its tenuous blood supply. A fresh full-thickness skin graft is often preferred.

Because many of these fingers are short, the surgeon and parents often want to preserve as much length as possible. It is often better to form a shorter, well-padded fingertip instead of a longer one that ends in a sharp point with an overlying callus. Many short digits with transverse amputation at the proximal half of the proximal phalanx are often best left unseparated within a common soft tissue envelope.

A wide, well-lined first web space is crucial for the function of these hands. For mild or moderate deficien-

cies, local flaps are used. For severe deficiencies, tissue must be added before any required thumb reconstruction. In all three, dense fibrous bands will be found that may extend to the carpometacarpal joint level. The options for skeletal reconstruction are covered in Chapter 208. Under ideal conditions, it is preferable to use toe transfers for thumbs with no phalangeal components and full-thickness tissue within the first web (Fig. 204-29).

OUTCOMES

The outcomes in these patients are covered in Chapter 205. Adrian Flatt's description of the typical cleft hands with a deep central deficiency as "functional triumphs, but aesthetic disasters"[9] would certainly apply to many of these hands. There are no long-term follow-up evaluations that focus on both aspects. Any surgeon, critical of his or her work, will not be satisfied with the

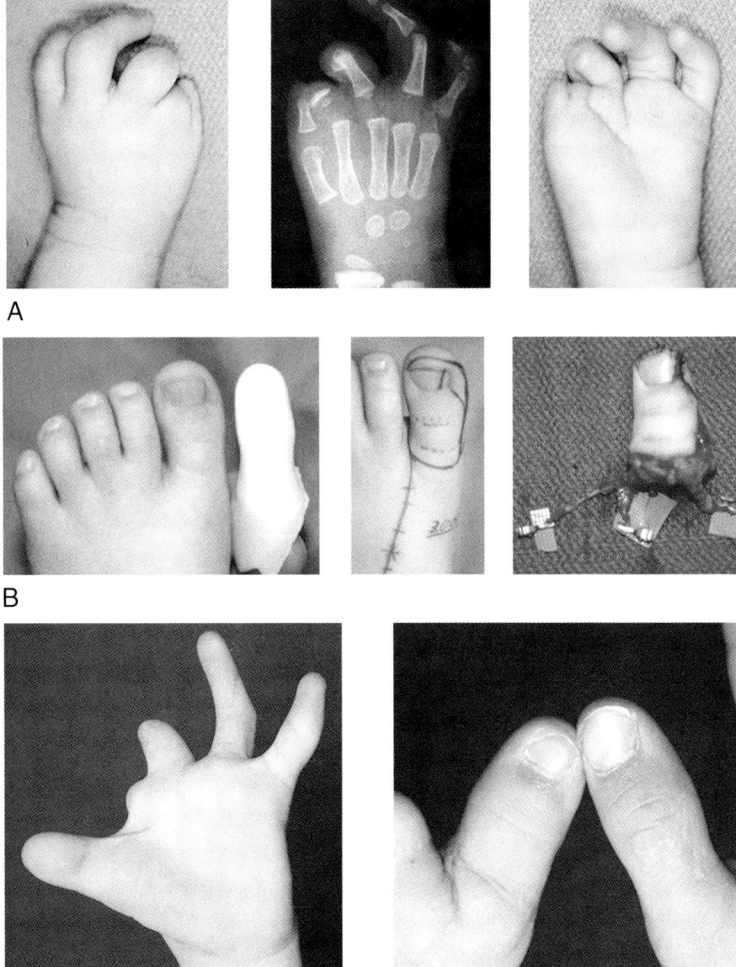

FIGURE 204-29. Acrosyndactyly (constriction ring syndrome) toe transfer. *A,* This child with the constriction ring syndrome was born with an acrosyndactyly involving the thumb, index, and long digits. Small soft tissue bridges were released in the newborn nursery. There is no first web space, and the distal phalangeal segment of the thumb is missing. *B,* A methyl methacrylate mold and model of the normal thumb have been used to measure the dimensions and to mark the incisions for a modified ipsilateral great toe to thumb (toe) transfer. The soft tissue surgery has been completed on the toe before it has been detached from the foot. This is similar to a type II thumb duplication correction. *C,* The thumb-index (first) web space has been augmented with a distally based radial forearm flap. The parents did not want the index ray to be removed. The toe is seen 2 years after transfer. Sensation of the left thumb is normal at 3 mm, and there is 45 degrees of flexion at the interphalangeal joint. A deep constriction ring on the right thumb at the level of the proximal phalanx had been corrected within the first year of life.

appearance and limited function of an acrosyndactyly hand with multiple transverse losses, hyperpigmented grafts, conspicuous incisions, tight web spaces, and tapered fingers with irregular contours shaped more like lollipops than digits. The technique of constriction ring correction outlined in Chapter 208 is strongly recommended because it places emphasis on the long-term contour correction. The use of local flaps or any method to improve contour pays tremendous dividends in these hands. With the presence of a thumb or first ray with an intact carpometacarpal joint, almost all of these hands are remarkably functional. Thumb elongation with either toe transfer or distraction lengthening is strongly recommended in these patients.

REFERENCES

1. Goldberg M, Bartoshesky L: Congenital hand anomaly: etiology and associated malformations. Hand Clin 1985;1:405-415.
2. Goldberg M: Syndactyly and polydactyly. In Goldberg M: The Dysmorphic Child: An Orthopedic Perspective. New York, Raven Press, 1987:264.
3. Blauth W: Syndaktylien der Hand. Dtsch Arztebl 1972;69:2013-2021.
4. Littler J: Principles of reconstructive surgery of the hand. In Converse JM, ed: Plastic and Reconstructive Surgery, 2nd ed. Philadelphia, WB Saunders, 1977:3103-3153.
5. Dobyns J: Syndactyly. In Green DP, ed: Operative Hand Surgery. New York, Churchill Livingstone, 1982:281-301.
6. Upton J: Congenital anomalies of the hand and forearm. In May JW Jr, Littler JW, eds: The Hand. Philadelphia, WB Saunders, 1990:5213-5398. McCarthy JG, ed: Plastic Surgery; vol 8.
7. Kelikian H: Congenital Deformities of the Hand and Forearm. Philadelphia, WB Saunders, 1974:330-407, 902-938.
8. Woolf C, Woolf R: A genetic study of syndactyly in Utah. Soc Biol 1973;20:335-346.
9. Flatt A: The Care of Congenital Hand Anomalies. St. Louis, CV Mosby, 1977:99-117, 228-248.
10. Temtamy S, McKusick V: Syndactyly as an isolated malformation. Birth Defects Orig Artic Ser 1978;14:302-322. The Genetics of Hand Malformation.
11. Goodman FR, Mundlos S, Muragaki Y, et al: Synpolydactyly phenotypes correlate with the size of expansion of HOXD13 polyalanine tract. Proc Natl Acad Sci USA 1997;94:7458-7463.
12. Posch J, Dela Cruz-Saddul FA, Posch JL Jr: Congenital syndactylism of fingers in 262 cases. Orthop Rev 1981;10:23-32.
13. Poznanski A: The Hand in Radiologic Diagnosis, with Gamuts and Pattern Profiles, 2nd ed, vol 1. Philadelphia, WB Saunders, 1984:232-235.
14. Ravitch M: Poland's syndrome—a study of an eponym. Plast Reconstr Surg 1977;59:508.
15. Golladay E, Golladay GJ: Chest wall deformities. Indian J Pediatr 1997;64:339-350.
16. Clarkson P: Poland's syndactyly. Guys Hosp Rep 1962;111:335-346.
17. Epstein L, Bennett J: Syndactyly with ipsilateral chest deformity. Plast Reconstr Surg 1970;46:236-240.
18. Ireland D, Takayama N, Flatt A: Poland's syndrome. A review of forty-three cases. J Bone Joint Surg Am 1976;58:52-58.
19. Goldberg M, Mazzei R: Poland syndrome: a concept of the pathogenesis based on limb bud embryology. Birth Defects Orig Artic Ser 1977;8:103-115.
20. Poland A: Deficiency of the pectoral muscles. Guys Hosp Rep 1841;6:191-194.
21. Senrui H, Egawa T, Horiki A: Anatomical findings in the hands of patients with Poland's syndrome. J Bone Joint Surg Am 1982;64:1079-1082.
22. Bouvet J, Maroteaux P, Briard-Guillemot M: Le syndrome de Poland. Etudes clinique et genetique—considerations physiopathologiques. Nouv Presse Med 1976;5:185-190.
23. Bouvet J, Leveque D, Bernetieres F, Gros JJ: Vascular origin of Poland syndrome: a comparative rheographic study of the vascularisation of the arms in eight patients. Eur J Pediatr 1978;128:17-26.
24. Bouwes-Bavinck J, Weaver D: Subclavian artery supply disruption sequence: hypothesis of a vascular etiology for Poland, Klippel-Feil, and Mobius anomalies. Am J Med Genet 1986;23:903-918.
25. Prati R, Vandelli C, Prosdocimo M, Piacentini F: Poland syndrome associated with Moebius syndrome. Pediatr Med Chir 1985;7:901-903.
26. Wood VE: The hand in the Pierre Robin syndrome. J Hand Surg 1983;8:273-276.
27. Blauth W, Gekeler J: Zur Morphologie und Klassifikation der Symbrachydaktylie. Handchirurgie 1971;3:123-128.
28. Blauth W, Gekeler J: Symbrachydaktylien. Beitrag zur Morphologie, Klassifikation und Therapie. Handchirurgie 1973;5:121-171.
29. Miura T, Nakamura R, Horii E: The position of symbrachydactyly in the classification of congenital hand anomalies. J Hand Surg Br 1994;19:350-354.
30. Foucher, G, Medina, J, Navarro R, et al: Apport d'une nouvelle plastic a la reconstruction de la previere commissure dans les malformations congenitales. A propos d'une serie de 54 patients. Chir Main 2000;19:152-160.
31. Beals R, Crawford S: Congenital absence of the pectoral muscles. A review of twenty-five patients. Clin Orthop 1976;119:166-171.
32. Ohmori K, Takada H: Correction of Poland's pectoralis major muscle anomaly with latissimus dorsi musculocutaneous flaps. Plast Reconstr Surg 1980;65:400-404.
33. Wilson M, Louis DS, Stevenson TR: Poland's syndrome: variable expression and associated anomalies. J Hand Surg Am 1988;13:880-882.
34. Blank C: Apert's syndrome (a type of acrocephalosyndactyly)—observations on a British series of thirty-nine cases. Ann Hum Genet 1960;24:151-164.
35. Slaney S, Oldridge M, Hurst JA, et al: Differential effects of the FGFR2 mutations on syndactyly and cleft palate in Apert syndrome. Am J Hum Genet 1996;58:923-932.
36. von Gernet S, Golla A, Ehrenfels Y, et al: Genotype-phenotype analysis in Apert syndrome suggests opposite effects of the two recurrent mutations on syndactyly and outcome of craniofacial surgery. Clin Genet 2000;57:137-139.
37. Hoover G, Flatt A, Weiss M: The hand and Apert's syndrome. J Bone Joint Surg Am 1970;52:878-895.
38. Mah J, Kasser J, Upton J: Foot, shoulder and elbow in Apert's syndrome. Clin Plast Surg 1991;18:391-397.
39. Journeau P, Lajeunie E, Renier D, et al: Syndactyly in Apert syndrome; the utility of a prognostic classification. Ann Chir Main Memb Super 1999;18:13-19.
40. Van Heest A, House JH, Reckling WC: Two-stage reconstruction of Apert acrosyndactyly. J Hand Surg Am 1997;22:315-322.
41. al-Qattan M, al-Hussain MA: Classification of hand anomalies in Apert's syndrome. J Hand Surg Br 1996;21:266-268.
42. Anderson P, Smith PJ, Jones BM: New classification for the hand anomalies in Apert's syndrome [letter, comment]. J Hand Surg Br 1997;22:140-141.
43. Chang J, Danton A, Ladd AL, Hentz R: Reconstruction of the Apert syndrome: a simplified approach. Plast Reconstr Surg 2002;109:465-470.

44. Upton J: Discussion of the management of the hands and feet in the Apert syndrome. Plast Reconstr Surg 2003;112:13-19.

45. Feron J: Treatment of the hands and feet in Apert syndrome: an evolution of management. Plast Reconstr Surg 2003;112:1-12.

46. Upton J: Early intervention in Apert's syndactyly: a discussion. Plast Reconstr Surg 1986;77:286.

47. Green S: Pathological anatomy of the hands in Apert's syndrome. J Hand Surg Am 1982;7:450-453.

48. Fereshetian S, Upton J: The anatomy and management of the thumb in the Apert syndrome. Clin Plast Surg 1991;18:365-380.

49. Anderson P, Hall R, Smith PJ: Finger duplication in Apert's syndrome. J Hand Surg Br 1996;21:649-651.

50. Losch G, Duncker H: Acrosyndactylism. Transactions of the International Society of Plastic and Reconstructive Surgeons, 5th Congress. Melbourne, Australia, Butterworth Pty, 1971.

51. Patterson T: Congenital ring constrictions. Br J Plast Surg 1961;14:1-31.

52. Torpin R, Faulkner A: Intrauterine amputation with the missing member found in the fetal membranes. JAMA 1966;198:185-187.

53. Granick M, Ramasastry S, Vries J, Cohen MM: Severe amniotic band syndrome occurring with unrelated syndactyly. Plast Reconstr Surg 1987;80:829-832.

54. Walsh R: Acrosyndactyly. A study of 27 patients. Clin Orthop 1970;71:99-111.

55. Maisels D: Acrosyndactyly. Br J Plast Surg 1962;15:166-172.

56. Upton J, Tan C: Correction of constriction rings. J Hand Surg Am 1989;16:947-953.

57. Losch G, Duncker H: Anatomy and surgical treatment of syndactyly. Plast Reconstr Surg 1972;50:167-173.

58. Call W, Strickland J: Functional hand reconstruction in the whistling-face syndrome. J Hand Am Surg 1981;6:148-151.

59. Zancolli E, Zancolli EJ: Congenital ulnar drift of the fingers. Hand Clin 1985;1:443-456.

60. Burian F: The whistling face characteristic in a compound cranio-facio-corporal syndrome. Br J Plast Surg 1963;16:140.

61. Flatt A: Practical factors in the treatment of syndactyly. In Littler J, Cramer L, Smith J, eds: Symposium on Reconstructive Hand Surgery. St. Louis, CV Mosby, 1974:144-156.

62. Losch S: Connective tissue structures in the first intermetacarpal space in case of malformations of the hand with and without syndactyly. Chir Plast (Berl) 1978;4:145-149.

63. Verdan C: The thumb in syndactyly. Ann Chir Main 1982;1:29-39.

64. Mantero R, Ferrari GL, Ghigliazza GB, Auxilia E: Syndactyly: an angiographic study. Ann Chir Main 1983;2:62-65.

65. Micali G, Di Bennedetto A, Leofreddi L: Angiographic findings in hand malformations. Chir Ital 1968;20:1333-1444.

66. Inoue G: An angiographic study of congenital hand anomalies. Nippon Seikeigeka Gakkai Zasshi 1981;55:183-197.

67. Flatt A: The Care of Congenital Hand Anomalies, 3rd ed. St. Louis, Quality Medical Publishing, 1992.

68. Gesell A: The First Five Years of Life: A Guide to the Study of the Preschool Child. New York, Harper & Row, 1940.

69. Jones N, Upton J: Early release of syndactyly within six weeks of birth. Orthop Trans 1992;17:360-361.

70. Reuss E: Repair of simple syndactylism in the healthy neonewborn. Orthop Rev 1984;13:33-37.

71. Allard T, Clark SA, Jenkins WM, Merzenich MM: Reorganization of somatosensory area 3b representations in adult owl monkeys after digital syndactyly. J Neurophysiol 1991;66:1048-1058.

72. Merzenich M, Jenkins WM: Reorganization of cortical representations of the hand following alterations of skin inputs induced by nerve injury, skin island transfers, and experience. J Hand Ther 1993;6:89-104.

73. Rolle A, Wilhelm K: Syndactylia results. Handchir Mikrochir Plast Chir 1984;16:52-55.

74. Kettelkamp D, Flatt A: An evaluation of syndactylia repair. Surg Gynecol Obstet 1961;113:471-478.

75. Ebskov B, Zachariae L: Surgical methods in syndactylism. Evaluation of 208 operations. Acta Chir Scand 1966;131:258-268.

76. De Smet L, Van Ransbeeck H, Deneef G: Syndactyly release: results of the Flatt technique. Acta Orthop Belg 1998;64:301-305.

77. Brown P: Syndactyly: a review and long term results. Hand 1977;9:16-27.

78. Keret D, Ger E: Evaluation of a uniform operative technique to treat syndactyly. J Hand Surg Am 1987;12:727-729.

79. Percival N, Sykes PJ: Syndactyly: a review of the factors which influence surgical treatment. J Hand Surg Br 1989;14:196-200.

80. Toledo L, Ger E: Evaluation of the operative treatment of syndactyly. J Hand Surg Am 1979;4:556-564.

81. van der Biezen J, Bloem JJ: The double opposing palmar flaps in complex syndactyly. J Hand Surg Am 1992;17:1059-1064.

82. Dobyns J: Problems and complications in the management of upper limb anomalies. Hand Clin 1986;2:373-381.

83. Boyes J: Syndactyly. In Boyes J, ed: Bunnell's Surgery of the Hand. Philadelphia, JB Lippincott, 1970:59-107.

84. Davis JS: Plastic Surgery. Philadelphia, Blakiston, 1919:239-245.

85. Deutinger M, Mandl H, Frey M, et al: Late results following surgical correction of syndactyly and symbrachydactyly. Z Kinderchir 1989;44:50-54.

86. Meissl G, Millesi H, Piza-Katzer H: Critical considerations of various surgical methods for correction of syndactylia (report on an observation period of 10-20 years). Handchirurgie 1975;7:69-75.

87. Bunnell S: Surgery of the Hand. Philadelphia, JB Lippincott, 1944:609-647.

88. Upton J: Early surgical intervention in Apert's syndactyly: a discussion. Plast Reconstr Surg 1986;77:286-287.

89. van der Biezen J, Bloem JJ: Dividing the fingers in congenital syndactyly release: a review of more than 200 years of surgical treatment. Ann Plast Surg 1994;33:225-230.

90. Velpeau A: New Elements of Operative Surgery, vol 1. New York, Samuels & Wood, 1847:385-387. Cited by Kelikian, 1974.

91. Zeller S: Abhandlung über die ersten Erscheinungen venerischer Lokal-Krankheits-Formen und deren Behandlung, sammt einer kurzen Anzeige zweyer neuen Operazions—Methoden, nahmlich: die angebornen verwachsenen Finger und die Kastrazion betreffend. Wien, Binz, 1810:107-111.

92. Nelaton A: Elements de Pathologie Chirurgicale, vol 16. Paris, G. Bailli, 1884.

93. Didot A: Note sur la separation des doigts palmes, et sur un nouveau procede anaplastique destine a prevenir la reproduction de la difformite. Bull Acad Roy Med Belg 1849/50;9:351-356.

94. Bierens de Haan J: Aangeboren ontbreken van de groote borstspier met syndactylie. Leiden, Rosenstein, 1902.

95. Agnew D: The Principles and Practice of Surgery: Being a Treatise on Surgical Diseases and Injuries, vol 3. Philadelphia, JB Lippincott, 1883.

96. Davis JS, German W: Syndactylism. Coherence of the fingers or toes. Arch Surg 1930;21:32-75.

97. Felizet G: Operation de la syndactylie congenitale (procede autoplastique). Rev Orthop 1892;10:49-61.

98. Faniel H: Syndactylie: modification du procede de Didot. Le Scalpel 1911;64:254-258.

99. Dieffenbach F: Chirurgische Erfahrungen besonders über die Wiederherstellung zerstörter Theile des menschlichen Körpers nach neuen Methoden. Berlin, TCF Enslin, 1834.

100. Forgues L: Syndactylie membraneuse congenitale du medius et de l'annnulaire de deux main: operation. Arch Med Pharm Mil 1896;27:128-133.

101. Kummer E: Syndactylie congenitale. Anaplastie d'apres la methode italienne. Rev Orthop Chir Paris 1891;2:129-133.

102. Lennander K: Fall af kongenital syndaktyli operadt med hjelp af Thiersch's hudtransplantationsmetod. Upsala Lak Foren Forh 1891;26:151-152.

103. Norton A: A new and reliable operation for the cure of webbed fingers. Br Med J 1881;2:931-932.

104. Rudtorffer F: Abhandlung über die einfachste und sichereste Operations—Methode eingesperrter Leisten und Schenkel-brücke. Band 11. Vienna, JU Degan, 1808:472-487.

105. Hentz V, Littler J: Abduction-pronation and recession of second (index) metacarpal in thumb agenesis. J Hand Surg Am 1977;2:113-117.

106. Pieri G: Plastica cutanea per le retrizioni cicatriziali ditta. Chir Organi Mov 1920;4:303-306.

107. Cronin T: Syndactylism: results of zigzag incision to prevent postoperative contracture. Plast Reconstr Surg 1956;18:460-468.

108. Tubby A: An operation for webbed fingers. Br Med J 1912;2:1464-1466.

109. Blauth W: Das Syndaktylie—Rezidiv. Handchirurgie 1970;2:95-101.

110. Blauth W: Syndaktylie und Rezidiv. Fingersyndaktylien und ihre Behandlung. Z Orthop 1979;117:523-530.

111. Blauth W, Schneider-Sickert F: Congenital Deformities of the Hand: An Atlas of Their Surgical Treatment. Berlin, Springer-Verlag, 1981:10-72.

112. Barsky A: Congenital anomalies of the hand. J Bone Joint Surg Am 1951;33:35-64.

113. Blackfield H, Hause D: Syndactylism. Plast Reconstr Surg 1955;16:37-46.

114. Cronin T: Syndactylism. Experiences in its correction. Tri State Med J 1943;15:2869-2871, 2884.

115. Cogswell H, Trusler HM: A modified Agnew's operation for syndactylism. Surg Gynecol Obstet 1937;64:792-795.

116. Bauer T, Tondra J, Trusler H: Technical modification in repair of syndactylism. Plast Reconstr Surg 1956;17:385-392.

117. Zachariae L: Syndactylia. J Bone Joint Surg Br 1955;37:356.

118. Velasco J, Broadbent T, Woolf R: Syndactylism. Br J Plast Surg 1967;20:364-368.

119. Rypalkova B: Dnesmi stav operaci syndaktylie. Cas Lek Ces 1951;90:1081-1084.

120. Stucke K: Über die Erscheinungsformen der Syndaktylie und ihre operative Behandlung. Langenbecks Arch Klin Chir 1940;261:215-232.

121. Stucke K, Gansmuller O: Zur Klassifizierung, Klinik und Behandlung der Syndaktylie. Langenbecks Arch Klin Chir 1947;260:77-108.

122. Skoog T: Syndactyly. A clinical report on repair. Acta Chir Scand 1965;204:537-549.

123. Shaw D, Li CS, Richey DG, Nahigian SH: Interdigital butterfly flap in the hand (the double opposing Z-plasty). J Bone Joint Surg Am 1973;55:1677-1679.

124. Savaci N, Hosnuter M, Tosun Z: Use of triangular V-Y flaps to create a web space in syndactyly. Ann Plast Surg 1999;42:540-544.

125. Schatzki P: Über verdeckte Syndaktylie Polydaktylie und über "Triangelbildung" in der menschlichen Mittelhand. Arch Orthop Unfallchir 1934;34:637-652.

126. Schickedanz H, Adam G: Korrektur der hautigen Fingersyndaktylie. Zentralbl Chir 1969;94:187-193.

127. Schulstad I, Skoglund K: Surgical treatment of simple syndactyly. Scand J Plast Reconstr Surg 1977;11:235-237.

128. MacCollum D: Webbed fingers. Surg Gynecol Obstet 1940;71:782-789.

129. Oldfield M: The "horse-shoe" web flap in the treatment of syndactyly. Br J Plast Surg 1948;1:69-72.

130. Nylen B: Repair of congenital finger syndactyly. Acta Chir Scand 1957;113:310.

131. Mansfield O: Syndactyly. Br J Plast Surg 1961;13:249.

132. Millesi H: Kritische Betrachtungen zur Syndaktylie—Operation. Chir Plast Reconstr 1970;7:99-116.

133. Nakamura J, Yanagawa H, Kubo E, Endo T: New modified method for the surgical treatment of syndactyly. Ann Plast Surg 1989;23:511-518.

134. Karacaoglan N, Velidedeoglu H, Cicekci B, et al: Reverse W-M plasty in the repair of congenital syndactyly: a new method. Br J Plast Surg 1993;46:300-302.

135. Lewis R, Nordyke M, Duncan K: Web space reconstruction with a M-V flap. J Hand Surg Am 1988;13:40-43.

136. Kanavel A: Congenital malformations of the hands. Arch Surg 1932;28:282-320.

137. Hentz V, Littler J: The surgical management of congenital hand anomalies. In Converse JM, ed: Plastic and Reconstructive Surgery, 2nd ed. Philadelphia, WB Saunders, 1977:3325.

138. Heinrick R, Vavuras E: Zum Problem der Syndaktylie der Kinderhand. Z Kinderchir 1968;6:216.

139. Ladd A, Hentz V: Congenital malformations. In Herndon J, ed: Surgical Reconstruction of the Upper Extremity. Stamford, CT, Appleton and Lange, 1998:895-922.

140. Iselin M: Chirurgie der Hand: Atlas der Operationstechnik. Stuttgart, Georg Thieme Verlag, 1959.

141. Buck-Gramcko D: Fehlbildungen der Hand. Einfuhrung und Grundsatze der operativen Behandlung. Österreichische Gesellschaft für Chirurgie, 11th meeting, Wien, 1970. Wien, Verlag Wiener Medizinische Akademie, 1971.

142. Bandoh Y, Yanai A, Seno H: The three-square-flap method for reconstruction of minor syndactyly. J Hand Surg Am 1997;22:680-684.

143. Upton J: Treatment of congenital forearm and hand anomalies. In May JW Jr, Littler JW, eds: The Hand. Philadelphia, WB Saunders, 1990:5352-5356. McCarthy JG, ed: Plastic Surgery; vol 8.

144. Gilbert A: Toe transfers for congenital hand defects. J Hand Surg Am 1982;7:118-124.

145. Quaba A, Davidson PM: The distally-based dorsal hand flap. Br J Plast Surg 1990;43:28.

146. Colville J: Syndactyly correction. Br J Plast Surg 1989;42:12-16.

147. Earley M, Milner RH: Dorsal metacarpal flaps. Br J Plast Surg 1987;40:333-341.

148. Foucher G, Medina J, Pajardi G, Navarro R: Classification and treatment of symbrachydactyly. Chir Main 2000;19:161-168.

149. Maruyama Y: The reverse dorsal metacarpal flap. Br J Plast Surg 1990;43:24-27.

150. Sherif M: V-Y dorsal metacarpal flap: a new technique for the correction of syndactyly without a skin graft. Plast Reconstr Surg 1998;101:1861-1866.

151. Yao J, Shong JL, Sun H, et al: Repair of incomplete syndactyly by a web flap on a subcutaneous pedicle. Plast Reconstr Surg 1997;99:2079-2081.

152. Richterman I, DuPree J, Thoder J, Kozen SH: The radiographic analysis of web height. J Hand Surg Am 1998;23:1071-1076.

153. Brody G: Immobilization of tiny hands. Hand 1971;3:97-100.

154. Leung P, Hui KM: A simple splint for the intraoperative and early postoperative separation of fingers in syndactylia. J West Pac Orthop Assoc 1981;18:22-26.

155. Upton J: The Apert hand. In Gupta A, Kay SPJ, Scheker LR, eds: The Growing Hand: Diagnosis and Management of the Upper Extremity in Children. London, CV Mosby, 2000:345-362.

156. Buck-Gramcko D: Skin loss in the palm and web spaces. In Evans D, ed: The Hand and Upper Limb, vol 9. Edinburgh, Churchill Livingstone, 1992:159-180.

157. Buck-Gramcko D: Syndactyly between the thumb and index finger. In Buck-Gramcko D, ed: Congenital Malformations of the Hand and Forearm. London, Churchill Livingstone, 1998:141-148.

158. Kozin S: Congenital anomalies. Hand Surgery Update 3, vol 1. Rosemont, Ill, American Society for Surgery of the Hand, 2003:616.

159. Furnas D, Fischer G: The Z-plasty: biomechanics and mathematics. Br J Plast Surg 1971;24:144-160.

160. Woolf R, Broadbent T: The four-flap Z-plasty. Plast Reconstr Surg 1972;49:48-51.

161. Ostrowski D, Feagin CA, Gould JS: A three-flap web-plasty for release of short congenital syndactyly and dorsal adduction contracture. J Hand Surg Am 1991;16:634-641.

162. Hirshowitz B, Karev A, Rousso M: Combined double Z-plasty and Y-V advancement for thumb web contracture. Hand 1975;7:291-293.

163. Emmett A, Morris A: Ring constriction syndrome. In Buck-Gramcko D, ed: Congenital Malformations of the Hand and Forearm. London, Churchill Livingstone, 1998:169-182.

164. Ezaki M, Kay SPJ, Light TR, et al: Congenital hand deformities. In Green D, Hotchkiss RN, Pederson WC, eds: Green's Operative Hand Surgery, 4th ed, vol 1. New York, Churchill Livingstone, 1999:324-551.

165. Strauch B: Dorsal thumb flap for release of adduction contracture of the first web space. Bull Hosp Joint Dis 1975;36:34-39.

166. Tajima T: Classification of thumb hypoplasia. Hand Clin 1985;1:577-594.

167. Foucher G, Medina J, Navarro R, Khouri R: Correction of the first web space deficiency in congenital deformities of the hand with the pseudo-kite flap. Plast Reconstr Surg 2001;107:1458-1463.

168. Foucher G, Braun JB: A new island flap transfer from the dorsum of the index to the thumb. Plast Reconstr Surg 1979;63:28-31.

169. Flatt A, Wood VE: Multiple dorsal rotation flaps from the hand for thumb web contractures. Plast Reconstr Surg 1970;45:258-262.

170. Buck-Gramcko D: Angeborene Fehlbildungen der Hand. In Nigst H, Buck-Gramcko D, Millesi H, eds: Handchirurgie. New York, Thieme, 1988:12.1-12.

171. Brown P: Adduction-flexion contracture of the thumb: correction with dorsal rotation flap and release of contracture. Clin Orthop 1972;88:161-168.

172. Caroli A, Zanasi S: First web space reconstruction by Caroli's technique in congenital hand deformities with severe thumb ray adduction. Br J Plast Surg 1989;42:653-659.

173. Sandzen S: Dorsal pedicle flap for resurfacing a moderate thumb index web contracture release. J Hand Surg Am 1982;7:24-27.

174. Friedman R, Wood VE: The dorsal transpositional flap for congenital contracture of the first web space: a 20-year experience. J Hand Surg Am 1997;22:664-670.

175. Tijima T: Dorsal sliding flap for adduction contracture of the thumb. Seikeigeka (Orthop Surg) 1965;16:935-938.

176. Spinner M: Fashioned transpositional flap for soft tissue adduction contracture of the thumb. Plast Reconstr Surg 1969;4:345-348.

177. Buck-Gramcko D: Syndactyly and related deformities. In Nigst H, Buck-Gramcko D, Millesi H, Lister GD, eds: Hand Surgery. New York, Thieme, 1988:12.

178. Lister G, Milward T: Skin contracture of the first web space. Transactions of the Sixth International Congress of Plastic and Reconstructive Surgery, Paris, 1975.

179. Coombes C, Mutimer KL: Tissue expansion for the treatment of complete syndactyly of the first web. J Hand Surg Am 1994;19:968-972.

180. Smith P: Lister's The Hand: Diagnosis and Indications, 4th ed. London, Churchill Livingstone, 2002:457-522.

181. Upton J, Coombes CJ, Havlik RJ: Use of forearm flaps for the severely contracted first web space in children with congenital malformations. J Hand Surg Am 1996;21:470-477.

182. Zucker R, Cleland HJ, Haswell T: Syndactyly correction of the hand in Apert syndrome. Clin Plast Surg 1991;18:357-364.

183. Song R, Gao Y, Song Y, et al: The forearm flap. Clin Plast Surg 1982;9:21-26.

184. Masquelet AC, Penteado CV: Le lambeau interosseux posterieur. Ann Chir Main 1987;6:131-139.

185. Upton J: Classification and pathologic anatomy of limb anomalies. Clin Plast Surg 1991;18:321-356.

186. Kay S: Free tissue transfer in children. In Gupta A, Kay SPJ, Scheker LR, eds: The Growing Hand: Diagnosis and Management of the Upper Extremity in Children. London, CV Mosby, 2000:969-986.

187. Morgan R, Edgerton MT: Tissue expansion in reconstructive hand surgery: case report. J Hand Surg Am 1985;10:754-757.

188. Upton J: Apert bibliography. Clin Plast Surg 1991;18:417-431.

189. Flatt A: The Care of Congenital Hand Anomalies, 2nd ed. St. Louis, Quality Medical Publishing, 1994.

190. Pandya A, Belcher HJ: The Chevron technique for skin markings in syndactyly release. Plast Reconstr Surg 1998;101:808-809.

191. Hentz V: Correspondence Newsletter. Rosemont, Ill, American Society for Surgery of the Hand, 1985:65.

192. Sommerkamp T, Ezaki M, Carter PR, Hentz VR: A composite graft for complete syndactyly fingertip operations. J Hand Surg Am 1992;17:15-20.

193. Zoltie N, Verlende P, Logan A: Full thickness grafts taken from the plantar instep for syndactyly release. J Hand Surg Br 1989;14:201-203.

194. Johannson S: Nagelwallbildung durch Thenarlappen bei kompletter Syndaktylie. Handchirurgie 1982;14:199.

195. Johannson S: Nail folds in total syndactyly. Paper read at the First Congress of the International Federation of Societies for Surgery of the Hand, Rotterdam, 1980.

196. Greuse M, Coessens BC: Congenital syndactyly: defatting facilitates closure without skin graft. J Hand Surg Am 2001;26:589-594.

197. Buck-Gramcko D: Correspondence Newsletter. Rosemont, Ill, American Society for Surgery of the Hand, 1985:47.

198. Chiu D: Staged separation of complex syndactyly in the Apert hand. American Association of Plastic and Reconstructive Surgeons, Vancouver, BC, 1994.

199. Gundushauri O, Tvaliashvili LA: Local epidermoplasty for syndactyly. Int Orthop 1991;15:39-43.

200. Lundkvist L, Barfred T: A double pulp technique for creating nail folds in syndactyly release. J Hand Surg Br 1991;16:1991.

201. Sugihara T, Ohura T, Umeda T: Surgical method for treatment of syndactyly with osseous fusion of the distal phalanges. Plast Reconstr Surg 1991;87:157-164.

202. Millard D: Principlization of Plastic Surgery. Boston, Little, Brown, 1986:191-228.

203. Fontenot C, Ortenberg J, Faust D: Hypospadiac or intact foreskin graft for syndactyly repair. J Pediatr Surg 1999;34:1826-1828.

204. Oates S, Gosain AK: Syndactyly repair performed simultaneously with circumcision: use of foreskin as a skin-graft donor site. J Pediatr Surg 1997;32:1482-1484.

205. Withey S, Kangesu T, Carver N, Sommerlad BC: The open finger technique in the release of syndactyly. J Hand Surg Br 2001;26:4-7.

206. Habenicht R: The open finger technique for release of syndactyly. J Hand Surg Br 2001;26:3.

207. Eaton C, Lister GD: Syndactyly. Hand Clin 1990;6:555-575.

208. Rowsell A, Godfrey A: A fortuitous donor site for full thickness skin grafts in the correction of syndactyly. Br J Plast Surg 1984;37:31-34.

209. Park S, Hata Y, Ito O, et al: Full-thickness skin graft from the ulnar aspect of the wrist to cover defects on the hands and digits. Ann Plast Surg 1999;42:129-131.

210. Ekerot L: Syndactyly correction without skin grafting. J Hand Surg Br 1996;21:330-337.

211. Ogawa Y, Kasai K: The preoperative use of extra-tissue expander for syndactyly. Ann Plast Surg 1989;23:552-559.

212. Ashmead D, Smith PJ: Tissue expansion for Apert's syndactyly. J Hand Surg Br 1995;20:327.

213. Austad E, Thomas S, Pasyk K: Tissue expansion: dividend or loan? Plast Reconstr Surg 1986;78:63-67.

214. Van Beek A, Adson MH: Tissue expansion in reconstructive hand surgery. Clin Plast Surg 1987;14:535-542.

215. Moss A, Foucher G: Syndactyly: can web creep be avoided? J Hand Surg Br 1990;15:193.

216. Marumo E, Kojima T, Suzuki S: An operation for syndactyly, and its results. Plast Reconstr Surg 1976;58:561-567.

217. Neff G, Plaue R, Aulbach D: Results of various operations for syndactylia (follow-up studies and statistical evaluation of 101 primary operations). Handchirurgie 1978;10:21-30.

218. Brauer R, Cronin T, Smoot W: Treatment of syndactylism. In Goldwyn R, ed: Long-term Results in Plastic and Reconstructive Surgery. Boston, Little, Brown, 1980:812-835.

219. Eslov B, Zachariae L: Surgical methods in syndactylism. Acta Chir Scand 1966;131:258-268.

220. Bastian H, Schutze C: Results of surgical treatment of syndactylia of the hand. Beitr Orthop Traumatol 1989;36:267-274.

221. Bensahel H, Boureau M: Medecine pratique et syndactylies. Rev Prat 1972;22:3265-3274.

222. Helbig B, Hippe P: Preliminary report of the results of syndactyly surgery. Handchir Mikrochir Plast Chir 1984;16:44-47.

223. Johne B: Operative Behandlung der Syndaktylie: Zeitpunkt—Technik—Ergebnisse [thesis]. Hamburg, Hamburg University, 1979.

224. Kramer R, Hildreth DH, Brinker MR, et al: A comparison of patients with different types of syndactyly. J Pediatr Orthop 1998;18:233-238.

225. Ruby L, Goldberg M: Syndactyly and polydactyly. Orthop Clin North Am 1976;7:361-374.

226. Schrader M, Losch G: Differential diagnosis, operative treatment, and prognosis of complicated syndactylies. Handchir Mikrochir Plast Chir 1985;17:122-128.

227. Upton J, Murray J: Classification and treatment of deformities in Apert's syndrome. Presented at the 31st annual meeting of the American Society for Surgery of the Hand, New Orleans, 1976.

228. Holten W, Smith AW, Isaacs JL, et al: Imaging of the Apert syndrome hand using three-dimensional CT and MRI. Plast Reconstr Surg 1997;99:1675-1680.

229. Barot L, Caplan H: Early surgical intervention in Apert's syndactyly. Plast Reconstr Surg 1986;77:282-287.

230. Noguchi M, Iwasawa M, Matsuo K, Kondoh S: A four-pulp flap technique for creating nail folds in the separation of a mid-digital mass in a patient with Apert's disease. Ann Plast Surg 1996;37:444-448.

231. Golash A, Watson JS: Nail fold creation in complete syndactyly using Buck-Gramcko pulp flaps. J Hand Surg Br 2000;25:11-14.

232. Guzanin S, Zabavnikova M, Kacmar P, et al: Surgical treatment of hand syndactyly in Apert syndrome. Act Chir Orthop Traumatol Cech 2001;68:249-255.

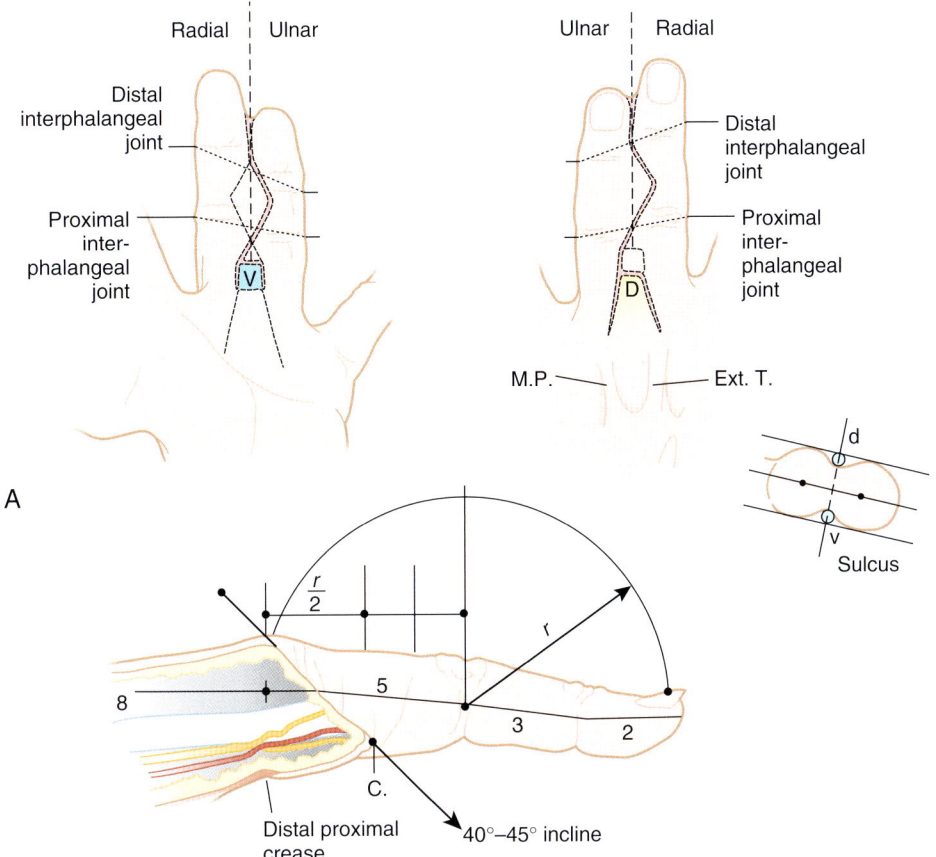

COLOR PLATE 204-1. Normal anatomic relationships. *A,* These original sketches by J. William Littler demonstrate the hourglass configuration of the interdigital web space. Dorsal nonglabrous skin without hair extends into the commissure region and gradually blends with the glabrous skin from the palmar surface. The dorsal (D) and palmar (V) flaps outlined, when joined at the base of the new commissure, will simulate the normal hourglass configuration. M.P., metacarpophalangeal joint; Ext. T., extensor tendon. *B,* This side view of a digit pinpoints the level of the commissure base at the midportion of the proximal phalanx. The normal slope of the commissure subtends a 40- to 45-degree incline from proximal to distal. The relative lengths of the skeletal segments relate to the Fibonacci sequence (1, 1, 2, 3, 5, 8, 13, 21 . . .), in which the length of a given segment is the sum of the two preceding segments. C, digitopalmar flexion crease.

Constriction Ring Syndrome

JOSEPH UPTON III, MD

TERMINOLOGY

When the etiology of a condition is not known, there are almost as many theories of origin as there are hand surgeons—hence the large array of eponyms associated with this fascinating condition, which does not fit into any other classification. Consequently, it has been designated a category of its own, the constriction ring syndrome (CRS). Other terms used in the literature include annular band, constriction band or ring, Streeter dysplasia, intrauterine or congenital amputations, acrosyndactyly, and fenestrated syndactyly. Because these hands demonstrate no failure of formation or differentiation and no overgrowth or undergrowth, a special designation within the International Federation of Societies for Surgery of the Hand classification has been applied (Table 205-1).[1]

The dysmorphologists have properly recognized that the deformities seen are the result of a cascade of events that follow an intrauterine disruption (see Chapter 201).[2,3] Many theories attempt to explain the specific cause of the disruption, and they are discussed.

CLASSIFICATION

As defined by Patterson,[4] the congenital hand differences associated with CRS contain one or more of the following characteristics:

1. simple constriction rings;
2. constriction rings accompanied by deformity of the distal part, with or without lymphedema;
3. constriction rings accompanied by fusions of distal parts, ranging from mild to gross acrosyndactyly;
4. intrauterine amputations.

These groups are clinically useful because they require different treatments. Other clinicians have amended this scheme by separating the depth of the ring into mild, moderate, severe, and amputation[5-7] and by further defining the presence or absence of lymphedema or soft tissue loss distal to the ring.[8] For practical considerations, I do not further subdivide the rings by their depth because the principles of treatment and technique for correction are the same. Great variations do exist because most constriction rings of the hand and wrist are incomplete or shallow and are located on the dorsal surfaces.

The absence of a digit or thumb in CRS is termed an intrauterine amputation. These are transverse amputations at the level of a deep constricting ring that has cut off the vascular supply to the developing portion of the extremity, usually a digit or toe. A congenital amputation, or aplasia, is a developmental malformation in which the deficient part does not develop. In contrast to congenital deficiencies, an amputation in CRS may often be found as a dismembered part within the placenta or amniotic fluid[9-13] or even engrafted somewhere on the fetus.[14,15]

TABLE 205-1 ✦ TERMS USED FOR THIS CONDITION

Streeter dysplasia
Torpin dysplasia
Annular band syndrome
Constriction ring syndrome*
Amniotic band syndrome
Amniotic band disruption sequence
Acrosyndactyly
Congenital amputation syndrome
Fenestrated syndactyly

*Term that has been adopted by the Committee on Congenital Differences of the International Federation of Societies for Surgery of the Hand.

INCIDENCE

The incidence of this entity varies. Patterson[4] from England reported an occurrence of 1 per 15,000 live births. However, Pillay[16] from Singapore noted that it was 1 per 4000 live births in the Malay population, which he thought was related to general dietary deficiencies and frequent pregnancy-related illnesses that occurred in 60% of mothers with CRS babies. A much lower prevalence of 0.19 per 50,000 live births has been reported in British Columbia from a registry of more than 1.2 million live births[17] and of 2.03 per 10,000 live births in Western Australia.[18] Clearly, environmental conditions, nutrition, and access to proper prenatal medical care are significant. Some surgeons who have long experience with CRS think that it is becoming more frequent with the rise of abnormal gestational histories in the lower socioeconomic groups of populations.[19] I agree with this but also realize that my experience in a tertiary children's hospital in the New England states is quite skewed.

INHERITANCE

No positive relationship between CRS and genetic inheritance has been reported. There is one case report of twins with asymmetric constriction rings,[20] and there are some cases within a single pedigree.[21] There are a number of reports of CRS in twin gestations associated with teratogens, lysergic acid diethylamide (LSD),[22] and monozygotic twins.[23] Throughout $2^{1}/_{2}$ decades of practice, I have treated six sets of twins, one monozygotic and five dizygotic, with one partner affected with CRS (Fig. 205-1).

ASSOCIATED MALFORMATIONS

The percentage of associated anomalies varies from 40% to as high as 80% (Table 205-2).[24-26] Constric-

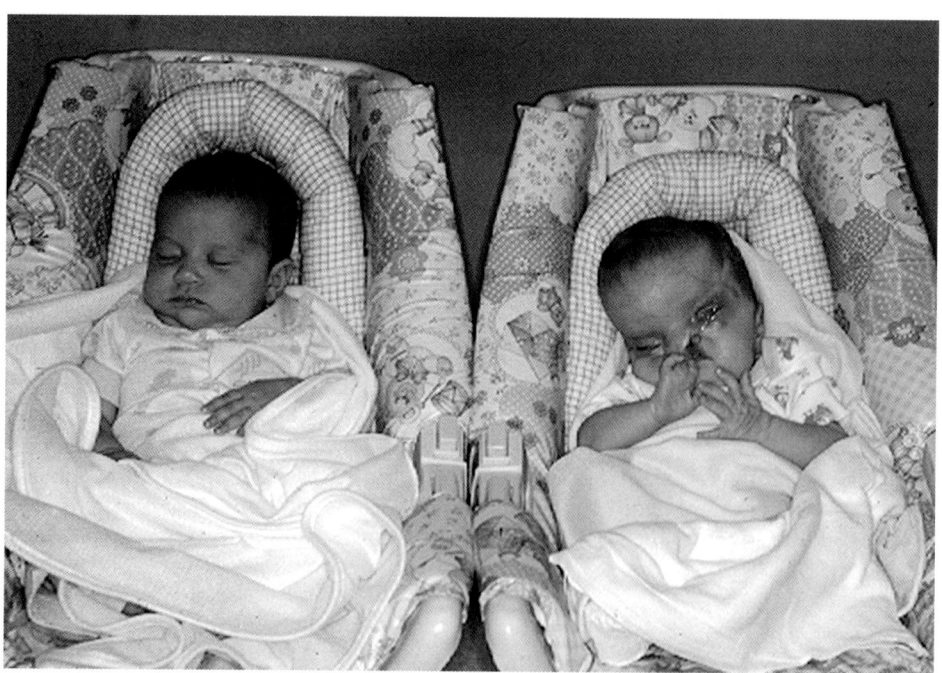

FIGURE 205-1. CRS and twinning. In a set of monozygotic twins, the baby on the right has an acrosyndactyly of the right hand, a characteristic wide bilateral cleft of the lip and palate, and associated hypertelorbitism. Multiple toes were also missing. Constriction rings and congenital amputations are present on the right hand.

TABLE 205-2 ✦ MALFORMATIONS ASSOCIATED WITH THE CONSTRICTION RING SYNDROME

Anencephaly
Unusual, wide paramedian facial clefts
Ocular and orbital defects, encephalocele
Cleft lip and cleft palate
Choanal atresia
Cleft palate as part of Pierre Robin sequence
EEC syndrome
Ear deformations
Upper and lower limb malformations
  Acrosyndactyly
  Syndactyly
  Amputations
  Lymphedema
  Clubfoot
  Pseudarthrosis of the tibia and fibula
  Ulnar dysplasias
  Radial dysplasias
Abdominal wall defects
Thoracic wall defects
Scoliosis and kyphosis
Omphalocele
Absent or dysplastic kidneys
Diaphragmatic abnormalities
Imperforate anus
Cutis aplasia of the scalp
Anemia
Congenital heart defects

tion ring deformities are as common on the lower extremity as on the upper. Almost all of these involve the musculoskeletal system, with clubbed feet being most common.[19,25,27] The coincidence of clubfoot, reported in up to 30% of most series, and cleft palate (similar to the Pierre Robin sequence) and CRS is thought to be secondary to oligohydramnios and increased uterine pressure on the fetus[28] and has been attributed to amniocentesis.[29] Unrelated syndactyly[30] and ulnar dysplasia[31] have been reported in addition to many incidental findings, such as anemia and congenital heart disease.

Large reported series reveal an incidence between 5% and 15% of craniofacial malformations with clefting of the lip or palate.[32-38] The clefting often appears in paramedian locations and can be wide and disfiguring. These "monstrosity" clefts comprise one of the most complex craniofacial problems treated today (Fig. 205-2). The common association of these limb defects and certain craniofacial clefts[33,39,40] has been termed the ADAM complex (amniotic deformity, adhesions, mutilations), which some think is the result of early amnion rupture.[37,41,42]

Syndromic designations can be confusing. Those with the manifestations of CRS in the limbs have the amniotic band disruption sequence, and those with concomitant limb and craniofacial malformations have the ADAM sequence.[43] Those with another entity, the Adams-Oliver syndrome (Fig. 205-3), have the co-occurrence of paramedian scalp aplasia and acral limb defects similar to those described.[44] Upper and lower limb defects identical to those seen in CRS are also described in association with exencephaly-encephalocele, facial clefting, and thoracoschisis or abdominoschisis, a combination that pathologists term the "limb–body wall complex."[37,41,45]

The association of facial clefts, central nervous system malformations, and thoracic or abdominal

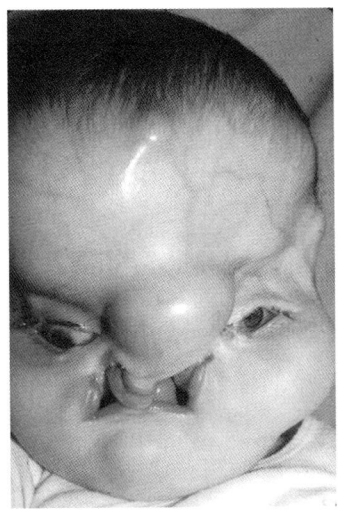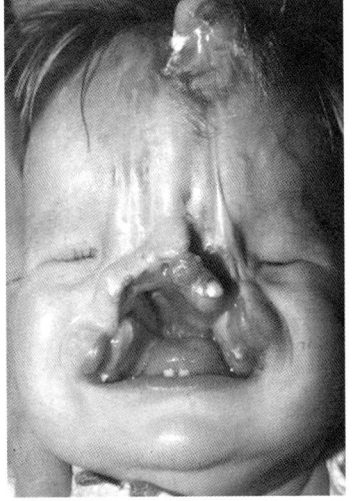

FIGURE 205-2. Facial clefts. *A,* This CRS infant with a double cleft of the lip and palate demonstrates the path of a band present at birth that extended across the nasal dorsum and the left supraorbital ridge into the left temporal scalp. The mother's pregnancy was complicated by poor nutrition and oligohydramnios. *B,* In another CRS baby, a large paramedian cleft extends upward medial to the left eye into the forehead. All four extremities contained constriction rings and congenital amputations. These are some of the most extensive clefts seen by the craniofacial surgeon.

A   B

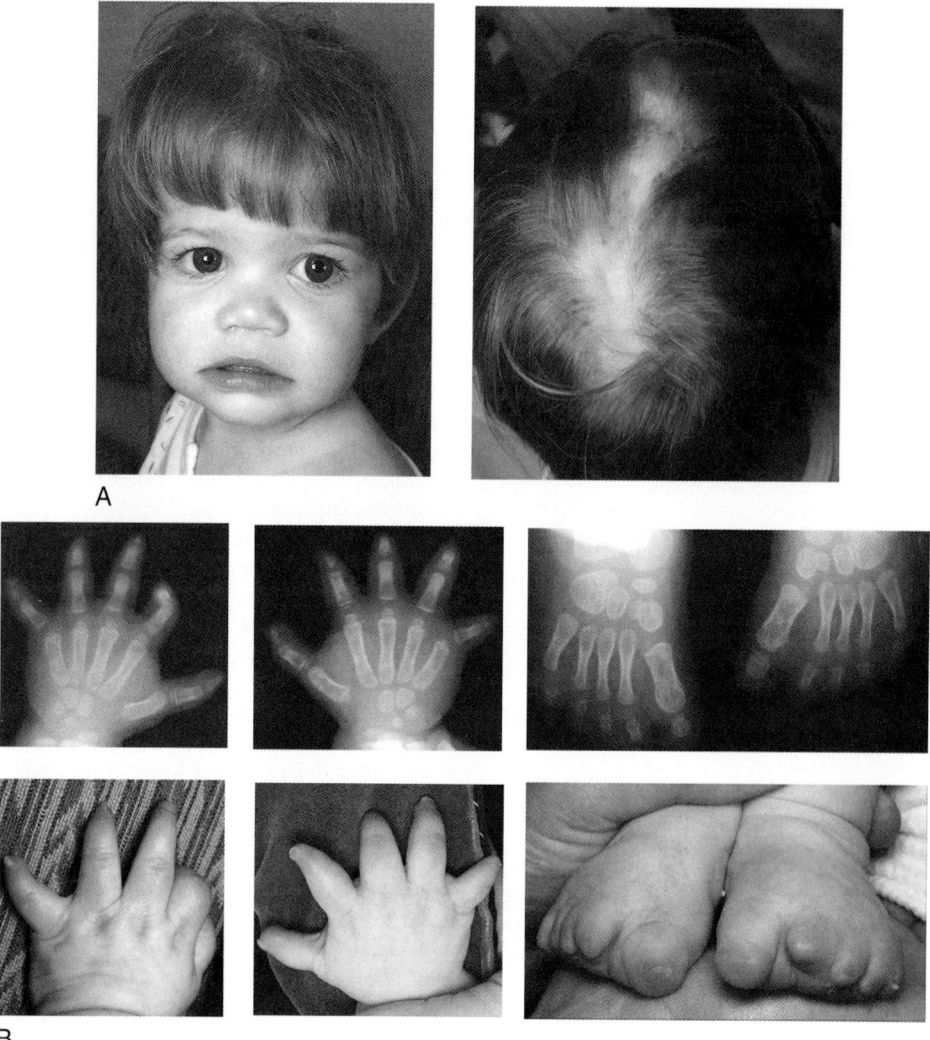

FIGURE 205-3. The Adams-Oliver syndrome. *A,* The Adams-Oliver syndrome is often misla-beled as CRS and consists of cutis aplasia of the scalp in which a longitudinal defect can vary in size and can often be associated with full-thickness calvarial loss. *B,* The distal digital or toe hypoplasia-aplasia is often confused with CRS. Constriction rings with or without edema are not present. The digital or toe hypoplasia-aplasia usually contains diminutive nails or nail folds. This child also has a camptodactyly of the left index finger.

anomalies has been discussed. These patients do not fall into the normal CRS or amniotic band disruption sequence. Most large series quote associated defects ranging from 40% to 56%.[7,25,46-49] Eighty percent have concomitant hand and foot defects, the most frequent being a hand syndactyly and a clubfoot.[6,7,50]

Deep constriction rings can be accompanied by neurologic deficits that are often overlooked in the distal portions of the extremities during clinical examination. Although the depth of most rings is maximal on the dorsal surfaces, they can penetrate to and compress digital neurovascular structures on the palmar surfaces of the digits and thumb. Deep rings of the arm or axillary regions do not have a predilection for the dorsal surfaces and can cause severe motor and sensory deficits or neurologic palsies.[51-54] The postoperative course after nerve grafting in these patients is not encouraging (Figs. 205-4 and 205-5).[51]

Those with deep rings have a predictable temperature gradient across the level of the ring, even after surgical correction. The 11% to 16% incidence of edema and decreased capillary refill distal to the ring[50,53,55] is probably low. Almost all of the children living in the New England climate demonstrate peripheral cyanosis, cold digits, and a marked decrease in capillary refill after they have been playing outside in the cold winter temperatures. However, few of these youngsters complain of pain.

Hand anomalies that have been described and bear no apparent association with amniotic bands include nonadjacent simple syndactyly,[56] the EEC syndrome,[57] ulnar clubhand,[31] and hypoplasia of the radius. A clear distinction can be made between the terminal hypoplasias or absence of portions of the hand in the chorionic villus sampling and CRS patients.[58] In chorionic villus sampling, no constriction rings or bands are seen proximal to the levels of congenital amputation. The proximal anatomy in both conditions is normal.

PATHOGENESIS

The etiology of this condition has been both speculative and controversial. The implications of different theories for guilty parents can be significant. Three positions have been described and are still supported by clinical findings and experimental models. After the extensive literature is read, it becomes clear that manifestations of CRS can be caused in a number of ways.

Intrinsic Theory

The earliest theory stated that these deformities were the result of a "defective germ plasm" within the embryo.[59] Others have pointed out that the localized areas of involvement within the limb might best support this theory.[4,60,61] Streeter thought that the bands represented macerated sheets of epidermis and the residual of defective local tissue. The presence of systemic and internal visceral anomalies could only be explained by this theory.[62] Clavert's experimental model of injecting hypertonic solutions into the amniotic sac demonstrated that injury to the ectoderm and mesoderm of the developing limb at critical periods sets the stage for band formation.[63-66] Kino's experimental model in the rat demonstrated that hemorrhages along the marginal sinuses of the digital rays were precursor lesions to the development of congenital amputations and acrosyndactyly identical to those seen in CRS.[67] Intrinsic abnormalities would also

CONSTRICTION RING VARIATIONS

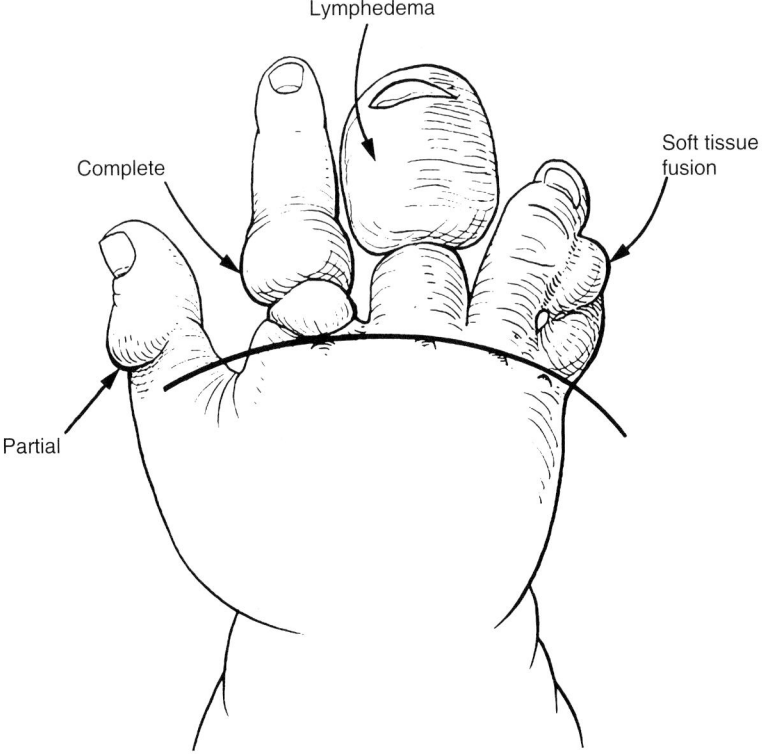

FIGURE 205-4. Constriction rings. The configuration of rings may be partial (usually on the dorsal surfaces) or complete with or without distal swelling or lymphedema. The distal fusion between digits or toes never initially involves a skeletal coalition, and there are dorsal to palmar sinuses proximal to these fusions. The level of these epithelialized tracks is characteristically more distal than the usual level of the commissure. No two patients, and no two hands for that matter, are exactly the same.

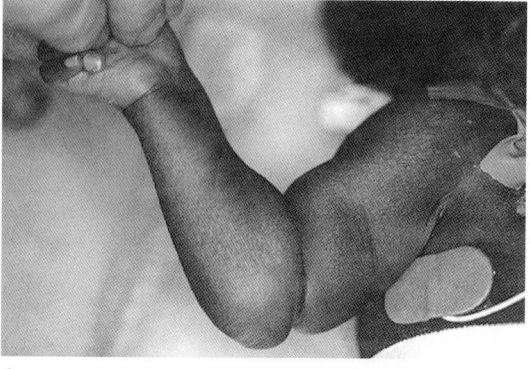

A

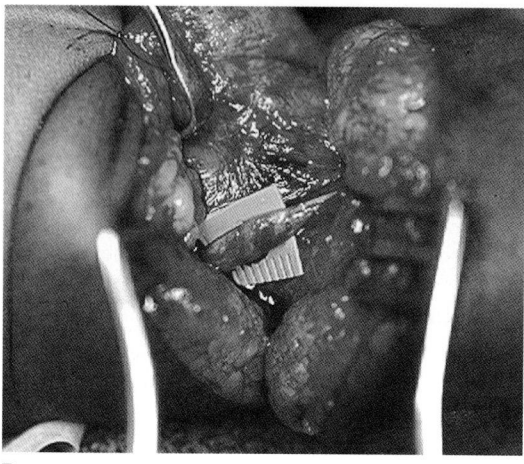

B

FIGURE 205-5. Deep rings with neurologic impairment. *A,* This newborn with a deep ring at the supracondylar level of the arm had an associated facial cleft, omphalocele, and acrosyndactyly. All three nerves of the upper limb, the median seen in *B,* contained compression lesions but were in continuity. Twenty years later, all three nerves are functional, although the patient has limited function because of central nervous system deficits related to her prematurity. *B,* A significant flattening of the median nerve is seen at the site of compression beneath the depth of the groove. There is a broad, flat neuroma proximal to the level of the compression. At no time was there any venous compromise in this limb, which contained only a deep venous drainage system.

help explain the internal visceral abnormalities, such as imperforate anus, ectopic gallbladders, diaphragmatic abnormalities, and the like.

Extrinsic Theory

The second theory was first described by Torpin,[11,68] who exhaustively studied the placentas and malformations of these babies. Early rupture of or damage to the amnion could cause oligohydramnios, which in turn would result in tears in the placental amnion and the formation of amniotic bands within the sac. Subsequently, developmentalists invoked the concept of an intrauterine "disruption," which would trigger a sequence of events resulting in malformations.[2,3,30] Oligohydramnios could produce abnormal pressure on the developing extremities (including clubfeet), and the bands result in both rings and amputations. Mounting evidence supporting this theory includes the high rate of involvement of the longer central digits and longer great toe,[69] delivery of amputated parts,[10,13,49,69,70] engrafting of amputated parts (Fig. 205-6),[15,71] peripheral neural defects with and without vascular compromise distal to the constriction ring,[6,51,54] and fibrous strings within the band at birth.[25,42,49,72-75]

Additional experimental evidence has demonstrated that amniotic pressure changes in rats[28] and application of ligatures around developing avian extremities[76-78] will produce the whole spectrum of constriction rings. Perhaps the most compelling evidence is the ultrasonic documentation of the poor growth, diminishing blood flow, and ultimate resorption of a leg in a fetus with below-knee amniotic band formation.[79]

Intrauterine Trauma Theory

The third postulation was made by Kino,[67] who demonstrated in a rat model that intrauterine trauma could cause hemorrhage of the marginal sinuses of the hand plate, which would lead to digital fusion identical to that seen in acrosyndactyly. In utero, amniotic bands attached to limbs have been observed on sonography as early as the first trimester,[80-82] and one paper describes the "cobweb syndrome" of multiple amniotic bands confirmed by fetoscopy.[80] Amniotic bands have been demonstrated by sonography to follow chorioamniotic membrane separation after fetal surgery in 5 of 40 cases.[81] In one of these cases, a constricting band around the umbilical cord was responsible for a fetal death.

Today, most agree that there is no genetic predisposition to this condition, which appears to be the result of an "early amnion rupture sequence." (See Chapter 201.) All experienced clinicians—especially those who have performed toe transfer reconstructions on these children—know that the anatomy proximal to the site of constriction (or amputation) is completely normal.[72,83]

CLINICAL PRESENTATION

These deformities are always present at birth. On occasion in the neonatal nursery, drying, desiccated bands can be seen within the depth of the grooves in the skin

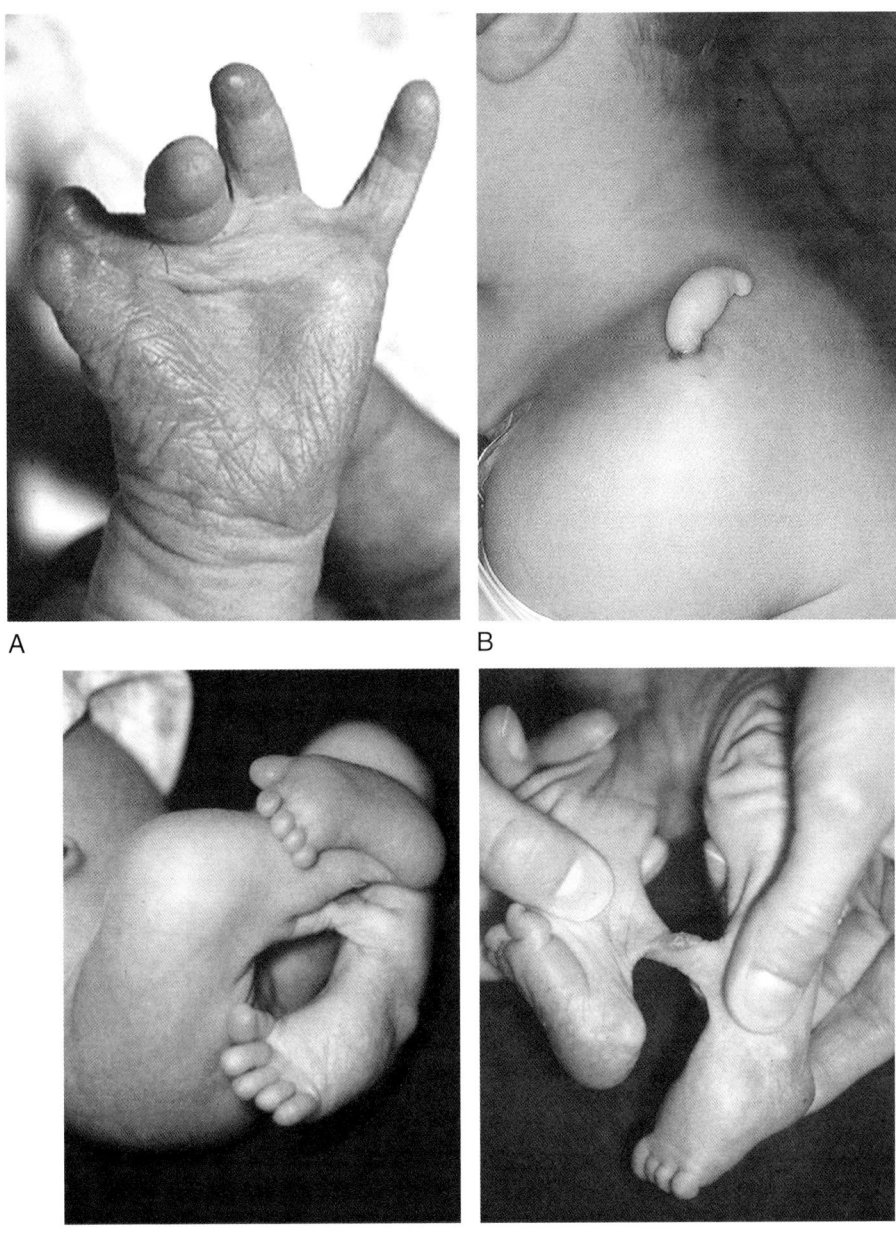

A

B

C

D

FIGURE 205-6. Engrafting of amputated parts. *A,* This child with CRS was delivered with an acrosyndactyly of the right hand with congenital amputations of all but the fifth finger and a complete syndactyly of the thumb and index rays. *B,* One dislodged digit became engrafted in the left supraclavicular region. Histologic examination showed little cartilage in the phalanx and a rudimentary nail on the distal portion of the amputated part. Examination of the whorl pattern of the tip did not enable accurate determination of the digit of origin. *C,* The lower extremities of this CRS child are joined by a soft tissue bridge at the distal tibial level; a severe clubfoot is present on the right side. *D,* At birth, there was evidence of ulceration and healing across this bridge. Pregnancy was complicated by poor nutrition and oligohydramnios.

(Fig. 205-7). Tight constriction rings (annular bands) may be found around any part of the upper or lower extremity and have a predilection for the longer central three digits of the hand and the great toe of the foot. More than one extremity is usually affected, and it is rare for only one ring to present as an isolated malformation with no other manifestation of this syndrome.[4,6,7,50,84,85] Bilateral hand anomalies are common and are usually accompanied by one or more foot deformities (Fig. 205-8). The precise configuration of the bands, lymphedema, and character of the amputations are not predictable and vary with each individual patient. No two patients are identical. No two affected limbs are enantiomorphic. There is no direct relationship of the severity of the deformity from one limb to another. However, patients with severe bilateral upper limb constriction rings with multiple amputations often have few available toes for microvascular reconstruction (see Fig. 205-8).

The depth of the groove may vary, resulting in anything from a partial defect with a mild deficiency in the subcutaneous tissue to an extensive circumferential indentation that may interrupt or obstruct nerves, veins, or lymphatic channels in the areolar plane or tendons, muscles, or major motor or sensory nerves (Figs. 205-9 and 205-10).[6,51,52,54,86,87] The rings are typically more pronounced on the dorsal surfaces of the hand and foot (see Figs. 205-4, 205-7, 205-9, and 205-

10). Deeper indentations on the palmar surfaces are often accompanied not only by flexion contracture of the local joint but also by contracture of the glabrous tissue—with or without a deformity of the nail.

The deepest rings, which extend into the bone, are rarely seen because the digits or other limb parts involved have autoamputated. On occasion, at birth, these disconnected parts may be recovered with the placenta during delivery.[25,72,88] However, most are resorbed during intrauterine development.[79] The author has seen four cases of engraftment of these floating parts elsewhere on the cutaneous surface (see Fig. 205-6). This phenomenon has been reported by others.[14,15]

Both deep and more superficial bands are not restricted to the distal portion of the upper and lower limbs. They are frequently found wrapped around one or both legs, ankles, and feet. Clubfeet are the most frequently associated malformation in the lower extremity (Fig. 205-11). Deeper rings have the same sequelae of mild to moderate to deep distal swelling or lymphedema. A congenital tibial pseudarthrosis or below-knee amputation is often associated with a deep constriction ring. Superficial or deep rings appear at the humeral, forearm, femoral, and tibial levels with much less frequency.

When spontaneous rupture of the amnion occurs early in the second trimester, the separation of amnion

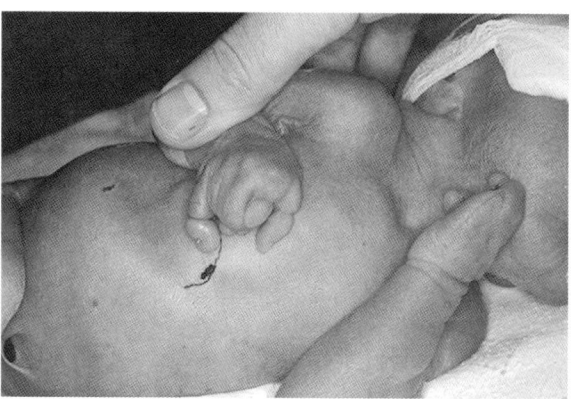

A

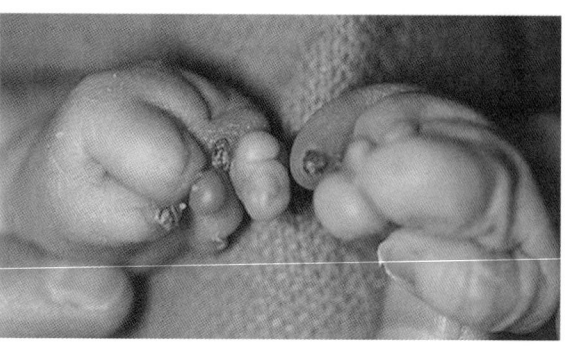

B

FIGURE 205-7. Neonatal bands. *A,* A dry desiccated amniotic band is seen within a deep ring in a premature newborn. The bands around the thumb and index ray were removed by a nurse at the time of delivery. The histologic features were consistent with amniotic membrane. *B,* The stumps of similar rings are often seen at the juncture of coalesced digits in acrosyndactylies. The side-to-side fusion of these digits is marked by a fibrous (scar) union in contrast to a skeletal union.

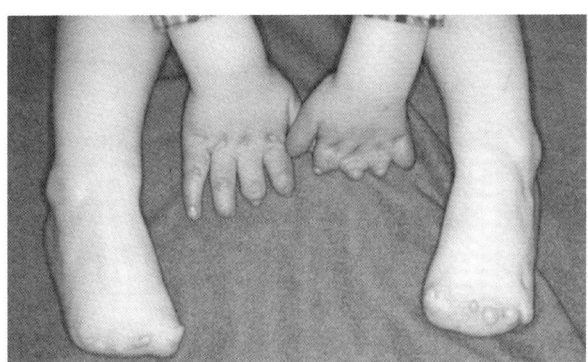

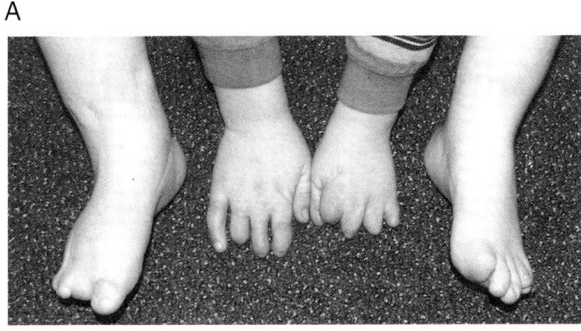

FIGURE 205-8. Extremity involvement. *A,* This youngster with CRS has congenital amputation of all toes and 9 of his 10 fingers, so microvascular toe transfer is not an option for reconstruction. It is not uncommon to find involvement of three limbs or of all the limbs in this syndrome. Despite these limitations, his hand function is remarkably good, and his lower extremity function is normal. *B,* The second youngster shows a similar clinical pattern and does have some toes, but they are not amenable for transfer to the hand.

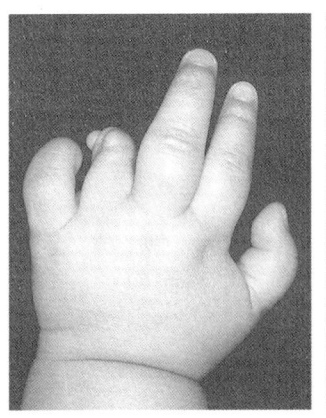
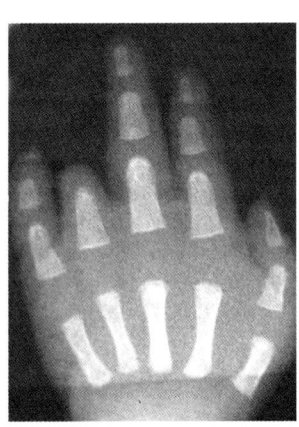

A

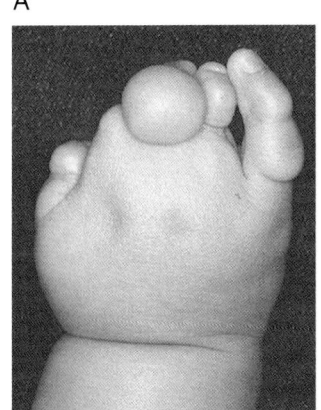
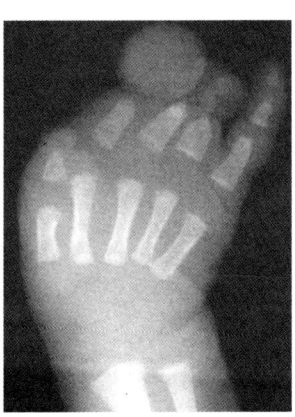

B

FIGURE 205-9. Constriction rings. *A,* All variations of constriction ring involvement are seen in this newborn. The left hand has a deep ring and congenital amputation at the proximal interphalangeal joint level of the ring finger; the distal segment of the ring is flexed and floppy without any skeletal stability; and the distal phalangeal segments are hypoplastic on all intact digits. *B,* The right thumb is amputated at the proximal interphalangeal joint. The index finger and ring finger have deep rings at the proximal interphalangeal joints with significant distal swelling. Hypoplastic nails are present. The fifth finger has shallow rings with minimal to moderate swelling at the proximal and middle phalanx levels. The nail approaches normal. The central three digits are joined by a side-to-side fibrous union in an acrosyndactyly.

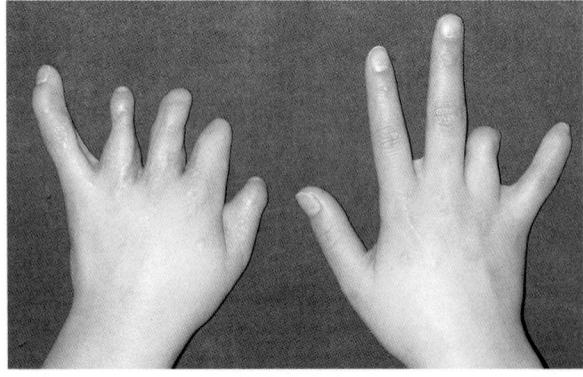

A

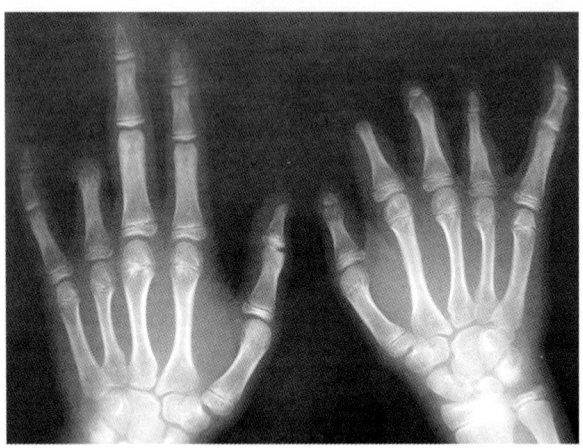

B

FIGURE 205-10. Constriction rings. *A* and *B,* The clinical appearance and radiographs of the same patient as in Figure 205-9 are seen 16 years later. In multiple stages, the acrosyndactyly on the right side has been separated and the extra bulbous skin used as either a pedicle flap or skin graft. The floppy ring tip has been amputated. After release of the left first web space, the patient did not want any thumb lengthening either with distraction or by microvascular transfer. The development of the hypoplastic distal segments has not been the same as that of the more proximal skeletal parts, and these hypoplastic fingertips and amputation stumps become more obvious with growth.

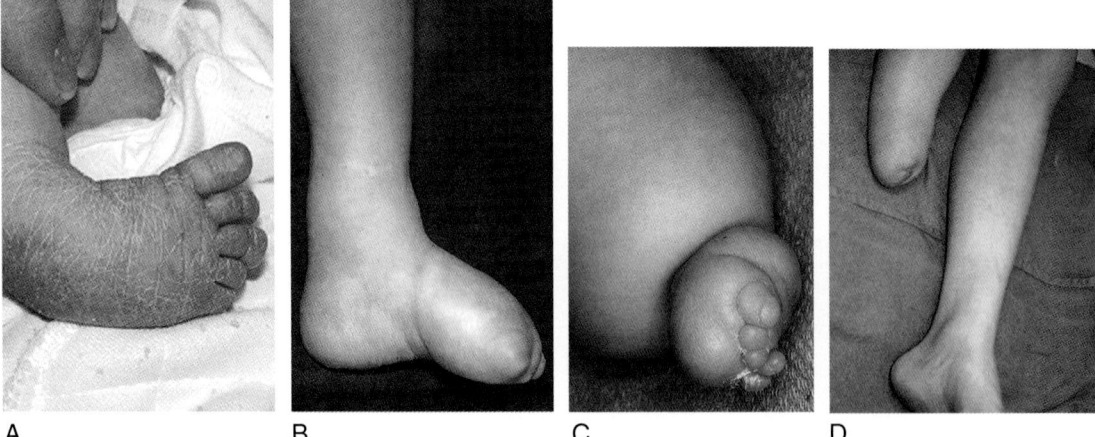

A   B   C   D

FIGURE 205-11. Lower extremity. In addition to constriction rings and amputations involving the toes, common lower extremity findings include these: *A,* a clubfoot, the most common; *B,* a hypoplastic foot associated with a midtarsal constriction ring; *C,* a hypoplastic foot without skeletal attachment to the tibia; *D,* a right below-knee amputation.

from chorion produces many small, hair-like strands that can become entangled within digits and toes. The longer central digits of the hand are most likely to become entangled, and the thumb, which the fetus often holds in tight adduction and flexion, is the least likely to become involved. As the pregnancy continues, the amnion thickens. When it separates from the chorion, it can roll up on itself and form a much thicker, longer cord, which can be swallowed by the fetus to produce facial clefts[68,89]; encircle the umbilical cord to produce fetal death; or constrict the arm, forearm, or torso, where deep bands frequently result in neurologic impairment (see Fig. 205-5).

The congenital amputations are classified as transverse and occur at all levels.[90] The tip often tapers to a point that may or may not have been connected to an amputation of an adjacent digit at the same level as part of an acrosyndactyly. Often at birth, the stump may be edematous and not completely covered with epithelium (Fig. 205-12).[73] Some isolated thumb, digital, or leg amputations do have a well-padded mobile stump, but most at the phalangeal level taper to a sharp tip. Sensation is always normal in these stumps. Although neuromas are found surgically within these stumps, patients are never symptomatic. Despite the diminutive digital length of proximal digital amputations, function is usually good (see Fig. 205-12).

The specific character of the acrosyndactyly is discussed in more detail later. The soft tissue webbing between digits is always simple and usually incomplete. Extra skeletal parts are never present, but adjacent digits and thumb can be joined side by side, either by a common scar or by bone. This site of fusion also corresponds with an external band, which may still be present at birth and often causes the most significant scarring and disfigurement. Various digital overlapping combinations may be seen in hands, which resemble a "bundle of grapes."[50] In these cases, the long and fifth fingers are usually palmar.[72,91]

In most hands, the level of intrauterine disruption is clear. Fortunately for the reconstructive surgeon, soft tissue and skeletal structures are always normal proximal to this level. Dimpling and soft tissue dorsal to palmar sinuses are characteristic within the syndactyly. These result from apoptosis and re-epithelialization as the digital rays began to separate normally. Most sinuses are easily probed, but those at the base of dorsal dimples must be opened by smaller probes. The location of these sinuses can help determine which distal digital parts match the appropriate proximal skeletal structures, which are often coalesced by scar or bone. When they are blocked, epidermal inclusion cysts may form.[62]

The swollen soft tissue distal to the constriction ring presents with all degrees of induration. A

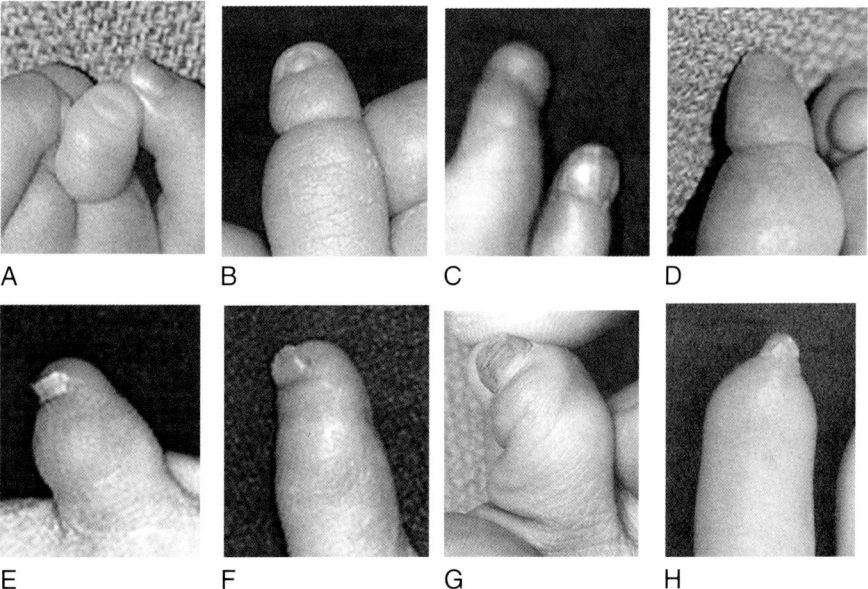

FIGURE 205-12. Stumps and nails. *A* to *H,* Small nails with much less vertical height than width are attached to hypoplastic distal phalanges. Despite limited usefulness, patients become emotionally attached to them and learn to use them in many ingenious adaptive maneuvers. Nail plates not adherent to the underlying sterile matrix often have chronic subungual fungal infections (*E, F, G,* and *H*). The growth of these nails is delayed in comparison to growth of those on normal digits or toes. Like the underlying skeletal segments, these nails do not "catch up" to the normal nails as far as growth is concerned.

TABLE 205-3 ◆ DIFFERENTIAL DIAGNOSIS FOR THE HAND SURGEON

Constriction ring syndrome
Symbrachydactyly
Chorionic villus sampling
Congenital amputations
Hypoplasias of hand, digit, thumb
Adams-Oliver syndrome
ADAM complex

massively swollen part at birth is often filled primarily with fluid, but most smaller parts are indurated and contain interstitial fluid and swollen adipose tissue, which often has a lighter color than the normal fat seen on the dorsum of the same hand (see Fig. 205-5). With compromise of neurovascular structures, sensation may be diminished, but it is rarely absent, although the distal parts may be blue. Capillary refill may be decreased, and acral temperatures are less than in unaffected digits. Throughout life, these hands and digits will show characteristic vascular impairment on exposure to cold temperatures.[25,55,92,93]

The differential diagnosis for this condition is confusing, and almost half of infants are referred with a wrong diagnosis—often a syndromic designation (Table 205-3). The most frequent mislabels are given to patients with symbrachydactylies containing rudimentary central digits or nubbins narrowed at their bases. These are not constriction rings. One sure cue to the difference is that symbrachydactylies, previously called atypical cleft hands, are unilateral; they are usually isolated to one extremity and do not have congenital amputations without distal nail parts or remnants. Syndromologists may include patients with facial clefting and trunk and torso malformations as variants within the spectrum of the amniotic disruption sequence. When asked specific information about heredity, the hand surgeon should defer to them. In determination of this syndrome, the author has adhered to Patterson's criteria and insisted that distinct constriction rings be present.[72]

TREATMENT

Timing

The parents of these newborn infants are often devastated by the appearance and apparent lack of function of these hands and feet. Thorough initial evaluation, formulation of surgical goals, and outline of a long-term plan are helpful for both the patient's family and the surgeon.[49,94,95] These babies often need staged corrections on the same digit or thumb and multiple procedures on the same limb. During this initial consultation, making the correct diagnosis will benefit everyone involved.

Within the neonatal period, the surgeon should take time to discuss both the etiology and the treatment of CRS with the parents. The only surgery that is necessary within the neonatal period is the release of small soft tissue bridges between digits and thumb to allow their unrestricted growth. These bridges can often be snipped under local anesthesia in the nursery (Fig. 205-13). In utero lysis of amniotic bands is possible and has been successfully performed for release of bands around limbs that could be monitored by Doppler examination. However, before "minimally invasive" fetal surgery is performed, the surgeon must be certain of the diagnosis. In one child, an isolated large lymphatic malformation of the hand was misdiagnosed as a constriction ring and "decompressed" with fetal surgery, which resulted in a premature birth (Fig. 205-14). Fortunately, the baby was otherwise normal and healthy.

The massively swollen lymphedematous parts are more easily decompressed during infancy because they are filled with fluid and have not yet become indurated by scar. At this time, the surgeon may take advantage of the extra skin with judicious excision of proximal scarred areas and resurfacing. Often, most of this skin is discarded (see Fig. 205-5). On occasion, a hypoplastic hand or foot will remain distal to what normally would be a below-elbow or below-knee amputation. These are best removed unless they can be effectively used to lengthen an otherwise short amputation stump (Fig. 205-15).

The correction of the constriction rings and separation of digits are best initiated within the first year of life, preferably as close to 1 year as possible. Simultaneous hand and foot procedures are best performed before the child begins to walk and explore the environment with his or her hands. Caring for a child with bilateral upper limb restraints in the form of casts can be challenging for busy parents but will become impossible once the youngster begins to ambulate. Complex procedures such as digital transposition, toe transfer, skeletal lengthening, and bone grafts should be delayed until the child is much older and the surgeon is comfortable with the size of the hand and the structures to be dissected. However, all the major reconstructive work should be completed by school age.

In those with extensive and complex rings, amputations, syndactylies, digital fusions, and web space contractures, many staged procedures will be necessary. Here, one can operate on both hands (and feet) simultaneously before 12 to 14 months of age.

Principles of Correction

The principles of digital and thumb constriction ring correction are the following:

- Excision of the central scarred region and atrophic skin and replacement with normal skin flaps.

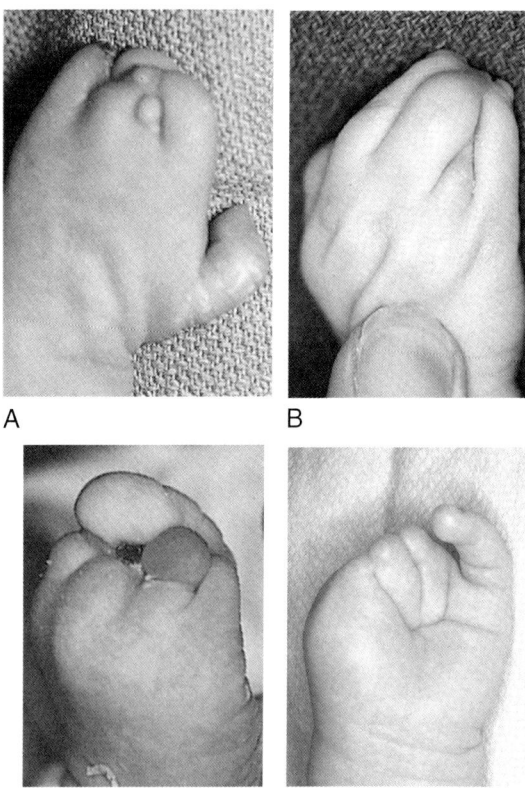

FIGURE 205-13. Bands in newborn nursery. *A* to *D,* All of these infants show some form of acrosyndactyly and had large intradigital sinuses and small distal soft tissue connections, which were conveniently released in the newborn nursery under local anesthesia. Adjacent digits were then allowed unrestricted growth. If the bands are more than 1.0 cm in width, release may be more appropriately performed in operating room conditions.

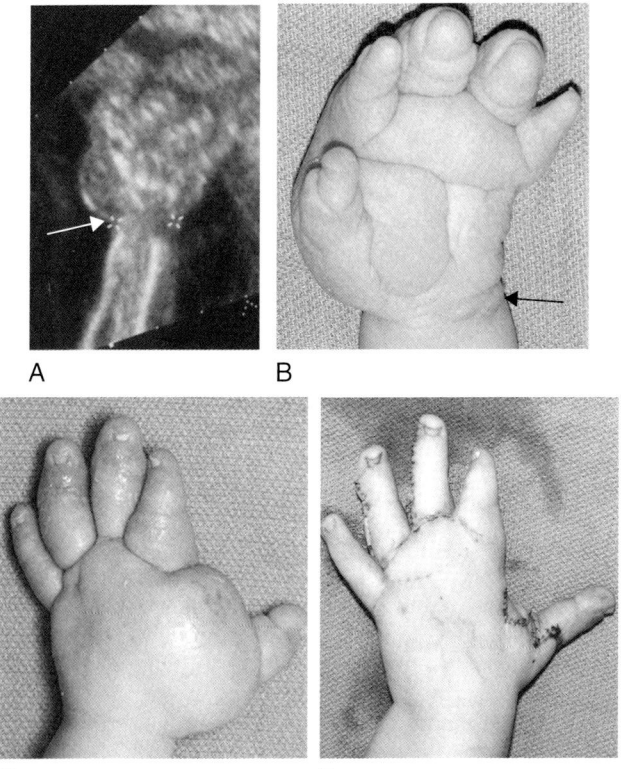

FIGURE 205-14. Fetal surgery and misdiagnosis. *A,* The diagnosis of CRS was made from this fetal ultrasound study, which showed excessive swelling of the wrist and hand distal to an area of presumed constriction *(arrow). B* and *C,* The clinical appearance of the hand at birth was more consistent with a lymphatic malformation. The scar along the wrist flexion crease *(arrow)* is secondary to an open release performed during the third trimester. Most of the swelling noted at birth was on the dorsal surfaces. *D,* Clinical appearance after multiple debulkings. All incisions have been placed in the midaxial line of either the digit or the hand.

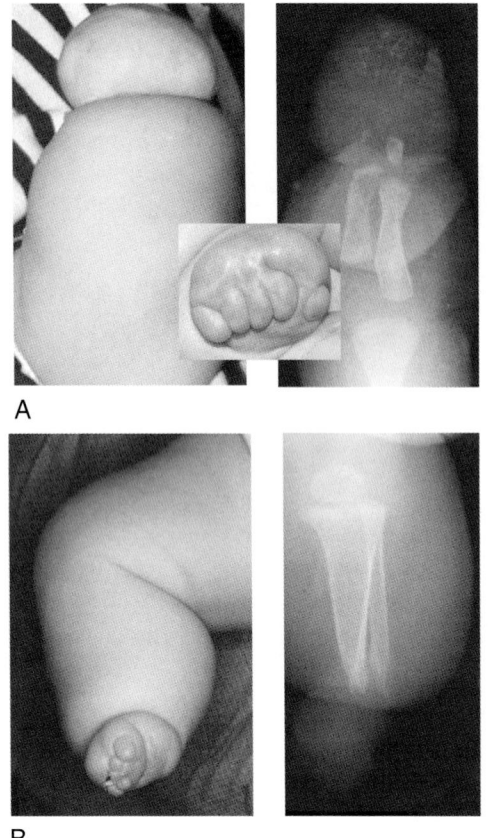

A

B

FIGURE 205-15. Diminutive hands and feet. *A,* Rarely, a diminutive hand or foot is found distal to a constriction ring. The parents of this baby refused to have the floppy hand amputated. The ring was corrected in two stages and the distal part bone grafted to the residual radius to lengthen a short below-elbow amputation stump. *B,* The small mobile foot remnant without much skeletal development was amputated so that this child could be fitted early with a below-knee prosthesis.

- Maintenance of digital length and joint mobility, especially of the thumb.
- Separation of digits and thumb to allow unrestricted growth.
- Design of well-padded, sensate, scar-free amputation stumps.
- Design of scar-free first web space lined by full-thickness flaps.
- Orientation of incisions along the sides of digits or thumb and the borders of the hand.

For correction of the simplest shallow bands, linear closures with Z-plasties are sufficient. In such cases, most authors have recommended release of only half of the circumference of the digit, forearm, arm, leg, or foot at one time,[86,91,96,97] whereas others do not hesitate to perform a one-stage total release.[46,72,87,94,98-103] Thirty years ago, general opinion held that not more than 50% of the circumference should be dissected at

one time and that a staged reconstruction should always be performed. Although I and many others frequently perform single-stage corrections, staged procedures are safe for patients with deep rings or significant amounts of distal swelling.[50]

A number of techniques have been described for release of the deeper rings. Most of the traditional explanations describe making a series of Z-plasties or W-plasties but make little mention of the tight scar band at the depth of the groove or the atrophic tissue along the sidewalls and the indurated fatty tissue within the distal swollen part. A good release should deal with all three.

Technique of Correction of Constriction Ring

Both shallow and deep constriction rings can be corrected with this method, which is designed to minimize conspicuous, depressed dorsal scars (Figs. 205-16 and 205-17) and to correct the contour deficiency. With distal and sometimes with proximal soft tissue swelling, there is an excess of skin. Transverse incisions are outlined dorsally on both sides of the depressed ring by use of a pen to mark one side of the groove. Simple compression of the soft tissue will leave a matching mark on the opposite side (Figs. 205-18 and 205-19). On the sides of the digit, thumb, wrist, or arm, all skin is saved.

Incisions are made proximally and distally, and all skin within the sidewalls is excised. Two layers of tissue are elevated: first, the skin and some superficial fat; and second, the deep fat and areolar tissue, which is easily mobilized above the extensor tendons dorsally or the flexor sheath palmarly. Excess deep fat is excised, and the flaps are advanced to fill the contour defect. The outer skin flaps are then advanced over this closure, appropriately trimmed, and sutured. The excess tissue on either side of the digit or thumb is also mobilized, advanced, trimmed, and closed so that the transverse incision of the Z-plasty corresponds with the midlateral line of the digit or thumb. A simple everted 6-0 mild chromic skin closure of the transverse incision is all that is visible dorsally. Subcuticular closures are used for larger surfaces on a leg, thigh, arm, trunk, or abdomen. Over time, Z-plasties, bilobed flaps, W-plasties, and other local transposition flaps on these surfaces become depressed; however, transverse incisions with contour beneath do not.

All scarred tissue within the depth of the ring must be excised, and concerted effort should be made to preserve large dorsal veins and palmar nerves, arteries, and flexor tendons (see Fig. 205-18). In the correction of deep rings, the most harm can be inflicted distal to the proximal interphalangeal joints, where the neurovascular structures are normally located in the subcutaneous tissue just below the dermis (see Fig. 205-17).

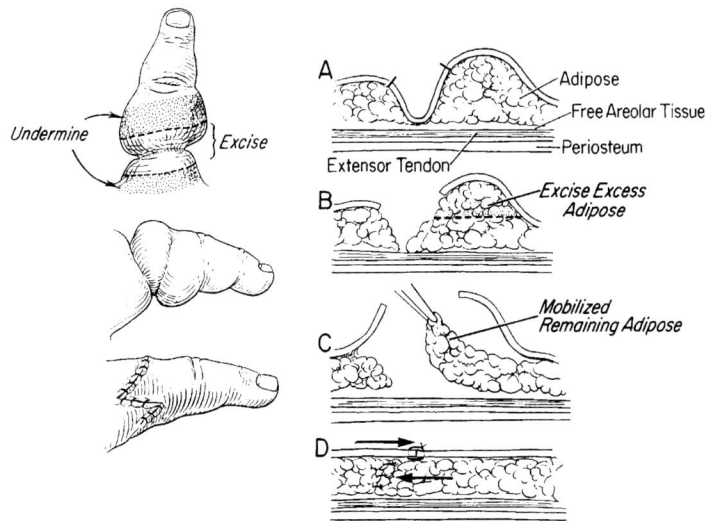

FIGURE 205-16. Technique of shallow or deep ring correction.[72] Excision and restoration of contour involve more than a simple series of Z-plasties. *A* and *B,* A complete excision of skin within the entire depth of the groove is usually possible because excess tissue is present. *C,* Dorsal and distal adipose tissue is debulked while a tongue is retained and mobilized into the defect made by the groove. *D,* Differential closures of the skin and underlying fat will help minimize a residual groove or ring. Z-plasties in the midlateral or midaxial lines of the digit conform better than do multiple smaller Z-plasties around the entire circumference of a digit or thumb.

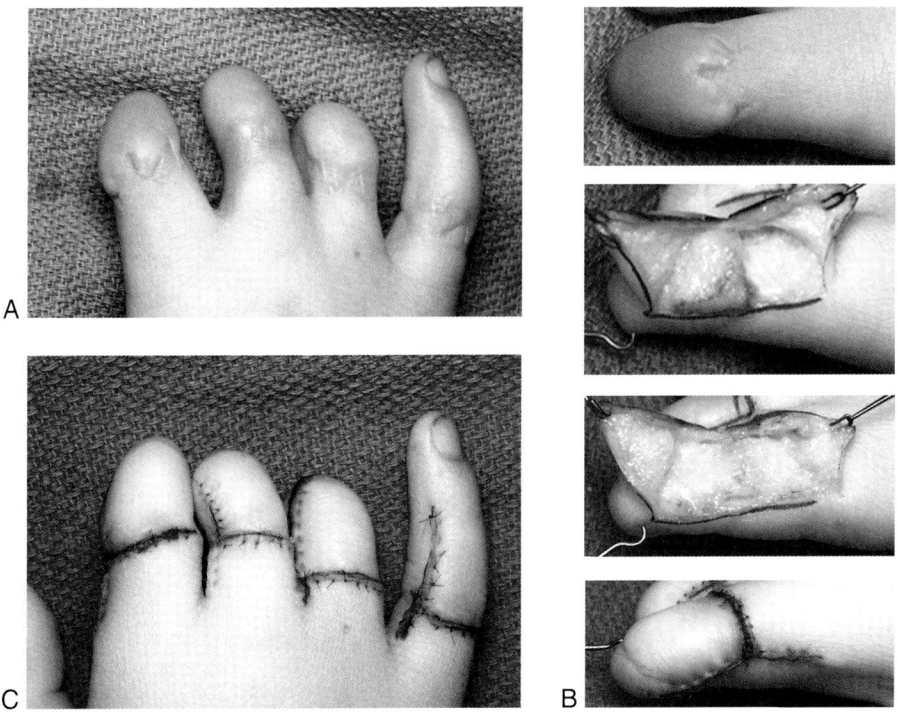

FIGURE 205-17. Constriction ring release. *A,* Depressed, conspicuous, "sawtooth" scars are seen after a circumferential ring release with multiple Z-plasties. Distal swelling of all four digits is present. With time, the scars become depressed and experience increased distal swelling. *B,* Correction consisted of scar excision, contouring of distal fat tissue, flap advancement, and closure with a transverse dorsal incision. Redundant tissue is easily excised through midaxial incisions. A Z-plasty or local rotation or transposition flap is best located along the side of the digit or thumb. Straight-line closures were all that was necessary here. *C,* Multiple digits can be corrected during the same tourniquet run of 90 minutes.

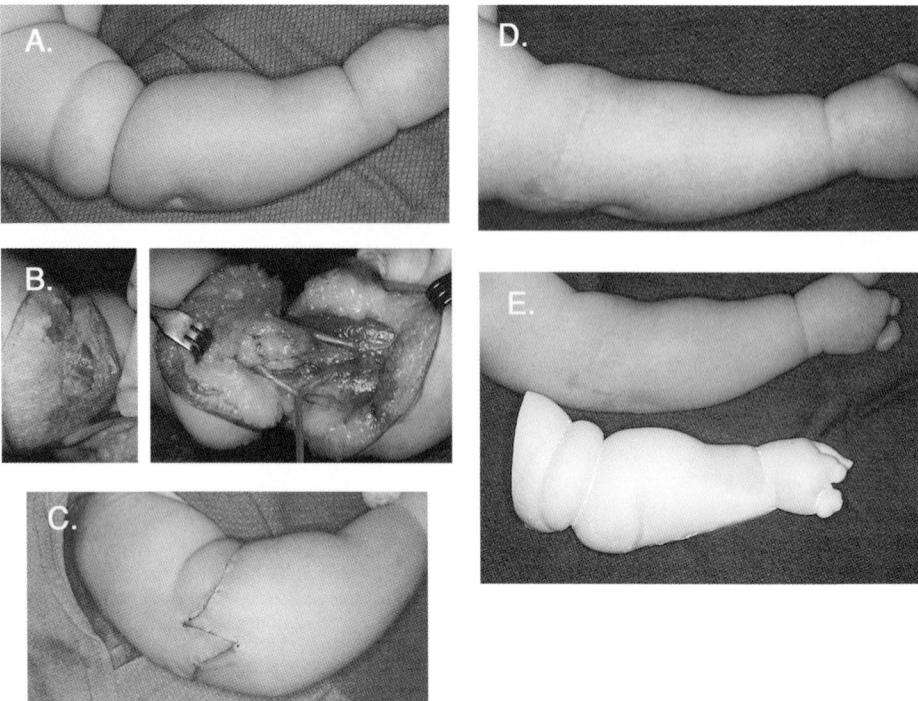

FIGURE 205-18. Constriction ring correction. *A,* A deep circumferential ring is present in the proximal forearm-elbow level. *B,* The ring depth typically extends to the tight muscular fascia. No veins have been encountered. After fascial excision, the median and radial nerves have been released and the muscle compartments decompressed. *C,* With layered closure, the Z-plasty has been positioned on the posterior surface. *D,* Two years later, the contour improvement has been maintained. *E,* The growth of the arm at age 23 months compared with the preoperative mold made at age 3 months.

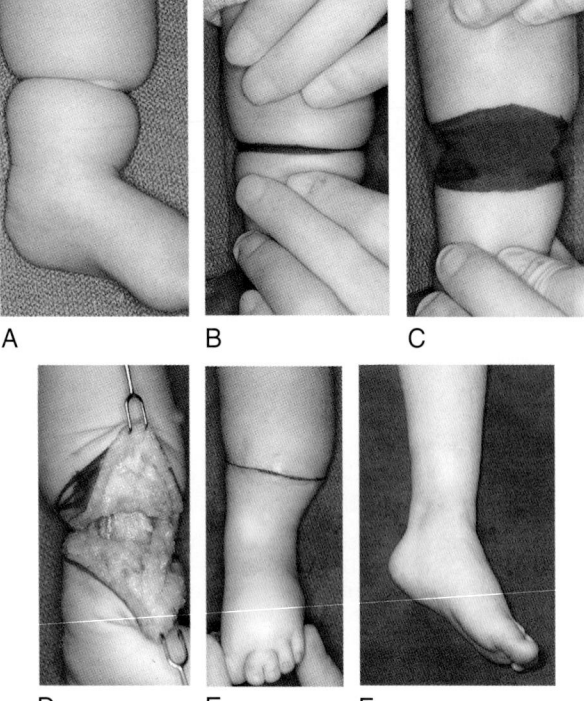

FIGURE 205-19. One-stage CRS correction. *A,* A deep constriction ring in the midtibial region is marked by pressing the opposite sidewalls together. *B,* The amount of skin to be excised is always greater than anticipated when it is marked out. *C,* This is extra skin. *D,* No superficial draining veins were noted above the dense muscular fascia. The deep venous system is intact and runs parallel to the three axial arteries to the foot and ankle. *E,* Subcutaneous adipofascial flaps are approximated across the defect, and Z-plasties are made on the sides of the leg (if necessary). *F,* Clinical appearance of the same leg 11 years later. No revisions have been necessary.

Specific Clinical Problems

ACROSYNDACTYLY

The principles of syndactyly releases are covered in Chapter 204. However, the morphologic appearance in CRS goes well beyond the incomplete and complete simple syndactylies seen in most conditions and has

acquired the name acrosyndactyly (Greek *akros*, peak, summit, topmost) (Fig. 205-20). A large number of unique problems are seen within these variations of syndactyly and require both ingenuity and meticulous technique if a satisfactory surgical outcome is to be achieved. When multiple digits are involved with a common ring or scar, the digits are usually hypoplas-

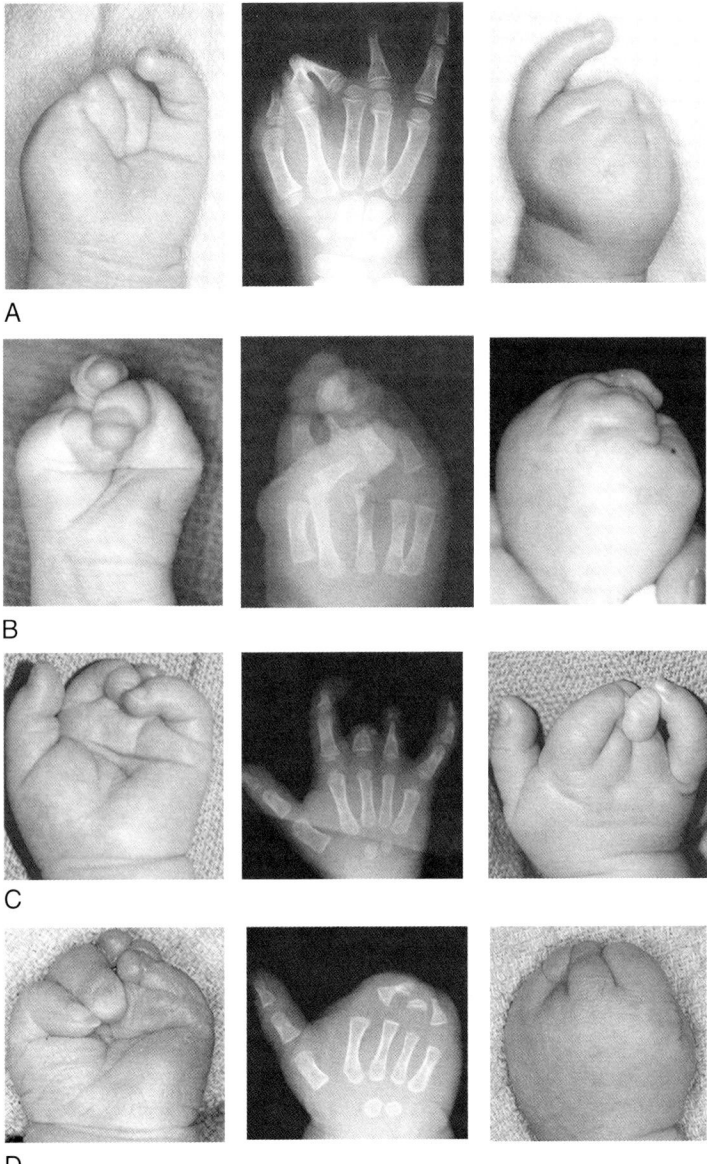

FIGURE 205-20. Acrosyndactyly. There are many variations in the definition of acrosyndactyly, which refers to a characteristic distal coalition of digits resembling a summit or peak. *A,* Clinical appearance and radiograph show a coalescence of the thumb-index-long rays at the proximal phalangeal level. Sinuses are present between all three digits. *B,* The thumb in this infant is free of the index-long-ring fibrous union within another acrosyndactyly. *C,* The central three rays in this acrosyndactyly contain one well-formed distal part. *D,* All four digits are joined in this acrosyndactyly. The thumb and first web space (not shown) were normal.

tic, and there is only a fibrous union at the site of digital coalition. When the constriction cuts off the blood supply to distal parts, the hand resembles a peak, and when remnants of digital tips remain, the appearance is similar to a bunch of grapes, in which the most palmar digit is the index finger (Fig. 205-21). These hands with fused digits need to be released in stages to preserve blood supply to distal parts. Normal neurovascular bundles are not present in the distal parts. I have often excised the central scar and advanced proximal undisturbed skin across the gap before digital separation. In these cases, the most palmar distal parts have been positioned on top of the index proximal phalanx, where a fibrous union with angulation develops instead of a solid skeletal union. These separated digits are always short and thin.

Because no two cases are identical, the hand surgeon must use both caution and creativity during these separation procedures. Neurovascular structures must be identified proximal to the fibrous union, and dissection on both sides of a digit should be avoided. Discarded skin may be used as a de-epithelialized spacer to improve contour defects. Although a full thickness of skin within epithelialized sinus tracks may be used as a local pedicle flap, the tissue is often unsuitably located or too macerated to be effective. The advancement of undisturbed or relatively normal full-thickness skin flaps across this fibrous track will often improve both venous and lymphatic drainage of the distal part, and it is wise to complete this stage before the separation of the coalesced digits.

BALLOON DIGITS OF THE NEWBORN

Rarely, a newborn will present with a tight constriction ring associated with excessive distal swelling and cyanosis (Fig. 205-22). The most common presentation is of a massively swollen digit or toe distal to a

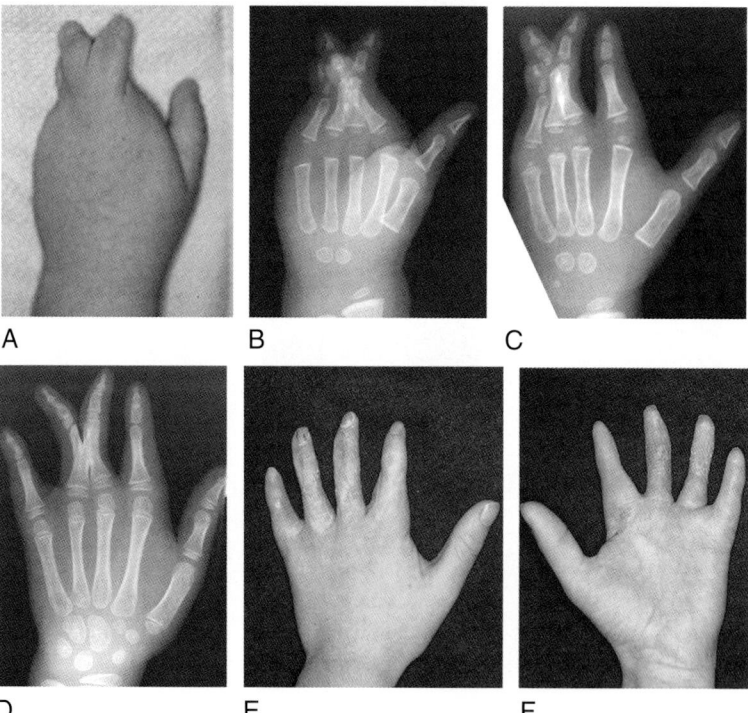

FIGURE 205-21. Acrosyndactyly. *A,* The clinical appearance at age 1 year of the left hand of a baby with distal coalition of all four digits at the level of the proximal and middle phalanges. *B,* The radiographic appearance does provide important information about the identification of the bunched distal digital parts. The tip of the index finger is usually palmar. *C,* The first procedure was to liberate the index ray. Further dissection of the fifth finger at this time would have placed the other tips in jeopardy because the blood supply at the level of fibrous union can be marginal. *D,* The fifth finger was released next. *E* and *F,* Clinical appearance at age 4 years after release of the central two digits combined with osteotomies for correction of lateral deviation. The patient is now 25 years old. No further revisions have been necessary. Growth of all digits has occurred, but they are shorter than on the uninvolved side.

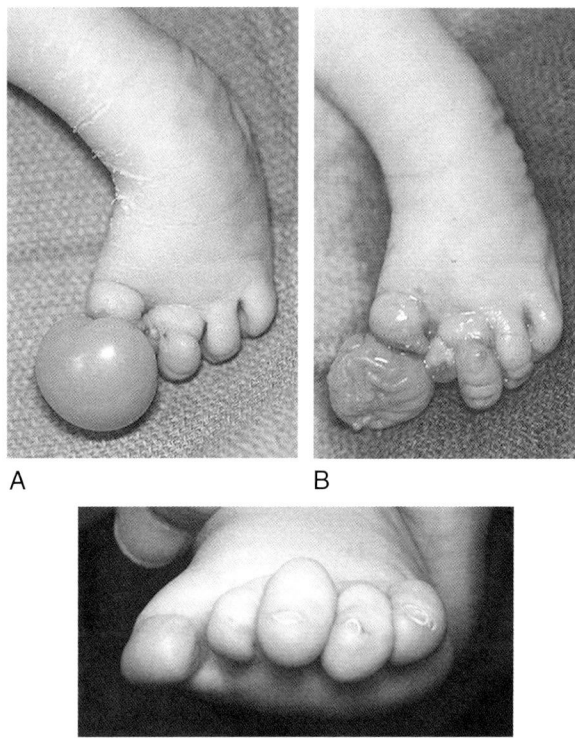

FIGURE 205-22. Massive distal swelling. *A,* The massive swelling distal to a deep circumferential constriction ring represents a fluid-filled cyst. *B,* Immediate decompression will effectively relieve the pressure and decrease the potential for infection. Excessive distal soft tissue is débrided and best contoured to the defect, and the soft tissue is used to bridge the defect. Most of the extra tissue is closed in the midaxial lines of the toe. *C,* Clinical appearance at age 11 months when the child began to walk.

tight constriction ring, although entire feet or hands can be involved. Immediate decompression of the distal fluid-filled cyst and release of the ring are indicated. I excise at least 50% of the ring and use the distally based tissue excess to resurface and to recontour the region of the constriction. Nerve injuries are frequent when these rings are proximal in the wrist, arm, leg, or foot. It is not necessary to decompress lymphedematous masses with good capillary reflow during the neonatal period. These less ballotable masses contain fibrous adipose tissue and are best trimmed down during the definitive ring correction.

When an entire hand or foot is involved, it may be salvageable if the distal part is of normal size and contains at least one major artery and has intact sensory nerves. Midforearm tight constrictions are more often associated with congenital below-elbow amputations. On occasion, a hypoplastic nonfunctional hand will be attached by a soft tissue bridge (see Fig. 205-15).

SINUSES

Sinuses seen with acrosyndactyly are well epithelialized dorsal to palmar conduits that represent the level of the initial separation of digits. They do not represent the appropriate level of new commissure placement. Treatment is discussed in Chapter 204 (see section on acrosyndactyly). Because these sinuses are normally located distal to the normal commissure depth and consist of macerated tissue, excision of the entire sinus is the preferred treatment.[50,55,104] On occasion, these small sinuses may become walled off early in life and become the nidus for the development of an epidermal inclusion system that may present any time later in life as a painless mass with or without infection.[62,72,105] I have encountered these cysts on eight hands during the past 25 years (Fig. 205-23).

SHORT THUMB AND DIGITS

Isolated transverse amputations of digits at the proximal phalangeal level are not treated unless a ray resection has been requested for aesthetic reasons or the ray is transposed to construct a thumb. Separation of two proximal phalanges joined distally in an acrosyndactyly will produce very short and thin stumps that may not function as well as the original coalition (Fig. 205-24). These transverse amputations of the thumb or digits at the phalangeal level are ideal candidates for toe to hand transfers, primarily because all the proximal anatomy is normal. I prefer a modified great-toe transfer[106,107] instead of the second toe for the prime thumb position and like to transfer the second and

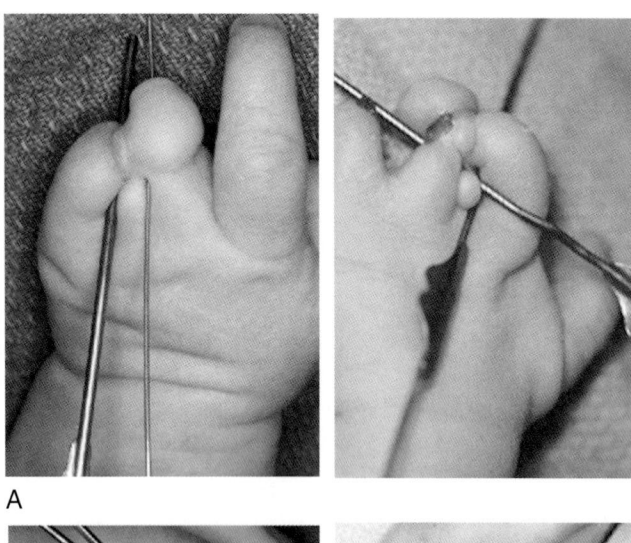

A

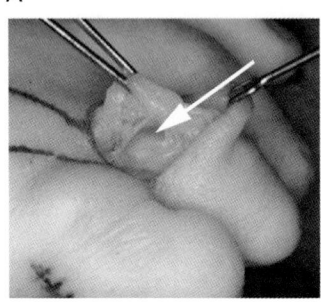

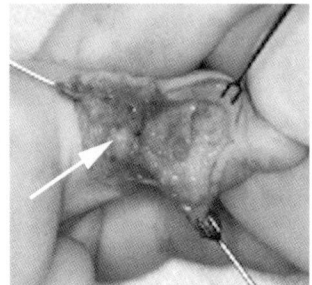

B

FIGURE 205-23. Sinuses and inclusion cysts. *A,* Dorsal to palmar epithelium-lined sinuses are present in most acrosyndactylies. The location and orientation of the probes can provide information as to which distal part matches the appropriate proximal part. Unfortunately, they are more distal than the normal commissure location. The sinus tissue can be used as a local flap for reconstruction of a normal commissure. *B,* During the separation of these digits, epidermal inclusion cysts may be encountered *(arrows).*

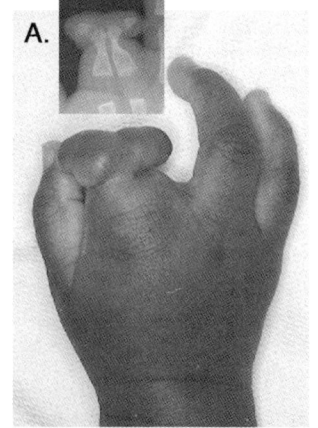

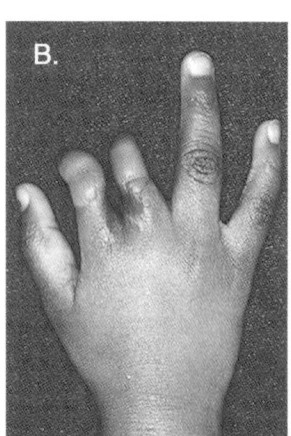

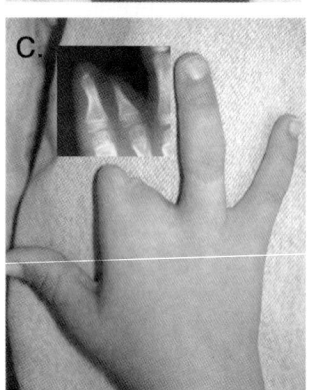

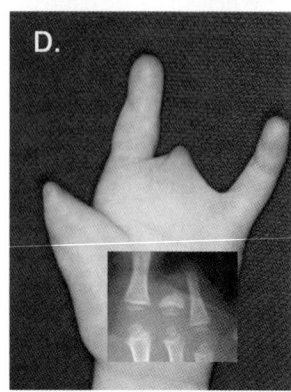

FIGURE 205-24. CRS: the short "double digit." *A,* The short index and long digits are joined at birth by a fibrous union of the outward deviation of middle phalangeal segments. Treatment consisted first of advancement of good proximal tissue across the fibrous band and realignment of the phalangeal segments followed by a formal syndactyly release with commissure flaps and skin grafts. *B,* The same hand is seen 20 years later. The tips of the index and long fingers remain bulbous but actually are quite functional. As a teenager, this patient obtained digital prostheses to be worn at important social functions. *C,* The proximal index-long union in this patient was treated as a single digit that the patient did not want to lose. It functioned well with a thumb to index key pinch. *D,* The central two digits were left as a single digit because of the proximal level of this fibrous union.

third toes (double toe transfer) whenever possible for central digit losses. These microvascular procedures are labor-intensive but well worth the effort.[83,107-110] An adequate first web space construction with full-thickness flap tissue should be completed before the toe to thumb transfer.

A second option for treatment of thumb losses at the metacarpal or phalangeal level is distraction lengthening.[72,111-114] The original applications of these methods in the hand were for post-traumatic amputations in adults. In these cases, the external fixators were left for many months until the bone regenerate became solid. The bone, which develops by "callotasis," originates from both periosteum and the medullary canal and moves from both ends of the osteotomy site toward the central portion of the gap. Healing is much better at the forearm and metacarpal levels, where the distracted gap is surrounded by well-vascularized muscle.[72] In young children, it is best to distract the ray to the desired length, remove the external fixation apparatus, and fill the intercalated gap with a bone graft held with an internal plate.[49,115] The complication rate is directly proportional to the length of time the child wears the cumbersome apparatus. Many prefer to leave the apparatus on until adequate bone fills the gap,[113,114] to hold the position with a longitudinal C wire during callotasis,[90,114,116,117] or to distract as much as possible

during one anesthetic and fill the gap with an intercalated bone graft.[115] Most of these approaches will work at the forearm or metacarpal level, but the rate and quality of new bone formation dramatically decrease at the digital level.

Because of disappointing outcomes with distraction lengthening at the phalangeal level of digits, it is not recommended. The skeletal stock is characteristically thin and tapered; therefore, the lengthened digit is very thin, and a nonunion often occurs at the juncture between the bone graft and the distal phalangeal segment (Figs. 205-25 and 205-26).

A third application in the patient with a constriction ring is the use of these techniques both to lengthen and to move a skeletal segment as part of a digital transposition (Fig. 205-27). When this is performed, it is best to disarticulate the proximal portion at a joint space (carpometacarpal or metacarpophalangeal joints) instead of making an osteotomy because a solid segment of bone will develop along the entire path of the transposed segment.

THE TWO-FINGERED HAND

An acrosyndactyly may occasionally be so severe that the digits are represented by hypoplastic nubbins with or without nail remnants. Three or more metacarpals

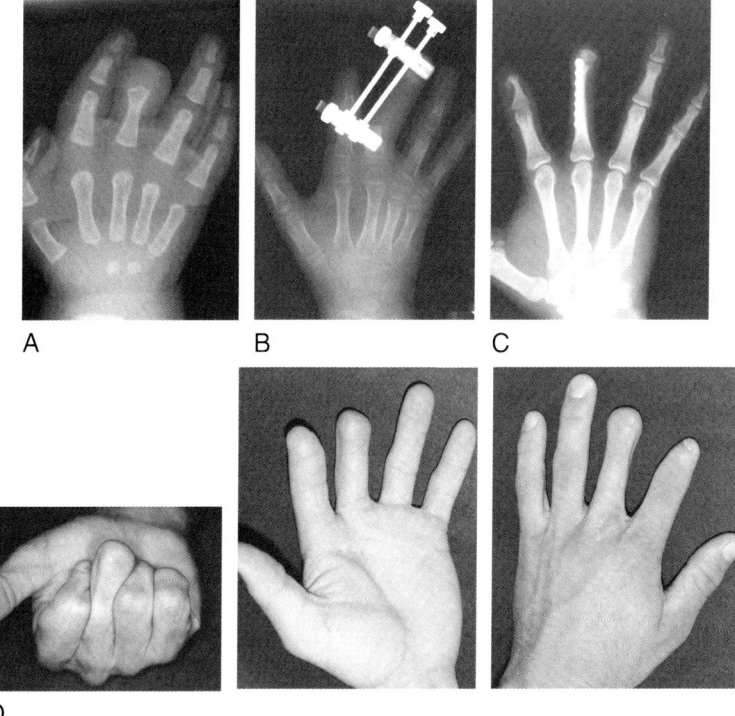

FIGURE 205-25. Digital lengthening. *A,* Radiographs of an acrosyndactyly that was treated with the usual soft tissue web and ring corrections. A transverse amputation is present at the level of the proximal interphalangeal joint of the long digit. As a teenager, he returned and requested digital lengthening for aesthetic reasons. *B,* The first stage of the lengthening consisted of mid-diaphyseal osteotomy and application of the external apparatus. The digit was purposely lengthened longer than the ring finger, which still contained some anticipated growth. *C,* Six weeks later, a bone graft was placed within the intercalated gap and fixed with a miniplate. *D,* The desired length has been achieved, but the long finger is still narrow and lacks interphalangeal motion. The patient, shown here 10 years later, has been happy with the appearance.

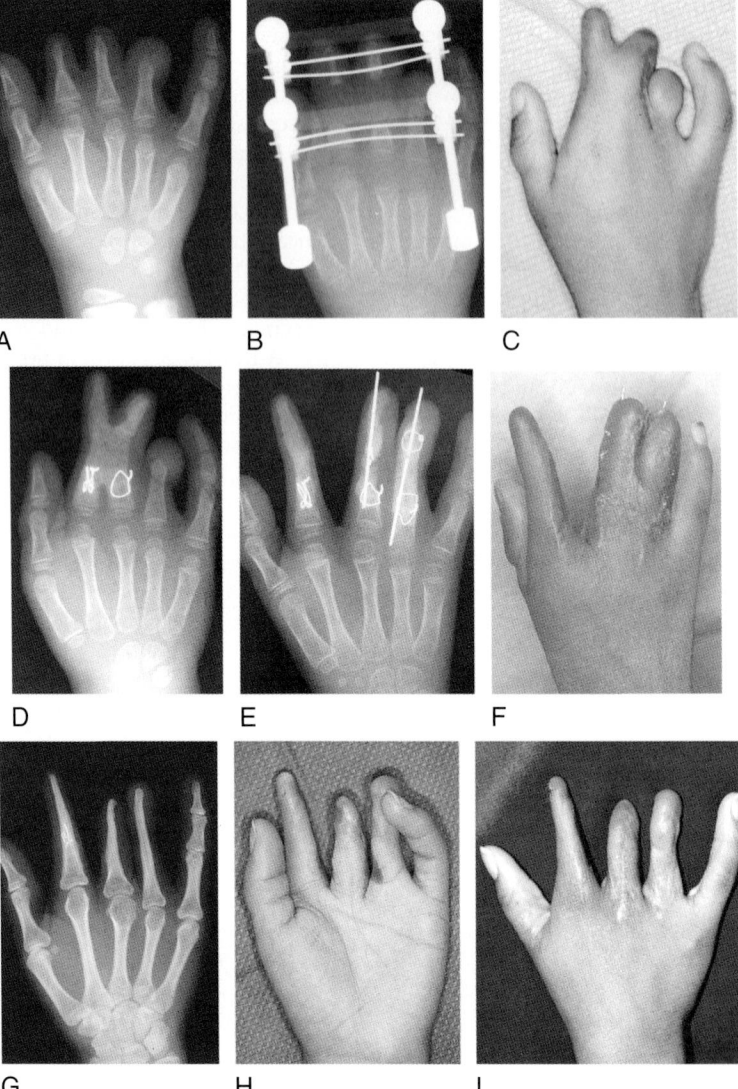

FIGURE 205-26. Digital lengthening. *A,* The radiographic appearance of the right hand of a 4-year-old child with a central acrosyndactyly that had been released during infancy. *B,* The distractor has been applied to the index and long digits. Note the tapered bone stock of the phalanges being lengthened. *C,* The clinical appearance at the end of distraction. The simple syndactyly has been made. *D,* A corticocancellous iliac bone graft was used to fill both intercalated gaps. *E,* During the next stage, the ring digit was lengthened, and a nonunion of the tip of the long ray needed to be regrafted. When this case was performed in the late 1970s, miniplates and screws were not available. Instead, intraosseous wiring techniques were popular. *F,* The incomplete simple syndactyly was then separated with the usual commissure flaps and full-thickness skin grafts. *G,* Twenty-five years later, the lengthened three digits are thin and narrow with no interphalangeal motion. *H,* She has adapted well and does not complain of the stiffness or lack of motion. Sensation on the tips is narrow. *I,* To the surgeon, the dorsal scars and hyperpigmented skin grafts are conspicuous. However, as a young mother, this patient continues to teach elementary school.

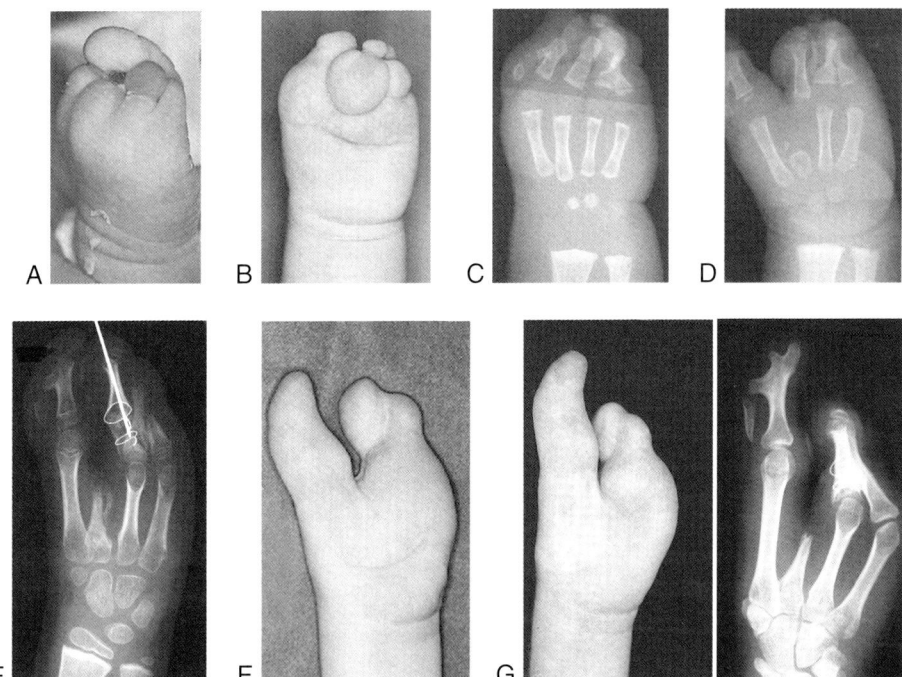

FIGURE 205-27. CRS: the "two-fingered hand." *A,* This child with acrosyndactyly had four metacarpals and hypoplastic phalangeal remnants of all digits and the thumb. The desiccated remains of an amniotic band are seen. *B,* Hidden dorsal to palmar sinuses are present between digital segments. *C,* The radiograph shows the presence of all five proximal phalanges. *D,* At 6 months of age, the long metacarpal was partially excised to form a web space, and the adductor pollicis was attached directly to the index proximal phalanx. *E,* At age 2 years, the proximal phalanx of the long finger was distracted and placed on the distal portion of the ring to fifth digit proximal phalanges. *F,* At age 10 years, he had maintained a strong pinch and did not want any more surgery. *G,* The clinical appearance and radiograph at age 20 years show the continued growth of the new thumb in comparison to the rest of the hand. Despite his limitation in grip strength, he has functioned well.

may be present in these hands, which are distinctly different from symbrachydactyly. Both hands are usually severely affected, and unfortunately, most or all of the toes are absent. Design of a basic hand with a rudimentary pinch and grasp can be beneficial for these children. The components consist of a mobile thumb on the radial side, a well-surfaced web space, and at least one finger or a post on the opposite side of the hand. An intact third metacarpal indicates that a strong adductor pollicis will be present for pinch. I have not embraced the concept of "phalangealization" or deepening the intermetacarpal space too aggressively because of the potential damage to the intact intrinsic muscles, which in this condition are normal proximal to the level of amputation. Distraction lengthening of metacarpals (Fig. 205-28) and distraction-transposition of skeletal segments on top of one another to gain length are both effective. However, damage to the growth plates and stiffness are potential complications.

In the author's series of more than 300 patients with constriction rings seen during the past 25 years, only 12 patients were born with severe acrosyndactyly without functional digits. These have been treated with construction of a basic hand that consists of a mobile thumb in the radial position, a web space, and at least one digit or post on the opposite side. The presence of a third (long) metacarpal indicated the presence of an adductor pollicis muscle, which could be used to provide an effective pinch. In addition, the extrinsic flexor tendons, which extended to the distal common scar of the acrosyndactyly, could be used for the same purpose. Unfortunately, most of these patients had no toes available for transfer (see Figs. 205-27 and 205-28).

SIDE-BY-SIDE SHORT DIGITS

After release of distal acrosyndactylies, two digits often remain connected by scar tissue at the end of thin, tapered diaphyses. All combinations (index-long, long-ring, ring-small) may present, but central digit coalitions are most common. When these are separated surgically, the end result is often disappointing.

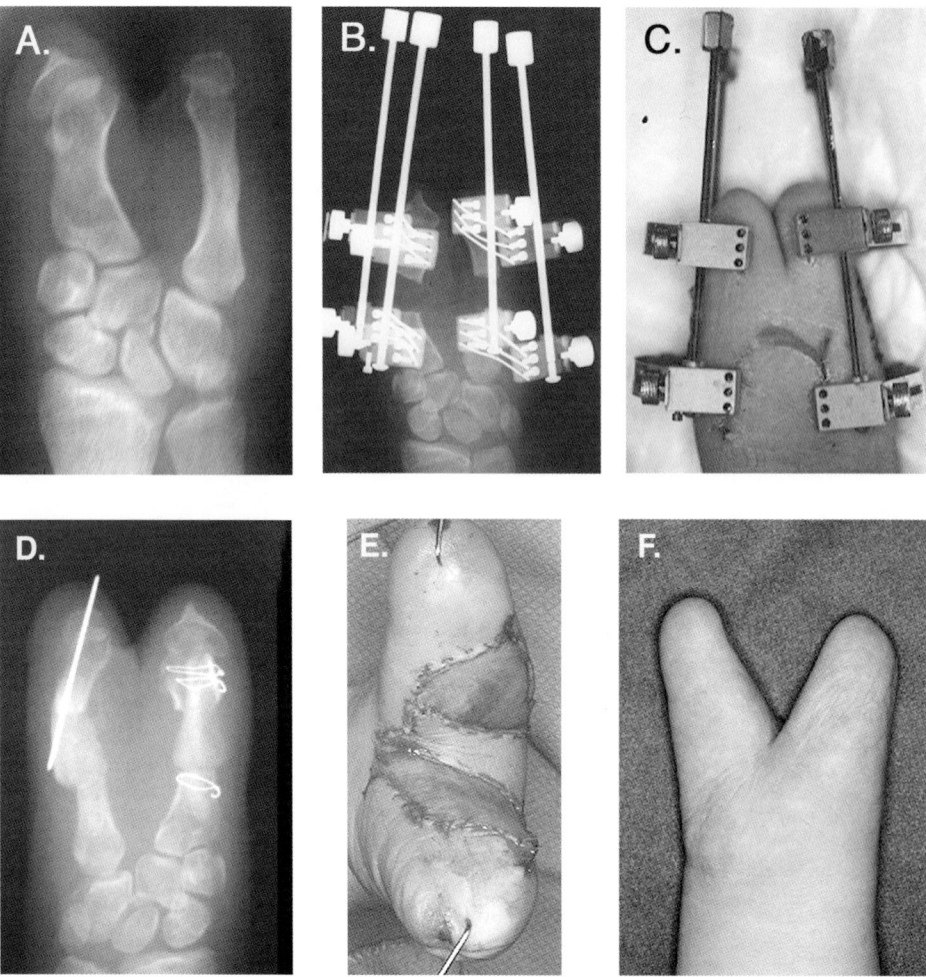

FIGURE 205-28. Two-fingered hand (Clark). *A,* A CRS patient from the mid-1970s is seen with a two-metacarpal and no-digit hand. On the opposite lower limb, she had below-knee amputation. No toes were present on the other lower extremity. Possible allograft transfer was discussed at the time but rejected by the family. *B,* The radiograph shows the distractors in place. The webbing between the rays had not been released. *C,* The clinical appearance of the Cowen apparatus used at that time. *D,* When the desired length had been obtained, the intercalated gaps were filled with corticocancellous iliac bone grafts. *E,* The syndactyly was released with a large commissure flap and full-thickness skin grafts. *F,* A functional pinch was possible after the web space deepening.

The phalangeal stock is usually inadequate for lengthening, and the author's preference after years of all types of treatment is to leave them alone to function as a single digit. The only procedure necessary is local soft tissue stump revision.

THE "FLOPPY" INDEX FINGER

Another problem encountered in severe central digit acrosyndactylies is the assignment of distal fingertips with nails to the available proximal phalanges with intact metacarpophalangeal joints. When there is an intact thumb and a good first web space, the priority solution is to transpose one of the best distal segments into the index position. The index finger

is usually the most palmar on the radial side of the coalition, and its corresponding distal tip is the most radial. This is accomplished well in stages, but instability of the index tip or residual malunion with ulnar deviation often results (Fig. 205-29). This surgery must be completed within the first 5 years of life, but secondary procedures for stabilization are necessary.

FLEXED DIGITS

In complex acrosyndactylies and cases with multiple side-to-side fusion of digits, proximal or middle phalangeal segments are positioned in a flexed position, which is not originally appreciated because of the

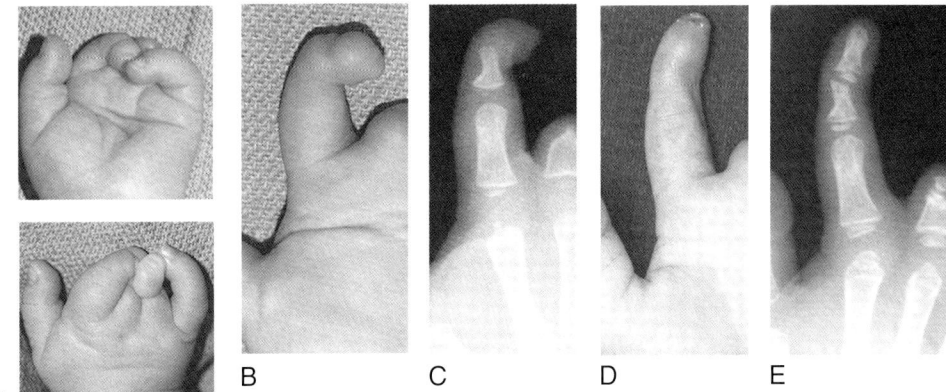

FIGURE 205-29. The "floppy" index finger. *A,* Dorsal and palmar views of an acrosyndactyly at birth. The instinct of the reconstructive surgeon is to save the floppy central fingertip, which is blanched in this view. *B,* The tip was saved and positioned on top of the index digit. *C,* The radiograph at age 18 months shows that it contained no significant bone. *D,* This tip was stabilized with a nonvascularized toe phalangeal transfer. The characteristic ruddy hue is present whenever the hand is cold. There is no perceived pain by the child. *E,* Radiograph shows that the growth plate is open 4 years later.

delayed ossification of these small tapered bones. This is not appreciated during childhood because these digits are often encased by bulbous soft tissue envelopes. Later in childhood or during adolescence, they can be repositioned with joint releases followed by digital separations. On the ulnar side of the hand, these realigned joints can become functional.

SOFT TISSUE ASYMMETRIES

The abnormal bulk of soft tissue, the location distally within the digit, and the marginal blood supply of the distal lymphedematous parts all conspire to make final outcomes frustrating from an aesthetic standpoint (Fig. 205-30). Frequently, these outcomes are more both-

FIGURE 205-30. Disappointing outcomes. *A,* The appearance of a hand with superficial and deep constriction rings with and without lymphedema. Multiple-staged ring corrections combined with syndactyly releases were completed within the first few years of life, and the child's hand functioned well. *B,* The clinical appearance 10 years later demonstrates many of the common aesthetic problems, which include the atrophic, infected nail; a rotated floppy tip of the index finger; hyperpigmented scars along the sides of the released digits; a bulbous long fingertip distal to a narrow contracted finger; and the absence of normal fingertips and nails with transverse amputations. Despite these differences, most children adapt and use these hands effectively. *C,* The short ulnar two digits in this hand are conspicuous because of the excessive deepening of the web space and the bulbous palmar surface of the long finger. *D,* Despite some correction, the hypoplastic index and long finger nails, irregular web spaces, and redundant tissue along the sides of all digits are obvious. With soft tissue refinements, this hand would be much more acceptable to the surgeon, but the patient had no complaints.

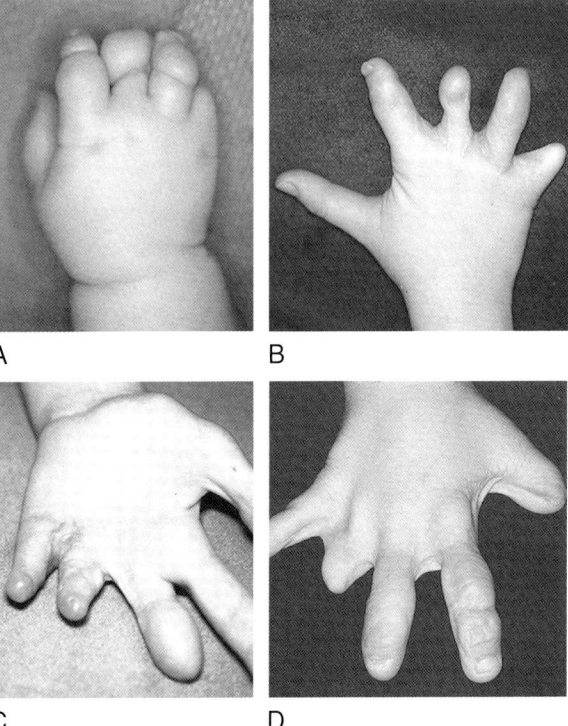

ersome to the critical surgeon than to the patient and family. Despite aggressive defatting, distal soft tissues may remain bulky, and the irregularities can be accentuated by contracted or *biscuited* scarring along suture lines. The best way to avoid these problems is to advance the normal proximal skin flaps as far distally as possible while the distal tissue is debulked. Initially, I tried to incorporate as much of the distal soft tissue into the correction as possible. With time, I realized that this is not normal tissue and is preferably excised and replaced by normal proximal tissue (if possible). When the distal parts are defatted and inset, every effort must be made to make the closures in the high midlateral or midaxial line along the sides of the digits. Achieving the goal of a symmetric digit with normal contour at the site of the previous constriction ring can become a formidable task.[49,50]

POINTED AMPUTATION STUMPS AND HYPOPLASTIC NAILS

After separation, the tips of shortened digits often have pointed, painful, hypermobile tips, which are best treated with skeletal shortening and advancement of full-thickness skin flaps. The nail plates of distal digital parts in severe acrosyndactyly deformities are often deficient and grow slowly. These nails are not functional. If recurrent infection or pain is present within the first few years of life, excision and closure with good full-thickness tissue are preferred. If these digits are left until the child and parents become psychologically attached to them, they may remain prob-lematic for life. On-top-plasty of local tissue with skeletal elements is an option both to maintain length and to improve appearance, but after multiple procedures, the final outcomes are often more disappointing to the self-critical surgeon than they are to the functional patient.[118,119]

MICROVASCULAR THUMB AND DIGIT TRANSFER

These procedures are covered in Chapter 208. The distinguishing feature of CRS thumbs is that all of the anatomy proximal to the level of the ring or transverse amputation is normal.

Complications

There are few large series of constriction ring patients and even fewer with a discussion of complications. In the past 25 years, data have been obtained for more than 300 patients, not all of whom I have operated on. As adults, they are resourceful and grateful patients who do not remember many of the problems encountered during their reconstructions, such as infection, hematoma, flap necrosis, distal circulatory failure, sensory loss, and skeletal malunion and nonunion.

The early problems, such as maceration, infection, and graft loss, relate primarily to inadequate immobilization of the active child. Flap necrosis, distal circulatory compromise, and distal digital loss are all secondary to the interruption of adequate flow to the parts distal to the constriction. Sensory losses are subtle

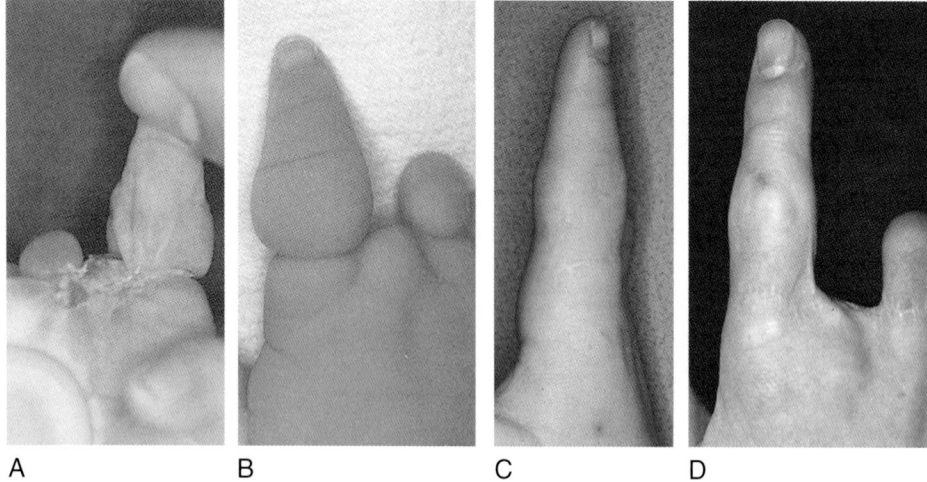

A   B   C   D

FIGURE 205-31. Growth. *A,* The remnants of an amniotic band at the base of an index digit are seen in a newborn. *B,* As the baby grew, the distal swelling and lymphedema became more prominent. The digit was never compromised. A two-stage ring correction was performed at the time. *C,* The Z-plasty along the side of the digit is seen at age 19 years. *D,* The growth of the phalangeal segments has not been proportional. The proximal phalanx of the index grew more than that of the ring, and the small proximal phalanx of the long ray did not grow at all.

and are not recognized until the child is older and able to communicate during sensory testing. In the younger child, the digit or hand that does not wrinkle after 5 to 10 minutes of water immersion is usually an insensate part. Skeletal malunion and more commonly nonunion occur frequently in CRS when phalanges in particular with poor skeletal stock are either manipulated with osteotomies or lengthened by distraction techniques (see Fig. 205-30).

GROWTH

With most congenital differences, the hypoplastic hand usually grows proportionally with the rest of the limb or body. In CRS, the growth centers distal to and just proximal to the constriction ring may be injured (Fig. 205-31; see also Fig. 205-30). Often, the hypoplastic phalanges with atrophied parts such as nails do not grow. Parents commonly ask (and children often fantasize about) whether the abnormal parts will "catch up" and reach normal size and contour. The answer is an emphatic no.

REFERENCES

1. Swanson A: A classification for congenital limb malformations. J Hand Surg Am 1976;1:8-22.
2. Smith D: Recognizable Patterns of Human Malformation. Philadelphia, WB Saunders, 1982:1-9.
3. Jones M: The spectrum of structural defects produced as a result of amnion rupture. Semin Perinatol 1983;7:281.
4. Patterson T: Congenital ring constrictions. Br J Plast Surg 1961;14:1-31.
5. Hall EJ, Johnson-Giebink R, Vasconez LO: Management of the constriction ring syndrome: a reappraisal. Plast Reconstr Surg 1982;69:532-536.
6. Moses J, Flatt AE, Cooper R: Annular constricting bands. J Bone Joint Surg Am 1979;61:562-565.
7. Ogino T, Saitou Y: Congenital constriction band syndrome and transverse deficiency. J Hand Surg Br 1987;12:343-348.
8. Weinzweig N, Barr A: Radial, ulnar, and median nerve palsies caused by a congenital constriction band of the arm: single-stage correction. Plast Reconstr Surg 1994;94:872-876.
9. Montgomery W: Observations on the spontaneous amputation of the limbs of the fetus in utero with an attempt to explain the occasional cause of its production. Dublin J Med Chem Sci 1832;1:140.
10. Lennon G: Some aspects of fetal pathology (with special reference to the role of amniotic bands). J Obstet Gynecol Br Empire 1947;54:830.
11. Torpin R: Fetal Malformations Caused by Amnion Rupture During Gestation. Springfield, Ill, Charles C Thomas, 1968.
12. Torpin R, Faulkner A: Intrauterine amputation with the missing member found in the fetal membranes. JAMA 1966;198:185-187.
13. Glessner J: Spontaneous intra-uterine amputation. J Bone Joint Surg 1963;45:351.
14. Inoue G, Inagaki Y: Extra digit arising from the forearm. J Hand Surg Am 1991;16:650-652.
15. Rayan GM: Ectopic implantation of constriction band intrauterine digital amputation. Plast Reconstr Surg 2001;107:1000-1002.
16. Pillay V: Congenital constriction bands in Singapore. Singapore Med J 1964;5:198-202.
17. Froster UG, Baird PA: Amniotic band sequence and limb defects: data from a population-based study. Am J Med Genet 1993;46:497-500.
18. Bower C, Norwood F, Knowles S, et al: Amniotic band syndrome: a population-based study in two Australian states. Paediatr Perinat Epidemiol 1993;7:395-403.
19. Foulkes GD, Reinker K: Congenital constriction band syndrome: a seventy-year experience. J Pediatr Orthop 1994;14:242-248.
20. Zionts LE, Osterkamp JA, Crawford TO, Harvey P: Congenital annular bands in identical twins. J Bone Joint Surg Am 1984;66:450-453.
21. Lubinsky M, Sujansky E, Sanger W, et al: Familial amniotic bands. Am J Med Genet 1983;14:81-87.
22. Lockwood C, Ghidini A, Romero R: Amniotic band syndrome in monozygotic twins: prenatal diagnosis and pathogenesis. Obstet Gynecol 1988;71:1012-1016.
23. Blanc WA, Mattison DR, Kane R, Chauthan P: L.S.D., intrauterine amputations, and amniotic-band syndrome. Lancet 1971;2:158-159.
24. Temtamy SA, McKusick V: Digital and other malformations associated with congenital ring constrictions. Birth Defects Orig Artic Ser 1978;14:547.
25. Light TR, Ogden JA: Congenital constriction band syndrome. Pathophysiology and treatment. Yale J Biol Med 1993;66:143-155.
26. Garza A, Cordero JF, Mulinare J: Epidemiology of the early amnion rupture spectrum of defects. Am J Dis Child 1988;142:541-544.
27. Pillay VK: Intrauterine amputations and annular limb defects in Singapore. J Bone Joint Surg Am 1965;47:514-519.
28. Poswillo D: Observation of fetal posture and causal mechanisms of congenital deformity of palate, mandible, and limbs. J Dent Res 1966;45:584-596.
29. Rehder H: Fetal limb deformities due to amniotic constrictions (a possible consequence of preceding amniocentesis). Pathol Res Pract 1978;162:316-326.
30. Granick M, Ramasastry S, Vries J, Cohen MM: Severe amniotic band syndrome occurring with unrelated syndactyly. Plast Reconstr Surg 1987;80:829-832.
31. Malpas T, Anderson N, Langley S: Ulnar club-hand and constriction-ring syndrome. Pediatr Radiol 1995;25:233-234.
32. Casaubon J: Congenital band about the pelvis. Plast Reconstr Surg 1983;71:120-122.
33. Coady MS, Moore MH, Wallis K: Amniotic band syndrome: the association between rare facial clefts and limb ring constrictions. Plast Reconstr Surg 1998;101:640-649.
34. Eppley BL, David L, Li M, et al: Amniotic band facies. J Craniofac Surg 1998;9:360-365.
35. Hudgins RJ, Edwards MS, Ousterhout DK, Golabi M: Pediatric neurosurgical implications of the amniotic band disruption complex. Pediatr Neurosci 1985-1986;12:232-239.
36. van der Meulen J: The amniotic band syndrome. Plast Reconstr Surg 1999;13:1087-1090.
37. Van Allen MI, Curry C, Gallagher L: Limb body wall complex: I. Pathogenesis. Am J Med Genet 1987;28:529-548.
38. Jones K, Smith DW, Hall BD, et al: A pattern of craniofacial and limb defects secondary to aberrant tissue bands. J Pediatr 1974;84:90-95.
39. Keller H, Neuhauser G, Durkin-Stamm MV, et al: "ADAM complex" (amniotic deformity, adhesions, mutilations)—a pattern of craniofacial and limb defects. Am J Med Genet 1978;2:81-98.
40. DeMeyer W, Baird I: Mortality and skeletal malformations from amniocentesis and oligohydramnios in rats: cleft palate, clubfoot, microsomia, and adactyly. Teratology 1969;2:33-37.
41. Van Allen MI, Curry C, Walden CE, et al: Limb-body wall complex: II. Limb and spine defects. Am J Med Genet 1987;28:549-565.

42. Yang SS: ADAM sequence and innocent amniotic band: manifestations of early amnion rupture. Am J Med Genet 1990;37:562-568.

43. Day-Salvatore DL, Guzman E, Weinberger B, et al: Genetics casebook. Amniotic band disruption sequence. J Perinatol 1995;15:74-77.

44. Keymolen K, De Smet L, Bracke P, Fryns JP: The concurrence of ring constrictions in Adams-Oliver syndrome: additional evidence for vascular disruption as common pathogenetic mechanism. Genet Couns 1999;10:295-300.

45. Der Kaloustian V, Hoyme HE, Hogg H, et al: Possible common pathogenetic mechanisms for Poland sequence and Adams-Oliver syndrome. Am J Med Genet 1991;38:69-73.

46. Emmett AJ: The ring constriction syndrome. Handchir Mikrochir Plast Chir 1992;24:3-15.

47. Emmett AJ, Morris A: Ring constriction syndrome. In Buck-Gramcko D, ed: Congenital Malformations of the Hand and Forearm. London, Churchill Livingstone, 1998:169-182.

48. Tada K, Yonenobu K, Swanson AB: Congenital constriction band syndrome. J Pediatr Orthop 1984;4:726-730.

49. Upton J: Treatment of congenital forearm and hand anomalies. In May JW Jr, Littler JW, eds: The Hand. Philadelphia, WB Saunders, 1990:5352-5356. McCarthy J, ed: Plastic Surgery; vol 8.

50. Flatt A: The Care of Congenital Hand Anomalies, 2nd ed. St. Louis, Quality Medical Publishing, 1994:292-314.

51. Uchida Y, Sugioka Y: Peripheral nerve palsy associated with congenital constriction band syndrome. J Hand Surg Br 1991;16:109-112.

52. Jones NF, Smith AD, Hedrick MH: Congenital constriction band syndrome causing ulnar nerve palsy: early diagnosis and surgical release with long-term follow-up. J Hand Surg Am 2001;26:467-473.

53. Askins G, Ger E: Congenital constriction band syndrome. J Pediatr Orthop 1988;8:461-466.

54. Weeks P: Radial, median and ulnar nerve dysfunction associated with a congenital constricting band of the arm. Plast Reconstr Surg 1982;69:333-336.

55. Flatt A: The Care of Congenital Hand Anomalies. St. Louis, CV Mosby, 1977:99-117, 228-248.

56. Moore MH: Nonadjacent syndactyly in the congenital constriction band syndrome. J Hand Surg Am 1992;17:21-23.

57. Guion-Almeida ML, Rodini ES, Pereira SC, Richieri-Costa A: Amniotic bands and the EEC syndrome. Birth Defects Orig Artic Ser 1996;30:171-177.

58. Boyd PA, Keeling JW, Selinger M, Mackenzie IZ: Limb reduction and chorion villus sampling. Prenat Diagn 1990;10:437-441.

59. Streeter G: Focal deficiencies in fetal tissues and their relation to intrauterine amputation. Contrib Embryol Carnegie Inst 1930;22:1-44.

60. Maisels D: Lobster-claw deformities of the hands and feet. Br J Plast Surg 1970;23:269-282.

61. Maisels D: Lobster-claw deformities of the hand. Hand 1970;2:79-82.

62. Lechner CT, Greene WB, Hill N: Acrosyndactyly with epidermoid inclusion cysts: evidence for the extrinsic theory. J Hand Surg Am 1993;18:842-846.

63. Clavert J, Berlizon A, Clavert A, Buck P: Etude experimentale: les amputations de membre obtenues par injection intra-annexielle de glucose chez le foetus de lapin. Ann Chir Infant 1977;18:405-411.

64. Clavert J, Clavert A, Berlizon A, Buck P: Abnormalities resulting from intra-adnexal injection of glucose in rabbit embryo—an experimental model of "amniotic disease." In Rickham P, Hecker W, Prevot J, eds: Progress in Pediatric Surgery. Baltimore, Urban & Schwarzenburg, 1978:143-164.

65. Clavert J, Clavert A, Issa WN, Buck P: Experimental approach to the pathogenesis of the anomalies of amniotic disease. J Pediatr Surg 1980;15:63-67.

66. Bokmand S, Bangsboll S, Ornvold K: Early amnion rupture or amniotic band syndrome [in Danish]. Ugeskr Laeger 1991;153:1846-1848.

67. Kino Y: Clinical and experimental studies of the congenital constriction band syndrome, with an emphasis on its etiology. J Bone Joint Surg Am 1975;57:636-643.

68. Torpin R: Amniochorionic mesoblastic fibrous strings and amniotic bands. Associated fetal malformation or fetal death. Am J Obstet Gynecol 1965;91:65-75.

69. Browne D: The pathology of congenital ring constrictions. Arch Dis Child 1957;32:517-519.

70. Torpin R, Faulkner A: Intrauterine amputation with the missing member found in the fetal membranes. JAMA 1966;198:185-187.

71. Inoue G, Inagaki Y: Extra digit arising from forearm. J Hand Surg Am 1991;16:650-652.

72. Upton J, Tan C: Correction of constriction rings. J Hand Surg Am 1991;16:947-953.

73. Weinzweig N: Constriction band–induced vascular compromise of the foot: classification and management of the intermediate stage of constriction ring syndrome. Plast Reconstr Surg 1995;96:972-977.

74. Baker C, Rudolph A: Congenital ring constrictions and intrauterine amputations. Am J Dis Child 1971;121:393-400.

75. Nagore E, Sanchez-Motilla JM, Febrer MI, et al: Radius hypoplasia, radial palsy, and aplasia cutis due to amniotic band syndrome. Pediatr Dermatol 1999;16:217-219.

76. Rowsell A: The amniotic band disruption complex. The pathogenesis of congenital limb ring-constrictions; an experimental study in the foetal rat. Br J Plast Surg 1988;41:45-51.

77. Rowsell AR: The amniotic band disruption complex. The pathogenesis of oblique facial clefts; an experimental study in the foetal rat. Br J Plast Surg 1989;42:291-295.

78. Rowsell A: The intra-uterine healing of foetal muscle wounds: experimental study in the rat. Br J Plast Surg 1984;37:635.

79. Tadmor OP, Kreisberg GA, Achiron R, et al: Limb amputation in amniotic band syndrome: serial ultrasonographic and Doppler observations. Ultrasound Obstet Gynecol 1997;10:312-315.

80. Schwarzler P, Moscoso G, Senat MV, et al: The cobweb syndrome: first trimester sonographic diagnosis of multiple amniotic bands confirmed by fetoscopy and pathological examination. Hum Reprod 1998;13:2966-2969.

81. Graf JL, Bealer JF, Gibbs DL, et al: Chorioamniotic membrane separation: a potentially lethal finding. Fetal Diagn Ther 1997;12:81-84.

82. Laberge LC, Ruszkowski A, Morin F: Amniotic band attachment to a fetal limb: demonstration with real-time sonography. Ann Plast Surg 1995;35:316-319.

83. Gilbert A: Toe transfers for congenital hand defects. J Hand Surg Am 1982;7:118-124.

84. Feingold M: Picture of the month. Amniotic constriction bands (Streeter dysplasia, ring constrictions). Am J Dis Child 1984;138:199-200.

85. Wiedrich TA: Congenital constriction band syndrome. Hand Clin 1998;14:29-38.

86. Farmer A: Congenital elephantiasis associated with constriction by anomalous bands. J Bone Joint Surg Br 1948;30:606-612.

87. Di Meo L, Mercer DH: Single-stage correction of constriction ring syndrome. Ann Plast Surg 1987;1:469-474.

88. Field J, Krag D: Congenital constricting band and congenital amputation of the fingers: placental studies. J Bone Joint Surg Am 1973;55:1035-1041.

89. Mayou BJ, Fenton OM: Oblique facial clefts caused by amniotic bands. Plast Reconstr Surg 1981;68:675-681.

90. Ogino T, Saitou Y: Congenital constriction band syndrome and transverse deficiency. J Hand Surg Br 1987;12:343-348.

91. Fischl R: Ring construction syndrome. Transactions of the International Society of Plastic and Reconstructive Surgeons, 5th Congress. Melbourne, Australia, Butterworth Pty, 1971.

92. Dobyns JH: Problems and complications in the management of upper limb anomalies. Hand Clin 1986;2:373-381.

93. Dobyns JH: Congenital ring syndrome. In Green DP, ed: Operative Hand Surgery, 2nd ed. New York, Churchill Livingstone, 1988:503-509.

94. Buck-Gramcko D: Hand surgery in congenital malformations. In Jackson I, ed: Recent Advances in Plastic Surgery. London, Churchill Livingstone, 1981:115-129.

95. Buck-Gramcko D: Constriction ring complex. In Nigst H, Buck-Gramcko D, Millesi H, Lister GD, eds: Hand Surgery. New York, Thieme, 1988:12.42-12.48.

96. Blackfield H, Hause D: Congenital constricting bands of the extremities. Plast Reconstr Surg 1951;8:101-109.

97. Stevenson T: Release of circular constricting scar by Z flaps. Plast Reconstr Surg 1946;1:39-42.

98. Greene WB: One-stage release of congenital circumferential constriction bands. J Bone Joint Surg Am 1993;75:650-655.

99. Muguti GI: The amniotic band syndrome: single-stage correction. Br J Plast Surg 1990;43:706-708.

100. Visuthikosol V, Hompuem T: Constriction band syndrome. Ann Plast Surg 1988;21:489-495.

101. Bourne MH, Klassen RA: Congenital annular constricting bands: review of the literature and a case report. J Pediatr Orthop 1987;7:218-221.

102. Bouche-Pillon M, LeFort G, Daoud S: Amniotic disease. Apropos of a series of 20 cases. Chir Pediatr 1987;28:235-239.

103. Miura T: Congenital constriction band syndrome. J Hand Surg Am 1984;9:82-88.

104. Walsh R: Acrosyndactyly. A study of 27 patients. Clin Orthop 1970;71:99-111.

105. Tanabe Y, Kikuchi Y, Nozaki M: Case of constriction band syndrome with annular epidermal cyst. Ann Plast Surg 2002;48:312-314.

106. Wei F, Chen HC, Chuang CC, Noordhoff MS: Reconstruction of the thumb with a trimmed-toe transfer technique. Plast Reconstr Surg 1988;82:506-513.

107. Upton J, Mutimer K: A modification of the great-toe transfer for thumb reconstruction. Plast Reconstr Surg 1988;82:535-538.

108. Yoshimura M: Toe-to-hand transfer. Plast Reconstr Surg 1980;66:74-83.

109. Lister G, Scheker L: The role of microsurgery in the reconstruction of congenital deformities of the hand. Hand Clin 1985;1:431-442.

110. Foucher G, Greant P, Merle M, Michon J: Congenital abnormalities of the thumb. Contribution of microsurgical technics [in French]. Chirurgie 1988;114:60-66.

111. Matev I: Thumb reconstruction through metacarpal bone lengthening. J Hand Surg Am 1973;5:482-487.

112. Seitz WH Jr, Froimson AI: Callotasis lengthening in the upper extremity: indications, techniques, and pitfalls. J Hand Surg Am 1991;16:287-294.

113. Cowen N, Loftus J: Distraction augmentation manoplasty technique for lengthening digits or entire hands. Orthop Rev 1978;7:45-53.

114. Kessler I, Baruch A, Hecht O: Experience with distraction lengthening of digital rays in congenital anomalies. J Hand Surg Am 1978;2:394-401.

115. Fultz C, Lester D, Hunter J: Single stage lengthening by intercalary bone graft in patients with congenital hand deformities. J Hand Surg Br 1986;11:40-46.

116. Wenner SM: Angulation occurring during the distraction lengthening of digits. Orthop Rev 1986;15:177-179.

117. Foucher G, Pajardi G, Lamas C, et al: L'allongement par distraction progressive squelette de la main dans les malformations congenitales. A propos de 41 observations. Rev Chir Orthop Reparatrice Appar Mot 2001;87:451-458.

118. Soiland H: Lengthening a finger with the "on the top" method. Acta Chir Scand 1961;122:184-186.

119. Peacock EJ: Metacarpal transfer following amputation of a central digit. Plast Reconstr Surg 1962;29:345-355.

Disorders of Duplication

Joseph Upton III, MD

RADIAL (THUMB) DUPLICATION

Terminology

In the past, polydactyly has been broadly classified as either preaxial or postaxial. Because duplications involving the central three rays of the hand were not accurately described, hand surgeons have preferred the terms of radial, central, and ulnar to designate the location of the duplicated parts.[1]

Glossary of Terms

Duplication. A number of authors have correctly observed that extra parts are not really exact replicas and that the extra part, wherever it exists within the hand, is abnormal both in size and shape.[1-3] Polydactyly is the term preferred by most surgeons.

Preaxial and Postaxial. Polydactyly has been further subdivided by the location within the hand.

Preaxial and postaxial have commonly been designated to be the thumb and fifth borders of the hand. The true "axis" along which the limb bud and hand develop runs through the humerus, ulna, and fifth finger. Consequently, the embryologic preaxial portions of the hand include the thumb, index, long, and ring rays.[1,2]

Radial, Central, and Ulnar. These are more descriptive designations of the location of polydactyly. Radial refers to the thumb ray; central to the index, long, and ring rays; ulnar to the fifth ray.[4,5] The Congenital Hand Committee for the International Federation of Societies for Surgery of the Hand decided to use these terms instead of preaxial and postaxial. Within each of these three regions, there may be separate classifications and designations for the level of the duplication (Fig. 206-1).

Balanced and Unbalanced. These terms have been used by many authors to describe the skeletal

215

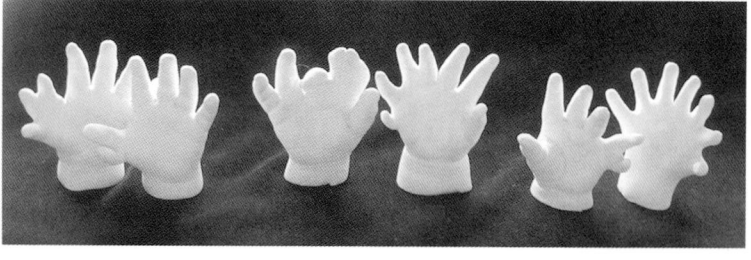

FIGURE 206-1. Duplications may occur in any region of the hand and at any level along the axial ray. These molds of individual hands illustrate a spectrum of duplications. On the radial side are examples of a double and triple thumb; in the central hand are complex duplications involving the index, long, and ring rays alone or in combination; and on the ulnar side are examples of the common phalangeal duplication of the fifth digit and the rare mirror hand with seven digits.

and soft tissue structures of each thumb relative to one another. Balanced thumbs are identical or "duplicate" partners. The overwhelming majority of thumb polydactylies are unbalanced, with the radial partner being the most deficient.

Biphalangeal and Triphalangeal. This designates the number of phalanges within the duplicate partner.

Distal, Proximal, or Metacarpal. Some authors refer to the skeletal part at which the duplication occurs with no particular designation of the joint space or bone itself.[2,6-23]

Rudimentary, Floating, or Supernumerary. This small type does not have any skeletal connection to the more normal thumb and is usually the radial of the two partners.[24] This type is often not included in many schemes of radial or thumb duplication. These types can range in size from a well-formed thumb with a phalanx to a small bulge on the radial side of the existing thumb.

Classification

With time, each classification has been refined. Present-day surgeons have used the Iowa system, which designated the type of thumb polydactyly along a longitudinal axis, divided into six levels: one for each bone and one for each joint (Fig. 206-2).[25] This system was then expanded to include a seventh category of triphalangeal duplicated and triplicated thumbs.[26] A separate subclassification of the most common site of duplication at the metacarpophalangeal (MP) joint into four specific types has been proposed.[27]

Several generations of German surgeons then provided an expanded classification organized along both longitudinal and transverse axes (Fig. 206-3).[24,28] Within this comprehensive system, the longitudinal axis is divided into 10 levels. On the transverse axis, there are individual designations for the digit involved (I to V), absent phalanx (−), partially absent phalanx (PART −), additional phalanx (+), rudimentary digit (RUD), triplication (Tr), and hand or foot. This system, although cumbersome, is logical. It can be applied to all portions of the hand.

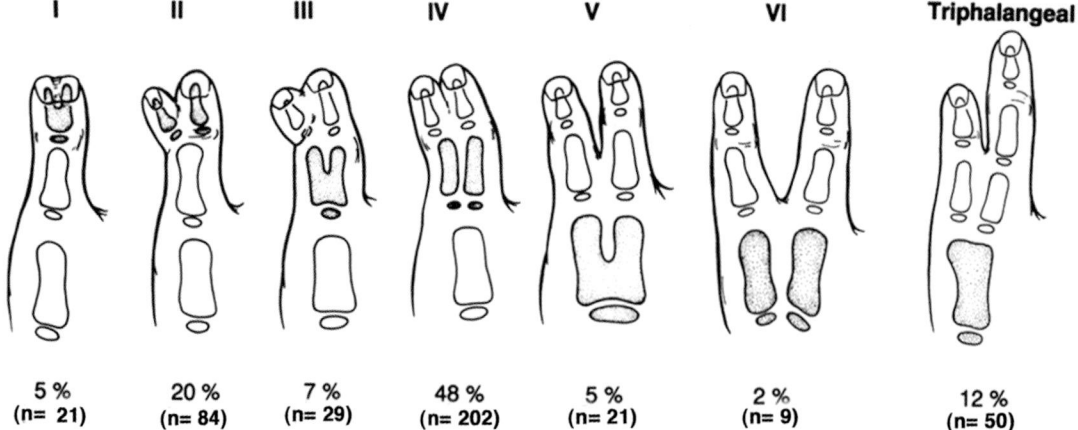

I	II	III	IV	V	VI	Triphalangeal
5 % (n= 21)	20 % (n= 84)	7 % (n= 29)	48 % (n= 202)	5 % (n= 21)	2 % (n= 9)	12 % (n= 50)

FIGURE 206-2. The Iowa system[25] is the most commonly used by hand surgeons. The level of duplication is designated by either the bone or joint of arborization. Group VII consists of unusual proximal types with and without triphalangeal components. The relative frequency of each type in our series of 416 radial (thumb) polydactylies is reflected in other large series. Duplications at the MP joint (type IV) and at the IP joint (type II) are the two most commonly treated by the hand surgeon.

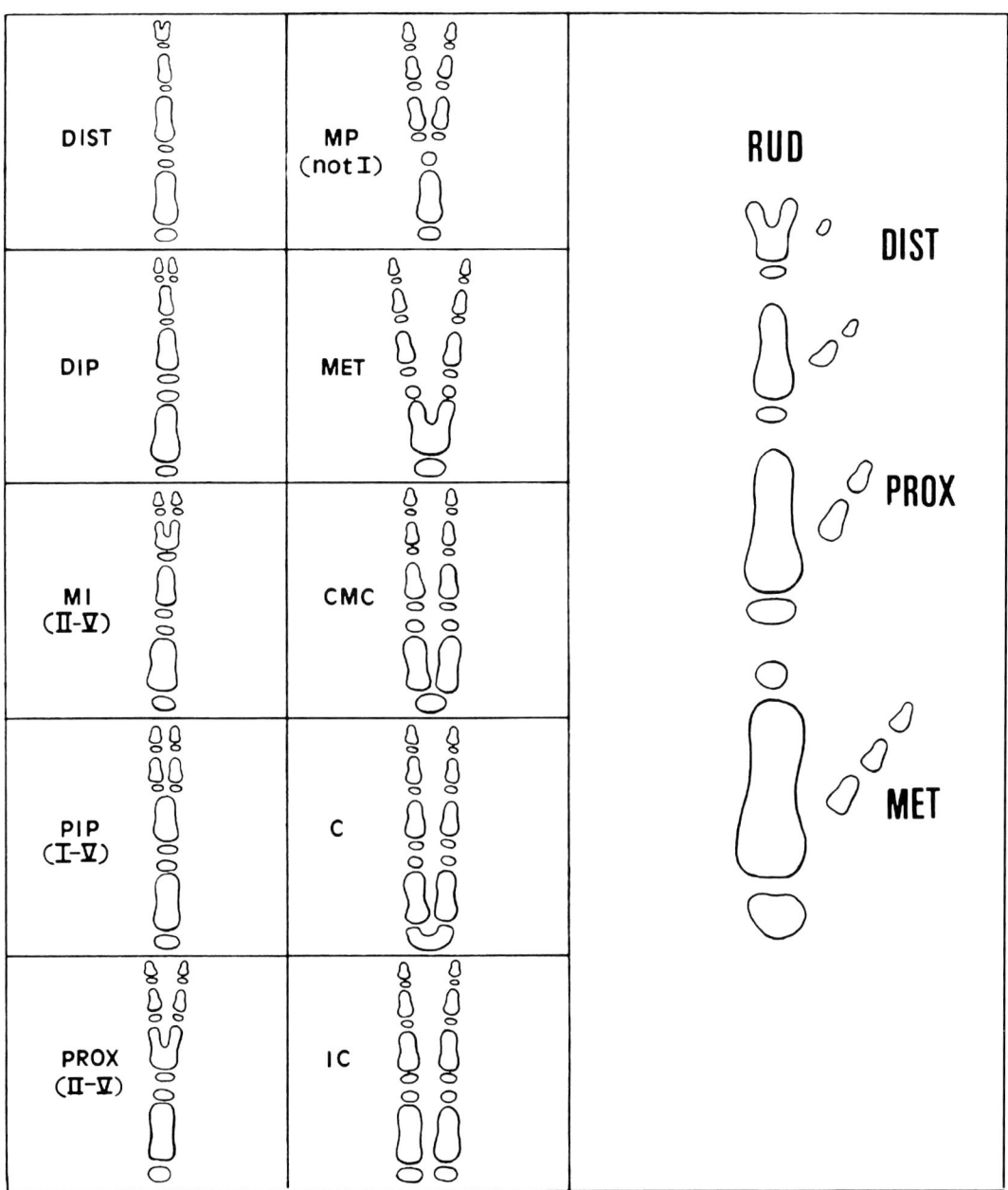

FIGURE 206-3. Illustration of the German system.[24] Each ray is designated by a Roman numeral, I (thumb) through V (fifth digit). Each digit is divided into 10 levels: DIST (distal phalanx), DIP (distal interphalangeal) joint, MI (middle phalanx), PIP (proximal interphalangeal) joint, PROX (proximal phalanx), MP (metacarpophalangeal) joint, MET (metacarpal), CMC (carpometacarpal) joint, C (carpal), and IC (intercarpal) joint. The prefix RUD is used to designate rudimentary digits or thumbs. An extra or triphalangeal component is represented by a plus sign, and an absent or partially deficient part by a minus sign. For unusual rays with three differing components, the subscript Tr is used. For foot polydactylies, the C (carpal) is changed to T (tarsal) and M (metacarpal) becomes TM (metatarsal). Hand is designated by H and foot by F.

Light[3] has also demonstrated the change in radiologic features of these thumbs from the appearance of secondary ossification centers through their closure at skeletal maturity. Radiographs obtained during the first few years of life do not give an accurate indication of the joint contour or configuration.

During the past 3 decades, hand surgeons have used the Iowa system; most have added an extra category VII for the rare and unusual types of duplications of two or more metacarpals with and without triphalangeal components.[9,26,29] Those systems proposed by geneticists[30] have not been particularly useful to the hand surgeon.

Incidence

Polydactyly, defined as an excess of digits or parts in the hand or foot, is the most common type of congenital anomaly in the upper limb. In white and Asian populations, thumb or radial polydactyly occurs more commonly than ulnar polydactyly with an incidence of 1 in every 3000 live births.[31,32] In contrast, in African American populations, ulnar polydactyly was noted in approximately 1.3% of all live births or in 13 of 1000 births,[33] and in Mexican populations, it was noted in 1 of 1000 live births.[34] Nonsyndromal thumb duplications occurred in 2.08 per 10,000 live births in a large collaborative study from Latin America.[35] Because of this variation, the overall incidence of polydactyly in the general population is estimated to occur between 2 and 19 times per 10,000 live births. When there is a positive family history suggesting autosomal dominant inheritance, up to one third have an associated congenital anomaly.[36]

The frequency of duplication at the different skeletal levels is compared in Table 206-1. Types II and IV at the distal and interphalangeal levels are the most common in all large series within the literature.

Etiology

The genetics and cause of radial polydactyly have not been precisely defined. Most reports suggest an imbalance between the apical ectodermal ridge and the underlying mesoderm. Rats given cytosine arabinoside on day 11 of their pregnancies may develop radial polydactyly.[37] In human embryos, Yasuda[38] noted a persistent folding of the apical ectodermal ridge and a notch within the first ray of the hand plate. In both human and experimental systems, there is an imbalance between cell division and programmed cell death.

A gene responsible for certain types of radial polydactyly with triphalangeal thumb and for triphalangeal thumb alone has been localized to chromosome 7q36.[39,40]

Clinical Presentation (by skeletal level of duplication)

No two polydactyly thumbs are exactly alike![41] However, the position of the skeletal elements and resting posture of the two duplicates will provide excellent clues to the underlying soft tissue abnormalities.

DISTAL PHALANX (IOWA TYPES I, II; GERMAN TYPES I DIST, I DIP)

The nail may be either fused with a longitudinal ridge or separated with the soft tissues joined at the metaphyseal level. Although the radial partner is usually the most deficient in the unbalanced types, the ulnar partner is smaller than normal. The volar pulp tissue is broad with no redundancies. The nail plate may have many configurations, depending on the amount of divergence of the diaphyseal portions of each partner. Duplicates close to one another will have a flat or convex configuration with a longitudinal ridge. In contrast, divergent type II duplicates may share a wide nail with a central concave depression. The shape of the nail is important if a sharing type of procedure is chosen for correction. The princeps pollicis artery is always the major arterial conduit.[42] Interphalangeal (IP) joint motion is present but often deficient with a broad articular surface in type II thumbs (Figs. 206-4 and 206-5).

TABLE 206-1 ✦ RELATIVE INCIDENCE OF DIFFERENT TYPES OF THUMB (RADIAL) POLYDACTYLY

Type	Chicago[3]	Boston[3]	Iowa[25]	Hong Kong[7]	Hiroshima[15]	Paris[80]
I	6	2	6	5	2	5
II	12	15	17	20	18	23
III	10	6	9	5	8	6
IV	44	43	46	32	52	39
V	4	10	12	4	0	6
VI	6	4	3	9	4	3
VII	18	20	6	14	16	18
Total	50	70	95	267	50	418

Type I

A.

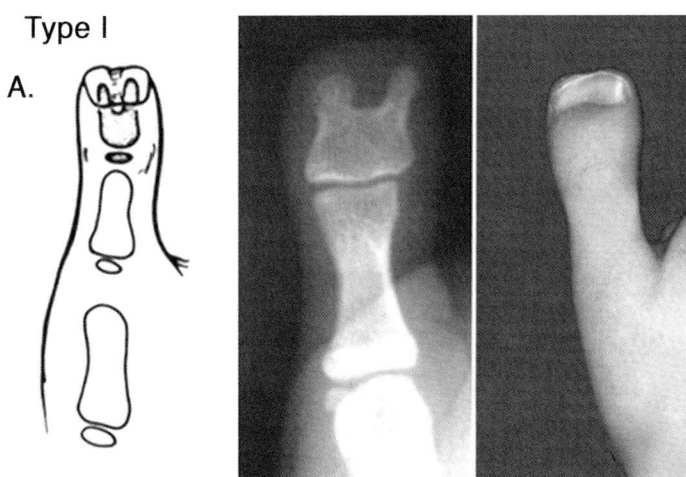

FIGURE 206-4. Distal phalangeal level thumb polydactyly. *A*, The clinical and radiologic appearance of a type I duplication within the distal phalanx. *B*, The variation sequence of duplications of the distal phalanx of a right thumb seen from a dorsal view. The example on the far left would be designated a rudimentary digit by some. The radial of the two partners is usually the most hypoplastic.

B.

Type II

A.

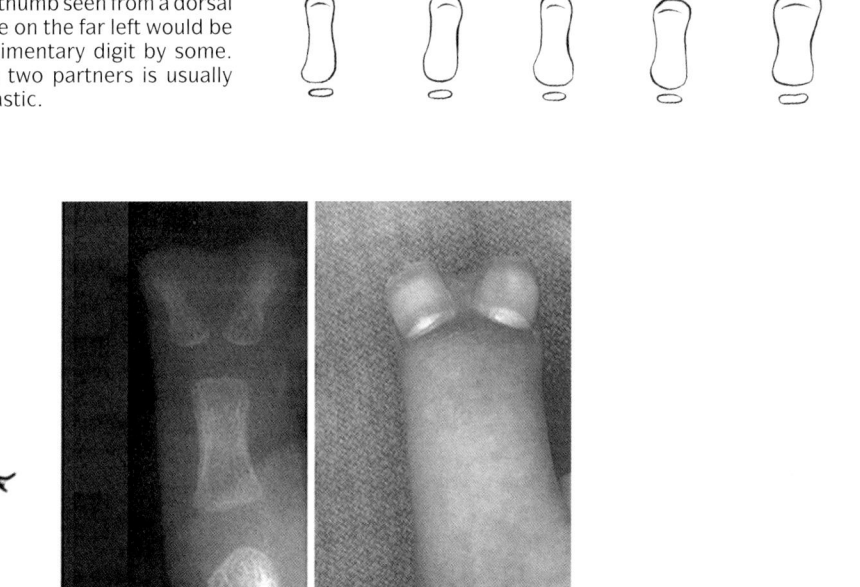

B.

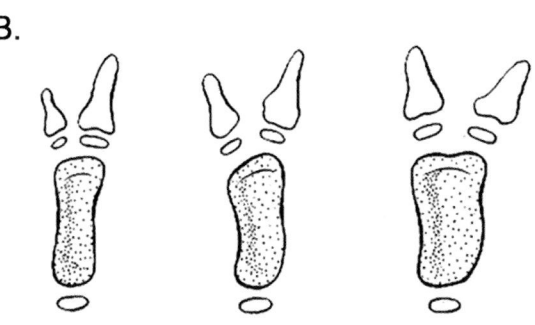

FIGURE 206-5. Distal phalangeal level thumb polydactyly. *A*, The clinical and radiologic appearance of a type II duplication at the IP joint level. *B*, The common variations seen at the IP joint level.

PROXIMAL PHALANX (IOWA TYPES III, IV; GERMAN TYPES I PROX, I MP)

In all cases, an IP joint is intact and the distal phalanx contains a separate nail. The radial thumb is invariably the most deficient partner, and more than 90% are unbalanced thumbs. Those thumbs that diverge at the proximal phalangeal level (Iowa type III; German I PROX) are usually more parallel in alignment (Fig. 206-6). The thumbs separating at the MP joint level are in *all* series the most common form of thumb duplication (see Table 206-1). All are slightly different (Fig. 206-7). The metacarpal head is broad with bifid condyles. The shape of the articular surface cannot be predicted from early radiographs. When the metacarpal head is more flat and round, the duplicates are parallel to one another. When the metacarpal head is more steep and V shaped, the thumbs diverge, sometimes greatly. They have been called pincer thumbs. Although it is smaller, the radial thumb commonly shares the extrinsic flexor and extensor with its partner. The base of the soft tissue bridge between the two marks the point at which the common flexor tendon splits toward each partner. When the proxi-

mal phalanx diverges and the distal phalanx converges, an asymmetric distal insertion of both flexor and extensor tendons can be found. Because this relationship has been present during growth and development, asymmetric, canted joint surfaces will result. The configuration of these joint may *not* change despite reinsertion of these balancing forces (Fig. 206-7*B*).

A small number of these thumbs will be balanced in terms of size and length. The same anatomic relationships described with the parallel and angulated (pincer) thumbs exist. Both polydactyly partners are much smaller than normal. One thumb may be triphalangeal with an extra phalanx. This is described in more detail later.

In all of these varieties, the ulnar thumb contains a strong ulnar collateral ligament at the MP joint level, and a normal adductor aponeurosis can be expected. On the radial side, the radial collateral ligament, abductor, and flexor pollicis brevis muscle articulate with the radial thumb unless this partner is rudimentary.

The first web space may be tight and is often overlooked with divergent type IV (German I MP) thumbs. A fibrous band is often present between the first two metacarpal heads, and the investing fascia of the first

Type III

A.

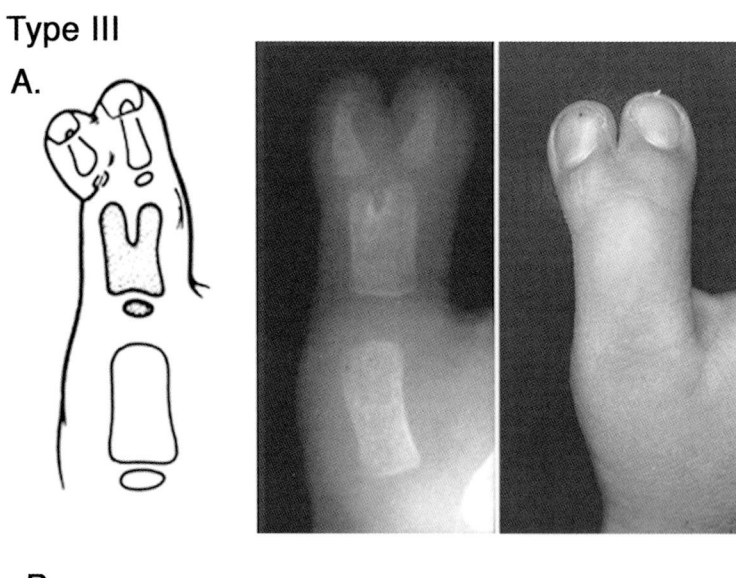

B.

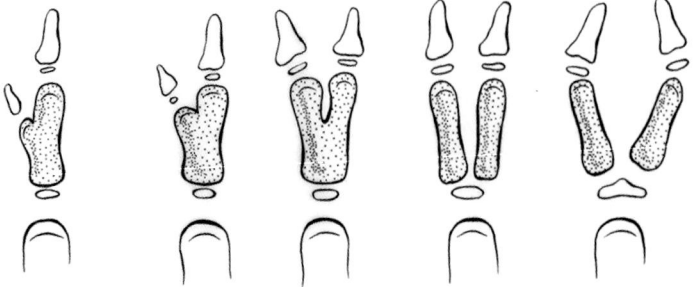

FIGURE 206-6. Proximal phalangeal level thumb polydactyly. *A,* Type III polydactylies can arise at any level of the phalanx. Both partners share a common growth plate and articular surface. *B,* A wide sequence of variation is seen; both partners may be of equal or unequal size with or without deviation from one another. The base of the proximal phalanx is usually broad.

Type IV

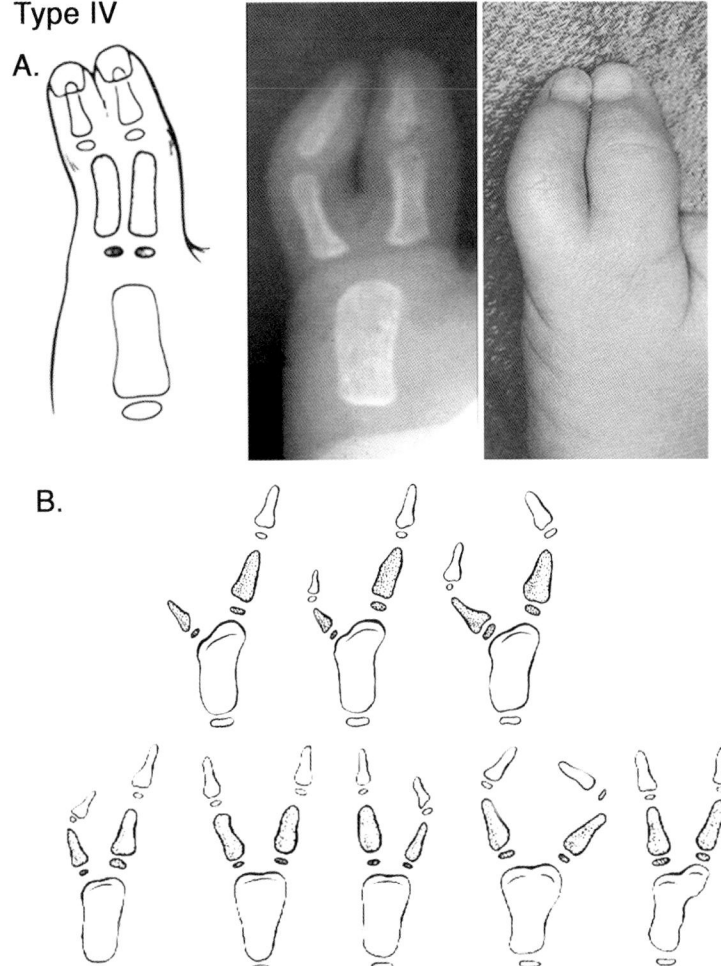

FIGURE 206-7. Proximal phalangeal level thumb polydactyly. *A,* Type IV poly-dactylies arborize at the IP joint, which creates a broad metacarpal bifid head with asymmetric condyles. *B,* A much larger sequence of eight common variations is seen, and the radial partner is deficient in all but a few cases. No two clinical cases are identical. The skeletal appearance, including the deviation and rotation of the partners, does give important clues about the soft tissue abnormalities.

dorsal interosseous and adductor pollicis muscles is abnormally thick. These fascial bands may originate both dorsal and palmar to the neurovascular bundle along the sides of each thumb.

METACARPAL (IOWA TYPES V, VI; GERMAN TYPES I MET, I CMC)

With more proximal separation, the anatomic variations with thumb polydactyly become infinitely greater and more complicated (Fig. 206-8).

A rudimentary or accessory thumb will often attach to the radial side of the first metacarpal. Thenar intrinsic muscles do not attach to this nubbin. One interesting variant is the biphalangeal thumb with a hypoplastic metacarpal positioned but not attached ulnar to the normal thumb. Because there is a metacarpal remnant, these are usually included within the type V category. Flexor and extensor tendons are shared, and intrinsic muscles attach individually to each of the proximal phalanges.

The thenar intrinsic muscles are never normal in size, and their insertions are unpredictable. Consequently, these thumbs may lack the proper pronation or palmar abduction because of their lack of proper intrinsic support. The first web space is small and in some hands nonexistent. With some type VI (German I CMC) thumbs, the ulnar partner with the best metacarpal is positioned parallel to the second metacarpal. The proximal phalanx is angulated 90 degrees at the MP joint, which has no collateral ligament stability. A deviated proximal phalanx often masks the true soft tissue deficiency within the first web space. The tight thumb-index web space must also have a tight adductor pollicis muscle and medial short flexor. The lack of normal intrinsic support often places one or more of these thumbs in the same plane as the rest of the hand.

At the phalangeal level, deviation is variable but is always present in unbalanced thumbs. This also means that joint configuration will be abnormal and range of motion usually decreased. Many types of bizarre

Type V

A.

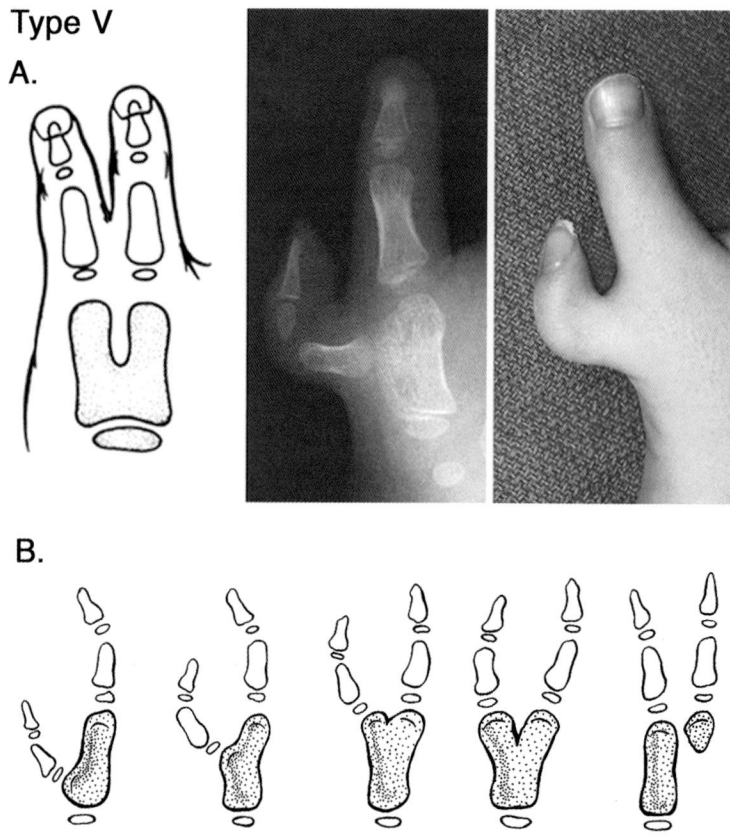

B.

FIGURE 206-8. Metacarpal level thumb polydactyly. *A*, The clinical and radiologic presentation of these less common type V forms is usually with a hypoplastic radial thumb and an intact ulnar thumb. The radial thumb in this illustration has three phalanges. *B*, Five common variations are seen. The most controversial is on the far right, in which the metacarpal head of the ulnar thumb is not attached to the radial metacarpal. The German classification describes this type as a CMC level polydactyly with a partially missing (–) metacarpal. Most common variations present a hypoplastic radial thumb with phalangeal deviation toward the ulnar partner.

configurations present at the carpometacarpal (CMC) joint level, in which the radial partner is the most hypoplastic (Fig. 206-9). Both extrinsic flexor and extensor tendons are shared and have abnormal insertions. Often overlooked are the lax or absent normal flexor retinaculum and sagittal shroud portion of the extensor mechanism at the MP joint level.

Because these metacarpals are smaller and the phalangeal segments deviated, these thumbs are much shorter than normal. Even those rare balanced duplicates at this level (Iowa V, VI; German I MET, I CMC) are short and thin. The exception, of course, is the triphalangeal partner, which commonly occurs with thumb polydactyly at the metacarpal level.

In thumbs with eccentric tendon insertions and phalangeal deviation, usually radial, one must look for the pollex abductus[13,43] anomaly, which consists of tendinous interconnections between the common flexor and extensor tendons. Held together, these extrinsic flexor and extensor muscle tendon units can function only as deviators. On the ulnar side of these thumbs, one may occasionally see a small lumbrical muscle, which may originate from the thumb and attach to the index proximal phalanx and contribute to abnormal MP flexion and supination.[44] Sheet-like connections between common extensor tendons can

often be found in the more proximal levels of duplication. These can be larger than the normal tendon.

The CMC joint may have an unusual configuration in the type VI variants. The trapezial surface is often flat instead of saddle shaped. The position of the radial duplicate surface will determine the amount of adduction-abduction as well as rotation of the retained metacarpal.

Treatment

DISTAL PHALANX (IOWA TYPES I, II; GERMAN TYPES I DIST, I DIP)

These are the easiest groups to treat. Incisions must be kept high in the axial line at the juncture of the glabrous and nonglabrous dorsal skin. In the unbalanced groups, the radial distal phalanx is trimmed, the collateral ligament constructed from local tissue, and soft tissue contoured to make a symmetric thumb tip. A broad condyle may need to be trimmed and joint deviation corrected with a closing wedge osteotomy (Fig. 206-10). The joint configuration will not change with growth and motion (Fig. 206-11). During the past 2 decades, most surgeons have included skeletal correction as part of their initial procedure.

Type VI

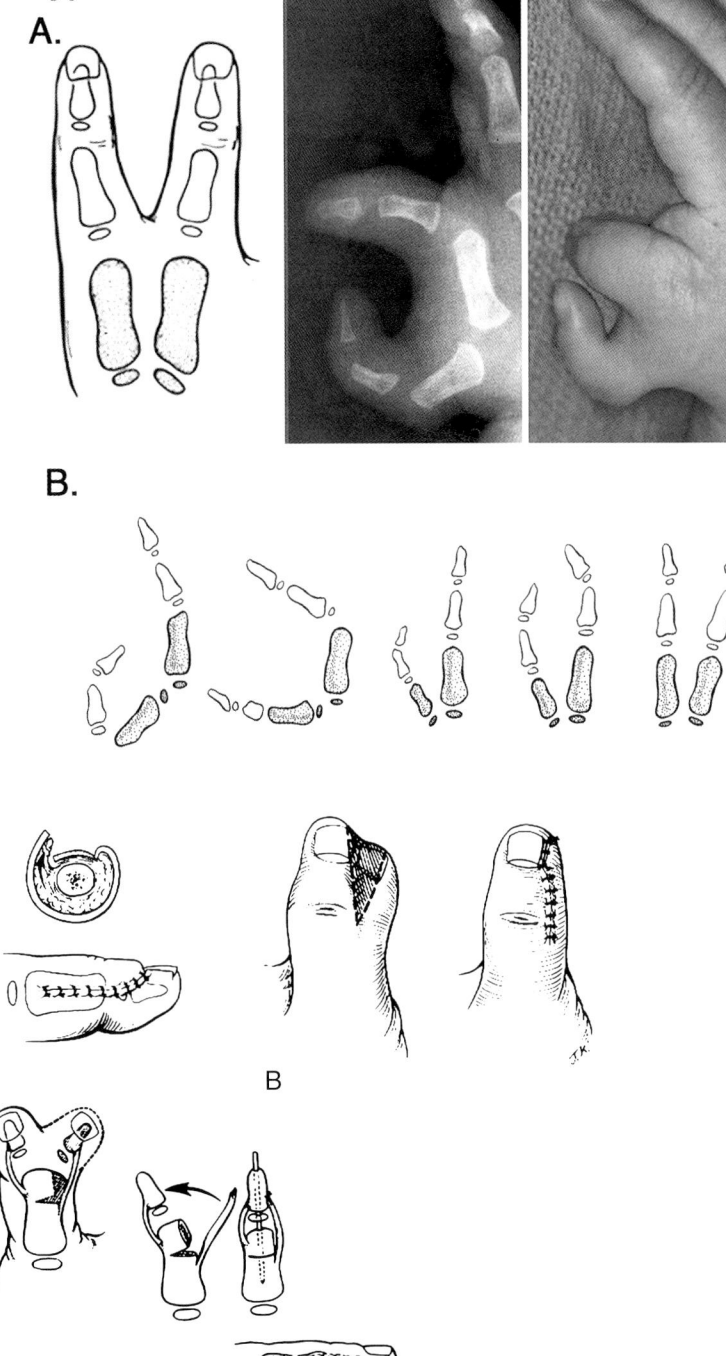

A.

B.

FIGURE 206-9. CMC joint level poly-dactyly. *A*, Type VI duplications share a common and asymmetric CMC joint with all possible levels of divergence and convergence of the metacarpals. *B*, Although a wide variety of examples are imaginable, five common variations are usually seen ranging from complete divergence of the metacarpals to a parallel positioning of equal-sized metacarpals.

A

B

C

FIGURE 206-10. Treatment of distal phalangeal types. *A*, The skeletal portion of the radial partner of a left thumb is excised and the soft tissue debulked and attached to the nail plate to construct a radial paronychial fold. *B*, The radial flap is advanced 2 to 3 mm above the nail plate and its raw edge left to epithelialize. With normal healing and contracture, a rounded, contoured nail fold will result. *C*, The broad radial condyle in type II thumbs must be excised and in some cases combined with a closing wedge osteotomy to correct excessive deviation of the retained ulnar thumb. The collateral ligament is raised on a periosteal sleeve *(arrow)*, and skin redundancies are hidden with incisions within the existing flexion creases.

A

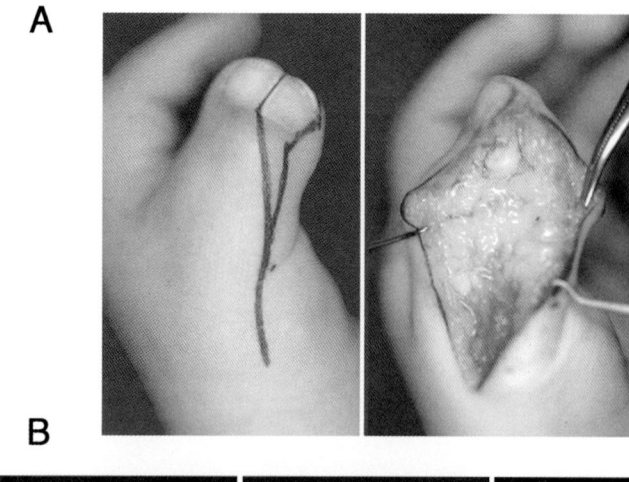

B

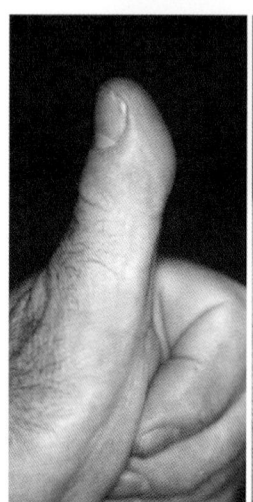
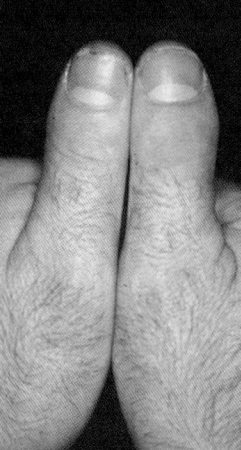
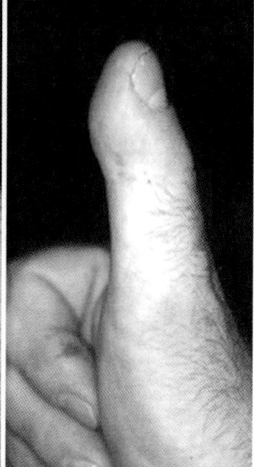

FIGURE 206-11. Type I thumb polydactyly correction. *A,* Incisions are outlined just above the juncture of the glabrous (palmar) skin and dorsal skin. The broad condyle has been trimmed and the collateral ligament resutured to the distal phalanx of the ulnar thumb. *B,* Twenty-four years later, the constructed thumb is still smaller, the pulp symmetric, and the paronychial fold well contoured without a vertical notch at its base.

In balanced thumbs of equal size, most authors prefer to excise the radial partner and to contour the soft tissue as outlined. Some prefer the Bilhaut operation,[45-47] in which the outer portions of each partner are shared to form a larger thumb. Although this reconstruction is not preferred by the inexperienced surgeon, some authors have refined their methods to achieve excellent functional and aesthetic outcomes. Most techniques save the ulnar IP joint and create a side-to-side skeletal union at the diaphyseal level. The nail matrix is repaired under magnification. Manipulation of the growth plate will affect growth. The major indication is for the thumb with small but identical partners (Fig. 206-12 and Table 206-2).

PROXIMAL PHALANX (IOWA TYPES III, IV; GERMAN TYPES I PROX, I MP)

The goal is to correct both soft tissue and skeletal structure in one operation at or before 1 year of age. The best phalangeal portions of both thumbs are incorporated to make the best thumb possible. Because the

TABLE 206-2 ✦ TREATMENT OF DISTAL PHALANGEAL DUPLICATIONS

Problems

Small nail and thumb in transverse dimension
Notch in eponychial fold
Bulge of pulp flap on radial side
Uncorrected deviation at IP joint
Conspicuous scars
Bilhaut correction: broad, flat nail with longitudinal ridge; decreased IP joint motion (see Fig. 206-12)

Caveats

Spend time narrowing the nail and reconstructing the paronychial fold.
Correct skeletal deviation initially.
An asymmetric secondary ossification center may cause deviation later in childhood. Correct this at a later date.
Avoid saving excess bulk from the excised radial partner.
Carefully document the abnormal preoperative IP joint motion.

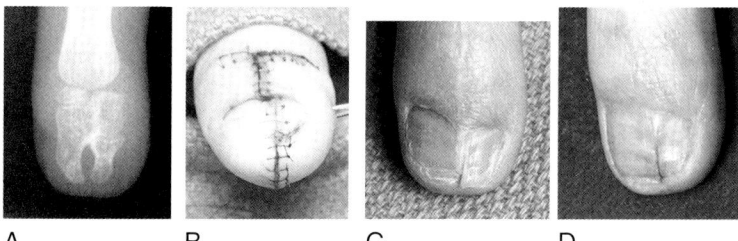

A   B   C   D

FIGURE 206-12. Correction of small identical thumbs. *A,* A thumb radiograph shows a type I polydactyly. *B,* At surgery, the longitudinal ridge between the two segments of the conjoined nail was divided, the two tufts were brought together, and the nail matrix was sutured under magnification. A concave contour was held with transverse pins. *C,* Six months later, the contour is improved, but there is a web in the eponychial fold. *D,* Four years later, the contour is maintained, the fold is improved, but a ridge still remains within the nail plate.

Iowa type IV polydactyly is the most common in the thumb, it is described in detail.

Technique of Correction (thumb polydactyly at MP joint level)

INCISION. The incision courses around the thumb (usually the radial) to be ablated at the proximal phalangeal level, leaving extra tissue for closure on both dorsal and palmar surfaces. This incision is extended in the midaxial line of the ulnar thumb proximal phalanx and along the metacarpal, 1.0 mm above the juncture between the glabrous and nonglabrous skin (Figs. 206-13 and 206-14).

DISSECTION. Dorsal and palmar flap dissections expose the extensor and flexor mechanisms, dorsal veins, and palmar neurovascular bundles of the radial thumb. The periosteum on the radial side of the radial proximal phalanx is raised with the collateral ligament, which is then isolated on a periosteal sleeve from the metacarpal. Next, thenar intrinsic muscles are detached from both bone and the extensor mechanism. The

digital artery, usually on the radial side, is cauterized. The flexor tendon is then cut sharply at the point of arborization. The retinacular sheath on the ulnar thumb is left intact, and the digital nerve is left in the palmar flap and not buried. The radial thumb is then disarticulated.

SKELETAL CORRECTION. The proximal phalanx is shifted radial at the MP joint level. The cartilage on the radial portion of the bifid first metacarpal head is incised with a knife, and the underlying bone is removed with saw or osteotome. This includes some ulnar cortex of the metacarpal. If necessary, a greenstick osteotomy is made in the metacarpal to correct angulation that cannot be corrected by advancing the ulnar proximal phalanx and reattaching the collateral ligament. Failure to remove this facet from the broad metacarpal head will result in a large radial bulge as the hand grows. Reciprocal deviation at the phalangeal level is simultaneously corrected with an osteotomy through a high midaxial incision on the distal portion of the proximal phalanx. A single 0.028 C wire can be

FIGURE 206-13. Type IV thumb polydactyly correction. *A,* The adductor pollicis brevis muscle and medial head of the flexor pollicis brevis muscle will attach to the ulnar thumb. *B,* The abductor pollicis brevis muscle and lateral head of flexor pollicis brevis muscle will be detached from the radial thumb, and the bifid metacarpal head on the radial side must be trimmed. *C,* After ablation of the radial thumb, the abductor pollicis and lateral head of the flexor pollicis brevis are attached to both bone and the extensor mechanism. If only one muscle is present, skeletal insertion is preferred. The adductor remains in its normal position.

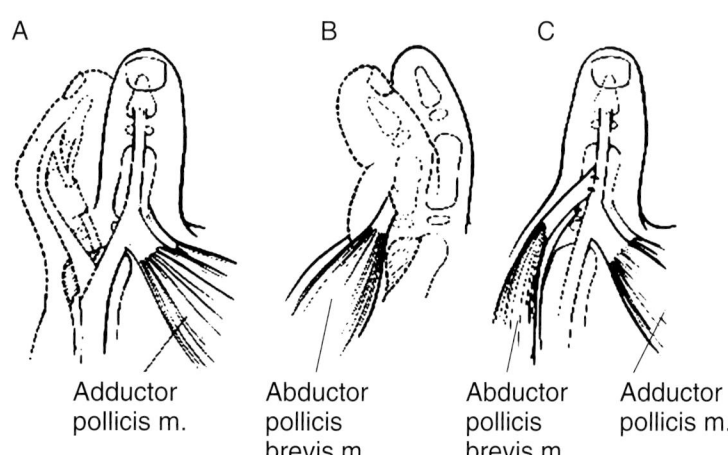

A   B   C

Adductor pollicis m.   Abductor pollicis brevis m.   Abductor pollicis brevis m.   Adductor pollicis m.

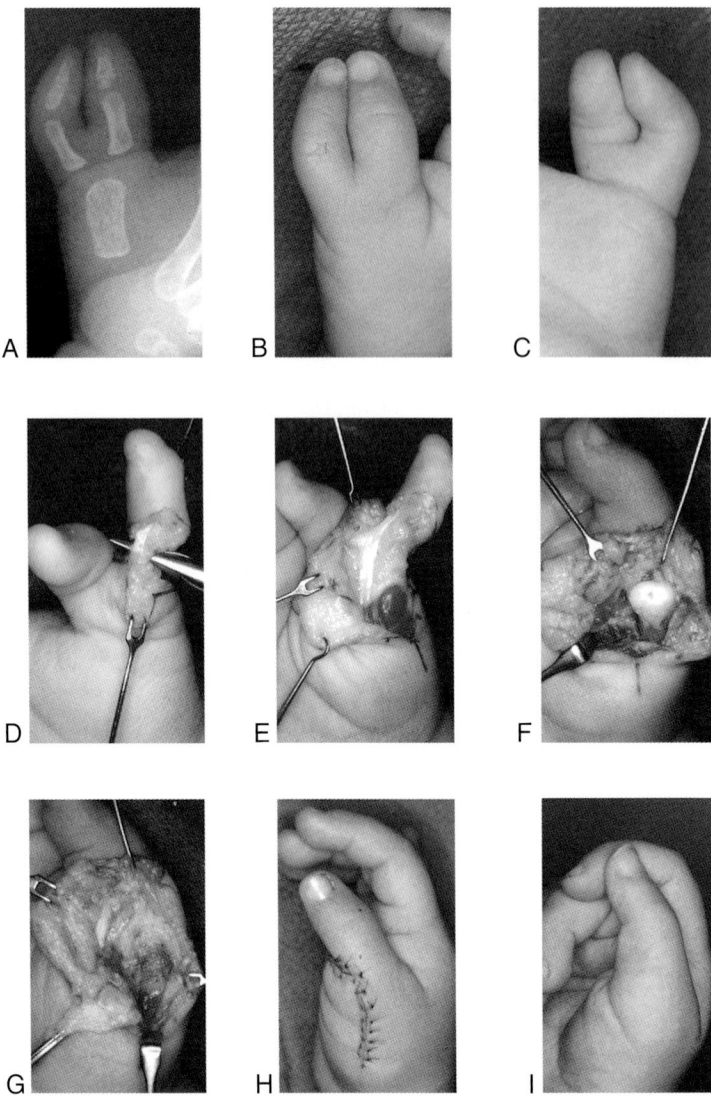

FIGURE 206-14. Type IV thumb polydactyly correction. *A to C,* The dorsal and palmar appearance and radiograph of a typical type IV thumb polydactyly. *D* and *E,* The flexor to the radial partner is identified and followed to its eccentric distal insertion, which creates the abnormal deviation and rotation seen in the radial thumb preoperatively. *F,* After disarticulation of the radial thumb, the bifid condyle of the metacarpal head is ablated. *G,* The radial collateral ligament is part of the periosteal flap, which is held to the left before it is reattached to the retained proximal phalanx. *H* and *I,* The immediate closure is contrasted with the appearance 5 years later.

placed across both osteotomies parallel to the growth plates. In most thumbs, these osteotomies are not needed.

REATTACHMENT. The radial collateral ligament is reattached to the radial base of the proximal phalanx. Periosteal flaps are approximated over the exposed metacarpal. Portions of the extensor mechanism are *not* used to reinforce the collateral ligament closure. The thenar intrinsic muscles are attached to the base of the proximal phalanx, and the extensor mechanism is attached with preference to the bone if only one muscle is available. Distally, the attachments of the flexor pollicis longus and extensor pollicis longus are inspected and centralized if necessary. The flexor sheath is checked to make sure there is no impingement at the point where the extra flexor tendon was cut sharply

from the retained flexor. A portion of the extra extensor tendon can be used to construct a shroud for the extensor pollicis longus.

CLOSURE. The closure is kept 1.0 mm above or dorsal to the line of demarcation of the two types of skin on the radial side of the digit. Cutback incisions within the normal flexion creases (IP joint, MP joint, and thenar) on the radial side of the thumb are all that is needed to correct tissue redundancies. Z-plasties should not be necessary. These incisions are closed with 6-0 or 7-0 mild chromic sutures, and the longitudinal incision is closed by a subcuticular technique with an absorbable suture.

DRESSING. A carefully applied soft hand dressing is covered with a long-arm cast extending well past the

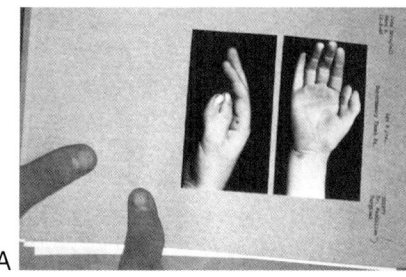

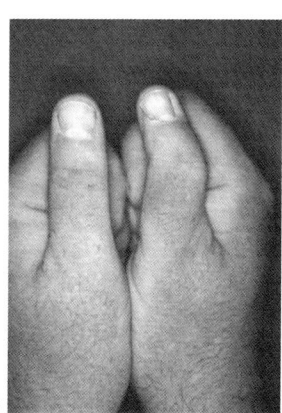

Five-decade follow-up

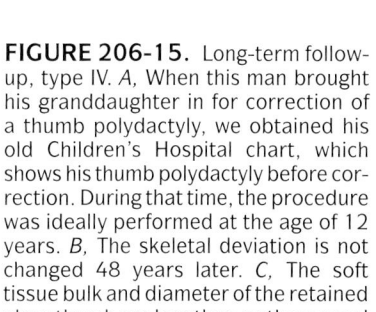

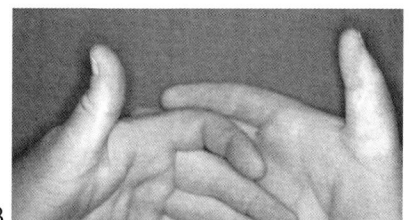

FIGURE 206-15. Long-term follow-up, type IV. *A,* When this man brought his granddaughter in for correction of a thumb polydactyly, we obtained his old Children's Hospital chart, which shows his thumb polydactyly before correction. During that time, the procedure was ideally performed at the age of 12 years. *B,* The skeletal deviation is not changed 48 years later. *C,* The soft tissue bulk and diameter of the retained ulnar thumb are less than on the normal side. IP joint motion is also reduced. He has reported no functional problems.

elbow, which should be flexed 90 degrees. Only the thumb tip is visible. Three weeks later, the cast and sutures are removed with the child sedated (Table 206-3). Circumstances allowed us to examine the result of surgery performed almost 50 years earlier (Fig. 206-15).

TABLE 206-3 ✦ TREATMENT OF PROXIMAL PHALANGEAL DUPLICATIONS

Problems

Limited range of motion at MP and IP joints (see Fig. 206-15)
Uncorrected angulation at proximal phalangeal level
Weak intrinsic muscles
Radial bulge of metacarpal
Unrecognized deficient first web space
Limited extensor tendon excursion from checkrein effect of scar
Narrow appearance
Bilhaut correction: broad, flat nail with longitudinal ridge; decreased MP range of motion

Caveats

Do not use the extensor mechanism for collateral ligament reconstruction. A checkrein effect will result.
Keep nontraumatized periosteum beneath extensor tendon so that the extensor glides on a smooth areolar layer.
Use periosteal sleeve attached to collateral ligament.[48]
Reattach the best thenar intrinsic muscle to bone.
Look for pollex abductus! When present, make sure it is completely released proximally.[13]
Closing wedge osteotomy is safer and heals more predictably than an opening wedge plus bone graft.

METACARPAL (IOWA TYPES V, VI; GERMAN TYPES I MET, I CMC)

Because of the extreme degree of anatomic variation, each correction must be considered one tissue at a time. The basic principles are identical to those outlined. The radial thumb is usually the most deficient, and the ulnar metacarpal is tightly adducted in the same plane as the digits. The preferred incision is to encircle both thumbs at the MP joint level and to raise equal dorsal and palmar flaps (Fig. 206-16). With this wide exposure, the retained thumb can be transposed into a position of palmar abduction, the intrinsic muscles including the adductor pollicis can be carefully repositioned, collateral ligaments can be tightened, and extrinsic tendons can be realigned. Fibrous bands within the first web space must be released and excised. A short metacarpal often contributes to the tight first web space. This can be lengthened with an osteotomy and use of excised bone (with periosteum) as an intercalated graft. With Iowa type VI variants, the CMC joint anatomy may be bizarre. In all reconstructions, the joint contour should be shaved so that the retained thumb metacarpal is in a position of palmar abduction. In rare Iowa type V duplications (see Fig. 206-8*B,* far right), the same incision can be used to transpose the better phalangeal components from the ulnar thumb "on top" of the radial thumb with an intact metacarpal and MP joint. Once the skeletal and muscle components are repositioned, the soft tissue flaps can be redraped to make a good web space. At this point, appropriate Z-plasties or other transposition flaps may be performed. If this type of incision is used, the surgeon can take full advantage of all of the skin available. All too often, the entire deficient radial thumb is excised and usable skin discarded. Chondrodesis at the MP joint may provide the much

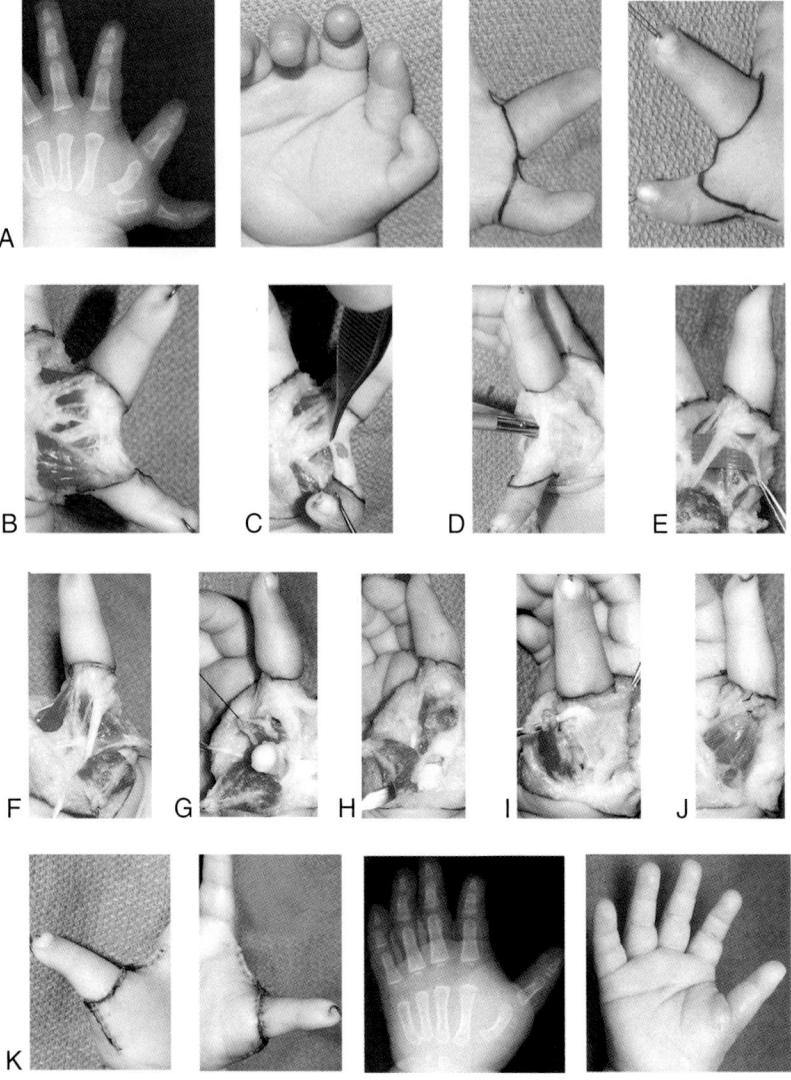

FIGURE 206-16. Type VI metacarpal level correction. *A,* Clinical appearance and radiograph of a type VI polydactyly originating at the CMC joint. The real deficiency of the first web space is masked by the radial deviation of the ulnar thumb at the MP joint. The radial thumb shares a common CMC joint. The dorsal and palmar incisions encircle both thumbs at the MP level. Extra skin has been saved on the radial thumb. *B,* A common flexor is seen with arborization to the individual thumbs. *C,* Pulling on the radial thumb flexor causes the clinical deviation of the radial thumb due to the eccentric flexor insertion. *D,* A tight fibrous band is usually present between the two thumbs. *E,* Less frequent is the common band to both the flexor and extensor tendons, which compose the "pollex abductus" anomaly. *F,* The radial thumb has been removed, and the extra adductor pollicis muscle is saved and reflected with a suture. *G,* The thenar intrinsic muscles (abductor pollicis brevis, flexor pollicis brevis) have been detached from the radial metacarpal. *H,* The CMC disarticulation has been completed. Transposition of the ulnar metacarpal into the radial CMC position will achieve more palmar abduction of the retained thumb and broaden the first web space. *I,* The lateral bands of the extensor mechanism are used for intrinsic muscle reattachment. *J,* Both bone and tendinous insertions have been completed. *K,* After the thumb has been placed in optimal position, the dorsal and palmar flaps are draped over it and used to make a much wider first web space. The radiograph and clinical appearance of the hand 1 year later. The metacarpal is still short in comparison to the opposite side.

TABLE 206-4 ✦ TREATMENT OF METACARPAL DUPLICATIONS

Problems

Same as those outlined in Iowa type IV
Unrecognized multiple factors in first web space deficiency: intrinsic muscles, tight fibrous bands, abnormal CMC joint, and skin
Extensor tendon adherence
Ulnar collateral ligament reconstructions must be anchored to bone or subperiosteal tunnels. Suturing alone is not sufficient. Imbrication of local tissue often attenuates with growth and results in a lax ligament.
Collateral ligament reconstructions without a volar accessory portion may result in MP hyperextension.

Caveats

Enough skin is present if the preferred incision is used.
A short thumb with a good web space functions well.
With growth, revision of both soft tissue and skeletal components may be required.
Use all available spare parts.
These are never normal thumbs!

needed stability in type VI variants in which both CMC and MP joints are abnormal. In this procedure, the articular hyaline cartilage is shaved to bleeding surfaces, and the epiphyses are left intact.

The intrinsic muscle anatomy requires careful inspection. Recession of the first dorsal interosseous muscle and lengthening of the adductor pollicis muscle are necessary for adequate repositioning of the thumb metacarpal. Ulnar deviation of the proximal phalanx of the ulnar thumb is indicative of an absent ulnar collateral ligament at the MP joint. This important ligament can be constructed with portions of the excised thumb. However, bone to bone fixation without injury to growth plates can be challenging (Table 206-4).

THUMB POLYDACTYLY WITH TRIPHALANGEAL COMPONENTS

The association of thumb polydactyly with extra or triphalangeal components has long been recognized as rare.[49,50] The morphologic appearance of all patients is different, and the construction of one good thumb must be individualized. These triphalangeal parts are most commonly seen with the most frequent form of thumb polydactyly, Iowa type IV at the MP joint level.

Inheritance

In contrast to isolated thumb polydactyly, the occurrence of triphalangeal components is not purely spo-

radic.[4,5,26,51,52] The author notes that approximately half of the triphalangeal thumbs recorded in our registry are associated with thumb polydactyly.[53]

Classification

In an attempt to further standardize and categorize these unusual duplicated and triplicated thumbs, Wood[26] added additional categories to the existing Iowa system. Type IV thumbs with a triphalangeal component were further subdivided into IVA and IVB. An additional group VII was created for those type V and type VI polydactylies with one or more triphalangeal rays. Buck-Gramcko's newer system designates the presence of a triphalangeal component with a plus sign following the appropriate level.[24] A less detailed and more practical system has been used in which the level of duplication is followed by a notation of which component contains an extra phalanx (Fig. 206-17).[53] These systems deal only with those triphalangeal thumbs associated with polydactyly, and extended classification systems that take into consideration the exact shape of the extra phalanx have not been incorporated.

Associated Anomalies

Various forms of polydactyly of the great toe are frequently associated with these interesting thumbs.[26,51,52] This is consistent with the positive familial inheritance and the bilaterality of this anomaly. Because the lower extremity differentiates 2 to 3 days later than the upper, more proximal levels of branching are seen in the hand than in the foot. The only manifestation of a toe polydactyly will often be a short distal phalanx and a broad flat nail on the great toe.

Clinical Presentation

Thumbs with triphalangeal parts are seen in approximately one fifth of all radial polydactylies. With one exception, all of these thumbs have their level of duplication at or proximal to the MP joint. The largest single group are those originating at the MP joint (type IV Iowa classification), and one or both of the two thumbs may have an extra phalanx. The abnormal anatomy is similar to that described for the MP duplications. The triphalangeal rays can be either balanced when both partners have extra bones or unbalanced when only one side is abnormal. Extrinsic flexor and extensor tendons are commonly shared with eccentric distal insertions as described, and intrinsic muscles will insert into the nearest skeletal partner.

The next group includes thumbs originating at the metacarpal or CMC joint level. All permutations and combinations of tendon, muscle, and skeletal anatomy exist. Parts for two or three thumbs may be present. There is usually one ray with two or three relatively normal phalanges that is most suited to become the thumb. The ray with the best metacarpal and MP joint usually becomes the foundation for the constructed thumb. The phalanx with the most normal nail plate and nail folds is usually most suited to become the terminal portion of the thumb.

A final small group of thumbs with extra phalanges is not easily classified into any specific group. The hypoplastic hands usually have two functional digits. The thumb has a broad nail and many asymmetric phalanges with longitudinal epiphyseal brackets. These bones are positioned obliquely and are not rectangular. A broad conjoined nail is present distally. A simple syndactyly may span the distance between the two rays. The opposite fifth ray has a metacarpal and two or three phalanges in longitudinal orientation.

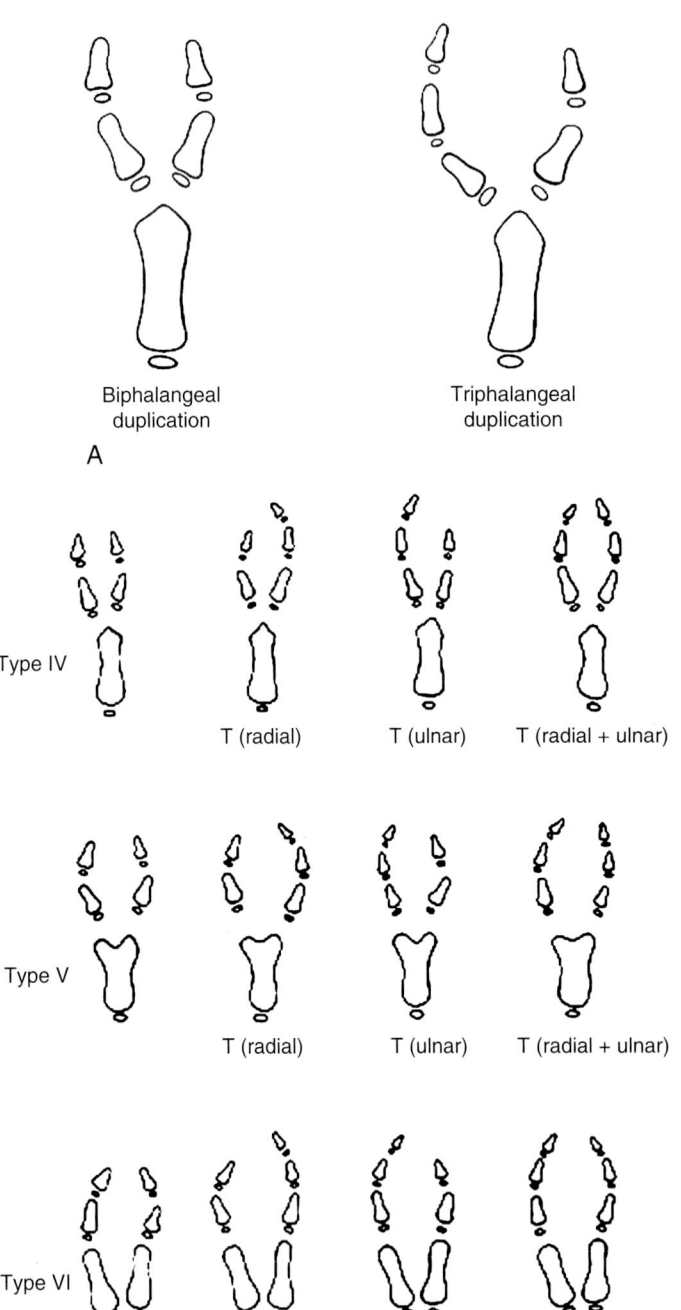

FIGURE 206-17. Radial polydactyly with triphalangeal components. *A,* A simple version of the German classification first identifies the thumb as either biphalangeal or triphalangeal. *B,* These thumbs all occur at or proximal to the MP joint at levels IV through VI in the Iowa classification. The position of the thumb with the extra phalanx is designated with a T for triphalangeal.

Treatment

The guiding principle is the same: make the best thumb from the available parts. In more than half of these hands, the triphalangeal thumb or portion thereof is discarded. If both thumbs are equal in size, appearance, and function, it is best to save that partner with a strong ulnar collateral ligament at the MP joint. If the triphalangeal thumb is well aligned, stable, and well positioned within the hand and the biphalangeal thumb is deviated, the longer triphalangeal thumb should be retained (Fig. 206-18).[31]

Outcomes

The outcomes of this group of duplications are similar to those described for radial duplication. Thumbs duplicated beyond the MP joint have a greater total active motion because the proximal two joints are normal or close to normal. This is not surprising because in at least half of all patients, the triphalangeal ray is ablated. There is much less extrinsic tendon adherence and joint instability. None of the complex thumbs with duplications at the metacarpal level is normal. In addition to associated tendon and muscle anomalies and joint instability, these metacarpals may be short

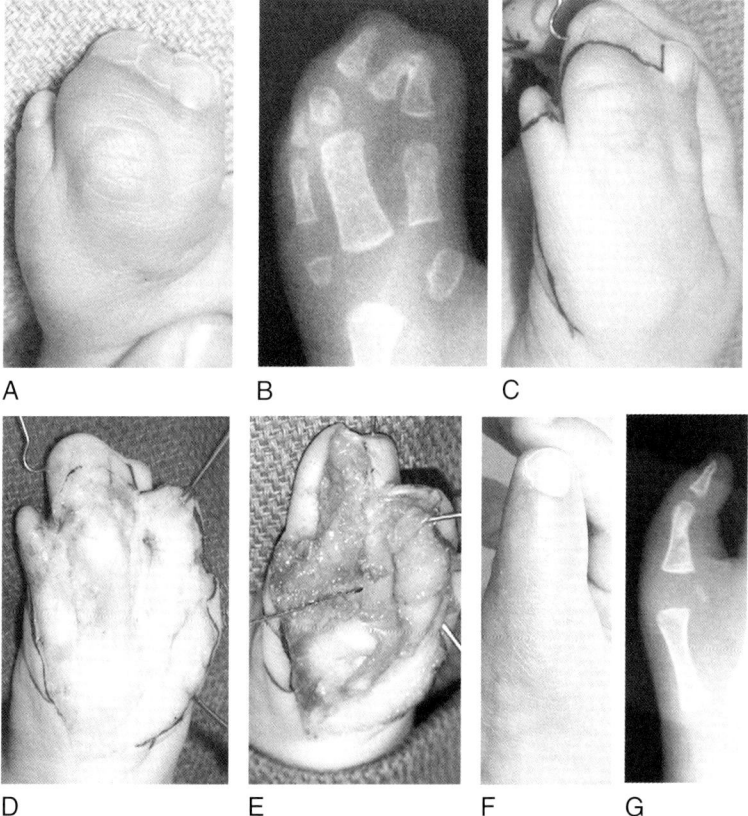

FIGURE 206-18. Complex thumb duplication with polydactyly. *A* and *B*, The clinical appearance and radiograph of a complex right thumb with four phalangeal components and a conjoined nail with three distal phalanges. Classification by any scheme would be quite difficult. The level of the duplication occurs at the MP joint level (level IV in the Iowa system). The radial and ulnar thumbs are triphalangeal, and the central thumb, the largest, is a "special thumb" with two well-formed distal phalanges. *C*, A fillet incision is outlined. The goal is to save as much tissue as possible and to construct one good thumb from the parts of four incomplete thumbs. *D*, The skeletal parts are exposed with reflection of the dorsal flap. The proximal portion of the central thumb with the intact MP joint will be saved and a ray resection of the radial thumb performed. *E*, The distal portion of the most ulnar thumb with the best nail is transposed on top of the central thumb and joined at the midportion of the proximal phalanx. *F*, A satisfactory paronychial fold has been made as described in Figure 206-10. Motion of the MP and IP joints is normal 1 year later. A piece of cortical bone was used as an intramedullary strut. *G*, Radiograph has the appearance of a normal proximal phalanx.

and require lengthening. The most commonly overlooked deficiency in the uncorrected thumb is the short first web space. The transfer of intrinsic muscles and extrinsic tendons, reconstruction of ligaments, and correction of skeletal deviation are the same as described in the preceding section. Treatment of the long extra phalanx with arthrodesis is described in a later section.

SPECIAL THUMBS (Fig. 206-19)

Inheritance

There is no inheritance pattern in this group of malformations.

Clinical Presentation

In the author's evaluation of more than 400 patients with radial thumb duplications, a small group of previously undescribed patients appeared. Many similar thumbs have been included in textbooks and articles on unusual instances that do not fit the standard classification systems.[54,55] All but three of these patients presented with a unilateral hypoplastic thumb in which the first two rays contained either one or two metacarpals with shared thumb phalangeal components. The duplication commonly started at the MP joint, which articulated with abnormally shaped phalangeal segments. None of these hands contained more than two additional digits, and the web space between the thumb and the next complete ray was always deficient when it was not absent. A complete syndactyly was present in six hands. The extra thumb phalangeal bone often articulated with an intact triphalangeal index ray within a complete, simple syndactyly. When two distal phalangeal bones were present, a common flexor pollicis longus was also present. The median-innervated thenar intrinsic

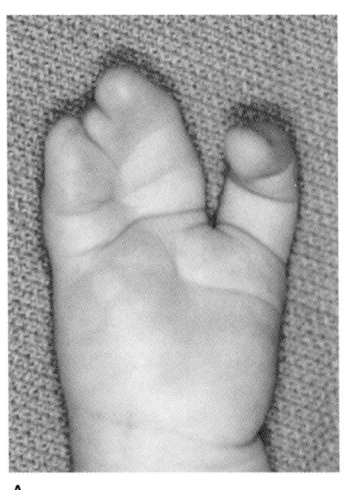

A

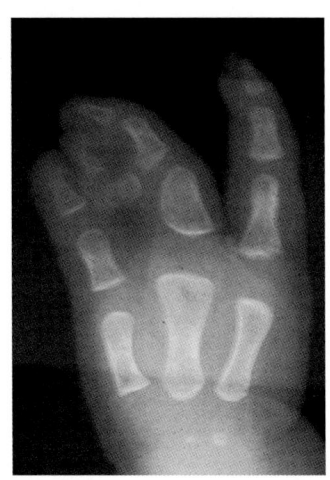

B

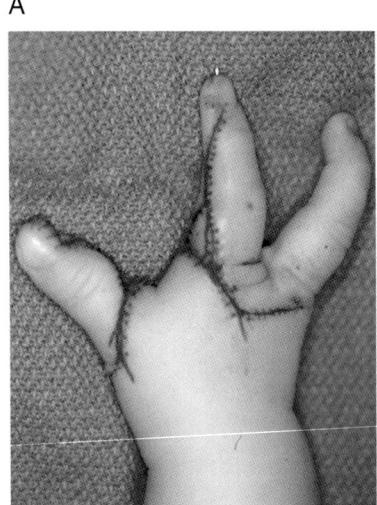

C

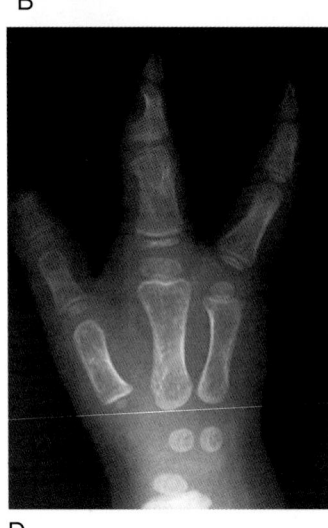

D

FIGURE 206-19. Special thumb. *A,* The clinical appearance of a complex thumb duplication that articulates with a bizarre index duplication at the level of the IP joint. *B,* Radiograph shows a duplicated distal phalanx and a shared rectangular bone with the index PIP joint. The proximal phalanx of the index has a longitudinal epiphyseal bracket. Treatment consisted of excision of the shared bone, osteotomy, and bone graft of the index proximal phalanx and a dorsal flap reconstruction for the first web space. No skin grafts were necessary. *C,* The dorsal flap has provided an excellent first web space lined with full-thickness tissue. *D,* Radiograph 1 year later demonstrates maintained longitudinal growth of both the thumb and oversized index rays.

muscles always attached to the most radial phalangeal bones, and the affected hand was always much smaller than the opposite hand.

Treatment

The treatment of these hypoplastic hands, which will always be used as helper hands, involves the construction of a wide first web space lined by full-thickness tissue, reduction of the thumb with preservation of motion, and positioning of the border rays for either a key or pincer pinch or rudimentary grip (see Fig. 206-19). Treatment of these patients needs to be carefully individualized. The Y to V principle has been effectively used to widen a thumb-index web space during a rotation-recession osteotomy of the ulnar metacarpal (Fig. 206-20).[56]

Outcomes

In those with unilateral deformities, the opposite limb was used as the master hand. A thumb with a full web space always had a much greater grip span than in those hands with one thumb and one finger. Rotation-recession osteotomies at the metacarpal level of one or both digits commonly improved the span and ability

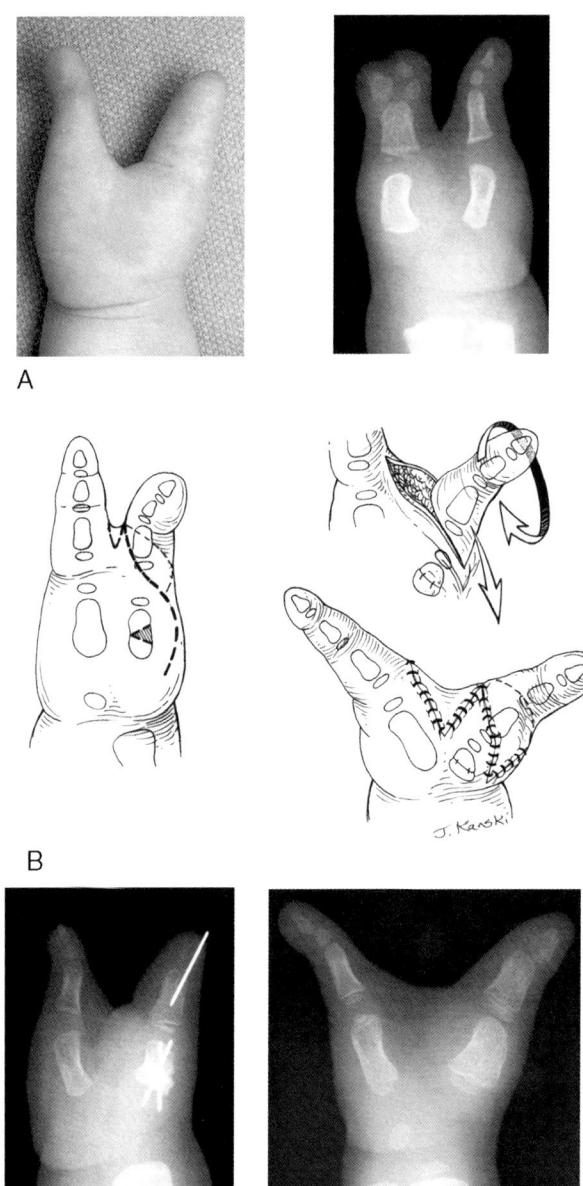

FIGURE 206-20. Special thumb, two-fingered hand. *A,* Radiograph of a hand with two rays. The radial ray is designated a thumb with a broad proximal phalanx and two sets of distal phalanges. Both rays are oriented in the same plane. *B,* Illustrations show the incision marking for thumb repositioning; the thumb is moved in a Y to V after a closing wedge rotational osteotomy is made at the midmetacarpal level. *C,* The radiographic appearance is shown immediately after the procedure and 1 year later. The web space has been widened, and the two digits are not opposed to one another.

to hold objects but did not affect the weak pinch strength in all of these hands. Because the terminal flexor tendon to the thumb and index is commonly shared from one proximal muscle belly, these rays will pinch simultaneously with little individuality of function.

CENTRAL POLYDACTYLY (duplication of index, long, and ring rays)

Terminology

Central polydactyly is defined as duplications involving the central three rays of the hand: index,

long, or ring. The genetic literature uses the terms synpolydactyly and polysyndactyly for these hands. These are the most unusual types of duplications in the upper extremity, and that of the index finger is the rarest of all. Few papers have been published on this subject, in part because most of these patients have been described with complex or complicated syndactyly.

The author's experience is one of the largest recorded because of interest in the genetic cause and pursuit of many afflicted large family pedigrees (Fig. 206-21).[56,57] Our clinical experience with this condition is similar to that of others.[26,57-60] Perhaps another reason for the paucity of papers on this subject relates

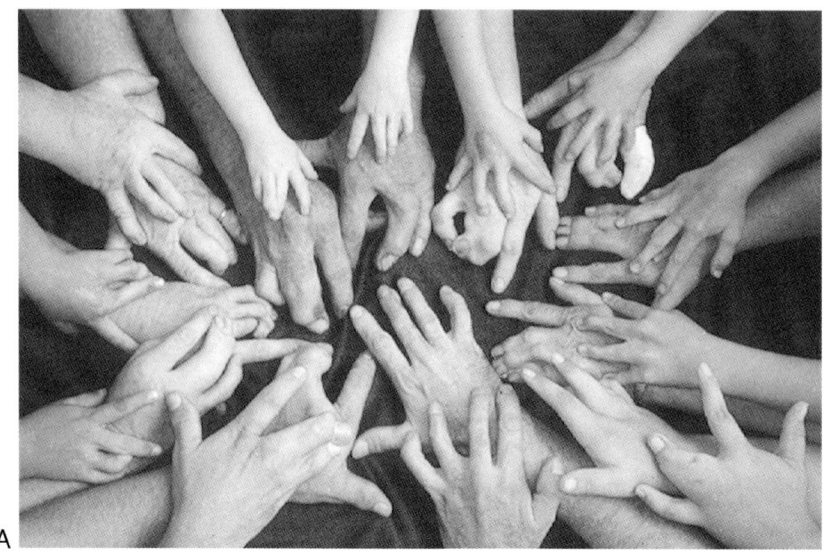

A

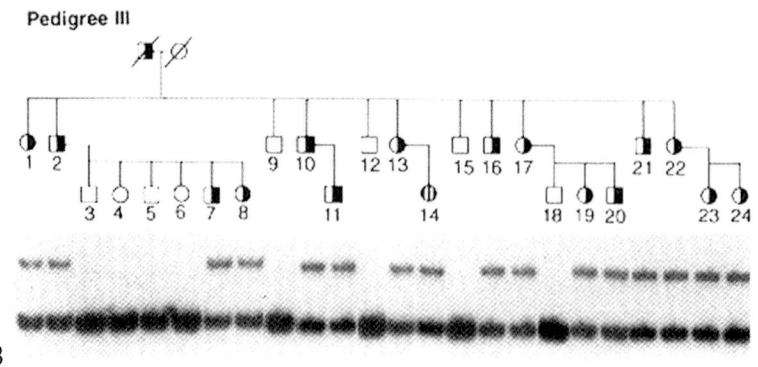

B

FIGURE 206-21. Central synpolydactyly. *A,* This photograph (taken by the author hanging from a tree) shows three generations of affected individuals with synpolydactyly during a midsummer family picnic. All descended from a single immigrant from Germany to western Pennsylvania in the middle 1880s. Many of the older individuals had no surgical corrections because of the poor results and complications encountered during the mid-1900s. *B,* Gel analysis of polymerase chain reaction–amplified polyalanine coding regions of *HOXD13* from these individuals. Nonpenetrant heterozygous individuals are indicated by a vertical stripe. There were no homozygous individuals. The young girl represented by number 14 in the third generation had a minimal incomplete simple syndactyly on one hand, and her analysis was positive.

to the high percentage of poor and fair surgical outcomes in these very complicated hands.

Incidence

A true incidence has never been reported. An isolated duplication involving the index ray is the most uncommon, and those duplications involving the long and ring rays are most common. In a series of 2500 patients, Buck-Gramcko[60] reports 7 true index duplications; the author's registry of 4500 patients contains 6, all unilateral and all associated with either hypoplasia of the thumb or a spoon hand, which was not associated with a craniosynostosis syndrome.

Duplications of the long finger are more commonly seen, but not as often as those of the ring ray.[48] Isolated duplication of the long finger metacarpal or phalanges is much less common than all forms of duplication involving the ring ray. Because of the obligatory soft tissue webbing associated with duplications at the phalangeal levels, most of these have been reported as synpolydactyly or "hidden polydactyly"[61-65] or "syndactylized polydactyly."[66] Incidence figures of one or all of these types have not been published. Our large experience with long and ring duplications is skewed because these patients were seen as part of ongoing genetic studies of large family pedigrees.

Inheritance

Most descriptions of isolated index or long digit polydactylies are part of large family pedigrees with a positive penetrance.[67,68] The author's experience is similar to that of Buck-Gramcko[60]: none of 4 patients with isolated index duplications and only 3 of the 18 patients with long finger polydactylies had a family pedigree positive for polydactyly. In an additional group of patients, combined index and long duplications were both unilateral and isolated (Fig. 206-22).

In contrast, a positive penetrance had been reported in more than 90% of the author's patients with the combined long-ring ray polydactyly.[56] The largest kindred study comes from Turkey,[69] where penetrance was estimated to be 96%. The gene responsible for this variant of synpolydactyly was first identified as a HOXD13 mutation[70] and subsequently confirmed by others.[71-73] The mutation consists of extra polyalanine expansions on the nonbinding portion of chromosome 2. Study of large pedigrees has shown a direct relationship between the level of duplication within the hand and foot and the size of the alanine expansion.[56]

Associated Anomalies

No significant malformations outside of the musculoskeletal system have been reported. Long and ring duplications occurring at either the metacarpal or proximal phalangeal level often have less severe foot malformations manifested by cutaneous syndactyly and duplication at the phalangeal level. The lateral three toes are more commonly affected than the great and second toes. Because development and differentiation in the foot occur approximately 3 days later than in the hand, metacarpal level duplications are rarely seen. Syndromic associations include the typical cleft hand, orofaciodigital type II, and Laurence-Moon-Biedl, among others.[54] The incidence of other limb anomalies is high, however; these include metacarpal synostoses, triphalangeal bones with longitudinal epiphyseal brackets, radial and ulnar polydactyly, cleft hands and feet, thump hypoplasia, and soft tissue and osseous syndactylies.

Classification

The author's classification system is a simplified version of the Buck-Gramcko and Behrens system in which the ray with its metacarpal and three phalanges is divided into eight levels. The most proximal level of the skeleton is noted at which evidence of a partial or complete branching is seen. This could include a longitudinal epiphyseal bracket, a bifid metacarpal head, or a transverse tubular bone spanning two adjacent rays (Fig. 206-23). Additional designations for transverse skeletal parts, such as tubular bones or "delta" phalanges with longitudinal epiphyseal brackets, have not been incorporated for simplicity's sake.

Clinical Presentation

The index polydactyly at the phalangeal level is the rarest within the hand but does occasionally occur (Fig. 206-24). In some instances, the distal parts are very small at the phalangeal level. However, more often, there is a combined duplication with the long ray that originates more proximally and reveals splitting of the extrinsic flexor and extensor tendons, abnormal insertions of proximal intrinsic muscles, and very distal bifurcation of the neurovascular structures. When the duplication starts at the MP joint, there is a double or split proximal phalanx. The most rudimentary form is the broad distal phalanx with a split or bifid tuft. Some form of cutaneous syndactyly is usually present.

Duplications involving the long ray and combined polydactyly of the index-long rays are more common. It is interesting that there are no papers in the literature devoted completely to this topic. Most are simple case reports.[61,65,74,75] The Japanese have stressed a developmental relationship between the distal duplication at the phalangeal level and the spectrum of typical cleft hands. They have speculated that the "cleft

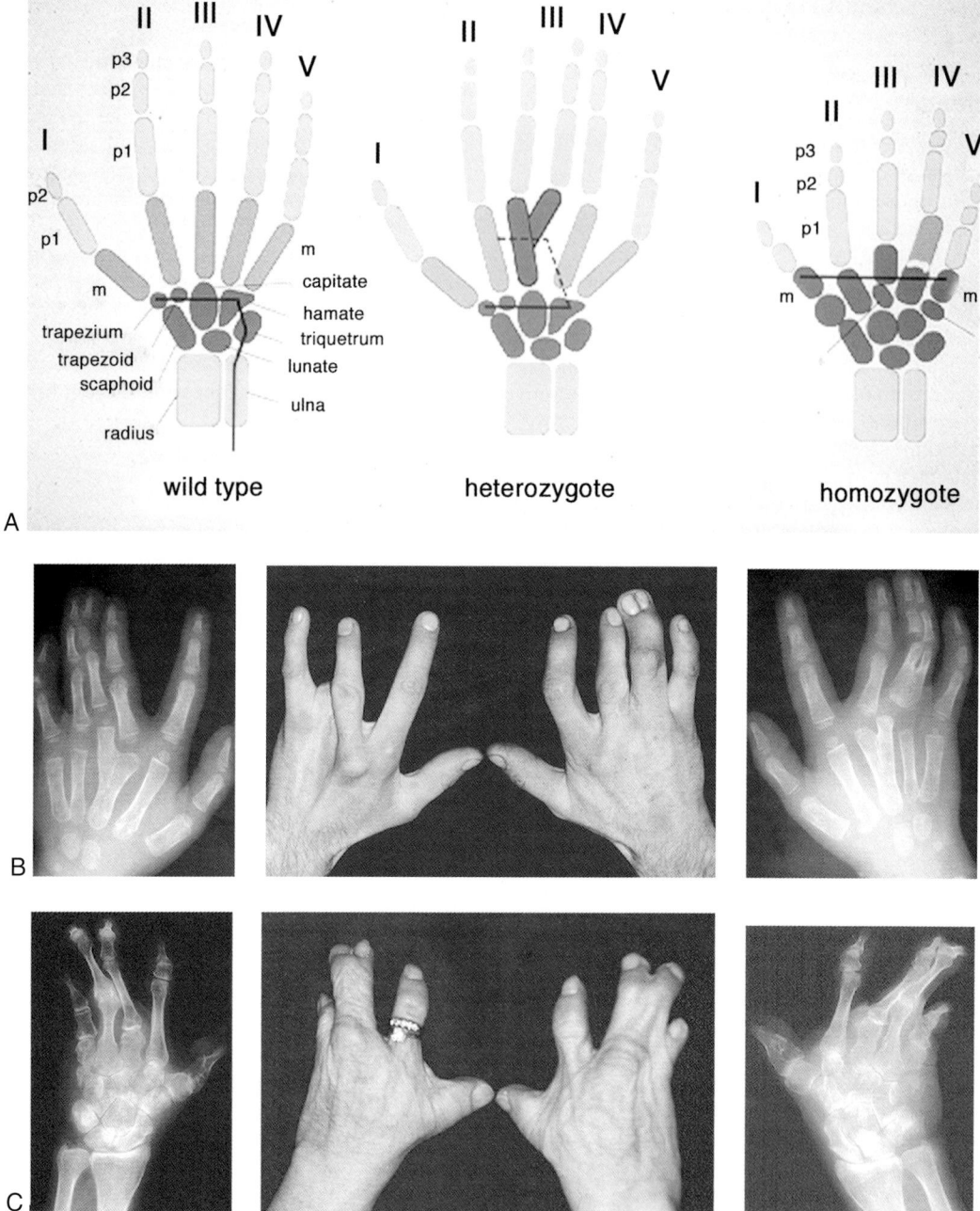

FIGURE 206-22. Synpolydactyly (see also Color Plate 201-2). *A,* Diagrams of the hand skeleton of heterozygous and homozygous individuals with synpolydactyly compared with a normal (wild-type) hand. The carpal pisiform is not shown. Digits are indicated by Roman numerals; metacarpals are indicated by the letter *m*; and the phalanges are indicated by p1, p2, and p3. In the heterozygote, metacarpal III is branched and gives rise to an extra digit IIIa. In the homozygote, the metacarpals are fully (metacarpals I, II, III, V) or partially (metacarpal IV) replaced by carpal-like bones. Two additional carpal bones are present. The trapezoid is absent. Note the short p2 in all digits. *B,* The clinical appearance and radiographs of a heterozygous individual. The left hand in the central frame is shown many years after a syndactyly release that resulted in ring finger loss due to compromised blood supply, a frequent complication after surgical correction during the 1950s. *C,* The mother of the patient in *B* was a homozygous individual. She has had no surgical correction. Her feet were more deformed than her hands.

Level of Duplication

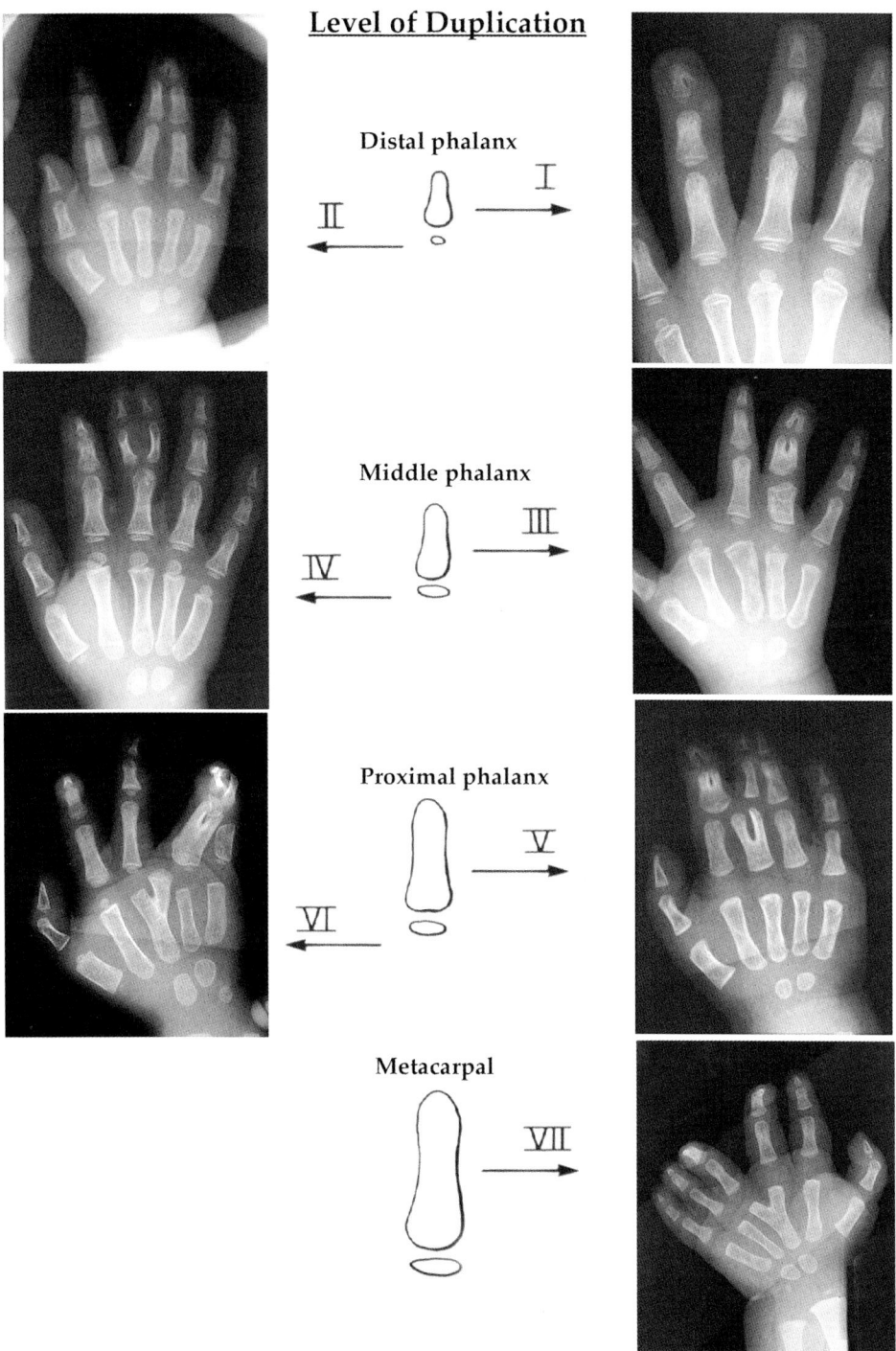

FIGURE 206-23. Author's central synpolydactyly classification. The simplified classification system designates the level of the duplication as it relates to the normal skeletal ray of one metacarpal and three phalanges. The level is determined by the most proximal point of divergence of the shared skeletal structures. No additional specifications have been made for the varied transverse and oblique phalanges connecting two rays of the hand or the abnormal phalanges with longitudinal epiphyseal brackets.

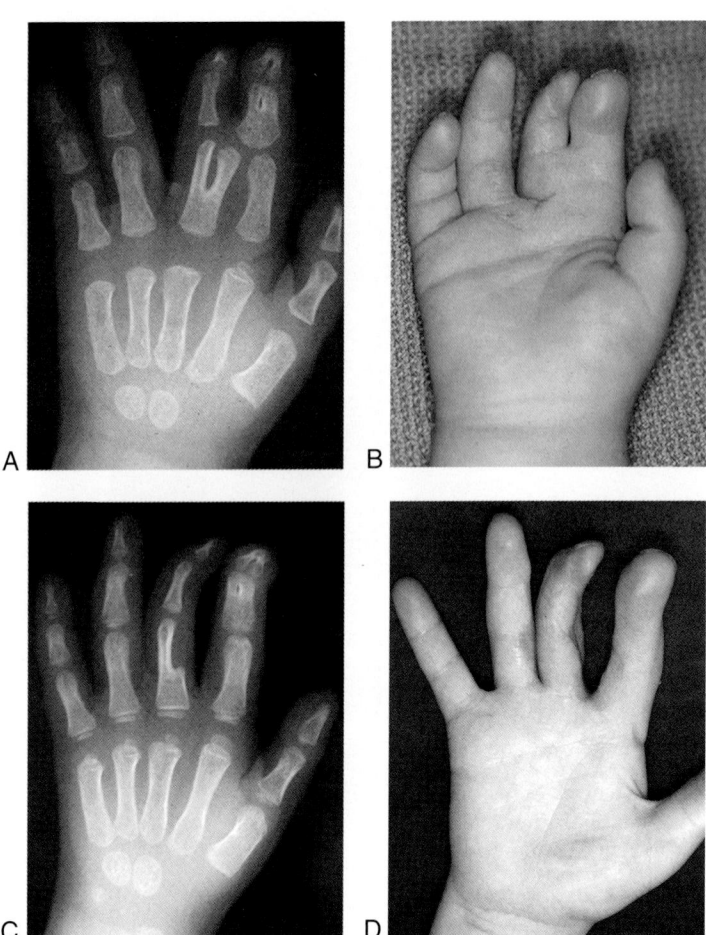

FIGURE 206-24. Index ray duplication. *A*, A radiograph of the polydactyly involving the index and long digits. The extra digit is shared between the middle and distal phalanges of the index finger and the proximal phalanx of the long finger. *B*, An incomplete simple syndactyly is present. *C*, Radiograph after release of complex syndactyly shows a much smaller long finger with deviation. *D*, With growth, the deviation and angulation have been accentuated and will require further correction.

hand complex"[76] starts as a distal duplication of the long ray and that there is a relationship with osseous syndactyly.[60] Experimentally, Ogino[77,78] has been able to reproduce these phenotypes in rats after the administration of busulfan during days 10 and 11 of gestation.

The clinical spectrum of long-ring and isolated ring duplication is varied (Fig. 206-25). Much more complex soft tissue and osseous anomalies are found at the more proximal levels, similar to the types IV to VI thumb polydactylies described earlier. All types of separate transverse or oblique skeletal parts may span the two rays at the level of the MP joint. Divergent and parallel metacarpal synostoses usually originate along the long metacarpal as the duplicate part joins the ring ray at the proximal phalangeal level. At the phalangeal level, divergent and parallel bifurcations of the proximal and middle phalanges are seen, with or without triangular bones with longitudinal epiphyseal bracketing. Fusion of distal phalanges near the tip of the conjoined digits

is common. The congruency and cant of the affected joints are abnormal (Fig. 206-26). Neurovascular structures are usually normal up to the level of the MP joints, where they can then be expected to have more distal bifurcations into individual digits. Extrinsic flexor and extensor tendons usually split at the level of bifurcation and have abnormal distal insertions. However, interosseous muscles have their normal proximal origins and typically insert into the transverse or oblique phalanges at the MP joint or into the base of the duplicate part at the proximal phalangeal level (Figs. 206-27 and 206-28).

Treatment

It is not surprising that there are so few publications that devote more than a few sentences to these very difficult surgical problems.[41,58-60,62,79] The more complete descriptions[41,58,60] all stress the complex anatomy, the high incidence of potential complications, and the

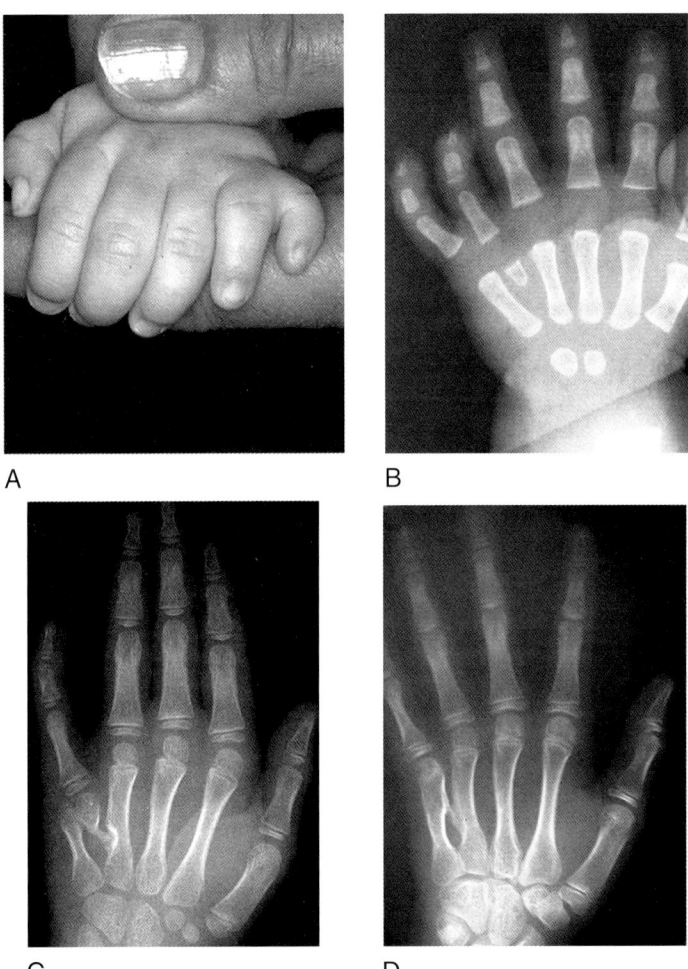

FIGURE 206-25. Hidden polydactyly. *A,* The clinical appearance of a baby with what appears to be a fifth finger duplication. *B,* The radiograph shows an incomplete ray between the ring and fifth fingers. *C,* The radiograph and picture shown in *A* and *B* were obtained after the patient was first seen with this radiograph. Shortly after birth, the complete fifth finger was excised and the incomplete ray was mistakenly retained. *D,* With distraction lengthening techniques, the incomplete polydactylous ray was transposed on top of the fifth metacarpal.

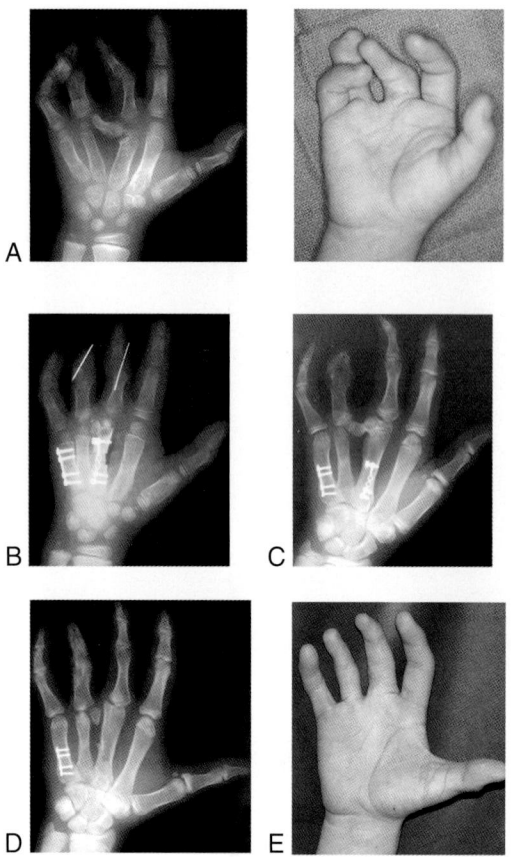

FIGURE 206-26. Central synpolydactyly, natural history. *A,* Clinical appearance and radiograph of a young boy who presented several years after correction of a syndactyly. He complained of scissoring of his ulnar three digits with flexion. He was a member of a large pedigree with synpolydactyly. The initial separation of the long and ring fingers did not include any skeletal corrections. *B,* Treatment consisted of PIP joint releases of the long and ring fingers, excision of the transverse phalanx at the metacarpal level, lengthening and bone grafting of the short metacarpal of the long finger, and rotational osteotomy of the fifth metacarpal. *C,* Within 3 years, the transverse bone had regenerated because portions of the original bone were left to avoid MP joint deviation. *D,* In the final stage, this bone was again partially excised, and the ring finger was lengthened with distraction techniques. *E,* The clinical appearance shows well-aligned digits with intact MP joint motion. IP joint motion is limited but does not hinder this youngster who is an all-star collegiate hockey player. His grip strength is 70% of the opposite hand. Thumb to fifth finger pinch is not affected.

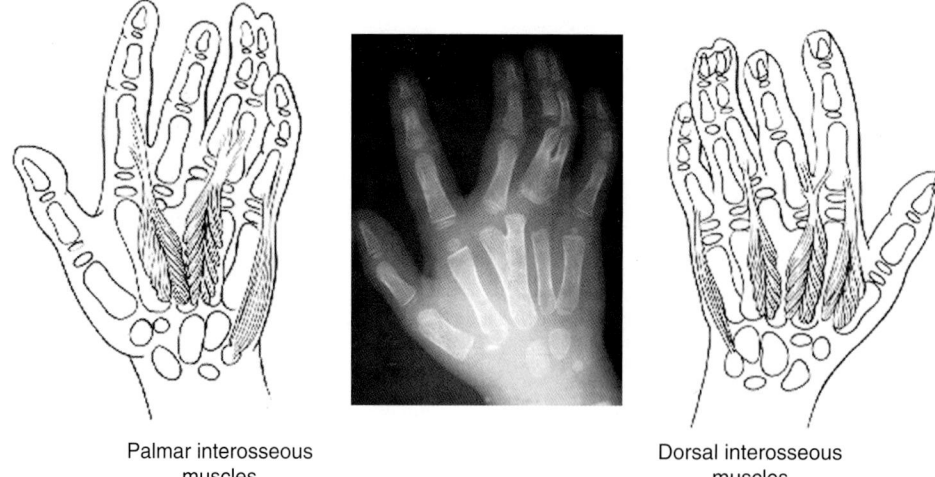

Palmar interosseous
muscles

Dorsal interosseous
muscles

FIGURE 206-27. Intrinsic muscle insertions in synpolydactyly. The intrinsic muscles in these synpolydactyly hands develop normally in the uninvolved proximal portions of the hand. This illustration demonstrates the distal insertions of both palmar and dorsal interosseous muscles in the area of central polydactyly. There is no selective attachment to bone or extensors. These muscles are noted at surgery to attach to the nearest skeletal structure, and in this hand, they have no functional value. For this child, all thenar (including the adductor pollicis muscle) and hypothenar musculature was normal.

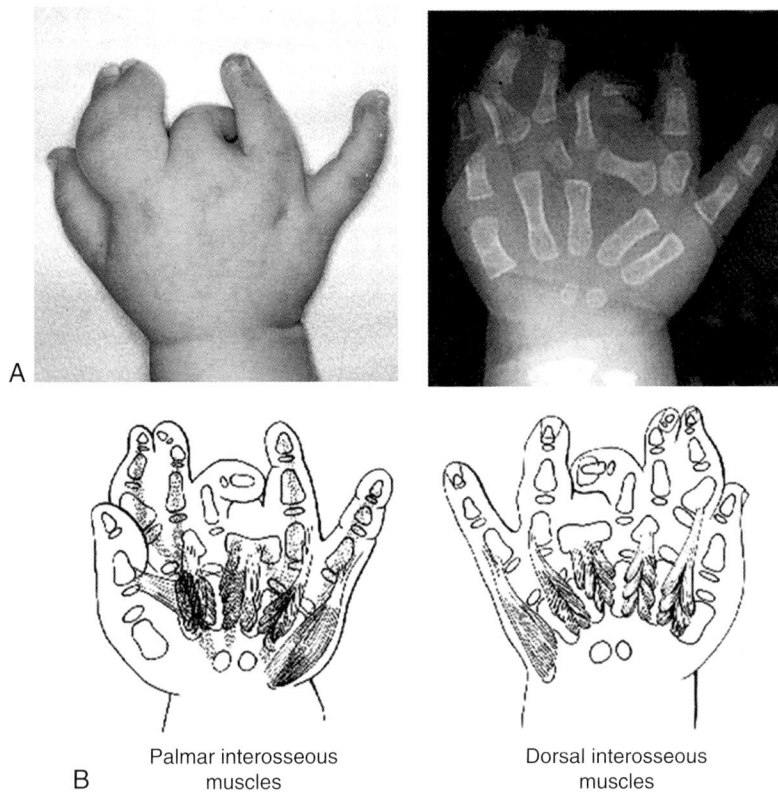

FIGURE 206-28. Complex, complicated central polydactyly (synpolydactyly). *A,* The clinical appearance and radiograph of a baby with a unilateral polydactyly involving all three central rays of the hand. The foot on the same side was abnormal. Family history was negative. *B,* The clinical anatomy observed during multiple staged operations (see Fig. 206-29) is shown from both the dorsal and palmar sides of the hand. All dorsal and palmar interosseous muscles had normal origins at the proximal metacarpal level. The distal insertion was to the nearest skeletal structure. Despite the preservation and reattachment of the individual intrinsic muscles during correction, this boy had no functional abduction-adduction of the involved rays of the hand.

less than optimal outcomes in the majority of patients (Table 206-5 and Fig. 206-29).

SYNDACTYLY

The principles of management are identical to those outlined in Chapter 204. Full-thickness skin grafts are always needed. Commissures should always be lined with full-thickness flaps. Either the large dorsal rectangular flaps or interdigitating dorsal and palmar triangular flaps are preferred. Osseous correction is completed at the same time as syndactyly release. It is useful to specifically identify and photograph the neurovascular structures and anomalies at this point because they may be useful if any further treatment is required at a later date. Pulp-plasties and paronychial fold construction should be used to contour these fingertips as normally as possible.[5] In some children with a longitudinal epiphyseal bracket along the radial

TABLE 206-5 ✦ TREATMENT PRINCIPLES FOR ASSOCIATED ANOMALIES

Maintain digital length without significant rotation or angulation in both flexion and extension.
Preserve motion at the MP joint.
Remove abnormal transverse phalanges with attached intrinsic muscles.
Ablate or transpose rays without enough skeletal parts to construct a digit of normal length.
Keep central rays from obstructing thumb–fifth finger pinch or grasp.
Construct interdigital web spaces at normal levels by use of the principles outlined. Reconstruct nails and nail folds and contour as close to normal as possible.

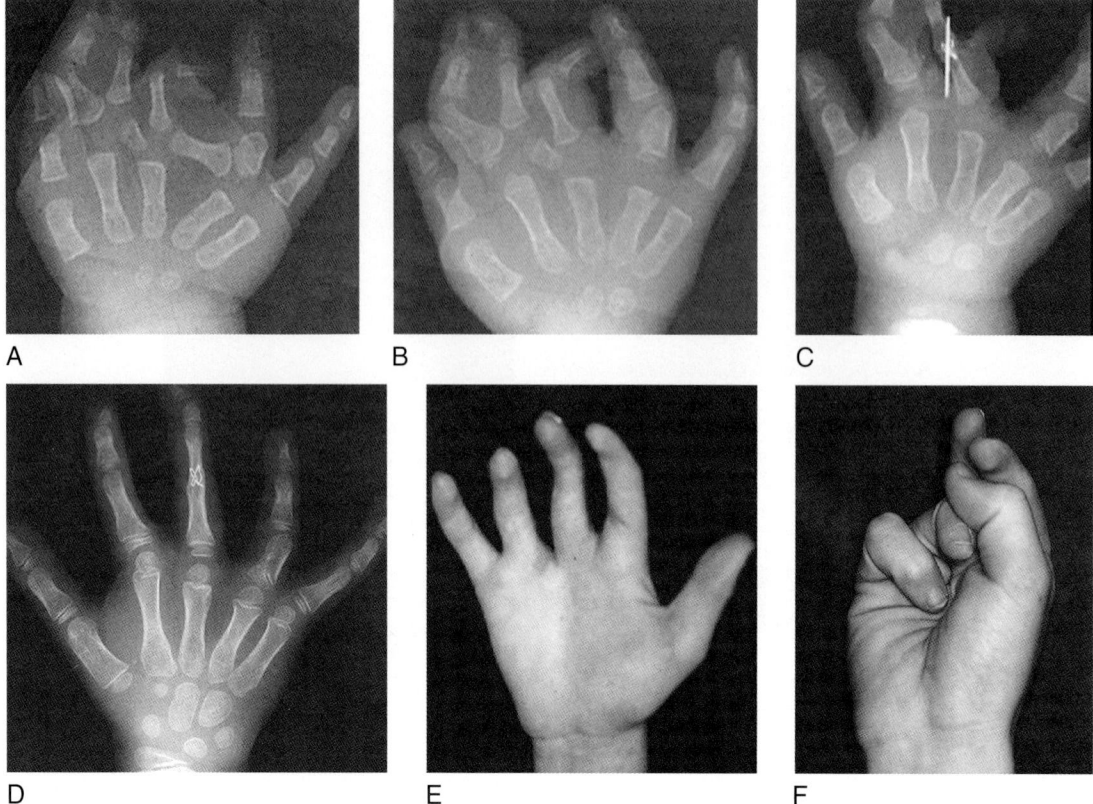

FIGURE 206-29. Surgical correction. *A,* The initial radiograph of the hand illustrated in Figure 206-28. *B,* During the first procedure, the transverse phalanx between the long and ring MP joints was excised and the web space deepened to normal level. *C,* Next, the oblique phalanx between the index and long MP joint was excised, and the proximal phalanx of the long finger, which contained a good MP joint and metacarpal, was fused to the proximal phalanx of the ulnar index finger polydactyly, which contained a good distal nail segment. *D,* Six months later, the PIP joint of the radial index polydactyly was straightened during a formal soft tissue separation of the two index digits. The four metacarpals are well aligned, and motion has been preserved. *E,* The hand is seen 19 years later. The long finger is very long with no IP motion. He has fractured the long and index digits twice while playing football. *F,* Despite obvious limitation with flexion and a weak grasp, he has maintained a functional hand and is pleased with the appearance. The central three digits do not interfere with the thumb to fifth finger pinch or grasp.

side of the ring proximal phalanx, opening wedge osteotomy and bone grafting are performed before syndactyly release (see Fig. 206-29).

ACCESSORY BONES

Extra phalanges in the midline of the "hidden syndactyly" (see Fig. 206-25) and not fused to the proximal or middle phalanges are simply excised at the time of syndactyly release. Transverse and oblique skeletal parts at the level of the metacarpal heads or MP joints must be excised if the commissures are to be placed at the appropriate level. The intrinsic muscle insertions with the proximal muscles are excised at the same time. These muscles have little excursion and balance and will cause a deforming force if they are reattached to retained proximal phalanges. When portions of these bones are left for the purpose of MP joint stability, excessive bone growth will usually account for a distal "creep" of the syndactyly. Synostoses between duplicated proximal or middle phalanges are usually left alone during childhood and trimmed at the time of skeletal maturity if excessive width is to be reduced.

INTRINSIC MUSCLES

Proximal intrinsic muscles are normal when the polydactyly does not involve the metacarpals or the MP joints. With proximal levels of duplication, these muscles have proximal origins from either the proximal portion of the metacarpal or the synostosis. Muscle origins within the divergence of a split metacarpal are rare. These muscles insert directly into the next more distal phalangeal structure, which could include a transverse phalanx, a fused proximal phalanx, a longitudinal epiphyseal bracketed phalanx, or a fused middle phalanx. Separate insertions into the central extensor mechanism should not be expected in these proximal synpolydactylies (see Fig. 206-27).

FUSED BONES

Fusion of duplications at the middle or distal phalangeal level, particularly with isolated index or long digit polydactylies, may be indicated when both partners are much smaller than normal. The Bilhaut operation, or one of the many modifications, does have limitations. The short ring proximal phalanx with a longitudinal bracket can be corrected with excision of the bracket (typically on the radial side of the phalanx), opening wedge osteotomy, and bone graft several months before the formal syndactyly release (see Fig. 206-12). When phalangeal fusions are associated with parallel distal segments, nothing needs to be done, and a wider than normal phalanx is acceptable. Osteotomies through the fused portion can be done to correct abnormal rotation or angulation that may become accentuated with growth. When one portion of a divergent segment of a middle phalangeal duplication is excised, the unsupported distal phalanx will predictably deviate. When the proximal portion of an oblique phalanx originating from the MP joint of an adjacent ray is excised during a syndactyly release, the neurovascular structures should be carefully identified and preserved.

Duplications that originate at the metacarpal level result in a divergent duplicate part, which displaces the position of the long and ring metacarpal heads. Correction involves excision of the synostosis and repositioning of the MP joints in their proper location. If the metacarpal heads are too close together, the digits will diverge with growth. If too far apart, they will converge and scissor. Abnormal cants of the articular surface are best corrected with osteotomies in lieu of manipulation of the collateral ligaments and joint capsules. Because these digits with complex polydactylies ultimately have stiff IP joints, every effort should be made to reposition the MP joint and to maintain as much motion as possible.

The abnormally short digit, such as the ring finger in the combined long-ring polydactyly, can be lengthened and bone grafted during adolescence.

TENDON RECONSTRUCTION

With polydactylies of all three central rays, abnormalities of the extrinsic extensors are much more common than those on the flexor side. The intrinsic tendon insertions are abnormal with all metacarpal level duplications. It is difficult to rearrange the extensors at the phalangeal level with fused segments. These flat extensors have many attachments to the underlying bone and often do not glide freely. The flexor tendons simply bifurcate at the level of the duplication and are ensheathed within common broad pulleys. Construction of at least one pulley at the normal A2 level is important in digits that have both MP and some IP joint motion. Failure do this will contribute to an increased scissoring with growth of the ray. Reinsertion of the extrinsic flexor and extensor tendons is less predictable than arthrodesis at the proximal interphalangeal and distal interphalangeal joint levels. Extrinsic tendons can be transposed from excised accessory skeletal parts if there is some proximal excursion and free gliding. Intrinsic insertions should be excised.

DIGITAL TRANSPOSITIONS

At the phalangeal level, a transposition is usually obvious when one ray has an intact metacarpal and MP joint and an inadequate or missing distal part (see Fig. 206-29). It is often best to perform the skeletal transposition before an overlying soft tissue syndactyly is released. Transposition at the metacarpal level is a special situation. Both the length of the metacarpal and the location of the MP joint are critical during this procedure.

AMPUTATION

Either primary or secondary ray or isolated digital amputations have been recommended by experienced hand surgeons who are well aware of the limited function of the proximal level polydactylies.[62,79] A functional three-fingered hand can be more acceptable than a deformed four-fingered hand. It is preferable to construct four-digit hands whenever possible, but do not hesitate to sacrifice one ray, usually the ring, when there are not enough structures to construct a functional digit. A hand with a good thumb and five separate digits is acceptable in some cultures.[59]

More often, amputation is necessary after vascular compromise due to syndactyly release. The author has observed two large pedigrees in which the oldest child had required central ray amputation. Subsequently, none of the siblings had their complex duplications corrected.

OSTEOTOMIES

Osteotomies with and without appropriate arthrodeses can effectively correct significant deviations or rotational deformities that always increase with growth. The most difficult situations occur when the soft tissue joint laxities contribute to the abnormal rotation. Osteotomy combined with the excision of longitudinal brackets is effective early in life. These phalanges can be expected to grow normally if a good growth plate is retained at the base of the proximal or middle phalanx. Osteotomies through or distal to metacarpal synostoses can effectively reposition a functional MP joint in the proper location. I do not hesitate to combine these osteotomies with metacarpal lengthening with bone grafts in a single stage (Fig. 206-30).

COMPLICATIONS

The number of necessary operations per hand is much greater than for other types of congenital malformations. Wood[58] describes 15 surgeries in one patient, and the author has evaluated one man who had 23 procedures on his hands.[80] Early complications of graft or flap loss, digit loss, pulp loss, and infection are related to insufficient circulation or inadequate immobilization of the young child. Later problems include hypertrophic scars, flexion contractures, loss of the web space, and joint instabilities. With growth, patients with duplications arising at the distal metacarpal or proximal phalanx may demonstrate increased amounts of deviation or rotation due to the asymmetric growth from abnormal epiphyses. An acceptable result at age 3 or 4 years may evolve into an unacceptable functional result during adolescence. By that later time, a great

number of these patients benefit from soft tissue or skeletal revisions.[80] The most unacceptable results may be seen in the parents or grandparents of younger patients.

It is sometimes difficult to distinguish between a complication and an inevitable result from abnormal growth plate, canted articular surface, unstable joint, asymmetric growth, limited motion, or soft tissue anomalies. These patients have many of these conditions at the same time. Within the entire spectrum of congenital upper limb differences, there are few conditions with as many untoward results.

Outcomes

Similar to outcomes for radial polydactylies, the best results are obtained with the distal three types at the distal or middle phalangeal levels (types I to III) and the most proximal type at the CMC joint (type VIII), in which all that is needed is a simple ray resection (Fig. 206-31). Unfortunately, these are the least common forms.

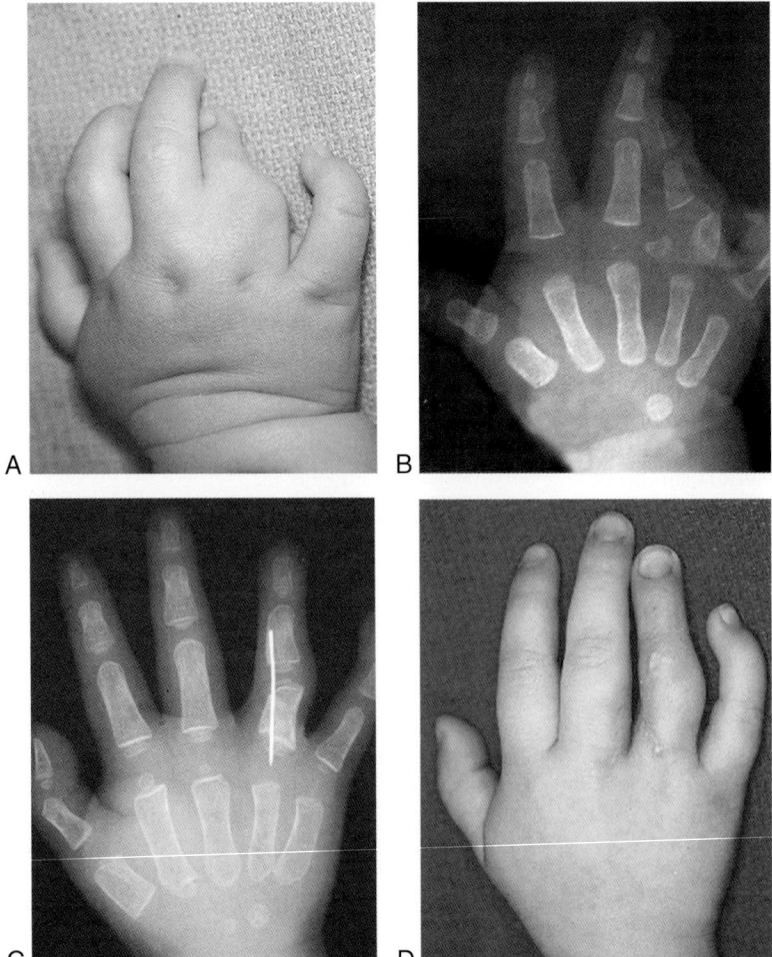

A

B

C

D

FIGURE 206-30. Syndactyly as "a blessing in disguise." *A,* The clinical appearance of the right hand shows a shortened, rotated ring finger. *B,* Within the incomplete syndactyly is a transverse bone articulating with a ring proximal phalanx with a longitudinal epiphyseal bracket. *C,* Before syndactyly release, an opening wedge osteotomy and bone graft were performed on the ring finger. *D,* Two months later, a formal syndactyly release and commissure construction were performed.

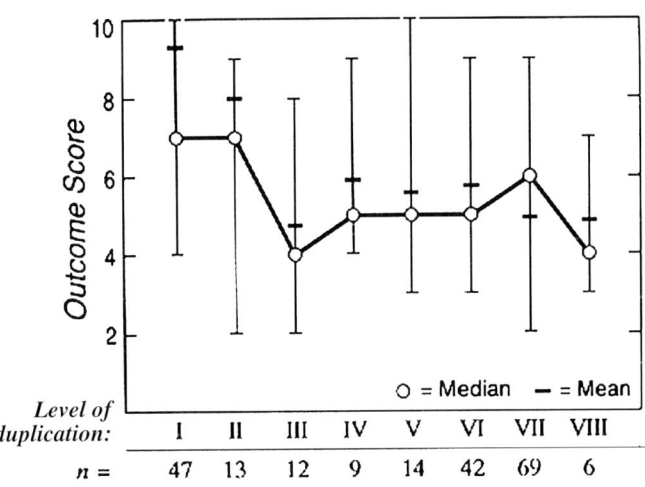

SYNPOLYDACTYLY
Level of Duplication vs. Outcome

FIGURE 206-31. Outcomes of synpoly-dactyly correction. The short- and long-term outcomes after correction of these central polydactylies are summarized in this graph, which correlates the outcome score (function: pinch and grasp = 2 points, appearance = 2 points, contour skeletal deviation and rotation = 2 points, range of motion = 2 points, and soft tissue coverage and contour = 2 points) with the level of branching. Only the most distal corrections are predictably better. There is a wide standard deviation to each level, and satisfactory or unsatisfactory results were noted at all levels. The correction of each hand must be carefully individualized.

ULNAR DUPLICATION

Terminology

Years ago, the small rudimentary form was known as pedunculated postminimus.[81] Duplication on the ulnar border of the hand is also called postaxial and fifth-finger duplication. The preaxial and postaxial terms are confusing because the true developmental axis of the hand runs down the humerus through the ulna to the fifth ray of the hand.[2] The fifth ray is the only postaxial digit, and by definition, the other three digits and the thumb are preaxial digits. Ulnar duplication is the preferred term.

Incidence

Duplication deformities are the most common of all congenital differences of the upper limb, and ulnar (postaxial) polydactyly is by far the most common duplication. In the United States, ulnar duplications are seen about 10 times more frequently in blacks, who show an incidence of 1 in 300,[82] than in whites (1 in 3000).[33,83,84]

Inheritance

Type I deformities, which represent rudimentary nubbins with soft tissue bridges duplicated at the proximal phalangeal level, are dominant with incomplete penetrance, but the whole spectrum exists.[85,86] In 37 affected individuals from 6 generations, Sverdrup and Odiorn have suggested that there is a genetic difference between type I and type II deformities. In contrast, type II and type III deformities carry a dominant inheritance.[87] Children born to parents with type II and type III duplications can produce progeny with all types of duplication, but children born to parents with type I duplications can have children with only the same types of polydactyly.

Syndromic Associations

Associations with ulnar duplication are common in whites and uncommon in blacks.[55,79,88,89] Rarely will a black individual with a type I ulnar duplication show any signs of an associated anomaly, but a white person with the same deformity should be evaluated for more than 40 syndromes that have been chronicled by geneticists. They involve abnormalities of almost all organ systems, including chromosomal syndromes (trisomy 13 and trisomy 18), bone dysplasias (achondroplasia, Ellis-van Creveld), syndromes involving eyes (Laurence-Moon-Biedl), those involving skin (Bloom, Goltz), orofacial syndromes (cleft lip, Meckel), and syndromes with mental retardation (Cornelia de Lange, Smith-Lemli-Opitz).

Classification

The extent of duplication varies from a completely formed digit to a single phalanx or skin tag. Surgeons prefer to classify these duplications by the level at which the malformation originates. The classification system of Temtamy[84] is similar to that outlined previously by Stelling[90] and Turek[91] (Fig. 206-32). In type I, a small, poorly formed digit is attached to the ulnar ray of the hand by a skin bridge of variable width that contains an intact neurovascular bundle. There is no skeletal articulation, and the rudimentary digit is devoid of bone in most instances. Type II involves a duplicated digit with normal components that usually articulates with a bifid metacarpal condyle.

Type I

Type II

Type III

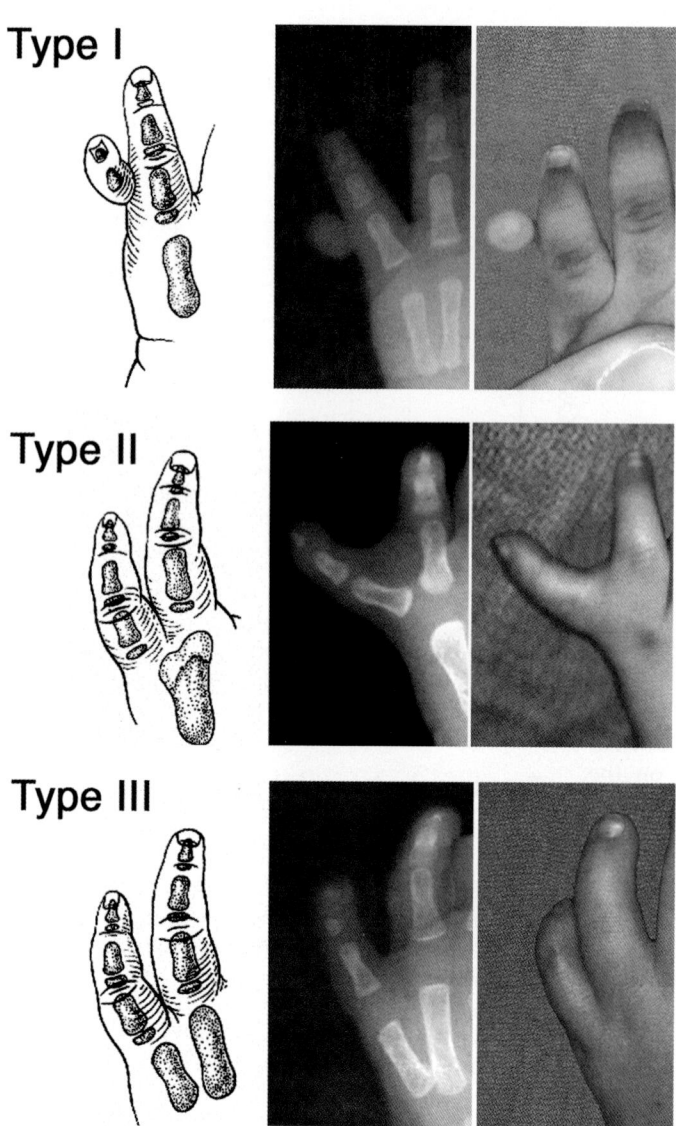

FIGURE 206-32. Ulnar polydactyly, classification. Ulnar polydactylies are classified into three separate groups: type I, simple skin bridge with no skeletal connection; type II, definite skeletal connection at a phalanx or joint; and type III, complete duplication of the entire ray.

The metacarpal may be thickened; a carpal coalition or duplication may occur. Type III, a complete duplication of the entire ray, is rare but does occur.

The system preferred by pediatricians and geneticists subdivides ulnar polydactyly into two broad groups: type A, a hypoplastic digit with well-formed parts and a skeletal connection to the fifth ray of the hand; and type B, rudimentary nubbins joined only by a soft tissue bridge. Type A and type B are terms used interchangeably with type I and type II by geneticists and pediatricians.

Clinical Presentation

The anatomic abnormalities of ulnar duplications parallel those seen with radial polydactyly. Absence and hypoplasias predominate. In type I deformities, only a small neurovascular bundle is present within the skin bridge. Type II duplications have hypoplastic or absent extrinsic and intrinsic muscles, abnormal and bifid articular surfaces, small phalanges with clinodactyly, and hypoplastic nails. In type III polydactyly, subtle changes in the tendons, intrinsic muscles, joint surfaces, and skeletal growth may not become evident until the child progresses through the adolescent growth spurt. After surgical correction and rebalancing of all muscle-tendon units, it is not common to see decreased motion at MP or IP joints and hypothenar muscle weakness.

Treatment

The management of polydactyly is surgical and varies from simple to complex, depending on the anatomic deformity. The timing of surgery also depends on the complexity of the deformity and the size of the child's hand. Type I nubbins can be treated expeditiously in the newborn nursery,[92] whereas a more complicated type II or type III polydactyly may require a well-planned, meticulously performed skeletal and soft tissue procedure (Fig. 206-33). Most ulnar duplications are corrected at or before the age of 12 months. The principles of correction of an ulnar duplication include

1. ablation of nonfunctional parts;
2. construction of the best possible digit from all available parts; and
3. preservation of skeletal length and joint stability without rotational deformity or angulation.

TYPE I. The treatment of the accessory digit is straightforward (Fig. 206-34). For type I deformities, excision of the digit at the base of the tissue bridge is easily done. Although suture ligation at the base of the pedicle may provide satisfactory results, this method often leaves small nubbins with retained cartilage that will grow and require removal during adolescence or adult life. Commonly, a young mother will bring her newborn to the surgeon because the gangrenous digit has not separated.[92,93] Flatt[93] has cited one example of death by exsanguination from a ligated pedicle in a child with an unrecognized coagulopathy. Simple suture ligation in the nursery is not recommended. Instead, the soft tissue pedicle can be effectively incised, the pedicle ligated or cauterized, and the incision closed in the newborn nursery or operating room.[93] Secondary scar contractures, especially

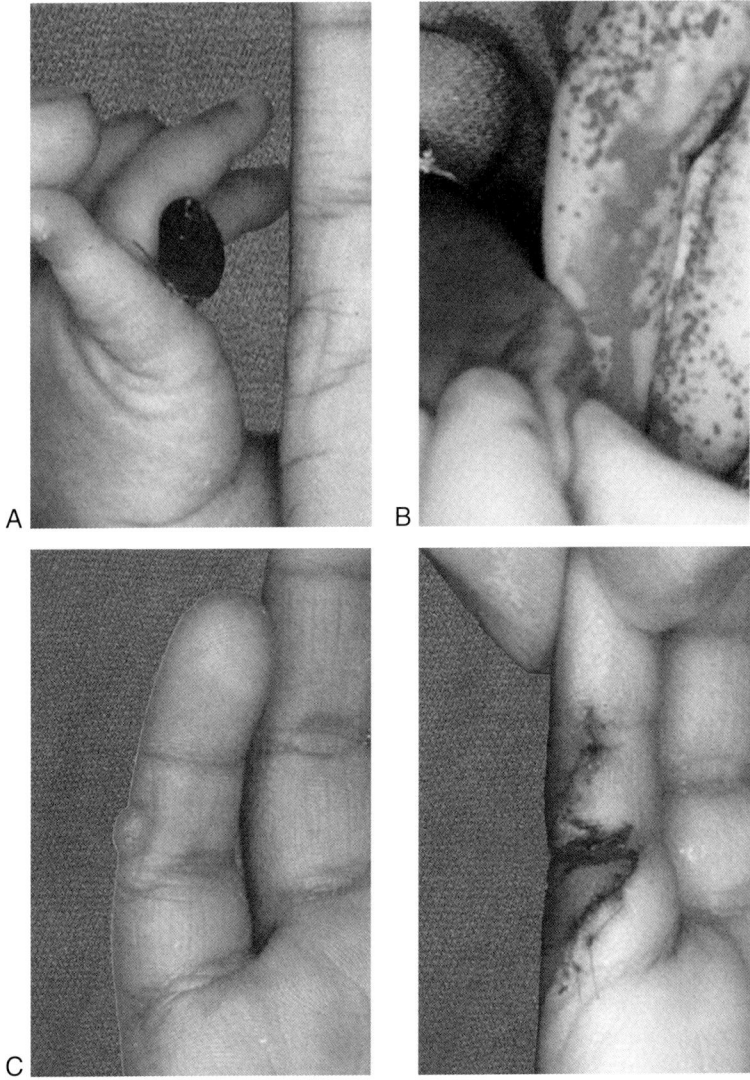

FIGURE 206-33. Type I ulnar polydactyly. *A,* Most pediatricians, obstetricians, and neonatologists "tie off" or ligate the pedicle of the nubbin and wait for it to fall off. *B,* When larger skin bridges are excised, a well-formed digital artery, shown here bleeding, must be either cauterized or ligated. *C,* This patient was referred from the dermatology clinic after she did not respond to wart medication. The polydactyly nubbin was excised, and the straight line was broken with a Z-plasty fashioned to the PIP flexion crease.

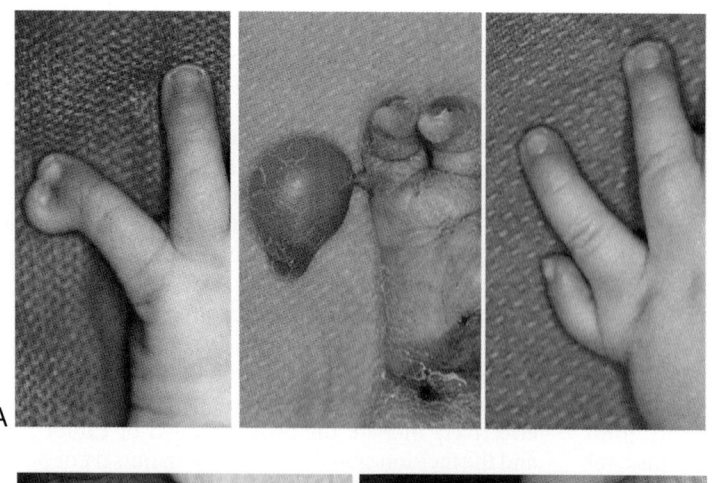

A

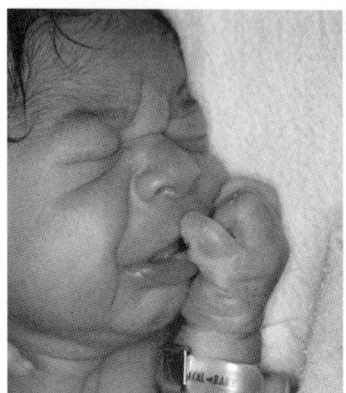
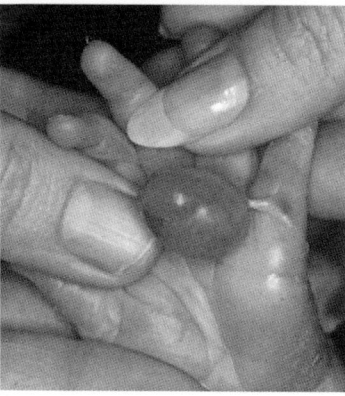

B

FIGURE 206-34. Type I ulnar polydactyly, presentation. *A,* Type I extra digits may present at any level along the digit with skin bridges of varying sizes. The digits on the left and right should be treated under optimal conditions surgically. *B,* This child with a type I "pacifier polydactyly" was sucking the nubbin in utero. The edematous extra digit had a matching contour to the lingual side of the hard and soft palate.

in darkly pigmented patients, may need secondary correction with Z-plasties. On occasion, teenage youngsters come to the clinic requesting revision of nubbins left after simple ligation. Although terminal neuromas are present on the ligated pedicle, a Tinel sign cannot be elicited.

TYPE II. Management of these duplications may be more complex and should be completed by 2 to 3 years of age (Fig. 206-35). The ulnar of the two partners is usually the most hypoplastic and is removed with retention of the hypothenar muscles and the ulnar collateral ligament at the MP joint. I do not agree with the statement that these corrections "require no ingenuity and create no problems."[55] Correction of some of these duplications may be difficult. At operation, incisions should be designed in the midaxial line, collateral ligaments reconstructed, broad metacarpal heads trimmed, hypothenar intrinsic muscles transferred, and dorsal capsules reconstructed to avoid postoperative problems.[94] Skeletal corrections should be performed at the same time as soft tissue surgery. On occasion, the more deformed of the two digits may function better than its partner. In this case, it is often better to reconstruct one good digit with use of the best structure of both, usually the flexor of the retained

digit and the extensor of the excised portion. It is difficult to transfer a flexor of one digit to another without causing tendon adherence. For this reason, the digit with the best intact flexor mechanism is preserved.

Secondary problems after ulnar polydactyly correction include the protuberant bifid fifth metacarpal head, retained bone or cartilage fragments, tight collateral ligament reconstructions, extensor tendon adherence or imbalance, and rotational deformities. Most are the result of incomplete initial surgery. Waiting later than the age of 3 years to correct the more severe deformities will accentuate the associated growth deformities (flexion contractures; skeletal angulation and rotation; tight hypothenar intrinsic muscles, collateral ligaments, and joint capsules—all of which may require additional surgery). MP joint motion is commonly decreased in type II duplications at the MP joint level.

TYPE III. The treatment of this unusual type of ulnar duplication is similar to that of the type II deformities. When both partners are of similar size and length, it is often best to retain the more ulnar ray with its intact complement of hypothenar muscles. Secondary problems are less frequent than those for type

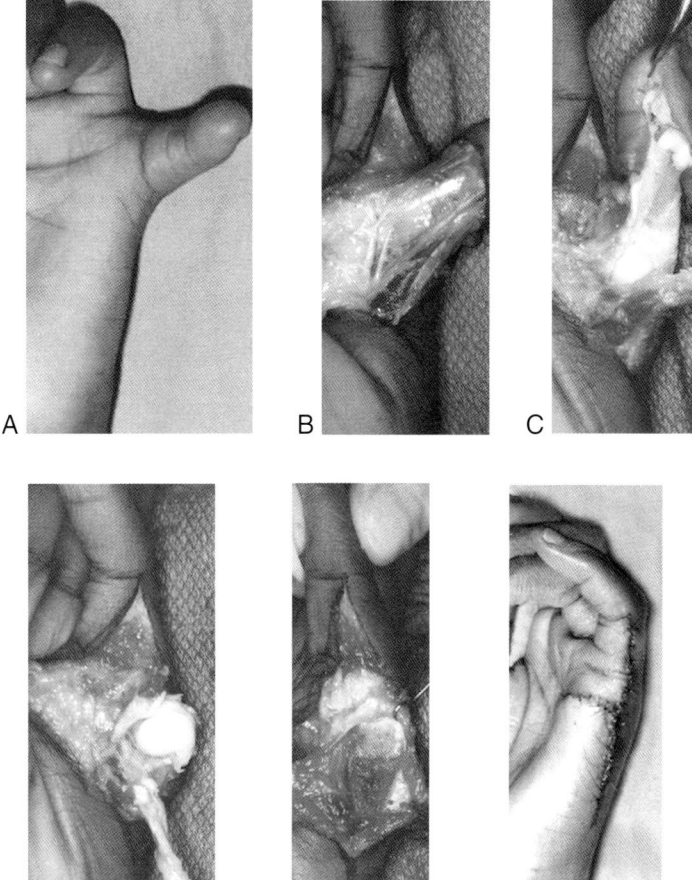

FIGURE 206-35. Type II ulnar poly-dactyly, treatment. *A,* Type II ulnar poly-dactylies are commonly connected at the MP joint level. *B,* After a fillet incision, the neurovascular structures and extrinsic tendons are identified. *C,* Hypothenar muscles are detached from the ulnar digit. A large sleeve of periosteum is retained with the tendon. *D,* The bifid condyle of the thumb metacarpal is exposed. The ulnar collateral ligament is attached to the proximal periosteal sleeve. *E,* Excision of the entire portion of the ulnar condyle exposes the growth plate. *F,* The hypo-thenar muscle and collateral ligament are reattached, and the skin is closed. Redundant skin is best excised through incisions in the normal flexion creases. Note that the MP motion of the radial fifth finger is still deficient.

II corrections. These patients will commonly have bilateral hand and foot duplications. Problems after foot correction become the patient's primary problem.

In rare instances, triplications of the fifth ray may present with extra phalanges, extra metacarpals, or metacarpal remnants,[94] which resemble the unusual configurations of triphalangeal thumbs. These are treated in the same fashion as the thumbs: construct the best possible digit from the available parts. Every deformity is different and requires an individualized reconstruction.

MIRROR HAND
Terminology

The patient with the classic ulnar dimelia will have duplication of the ulna with no radius bones, a hand with seven or eight fingers, and no thumbs, giving a bizarre appearance that is often called mirror hand. This rare entity is the most complete form of duplication in the upper extremity, and slightly more than 60 patients exist in the reported literature.[55] The term *mirror* has been used because the hand, wrist, and forearm on the ulnar side of the limb are reflected as symmetric opposites on the opposite side. Because the radius is absent, it is more appropriate to describe the components from the medial or lateral portion of the forearm, wrist, or hand.[95,96]

History

One of the first clinical descriptions with illustrations appeared in 1587, but the first well-documented case was presented by Jackson,[97] who had the opportunity to describe a mirror hand with duplicated ulnae at necropsy. His patient was a German machinist who found his extra digits and wide span useful while at work and playing the piano; the patient died in Boston in 1852. The dissection by Ainsworth and subsequent description by Jackson labeled the digits properly as little, ring, middle, index, accessory index, accessory middle, accessory ring, and accessory little.[97] The specimen is now in the Warren Museum at the Harvard Medical School (Fig. 206-36).

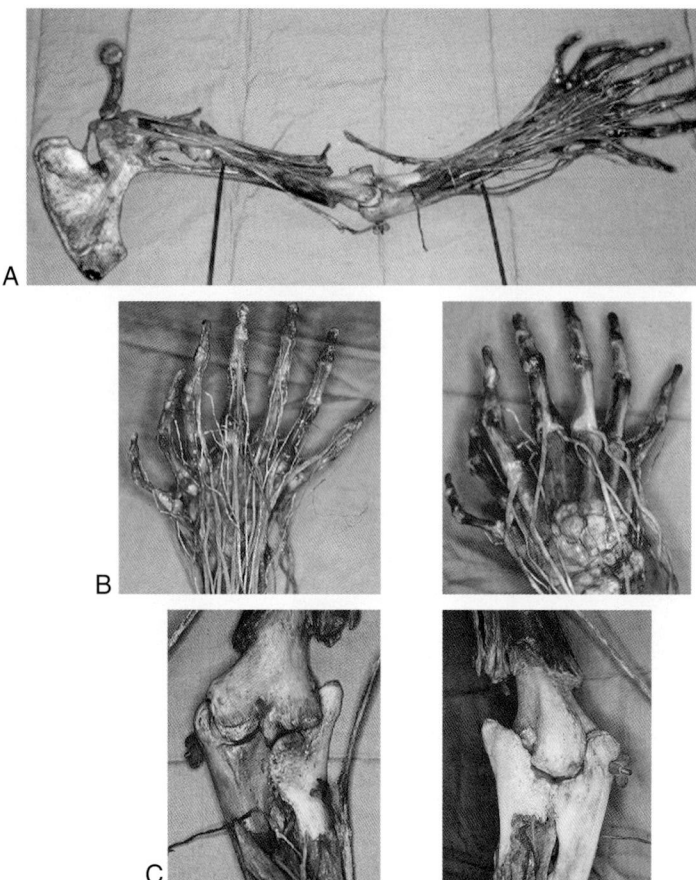

FIGURE 206-36. Mirror hand, anatomic specimen. *A,* The medial side of the arm, elbow, and forearm and palmar surface of the dissected specimen (ulnar dimelia) are demonstrated. Two ulnar arteries and a number of flexor tendons have been preserved. Large muscle bellies in the forearm and arm have not been preserved. *B,* Palmar (left) and dorsal (right) views of the hand. *C,* Anterior (left) and posterior (right) views of the elbow. (From Upton J: Congenital anomalies of the hand and forearm. In May JW Jr, Littler JW, eds: The Hand. Philadelphia, WB Saunders, 1990: 5213-5398. McCarthy JG, ed: Plastic Surgery; vol 8.)

Pathogenesis

Experimental embryologic studies correlate well with the varied soft tissue abnormalities observed by clinical hand surgeons.[96] Work with polarizing region grafts within the avian limb buds has shown that there are three planes of growth in the developing limb.[98] Cells that spend little time in the progress zone of the limb bud form proximal structures, such as the upper arm. The second plane is organized as a dorsoventral axis, which correlates with the flexor-extensor components of the arm. Seldom does orientation of this axis go awry. The third plane, radioulnar or preaxial-postaxial, is relevant to the mirror hand. In 1968, Saunders and Gasseling found that there is a zone of polarizing activity along the postaxial margin of the developing limb bud. Grafting experiments showed that these cells do not form parts but produce substances ("myofibrogens") that diffuse in gradients across the limb bud.[99] Wolpert[100] has produced "mirror hands" by grafting polarizing zones to different positions along the anteroposterior axis of the limb bud at specifically appropriate times. He speculates that

mirror hand may result from an additional polarizing region in the anterior margins of the limb.[96]

Inheritance

This, the rarest of all congenital upper limb differences, is not inherited but may occur with fibular dimelia of the lower extremity and absence of the tibia. There are no known associated malformations. Geneticists have described the cause as a spontaneous genetic mutation that can be transmitted as an autosomal dominant trait.[101] The embryology of this condition is unknown, but the mechanisms of duplication have great biologic significance. Several interesting theories relating to the inductive specificity of the apical ectodermal rings have been proposed.

Clinical Presentation

The clinical appearance varies between seven- and eight-fingered hands (Fig. 206-37). All elements are duplicated except those of the radial ray, including scaphoid, trapezoid, trapezium, metacarpal, and thumb

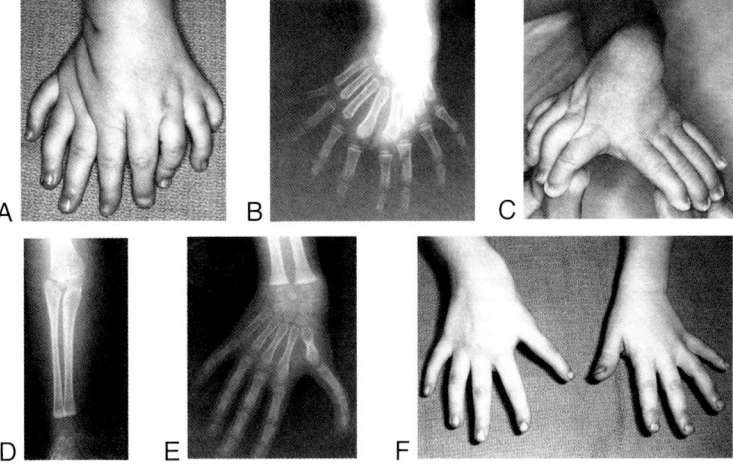

FIGURE 206-37. Mirror hand. *A,* The clinical appearance of a symmetric mirror hand (ulnar dimelia) is shown. *B,* The radiograph shows eight separate metacarpals with separate digits. *C,* The two sides of the hands are distinct and separate. Note the flexed posturing of the wrist. *D,* Two ulnae articulate with a single humerus. *E,* Radiograph after a pollicization of the index accessory digit. *F,* Clinical appearance shows a functional thumb, which is longer and more narrow than normal. The first web space is well maintained, and thumb motion is excellent. (Courtesy of V. R. Hentz, MD.)

phalanges. The hand is flexed at the wrist and may be deviated to one side, depending on the symmetry of existing carpal bones and the length of the two ulnae. There is a central axis and an exaggerated transverse metacarpal arch because the border digits oppose one another. Eight digits are usually present; the accessory index ray is often absent, hypoplastic, or webbed to its other index partner. Most digits are held in a flexed position because extensor muscles are often absent or hypoplastic.[96] The lateral (postaxial, ulnar) set of digits is usually more functional. A duplicated index ray on the radial side of the central hand axis may have either the scaphoid or trapezium missing. The distal articular surface of the medial (preaxial) ulna will usually broaden with growth. At the elbow level, the articular surface of each ulna is rotated so that the olecranon fossae face each other. The humerus lacks a normal capitellum and has two poorly developed trochleae.[102]

Function in mirror hands may be limited, especially when the forearm and elbow are severely affected. Elbow motion is often restricted, and the joint is held in an extended position. Poorly developed upper arm flexors (biceps and brachialis) frequently attach to the distal humerus and do not cross the elbow joint. Pronation and supination are limited, and muscles are often absent. There are weak extensors in a foreshortened forearm; the wrist is held in a flexed and, usually, ulnarly deviated posture (Figs. 206-38 and 206-39). Most digit function is achieved by the ulnar component of digits, and the radial three or four digits often obstruct the more functional ulnar digits in flexion. As expected, older patients with uncorrected deformities develop ingenious adaptive patterns.[97]

Treatment

Because ulnar dimelia usually involves the entire extremity, surgical management must start proximally. Limited shoulder motion, deficient elbow extension,

poor forearm pronation and supination, wrist flexion contractures, extra digits, no thumb, and syndactyly all conspire to make the mirror hand a helping extremity. There are reports of no treatment in individuals who have adapted and used these deformed limbs as 'helpers" and for special recreational activities such as playing the piano.[103] The bizarre appearance of these extremities alone dictates some type of treatment.[96]

ELBOW (FIG. 206-40)

Elbow motion is achieved by limited excision of one of the ulnae, usually the preaxial. Through a lateral incision, excision of as much as possible of the bulbous bone, including portions of the olecranon, lateral humeral condyle, and trochlea, while still allowing flexion-extension and pronation-supination movement is advocated.[102,104] The articulation of the ulna with the humerus is preserved by resecting the ulna proximal to the trochlear notch. The humeral epiphysis must remain unaltered if normal growth is desired. Instability of the elbow may require reconstruction of the collateral ligaments. Elbow motion becomes the next problem and can be achieved with an anterior transposition of the triceps, transfer of the biceps to the flexor carpi radialis,[102] or other transfers such as a Steindler flexor plasty. Improved active or passive motion of the elbow joint may not last, however.[96]

FOREARM

When the forearm and wrist are held in excessive pronation, derotational osteotomy of one or both ulnae may be helpful. Partial excision of one of the olecrana will improve this motion.

WRIST

Wrist flexion contractures present difficult problems and, in combination with a stiff elbow and pronated forearm, can severely limit function. Skin Z-plasty, cap-

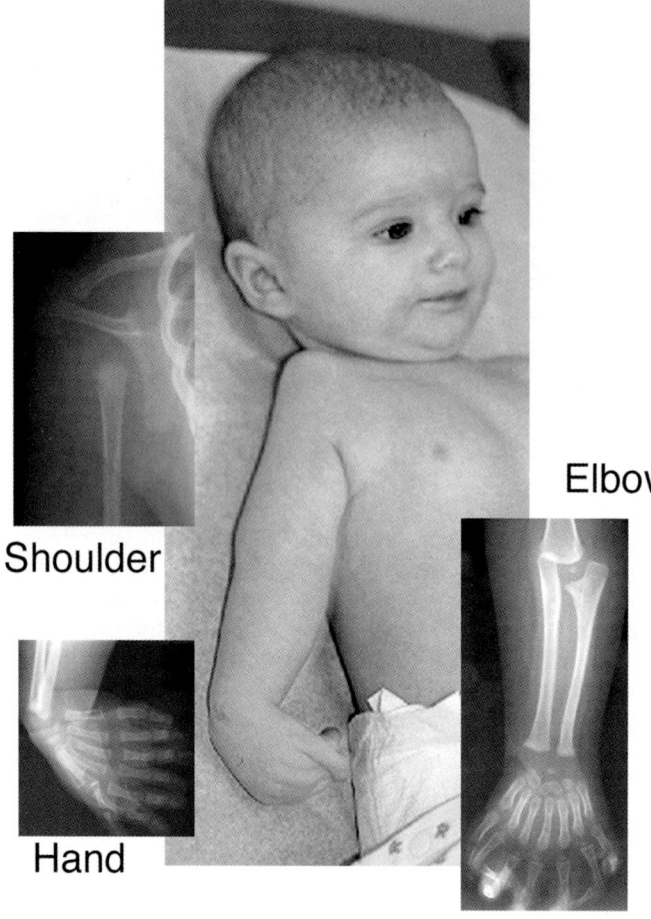

Elbow

Shoulder

Hand

FIGURE 206-38. Mirror arm. Another patient with an ulnar dimelia demonstrates the abnormal posturing and involvement of the entire upper limb. The glenohumeral joint is intact but hypoplastic with no abduction and little flexion or extension. The elbow is held in extension because of the absence of a flexor mechanism. The hand is held in tight flexion and ulnar deviation because of the overwhelming flexor forces on the hand and wrist. These deformities and possible correction at all three levels must be evaluated before any treatment of the hand. (Wagner clinical case.)

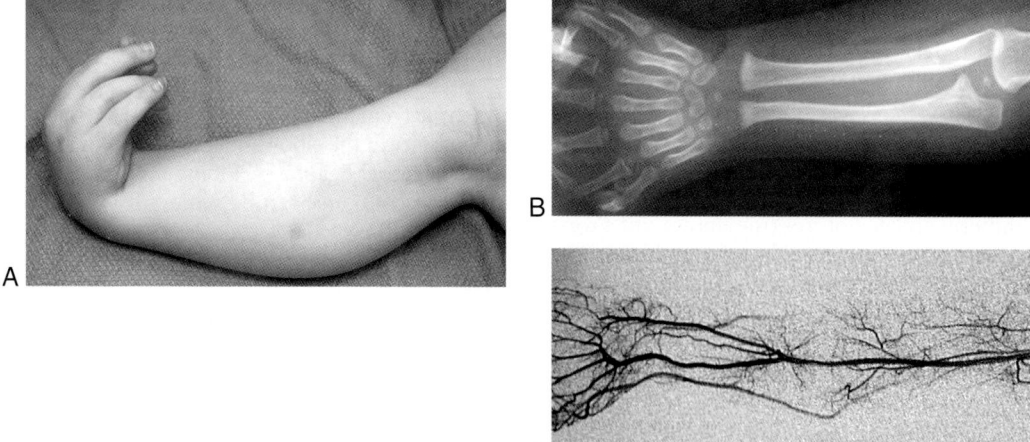

A

B

C

FIGURE 206-39. Mirror arm, anatomy. *A,* Since birth, the elbow was held tightly extended with the wrist flexed. No muscle mass could be palpated anterior or ventral to the humerus. Active digital flexion was much more prevalent in the ulnar four digits of this seven-digit hand. *B,* The radiograph of the forearm, wrist, and hand shows two ulnae articulating with a single humerus, multiple carpal coalitions, and seven metacarpals with triphalangeal digits. *C,* The angiogram demonstrates a single brachial artery branching into two ulnar arteries. The most prominent of the arteries is on the ulnar side of the limb and feeds into a prominent palmar arch, which connects to the lateral ulnar artery at the distal metacarpal level. This connection may be of importance during thumb construction.

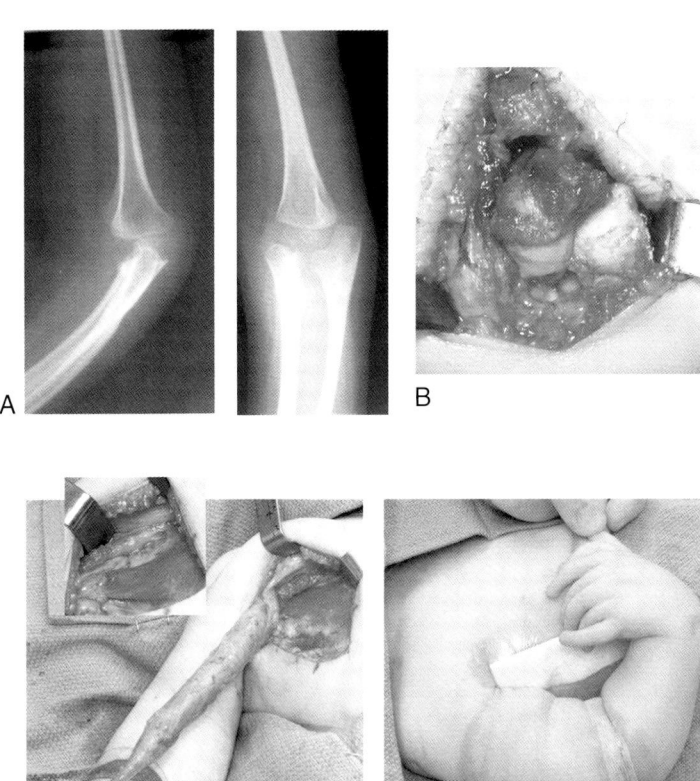

FIGURE 206-40. Mirror arm, elbow correction. *A,* Anteroposterior and true lateral radiographs of the ulna at the time of surgery show the site of resection of the medial portion of the lateral ulna. *B,* Bone was resected until unrestricted passive flexion of the elbow was possible. A vascularized local fasciocutaneous flap was interposed within this gap to prevent refusion. The trochlear notch is visible above as the elbow is best approached from posterior. The medial triceps tendon had a good passive excursion and was lengthened. A lateral triceps tendon was present with no excursion. Simple tenotomy was performed. *C,* Active elbow flexion was achieved with transfer of the sternocostal portion of the pectoralis major muscle (Clark transfer). The humeral origin was transferred to the acromion *(inset).* Tension on the transfer holds the elbow in flexion, which is maintained for 6 weeks postoperatively.

sulotomy, and division of contracted tendons may be required to centralize the hand on the ends of the forearm bones. Osteotomy of distal ulnae has been advocated.[105] Maintaining wrist extension, the next serious problem, can be accomplished with tendon transfers from the amputated digits[96,103,106] or of the flexor carpi ulnaris.[102] Proximal row carpectomy is another option.[102] The alternative approach is wrist arthrodesis.[107-109] All procedures designed to provide dynamic extension of the wrist will be ineffective if the elbow remains in a stiff, extended position. However, in this position, the appearance of the hand and function of the four medial digits are improved.

HAND: DIGITS

The last problem is that the hand has no thumb or thumb-index web space. Entin's procedure[108] has been most widely used; it consists of removing the accessory long and little digits and retaining the accessory ring ray that is in the best position to function as a thumb. A rotation osteotomy and bone block are then used to maintain opposition. Some have attempted to combine two accessory digits to make a single thumb.[110] More recently, those experienced in pollicization techniques have advocated repositioning the best of the accessory digits, usually the accessory index (if present)

or long finger, into a thumb position. Intrinsic muscle transfers convert the interossei of the amputated digits into thumb adductors and the hypothenar mass into the thenar intrinsic muscle mass. The new thumb is then shortened with either a rotation-recession metacarpal osteotomy or subtotal excision with preservation of the metacarpal head.[111]

HAND: THUMB

Despite these sophisticated reconstructions, thumb function is still limited, and additional procedures are required to restore adequate extension (Fig. 206-41). Some have considered complete ablation of all accessory digits and pollicization of the index ray as a more functional solution. The majority of hand surgeons advocate retaining the most normal accessory digit to construct a thumb. Preoperative evaluation, possibly including an angiogram, is critical to this decision and often requires prolonged observation of the child during play activities. No tissues from accessory digits should be discarded until their possible use in web space construction or for tendon transfers for wrist or thumb stabilization/dynamic balance has been ruled out. It is necessary to carefully watch the accessory medial digits function before the digit to be pollicized is chosen.[95]

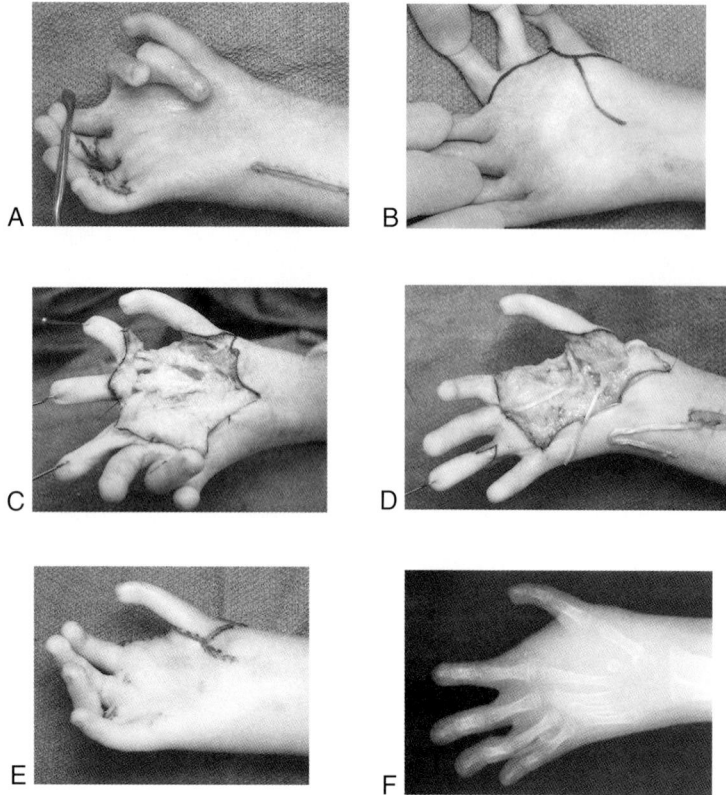

FIGURE 206-41. Mirror arm, pollicization operation. *A,* The first procedure was to release the flexion contracture of the wrist and transfer the flexor carpi ulnaris to the dorsum of the hand. At the same time, camptodactyly releases were performed on the ulnar three normal digits. Note the posturing of the accessory three digits. *B,* The outline of incision is similar to that of a normal pollicization. The most radial digit will be rotated and recessed. *C,* The accessory digits had a full complement of flexor tendons, lumbrical muscles, and digital nerves. The flexor tendons had no proximal excursion. *D,* After removal of the two accessory rays, flexor tendons were isolated. Only one, shown in the forearm, was suitable for transfer to the dorsal aspect of the hand. The patient had no extrinsic digital extensor muscles in the forearm. *E,* Appearance of the hand at the time of closure. *F,* Radiograph shows that the thumb has not been significantly shortened but has been moved over into the space left after ablation of a carpal bone.

Outcomes

Long-term follow-up of mirror hand reconstructions, presented primarily in single case reports or short series, documents far from normal thumb function and appearance in just about all cases. In addition, parents should be told that function of the original postaxial hand digits is not completely normal. Multiple operations are invariably required to achieve a maximal functional position and result.

TRIPHALANGEAL THUMB

Definition

A thumb with three phalanges, regardless of their shape, is considered a rare congenital difference. The earliest descriptions are found in the German and French literature. A report by Buck-Gramcko[112] indicates that this anomaly may not be as elusive as once thought. Well above half of all cases are part of a radial thumb polydactyly.

Incidence

The general incidence is reported as 1:25,000 live births[113] in an old reference. This figure changed dramatically in Europe with the introduction of thalidomide; this sedative, when taken during the first trimester of pregnancy, resulted in a large number of children with limb anomalies. Triphalangeal thumbs were common.[114] Most of the children with a positive family history have bilateral involvement, but some may demonstrate unilateral deformity.

Genetic analysis of multiple Dutch pedigrees with triphalangeal thumbs has localized this genetically transmitted malformation to the long arm of chromosome 7 (7q).[115] Clinical analysis of these families showed that there was a considerable amount of variation in degree among the affected individuals and a marked difference between the two thumbs of an affected child.[115]

Associated Anomalies

Thumb duplication is the most frequently associated anomaly. Great toe anomalies are common but do not consist of extra phalanges.[112] Typical cleft hands,[49,116] congenital heart disease, Holt-Oram syndrome,[117] radial dysplasias, blood dyscrasias,[118,119] gastrointestinal malformations,[52,120,121] absent tibia,[122] and the VACTERL association are less frequently encountered.

Classification

For decades, the triphalangeal thumb was classified into two types, brachymesophalangeal ("short, middle, phalanx") and dolichophalangeal ("long phalanx"), which in turn was subclassified into opposable and nonopposable.[123,124] Wood[52] then introduced the terms *delta, rectangular,* and *full* phalanges. In keeping with the German tradition, Buck-Gramcko[125] recognized other intermediate forms of phalanges and has described a teratologic sequence starting with the most rudimentary form and extending to a perfectly developed rectangular bone. This classification is much more comprehensive and follows a logical sequence. It is easy to understand and correlates well with the options for treatment.

Clinical Presentation

All degrees of development are seen (Fig. 206-42). Type I is the rudimentary form in which a small lucency on the radial side of the thumb IP joint is present at birth. With time, this cartilage will ossify. The distal portion of the thumb deviates in an *ulnar* direction. The proximal CMC and MP joints and thenar intrinsic muscles are normal. In type II, a short triangular bone also causes ulnar deviation of the distal portion of the thumb. The proximal joints and muscles are normal. The segmented interzone or joint space articulating with the distal portion of this bone usually has much less motion than the proximal joint. In type III, a much larger transitional bone is present. It is trapezoidal with two surfaces for articulation. The proximal CMC and MP joints are normal, but the thumb often lies supinated in the same plane as the digits. The thumb is longer. Thenar muscles are hypoplastic or absent, and the first web space is tight. In type IV, a long rectangular bone makes the thumb much longer. Many of these digits will resemble a digit more than a thumb. The distal portion is deviated ulnar; thenar intrinsic muscles are hypoplastic or aplastic, and the metacarpal is often short. The carpal trapezium and scaphoid may be hypoplastic. A perfectly formed middle phalanx is often referred to as the five-fingered hand. The interesting concept here is that it is really a digit, not a thumb. Two flexor tendons are present with a lumbrical originating from the radial side of the flexor digitorum profundus tendon. Type V constitutes a special group in which the entire ray, consisting of one metacarpal and three phalanges, is hypoplastic. All joints are abnormal, motion is limited, and intrinsic musculature is often absent. Joined to the index ray with a simple syndactyly, these thumbs are commonly seen in the Holt-Oram and thalidomide syndromes. Type VI triphalangeal thumbs are those associated with radial polydactyly. This is the largest group and is discussed in a previous section.

Treatment (Table 206-6 and Fig. 206-43)

TYPE I. At birth, the rudimentary middle phalanx may appear only as a widened lucent area on the radial side of the IP joint. No treatment is necessary if the deviation is less than 15 degrees. Some authors recommend early excision of these very small bones and tightening of the collateral ligament.[126,127] Others state that if the wedge-shaped bone is removed within the first year of life, the joint surface will remodel with motion and growth.[128] The author's experience indicates that the remodeling depends more on the size of the excised bone. Motion is usually diminished.

TYPE II. Simple excision of the small intermediate or short triangular middle phalangeal segment can be done within the first 12 months of life (Fig. 206-44). This segment is often much larger than appreciated on radiographs. The radial collateral ligament must be preserved and reattached to bone and periosteum and the joint immobilized with pin fixation for at least 4 weeks postoperatively. During the past 25 years, our positive outcomes have been related, in order of importance, to (1) size of the intermediate phalanx, (2) age at the time of correction, and (3) reconstruction of the collateral ligament. All IP joints can be preserved with a closing wedge osteotomy on the ulnar side of the proximal phalanx (Fig. 206-45).

TYPE III. The trapezoidal middle phalanx has two articulating surfaces and significant size, which makes

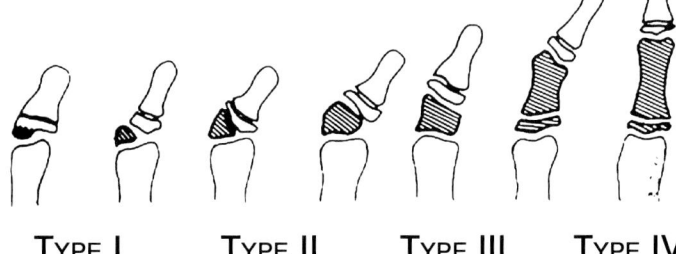

FIGURE 206-42. Triphalangeal thumb, teratologic sequence. A teratologic sequence for the triphalangeal thumb shows the possible variations: rudimentary triphalangism beneath one side of the epiphysis, short triangular bone, larger trapezoidal phalanx, and symmetric phalanx. These have been categorized into various types.

TYPE I
RUDIMENTARY
TRIPHALANGISM

TYPE II
SHORT TRIANGULAR
MIDDLE PHALANX

TYPE III
TRAPEZOIDAL
MIDDLE PHALANX

TYPE IV
LONG RECTANGULAR
MIDDLE PHALANX

TRIPHALANGEAL THUMBS

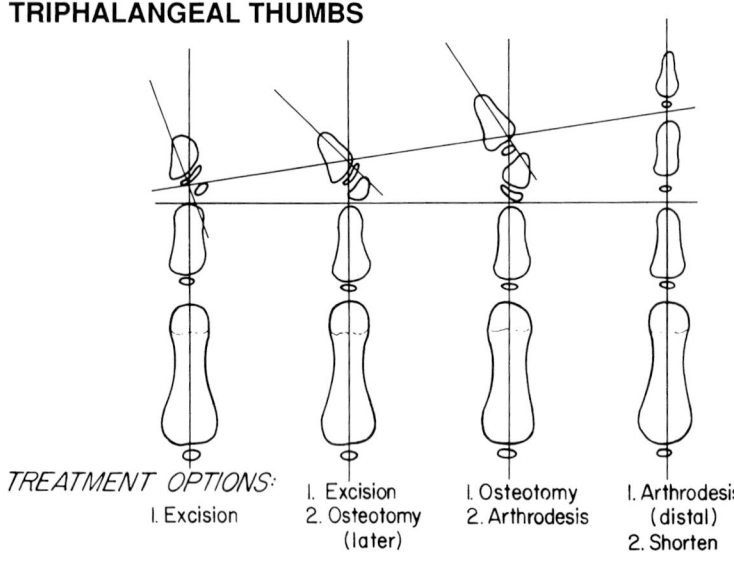

TREATMENT OPTIONS:

I. Excision	I. Excision 2. Osteotomy (later)	I. Osteotomy 2. Arthrodesis	I. Arthrodesis (distal) 2. Shorten

FIGURE 206-43. Treatment options. The treatment options vary with the size of the intermediate phalanx. It is important to determine clinically where motion exists on either side of this extra bone and to preserve as much motion as possible. With the larger phalanges, shortening and arthrodesis of the stiffer side and preservation of motion on the mobile side are preferred.

TABLE 206-6 ✦ TRIPHALANGEAL THUMB TREATMENT

Type	Characteristics	Treatment Options
I	Rudimentary phalanx Normal CMC, MP joints Normal thenar muscles Normal length	Nothing Excision with >15 degrees of deviation
II	Short triangular bone Normal CMC, MP joints Normal thenar intrinsics Ulnar > radial deviation	Excision Closing wedge osteotomy
III	Larger transitional bone Normal CMC, MP joints Thumb longer Palmar abduction absent Rotation in supination Tight first web space	Closing wedge osteotomy Partial resection, shortening Tendon transfer (flexor digitorum superficialis to abductor pollicis brevis) Metacarpal osteotomy Four-flap Z-plasty
IV	Long rectangular middle phalanx Restricted CMC, MP joints Excessive length Excessive deviation Hypoplastic, absent thenar muscles Deficient first web space Metacarpal hypoplastic Carpals hypoplastic, absent	Pollicization Same as with type III
V	Hypoplastic thumb Small phalangeal segments Syndactyly with index All joints abnormal Thenar muscles hypoplastic, absent Syndromic association: Holt-Oram, radial dysplasias, thalidomide, others	Ray resection Index pollicization Separation

VI	Associated with radial duplications
	
	All variations of middle phalanx
	
	Normal to absent CMC joint
	MP joint variable
	First web space often deficient
	Thenar muscles variable
		Depends on the thumb that is left after
		  duplication correction
		Goal: construct best thumb from all available
		  parts; preserve ulnar collateral ligament at
		  MP joint if possible

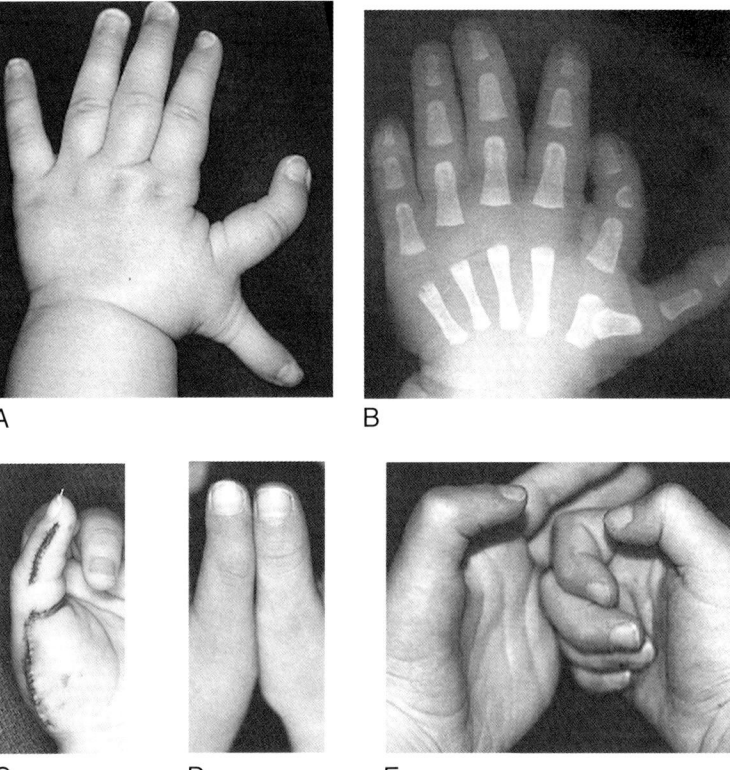

A   B

C   D   E

FIGURE 206-44. Type II, treatment. *A,* The clinical photograph shows a type VII polydactyly of the left thumb. *B,* The radiograph shows a short first metacarpal with branching at the mid-diaphyseal level. The extra phalanx on the ulnar thumb was trapezoidal and had more motion at the articulation with the proximal phalanx. *C,* A chondrodesis between the distal portion of this intermediate bone and the distal phalanx was performed through a midaxial incision at the same time as the resection of the radial thumb. *D,* The thumb contours and length are compared 12 years postoperatively. *E,* Full flexion has been maintained. Note that the triphalangeal left thumb is longer than the normal right side.

the thumb longer. Thenar intrinsic muscle deficiencies will place the thumb in a supinated position with a short first web space. Correction of the specific skeletal and soft tissue deficiencies can be performed in one or two steps. Skeletal revision should be completed first. The ray can be shortened by partial excision of the intermediate phalanx with or without partial metacarpal resection. With significant shortening, the intrinsic tendons must be advanced after reefing of the extensor mechanism at the MP joint, similar to an index pollicization. With a small middle phalanx, many prefer to perform a reduction osteotomy.[26,129-131] Most surgeons elect to resect a portion of this bone and fuse it to its articulating partner. The key to this procedure is the preservation of the joint with the greatest motion. Direct observation intraoperatively is the most accurate and practical test. The proximal joint is usually the most mobile, but not always![93] The soft tissue corrections include an adequate release of the first web space with a four-flap Z-plasty or other transposition flap technique. Local rotation flaps with dorsal unsightly skin grafts are to be discouraged. Thumb muscle balance and position can then be improved by a tendon transfer with use of the flexor digitorum superficialis, abductor digiti quinti minimi, or other muscle tendon motors (Fig. 206-46).

TYPE IV. Thumbs with the long rectangular middle phalanx are the most difficult to treat (Fig. 206-47). One should first determine whether the child is using this radial digit to a significant degree. Buddy taping of the index and long digits together is an important

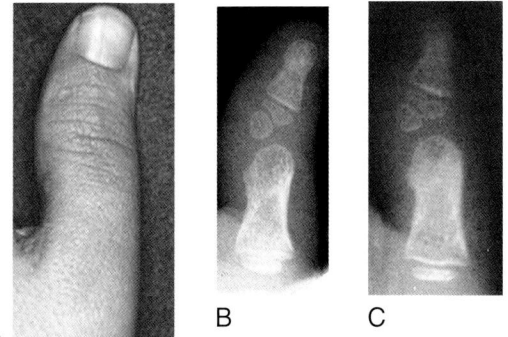

A   B   C

FIGURE 206-45. Type II, treatment. *A,* This thumb has the unusual radial deviation of the distal phalanx due to an extra bone. *B,* The radiograph shows a small ossified bone on the underside of the growth plate. There was normal IP joint motion. *C,* A closing wedge osteotomy of the proximal phalanx corrected the deviation and rotation with preservation of motion.

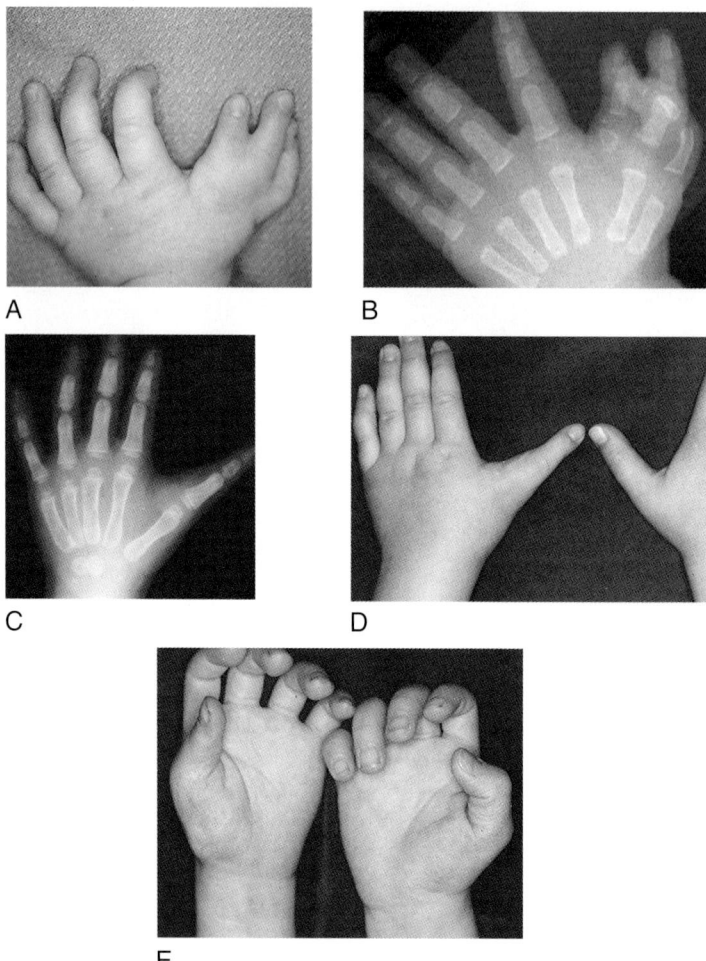

FIGURE 206-46. Polydactyly with triphalangeal thumb, treatment. *A,* The clinical appearance of a complex triplicated thumb and an adequate first web space. *B,* The radiograph shows three thumb rays. The ulnar is type V biphalangeal, the central and the radial rays are full triphalangeal rays (ulnar V; central T; radial T). *C,* In a single operation, the ulnar thumb was excised and the adductor pollicis transferred to the central thumb proximal phalanx. The ulnar collateral ligament of the MP joint was intact. The radial thumb was excised with transfer of the abductor pollicis brevis and flexor pollicis brevis to the radial side of the central thumb. The extra phalanx was not excised on the central thumb. *D,* Despite shortening of the middle phalanx and distal joint arthrodesis, the triphalangeal thumb is longer than normal. *E,* Although IP joint flexion is minimal, the patient has no functional or aesthetic complaints 21 years postoperatively.

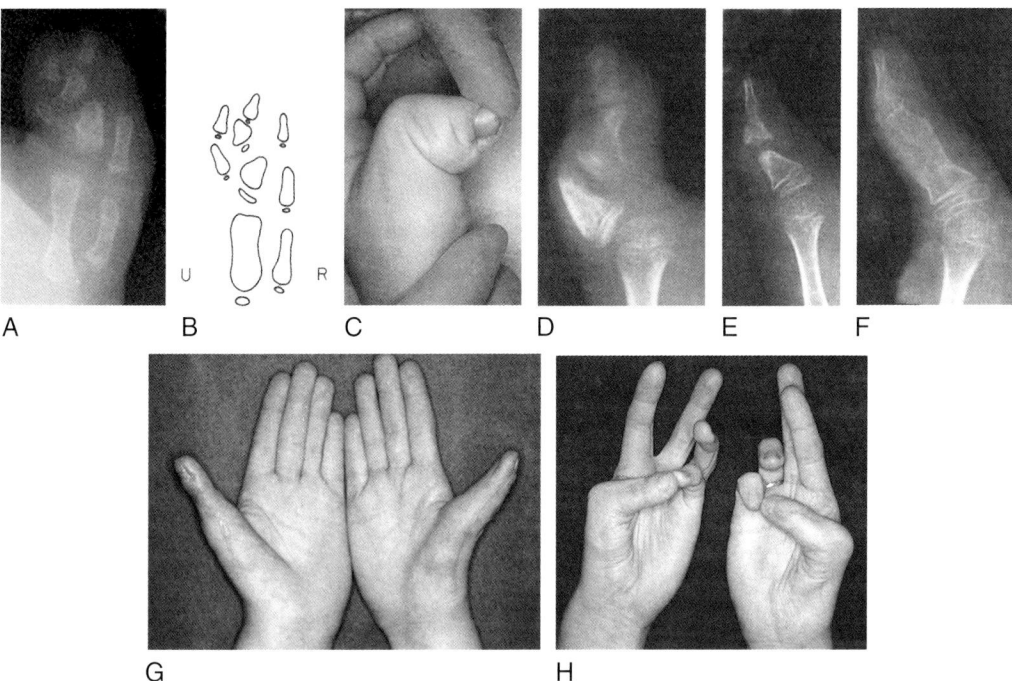

FIGURE 206-47. Complex polydactyly with triphalangeal thumb, treatment. *A,* The radiograph of one hand of a baby with complex, mirror image thumb polydactylies. All of the abnormal skeletal parts are within a single soft tissue envelope. *B,* An illustration shows an ulnar type IV triphalangeal radial thumb and a biphalangeal radial thumb. *C,* When the child was first examined at the age of 6 years, she had unstable thumbs. *D,* The radiograph at that time showed long, broad thumbs with three phalanges. *E,* Three years later, she presented with a nonunion after excision of the middle phalanx and chondrodesis of the remaining proximal and distal phalanges. *F,* After 3 weeks of distraction, optimal length was achieved, and the intercalated gap was bone grafted. *G,* At age 32 years, she has excellent function despite the deficiency of many thenar intrinsic muscles. *H,* The lack of IP joint motion with normal MP joint motion has not caused any functional problems. At this time, she brought in her first child with identical thumb malformations.

test. The first option is similar to that for the shorter trapezoidal phalanx, for example, to shorten the length with ostectomies, to rebalance intrinsic muscles, and to reposition the thumb in palmar abduction in one and preferably two operations. The second option is a formal pollicization of the radial digit. It is preferable to shorten the middle phalanx and fuse it to the distal phalanx with reinsertion of the extrinsic flexor and extensor tendons. When the new thumb is placed in proper position after an adequate web release, the soft tissue deficit requires more than local flaps can provide. Distally based fasciocutaneous flaps on either the dorsal interosseous arterial system or the radial arterial system are excellent sources of tissue.[132] A free transfer of a small fasciocutaneous flap in the small hand of a 1- to 2-year-old child is reasonable for an experienced pediatric microsurgeon. Tendon transfers for palmar abduction are then performed at a second stage. A simple rotation-recession

osteotomy with release of the first web space is a simpler option.[133]

TYPE V. This is the easiest group to treat. Every tissue within this ray is deficient, and the position of this thumb along the index finger will affect potential motion of the otherwise normal digit. The treatment of choice is early simple excision of the hypoplastic ray and index pollicization (Fig. 206-48). It is now preferable to combine both procedures in one operation ideally performed between 12 and 14 months of age. The decision to add tendon transfers for palmar abduction depends on the size and position of available intrinsic muscles and the thumb balance after skeletal repositioning (Fig. 206-49).

TYPE VI. The treatment of triphalangeal thumbs associated with radial duplications is covered in the section on radial polydactyly.

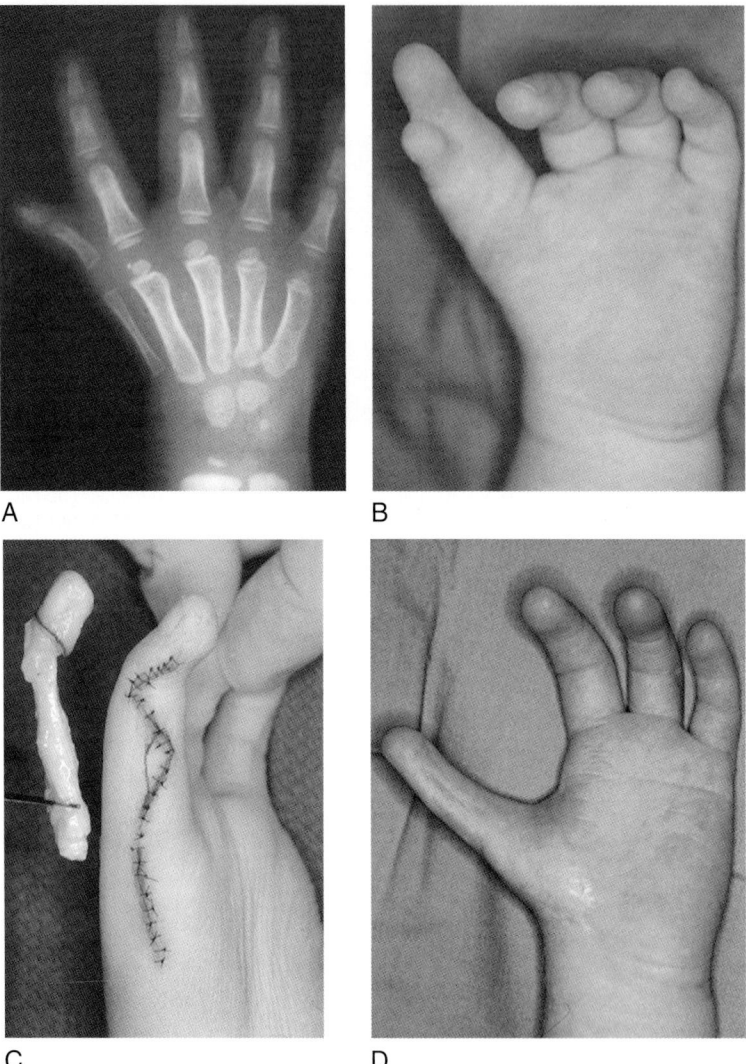

A

B

C

D

FIGURE 206-48. Type V, treatment. *A,* Radiograph of a hypoplastic thumb that is joined to a stiff index finger with the Holt-Oram syndrome. *B,* The clinical appearance of the hand shows a stiff index finger, which the child is trying to autopollicize. *C,* The mobility of the index finger is improved after resection of the hypoplastic thumb, which may be biphalangeal or triphalangeal. *D,* Clinical appearance several years after a pollicization of the index finger.

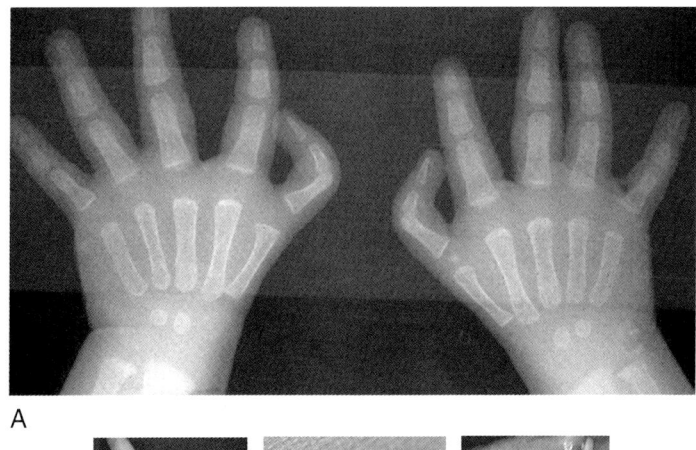

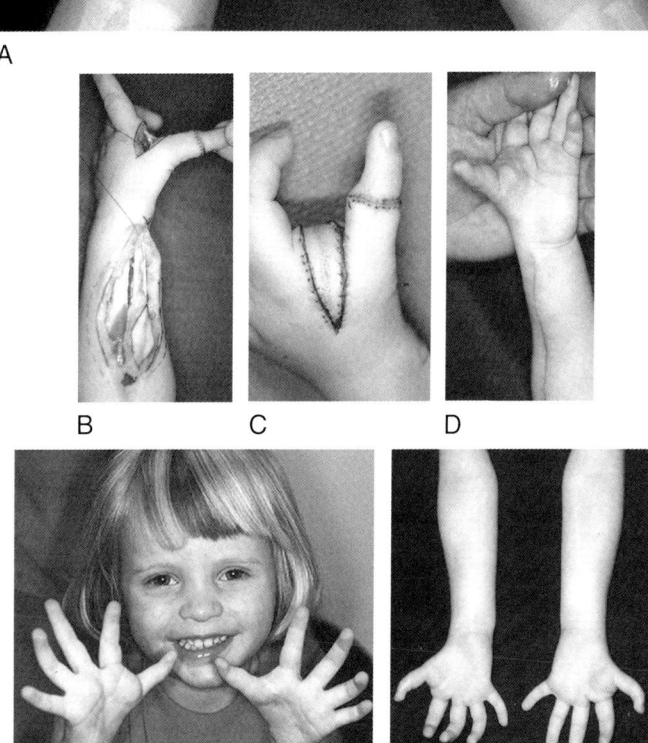

FIGURE 206-49. Type V, treatment. *A,* Radiographs of a child with bilateral five-fingered hands. The growth plate on both radial rays is at the distal metacarpal level. The PIP joints are flexed. *B,* Distally based radial forearm fasciocutaneous flaps were used to broaden the first web space on both hands. *C,* At the same time, the middle phalanx was shortened and fused to the proximal phalanx. *D,* The appearance of the thumb and forearm scar several months postoperatively. Note the absence of thenar muscles. *E,* Both thumbs have maintained their palmar abduction, and this child has been functional. *F,* Closed properly, the forearm scars are acceptable.

REFERENCES

1. Light T, Buck-Gramcko D: Polydactyly: terminology and classification. In Buck-Gramcko D, ed: Congenital Malformations of the Hand and Forearm. London, Churchill Livingstone, 1998:217-224.
2. Ezaki M: Radial polydactyly. Hand Clin 1990;6:577-588.
3. Light TR: Treatment of preaxial polydactyly. Hand Clin 1992;8:161-175.
4. Buck-Gramcko D: Congenital malformations of the hand: indications, operative treatment and results. Scand J Plast Reconstr Surg 1975;9:190-198.
5. Buck-Gramcko D: Congenital malformations. In Lister G, ed: Hand Surgery. Stuttgart, Thieme, 1988:12.1-12.115.
6. Andrew JG, Sykes PJ: Duplicate thumbs: a survey of results in twenty patients. J Hand Surg Br 1988;13:50-53.
7. Cheng J, Chan KM, Ma GF, Leung PC: Polydactyly of the thumb: a surgical plan based on 95 cases. J Hand Surg Am 1984;9:155-164.
8. Cohen MS: Thumb duplication. Hand Clin 1998;14:17-27.
9. Dobyns JH, Lipscomb PR, Cooney WP: Management of thumb duplication. Clin Orthop 1985;195:26-44.
10. Egawa T: Surgical treatment of the polydactyly of the thumb. Jpn J Plast Reconstr Surg 1966;9:97-105.
11. Ganley TJ, Lubahn JD: Radial polydactyly: an outcome study. Ann Plast Surg 1995;35:86-89.
12. Goffin D, Gilbert A, Leclercq C: Thumb duplication: surgical treatment and analysis of sequels. Ann Chir Main Memb Super 1990;9:119-128.
13. Graham TJ, Louis DS: A comprehensive approach to surgical management of the type IIIA hypoplastic thumb. J Hand Surg Am 1998;23:3-13.

14. Guero S, Haddad R, Glicenstein J: Surgical treatment of duplication of the thumb. Apropos of 106 cases [in French]. Ann Chir Main Memb Super 1995;14:272-283.

15. Ikuta Y: Thumb duplication. In Buck-Gramcko D, ed: Congenital Malformations of the Hand and Forearm. London, Churchill Livingstone, 1998:225-235.

16. Karchinov K: The treatment of polydactyly of the hand. Br J Plast Surg 1962;15:362-376.

17. Light T: Duplication du pouce: pathologie et traitement. In Gilbert A, Buck-Gramcko D, Lister G, eds: Les malformations congenitales du membre superieur. Paris, Expansion Scientifique Francaise, 1991:130-138.

18. Marks TW, Bayne LG: Polydactyly of the thumb: abnormal anatomy and treatment. J Hand Surg Am 1978;3:107-116.

19. Naasan A, Page RE: Duplication of the thumb. A 20-year retrospective review. J Hand Surg Br 1994;19:355-360.

20. Richard Y, Collin JP, Asencio JG, et al: Thirty cases of duplication of the thumb. Operative results. Ann Chir Main 1983;2:46-55.

21. Seidman GD, Wenner SM: Surgical treatment of the duplicated thumb. J Pediatr Orthop 1993;13:660-662.

22. Tuch BA, Lipp EB, Larsen IJ, Gordon LH: A review of supernumerary thumb and its surgical management. Clin Orthop 1977;125:159-167.

23. Townsend DJ, Lipp EB Jr, Chun K, et al: Thumb duplication, 66 years' experience—a review of surgical complications. J Hand Surg Am 1994;19:973-976.

24. Buck-Gramcko D, Behrens P: Klassifikation der Polydaktylie für Hand und Fuss. Handchir Mikrochir Plast Chir 1989;21:195-204.

25. Wassel H: The results of surgery for polydactyly of the thumb. Clin Orthop 1969;64:175-193.

26. Wood V: Polydactyly and the triphalangeal thumb. J Hand Surg Am 1978;3:436-444.

27. Hung L, Cheng JC, Bundoc R, Leung P: Thumb duplication at the metacarpophalangeal joint. Management and a new classification. Clin Orthop 1996;323:31-41.

28. Blauth W, Olason A: Classification of polydactyly of the hands and feet. Arch Orthop Trauma Surg 1988;107:334-344.

29. Dobyns J: Duplicate thumbs (split thumbs). In Green DP, ed: Operative Hand Surgery, 3rd ed. New York, Churchill Livingstone, 1993:440-450.

30. Temtamy S, McKusick V: The Genetics of Hand Malformations. New York, Alan R. Liss, 1978. Birth Defects: Original Article Series; vol 14.

31. Flatt A: The Care of Congenital Hand Anomalies, 2nd ed. St Louis, Quality Medical Publishing, 1994:292-314.

32. Yonenobu K, Tada K, Kurisaki E, et al: Polydactyly: an analysis of 232 cases. J Jpn Orthop Assoc 1980;54:121-134.

33. Woolf C, Myrianthopoulos N: Polydactyly in American Negroes and Whites. Am J Hum Genet 1973;25:397-404.

34. Perez-Molina JJ, Alfaro-Alfaro N, Lopez-Zermeno MC, Garcia-Calderon MA: Polidactilia en 26,670 nacimientos consecutivos: caracteristicas clinicas, prevalencia y factores de riesgo. Bol Med Hosp Infant Mex 1993;50:803-808.

35. Orioli IM, Castilla EE: Thumb/hallux duplication and preaxial polydactyly type I. Am J Med Genet 1999;82:219-224.

36. Castilla EE, Lugarinho da Fonseca R, da Graca Dutra M, et al: Epidemiological analysis of rare polydactylies. Am J Med Genet 1996;65:295-303.

37. Nogami H, Oohira A: Experimental study of pathogenesis of polydactyly of the thumb. J Hand Surg Am 1980;5:443-450.

38. Yasuda M: Pathogenesis of pre-axial polydactyly of the hand in human embryos. J Embryol Exp Morphol 1975;33:745-756.

39. Zguricas J, Baker WF, Heus H, et al: Genetics of limb development and congenital hand malformations. Plast Reconstr Surg 1998;101:1126-1135.

40. Zguricas J, Heus H, Morales-Peralta E, et al: Clinical and genetic studies on 12 preaxial polydactyly families and refinement of the localization of the gene responsible to a 1.9 cM region of chromosome 7q36. J Med Genet 1999;36:32-40.

41. Upton J: Congenital anomalies of the hand and forearm. In May JW Jr, Littler JW, eds: The Hand. Philadelphia, WB Saunders, 1990:5213-5398. McCarthy JG, ed: Plastic Surgery; vol 8.

42. Kitayama Y, Tsukada S: Patterns of arterial distribution in the duplicated thumb. Plast Reconstr Surg 1983;72:535-542.

43. Lister G: Pollex abductus in hypoplasia and duplication of the thumb. J Hand Surg Am 1991;16:626-633.

44. Lister G: Musculus lumbricalis pollicis. J Hand Surg Am 1991;16:622-625.

45. Light T: Duplication du pouce: pathologie et traitement. In Gilbert A, Buck-Gramcko D, Lister G, eds: Les malformations congenitales du membre superieur. Paris, Expansion Scientifique Francaise, 1991:130-138.

46. Bilhaut: Guerison d'un pouce bifide par un nouveau procede operatoire. Congr Franc Chir 1890;4:576-580.

47. Upton J: Duplicated thumb: discussion. Plast Reconstr Surg 1982;69:480-481.

48. Manske P: Treatment of the duplicated thumb using a ligamentous/periosteal flap. J Hand Surg Am 1989;14:728-733.

49. Barsky A: Congenital anomalies of the thumb. Clin Orthop 1959;15:96-110.

50. Muller W: Beitrage zur Kenntnis des dreigliedrigen Daumens. Langenbecks Arch Klin Chir 1936;185:337-386.

51. Nylander E: Pra-axial Polydactylie in fünf Generationen einer schwedischen Sippe. Upsala Lak Foren Forh 1931;36:275-292.

52. Wood V: Treatment of the triphalangeal thumb. Clin Orthop 1976;120:188-200.

53. Shoen S, Upton J: Classification and treatment of triphalangeal thumbs. Chief Residents Conference, Kansas City, Missouri, 1993.

54. Buck-Gramcko D: Teratologic sequences. In Buck-Gramcko D, ed: Congenital Malformations of the Hand and Forearm. London, Churchill Livingstone, 1998:17-20.

55. Kelikian H: Congenital Deformities of the Hand and Forearm. Philadelphia, WB Saunders, 1974.

56. Goodman FR, Mundlos S, Muragaki Y, et al: Synpolydactyly phenotypes correlate with the size of expansion of HOXD13 polyalanine tract. Proc Natl Acad Sci USA 1997;94:7458-7463.

57. DeSmet L, Fabry G: Type II syndactyly or synpolydactyly. Acta Orthop Belg 1992;58:209-212.

58. Wood V: Treatment of central polydactyly. Clin Orthop 1971;74:196-205.

59. Tada K, Kurisaki E, Yonenobu K, et al: Central polydactyly—a review of 12 cases and their surgical treatment. J Hand Surg Am 1982;7:460-465.

60. Buck-Gramcko D: Central polydactyly. In Buck-Gramcko D, ed: Congenital Malformations of the Hand and Forearm. London, Churchill Livingstone, 1998:237-264.

61. Bensahel H, Boureau M: Medecine pratique et syndactylies. Rev Pratt 1972;22:3265-3274.

62. Flatt A: Problems in polydactyly. In Cramer L, Chase R, eds: Symposium on the Hand, vol 3. St. Louis, CV Mosby, 1971:150-167.

63. Merlob P, Grunebaum M: Type II syndactyly or synpolydactyly. J Med Genet 1986;23:237-241.

64. Messina A, Pontini I: La polisindattilia centrale tipo III delle mani. Considerazoni clinico-genetiche e classificazione anatomo patologica delle lesioni. Riv Chir Mano 1984;21:203-215.

65. Tomsen O: Einige Eigentumlichkeiten der erblichen Poly- und Syndaktylie bei Menschen. Acta Med Scand 1927;65:609-644.

66. Schatzki P: Über verdeckte Syndaktylie, Polydaktylie und über "Triangelbildung" in dermenschlichen Mittelhand. Arch Orthop Unfall Chir 1934;34:637-652.

67. Manoiloff E: A rare case of hereditary hexodactylism. Am J Phys Anthropol 1931;15:503-508.

68. Schuler A: Zur Symptomatik und Genetik von Synpolydaktylie und Polysyndaktylie [dissertation]. Düsseldorf Universitäts, 1991.

69. Sayli BS, Akarsu AN, Sayli U, et al: A large Turkish kindred with syndactyly type II (synpolydactyly). Field investigation, clinical and pedigree data. J Med Genet 1995;32:421-434.

70. Muragaki Y, Mundlos S, Upton J, Olsen BR: Altered growth and branching patterns in synpolydactyly caused by mutations in HOXD13. Science 1996;272:548-551.

71. Bosse K, Betz RC, Lee YA, et al: Localization of a gene for syndactyly type I to chromosome 2q34-q36. Am J Hum Genet 2000;67:492-497.

72. Akarsu AN, Stoilov I, Yilmaz E, et al: Genomic structure of HOXD13 gene: a nine polyalanine duplication causes synpolydactyly in two unrelated families. Hum Mol Genet 1996;5:945-952.

73. Sarfarazi M, Akarsu AN, Sayli BS: Localization of the syndactyly type II (synpolydactyly) locus to 2q31 region and identification of tight linkage to HOXD8 intragenic marker. Hum Mol Genet 1995;4:1453-1458.

74. Messina A: Considerations cliniques, anatomo-pathologiques et chirurgicales sur la polysyndactylie centralie de type III des mains (systematisation et classification des lesions). Ann Chir Main 1989;8:135-145.

75. Manske P: Cleft hand and central polydactyly in identical twins: a case report. J Hand Surg Am 1983;8:906-908.

76. Tanabu S: Clinical and roentgenological study of the hands in symbrachydactyly, constriction band syndromes and cleft hand [in Japanese]. Nippon Seikeigeka Gakkai Zasshi 1985;59:167-182.

77. Ogino T: A clinical and experimental study on teratogenic mechanism of polydactyly, syndactyly and cleft hand. J Hand Surg Br 1990;15:201-209.

78. Ogino T: Clinical and experimental study on the teratogenic mechanisms of cleft hand, polydactyly, and syndactyly. J Jpn Orthop Assoc 1979;53:535-543.

79. Wood V: Postaxial polydactyly (little finger polydactyly). In Green DP, ed: Operative Hand Surgery, 3rd ed. New York, Churchill Livingstone, 1993:485-490.

80. Upton J: Classification, treatment and outcomes of 163 patients with central synpolydactyly. Plast Reconstr Surg; in press.

81. Cummins H: Spontaneous amputation of human supernumerary digits: pedunculated postminimi. Am J Anat 1932;51:381-416.

82. Frazier T: A note on race-specific congenital malformation rates. Am J Obstet Gynecol 1960;80:184-185.

83. Nathan P, Keniston R: Crossed polydactyly. J Bone Joint Surg Am 1975;57:847-849.

84. Temtamy S, McKusick V: Synopsis of hand malformations with particular emphasis upon genetic factors. Birth Defects 1969;3:125-184.

85. Sverdrup A: Postaxial polydactylism in six generations of a Norwegian family. J Genet 1922;12:217-240.

86. Odiorne J: Polydactylism in related New England families. J Hered 1943;34:45-56.

87. Barsky A: Congenital Anomalies of the Hand and Their Surgical Treatment. Springfield, Ill, Charles C Thomas, 1958:48-64.

88. Temtamy S, McKusick V: Polydactyly. Birth Defects 1978;14:364.

89. Ruby L, Goldberg M: Syndactyly and polydactyly. Orthop Clin North Am 1976;7:361-374.

90. Stelling F: The upper extremity. In Ferguson AB, ed: Orthopedic Surgery in Infancy and Childhood. Baltimore, Williams & Wilkins, 1963:282-402.

91. Turek S: Orthopaedic Principles and Their Application. Philadelphia, JB Lippincott, 1967:123.

92. Watson, B., Hennrikus WL: Postaxial type-B polydactyly: relevance and treatment. J Bone Joint Surg Am 1997;79:65-68.

93. Flatt A: The Care of Congenital Hand Anomalies. St. Louis, CV Mosby, 1977.

94. Light T, Buck-Gramcko D: Ulnar polydactyly. In Buck-Gramcko D, ed: Congenital Malformations of the Hand and Forearm. London, Churchill Livingstone, 1998:265-269.

95. Barton NJ, Buck-Gramcko D, Evans DM, et al: Mirror hand treated by true pollicization. J Hand Surg Br 1986;11:320-336.

96. Barton NJ, Buck-Gramcko D, Evans DM: Soft tissue anatomy of mirror hand. J Hand Surg Br 1986;11:307-319.

97. Jackson B: Malformation in an adult subject consisting of fusion of two upper extremities. Am J Med Sci 1853;25:91-93.

98. Wolpert L, Hornbruch A: Positional signalling along the antero-posterior axis of the chick wing: the effects of multiple polarizing region grafts. J Embryol Exp Morphol 1981;63:145-159.

99. Summerbell P: The zone of polarizing activity: evidence for a role in normal chick limb morphogenesis. J Embryol Exp Morphol 1979;50:217-233.

100. Wolpert L: Position and pattern formation. Dev Biol 1971;6:183.

101. Sandrow R, Sullivan R, Steel H: Hereditary ulna and fibular dimelia with peculiar facies. J Bone Joint Surg Am 1970;52:367-370.

102. Tsuyuguchi Y, Tada K, Yonenobu K: Mirror hand anomaly; reconstruction of the thumb, wrist, forearm and elbow. Plast Reconstr Surg 1982;70:384-387.

103. Harrison R, Pearson M, Roaf R: Ulnar dimelia. J Bone Joint Surg Br 1960;42:549-555.

104. Santero N: Dichiria con duplicata dell' ulna e assenza del radio. Arch Ital Chir 1936;43:173-193.

105. Zwierzchowski H, Komorowski T: Przyczynek do etiopato-genczy reki lustrzanej [contribution to the aetiopathogenesis of a mirror hand]. Chir Narzadow Ruchu Ortop Pol 1982;47:131-134.

106. Pintilie D, et al: Double ulna with symmetrical polydactyly. J Bone Joint Surg Br 1964;46:89-93.

107. Mukerji M: Congenital anomaly of the hand: "mirror hand." Br J Plast Surg 1956/57;9:222-227.

108. Entin M: Reconstruction of congenital anomalies of the upper extremities. J Bone Joint Surg Am 1959;41:681-701.

109. Gorriz G: Ulnar dimelia—a limb without anteroposterior differentiation. J Hand Surg Am 1982;7:466-469.

110. Davis RG, FA: Mirror hand anomaly; a case presentation. Plast Reconstr Surg 1958;21:80-83.

111. Beasley R: Reconstructive surgery in upper extremity anomalies. In Swinyard C, ed: Limb Development and Deformity. Problems of Evaluation and Rehabilitation. Springfield, Ill, Charles C Thomas, 1969:476-499.

112. Buck-Gramcko D: Triphalangeal thumb: a new classification depending on the operative treatment. Jpn J Surg Hand 1995;12:89-90.

113. Lapidus P, Guidotti F, Coletti C: Triphalangeal thumb: report of six cases. Surg Gynecol Obstet 1943;77:178-186.

114. Lenz W, Theopold W, Thomas J: Thiphalangie des Daumens als Folge von Thalidomidschadigong. Munsch Med Wochenschr 1964;106:2033-2041.

115. Zguricas J, Snijders P, Hovius S, et al: Phenotypic analysis of triphalangeal thumb and associated hand malformations. J Med Genet 1992;31:462-467.

116. Phillips R: Congenital split foot (lobster claw) and triphalangeal thumb. J Bone Joint Surg Br 1971;53:247-257.

117. Holt M, Oram S: Familial heart disease with skeletal malformations. Br Heart J 1960;22:236-242.

118. Aase JM, Smith D: Congenital anemia and triphalangeal thumbs. J Pediatr 1969;74:471-474.

119. Diamond L, Allen D, Magill F: Congenital (erythroid) hypoplastic anemia: a 25-year study. Am J Dis Child 1961;102:403-415.

120. Townes P, Brocks E: Hereditary syndrome of imperforate anus with hand, foot, and ear anomalies. J Pediatr 1972;81:321-326.

121. Chan KM, Lamb DW: Triphalangeal thumb and five-fingered hand. Hand 1983;15:329-334.

122. Lamb DW, Wynne-Davis R, Whitmore JM: Five-fingered hand associated with partial or complete tibial absence and pre-axial polydactyly. A kindred of 15 affected individuals in five generations. J Bone Joint Surg Br 1983;65:60-63.

123. Windle B: The occurrence of an additional phalanx in the human pollex. J Anat Physiol 1891;26:100-116.

124. Hilgenreiner H: Über Hyperphalangie des Daumens. Beitr Klin Chir 1907;54:585-629.

125. Buck-Gramcko D: Congenital and developmental conditions. In Bowers WH, ed: The Interphalangeal Joints. The Hand and Upper Limb, vol 1. Edinburgh, Churchill Livingstone, 1987:187-202.

126. Milch H: Triphalangeal thumb. J Bone Joint Surg Am 1951;33:692-697.

127. Cotta H, Jaeger M: Die operative Behandlung der angeborenen Daumenfehlbildung einschliesslich der Daumenaplasie. Arch Orthop Unfall Chir 1977;62:339-358.

128. Buck-Gramcko D: Handchirurgie, Band I. Allgemeines Wahloperationen. Stuttgart, Thieme, 1981: Chapter 12.

129. Malek R, Oger P: Les pouces a trois phalanges. Ann Chir 1976;30:849-854.

130. Peimer C: Combined reduction osteotomy for triphalangeal thumb. J Hand Surg Am 1985;10:376-381.

131. Jennings JF, Peimer C, Sherwin FS: Reduction osteotomy for triphalangeal thumb: an 11 year review. J Hand Surg Am 1992;17:8-14.

132. Upton J, Havlik R, Coombs C: The use of forearm flaps for the severely contracted first web space in children with congenital malformations. J Hand Surg Am 1996;21:470-477.

133. Hentz V, Littler LJ: Rotation-recession osteotomy. J Hand Surg Am 1977;2:113-120.

Failure of Differentiation and Overgrowth

JOSEPH UPTON III, MD

SKELETAL DEFORMITIES

Skeletal fusions occur at all levels of the upper limb skeleton and are classified separately and independently at each interval. No global classification exists, nor is one practical. These fusions may occur at more than one level, and they are often accompanied by overlying soft tissue anomalies.

The wide variety of individual skeletal parts that can cause abnormal rotation or angulation is too extensive to be considered here. Only the most common type, asymmetric shapes of the phalanges that cause clinodactyly, is discussed here.

Symphalangism

INCIDENCE

Because this is rarely a primary diagnosis and is usually seen in conjunction with another condition, the true incidence of symphalangism has never been determined.[1] True symphalangism accounts for 0.03% of all congenital differences of the upper limb in Flatt's series from Iowa[2] and 0% to 4% in Buck-Gramcko's reported series.[3]

GENETICS

For generations, failure of segmentation or incomplete segmentation with cavitation has been of great interest to geneticists. Cushing[4] noted that one of his patients with an intracranial glioma was unable to bend her proximal interphalangeal joints, and after 10 years of studying her kindred, he published a classic paper in which he introduced the term *symphalangism* to describe a family with 84 involved persons from a

kindred of 313 examined.[5] Strasburger et al[6] updated this family pedigree. The largest pedigree in the genetic literature involves the Talbot family of England, from the mid-1450s through the 20th century.[7]

Hereditary symphalangism (SYM or SYM1) is an autosomal dominant disorder characterized by multiple joint fusions of the fingers and toes.[4-6,8-12] Most forms are caused by mutations of the *NOG* gene or noggin gene, which maps to chromosome 17q22. So far, six independent *NOG* mutations have been identified.[13,14] Because the *NOG* gene is expressed in the ovary and interacts with bone morphogenetic proteins, which play an important part in ovarian function, *NOG* mutation may be important in the development of ovarian failure.[15] This may explain why acro-osteolysis is seen with symphalangism in some pedigrees. Bone morphogenetic proteins may be related to the association of SYM with abnormalities of the teeth[16] and hair,[17] conductive hearing loss,[10,18-24] osteoarthritis,[25] brachydactyly,[8,26-31] and abnormal facial appearance.[16,32]

The nonhereditary types often seen with symbrachydactyly are sporadic and usually associated with a deficient or absent middle phalanx in the involved digit or digits. Patients with Poland syndrome fall into this general group (Fig. 207-1).

CLASSIFICATION AND CLINICAL PRESENTATION

Various specialists have formulated different systems to classify at least 15 conditions in patients with stiff fingers. Flatt and Wood[2] classify the conditions as true symphalangism, in which digits have normal length; symbrachydactyly, in which digits are short as well as

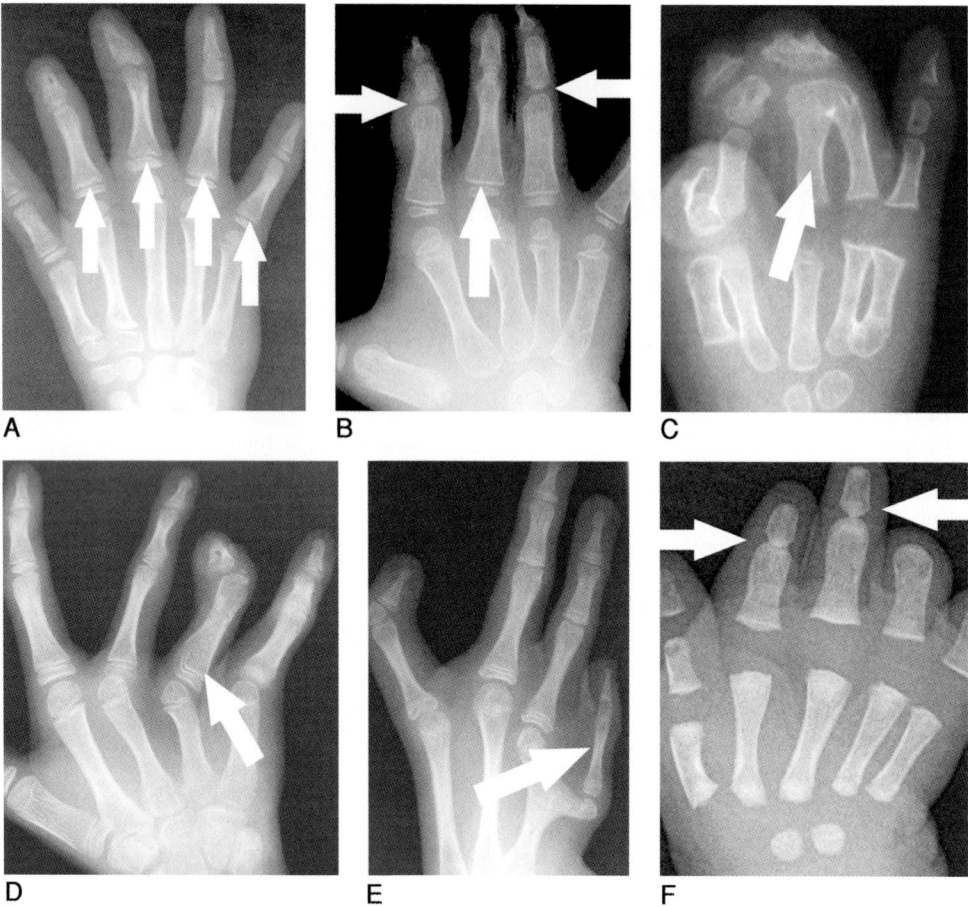

FIGURE 207-1. Examples of symphalangism. *A,* Symphalangism commonly occurs in the digits *(arrows)* of patients with brachysyndactyly associated with the Poland syndrome. Digital separations have been completed in this young patient. The ring ray shows a hypoplastic middle phalangeal segment. *B,* In another Poland syndrome child, narrow interzones demarcating PIP joints may be present early in childhood. However, by skeletal maturity, these cartilaginous bars will ossify, creating a true symphalangism. *C,* A coalition between the proximal and middle phalanges is common in the central three rays of children with the Apert syndrome. *D,* Symphalangism is commonly seen in the ring and, to a lesser extent, long ray in patients with central synpolydactyly. *E,* Phalangeal coalition is seen in the shorter of two digits that share a common metacarpal in this patient who also presents with a bizarre variation of an ulnar failure of formation. *F,* The two phalanges present in this child with brachydactyly D will fuse to form one bone with mobility only at the MP joint.

stiff; or symphalangism with associated anomalies. The majority of cases in the third group include syndactyly, and most are diagnosed within either Apert or Poland syndrome (see Fig. 207-1). Many other conditions with digital fusions, such as the Hurler syndrome (gargoylism), are not as frequently referred to the hand surgeon.

The proximal interphalangeal (PIP) joint is the most common site of involvement. In contrast, congenital fusion at the metacarpophalangeal (MP) joint is extremely rare; fusion of the distal interphalangeal (DIP) joint is seen with symbrachydactyly, in which other abnormalities of the digit exist. In very young children, physical findings may range from a well-

segmented but stiff joint space to a minimal space seen on radiographic examination. This is represented on gross examination by a solid cartilaginous bar joining articular surfaces. Initial radiographs of the infant's hand will appear normal because the cartilage representing the epiphysis and joint space is radiolucent. Therefore, early radiographic evaluations in these children may be confusing, with the middle phalangeal epiphysis mistaken for a joint space (see Fig. 207-1*B*).

When the PIP joint is primarily involved, a tremendous amount of compensatory motion in flexion is often present at the DIP joint, whereas MP motion in flexion is usually normal. Affected digits are more slender and lack normal flexion creases in the involved regions. The middle phalanx is usually deficient (see Chapter 204). Skin is often atrophic, but sensation is normal. One or more digits may be involved, but the thumb is rarely affected. Although the patient cannot make a full fist and power grip is deficient, use of the ulnar three digits may be effective despite the loss of normal flexion. The correct diagnosis should be made and often is made on physical examination of the hand (Fig. 207-2).

TREATMENT

Treatment of symphalangism is usually conservative. Early surgical misadventures failed because the normal intrinsic and extrinsic flexor and extensor motors are deficient. Efforts to supply functional motion with interposition arthroplasties with silicone caps[33] and with silicone implant arthroplasties[34,35] have produced unstable joints, despite attempts at collateral ligament construction. Perichondral arthroplasties have been successful at the MP joint level for post-traumatic conditions but have performed poorly at the interphalangeal (IP) joint level.[36] Repositioning the flexion position of the ulnar three fingers with either an angulation osteotomy or arthrodesis improves functional pinch and grip; however, such procedures are usually deferred until skeletal maturity has been reached. Recommended angles for fusion at the PIP joint level are

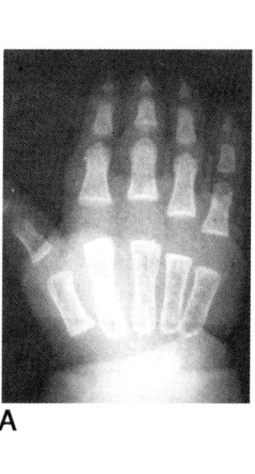

A

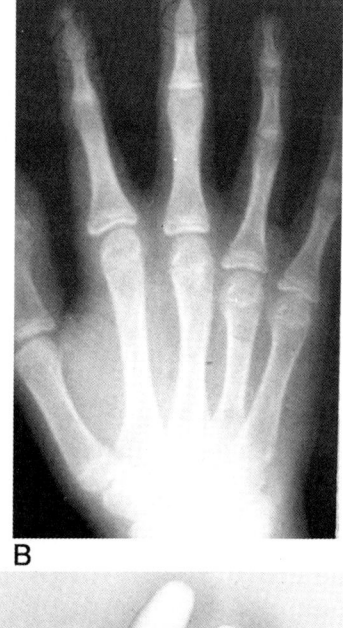

B

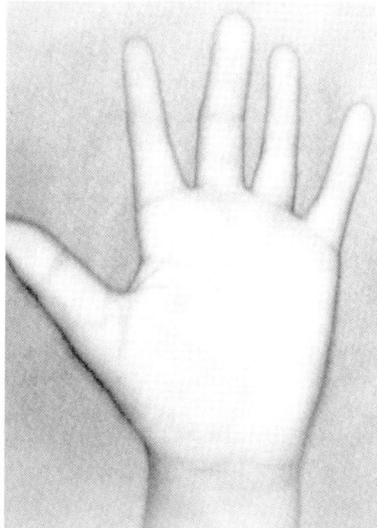

C

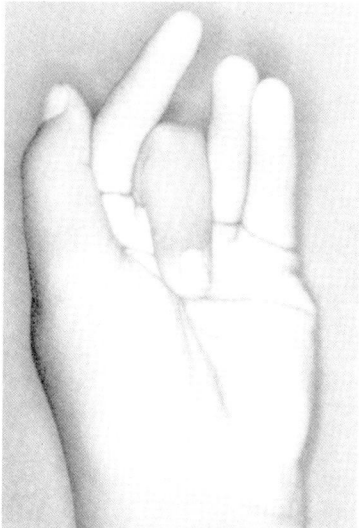

FIGURE 207-2. Physical examination of symphalangism. *A,* The radiograph of this child during the second year of life shows well-segmented interphalangeal joints in all digits. *B,* Ten years later, the long finger is the only digit with a mobile PIP joint. *C,* Note the slender appearance and absence of flexion creases in the index, ring, and small digits, which have not moved since birth.

20 degrees for the index, 30 degrees for the middle, 40 degrees for the ring, and 50 degrees for the small.[37]

In children younger than 2 or 3 years, exploration of a well-segmented joint space may be useful; in some cases, a solid cartilaginous bar is not present, and functional motion may be achieved by release of tight collateral ligaments and the dorsal capsule. When a segmented joint is visible on radiographic examination, early release may be worthwhile (Fig. 207-3). After soft tissue release and early passive motion, function may be maintained, although long-term results are less predictable. Excision of the cartilaginous bar, with con-

struction of concave-convex surfaces, and early postoperative motion can be frustrating, however, as these joints rapidly fuse. Methods of maintaining periodic distraction to these digits after release have not been reported.[2] The great challenge is to maintain motion and to prevent rapid re-fusion.

OUTCOMES

Premature surgery on these small digits will often lead to rapid re-fusion and may also run the risk of damage to epiphyses of already short and slender fingers.

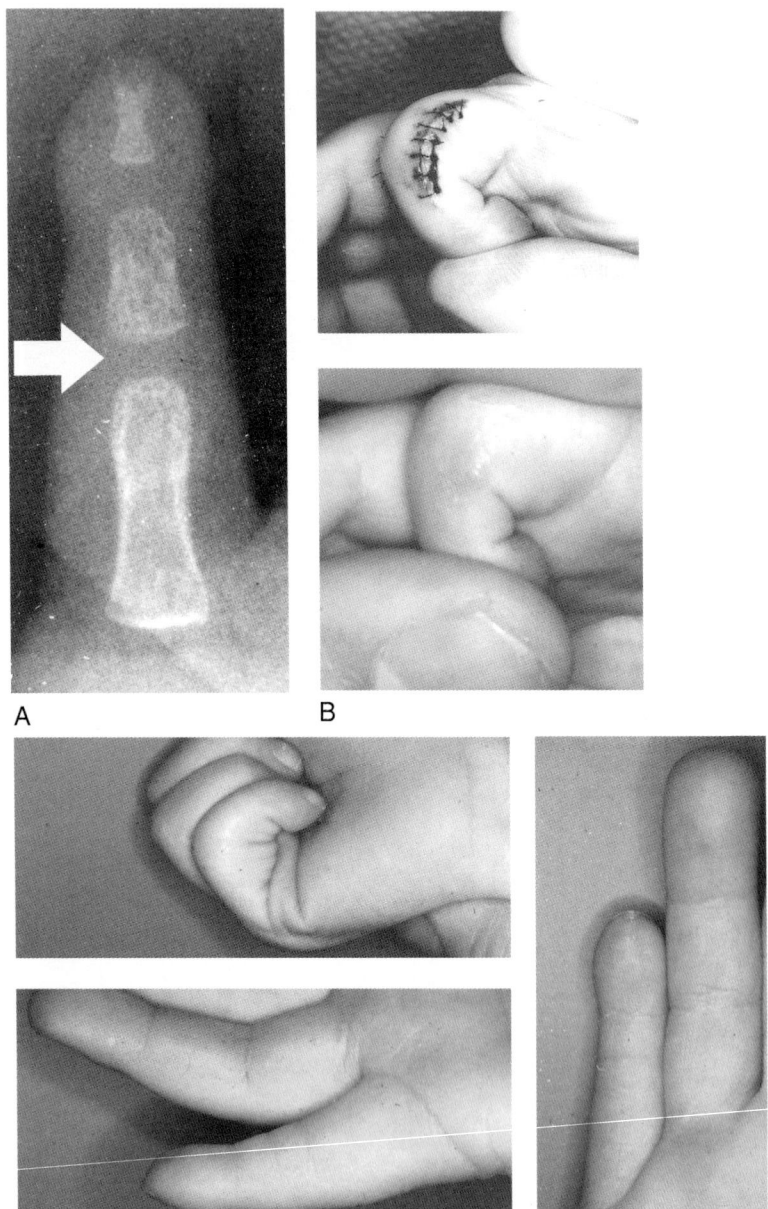

FIGURE 207-3. Early symphalangism release. *A,* The radiograph of this child with no motion at the interphalangeal joint clearly shows an interzone or lucent region between the proximal and middle phalanges. *B,* At 6 months of age, the cartilaginous bar was excised and early passive range of motion initiated and maintained. *C,* Ten years later, he still has 90 degrees of active flexion. Note the presence of both PIP and DIP flexion creases and the distal pulp atrophy so characteristic of digits with symphalangism.

Repositioning the PIP joint of one or more of the ulnar three digits may improve grip strength, but the percentage of improvement is unpredictable.[2,34,38] The majority of the literature on this condition deals almost exclusively with the diagnosis, genetics, and associated malformations. Outcome information is conspicuously absent. Distraction lengthening, described in multiple other chapters, is performed more for improvement in appearance. The lengthened digits and thumb are always thin and stiff. The major exceptions are for the improvement of pinch between the thumb and a short index finger.

Metacarpal Synostosis

INCIDENCE

The true incidence of this condition has not been determined, but it occurs more commonly than is appreciated, particularly in those with craniofacial and hand malformations such as the Apert syndrome, Crouzon syndrome, Pfeiffer syndrome, central synpolydactyly, syndactyly, and partial absences of the hand. In two large series of congenital hand anomalies, this malformation occurred in 0.02%[39] and 0.07%[3,40] of patients. In our series, the incidence is much higher, but the results may well be skewed because of the nature of the author's practice in collaboration with one of the larger craniofacial programs in the world. Approximately 120 patients with Apert syndrome and more than 200 children with central synpolydactyly have been evaluated.[3,40-43]

CLASSIFICATION

The classification used most frequently is that of Buck-Gramcko and Wood, which distinguishes three groups of patients according to the level of fusion.[40,44] In type I, the fusion is localized to the metacarpal base. Growth is normal, and there is minimal deformity and impairment. In type II, the fusion involves at least half of the metacarpals, and the affected two digits are close together. In type III, the fusion is complete, and there are two subtypes of MP joint configurations, IIIa with separate joints for each digit and IIIb with a common MP joint. Surgeons treating syndromic synostoses, such as in patients with the Apert syndrome, have used this classification (Fig. 207-4A).[43-49]

Foucher[50] has introduced another clinically useful system that is based on the curvature of the epiphysis, the discrepancy in length between the two metacarpals, and the shape of the two bones within the synostosis. These can be I shaped, U shaped, K shaped, and Y shaped. All of these categories contain subcategories (see Fig. 207-4B and C). This system is practical, intuitive, and clinically useful. For synostoses associated with central duplications, a classification based on the skeletal level of arborization is described in Chapter 206.

For the past 30 years, the author has used a system similar to both (see Fig. 207-4A). Three basic types of metacarpal synostosis are distinguished by the level of fusion as proximal, middle, and distal thirds. Within each level, three things are then considered: the relative length of the metacarpal segments, the position of the articulating digits, and the growth potential of the distal segments.

CLINICAL PRESENTATION

The fourth and fifth metacarpals are most frequently affected, and bilateral symmetric and asymmetric involvement occurs with equal frequency. Metacarpal fusions involving the radial three rays of the hand occur in the difficult to classify hand malformations associated with partial absence or reduction deformities of the upper limb. Synostoses within the central three rays of the hand are often associated with atypical cleft hands and synpolydactylies at the metacarpal level and polydactylies or superdigits[51-55] at the phalangeal level. The curvature of the two bones within the synostosis varies with the configuration of the growth plates within the metacarpal heads. The deviation of the digits is dependent on the location of the metacarpal heads and the cant of the joint space in both anterior-posterior and radioulnar planes. An abducted and short fifth finger is the most common variation seen in those with ring-small metacarpal synostoses (Fig. 207-5; see also Fig. 207-4B and C).

With the exception of the Foucher type K configuration, which usually presents as an isolated bilateral and asymmetric anomaly, the other I, Y, and U types are either associated with a syndrome or present as part of a more complex hand malformation. In the author's hospital, the Apert or synpolydactyly variants are the most common (see Fig. 207-4).[43] Synostosis between the thumb and index metacarpals is the most unusual and requires extensive reconstruction if a mobile thumb and adequate first web space are to be constructed.

The radiographic appearance of the skeletal structures gives clues about the abnormal anatomy seen, especially in synpolydactyly hands.[43] In a standard U metacarpal synostosis with metacarpals of equal length, the extrinsic flexor and extensor tendons are shared and probably split at the MP joint level and insert asymmetrically on the distal digits, which course toward one another. In an I pattern, the distal insertions are in their normal digital locations and intrinsic muscle balance is present. In the asymmetric U, Y, and K types, short and often deficient hypothenar muscles are accompanied by abnormal sharing of extrinsic tendons. The flexor retinaculum, which encases the flexor tendons in all of these variants, is abnormal at or distal to the level of arborization of the extrinsic flexor or extensor tendons. No generalizations can be made other than that the extrinsic musculotendinous systems appear to be normal proximal to the metacarpal synostosis.

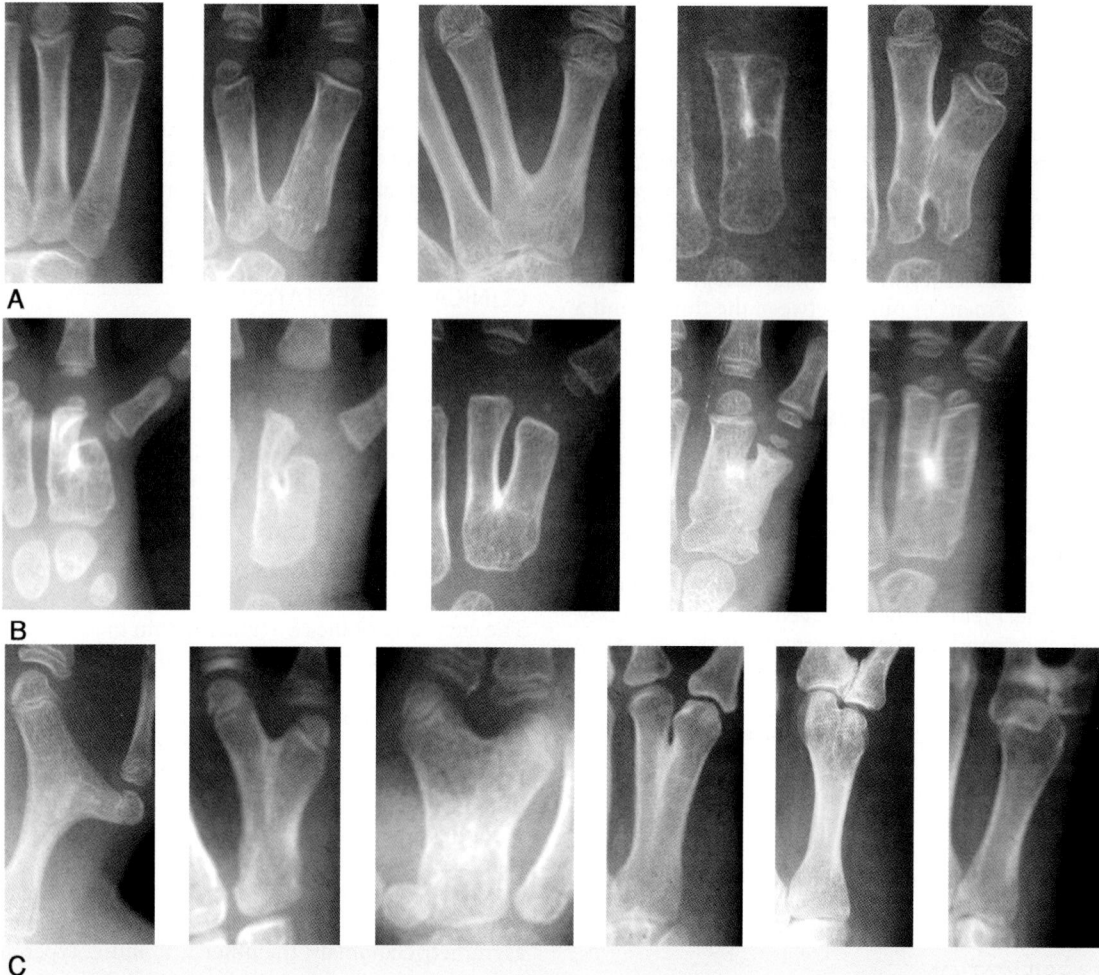

FIGURE 207-4. Metacarpal synostosis examples. *A,* From left to right, the progression from no skeletal fusion to complete fusion in the fourth frame is seen in various patients with the Apert syndrome. The image on the far right shows a re-fusion after release and interposition tendon arthroplasty at the age of 3 years. *B,* Synostoses with metacarpals of unequal lengths constitute the Foucher K types (frames one through four from left to right), and those of equal length form the U types. *C,* A progression is seen of an unequal K type to an I type, with a single metacarpal and bifid metacarpal head.

TREATMENT

For patients with metacarpals of equal length and minimal deformity, no treatment is necessary. For patients with hypoplastic fifth fingers, which often "get caught in pants pockets" and pose other functional problems, operations for the correction of length and rotation are often performed to improve appearance. These osteotomies are often accompanied by tendon and intrinsic muscle realignment.

Principles

The indications for surgical treatment are both aesthetic and functional. Realizing that total active motion of these digits may never be normal, the goals of surgery should be

- to construct a longitudinal, axial orientation of the ray;
- to place the MP joint in proper position relative to the other digits;
- to preserve MP joint motion and align joint surfaces;
- to correct angulation and rotation;
- to position less functional stiff, short, or rotated digits out of the way of thumb to fifth finger prehension; and
- to restore metacarpal descent of the fifth ray if possible.

In addition, it is absolutely necessary to observe these children through skeletal maturity because new problems with angulation, length, and rotation may

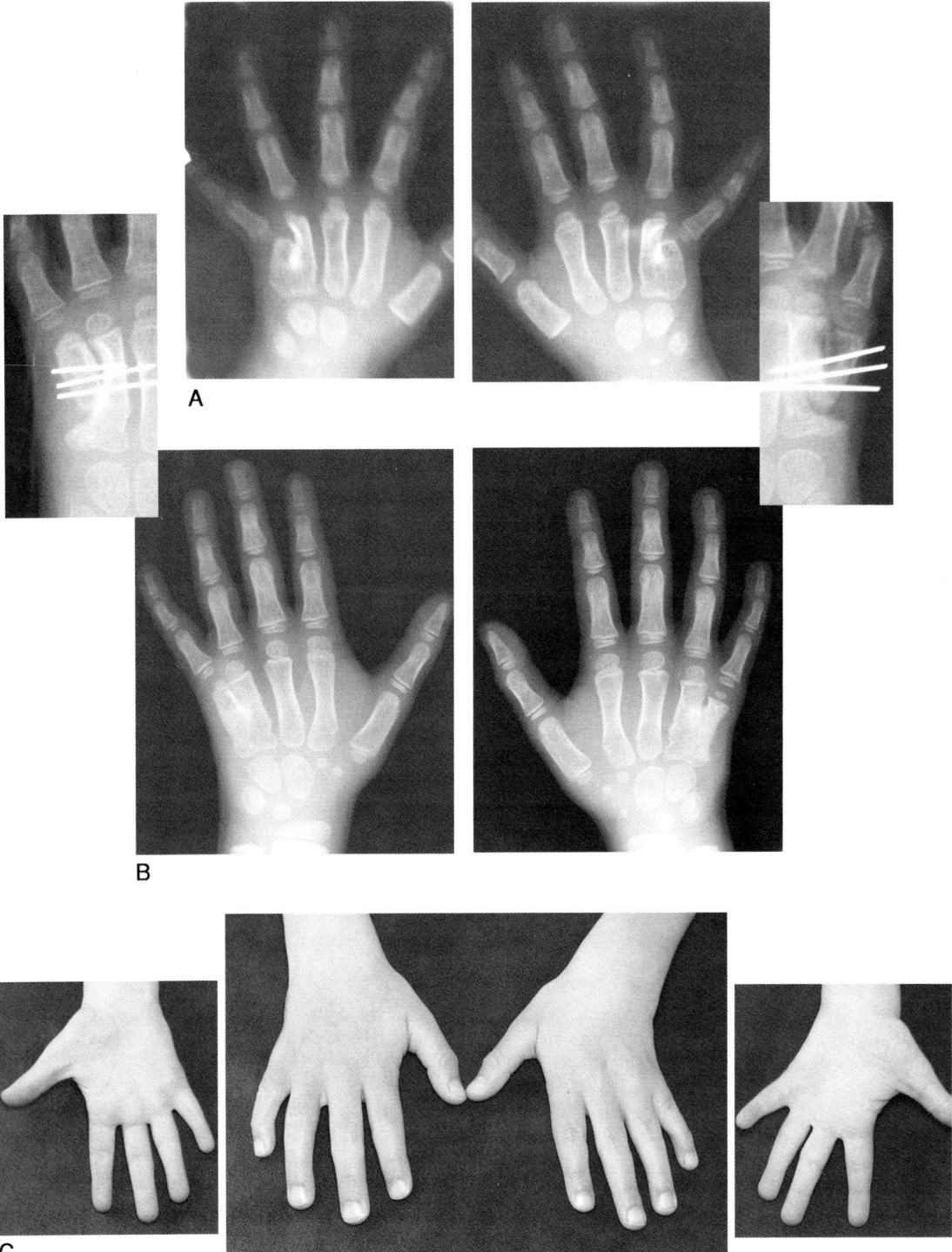

FIGURE 207-5. Correction of type K metacarpal synostoses. *A,* Radiographs of a 4-year-old child with bilateral metacarpal synostoses before surgery. Treatment consisted of oblique osteotomy and advancement of the shorter fifth metacarpal head to a length equal to the fourth. Fixation with multiple longitudinal C wires was maintained for 6 weeks. *B,* Hand radiographs of the same child 5 years later. Normal alignment with no rotational deformity has been maintained. *C,* The clinical appearance of both palmar and dorsal surfaces. Full range of motion of the initially stiff fifth finger MP joints was achieved.

develop as the children grow. Because the epiphyseal plates are abnormal, the effect of their growth on future problems cannot be precisely calculated at the time of initial correction. Deviation may recur or be persistent.

Procedures

For digits of equal length and for proximal fusions (Buck-Gramcko type I, Foucher type U), simple excision and placement of an interposition spacer will provide motion and metacarpal descent. Various types of spacers have included costal cartilage, silicone blocks,[56-58] silicone sheeting,[45] and cadaveric fascia lata[43] (Figs. 207-6 and 207-7). These procedures are particularly useful for Apert children, whose flexor function is compromised by symphalangism and short digits.

For configurations with asymmetry and digits of unequal length, combinations of osteotomy plus bone graft have been advocated.[40,56,58,59] Simple oblique osteotomy with advancement is another option.[47] For tightly spaced digits, simple splitting with widening of the synostosis plus bone graft has also been advocated (Fig. 207-8).[40,60]

Distraction has been effectively used to lengthen the deficient ulnar side of a synostosis and to reposition the MP joint. After the desired length has been achieved with distraction, two options are available. One can either let the gap fill with regenerated bone (callotasis)[49,61,62] or insert a bone graft and remove the apparatus early. My preference is the latter.[43,57] With gradual distraction not exceeding 1.0 mm per day, the hypothenar muscles do not need to be detached or lengthened. Some experienced authors prefer to complete the synostosis correction in a single stage.[40,44,47,56,63] In difficult cases with shortening, I prefer to use distraction and plan a two-stage procedure.[43,50]

For the distal Buck-Gramcko type III fusions with either separate (type IIIa) or shared (type IIIb) MP joints, a longitudinal split of the common metacarpal combined with an interposition bone graft, with or without additional transverse osteotomies as needed to correct rotation, is effective (see Fig. 207-8).[40,50,60]

The greatest short-term problem with all of these procedures is diminished MP joint motion, which is rarely normal preoperatively. The most predictable long-term problems relate to an increased angulation or rotation of the digit, usually the fifth finger, caused by abnormal growth. Longitudinal growth of the fifth finger is also diminished. When distraction techniques are used, MP joint release and rebalancing of appropriate motors are necessary.[64,65]

OUTCOMES

Fortunately, most metacarpal synostoses do not need surgical correction. MP joint motion is usually less than normal, and slight rotational deformities at the MP or

IP joint levels are most marked with flexion. After osteotomy through the synostosis and realignment of the MP joints, the appearance of the hand is usually improved. With correction of synostosis involving the ulnar three metacarpals of the hand, power grip is not significantly changed because MP joint motion is not normal despite secondary releases.[43] The most effective procedure is the release of small synostoses between the fourth and fifth metacarpals with interposition of fascia or other materials, which will prevent re-fusion. In Apert children, the construction of both a thumb to fifth finger pinch and grip can offer remarkable improvement in the function of severely compromised hands (see Fig. 207-7).

Carpal Coalitions

All permutations and combinations of carpal fusions have been described. The most frequent synostoses within the hand occur between the triquetrum and lunate and between the capitate and hamate. The latter is frequently seen in Apert children. Congenital fusion between the proximal and distal carpal rows is rare. The incidence in white populations is difficult to determine but has been described as 0% to 2% compared with a much higher prevalence in African populations, such as 9.5% in Nigeria.[66-68] These fusions are often seen in children with the Holt-Oram, Apert, Ellis-van Creveld, Cornelia de Lange, arthrogryposis, Nievergelt-Pearlman, and diastrophic dwarfism syndromes.[69]

Although these carpal coalitions may eliminate the 14-degree rotation between the triquetrum and lunate and the 25-degree rotation between the scaphoid and lunate, no significant functional impairment has been documented.[70] Pain from a fibrocartilaginous coalition should be treated with a surgical fusion. Congenital carpal coalitions are rarely if ever treated surgically.

Radioulnar Synostosis

INCIDENCE

This type of skeletal fusion occurs more commonly than is perceived by most hand surgeons and can be part of syndromes that may have skeletal coalitions at other levels, such as the Crouzon, Apert, and Poland syndromes,[71] Williams syndrome,[72,73] Antley-Bixler syndrome,[74] XYY chromosomal abnormalities,[75,76] Holt-Oram syndrome,[57] phocomelia,[77] and a variety of unnamed syndromes. However, the majority of patients have no syndromic association. The true incidence has not been reported but must be less than 1.0% of patients in large series of congenital hand differences.[2,33] Types of congenital forearm synostosis are much less commonly seen in the pediatric population than are the post-traumatic varieties, especially after

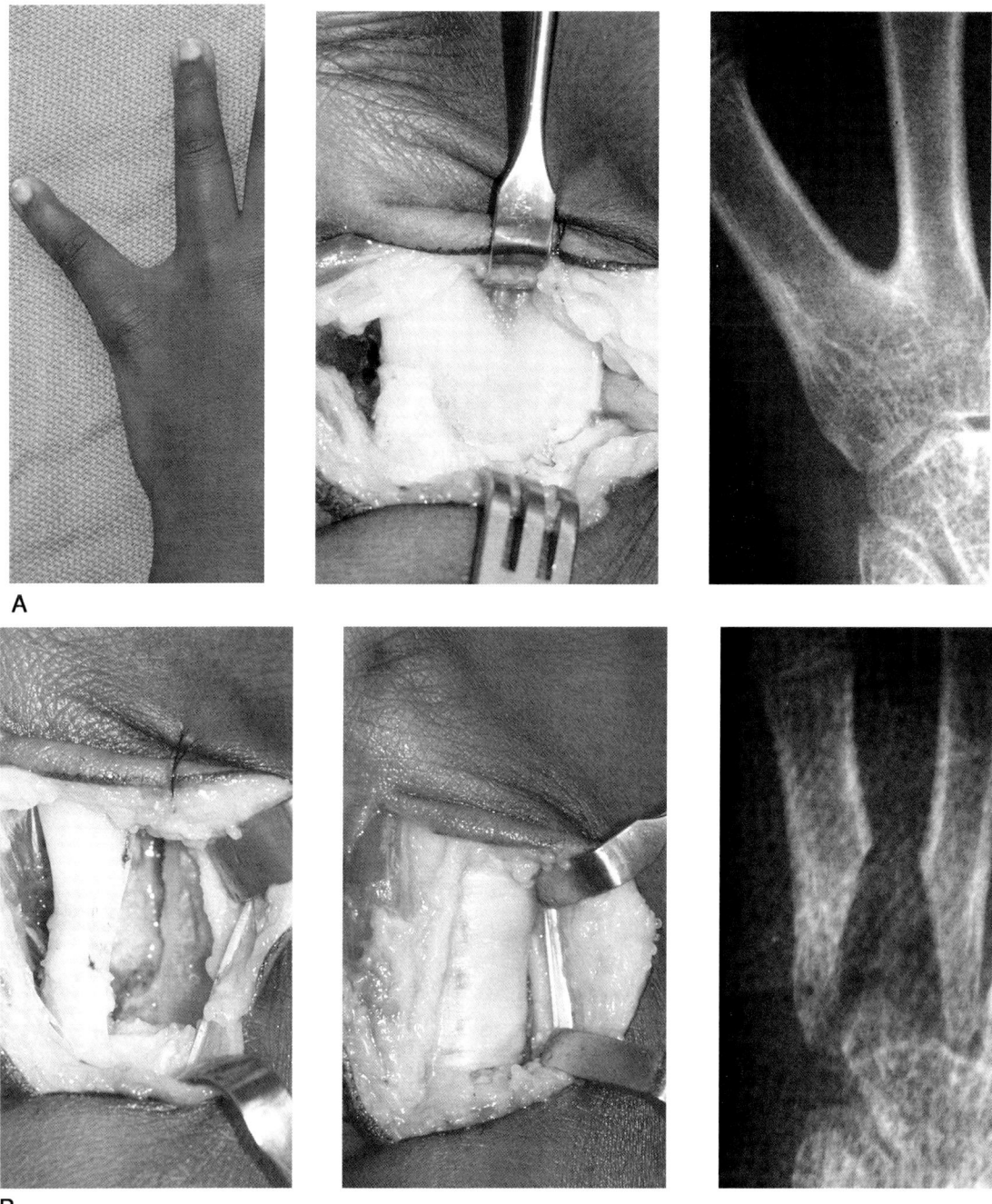

FIGURE 207-6. Correction of metacarpal synostosis with fascial interposition. *A,* The clinical appearance and radiograph of an older child with a proximal fourth-fifth metacarpal synostosis. *B,* The wide gap made by complete excision of the synostosis is seen. The palmar cortex and periosteum must be completely removed to prevent re-fusion at the metacarpal base. The center frame shows the rolled-up piece of hydrated cadaveric fascia lata obtained from the bone bank.

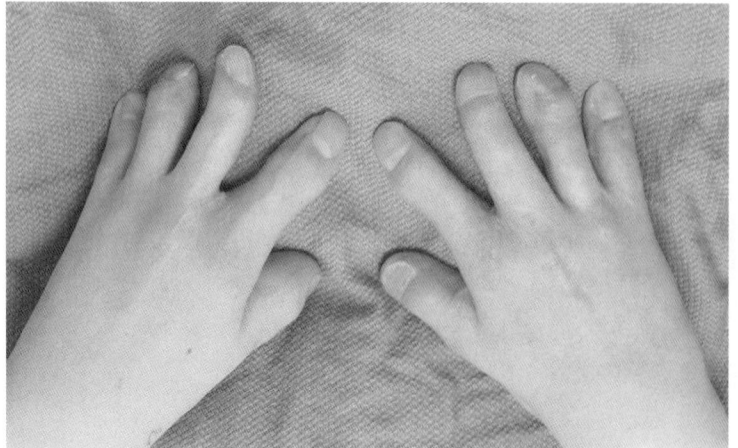

A

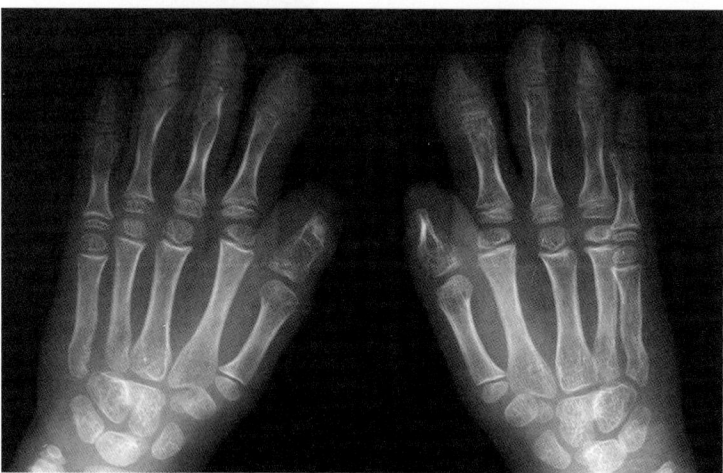

B

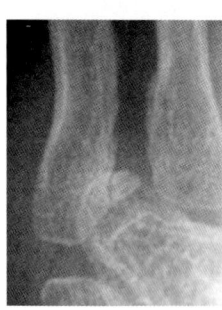

C

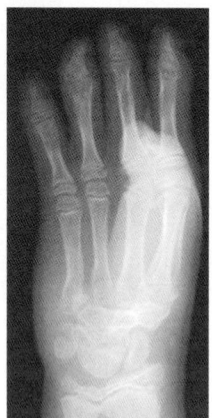

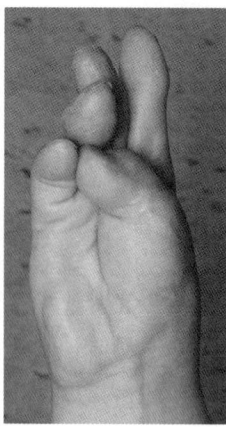

FIGURE 207-7. Thumb to fifth finger pinch and grip in the Apert patient. *A,* The clinical appearance of type I Apert hands is shown at the age of 12 years. Digital separations, thumb lengthening, and fascial interposition arthroplasties were completed by 5 years of age. The fingers are short with motion only at the MP joints and occasionally at the DIP joint of the fifth fingers. *B,* The radiographs demonstrate the symphalangism of all four digits, the longer index metacarpal, and the straightened thumbs. *C,* The gap after resection of the bone fusion between the fourth and fifth metacarpals has been maintained by the fascia and has permitted enough mobility and metacarpal descent to allow an effective thumb to fifth finger pinch and the ability to hold large objects, which previously required use of both hands together.

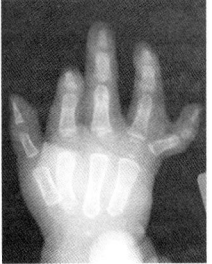

1 year

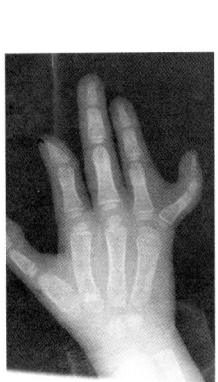

3 years

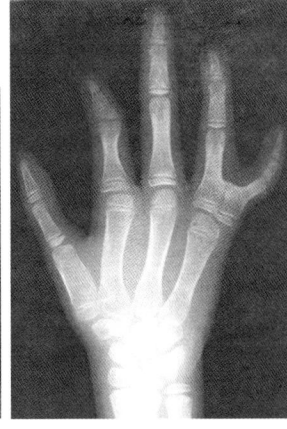

8 years

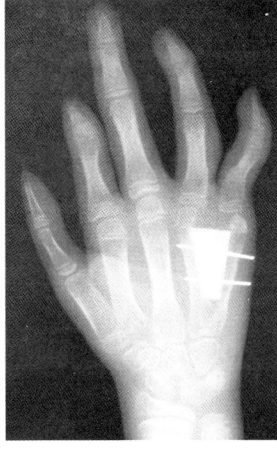

11 years

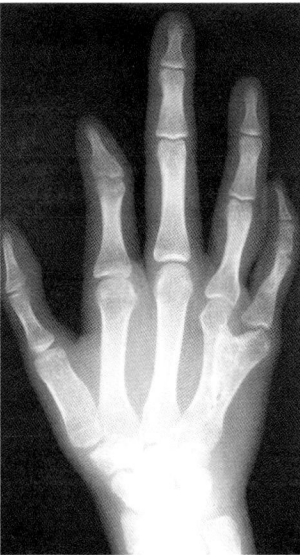

15 years

FIGURE 207-8. Correction of the rare type I metacarpal synostosis. This child with an I type of metacarpal syn-ostosis that contained a bifid metacarpal head supporting two phalanges was initially seen at 3 years of age. Three previous hand consultants had strongly recommended amputation, a reasonable option, but the parents refused. At the age of 3 years, the bases of the two ulnar digits were joined distal to the growth plates to prevent abduc-tion of the fifth finger. When next seen 8 years later, the common metacarpal was split to reposition the separate MP joints in a more correct alignment. By the age of 15 years, all epiphyses were closed, and she had maintained good stability and motion, although diminished in the fifth MP joint.

fractures or surgical manipulation of both bones of the forearm.

EMBRYOLOGY

The elbow joint is discernible at 34 days after fertil-ization, at which time the cartilaginous anlage repre-senting the humerus, radius, and ulna is present. Longitudinal segmentation between the radius and ulna starts distally and progresses proximally. If proper cavitation and segmentation between these forearm anlagen do not occur, the proximal radioulnar joint will not develop, and all degrees of synostosis may result. During this embryologic period, the forearm is in pronation, the position found with almost all radioulnar synostosis.[78,79]

CLINICAL PRESENTATION

The proximal third of the forearm is the most common site of involvement. About 60% of patients have bilat-eral involvement. Boys and girls are affected at an equal

rate.[80] Although these anomalies are not usually noted during infancy, most children present to the surgeon or pediatrician before the age of 3 years with prob-lems dressing, feeding, or holding objects two-handed. They are also often seen holding objects, such as coins, with a backhanded posture. Excessively pronated fore-arms cause these children to compensate by positioning their shoulders in hyperabduction. These strategies are most accentuated in cases of bilateral involvement or in children with more proximal limb anomalies at the elbow or shoulder level. Adaptive rotational hyper-mobility at the wrist occurs in most of these patients, who interestingly do not have a higher incidence of internal derangement of the wrist as adults do, despite the ligamentous laxity.[80,81]

Approximately one third of patients with radioul-nar synostosis have associated anomalies involving the cardiovascular, genitourinary, gastrointestinal, mus-culoskeletal, and central nervous systems. The patients seen most frequently in the author's center are those with congenital heart defects who fall into the

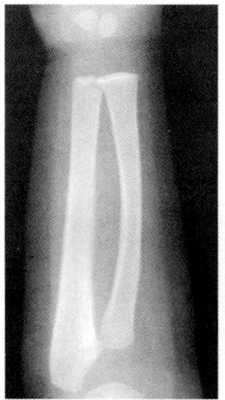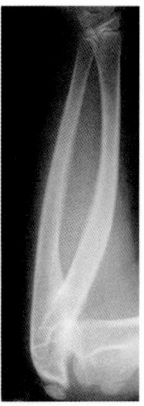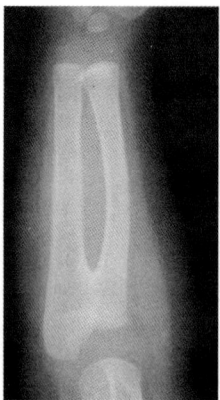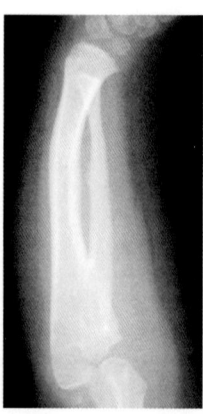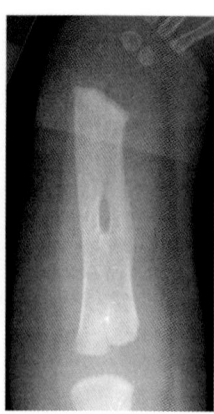

FIGURE 207-9. Radioulnar synostoses. The radius and ulna separate from one another in a distal to proximal direction. A variety of radiographs show that radioulnar synostoses occur most commonly in the proximal third of the forearm but can occur along the entire length of both radius and ulna. The forearm on the far right illustrates a patient with the Holt-Oram syndrome. Bowing of the longer radius will occur with growth when both ends of the radius are fixed to the ulna by cartilaginous or osseous unions. The radial head in these elbows is commonly fused to the ulna in a subluxed or dislocated position.

Holt-Oram syndrome[57] and have additional radial ray defects.

All levels of fixed pronation deformities occur, with approximately 40% of cases having less than 30 degrees of rotation, 20% between 31 and 59 degrees of rotation, and 40% more than 60 degrees of rotation. The radiographic analysis of this condition spans a wide spectrum from a complete fusion along the entire radius to a localized proximal synostosis, the most common type (Fig. 207-9).

TREATMENT

Few patients need surgery. Those with unilateral or bilateral deformities with less than 30 degrees of pronation generally do not need surgical correction[82] because they easily compensate. With 60 degrees or more of fixed pronation, there is obvious functional impairment in both unilateral and bilateral radioulnar synostosis cases. The dominant extremity should be given preference. For those with between 30 and 60 degrees of pronation, one must carefully individualize functional limitations, aesthetic needs, and degree of involvement. The most common clinical situation in which surgery is recommended is for the child with bilateral involvement of more than 40 to 50 degrees of fixed pronation. Derotational osteotomy through the area of synostosis is the treatment of choice, and the ideal time to complete surgery is before school age.[54,80,83-86] The recommended position after osteotomy varies between slight supination and 20 degrees of pronation, depending on the hypermobility of the wrist and other compensatory movements (Fig. 207-10).

The concept of resection of the synostosis and formation of a pseudarthrosis is not new. Most early attempts at resection of the synostosis and early motion failed because of rapid re-fusion. Fifty years ago, Kelikian[87] described the insertion of a swivel device within the radius to maintain motion after resection of the site of fusion. This procedure was combined with tendon transfers to improve supination and was performed between 12 and 16 years of age.[87] Unfortunately, others have not been able to repeat these results.[35,88,89] However, others have reported the use of Silastic[90] or the anconeus muscle[91] for interposition.

A more biologic approach is the use of nonvascularized fat,[92] vascularized pedicle fat or fascia flap,[93] vascularized free fat or fascia,[94] or fasciocutaneous flap[95] as an interposition barrier to block re-fusion across the osteotomy site. Kanaya's procedure involves a vascularized graft harvested from the lateral arm on the profundi brachii system, an osteotomy of the radius to relocate the radial head, and additional soft tissue procedures as needed to improve supination. I have used vascularized fat or fascial or fasciocutaneous flaps based on the radial artery or collateral vessels of the lateral elbow region. I have also routinely wrapped AlloDerm, an engineered dermal substitute, around both bones at the site of resection (Figs. 207-11 and 207-12). All of these procedures are most successful with small synostoses, which require less resection and have a lower potential for re-fusion. Osteotomy of the proximal radius is required to relocate the radial head, which in almost all of these elbows has a tremendous propensity for subluxation or dislocation.

OUTCOMES

Patients who do not have surgery continue to function well and develop new compensatory patterns for the remainder of their lives. After osteotomy,

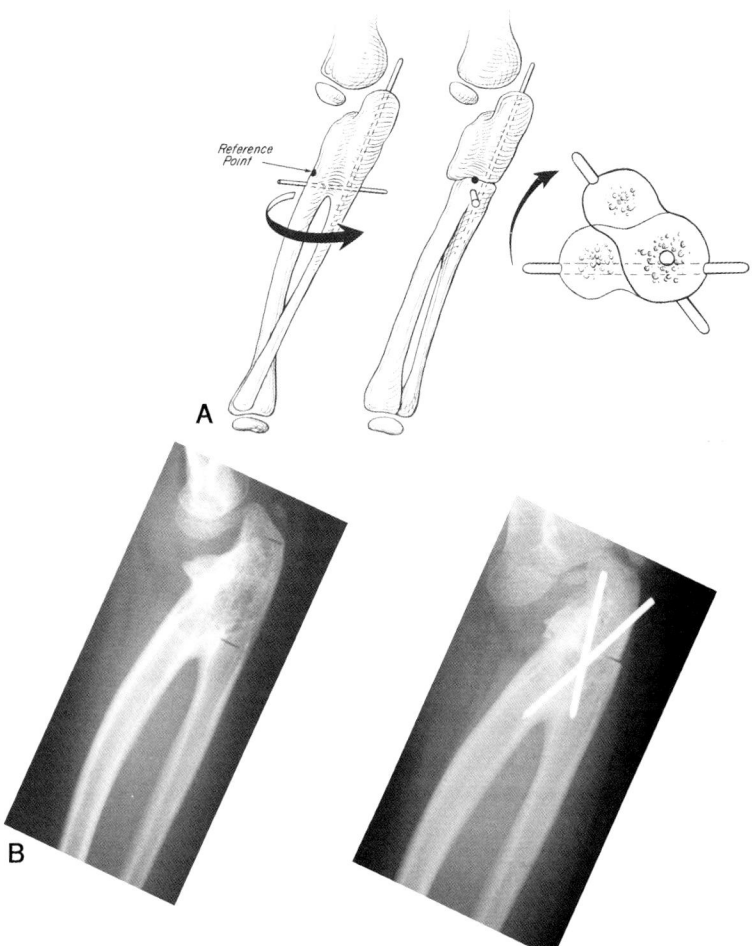

FIGURE 207-10. Osteotomy for radioulnar synostosis. *A,* A transverse osteotomy through the distal portion of the synostosis is the procedure most frequently performed for children with excessive fixed pronation. A transverse K-wire is used as a "joystick" to guide the forearm through the rotation, which should not exceed 45 to 55 degrees. Resection of 2.0 to 3.0 mm of bone will help prevent kinking of the vessels and vascular impairment, the most dreaded complication with this operation. *B,* Radiographs show the position of the osteotomy and K-wire fixation, which does not need to be maintained more than 6 to 8 weeks postoperatively. (Illustration by J. K. Biddl.)

however, good to excellent results are achieved in the majority of patients, who are surprised both by the improved function and by less musculoskeletal discomfort at other levels, such as the back, neck, and shoulders.

The author's short-term results in eight patients have been similar to those of the more complete follow-up studies by Kanaya, who achieved between 10 and 45 degrees of supination and 30 to 80 degrees of pronation without re-fusion in five patients observed for a minimum of 4 years. The average age of his patients at the time of surgery was 8 years. All patients demonstrated a marked improvement of function despite their preoperative compensatory movements.

The most common problem with any interposition procedure is loss of motion and reankylosis. The devastating complication of vascular compromise and Volkmann ischemic contracture after osteotomy on patients has been seen within the author's institution.[81] This can be avoided by monitoring the degree of rotation and by removing a segment of bone at the site of osteotomy.[89] Excessive swelling and wound

dehiscence are possible with any procedure, but the Ilizarov device has been effective in avoiding these complications.[96]

DIGITAL AND THUMB DEFORMITIES

The newborn infant will normally keep the thumb in a flexed-adducted position overlapped by the fingers until 3 to 4 months of age. The developmental reason for this is not well understood but may relate to the fact that the early flexor forces overpower the extensor muscle masses, which innervate later. The absence of independent extension after this period may be due to a number of conditions that may result in secondary fixed flexion contractures if they are not corrected. Although flexion deformities in the young child are relatively infrequent, the diagnoses and pathogenesis of each involved condition may be confusing.

MUSCULOTENDINOUS EMBRYOLOGY. During Streeter stage 18 at 44 days of gestation, the muscle-tendon

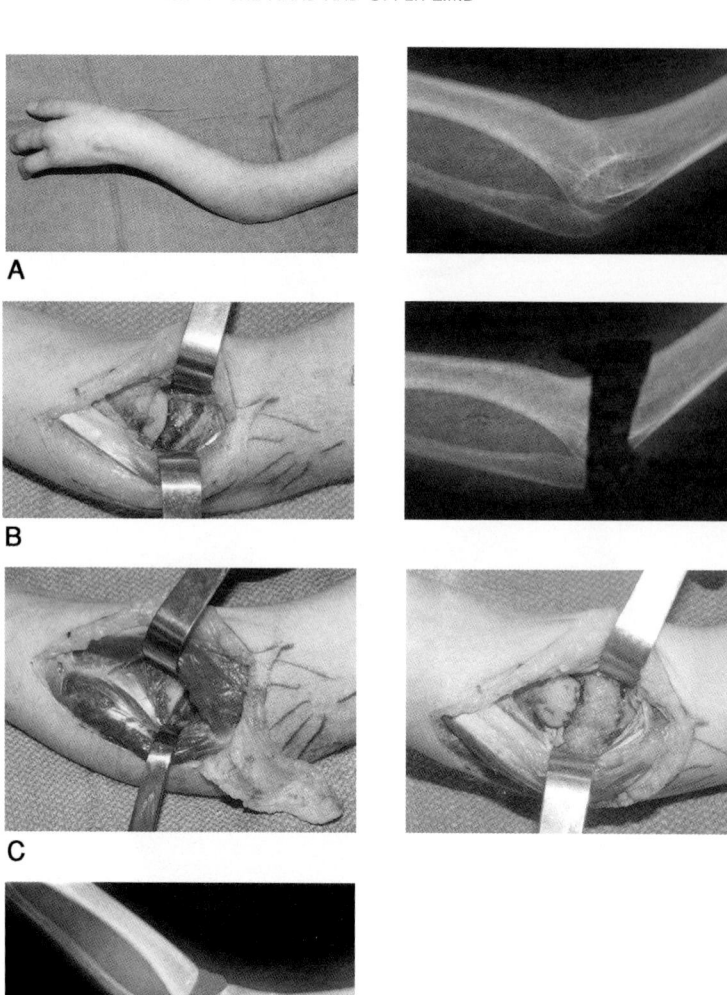

FIGURE 207-11. Vascularized flap arthroplasty. *A,* This child with bilateral elbow fusions incorporating humerus, radius, and ulna had severely limited upper limb function due to these skeletal fusions and the absence of the ulnar two digits of the hand. *B,* A generous resection of the majority of the synostosis has been completed. *C,* A proximally based fasciocutaneous flap including the terminal branches of the superior radial collateral arterial system to the lateral arm has been dissected, mobilized, and then used to fill this gap. Although much of her early postoperative motion has been lost, she has maintained a functional 35 degrees of motion in flexion and extension of her left elbow, which is now on her dominant upper limb. *D,* Postoperative x-ray demonstrating maintenance of pseudojoint.

unit in the upper limb arises from two distinct sources: the muscle from condensation of mesenchyme of somatic origin and the tendon (and bone) from somatopleure.[97,98] Although musculotendinous units present as a single entity, muscle and tendons can and do develop independently, then join in an integrated fashion.

Chick limb bud experiments have shed some light on this biology. When the distal portion of the bud is transplanted to the flank, tendons develop in the grafted segment and a muscle forms on the donor amputation stump.[99] When chick embryos are paralyzed by curare, muscle development is blocked while tendons initially develop distally for a short time.[100] The diameter of these tendons soon decreases when there is no proximal muscle to provide the requisite

motion and mechanical forces to promote growth. The mechanism of muscle and tendon attachment is unclear. When limb buds are amputated and rotated 180 degrees at the wrist level, dorsal tendons attach in a mismatched fashion to ventral muscles and vice versa.[101] Chiquet[102] has proposed the existence of a myotendinous antigen at the interface of muscle and tendon. At this juncture, there are large accumulations of muscle cells producing contractile substance and fibroblasts producing collagen.[103] Musculotendinous development and joint formation are as integrated as hand and glove. Joint formation will not progress without the stimulus of motion provided by the muscle-tendon movement. Symphalangism is the ultimate result of no motion, and the dorsal flattening of the condylar surfaces seen in severe campto-

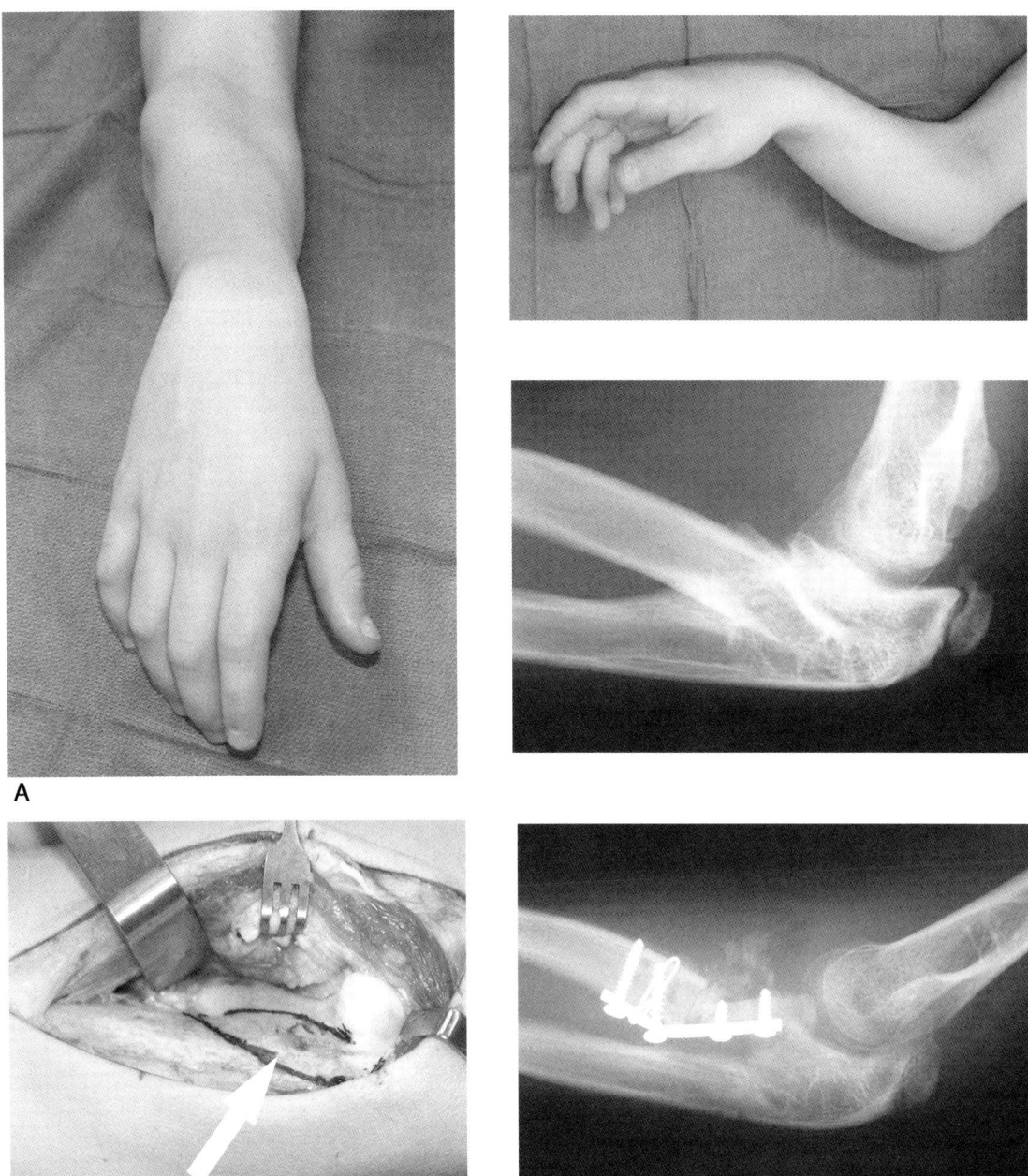

FIGURE 207-12. Radioulnar synostosis. *A,* This child has bilateral fixed forearm contractures in full pronation secondary to a proximal radioulnar synostosis. Although he compensates with hypermobility of the wrist and by changing his body position, this is a significant disability. *B,* The radius is bowed and the radial head lies in a dislocated position. The arrow marks the limit of the synostosis excision. In this patient, an osteotomy of the proximal radius was necessary for reduction after synostosis excision. A proximally based fasciocutaneous flap was interposed between the radius and ulna.

dactyly is caused by the lack of full dorsal motion by fixed flexion forces.

The clinical correlation of this embryology has been well documented in nature and humans[104] and is well known to any student of congenital hand differences.

In the hand and forearm, distal tendons preferably attach to their corresponding muscle belly and distally to bone. If that bone has not developed, the tendon will attach to an adjacent bone. If a bone is not available, the tendon will then attach to another tendon, local fascia, or an adjacent muscle. Graham[104] postulates that these proximal tendons reattach in a position of mechanical advantage. Our experience with the careful analysis of this hierarchy of reattachment substitution is that they realign with local adjacent structures. All of these combinations are seen in patients with the typical cleft hand (and foot) and symbrachydactyly (atypical cleft hand).

TERMINOLOGY. The clasped thumb of the young child was recognized as an entity more than 150 years ago.[105] The term *congenital clasped thumb* was coined by Weckesser[106] and has been cited frequently. The causes of the different forms of flexion postures seen in the young child cover a wide spectrum, and confusion over them stems from the many synonyms, which include trigger digit,[107] pollex varus,[108] pollex adductus, spastic thumb-in-palm,[109,110] thumb-in-palm, congenital flexion-adduction deformity of the thumb,[111] infant's persistent thumb–clutched hand, and congenital absence or hypoplasia of extensors. Instead, it seems most productive to view this group of patients as a heterogeneous group with a common clinical expression. Recognizable syndromes that present with a flexed and adducted thumb in the palm include the Freeman-Sheldon ("whistling face") syndrome, the Waardenburg syndrome, the windblown hand, and arthrogryposis.[57]

Camptodactyly refers to congenital flexion contractures of the digits and, to a lesser extent, the thumb. The secondary soft tissue anomalies are outlined in more detail. This condition is easily differentiated from clinodactyly, which is defined as a deviation in the radioulnar plane, in contrast to the flexion deformities in the opposite anteroposterior plane. Clinodactyly is usually secondary to skeletal abnormality.

DIFFERENTIAL DIAGNOSIS. For infants and young children presenting with flexion or adduction deformities of the thumb or flexion deformities of the digits, initial evaluation should consider trigger thumb or digit, cerebral palsy, congenital clasped thumb with extensor anomalies, camptodactyly, or a syndrome, the most common of which are arthrogryposis and the Freeman-Sheldon syndrome. In the absence of facial malformations, the term *congenital windblown hand* is often used. These hands, which present with all degrees of thumb adduction and digital MP flexion and ulnar deviation, are seen in a number of conditions and do not represent a specific condition with a specific cause. A thorough physical examination should provide grounds for the proper diagnosis in each case.

Trigger Digit or Thumb

INCIDENCE

Trigger thumb is common compared with the incidence of other congenital anomalies of the thumb and hand. Trigger digits are much less common in children than in adults and almost always involve the thumb.[112] In one series, there were 11 trigger digits released in comparison to 89 thumbs.[113] The true incidence of trigger digit or thumb in the pediatric age group has not been clearly established, although it is fairly well known and treatable. More than half of these children have bilateral involvement. Prospective screening of large numbers of newborns has failed to reveal many cases,[113,114] and although there have been isolated reports of trigger thumb between identical twins[115] and mother and child,[116] a true role for heredity has never been established.

Childhood trigger digit and thumb are common in patients with a diagnosis of mucopolysaccharidosis or collagen disease. In these patients, the stenosing tenosynovitis may cause flexor tendon impingement not only at the A1 pulley but also within the chiasm of Camper and the A2 and, to a lesser extent, A4 pulleys.[117]

CLINICAL PRESENTATION

Trigger digits are rarely present at birth. Instead, they are discovered by a parent while bathing the child.[57] Most trigger thumbs present as a palpable nodule or "Notta node"[118] and fixed flexion of the IP joint. The term *triggering* represents the snapping or popping experienced as the nodule passes beneath the first annular pulley.[119] Patients rarely experience pain from the triggering,[113,114,120,121] but children often avoid the strange sensation of triggering by maintaining the thumb or digit in extension.[122] Most of these digits are intractable and have developed a compensatory hyperextension of the MP joint (Figs. 207-13 and 207-14).

Few studies have documented the rate of spontaneous resolution, but the data so far suggest that 30% of children diagnosed between birth and 6 months resolve spontaneously compared with 12% of those diagnosed between 6 and 30 months.[107,123] However, this discrepancy could be explained by the difference of referral sources in the different studies.[124]

PATHOGENESIS

The exact origin of trigger thumb in children is not known, but three causes have been suggested.[125] A familial or congenital cause is the oldest proposed cause,[126-128] but there is little evidence now to support this line of thinking. Trauma has often been implicated, especially in young children, who may sustain minor injuries without complaint.[107,120] Other researchers have suggested that it is an acquired flexion deformity not necessarily associated with an injury.[129,130] The very low incidence of this condition in the newborn age group and in those up to 6 months of age suggests that in the majority, trigger digit or thumb is acquired.

The nodule starts out as the result of an intussusception of the peritendinous connective tissue beneath

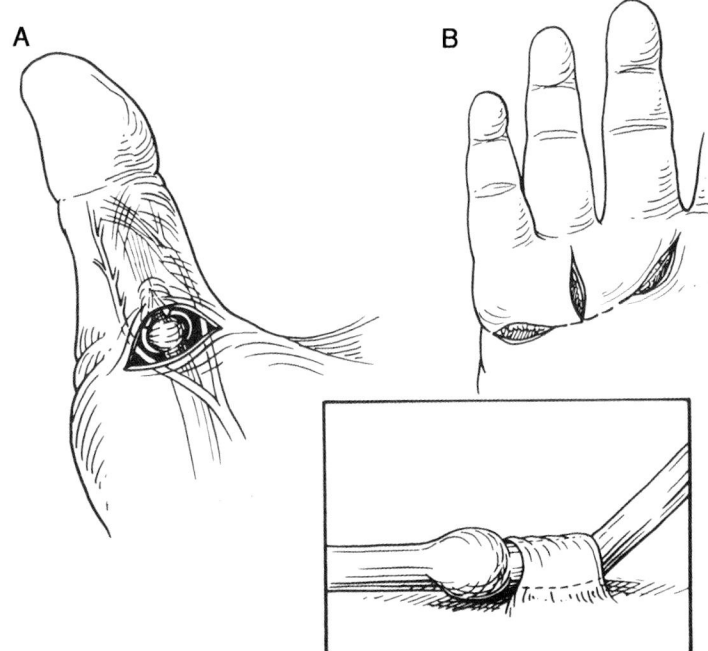

FIGURE 207-13. Technique of trigger release. *A,* A trigger thumb release is preferably made through an incision in the digitopalmar flexion crease directly over the palpable nodule or swelling within the flexor pollicis longus tendon. The proximity of the radial digital nerve to the thumb makes this structure vulnerable to injury. *Inset:* When size of the Notta node exceeds the space available beneath the pulley, locking occurs, usually in flexion. *B,* Alternative incisions for trigger digit release use normally existing skin creases, such as the distal palmar flexion crease at the base of the long and fifth digits or longitudinal creases distal to the palmar crease. (Illustration by J. K. Biddl.)

the leading edge of the A1 pulley. With repetitive flexion and swelling, a thickened nodule develops.[131] This concept is similar to the notion of buckling of peritendinous structures within the sheath.[132]

TREATMENT

When children present before the age of 1 year, I observe them for a minimum of 3 to 6 months and then recommend release if spontaneous resolution has not occurred. The time-honored treatment of trigger thumb or digit in children is surgical release of the first annular pulley (see Figs. 207-13 and 207-14).[57,107,128,133] However, in the past 5 years, a number of studies have proposed more conservative treatment, often espousing splinting, with full correction of a large number of patients after the age of 3 years.[130,134-137]

In the early 1990s, percutaneous release of the first annular pulley in trigger digits was performed with excellent results in a large series of adult patients. Percutaneous release is performed under local anesthesia with sedation in the outpatient surgery setting, which appeals to many parents.[138] Wang and Lin[139] have described this technique and have emphasized that there is an obligatory early learning curve; potential neurovascular injury can occur, especially to the radial digital nerve.[140] Steroid injection plus percutaneous release in the adult population has been reported to be twice as effective as injection alone.[141]

My preferred option is for surgical release in all children older than 2 years with fixed flexion contrac-

tures,[142-145] by use of an incision within the digitopalmar flexion crease, which heals well (see Fig. 207-13). I do not espouse the longitudinal incision advocated by Ger[121] or midlateral incisions[146] designed to minimize injury to the radial digital nerve. Complete release of the A1 pulley and unrestrained gliding of the nodular thickening must be observed under direct vision. It is not necessary to isolate and dissect either neurovascular bundle (see Fig. 207-14).

OUTCOMES

Splinting alone for 6 months at a time offers at best a 50% resolution.[107,121,135] Surgical release can result in a complete resolution of the problem but requires a short anesthetic for an outpatient procedure. Outcome studies show that there is a 100% success in the short term with surgical release, but residual limitation of IP joint motion or MP hyperextension may persist.[147] There are isolated cases of recurrence due to incomplete release of the A1 pulley or regrowth of fibrous tissue to reconstitute the pulley. Percutaneous release under local anesthesia is reported to give a 93% chance of success.[139] Although open surgical release by trained hand surgeons had a 100% chance of success,[57] release of the first annular pulley does not correct the MP hyperextension seen in long-standing cases.

In the author's experience, percutaneous release before open trigger release in 10 children has resulted in complete resolution of the problem with residual longitudinal scoring within the flexor, which did not have a deleterious effect on function. However, my

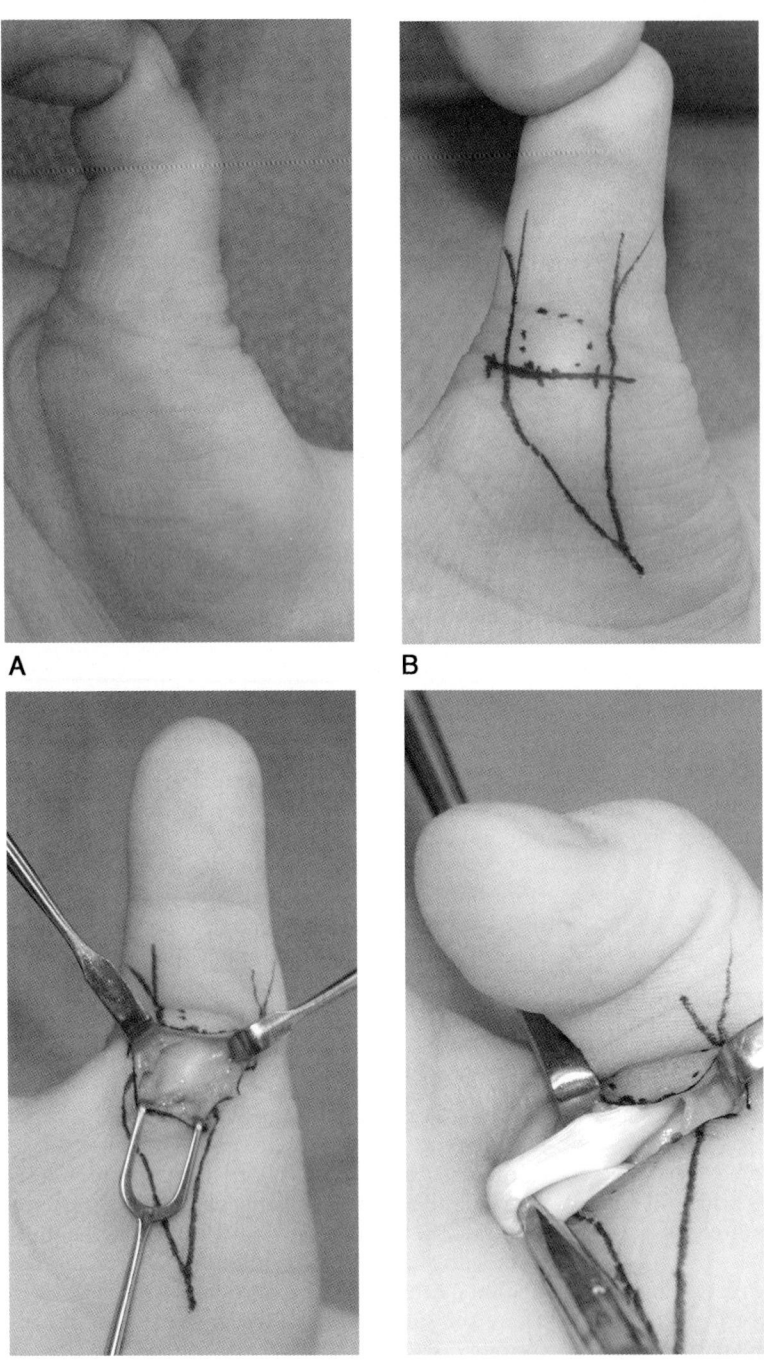

A

B

C

D

FIGURE 207-14. Trigger thumb release. *A,* This 2-year-old child presented with his right thumb locked in flexion and a palpable nodule proximal to the A1 pulley. The hyperextension at the MP joint allowed this youngster to adequately extend his thumb out of the palm. This compensatory hyperextension does not reverse itself after release. *B,* The proximity of the digital nerves of the thumb is outlined. The Notta node is outlined distal to the proposed incision in the proximal of two digitopalmar flexion creases. *C,* The A1 pulley is exposed with soft tissue dissection. The neurovascular structures on either side do not need to be individually exposed. *D,* The thickened region within the flexor pollicis longus tendon does not require any débridement once the pulley has been released.

preferred option is for surgical release in all children older than 2 years with fixed flexion contractures.[142,144,145,148] Either complete or partial transection of the radial digital nerve to the thumb[57] and incomplete release of the A1 pulley are the primary complications of this procedure, which is one of the safest and most predictable in pediatric hand surgery (see Fig. 207-13).

Congenital Clasped Thumb Deformity

CLINICAL PRESENTATION

These children are born with their thumbs flexed and adducted into the palm. It is more often bilateral and is seen in boys twice as often as it is seen in girls.[149] The thumb characteristically lies tightly flexed at both

MP and IP joints beneath the four digits (Fig. 207-15). Whereas all newborns show this posture at birth, babies with normal thumbs will start showing signs of extension by 3 to 6 months of age.[150]

Flexion deformity of the digits is rare and can occur as an isolated extensor loss to a single digit or as a common loss of extensors to two or more fingers. Patients with an isolated loss demonstrate good MP extension but lack adequate PIP joint extension. These anomalies are much less common than is thumb extensor loss, which causes the clasped thumb posture.[151,152] The extensor mechanism and often a lumbrical muscle can be deficient at the PIP joint level, and no functional central slip is present. The long and ring fingers are rarely involved, but patients with deficient thumb extensors often experience weakness or absence of common extensors to the index and occasionally long rays. In contrast, patients with multiple extensor deficiencies lack MP joint extension (with the wrist held in a dorsiflexed position) but do have good PIP and DIP joint extension through intact intrinsic muscles. Radiographic evaluation is not very helpful.

DIFFERENTIAL DIAGNOSIS

Trigger thumb can be eliminated by the absence of a nodule and full passive extension at the IP joint. The spastic thumb-in-palm occurs in patients with other features of cerebral palsy. Freeman-Sheldon patients have associated facial abnormalities, and patients with arthrogryposis multiplex congenita have associated lower extremity problems. Patients with distal arthrogryposis of the upper limbs will show signs of wrist flexion and ulnar deviation with or without ulnar deviation of the digits (Fig. 207-16). Similarly, the congenital windblown hand may have a tightly flexed and adducted thumb, but it occurs in combination with digital ulnar deviation with or without MP flexion.

CLASSIFICATION

Three classification systems have been widely used. The first system, developed by Weckesser,[149] designates three groups for thumbs, noting increasing degrees of severity of extensor and thenar hypoplasia, and a fourth group for all other cases, including syndromic hands. In contrast, McCarroll's system[153] recognizes only two groups: clasped thumbs that are passively correctable and those that are not. The third system is similar to McCarroll's but has a separate category for arthrogryposis multiplex congenita, which would be classified as group II or III by Weckesser and group II by McCarroll. However, it is not difficult to recognize arthrogryposis multiplex congenita clinically, and only those children with distal arthrogryposis and no lower extremity involvement would resemble a typical clasped thumb.

TREATMENT

In children with both passively correctable (group I in all three classifications) and fixed flexion contractures of the thumb or digits, initial splinting is the mainstay of treatment. Patients with passively supple thumbs or digits should wear splints day and night, keeping the MP and IP joints in complete extension. Passive stretching for recalcitrant contractures is performed five or six times per day, and this helps with sensory stimulation. In these cases, the splinting and stretching are effective, and surgery is usually not indicated as the dorsal soft tissue structures grow and mature without being pulled into flexion by the overpowering flexors.

More severe cases often do not respond to conservative measures, and surgery becomes necessary to restore extensor power to the digit and to provide an adequate web space (see Fig. 207-16). Many of these children initially start as group I patients at birth and become group II children as secondary soft tissue deformities develop. Some surgeons prefer to release and graft the contractures first and perform transfers as a secondary procedure. Others prefer to complete everything in a single stage.[153-155]

Aggressive surgery is needed in more contracted hands with a small first web space, absent extensors, and deficient thenar musculature. In thumbs, the extensor pollicis brevis is the most consistently absent structure. When it is absent, there is a high likelihood that the preferred tendon for restoration of thumb extension, the extensor indicis proprius, is also deficient or absent (see Fig. 207-15). Release or recession of the first dorsal interosseous muscle and adductor pollicis muscle must be done, and the thumb-index web space must be resurfaced with full-thickness skin flaps. Tendon transfers must be used to restore thumb extension, thumb metacarpal abduction, and palmar abduction (opposition) of the first ray. Threaded C wires are used to maintain the web for 3 weeks and are followed by night splinting for many months.

I prefer to avoid MP or IP joint chondrodesis in young children because of the high nonunion rate. Children with severe arthrogryposis multiplex congenita, Freeman-Sheldon syndrome, and windblown hands fall into this category.

Treatment is difficult in both isolated and multiple flexion deformities of the digits. At a young age, splinting and passive exercises should be used to maintain passive correction and to avoid contractures. If flexion contractures have occurred, soft tissue releases of skin, palmar plate, and collateral ligaments may be necessary before tendon transfers. Patients with isolated extensor losses can undergo reconstruction either by transfer of a lateral band from an adjacent normal digit[156] or by transfer of the flexor digitorum superficialis to the same finger.[87] In either case, incomplete palmar release will result in a residual flexion

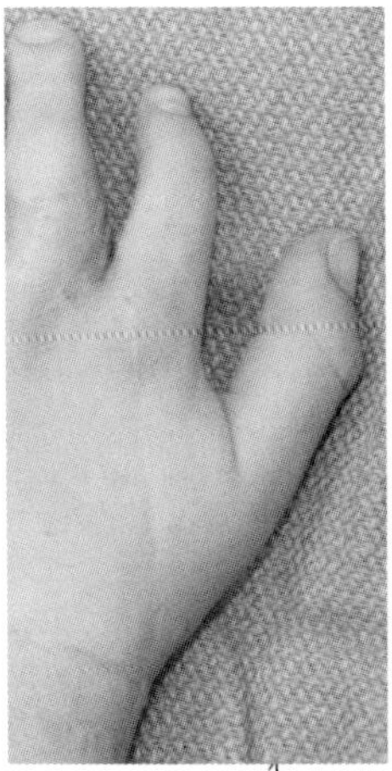

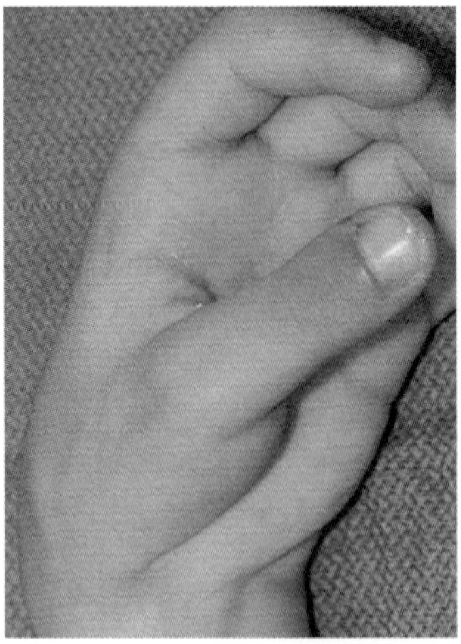

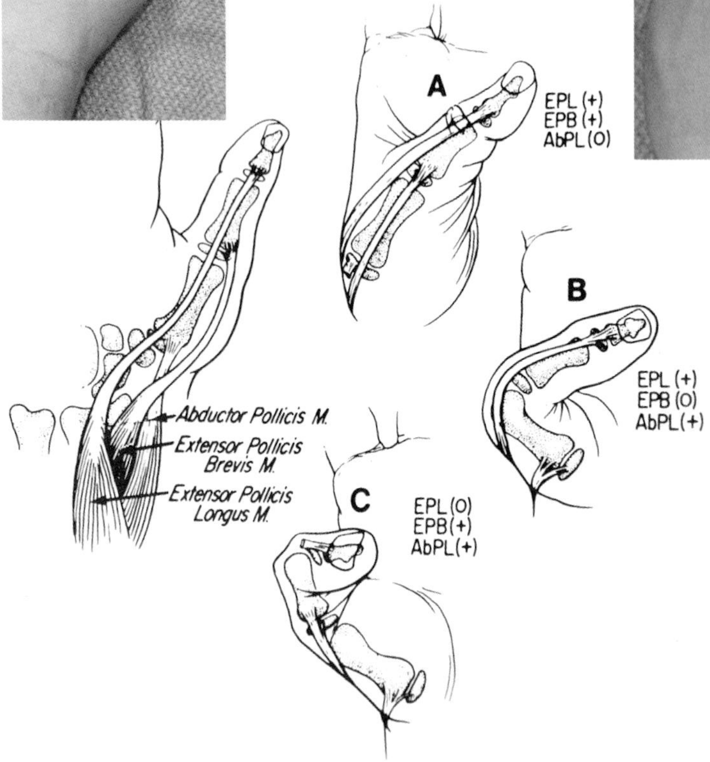

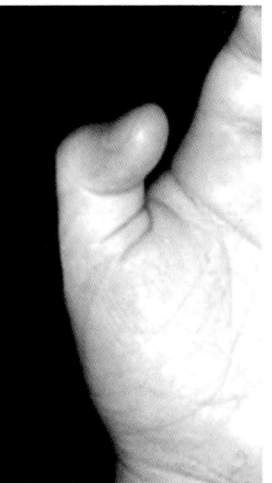

EPL (+)
EPB (+)
AbPL (O)

A

EPL (+)
EPB (O)
AbPL (+)

B

Abductor Pollicis M.
Extensor Pollicis Brevis M.
Extensor Pollicis Longus M.

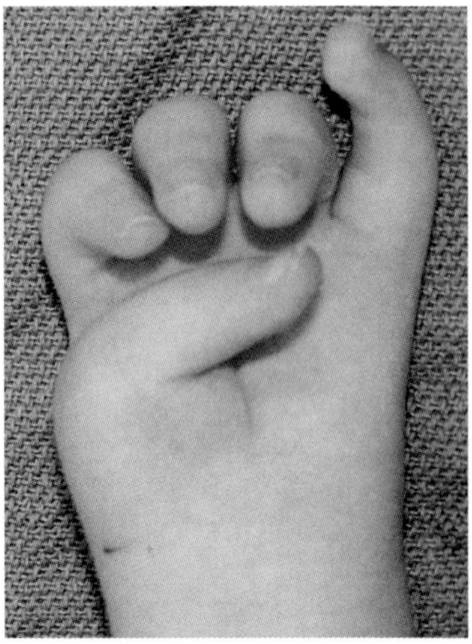

EPL (O)
EPB (+)
AbPL (+)

C

FIGURE 207-15. Clasped thumb postures. On the left, the normal resting posture of a child's thumb is seen from the dorsal surface. The extrinsic extensors include the abductor pollicis longus (AbPL), extensor pollicis brevis (EPB), and extensor pollicis longus (EPL), which attach to the dorsal base of the metacarpal, proximal phalanx, and distal phalanx, respectively. A deficiency in one or more of these extensors is reflected by the resting attitude of the thumb. The pathologic process on the extensor side of the thumb is clearly reflected by a careful physical examination. *A,* The thumb lies more in the palm because of an absence or weakness of the AbPL. *B,* In this common posture, the carpometacarpal and interphalangeal joints are extended, but the absence of the EPB places the thumb tightly flexed and in the way of other digits. *C,* The carpometacarpal and metacarpophalangeal joint postures are normal and the interphalangeal joint is flexed due to an absence of the EPL. In older children and adolescents, this mallet thumb posture is usually secondary to a traumatic rupture or laceration of the EPL. (Illustration by J. K. Biddl.)

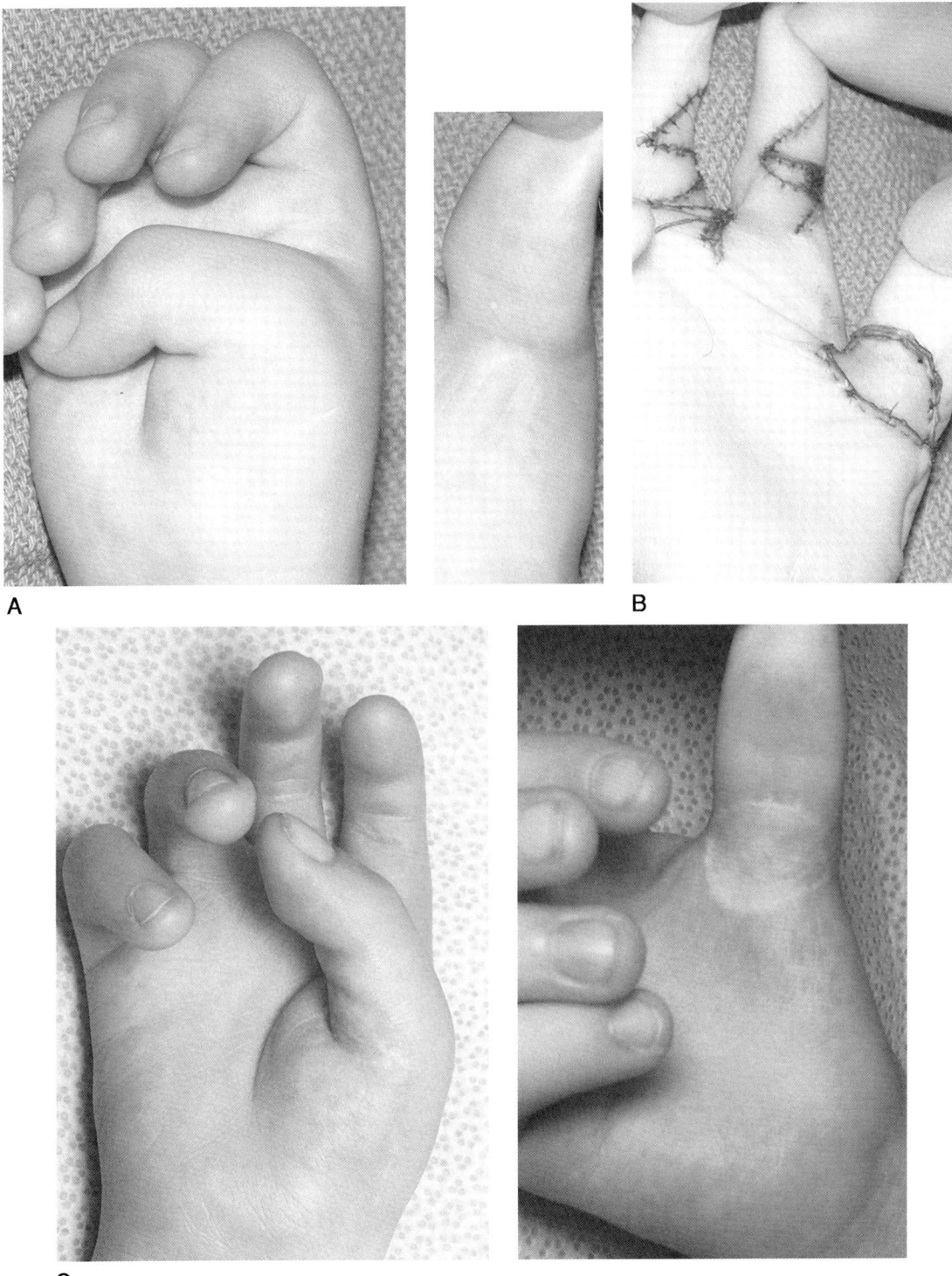

A

B

C

FIGURE 207-16. Congenital clasped thumb. *A,* This child with distal arthrogryposis presented late at 4 years of age with a tightly clasped thumb associated with a stretched or deficient extensor pollicis brevis. A severe skin contracture had developed despite early splinting. He did not use this hand. *B,* A palmar release and full-thickness skin graft were combined with a tendon transfer into the extensor pollicis brevis. Digital PIP joint releases with either a single Z-plasty (long finger) or Z-plasty plus skin graft (index) were also performed. *C,* The supple skin graft and much improved position of the thumb, index, and long fingers are seen 2 years later. He is actively using the hand and has become left-hand dominant.

contracture (Fig. 207-17). Extensor loss in multiple fingers can be corrected by transfer of the extensor carpi radialis longus plus a many-tailed graft[33,157] or by rerouting one or two of the superficial finger flexors around the ulnar border of the hand beneath the dorsal retinaculum with transfer into the common extensors to the individual digits (see Fig. 207-17). The deficient extensor tendons are usually present distally, the major abnormality existing in the proximal muscles.[158] Most surgeons prefer the latter procedure because these tendons have sufficient length, more excursion, and independence of motion. The major prerequisite to all these transfers is full passive extension and adequate release of tight palmar skin and other contractures. Any skin graft thinner than a full-thickness graft will contract with growth, particularly at the MP joint level (see Fig. 207-16).

OUTCOMES

Formal assessment of outcomes with objective documentation of correction is included in three series.[154,159,160] These reports agree that the majority of group I patients in all three classification systems resolve within 6 months of adequate splinting. If they are untreated, however, many of these children will develop more severe contractures and demonstrate continued disuse and neglect of this portion of the hand, particularly if the thumb is tightly clasped within the palm.[127,149,153] In all other groups, the quality of the long-term outcomes was proportional to the extent of the preoperative contracture and the amount of surgery required for correction. When treatment consisted of palmar release and skin graft with or without a transfer for extension, 12 of 16 hands were reported to have satisfactory results.[159] This result is standard in most series.

More variable outcomes are reported in the most severely contracted thumbs and hands, most notably in patients with arthrogryposis multiplex congenita. Children with arthrogryposis multiplex congenita or the lesser form termed distal arthrogryposis along with their first-cousin entities, Freeman-Sheldon syndrome, windblown hand, and MASA syndrome,[161] should fall into a special category because of the additional digital contractures, lower extremity involvement, and associated malformations that must be considered in any treatment plan for the thumbs or hands.

Camptodactyly

INCIDENCE AND CLASSIFICATION

Camptodactyly accounts for at least 5% of congenital hand anomalies in most studies and may occur in up to 1% of the white population.[162] A true incidence is difficult to establish because contractures of 20 degrees or less are rarely symptomatic and therefore go unrecorded.

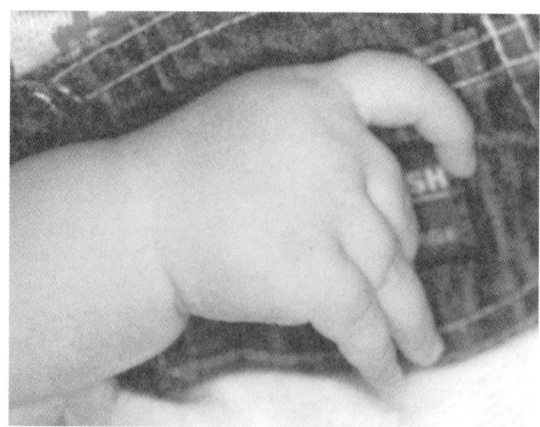

A

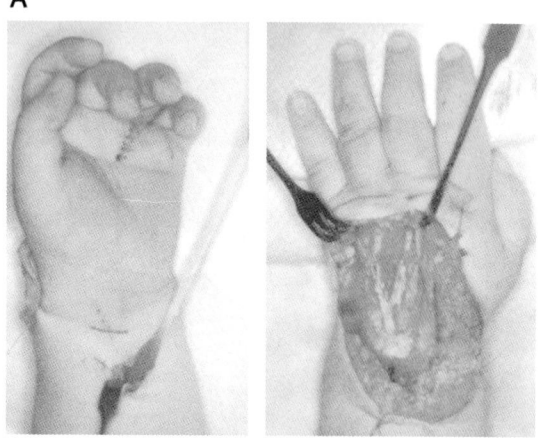

B

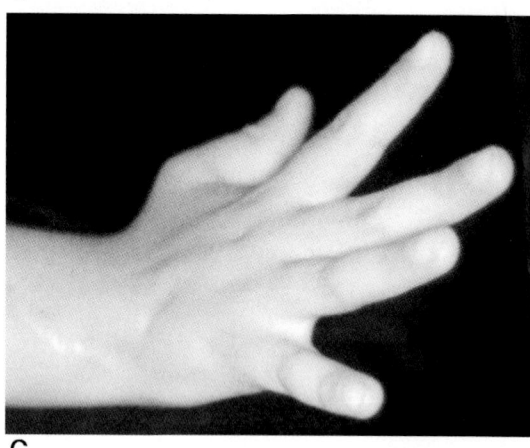

C

FIGURE 207-17. Extensor hypoplasia of the digits. *A,* This 1-year-old child had never been able to extend the ulnar three digits. He did have good independent extension of the thumb and index finger. *B,* The flexor digitorum superficialis muscle-tendon unit to the ring finger has been harvested through a trigger-type incision, isolated through a small forearm incision, rerouted around the ulnar side of the wrist, and then inserted into the common extensors of the three digits. *C,* Ten years later, he demonstrates excellent active extension with the wrist extended.

The majority of cases (84%) fall into the "congenital" group. These are noted within the first year of life and occur in boys and girls equally. The "noncongenital" group, patients who manifest after 10 years of age, is primarily female.[163,164]

Most reported cases are sporadic in distribution, but when a familial pattern is noted, it is autosomal dominant. Camptodactyly is not a disease but rather an individual defect. It is nonspecific and frequently occurs with associated anomalies as part of many syndromes (Fig. 207-18).[69,165-167]

PATHOGENESIS

Normal Intrinsic Muscle Anatomy

The lumbrical muscles originate from the flexor digitorum profundus and insert into another tendon, the extensor aponeurosis. All four pass radially to the MP joint. Innervation, origins, and insertions are variable in the third and fourth lumbricals; the first (index) lumbrical is most consistent (Fig. 207-19).[168,169]

Each finger has two interossei, with the exception of the fifth finger, which has the abductor digiti quinti minimi. Three palmar interosseous muscles adduct the long, ring, and small fingers toward the index, and four dorsal interosseous muscles abduct the digits. Distal insertions can be classified either as superficial (into the extensor aponeurosis) or deep (into bone)[170] or as proximal (into bone) or distal (into the extensor aponeurosis).[171] The first dorsal interosseous muscle inserts into bone (i.e., proximal or deep). The third inserts primarily into the extensor, whereas the second and fourth have mixed insertions. The palmar interosseous muscles have

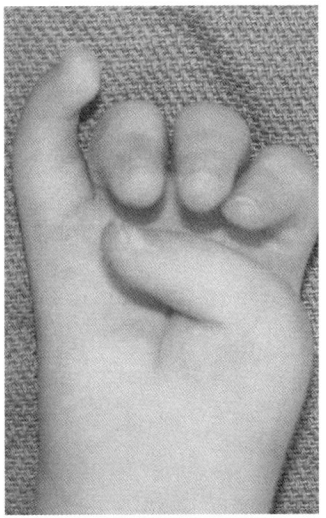
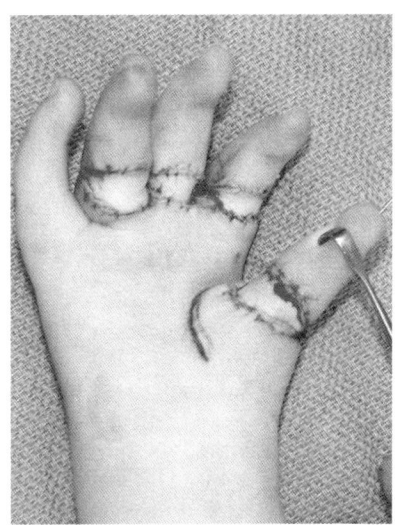

A

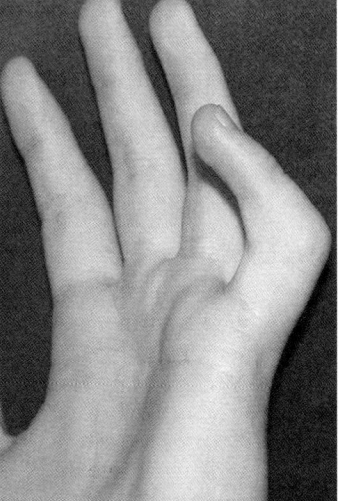
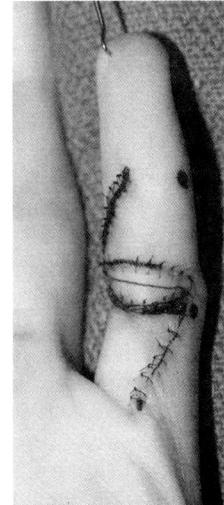

B

FIGURE 207-18. Camptodactyly. *A,* Although camptodactyly can be seen in many individual clinical situations, it usually presents at birth in syndromic patients. Multiple digits are involved in this child with arthrogryposis. Surgical release and skin grafting were necessary after a failed course of splinting. *B,* The second large group is adolescent boys and girls, who present with progressive flexion contractures of both fifth digits. Splinting is usually successful. A release, Z-plasty, and full-thickness hypothenar graft were used in this patient with a moderate to severe contracture.

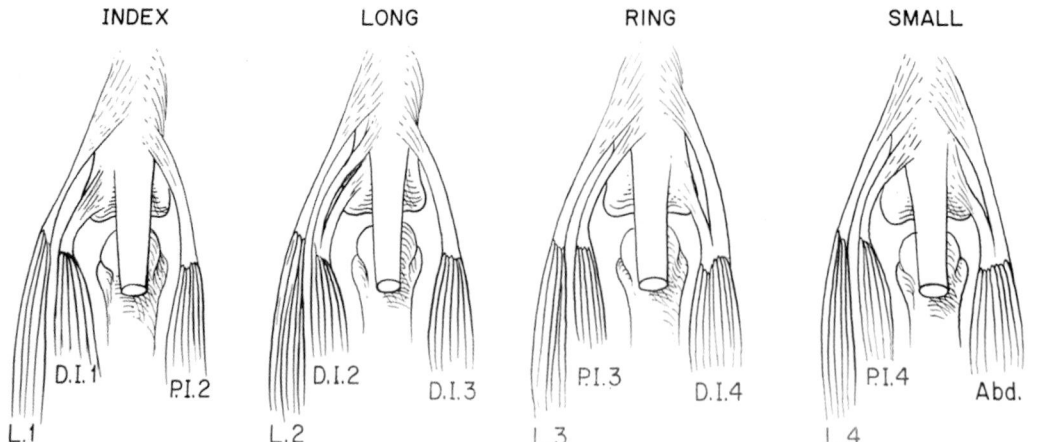

FIGURE 207-19. Normal intrinsic anatomy. The normal digital intrinsic anatomy is seen for the four digits. Only the most common variations are depicted here. L, lumbrical muscle; DI, dorsal interosseous; PI, palmar interosseous; Abd, abductor digiti minimi; 1, index finger; 2, long finger; 3, ring finger; 4, small finger. (Illustration by J. K. Biddl.)

predominant superficial insertions into the extensor aponeurosis on the ulnar side of the index finger and the radial sides of the ring and small fingers (see Fig. 207-19).

Abnormal Intrinsic Muscle Anatomy

The etiology of camptodactyly is confusing, and virtually every structure surrounding the PIP joint has been implicated in its pathogenesis.[172] Most authors emphasize the dynamic imbalance due to abnormal intrinsic muscle anatomy as the primary cause of these flexion contractures. Currently, the most culpable factor is thought to be an abnormal lumbrical insertion either into the superficialis tendon just distal to the MP joint[173] or into the fibrous flexor sheath or the capsule of the MP joint instead of into the lateral band.[174,175] Abnormal lumbrical and interosseous anatomy is common, more so on the radial side of the hand. The high frequencies of anomalous anatomy between the fourth lumbrical and fourth palmar interosseous insertions have consistently been implicated (Fig. 207-20).[174,176-178]

Other abnormal anatomic findings are tight superficialis muscle-tendon unit,[179] absent or hypoplastic flexor digitorum superficialis with abnormal insertions (Fig. 207-21),[180] contracture of collateral ligaments and palmar plate,[181] tight palmar skin,[182] slowly retracting flexor tendon,[183] deficient extensor tendons over the PIP joint,[184] including palmar interossei, and "fibrous substrata" beneath the skin.[166,185] In patients who report relief while flexing the MP joint and have active PIP joint extension against resistance, the primary cause probably lies on the palmar aspect.[163] Miura[186] postulated that the flexion-extension imbalance is the result of malposition of the extensor lateral slips due to anchoring of the middle phalanx in the

flexed position by fibrous substrata, abnormal shortening of the superficialis tendon, or abnormal insertion of the lumbrical muscle into the superficialis tendon. Ochi et al[187] reported two cases of camptodactyly that they attributed to intrauterine tenosynovitis. It is difficult to separate the primary from the secondary deformities, but most authors agree that capsular, ligamentous, and skeletal changes are secondary and that the dynamic muscle imbalance precipitates these changes.

CLINICAL PRESENTATION

The term *camptodactyly*, introduced by Tamplin,[105] comes from Greek derivatives and translates to "bent finger." It is used to describe a flexion deformity of the PIP joint in an anteroposterior direction. This deformity should be clearly distinguished from clinodactyly, in which there is a deviation in the radioulnar plane.[166]

Camptodactyly is seen in two distinct age groups, infants and adolescents (see Fig. 207-18). Within both groups, the flexion deformity may become dramatically worse during the adolescent growth spurt and does not resolve spontaneously. The deformity is usually bilateral and is most commonly seen in the small (fifth) finger. In some children, however, the fifth digit may not be involved at all.[188] Camptodactyly can occur, in decreasing order of frequency, in the ring, long, and index fingers. This finding parallels the incidence of anomalous intrinsic muscles in the hand.[174,175,189,190] Only 20% of patients show involvement of more than one digit. The degree of contracture in the other hand is not necessarily symmetric, and the severity and incidence of contractures are greater on the ulnar side of the hand.

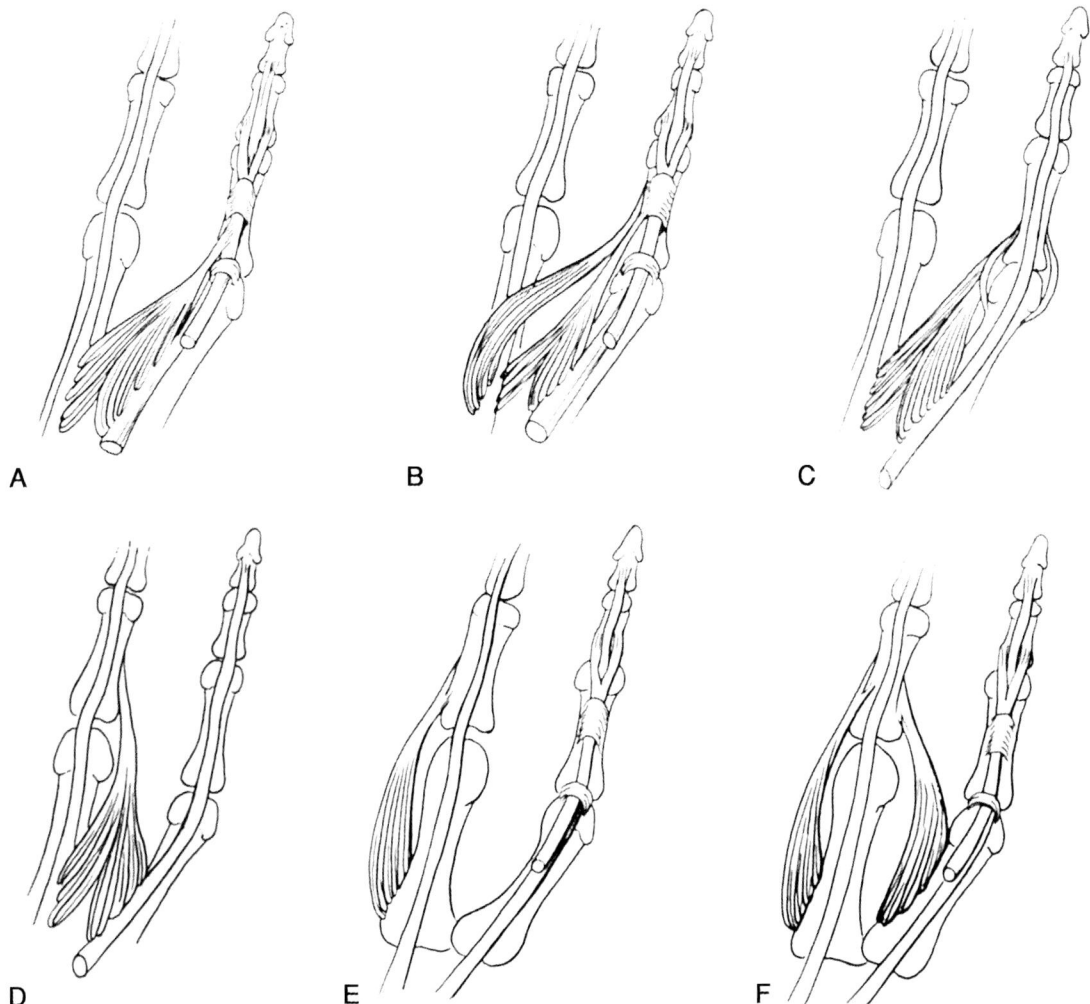

FIGURE 207-20. Abnormal lumbrical anatomy. Many common variations of muscle origin and insertion include the following: *A,* a bipennate origin with insertion into the flexor tendon and sheath; *B,* an extra muscle from the ring profundus origin with insertion into the flexor sheath; *C,* a bipennate origin with insertion into the collateral ligament of the MP joint; *D,* a bipennate muscle inserting only into the ring finger; *E,* an absent L4 muscle with intact extrinsic flexor tendons; *F,* a unipennate muscle with insertion into the ulnar side of the ring proximal phalanx. (Illustration by J. K. Biddl.)

Most flexion deformities are slight and are ignored by parents since children may compensate by hyperextending the MP joint of the same digit. Contractures range from 20 degrees to 100 degrees, and surprisingly little functional impairment is seen even in the most marked deformities, so appearance is what prompts many affected teenagers to see the hand surgeon. Only in severe cases will these children complain of functional problems.

RADIOLOGY

Long-standing or well-established cases show subtle radiologic changes on *true lateral* view. Careful scrutiny reveals a dorsal and palmar flattening of the normal circular surface of the condyle of the proximal phalanx, a narrowing of the joint space, and an indentation in the neck of the proximal phalanx corresponding to the anterior (palmar) lip of the middle phalanx. In addition, the base of the middle phalanx may be broad in teenagers or adults with fixed contractures[172,177,191] and may show greater subchondral bone density. These changes are thought to be the result, not the cause, of the contractures (Figs. 207-22 and 207-23).

DIFFERENTIAL DIAGNOSIS

Camptodactyly is differentiated from a traumatic boutonnière deformity by the lack of DIP joint hyperextension and an appropriate history. It is differentiated

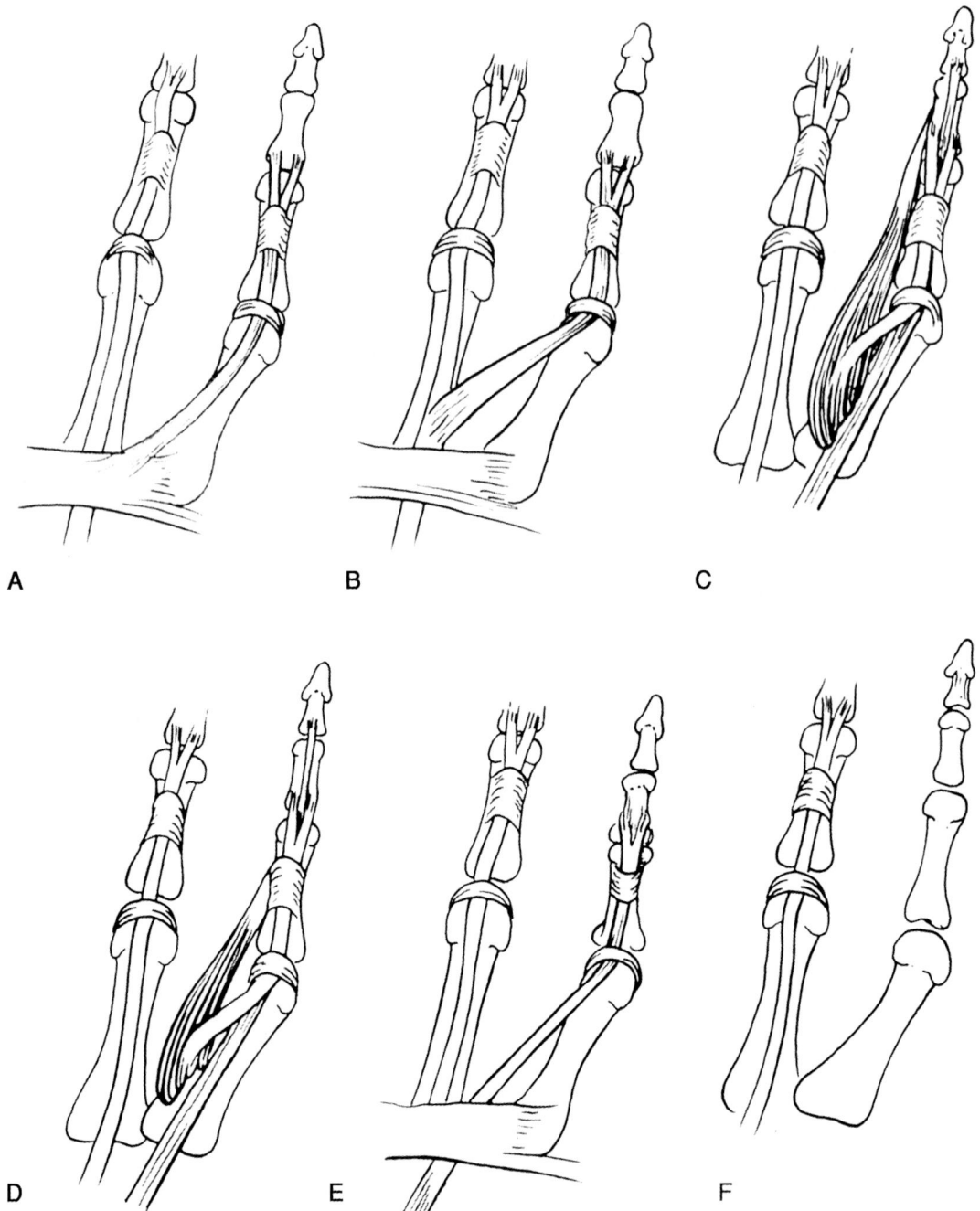

FIGURE 207-21. Abnormal flexor digitorum superficialis anatomy. Some variations of flexor digitorum superficialis anatomy seen in the hand include the following: *A,* an origin from the transverse carpal ligament; *B,* an origin from the adjacent ring profundus tendon; *C,* an origin from the normal lumbrical to the fifth digit; *D,* an origin of both lumbrical and flexor digitorum superficialis from the radial base of the fifth metacarpal; *E,* an origin proximal to the transverse carpal ligament in the distal forearm; *F,* a complete absence of the flexor digitorum superficialis. (Illustration by J. K. Biddl.)

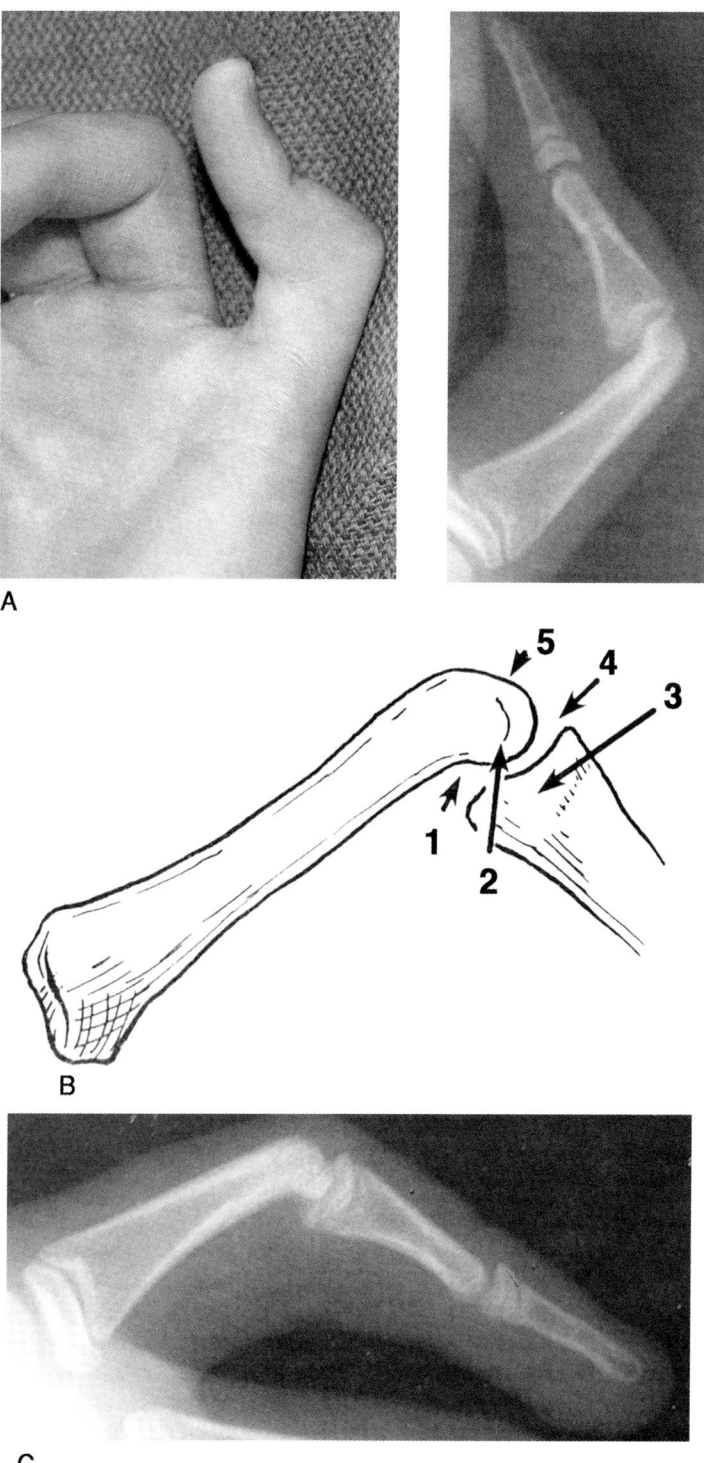

FIGURE 207-22. Radiology of camptodactyly. *A,* The clinical appearance and true lateral radiograph of a young adult with a long-standing severe PIP flexion contracture, which had progressed during his adolescent years. *B* and *C,* The characteristic radiographic findings include a narrowed retro-condylar recess (1), greater subchondral bone density (2), broader base of the middle phalanx (3), narrowed joint space (4), and flattening of the dorsal aspect of the head of the proximal phalanx (5). (Illustration by J. K. Biddl.)

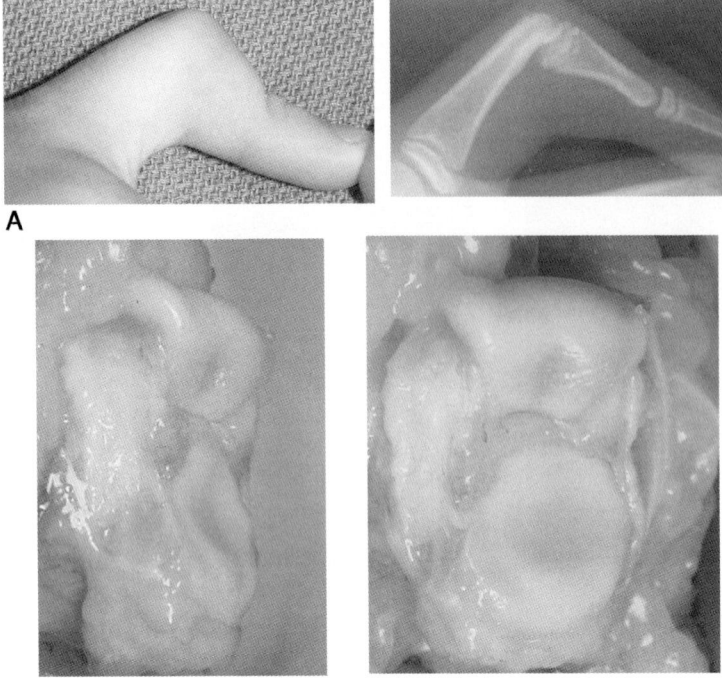

FIGURE 207-23. Camptodactyly. *A,* The appearance and true lateral radiograph in another patient who had a fixed 90-degree contracture from early childhood. *B,* During a release procedure, the jackknifed joint shows the widened base of the middle phalanx below and the eburnation that has occurred on the inferior portion of the condyle of the proximal phalanx above. The flattened articular surface of the middle phalanx is the result of a lack of motion during growth.

from trigger finger by the constant nature of the contracture and from Dupuytren contracture by the absence of palmar nodules and subcutaneous bands.[166] Rarely, Dupuytren contractures involve just the palmar aspect of the PIP joint, and in the young patient, this distinction can be confusing.[192] In congenital absence of central extensor tendons, there is a lack of extension at the MP joint and normal passive PIP joint motion with the MP joint held in flexion or extension. The same findings are present with a chronic attenuation of the central slip.[193] Syndromic flexion contractures are usually present at birth and are characterized by a lack of full passive extension.

TREATMENT

The correct treatment is as difficult to establish as the pathogenesis, but splinting is the hallmark for initial intervention in young patients.[164,174,177,194,195] In conjunction with passive stretching exercises, splinting may, in fact, obviate the need for surgery entirely if it is maintained religiously. The best advice is to encourage the patient and parents to accept the deformity for as long as possible, with the knowledge that it may worsen during the adolescent growth spurt and that aggressive surgery may further compromise the function of the finger.

This conservative approach is much less successful in adolescents, however. Splinting, of course, should be used first in adolescents with symptomatic, pro-

gressive contractures, but only about 50% of cases improve with conservative treatment, and the rest progress with growth. When the deformity has progressed or has stabilized, some form of surgical correction is generally advised.[163,164,172,175-177,186,194-196]

These older children and adults with contractures of 50 to 70 degrees or more may benefit from surgical correction (Fig. 207-24). If the joint can be actively extended with the MP joint and wrist flexed, release of the flexor superficialis alone is indicated.[172] The operation for significant contractures involves four logical steps: the incision; the examination of abnormal lumbrical, interosseous, and superficial flexor tendon anatomy; the release of secondary contractures; and the rebalancing with tendon transfer, if necessary. A longitudinal palmar approach in the distal palm with extension to the digit provides access to abnormal muscles and allows Z-plasty closure at several levels. More aggressive soft tissue release, Z-plasties, and skin grafts may be necessary with patients who have more than 40 degrees of contracture. In patients with established skeletal changes, the results of shaving of the joint articular surface are remarkably poor, and this is not recommended.

If an anomalous lumbrical can be released[174,175] or a tight superficialis lengthened[171] or released,[172] correction may be achieved. The chances of success may be improved if the tight flexor can be converted into a PIP joint extensor by transferring the two slips of the superficialis to the lateral band and the central slip via

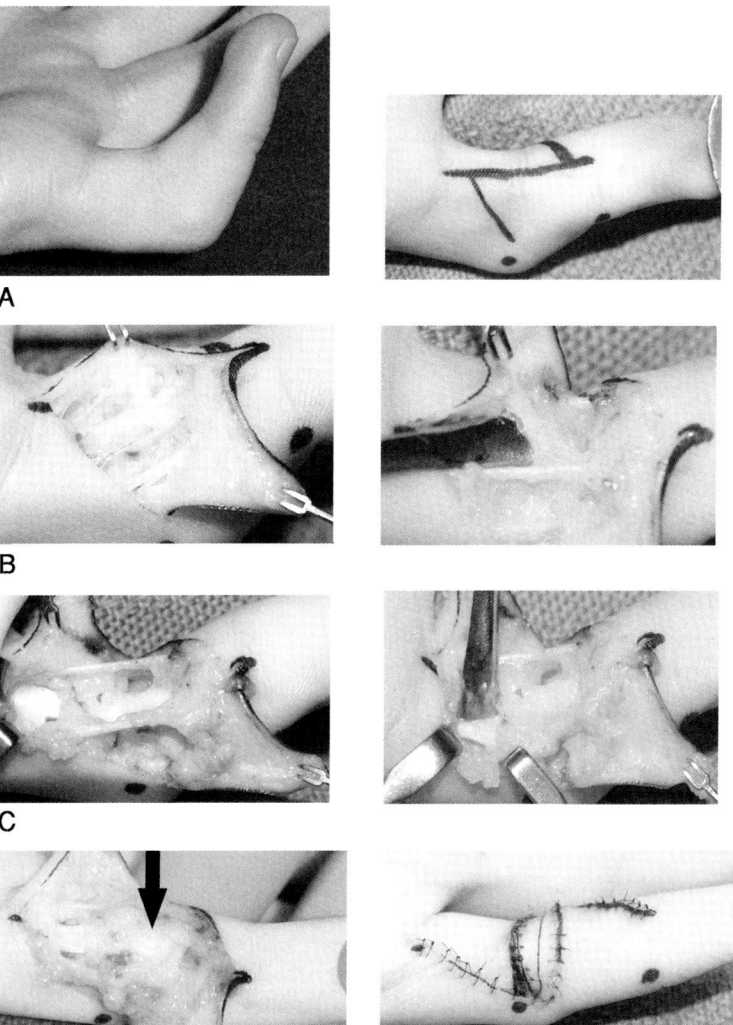

FIGURE 207-24. A technique of camptodactyly release. *A,* The markings for this 75-degree PIP joint flexion contracture start with a midline palmar incision perpendicular to the flexion creases. The Z-plasty transposition flaps are marked so that after transposition, the transverse component corresponds with the flexion crease. *B,* The fibrous bands within the connective tissue (fibrous substrata) are dissected and excised. The elevator is under a large one. *C,* The neurovascular bundles are identified but not skeletonized. They are more mobile once the bands have been excised. The flexor sheath is next incised and partially excised within the cruciate portion. The flaps have been turned back, and the volar plate is released next. *D,* Areolar tissue covers the flexor tendon in the flexion crease region in case a full-thickness skin graft is needed. A hypothenar graft was used in this digit.

the lumbrical canal.[197] This may be particularly effective if the MP joint has been held in hyperextension for a long time. In long-standing cases, it is generally necessary to correct secondary deformities, such as palmar plate and collateral ligament shortening. McFarlane et al[174] suggest that results are never as good when capsular or palmar plate release is necessary. They further suggest use of the ring finger flexor superficialis tendon rather than the little finger tendon, which may lack independence. For passively correctable joints, transfer of the extensor indicis proprius has been suggested to improve extension forces.[198]

Permanent correction of severe camptodactyly is unlikely without tendon transfer. For the best long-term results, small C wires are used to hold the PIP joint extended for 3 weeks, and night splints are worn for 3 to 6 months postoperatively. The distal phalanx should not be used as a pivot point in these splints because hyperextension may result. The three pressure points should be the dorsum of the PIP joint and the palmar aspects of the proximal and middle phalanges. These are difficult splints to maintain in children.

In older patients with significant bone changes and PIP contractures of 90 degrees that severely compromise function, a corrective osteotomy at the neck of the proximal phalanx may achieve PIP joint extension without loss of flexion.[199] If the severe contracture is fixed, arthrodesis and shortening in a more functional position should be considered. Established skeletal deformities are a contraindication to performing only soft tissue procedures.

OUTCOMES

Since there has been no universal classification system adopted for recording of outcome data, only broad generalizations can be made. Studies have stressed the importance of analyzing syndromic versus non-syndromic patients in one group and patients with fixed flexion versus mobile flexion deformities in another.[164,195] The dynamic imbalance between flexor and extensor forces at the joint space must be stressed. Surgery is generally reserved for progressive patients with 50- to 60-degree contractures.[177]

For the majority of patients with mild contractures of less than 45 degrees, splinting alone or in combination with release of a tight flexor digitorum superficialis tendon and other soft tissue structures provides improvement. With moderate contractures between 45 and 70 degrees, a much smaller number of patients achieve as much improvement, and many will lose some flexion as the PIP joint extension improves. For those with severe contractures of more than 80 degrees, less improvement is predictable, and good results are reported in only one third of patients. Preoperative complete passive mobility carries a more favorable prognosis than that of fixed contractures, and syndromic patients with multiple digital involvements rarely achieve the same results as nonsyndromic children do.[164,172,175,176,178,180,188,190,194,195,199-202]

Clinodactyly

INCIDENCE

Clinodactyly has been reported to occur in up to 1% of normal newborns and up to 10% of abnormal newborns.[203] Inward inclination of the border digits, particularly the fifth, is probably the most common congenital anomaly of the hand and has been noted to occur in up to 19.5% of nonwhite populations.[33,157] The proximal phalanx of the thumb is the second most common site of occurrence.

In most cases, there is a positive family history with an autosomal dominant pattern with variable penetrance,[203] but it can appear in a random occurrence. There can be a high correlation with mental retardation when clinodactyly is part of a syndrome; up to 79% of children with Down syndrome have clinodactyly. Males outnumber females, and bilateral involvement is most commonly seen.

CLINICAL PRESENTATION

Clinodactyly now denotes a deviation of a finger or thumb in a radioulnar or mediolateral direction, but when the term was used initially by Fort,[204] it meant deviation in any direction. The deviation is often the end product of an abnormally shaped bone, which may be triangular or trapezoidal instead of rectangular. Not all types of clinodactyly are caused by bone abnormalities, however; some involve soft tissue deficiencies. Progressive deviation of the distal phalanx at the DIP joint is inevitable when the middle phalanx is shorter on one side than on the other. Middle phalanges are the most commonly involved because they are the last bones of the hand to ossify (Fig. 207-25).[87] With large amounts of angulation, certain amounts of joint rotation and flexion will occur, making this a three-dimensional deformity. In such cases, the terms *clinodactyly* and *camptodactyly* are as related as hand and glove.

Because it has been described in association with more than 30 syndromes, clinodactyly is often an important symptom or indicator of an underlying malformation.[69] It is frequently associated with syndactyly, polydactyly, cleft hand, triphalangeal thumb, and symphalangism. Owing to its ubiquitous appearance in congenital hand anomalies, clinodactyly is often perceived as "background noise" or as a descriptive term that can be applied to identical deformities with different causes. The degree of deformity correlates directly with associated malformations, and a small amount of deviation is more likely to be an isolated anomaly.

Up to 10 degrees of deviation is considered normal in the thumb and fifth digit.[205,206] Abnormal deviation rarely exceeds 20 degrees in the finger or thumb and presents no functional problems. In cases of the rectangular middle phalanx, the phalanx can vary from being of normal length to being severely hypoplastic. Shortening of the phalangeal segment (brachyphalangia) is common and should be distinguished from the "delta" phalanx, which is discussed in the next section, and from an additional bone (triangular ossicle) that creates deviation, as seen in the triphalangeal thumb deformities (Fig. 207-26; see also Fig. 207-25).

Delta Phalanx

When it was first introduced, the term *delta phalanx* described a triangular bone with a C-shaped epiphysis running continuously along the shortened side of a phalanx.[207] It is an inaccurate term, however, because the bone may be either a metacarpal or a phalanx, and it is usually shaped more like a trapezoid than a delta or triangle.[44] Some authors have recommended the term *congenital triangular bone*.[208] In any case, these bones should be distinguished from those that do have a continuous epiphysis along one entire side. Theander and Carstam have described a C-shaped epiphysis extending along the short side of the diaphysis that accounts for the abnormal growth of this bone and have used the term *longitudinally bracketed diaphysis* to describe the phalanx.[209-211]

On histologic examination, the osseous bracket consists of trabecular bone with no periosteum that is entirely enclosed in hyaline cartilage in which there is active enchondral ossification. The long side of the bracketed diaphysis is the only part of the phalanx that has a cortex and periosteum.[210-212] Some authors

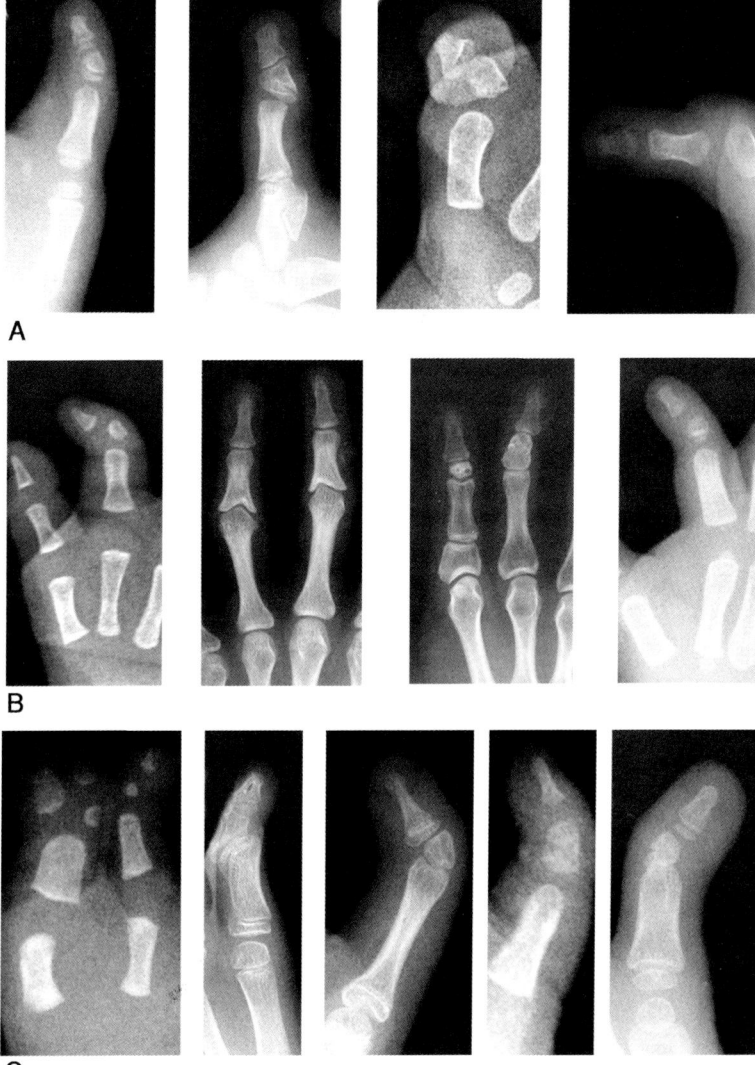

FIGURE 207-25. Examples of clinodactyly. Deviation in the radio-ulnar plane is diagnostic of clinodactyly. Innumerable examples exist in the congenital hand population. *A,* Thumb deformities are common as illustrated by (1) an intermediate phalanx in a triphalangeal thumb, (2) delta phalanges at the metacarpal and intermediate phalangeal level in a cleft hand deformity, (3) the radial clinodactyly of the Apert hand, and (4) the isolated radial clinodactyly in a symbrachydactyly. *B,* Clinodactyly of the index finger is the rarest occurrence and is seen (1) in isolated cases, (2) as slight ulnar deviation in congenital epiphyseal abnormalities, (3) as radial clinodactyly in hypersegmentation syndromes, or (4) as radial clinodactyly in the cleft hand-foot syndrome. *C,* Unusual clinodactylies in either direction are seen with (1) a two-digit hand with radial deviation of the thumb and ulnar deviation of the ulnar ray, (2) a fifth digit with a continuous longitudinal epiphyseal bracket, (3, 4) radial deviation of fifth digits with triangular or trapezoidal intermediate phalanges, and (5) ulnar deviation of a fifth digit with a symphalangism of proximal and middle phalanges.

believe that this represents a form of duplication.[213] The morphologic appearance of these bones runs a spectrum from trapezoidal to triangular to nearly round. Blevens and Light[214] have presented a five-part classification: two trapezoidal, two triangular, and one complex, almost round.

The distal phalanx is never involved. When a delta phalanx is present in the small finger, angulations of 10 to 50 degrees pose problems that are more cosmetic than functional. It is thought that this deformity may be an autosomal dominant trait with incomplete penetrance.[208] In most published series, the most common site of occurrence is the middle phalanx of the fifth digit, the last bone to ossify in the hand.[208] The next most common site is the proximal phalanx of the thumb or ring finger. The thumb radial clinodactyly of cra-

niofacial patients with the Apert, Pfeiffer, Crouzon, and Rubinstein-Taybi syndromes is a good example. The ulnar deviation of the congenital triphalangeal thumb and the deviation deformities seen in central polydactylies (central synpolydactyly) and the typical cleft hand all include these abnormal bones (see Fig. 207-25). Common to all is the abnormal epiphysis that surrounds one side of the bone like a staple. The three-dimensional character of these deformities is often overlooked as deviation in the radioulnar plane is commonly accompanied by a flexion deformity.

Kirner Deformity

The Kirner deformity is an unusual radial and volar curvature of the distal phalanx of the fifth digit.[215,216] With no dorsal support, the nail has the appearance

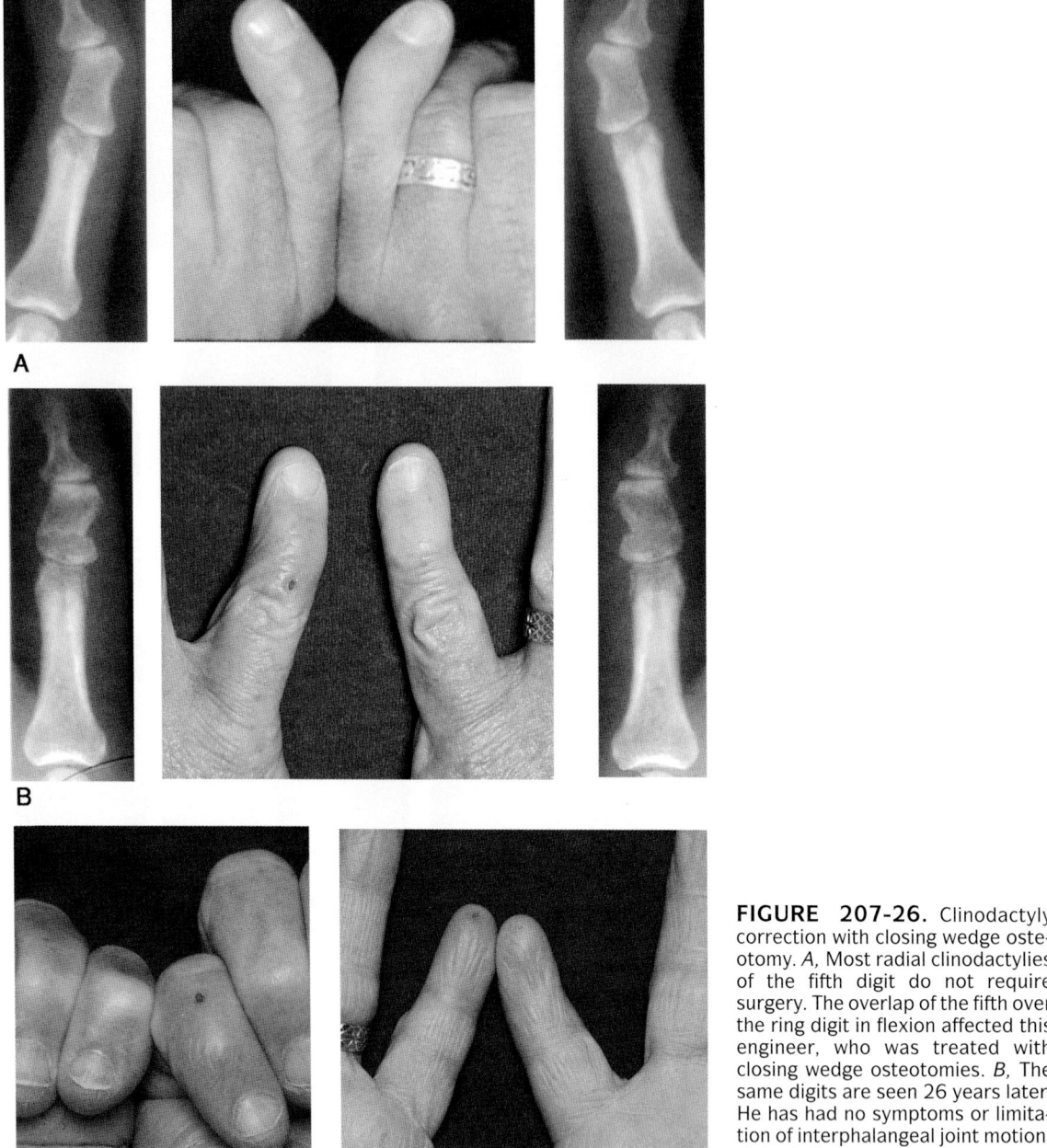

FIGURE 207-26. Clinodactyly correction with closing wedge osteotomy. *A,* Most radial clinodactylies of the fifth digit do not require surgery. The overlap of the fifth over the ring digit in flexion affected this engineer, who was treated with closing wedge osteotomies. *B,* The same digits are seen 26 years later. He has had no symptoms or limitation of interphalangeal joint motion. *C,* Both digits are straight, and there is no overlapping with flexion.

of a parrot's beak. The epiphysis and DIP joint are in normal position. There is association with a number of syndromes, including Turner, Down, and Cornelia de Lange.[217,218] Females outnumber males, and there may be some positive inheritance. Most cases are sporadic. Treatment is conservative. With extreme angulation, splinting is of little value and surgery is the most effective treatment.[219,220]

TREATMENT

Although some authors have recommended splinting, clinodactyly usually does not correct itself with growth. As most complaints are usually cosmetic rather than functional, surgery should be postponed until the child is older than 6 years. It should be reserved for cooperative patients who present with obvious cosmetic and functional problems.[221]

In cases of marked deviation, there are generally three surgical options: a closing wedge osteotomy, a reversed wedge osteotomy, or an opening wedge osteotomy with bone graft. A closing wedge osteotomy is usually performed for simple clinodactylies during late childhood or adolescence to improve function or appearance (see Fig. 207-26).[33,157] A reversed wedge osteotomy is technically demanding, requires precise judgment regarding the width of the wedge, and must be performed with osteotomes instead of electric saw blades, which remove small amounts of cortical bone.[222] An opening wedge osteotomy plus bone graft has the advantage of increasing length, leaving the longer cortical surface intact, and avoiding possible malrotation (Figs. 207-27 and 207-28). Results are generally excellent.

In the last two techniques, soft tissue releases (skin, fibrous tissue, extensor tendon) are occasionally required for simple clinodactyly but are more commonly employed for complex cases such as a delta phalanx. With all of these procedures, adequate bone stock should be present so that osteotomies do not injure the growth plates. A fourth option for correction, used for rare cases of more severe deviation, consists of excision of the midportion of the continuous epiphysis and underlying physis and replacement with a free fat graft.[223,224] These techniques are more frequently used with larger tubular bones such as the radius, humerus, and femur. Splinting does have a role in postoperative maintenance of correction for at least 3 to 6 months.

OUTCOMES

The outcomes of surgical procedures for clinodactyly with or without rotational impairment are good and predictable if the particular bone in question has reached skeletal maturity.[64,157,206,218,221,222] In young children with complex malformations involving more than one particular bone, the deformity may

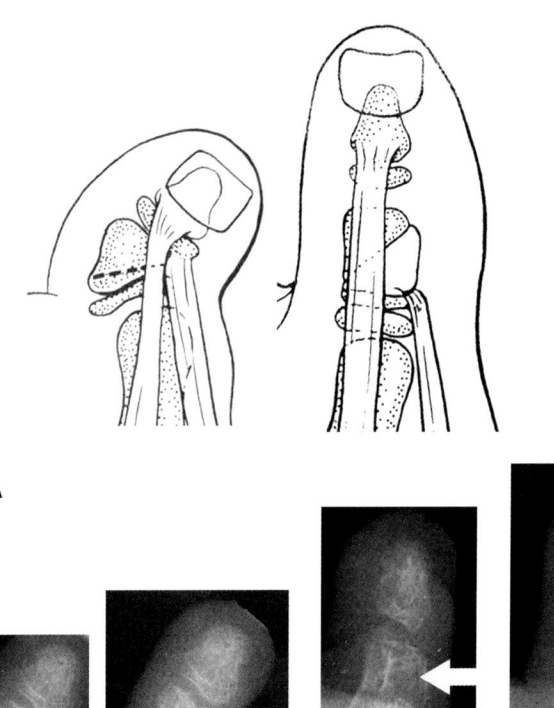

FIGURE 207-27. Clinodactyly correction with opening wedge osteotomy plus bone graft. *A,* The illustration shows the preoperative and postoperative alignment of the extensor pollicis longus (EPL) and abductor pollicis brevis (AbPB) tendons and their insertions in a thumb with radial clinodactyly of a left thumb, commonly seen in the craniofacial patients. *B,* Serial radiographs of the left thumb of this patient with Rubinstein-Taybi syndrome show the progression of the deformity between 1 and 2 years of age. An opening wedge osteotomy with bone graft was performed at the age of $3^{1}/_{2}$ years. Complete incorporation of the graft (*arrow*) is seen by her fourth birthday. The longitudinal growth of the phalanx progressed normally during the next 3 years. (Illustration by J. K. Biddl.)

A

B

1 year   2 years   4 years   7 years

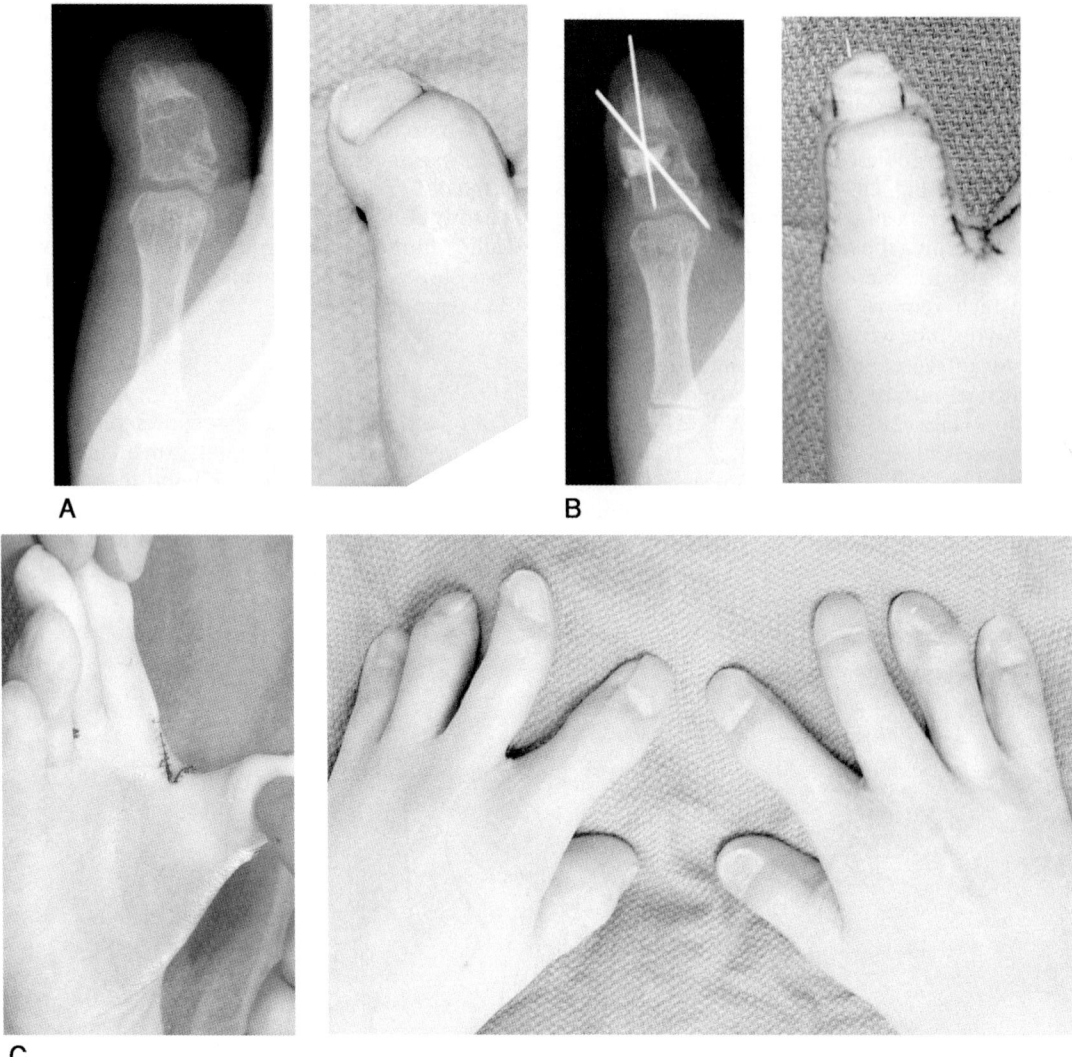

FIGURE 207-28. Apert thumb with recurrent clinodactyly. *A,* This Apert child had an osteotomy and bone graft at the age of 4 years for correction of the radial deviation. The deformity has recurred because the radial half of the epiphyseal plate closed prematurely. *B,* A second osteotomy and demineralized bone graft straightened the thumb. At the same time, the redundant radial soft tissue was debulked. *C,* Further deepening of the first web space effectively provides length to the thumb. Both hands are seen at 16 years of age.

recur as the child grows. This is often true, for example, with the Apert thumb if it has been corrected within the first few years of life (see Fig. 207-28). The major problem with an aggressive closing wedge osteotomy of the fifth digit, the most common site of clinodactyly in the hand, is the risk of causing a mallet deformity if too much shortening has occurred or with adherence of the extensor mechanism to the osteotomy site. The same is true for surgery on the intermediate bone of a triphalangeal thumb. Problems that can occur with the other techniques include malrotation, skin tightness and neurosis, and epiphyseal damage.

Overgrowth

DEFINITION

Depending on the location and degree of enlargement, overgrowth has been called many names. The term *macrodactyly* (Greek *makros*, large, and *daktylos*, digit) has been used most frequently, although the malformation is not restricted solely to digits.[33] Some authors prefer the term *digital gigantism* because it encompasses enlargement of all tissue elements, including the skeleton. Gigantism has simply been defined as "congenital pathologic enlargement of soft tissue parts with associated enlargement of the skeleton."[225]

Many of these conditions have been called hamartomas (Greek *hamartia,* to sin), malformed tissue that grows locally. In actuality, there is a wide spectrum of overlapping clinical presentations, some of which are described here. These are to be distinguished from other conditions that probably are related to failure of differentiation of certain elements: vascular malformations (arterial, venous, and lymphatic alone or in combination), enchondromatoses (Maffucci and Ollier syndromes),[226] osteoid osteoma,[33] fibrous dysplasia,[33] and lipomatoses. The term Klippel-Trénaunay is often incorrectly interchanged with any type of digital or limb overgrowth with or without abnormal amounts of fat.[227] To avoid confusion, common terms such as megalodactyly, macrodystrophia lipomatosa, macrodactylia fibrolipomatosis, dactylomegaly, gigantomegaly, and localized gigantism are best not used.

As a group, overgrowth or gigantism problems occupy a small portion of congenital hand deformities, but when present, they challenge even the most accomplished hand surgeon. They can involve all positions of the hand and upper limb (Fig. 207-29). Common to all types is overgrowth of one or more cell types, including the skeleton. It is not known whether enlargement is secondary to actual neoplasia or to enlargement of existing cells within the hand.

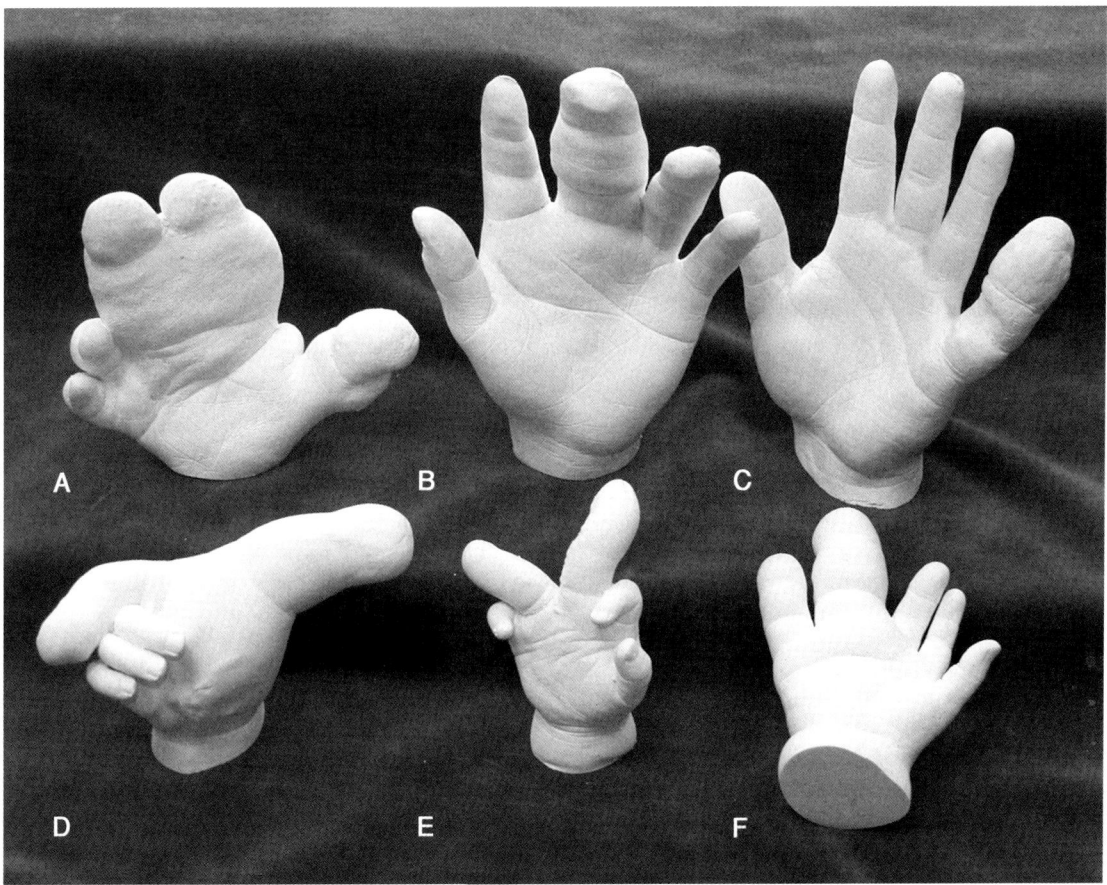

FIGURE 207-29. Macrodactyly hand patterns. Macrodactyly (*makros,* large, *daktylos,* digit) can occur in one or more digits in a number of specific clinical conditions that cannot always be identified by physical examination alone. However, some conditions, such as the Proteus syndrome, hyperostosis, and hemihypertrophy, are more easily identified. *A,* Massive overgrowth of soft tissue and bone is present in this child with nerve territory-oriented macrodactyly of the median nerve. The simple syndactyly has prevented the expected deviation of the index and long digits. *B,* Another child with nerve territory–oriented macrodactyly of nerves to second and third interdigital spaces demonstrates greatest involvement of the long digit and lesser soft tissue overgrowth on the ulnar side of the index and radial side of the ring digits. *C,* Both sides of the fifth digit are involved in this boy with neurofibromatosis, a diagnosis that must be confirmed with additional clinical findings. *D,* Massive hypertrophy and deviation are present in this child with lipomatous macrodactyly. No infiltration of nerves was seen. Her forearm, arm, and axilla contained additional fat deposits. *E,* Once the syndactyly of the long and ring digits was separated, the deviation in this child with nerve territory-oriented macrodactyly became progressively worse with growth. *F,* The ring and fifth rays are symmetrically enlarged in this child with lipomatous macrodactyly. Skeletal overgrowth was present in both metacarpals and all phalanges.

Seven distinct clinical entities are presented here, with the common characteristic being skeletal overgrowth of part or all of the hand. Clinical presentation, mode of inheritance, and treatment differ with each entity. Gigantism related to vascular anomalies is covered in the section on vascular malformations (see Chapter 209).

CLASSIFICATION

Because of the many variations and clinical presentations of overgrowth problems, several divergent classification systems have been proposed. The three systems presented have differentiated these patients by growth rate,[228] by affiliation with different syndromes,[66] or by specific disease entities.[33] My preference has been to use the last as it has proved to be the most useful to the clinical hand surgeon. Flatt[33] originally described four types as gigantism associated with lipofibromatosis (group I), neurofibromatosis (group II), hyperostosis (group III), and hemihypertrophy (group IV). I have also included additional conditions associated with overgrowth.[229]

COMMON TYPES

Nerve Territory–Oriented Macrodactyly

The initial descriptions of digital and hand enlargement were made in the 19th century by a number of authors who were specifically describing the disease neurofibromatosis.[230-232] For the next half-century, most researchers in the field thought that all forms of upper limb involvement were associated with neurofibromatosis. Kelikian[87] introduced the term *nerve territory–oriented macrodactyly,* which is useful because it emphasizes the relationship between enlargement and nerve distribution as part of a regional growth disturbance.

This common type of macrodactyly is unilateral in 90% of cases, has no familial inheritance pattern, and is not frequently associated with other malformations.[87,233,234] The normal stigmata of neurofibromatosis may not be present. Although the limb findings are similar, these patients do not have the specific finding sufficient for a diagnosis of neurofibromatosis. Males outnumber females by a 3:2 ratio. The median nerve region is most frequently involved, with the second web space predominantly affected. All digits and the thumb may be involved alone, but multiple digit involvement is three times more likely to occur than is single digit enlargement.

With severe enlargement, the involved digits deviate away from the involved interspace, which is webbed in 10% of patients and may restrict joint motion (see Fig. 207-29).[235] Overgrowth of all digits and the thumb is usually associated with gross overgrowth of the entire limb. In rare cases, the proximal portion including the brachial plexus may be involved.[236]

Affected thumbs have a characteristic extended, abducted posture.[237] The palm and wrist regions may primarily be involved, with large soft tissue masses but without significant digital gigantism. Carpal tunnel syndromes are common in older patients,[238-244] but normally, two-point discrimination and light touch are not impaired despite extensive enlargement.[245] As these children grow, however, the two-point discrimination is significantly impaired (Fig. 207-30).

Two types of growth patterns have been described by Barsky[237] and DeLaurenzi[228] and correspond with the author's clinical observations during the past 30 years of approximately 100 of these hands. In the *static type,* enlargement is present at birth, and growth of the limb is proportionate with that of the rest of the child. These patients tend to present for treatment with reasonably good function later in life, usually during adolescence.[228] In the *progressive type,* some overgrowth is obvious at birth, but around 2 years of age, there is slow, unrestricted, disproportionate digital or hand enlargement. Aggressive overgrowth in both length and circumferential width occurs, ceasing only after epiphyses have closed. Three-dimensional increases in palmar bulk and metacarpal enlargement with a progressive syndactyly between the involved digits characteristically extend into the palm.[237,246] Early in life, it may be difficult to differentiate static from progressive growth patterns. There is a small third group of these children. For them, significant overgrowth is present at birth, and the progressive enlargement continues in an unrestricted fashion. The disproportion is so great that most affected parts are amputated (Fig. 207-31).

The histology of involved nerves has been well documented and includes the presence of excessive fat[247,248] and distortion by a significant amount of epineural and perineural fibrosis[249,250] (see Fig. 207-30). These greatly distorted axons are, however, of normal size and caliber. The most impressive finding in these enlarged digits and palms is the markedly excessive fat infiltrating normal-appearing neural structures. Bone contains large numbers of osteoclasts and osteoblasts, and accelerated remodeling of bone at the periosteal level has been noted as the bone grows in length, width, and circumference.[57,250,251] In the immature skeleton, bone remodeling is normal but proceeds at an accelerated rate. Although there is no direct involvement of vascular structures, poor circulation and diminished temperature are common. Symptoms of vascular insufficiency are present in all patients with grotesquely enlarged hands or digits. In every case, comparison radiographs of both the patient's hands should be obtained periodically to document the growth. Accelerated osteoarthritis is common in older patients (see Fig. 207-31).

The cause of this condition is not known. An abundance of speculation as to cause ranges from localized

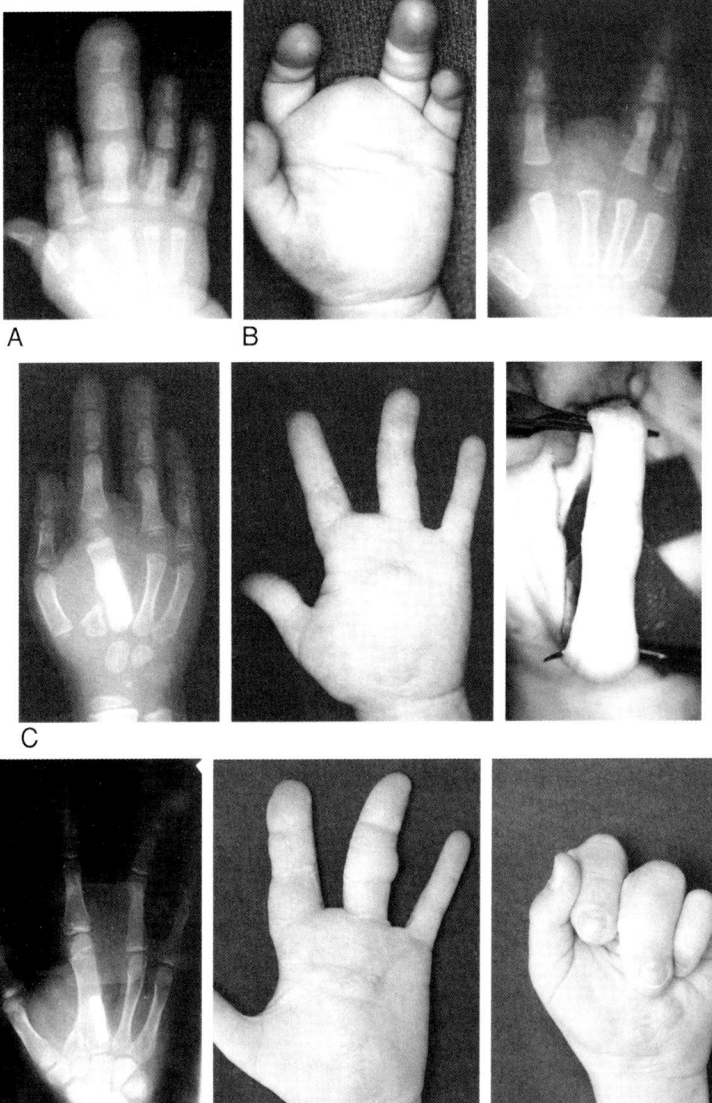

FIGURE 207-30. Compression neuropathy. *A,* The radiograph taken shortly after birth shows a massively hypertrophied long digit with skeletal overgrowth of all three phalanges and a normal metacarpal. The enlarged digit was amputated within the first 6 months of life. Clinically, the index and ring digits looked normal. *B,* At the age of 2 years, he was referred for follow-up care when his family moved. His hand functioned well, but massive lipomatous masses had developed within the palm. *C,* One year later, he could not feel the thumb, index, and ring digits because of an advanced carpal tunnel syndrome. A massively enlarged median nerve was demonstrated at the time of carpal tunnel release. Additional palmar and digital debulking along with ray transfer of the index to long metacarpals was performed at the same time. *D,* Growth has continued, and more digital debulkings have been required. At 17 years of age, he has good motion at MP and PIP joints, fused DIP joints, and new soft tissue irregularities. Light touch is present in the index and ring digits, but moving two-point discrimination is markedly increased to 8.0 mm (normal, 4.0 mm). His function remains excellent in this nondominant hand.

neurofibromatosis[252,253] to impairment of peripheral nerves,[253,254] local growth factor,[240,255] and defective germ plasm.[171,256] Tsuge and Ikuta[243] and others suggest that growth control is mediated through the nerve because, in isolated cases, incision or resection of the involved nerve has altered progressive growth.

Lipomatous Macrodactyly

This is the most common single group of overgrowth cases.[57,233] When more is learned about the genetic composition and molecular biology of this type, it may be turn out to be similar to nerve territory–oriented macrodactyly and neurofibromatosis. Common to all types is an abundance of fat, which probably contains the growth factors responsible for the skeletal and other

tissue overgrowth. One or both hands and sometimes feet are affected equally, and it is unusual for the enlargement to be confined to a single digit or thumb. There can also be significant palmar, forearm, and arm involvement.[2,233] Although most of the enlargement in the proximal portions of the upper limb is confined to the subcutaneous space, intermuscular and intramuscular infiltration may be seen. Muscle function may be surprisingly good despite extensive lipomatous infiltration, and the major functional deficit in these limbs is caused by their sheer size and weight.

This type is commonly confused with nerve territory–oriented macrodactyly and neurofibromatosis, but microscopic dissection of the neurovascular

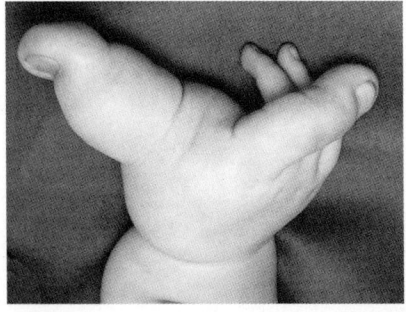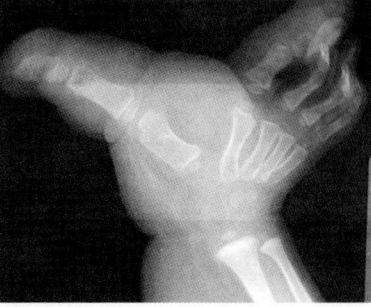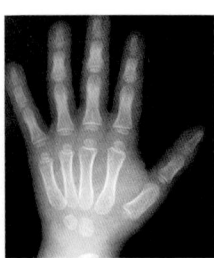

A

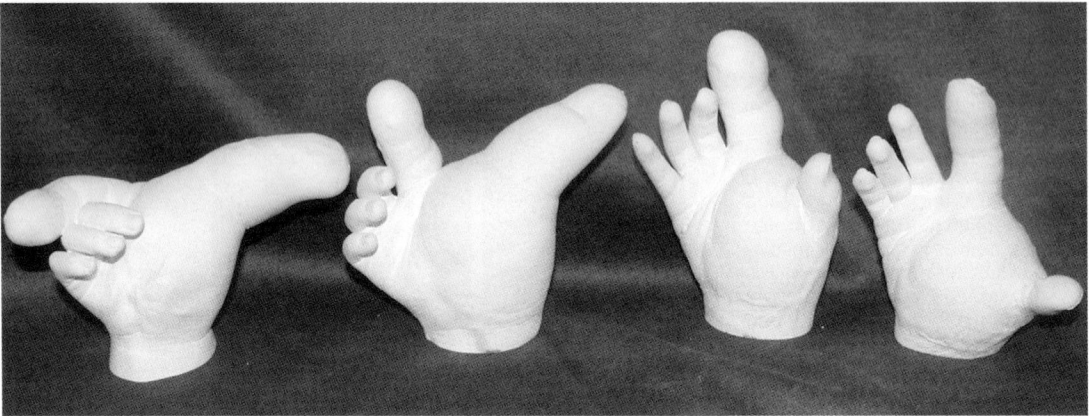

B

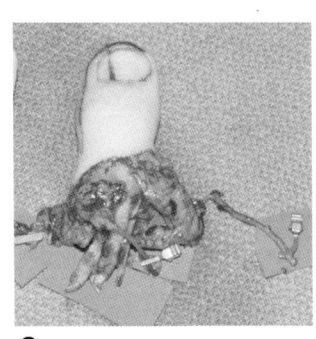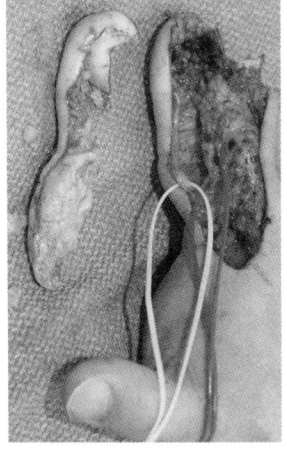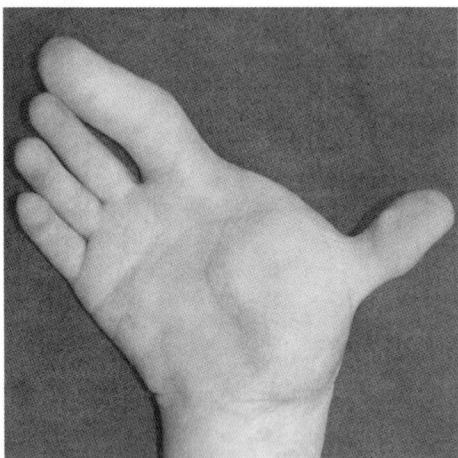

C

FIGURE 207-31. Massive, grotesque overgrowth. *A,* This 6-month-old child presented with massively enlarged thumb and index rays associated with large circumferential forearm, arm, and axillary fat deposits. The extent of the overgrowth is appreciated by comparison of the radiographs of her abnormal right hand and normal left hand. *B,* A number of staged operations were performed within the next 2 years as demonstrated by molds of her right hand. First, the index digit was debulked and straightened with an osteotomy and epiphyseal closure of the index ray (second from left). Next, the grotesquely enlarged thumb was amputated and replaced with an ipsilateral great-toe transfer at the age of 2 years (third from left). Soft tissue debulking of the radial side of the index digit followed (fourth from left). Circumferential debulking of the forearm, elbow, and arm fat was performed concomitantly. Liposuction was considered and not performed in the arm but done in the axilla. *C,* The great toe is seen en route to the hand. Although markings for a modified toe transfer had been made, no skeletal reduction was performed, nor has it been needed. The normal dorsal sensory nerves of the hand were used as recipient nerves for both digital nerves of the new "thoe." The aggressive soft tissue and skeletal reduction on the radial side of the index finger is demonstrated. The digital nerve and artery have been dissected and preserved out to the level of the distal pulp. On the far right, her hand is seen after her last procedure, an aggressive soft tissue debulking of the involved radial half of the palm. Sensation is normal in the thumb (3.0 mm of moving two-point discrimination) and abnormal in the index (8.0 mm). This is her dominant hand, and she has adapted well.

structures demonstrates no lipomatous infiltration of digital nerves (Fig. 207-32). Neurovascular structures are of normal caliber when they are dissected carefully under the operating microscope. All soft tissue structures are surrounded by an abundant amount of fat. At birth, many of the enlarged parts are gigantic and continue on a progressive growth pattern. However, there is a small group of patients who demonstrate a static growth pattern. All skeletal structures within the involved field have accelerated growth unless epiphysiodeses are performed (see Fig. 207-31).

An important previously unreported observation is that all of these patients have early onset of severe osteoarthritis or degenerative joint changes in the involved skeletal structures (Fig. 207-33; see also Fig. 207-31). This observation has been made by others in reflecting on other diagnoses,[257] and isolated reports in the literature do mention the treatment of degenerative joint problems and the appearance of abnormal calcifications with longer follow-up in these patients.[238,258] Early evidence in the author's patients also indicates that toe transfers placed into these fields also show an accelerated rate of osteophyte formation and joint space deterioration.

I disagree with previous reports that two-point discrimination is normal.[233,245] As with nerve territory–oriented macrodactyly, digital sensation measured by moving and static two-point discrimination and

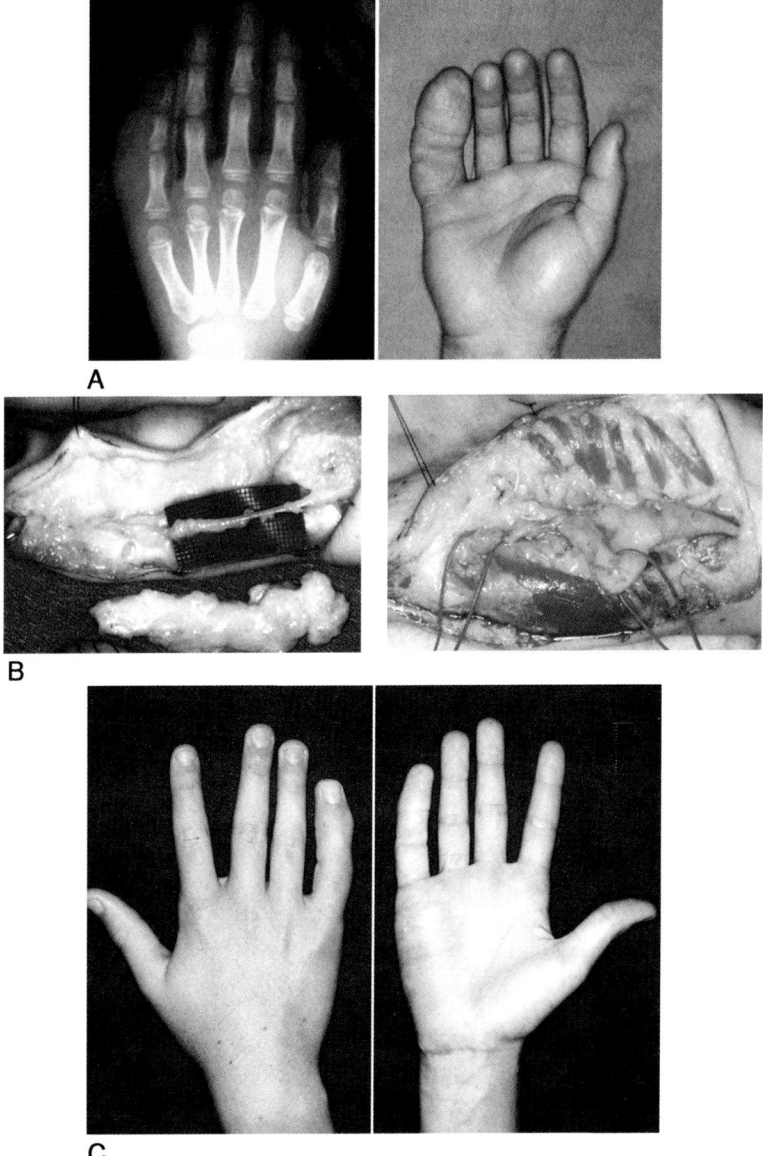

FIGURE 207-32. Isolated fifth digit macrodactyly. *A*, This teenager with neurofibromatosis presented with isolated soft tissue enlargement and no skeletal enlargement. Ray resection had been recommended by a number of hand surgeons, but the patient did not want to lose his digit. *B*, An aggressive debulking of the digit included a microscopic dissection and preservation of the digital artery (under the background) and digital nerve. The serpiginous common ulnar nerve with extensive intraneural fat infiltration is seen between the hypothenar muscles (below) and palmaris brevis muscle in the skin flap (above). *C*, Eighteen years after a two-staged debulking of the digit and palm, the contour has remained excellent, and he has not lost any range of motion. Two-point discrimination measured 6.0 mm (normal, 4.0 mm) on both sides of the digit.

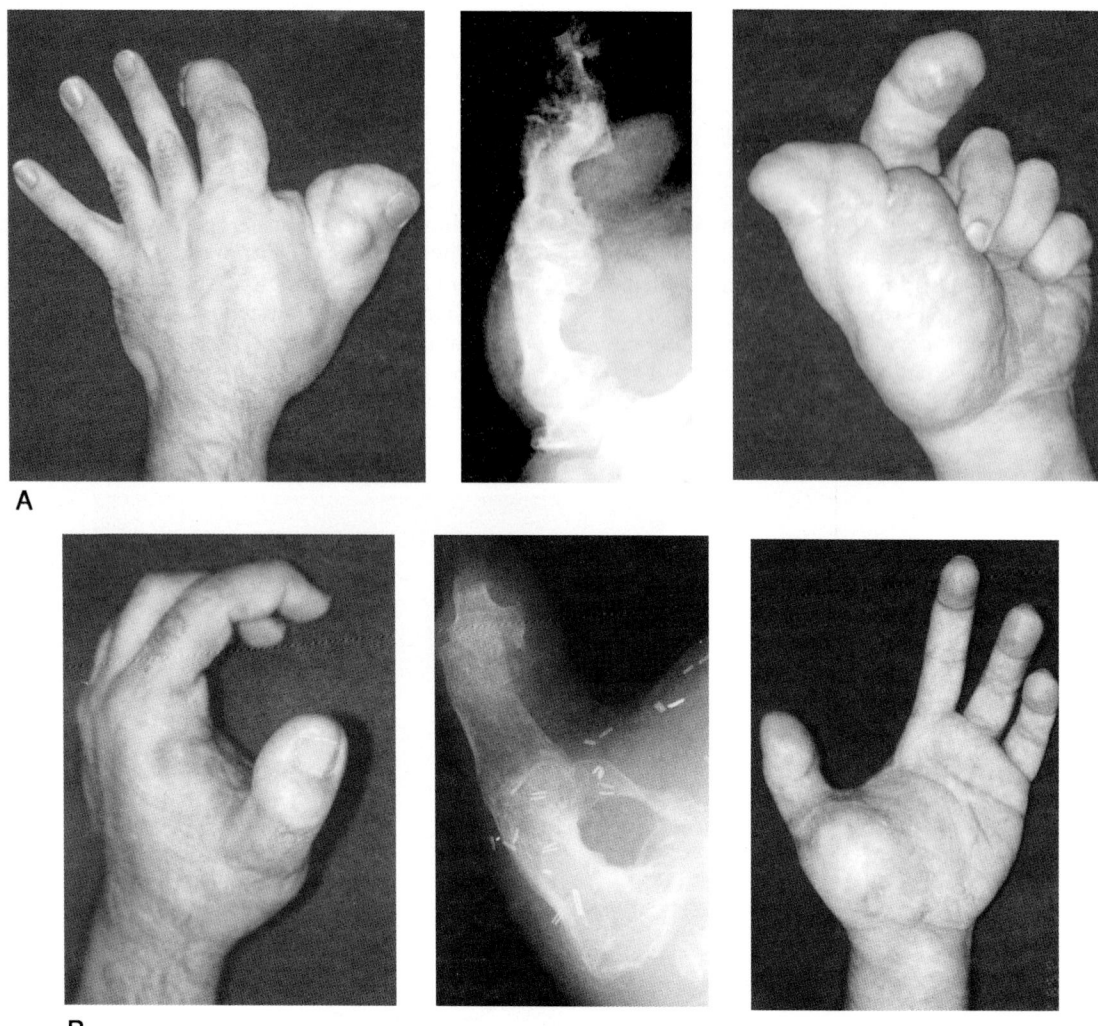

FIGURE 207-33. Macrodactyly and osteoarthritis. *A,* This 28-year-old librarian presented as a frustrated adult after multiple (>10) previous attempts to debulk a massive soft tissue and skeletal overgrowth. The radiographs of the thumb and index digits showed a marked amount of osteoarthritis at every joint level of both rays. The wrist was not involved. *B,* The surgical solution was an amputation of both rays and an ipsilateral great-toe transfer. As a second stage, an interpositional carpometacarpal joint arthroplasty was performed. Within 5 years, radiographs have begun to show signs of degenerative joint disease within the "thoe."

Semmes-Weinstein modalities reveals a progressive decrease with or without surgery. Longitudinal growth of the tubular bones can be stopped only by epiphyseal arrest, after which horizontal growth in width and circumference often continues. In contrast to previous reports,[237] the metacarpal of the involved ray is also enlarged (Fig. 207-34).

Neurofibromatosis

Digital, hand, and entire extremity gigantism are well-known sequelae of neurofibromatosis (von Recklinghausen disease), which has an autosomal dominant inheritance pattern and must contain the following clinical hallmarks: six or more areas of cutaneous pig-mentation (café au lait spots), pedunculated cutaneous tumors (molluscum fibrosum), and multiple tumors of peripheral nerves. The characteristic café au lait freckles are usually obvious at birth. A newborn patient with five of these freckles that exceed 1.5 cm in diameter is likely to receive a diagnosis of neurofibromatosis, which is a systemic disorder characterized by hyperplasia and neoplasia throughout the connective tissue of the nervous system.

Incidence is estimated to be 1 in every 3000 live births.[66] Neurofibromatosis has also been reported to be one of the most common spontaneously occurring mutations in humans. Digital enlargement is frequently bilateral and seldom unilateral (Fig. 207-35). The

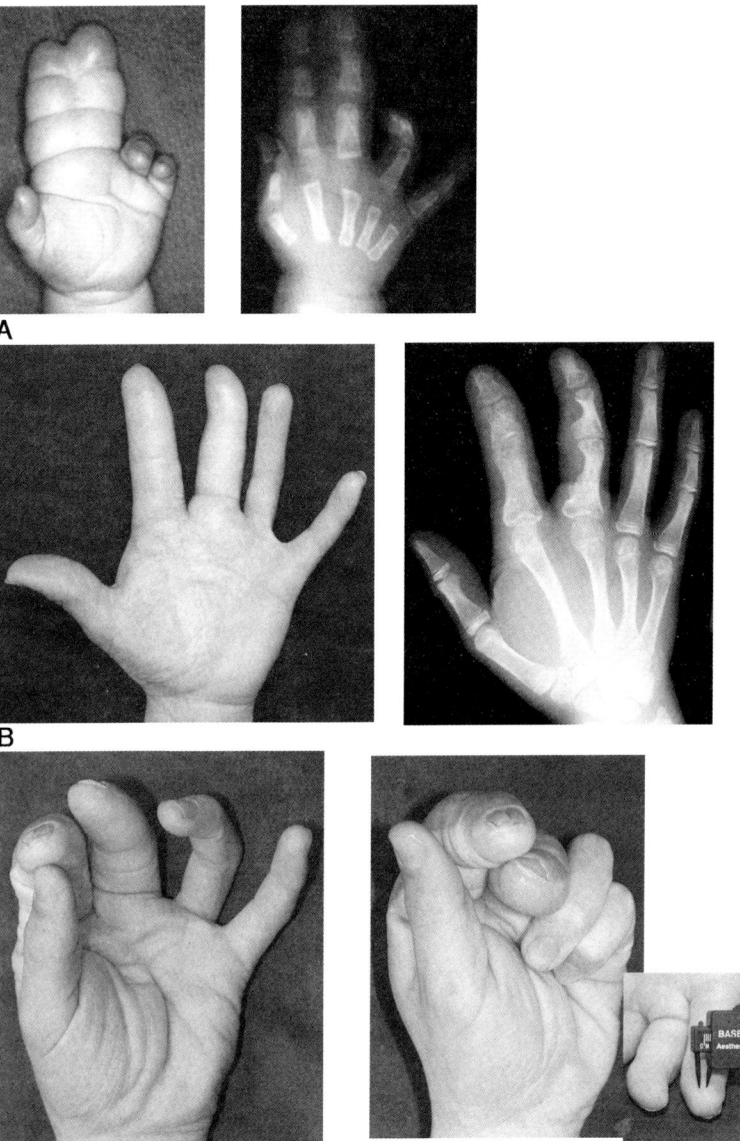

FIGURE 207-34. Lipomatous-type macrodactyly. *A,* The clinical appearance and radiograph of a young infant born with a lipomatous macrodactyly with associated syndactyly involving the index and long rays of the left hand. Within the first 6 months of life, the complete syndactyly was released, and the digits were debulked in separate procedures. *B,* At appropriate times, the growth plates of the phalanges were closed. The child and parents have been adamant in their desire to save these two digits. At the age of 14 years, these two digits are still enlarged, and radiographs show evidence of continued overgrowth. *C,* At 19 years of age, this patient has motion at the MP and PIP joints that has been preserved despite the soft tissue enlargement. Two-point discrimination of these digits approaches normal. These have been functional digits since the time of the original staged debulking procedures.

enlargement and curvature are similar to those seen in macrodactylies associated with nerve-oriented lipofibromatosis, except that osteochondral masses may be present around the epiphyses of phalanges and metacarpals,[234] which cause mechanical obstacles to joint motion and flexor tendon function. When large cartilaginous masses arise within the volar plate, digital flexion can be completely blocked and nerves, arteries, and flexor tendons significantly displaced.[259] Although Dell[234] includes gigantism in the neurofibromatosis group, it probably represents a completely different process and may fall into the hyperostosis group. The affected nerve may have the same size and tortuosity as those described.

On histologic evaluation, the same amount of epineural and perineural fibrosis and tortuosity is present, but there is no marked fatty infiltration of the involved nerves.[260,261] The presence of intracellular cytoplasmic granules and melanocytes staining positive to special dopamine stains suggests a primary disease of neural crest origin. Edgerton and Tuerk[247] have noted strong clinical similarities between the gigantism seen in lipofibromatosis and that seen in neurofibromatosis. Further, they believe that these two conditions may be part of the same disease process, neurofibromatosis. Fat infiltration is not predominant, as one sees an unorganized proliferation of epineurium, perineurium, and endoneurium.[260]

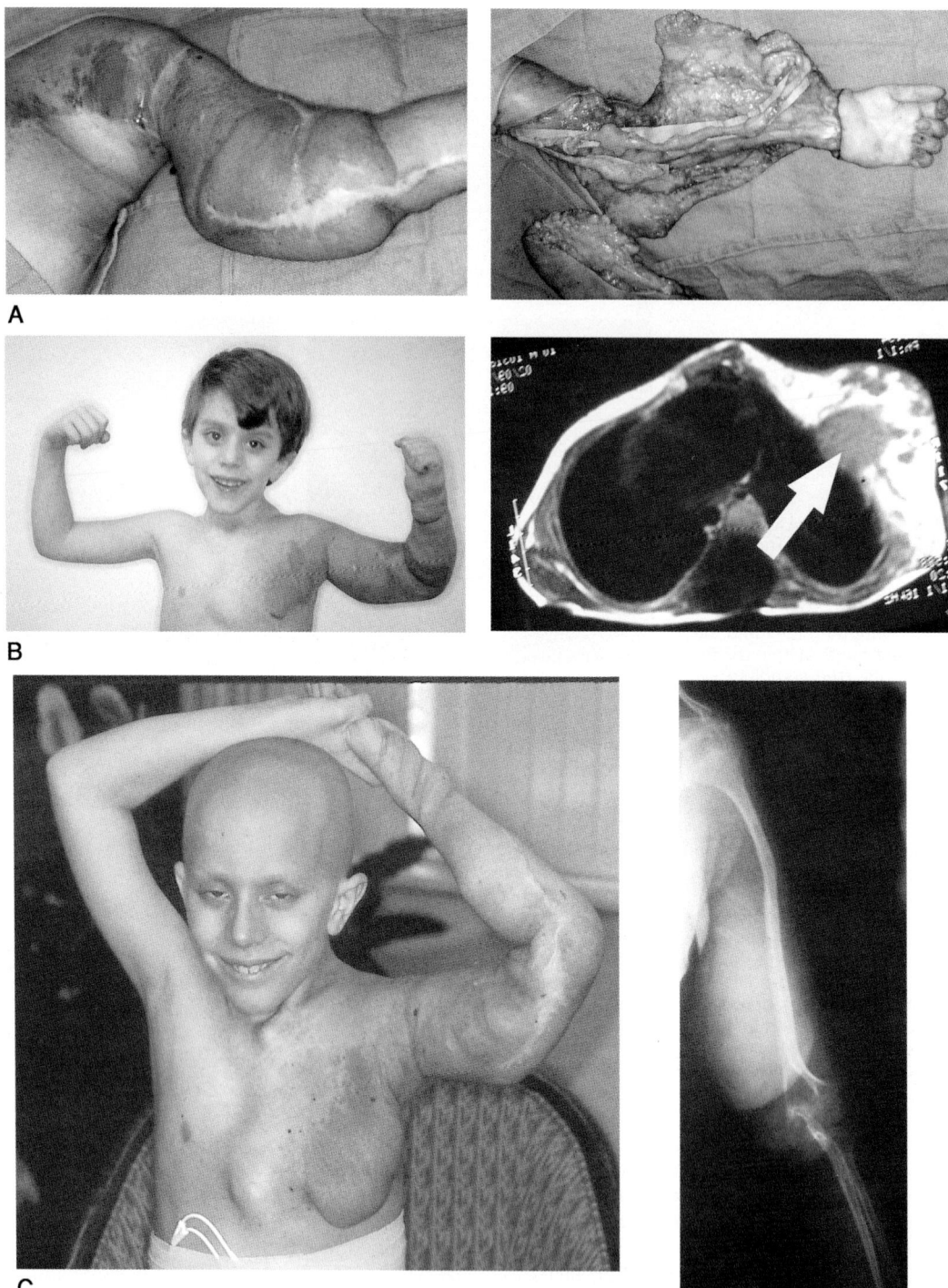

FIGURE 207-35. Neurofibromatosis and malignant degeneration. *A,* This 6-year-old child with a diagnosis of neurofibromatosis presented with an enlarging mass of the left upper extremity despite previous debulking procedures. Another aggressive soft tissue debulking was performed with isolation of the enlarged median nerve and medial antebrachial cutaneous nerve of the forearm (under the background). After this procedure, he retained excellent elbow, wrist, and hand function with two-point discrimination of 5.0 mm in the median nerve distributions. *B,* He functioned well for an additional 2 years, at which time he presented with a pain in the left upper chest region with radiation into the forearm and hand. *C,* Incisional biopsy confirmed the diagnosis of neurofibrosarcoma, and this young patient, always smiling, is seen with his portacath in place and well into chemotherapy. The radiograph of his left arm shows a significant amount of osteopenia and narrowing consistent with disuse atrophy. Unfortunately, he expired of his malignant disease several months later.

Associated features of neurofibromatosis make this entity easier to diagnose and categorize. Bone involvement may result in scoliosis, kyphoscoliosis, and pseudarthrosis of the tibia; seizures disorders; mental retardation; and nerve-related tumors, such as astrocytomas, gliomas, and pheochromocytomas. Bone may show either overgrowth or undergrowth patterns, as growth disturbances are common.[262] Peripheral nerve tumors are plentiful and are usually interpreted by pathologists as "plexiform neurofibromas."[260] These neurofibromas arise from both connective tissue and Schwann cells because both collagen and reticulin are seen with special stains. Multiple nodular thickenings may be seen along the course of an involved nerve.

Similar to the other types of overgrowth previously discussed, this type usually follows a nerve territory–oriented pattern. Simple resection of the involved nerves has been reported to limit the rapid rate of growth.[123,243,263] However, malignant transformation into neurofibrosarcoma does occur in the peripheral nerve system, whereas transformation of glial and astrocyte cells is common in the central nervous system (see Fig. 207-35).

Hyperostosis

This unusual type of gigantism is associated with local overgrowth of skeletal structures and symmetric enlargement of digits or the hand without gross hypertrophy of nerves. The lesions are present at or shortly after birth and enlarge progressively. The most remarkable findings are large osteochondral and osseous masses or growths adjacent to epiphyses and to the palmar plates of phalanges and metacarpals. Histologic analysis shows hypertrophic cartilage in normal-appearing bone. Ironically, these lesions have often been mislabeled as enchondromatoses,[259,264,265] hyperostotic lesions,[87] and multiple hereditary exostoses (Fig. 207-36). The last term is particularly confusing because there is little evidence to suggest that the lesions have a positive inheritance or represent true exostosis, although they are multiple. Further definition must await molecular analysis. My suspicion is that

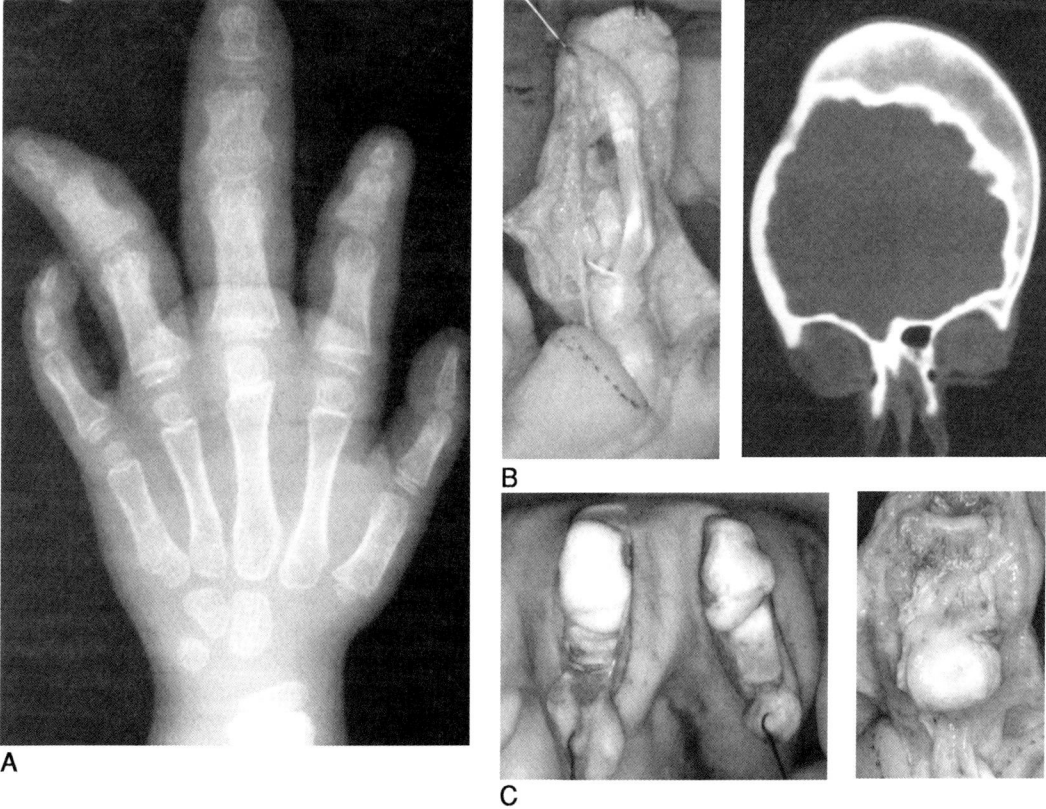

FIGURE 207-36. Overgrowth and hyperostosis. *A,* A radiograph of the right hand of a child with a diagnosis of hyperostosis demonstrates a premature appearance of all secondary ossification centers. There has been increased longitudinal and transverse overgrowth of the phalanges to the index, long, and ring digits and of the index and long metacarpals. *B,* Soft tissue structures such as tendons, retinacular sheath, and pulp tissues are also enlarged. Hyperostosis of the cranium is well demonstrated on this coronal view of the skull. *C,* Disarticulated MP and PIP joints show the cartilaginous hypertrophy of the metacarpal heads and the condyle of the proximal phalanx.

many of these hands may be closely related genetically to those with the Proteus label.

Gross enlargement of metacarpal heads and phalanges may occur without any obvious internal tumor, such as an enchondroma. Bilateral and asymmetric involvement is common, and associated problems in other musculoskeletal structures are present. Although there are no cutaneous manifestations of neurofibromatoses, linear nevi and plantar fibromatoses and hemihypertrophy have been noted in some patients with this unusual entity. Digital configuration may be bizarre and unpredictable, in contrast to that seen in the first two types of macrodactyly discussed. The median nerve distribution and the radial three digits and thumb are most commonly involved. Whole hands and digits may become grotesquely enlarged and small joint motion all but obliterated by the slowly expanding osteochondral masses, particularly within palmar plates at the MP and IP joints. The most striking clinical symptom is loss of joint motion due to the sheer size of the osteochondral lesions. Other symptoms are associated with the relative vascular insufficiency.

There appears to be no hereditary association in these patients. Approximately 17 patients with this syndrome have been described in the literature. The author's experience with 10 additional patients indicates that this entity is more common than has been assumed and that it has been classified in other categories. However, this is still a very rare hand disorder. The cause is unknown. On histologic examination, nerves are enlarged with all other structures in the involved digit or hand but do not contain fat infiltration, connective tissue, or Schwann cell proliferation.[57]

Hemihypertrophy

This category of macrodactyly is rare, difficult to describe, and impossible to find properly categorized in the hand literature. Affected patients usually present soon after birth with an enlargement of one extremity, and it is noted that half of the body is enlarged as well. In extreme cases, the hand is large and flexed at the wrist with severe ulnar deviation of the digits. They do not have vascular malformations, and the gigantism is not necessarily limited to a digit, hand, or single extremity, although certain areas may be more affected than others.

The palm and hand are less massive than in the types discussed previously, and there is commensurate enlargement of digits, which do not have the potential of reaching the grotesque proportions seen in other types of gigantism (Fig. 207-37). Early adduction thumb contractures and ulnar deviation of the digits may or may not be present during infancy. Cause is unknown. Involvement is unilateral. There is no known inheritance pattern. The association of hemihypertrophy with renal, adrenal, and brain tumors is well known.[266,267] Abdominal ultrasound examinations are commonly ordered by pediatricians to rule out these tumors.

At birth, all joints are supple, but severe flexion contractures and ulnar deviation of digits may occur during adolescence. Early surgery is performed to release individual contractures, and during surgery, it is common to find multiple abnormal atavistic intrinsic muscles and abnormal origins and insertions of both intrinsic and extrinsic muscles, which contribute to the contractures.[51,268-270] Wrist flexion contractures are associated with extra extrinsic superficial flexor muscle-tendon units that do not have normal passive stretch and become tighter with growth. Massive hypertrophy of thenar and hypothenar muscles is common, more often causing cosmetic concerns than functional problems. Forearms and upper arms may be massive in circumference. Patients' symptoms relate to the progressive adduction contractures of the thumb, flexion contractures at the MP joint, and ulnar deviation of digits. Vascular insufficiency is not seen. Function of these hands varies considerably but never approaches normal.

Proteus Syndrome

Wiedemann[271] described a new syndrome with a bizarre collection of soft tissue and skeletal malformations and variable phenotypes. He coined the term *Proteus syndrome,* named after the Greek god who was gifted with the power of prophecy and the ability to change his form at will. No two patients will present with the same morphologic features, but most will have overgrowth of the hands or feet, subcutaneous masses, linear nevi, long bone and skull overgrowth or protuberances, and a variety of visceral malformations.[272-275] The most definitive analysis of these cases has been performed by Biesecker[276,277] at the National Institutes of Health and by Cohen in Nova Scotia.

Specific to the hand surgeon are the asymmetric overgrowth seen in the digits and thumb, the cartilaginous masses that originate within or adjacent to the volar plates of the IP joints, and the often cerebriform, hyperkeratotic appearance of the glabrous skin of the soles or palms (Fig. 207-38).[275,278,279] Severe overgrowth and flexion contractures are the major deterrents to function, and the cerebriform hypertrophy of the glabrous skin on the palmar surfaces almost precludes functional use of these hands. Local maceration, infection, and drainage create almost parasitic hands. Within the overgrowth region, affected nerves, arteries, tendons, and skeletal structures may be much larger than normal. Lipomatous infiltration of neural structures is not present, but larger amounts of fat are present.

I do not agree with some authors[112,269,280,281] that the windblown hand posture is a variant of the Proteus syndrome. These hands are seen in patients with what

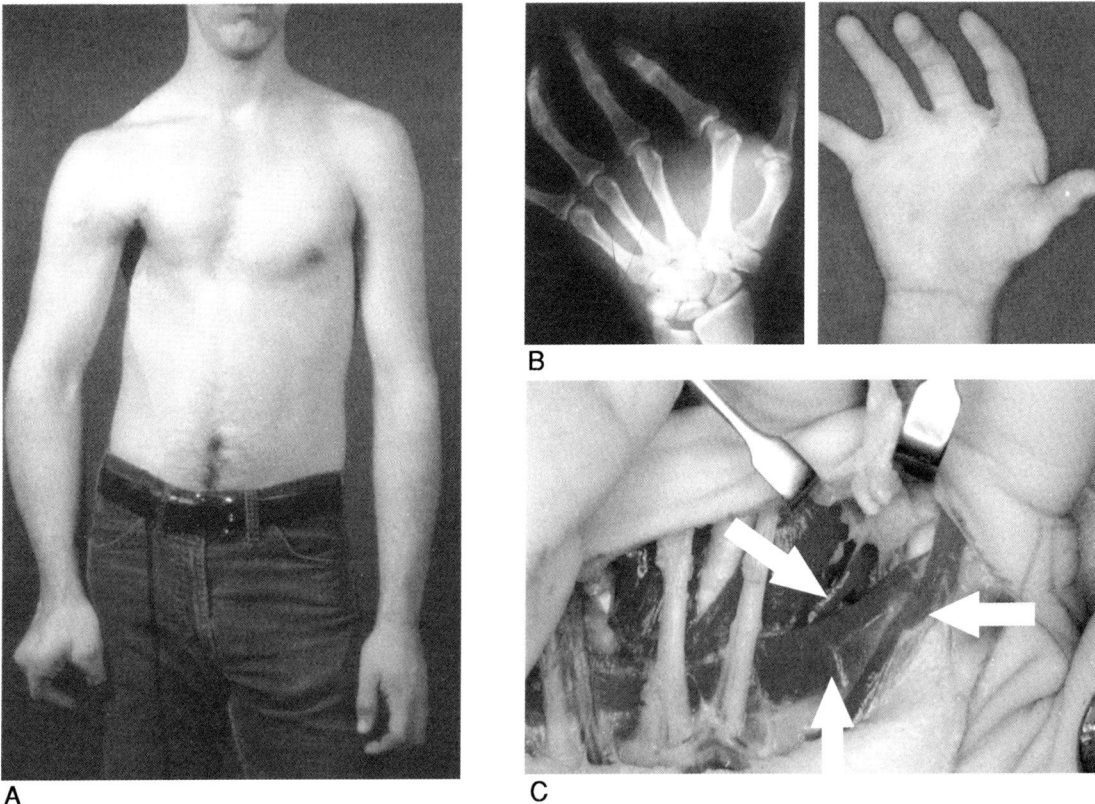

FIGURE 207-37. Hemihypertrophy. *A,* The soft tissue enlargement is much more striking in this teenaged boy with a diagnosis of hemihypertrophy, which was recognized early in childhood but became obvious during the adolescent growth spurt. A previous skin and muscle biopsy in the anterior deltoid region revealed normal skin and muscle. Elbow and wrist ranges of motion are compromised. *B,* By 7 years of age, a progressive widening of the right palm and progressive ulnar drift of all digits had developed. With time, the MP joints developed fixed flexion contractures as the intrinsic muscles tightened. *C,* Multiple abnormal atavistic intrinsic muscles coursing to the index muscle are seen. Distal attachments to the extensor mechanism and ulnar side of the proximal phalanx and flexor sheath have caused a flexion contracture. The soft tissue bulk of these redundant muscles within the intermetacarpal region has accentuated the broadening of the palm and exacerbated the ulnar drift of the index digit.

we presently call hemihypertrophy and various forms of vascular anomalies.[57,282] In fact, many of the examples of those conditions cited in textbooks of hand surgery[37,278] now appear to be hands with lipomatous-related overgrowth. As these children grow through adolescence and early adulthood, it will become important to screen for visceral malignant neoplasms. Carpal tunnel and other nerve compressions are often seen.[276,283,284]

Vascular Malformations

The Mulliken classification of vascular anomalies has been well accepted during the past 15 years.[285-287] This is explained in more detail in Chapter 106. Within this system, the malformations are identified by the endothelial cell type (C, capillary; V, venous; L, lymphatic; A, arterial) and also designated slow-flow or fast-flow lesions, the latter of which contain arteriovenous fistulas.

Syndromic. The hand and upper limb literature contains a number of confusing terms, including Klippel, Trénaunay, Parkes, and Weber, all of which we can now separate with some clinical relevance. The Klippel-Trénaunay syndrome represents a slow-flow capillary-lymphatic-venous malformation (CLVM). These lesions are more frequently seen in the lower extremity and may not have skeletal hypertrophy. When they are seen in the upper limb, the entire extremity is involved, and the windblown posture of the hand is often seen (Fig. 207-39). The Parkes Weber syndrome, in contrast, is a fast-flow capillary-arteriovenous malformation (CAVM) with arteriovenous fistula lesions. These lesions are much more commonly seen in the lower extremity; when they are present in the upper limb and hand, they are not always accompanied by skeletal overgrowth (Fig. 207-40). The Maffucci syndrome consists of multiple skeletal enchondromas and a specific type of venous malfor-

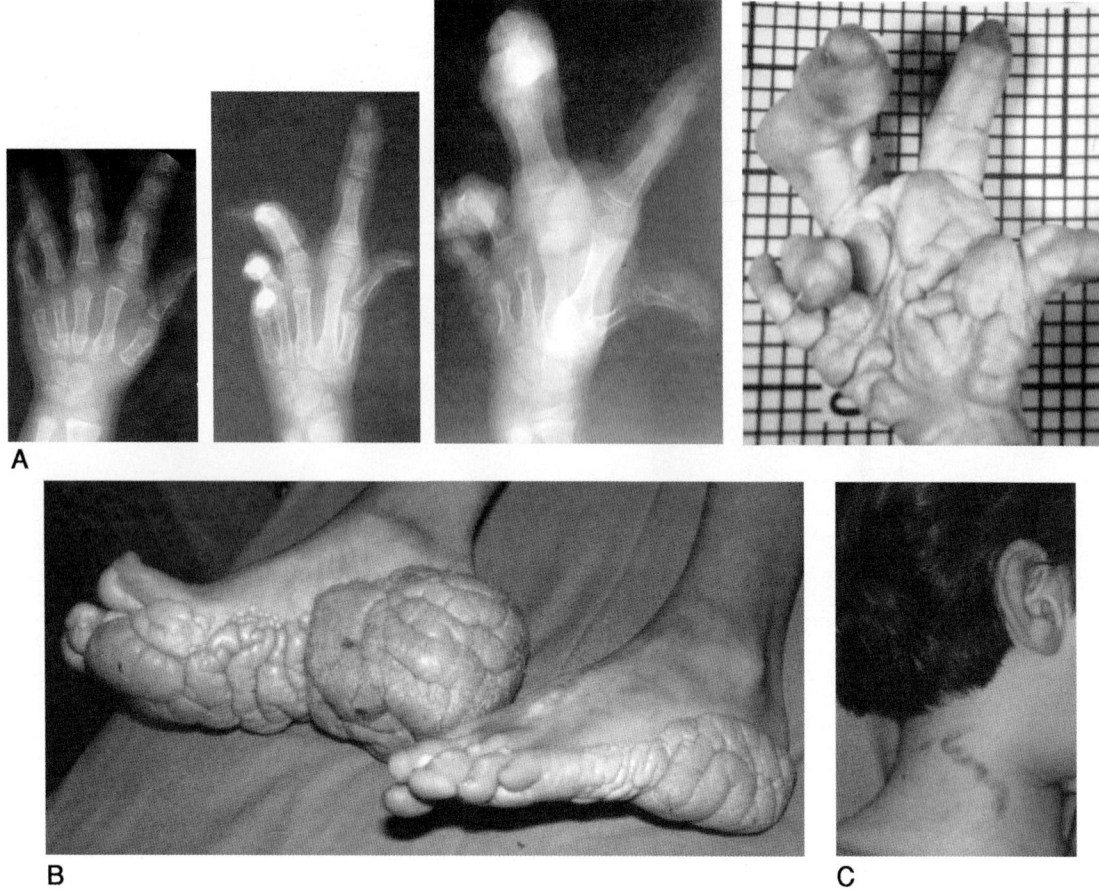

FIGURE 207-38. Proteus syndrome. *A,* Serial radiographs of the right hand between the ages of 4 and 17 years show a progressive, uncontrolled overgrowth of the central three rays in a child with the Proteus syndrome. The specialized glabrous skin of the palm may hypertrophy to form dense, immobile cerebriform mounds susceptible to maceration and infection. Both longitudinal and circular bone overgrowth results in flexion contractures (long and ring digits) and extension contractures (thumb) with or without rotational components. Cartilaginous overgrowth masses are also seen involving the volar plates of one or more joints. *B,* The same involvement of the glabrous skin of the foot can be disabling. *C,* In addition to the many musculoskeletal malformations and internal visceral problems, linear nevi of the skin are common and should alert one to this esoteric diagnosis. (Case demonstrated in *A* courtesy of M. Michael Cohen, MD.)

mation. These slow-flow lesions contain venous malformations (VMs) that occur in well-defined painful clusters in contrast to the more common diffuse venous lesions.

NONSYNDROMIC. Skeletal overgrowth is seen most commonly with isolated slow-flow lesions: VMs, lymphatic malformations (LMs), and combined lymphatic-venous malformations (LVMs). Osseous hypertrophy with fast-flow lesions does not occur as frequently as it does with the fast-flow lesions, as was commonly perceived. The mechanism of skeletal overgrowth is not well understood.[287,288] In fact, skeletal hypoplasia has been seen in the author's clinic with VMs and occasional LMs. It is not uncommon for a massive VM or CLVM limb and hand to demonstrate

undergrowth as these children grow into adulthood. As the soft tissue mass increases with progressive dilatation of the anomalous vessels, the axial skeleton shows signs of disuse (Fig. 207-41).

TREATMENT

General Principles

As a general rule in these cases, individualization of treatment is more important than in any other area of congenital limb surgery. The patient's age, digit involved, type of gigantism, progression, and rehabilitation potential must all be considered both individually and collectively. The major objectives should be to reduce length and circumferential bulk, to maintain sensation and circulation, and to preserve as much

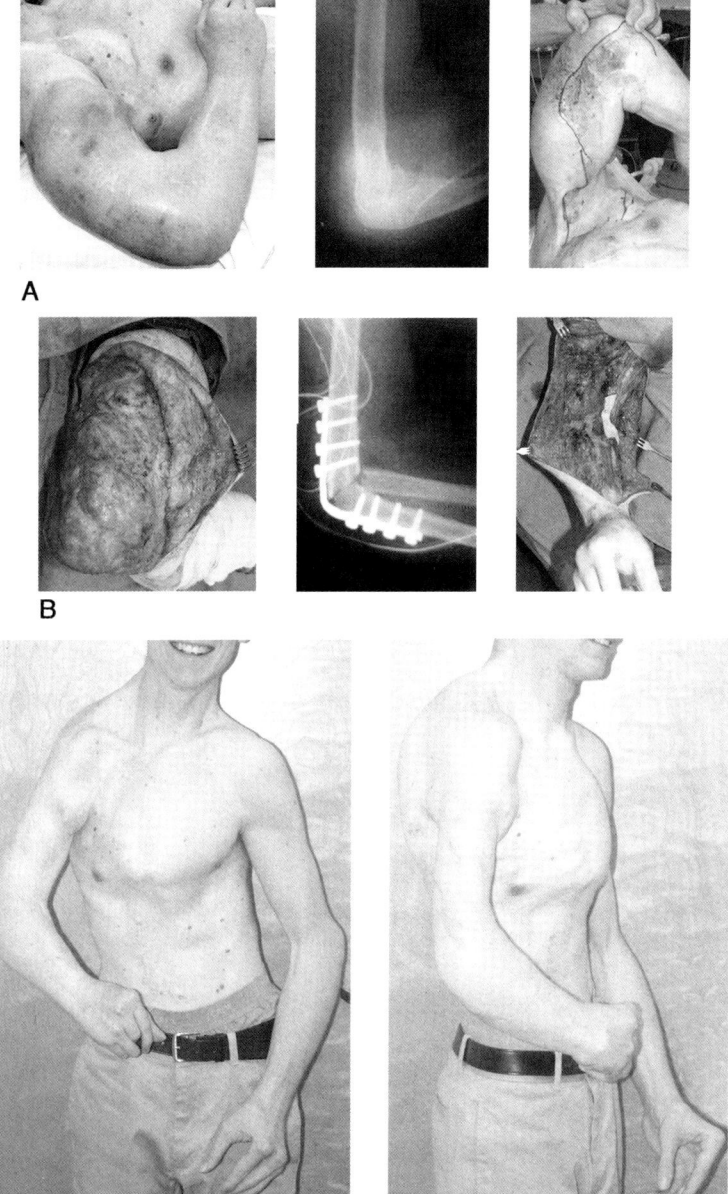

FIGURE 207-39. Klippel-Trénaunay malformation. *A,* This teenager with a combined capillary-lymphatic-venous malformation has the same lesion described by Klippel and Trénaunay. Multiple previous debulking procedures and a free tissue transfer had been performed to eliminate the chronically ulcerating skin. Although he still had problem ulcers on the median arm, excessive elbow flexion most severely restricted the function of this upper extremity. *B,* Multiple staged debulking and flap advancement of both the arm and forearm successively eliminated the problem skin lesions and improved the appearance of the limb. Repositioning of the elbow in more extension greatly enhanced function. *C,* Five years later, his primary problem was the progressive chest deformity and scoliosis, which have severely restricted his pulmonary function.

motion as possible. The patient should be observed carefully during infancy and early childhood, and a disproportionately large digit should *not* be allowed to go untreated through school ages. Digits with progressive types of gigantism are of primary concern.

Psychological Concerns

In addition to the obvious functional limitations of these various types of gigantism, the psychological effect on a small child and an entire family can be devastating.[247] There are no predictable ways to inhibit local growth, and surgery tends to be repetitive and

ablative. Multiple procedures are often done during a single operation, which can leave the patient and his or her family exhausted and discouraged. It is often important to make sure that the patients and family attend to the pressures and address ensuing psychological issues with a qualified therapist.

Nerve Decompression

Carpal tunnel release will relieve symptoms, but debulking of an enlarged nerve may result in a sensory deficit (see Figs. 207-30, 207-32, and 207-34). Despite the grotesque size of the nerves in the first two types

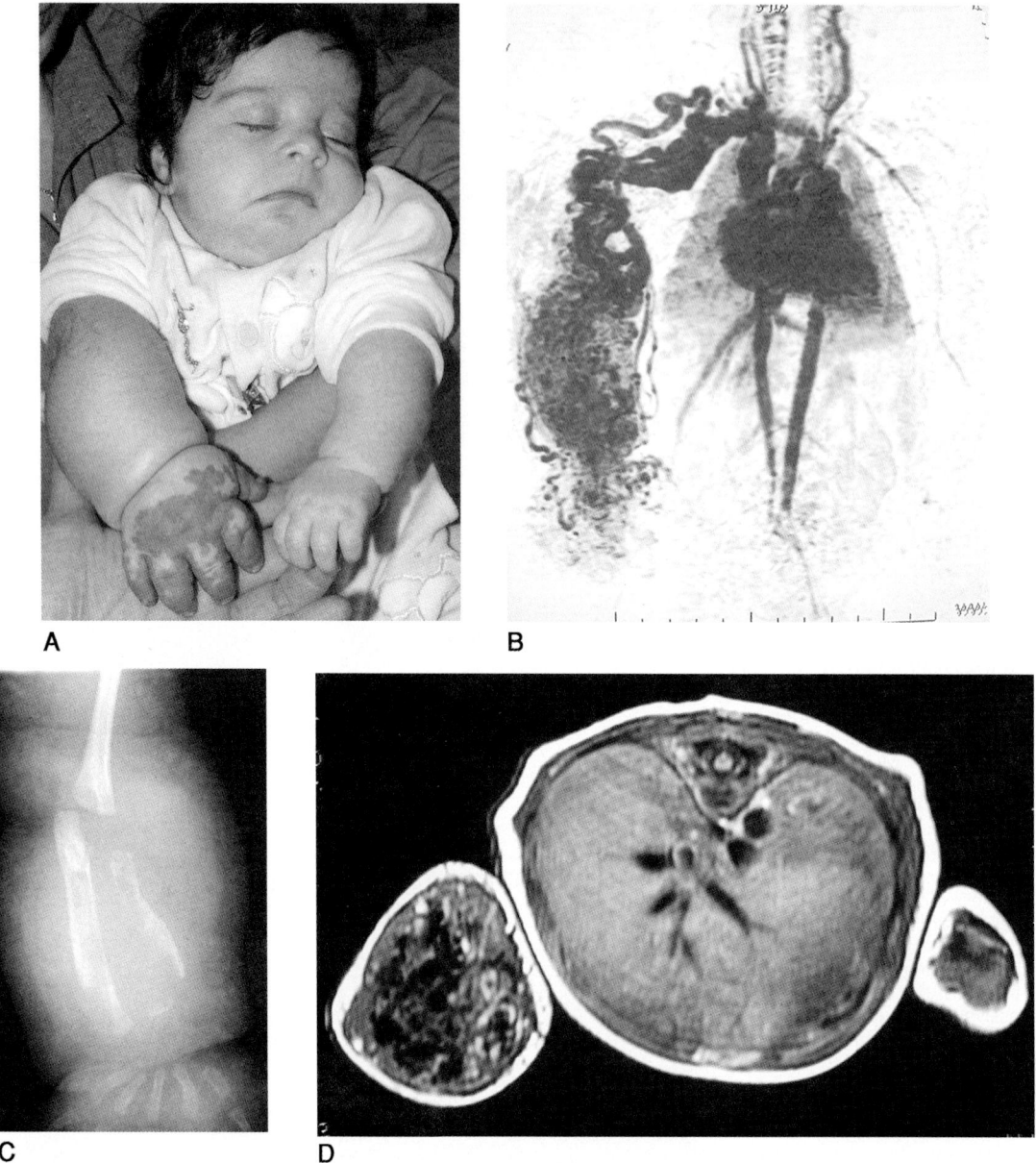

FIGURE 207-40. Parkes Weber malformation. The Parkes Weber malformation is a synonym for high-flow malformations with capillary stains: CAVMs with arteriovenous fistulas. They are most commonly seen in the lower extremity but do exist in the upper limb. *A,* This child was born with congestive heart failure and an enlarged, pulsating upper extremity. The capillary stain or malformation is seen in the digits and thumb. *B,* The myriad fistulas and enlarged vessels are spread diffusely throughout the upper limb. The subclavian and brachial arteries are four to five times normal size, and this limb consumes an inordinate amount of the cardiac output. *C,* Osteolysis is common. *D,* Coronal cuts on magnetic resonance imaging show the large flow voids involving both the flexor and extensor muscle groups. The uninvolved left arm is seen on the right side of the image. This particular child responded dramatically to prednisone therapy, and the lesion rapidly involuted during the next 2 years. She is no longer in congestive heart failure and has functional use of this extremity. The involution process indicates that this lesion should be diagnosed as a high-flow congenital hemangioma and not a malformation.

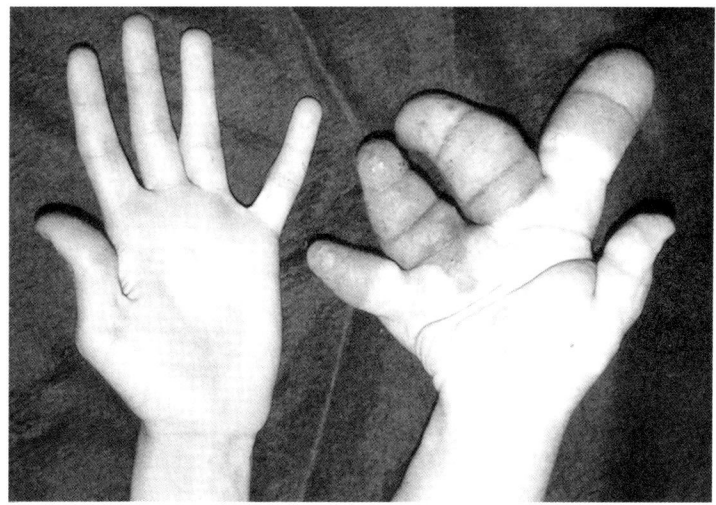

FIGURE 207-41. Venous malformation (VM) and overgrowth. *A,* Twenty years ago, this boy with multiple VMs was evaluated and treated in the author's clinic. Debulking of the large, diffuse lesion involving his right upper extremity was not performed because other VMs involving his feet and intra-abdominal region merited greater priority. At the age of 10 years, skeletal overgrowth of the index and, to a lesser extent, long digits is developing. *B,* The same hand with radiograph is seen at 32 years of age. The hand is clumsy and heavy and not even used as a helping hand. Disuse skeletal atrophy is marked in the ring and small rays. Regions of osteolysis demarcate intraosseous VM, and calcified phleboliths within the first web space are characteristic of VMs. Note the resorption of the distal radius and collapse of the wrist, which accounted for his primary complaint, wrist pain.

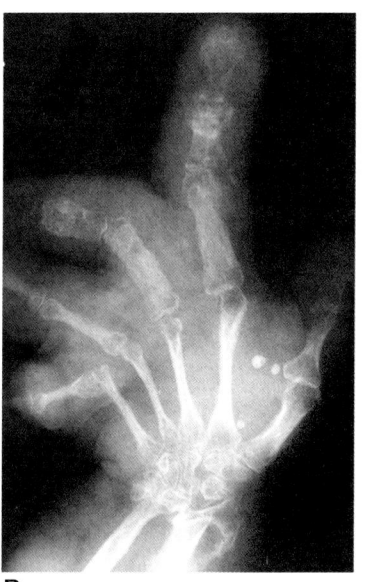
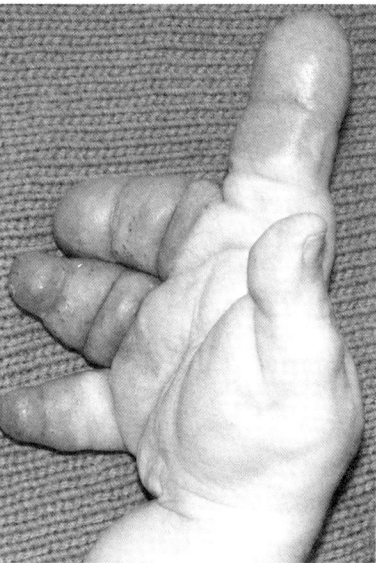

described, sensation is normal before treatment. The ulnar nerve at the elbow and median nerve within the forearm are rarely involved.

Epiphysiodesis

Epiphyseal arrest will control longitudinal growth if all growth centers are completely destroyed with a burr or osteotome. Frykman and Wood[289] emphasized that total excision of the epiphysis is an easier alternative and pointed out that this does not control circumferential growth or width, which can be reduced by a variety of maneuvers, all resulting in joint stiffness.

Soft Tissue Debulking

Staged debulking procedures at 3-month intervals have been recommended. They are effective but run the risk

of injury to neurovascular structures. Incisions made in the high mid to lateral line of the finger grow better and produce less scar hypertrophy and contractures than do palmar zigzag approaches. One side of the digit or hand should be treated at a time.

All neurovascular structures are isolated with use of the operating microscope, preserving, for example, vincular vessels at joint spaces and dorsal sensory nerves in the proximal portions of each involved digit (Fig. 207-42; see also Figs. 207-31 and 207-32). Patients with hyperostotic lesions, the Proteus syndrome, neurofibromatosis, and lymphatic malformations often form hypertrophic scars in incisions made in glabrous palmar surfaces. The digital nerves in these hands are often normal but displaced by the enlarged soft tissue and skeletal structures. Excess bone is usually

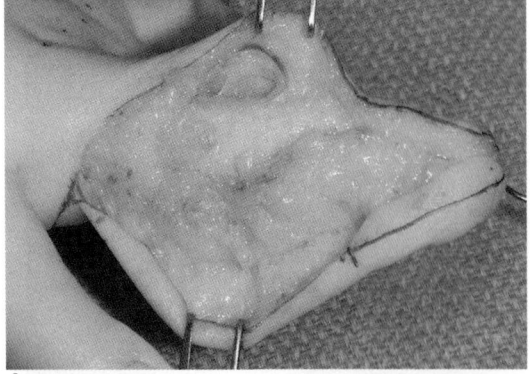

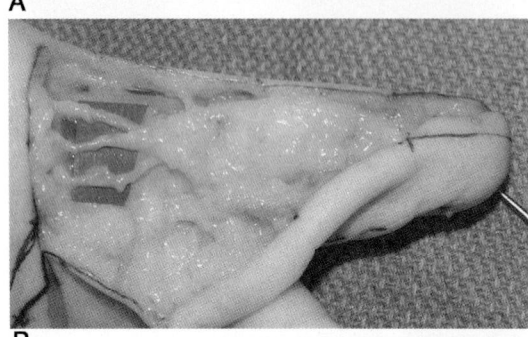

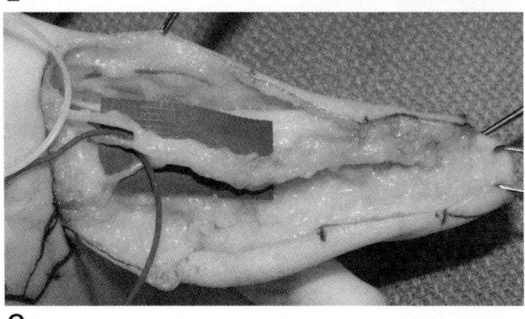

FIGURE 207-42. Nerve debulking—neurolysis. *A,* A high midaxial incision has been made along the side of a digit in a child with lipomatous overgrowth. Dorsal veins have been preserved as the adipose tissue is teased off the extensor mechanism. It will sometimes extend between the extensor mechanism and bone. Tissue on the palmar flap is dissected at the subdermal level. *B,* The digital artery, nerve, and dorsal sensory branch of the nerve are carefully identified. *C,* These neurovascular structures are kept together and not skeletonized as the bundle is dissected to the level of the distal phalanx. Vincular vessels at the joint space level are kept intact, if possible.

removed at the same time as soft tissue is debulked, particularly in the distal half of the digit or thumb.

Nerve Excision or Neurolysis

Tsuge and Ikuta[243] have recommended stripping the digital nerves and attempting to preserve the main nerve trunk to avoid major sensory deficits in the nerve-oriented and neurofibromatosis-related types of gigantism. Salon et al[290] reported the preservation of good sensation with neurolysis only. Kelikian[87] has recommended excision of the large tortuous segment of nerve, resection of redundancies, and end-to-end repair. Others have resected these nerves at very early ages, hoping to decrease the trophic influence on growth.[123,291] Nerve resection early in life will not predictably prevent overgrowth.[57,292] Clearly, these are difficult problems with no clear-cut solutions.

Skeletal Reduction

In the grotesquely enlarged digit, shortening or complete ablation may be the most practical treatment. The simplest method involves ablation of the distal phalangeal segment and debulking of the remainder of the digit. Others have retained a portion of this segment, making a dog-ear to be excised in a second stage.[237,243,293] Barsky[237] leaves the excess tissue on the palmar skin bridge, and Tsuge and Ikuta[243] prefer to leave it on the dorsal surface. There is a potential for nail deformities.

For correction of lateral deviation, closing wedge osteotomies through the metaphyses of the involved phalanges are effective, especially in the slowly progressing types of gigantism. If the phalanx has reached adult size, careful obliteration of the entire growth plate is necessary to control longitudinal growth. Arthrodeses of the proximal and middle phalanges are frequently done at the same time. Restoration of motion to stiff joints after multiple previous operations is impractical because of adherence of flexor and extensor tendons. Partial digital amputation or ray resection must always be considered in severe enlargement for grotesque deformities, after multiple failed previous operations, and in cases of an insensate digit (see Figs. 207-31 and 207-33).[233,294]

The enlarged thumb has evoked innovative alternative approaches. Millesi[184] has advocated a central en bloc resection of the distal phalangeal segment combined with an oblique skeletal shortening of the proximal phalangeal segment (Fig. 207-43). This principle can be applied further to central soft tissue and bone reduction in the grotesquely enlarged digit, where amputation with ray resection is the only other practical treatment. In all the radical resection procedures mentioned, skin and flap necrosis is the primary complication, coupled with loss of sensation. Some have even recommended removal of all marginal skin and replacement of the defatted tissue as a full-thickness skin graft so that it will survive as a graft rather than fail as a flap.[247] This tissue is not normal.

In the neurofibromatosis and hyperostotic forms, surgical resection of the large osteochondral masses should be performed before significant joint restriction has occurred. The palmar plate usually must be removed, and IP joint motion is often reduced after these resections. Early gains in motion after resection

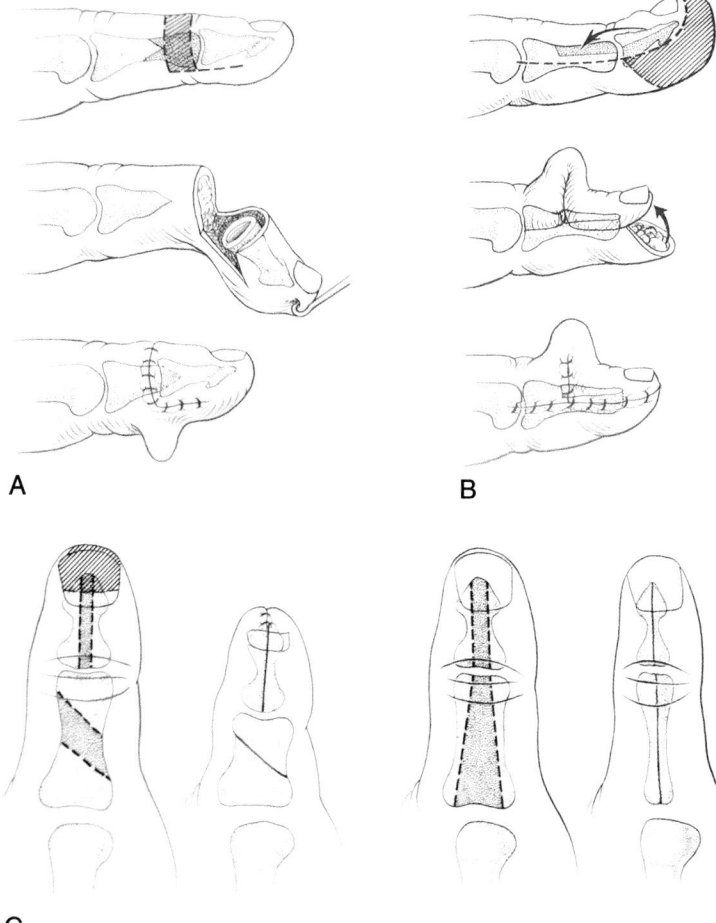

FIGURE 207-43. Skeletal and soft tissue debulking. In addition to staged soft tissue debulking along the side of involved digits and thumb, three excellent strategies for aggressive soft tissue and bone reduction depend on the relative amount of extra soft tissue. *A,* With satisfactory nail and distal soft tissue, a primary arthrodesis and bone resection at the middle phalangeal level leave a palmar soft tissue redundancy (dog-ear), which is corrected secondarily. *B,* With a gross excess of soft tissue and bone at the distal level, the entire nail complex is raised as a proximally based flap, including the dorsal cortex of the distal phalanx, and relocated over the middle phalanx. A fish-mouth closure leaves a dorsal redundancy, which is corrected secondarily. *C,* Midline skeletal reductions by either oblique or longitudinal ostectomies are effective for the enlarged thumb. IP joint motion is lost, and the split nail matrix often results in a longitudinal nail ridge (see Fig. 207-34*C*). These techniques are more useful in digits and thumbs of patients with Proteus syndrome or hyperostosis, in whom the skeletal overgrowth is much greater than soft tissue (see Fig. 207-36). (Illustration by J. K. Biddl.)

are often lost as the child grows. In adolescents and adults, arthrodesis is more practical. MP joint implant arthroplasty should be considered for preservation of motion at this level.

Patients with hemihypertrophy are difficult to treat. As long as the hand is functional and all joints are passively mobile, no surgery is recommended. If the patient is seen as an infant or during the first year of life, passive stretching exercises and static night splints should be started. The dynamic imbalance caused by abnormal intrinsic and extrinsic muscles combined with the abnormal bulk of these structures is the primary cause of the secondary contractures. Progressive ulnar drift and flexion of the digits may require centralization of the extensor mechanism and release of abnormal intrinsic muscles on the palmar side. Severe flexion contractures combined with ulnar drift are treated in stages. First, the splayed-out metacarpals are brought toward the midline of the hand with closing wedge osteotomies; as a second stage, deforming forces are released by excision of abnor-

mal intrinsic muscles, lengthening of extrinsic flexor tendons, and centralization of the extensors at the MP joint level. Debulking of massive thenar and especially hypothenar muscle masses can be done as a third stage and is often considered for aesthetic reasons. For gigantism recognized during infancy, passive range-of-motion exercises and night splinting have been recommended. On occasion, progressive, unrelenting contractures of the MP joint and wrist require early release and subsequent splinting.

OUTCOMES

None of the illustrations in current textbooks adequately portrays this deformity as it actually exists, and case reports and large series do not show long-term postoperative results, which are never normal.[234] All described series are small, and most contain a long list of different conditions as outlined before. No treatment is entirely satisfactory.[57,295] However, a number of useful techniques have been described for the treatment of these often conspicuous hands.[87,233,234,263,283,292,294,296-298] My experience with a large number of these patients treated during the past 30 years is summarized by specific condition.

Nerve Territory–Oriented Macrodactyly and Lipomatous Macrodactyly

The nerve territory–oriented macrodactyly with or without neural infiltration and lipomatous macrodactylies have similar outcomes. When motion is deficient because of sheer bulk, it is not improved postoperatively. Those with localized digit or thumb involvement will retain excellent sensation and will retain satisfactory motion.[157,233,292,296,299] Length is controlled with appropriate epiphyseal obliteration, but the circumference is always greater than in uninvolved digits. The skeletal deviation will recur unless the entire growth plate of the involved phalanx or metacarpal is obliterated.[57] Incisions in the glabrous skin of the digit are routinely more hypertrophied than high midaxial incisions. I disagree with those who advocate the use of palmar zigzag incisions.[233,278,293,299] Amputation of grossly enlarged digits or thumb is a good option. Microvascular great-toe transfer is preferable to multistaged debulking, but motion is diminished (see Fig. 207-31).

As these children are observed, attention must be directed to additional palmar, forearm, or arm enlargement, which may progressively increase as the child grows. There is a misconception that sensation is or can be normal in these patients. With the exception of those with minimal involvement, two-point discrimination is always increased. After repeated debulking and nerve manipulation, protective sensation, at best, will result. If they are observed long enough through adolescence into adulthood, clinical and radiologic signs of a progressive osteoarthritis in the involved portions of the hand will develop in the majority of these patients. We do not know if previous debulking or contouring can alter this process but are beginning to see early arthritis in toes transferred into these regions.

Neurofibromatosis

Neurofibromatosis represents a very small group of overgrowth patients. Minimal hand and forearm deformities should not affect existing hand function. Compression neuropathies at the wrist and elbow levels respond to appropriate decompression but are often overlooked in children, who have adapted and learned to avoid cuts, abrasions, and infections.[44,238,241-243,247,249,255,274,290,291] Extensive arm, forearm, and hand lesions can be debulked for functional reasons with predictable outcomes. Malignant degeneration is a concern in these extremities and has been seen in the author's practice five times during the last 30 years (see Fig. 207-35).

Hyperostosis and Proteus Syndrome

The hand deformities in those with Proteus syndrome and congenital hyperostosis are rare and have similar outcomes. The skeletal malformations and large cartilaginous masses that involve joint spaces are the cause of diminished motion and rotational or angulation deformities. Surgery along the digits or thumb invariably results in a loss of motion, which is proportional to the extent of the deformity. Incisions involving the glabrous skin become hypertrophic, and the cerebriform fibrous overgrowth must be removed and resurfaced if the digit, thumb, or hand is to be functional. Sensation is not normal in these hands because of the thickness of the outer skin layers.

Hemihypertrophy

Because there is such a wide variation of hand findings in those with hemihypertrophy, outcome studies do not exist. Most of these hands are amazingly functional despite the deformities caused by hypertrophic and atavistic muscle groups resulting in various flexion contractures of the forearm and hand and ulnar deviation of the digits (see Fig. 207-37). Every case must be carefully individualized.[269,276,282] Surgical decisions are dictated by functional and aesthetic needs. There is no loss of function with removal of hypertrophied muscle groups in the hand and forearm. Ulnar deviation of digits is not always reversed by early or late release of tight intrinsic muscles. Wrist and digital flexion contractures secondary to tight extrinsic flexor tendons are improved only by complete tenotomies instead of tendon lengthening. These muscles are nonfunctional and have little passive excursion. Excessive ulnar deviation and widening of the hand are best corrected with metacarpal osteotomies. Normal extrinsic and intrinsic muscles of the limb should be left untouched because diminution of excursion and weakness will invariably result from surgical manipulation. Progressive joint deformities will not be corrected with hand therapy and splinting alone.

Vascular Malformations

Outcomes of those with vascular malformations are summarized elsewhere.[286,287] The role of the interventional radiologist is crucial because more than 80% of these patients are treated with sclerotherapy, selective embolization, or other specialized technique before surgical resection. In general, venous malformations, which compose the largest group, are resectable, and results are proportional to the size and location of the malformation. Nerve-related problems predominate in untoward results. Large, diffuse lesions with or without lymphatic components seen in patients with the Klippel-Trénaunay syndrome (capillary-lymphatic-venous malformations) are the most difficult to treat, and results are never normal. Localized or high-flow lesions, fortunately, are rare. Embolization followed by complete excision and revascularization, if necessary, is effective in the short run. If observed long enough (>20 years), most of these lesions recur in adjacent regions and become problematic. Lymphatic malformations respond well to surgery, and function is not as severely affected as with other malformations primarily because most of these lesions are confined to the skin and subcutaneous tissue planes. Hypertrophic scars, continued swelling, and joint stiffness plague these patients. Small, localized lesions are easily removed without any loss of function.

REFERENCES

1. Goldberg M, Bartoshesky L: Congenital hand anomaly: etiology and associated malformations. Hand Clin 1985;1:405-415.
2. Flatt AE, Wood VE: Rigid digits or symphalangism. Hand 1975;7:197-214.
3. Buck-Gramcko D: Angeborene Fehlbildungen der Hand. In Nigst H, Buck-Gramcko D, Millesi H, eds: Handchirurgie. Stuttgart, Thieme, 1988:12.1-12.115.
4. Cushing H: Hereditary anchylosis of the proximal interphalangeal joints (symphalangism). Genetics 1916;1:90-106.
5. Cushing H: Hereditary anchylosis of the proximal phalangeal joints (symphalangism). 1915. Clin Orthop 2002;401:4-5, discussion 4.
6. Strasburger A, et al: Symphalangism: genetic and clinical aspects. Bull Johns Hopkins Hosp 1965;117:108-127.
7. Elkington SG, Huntsman RG: The Talbot fingers: a study in symphalangism. Br Med J 1967;1:407-411.
8. Castle JE, Bass S, Kanat IO: Hereditary symphalangism with associated tarsal synostosis and hypophalangism. J Am Podiatr Med Assoc 1993;83:1-9.
9. Gaal SA, Doyle JR, Larsen IJ: Symphalangism in Hawaii: a study of three distinct ethnic pedigrees. J Hand Surg Am 1988;13:783-787.
10. Perme CM, Johnson SP, Weinstein AS: Case report 857: hereditary symphalangism with carpal and tarsal fusions and deafness. Skeletal Radiol 1994;23:468-470.
11. Moumoumi H, Mayelo V, Anthonioz P: Familial symphalangism syndrome transmitted through five generations. Genet Couns 1991;2:139-146.
12. Takahashi T, et al: Mutations of the NOG gene in individuals with proximal symphalangism and multiple synostosis syndrome. Clin Genet 2001;60:447-451.
13. Mangino M, et al: Identification of a novel NOG gene mutation (P35S) in an Italian family with symphalangism. Hum Mutat 2002;19:308.
14. Polymeropoulos MH, et al: Localization of the gene (SYM1) for proximal symphalangism to human chromosome 17q21-q22. Genomics 1995;27:225-229.
15. Kosaki K, et al: Premature ovarian failure in a female with proximal symphalangism and Noggin mutation. Fertil Steril 2004;81:1137-1139.
16. Kantaputra PN, et al: A Thai mother and son with distal symphalangism, hypoplastic carpal bones, microdontia, dental pulp stones, and narrowing of the zygomatic arch: a new distal symphalangism syndrome? Am J Med Genet 2002;109:56-60.
17. Morimoto J, et al: Proximal symphalangism with "coarse" facial appearance, mixed hearing loss, and chronic renal failure: new malformation syndrome? Am J Med Genet 2001;98:269-272.
18. McKusick VA: Symphalangism and deafness. Birth Defects Orig Artic Ser 1971;7:124.
19. Makowski A, Latkowski B, Bieganski T: Dominant symphalangism and conductive hearing loss [in Polish]. Otolaryngol Pol 1995;49:57-63.
20. Hurvitz SA, et al: The facio-audio-symphalangism syndrome: report of a case and review of the literature. Clin Genet 1985;28:61-68.
21. Higashi K, Inoue S: Conductive deafness, symphalangism, and facial abnormalities: the WL syndrome in a Japanese family. Am J Med Genet 1983;16:105-109.
22. Gloede JF, Stenger HH: Symphalangism, strabism, and anomaly of the middle ear [author's transl; in German]. Humangenetik 1974;22:23-32.
23. Gorlin RJ, Kietzer G, Wolfson J: Stapes fixation a proximal symphalangism. Z Kinderheilkd 1970;108:12-16.
24. Akama H, Kiyotaki M, Motojima S: Proximal symphalangism associated with conductive hearing loss. Arthritis Care Res 2000;13:333-334.
25. Krohn KD, et al: Hereditary symphalangism. Association with osteoarthritis. J Rheumatol 1989;16:977-982.
26. Herrmann J: Symphalangism and brachydactyly syndrome: report of the WL symphalangism-brachydactyly syndrome: review of literature and classification. Birth Defects Orig Artic Ser 1974;10:23-53.
27. Kassner EG, Katz I, Qazi QH: Symphalangism with metacarpophalangeal fusions and elbow abnormalities. Pediatr Radiol 1976;4:103-107.
28. Siemian WR, Greider JL Jr: Symphalangism associated with constriction rings: syndactyly and brachytelophalangy in a black patient. J Hand Surg Am 1986;11:841-843.
29. Sugiura Y, Inagaki Y: Symphalangism associated with synostosis of carpus and/or tarsus. Jinrui Idengaku Zasshi 1981;26:31-45.
30. Walbaum R, Hazard C, Cordier R: Brachydactylia with symphalangism, probably autosomal recessive. Hum Genet 1976;33:189-192.
31. Zavala C, Hernandez-Ortiz J, Lisker R: Brachydactyly type B and symphalangism in different members of a Mexican family. Ann Genet 1975;18:131-134.
32. Poush JR: Distal symphalangism: a report of two families. J Hered 1991;82:233-238.
33. Flatt A: The Care of Congenital Hand Anomalies. St. Louis, CV Mosby, 1977:170-212.
34. Palmieri TJ: The use of silicone rubber implant arthroplasty in treatment of true symphalangism. J Hand Surg Am 1980;5:242-244.
35. Dobyns J: Synostosis. In Green DP, ed: Operative Hand Surgery. New York, Churchill Livingstone, 1993:321-326.
36. Upton J, Sohn S, Glowacki J: Neocartilage derived from transplanted perichondrium: what is it? Plast Reconstr Surg 1981;68:166-172.
37. Smith P: Congenital. In Smith P, ed: Lister's The Hand: Diagnosis and Indications. London, Churchill Livingstone, 2002:457-522.
38. Marumo E, et al: Surgery of symphalangism [in Japanese]. Shujutsu 1970;24:1002-1006.
39. Buckwalter J, et al: The absent fifth metacarpal. J Hand Surg 1981;6:364-367.
40. Buck-Gramcko D, Wood VE: The treatment of metacarpal synostosis. J Hand Surg Am 1993;18:565-581.
41. Goodman F, Mundlos S, Muragaki Y, et al: Synpolydactyly phenotypes correlate with size of expansions in HOXD 13 polyalanine tract. Proc Natl Acad Sci USA 1997;94:7458-7463.
42. Muragaki Y, Mundlos S, Upton J, Olsen BR: Altered growth and branching patterns in synpolydactyly caused by mutations in HOXD 13. Science 1996;272:548-551.
43. Upton J: Discussion of metacarpal synostosis. Plast Reconstr Surg 2001;108:1232-1234.
44. Wood VE: Metacarpal synostosis. In Green DP, ed: Operative Hand Surgery. New York, Churchill Livingstone, 1993:326-338.

45. Dao KD, et al: Synostosis of the ring-small finger metacarpal in Apert acrosyndactyly hands: incidence and treatment. J Pediatr Orthop 2001;21:502-507.

46. Guero S, Vassia L, Renier D, Glorion C: Surgical management of the hand in Apert syndrome. Handchir Mikrochir Plast Chir 2004;36:179-185.

47. Hooper G, Lamb DW: Congenital fusion of the ring and little metacarpal bones. Hand 1983;15:207-211.

48. Hoover GH, Flatt AE, Weiss MW: The hand in Apert's syndrome. J Bone Joint Surg Am 1970;52:878-895.

49. Pensler J, Carroll NC, Cheng LF: Distraction osteogenesis in the hand. Plast Reconstr Surg 1998;102:92-95.

50. Foucher G, et al: Metacarpal synostosis: a simple classification and a new treatment technique. Plast Reconstr Surg 2001;108:1225-1231, discussion 1232-1234.

51. Wood V: Super digit. Hand Clin 1990;6:673-684.

52. Upton J: Simplicity and treatment of the typical cleft hand. Handchir Mikrochir Plast Chir 2004;36:152-160.

53. Tada K, Yonenobu K, Swanson AB: Congenital central ray deficiency in the hand—survey of 59 cases and subclassification. J Hand Surg Am 1981;6:434-441.

54. Ogino T: Cleft hand. Hand Clin 1990;6:661-671.

55. Nutt JI, Flatt AE: Congenital central hand deficit. J Hand Surg Am 1981;6:48-60.

56. Ueba Y, Seto Y: Congenital metacarpal synostosis treated by longitudinal osteotomy and placement of a silicone wedge. Handchir Mikrochir Plast Chir 1997;29:297-302.

57. Upton J: Congenital anomalies of the hand and forearm. In May JW Jr, Littler JW, eds: The Hand. Philadelphia, WB Saunders, 1990:5213-5398. McCarthy JG, ed: Plastic Surgery; vol 8.

58. Horii E, et al: Surgical treatment of congenital metacarpal synostosis of the ring and little fingers. J Hand Surg Br 1998;23:691-694.

59. Miura T: Congenital synostosis between the fourth and fifth metacarpal bones. J Hand Surg Am 1988;13:83-88.

60. Hikosaka K, Yabe Y: Treatment for fourth and fifth metacarpal synostosis with abduction deformity of the little finger. Seikeigeka 1981;32:1682-1684.

61. Yamamoto N, Endo T, Nakayama Y: Congenital synostosis of the fourth and fifth metacarpals treated by free bone grafting from the fusion site. Plast Reconstr Surg 2000;105:1747-1750.

62. Kawabata H, Yasui N, Che YH, Hirooka A: Treatment for congenital synostosis of the fourth and fifth metacarpals with the hemicallotasis technique. Plast Reconstr Surg 1997;99:2061-2065.

63. Foucher G, Medina J, Bollecker V, Lorea P: The "candlestick" technique for the correction of certain types of congenital metacarpal synostosis. Chir Main 2002;21:288-292.

64. Upton J, Clarke H: Allongement progressif des membres. In Gilbert A, Buck-Gramcko D, Lister G, eds: Les malformations congenitales du membre superieur. Paris, Expansion Scientifique Française, 1991:117-129.

65. Seitz W Jr: Distraction treatment of the hand. In Buck-Gramcko D, ed: Congenital Malformations of the Hand and Forearm. London, Churchill Livingstone, 1998:119-130.

66. Temtamy SA, McKusick V: Carpal/tarsal synostosis. Birth Defects 1978;14:503.

67. Minaar A: Congenital fusion of the lunate and triquetral bones in the South African Bantu. J Bone Joint Surg Br 1952;34:45-58.

68. Gross S, Watson HK, Strickland JW, et al: Triquetral-lunate arthritis secondary to synostosis. J Hand Surg Am 1989;14:95-102.

69. Poznanski A: The Hand in Radiologic Diagnosis with Gamuts and Pattern Profiles, 2nd ed. Philadelphia, WB Saunders, 1984:2-10.

70. Ruby L, Cooney WP, An KN, et al: Relative motion of selected carpal bones: a kinematic analysis of the normal wrist. J Hand Surg Am 1988;13:1-10.

71. Wynne-Davies R: Heritable disorders in orthopedic practice. Oxford, Blackwell Scientific, 1973.

72. Bzduch V, Spissak L: Radioulnar synostosis in Williams syndrome. J Pediatr 1989;115:165.

73. Bzduch V: Radioulnar synostosis in Williams syndrome: a historical overview. Am J Med Genet 1994;50:386.

74. Hurley ME, et al: Antley-Bixler syndrome with radioulnar synostosis. Pediatr Radiol 2004;34:148-151.

75. James C, et al: 46,XY/47,XYY/48,XYYY karyotype in a 3-year-old boy ascertained because of radioulnar synostosis. Am J Med Genet 1995;56:389-392.

76. Cleveland WW, Arias D, Smith GF: Radioulnar synostosis, behavioral disturbance, and XYY chromosomes. J Pediatr 1969;74:103-106.

77. Thapar RK, Grewal HS, Kalra K: Phocomelia with radioulnar synostosis. Report of a case with review of the literature. Indian J Pediatr 1966;33:85-87.

78. Lewis W: The development of the arm in man. Am J Anat 1901-1902;1:146.

79. Wilkie D: Congenital radio-ulnar synostosis. Br J Surg 1914;1:366-375.

80. Mital MA: Congenital radioulnar synostosis and congenital dislocation of the radial head. Orthop Clin North Am 1976;7:375-383.

81. Simmons BP, Southmayd WW, Riseborough EJ: Congenital radioulnar synostosis. J Hand Surg Am 1983;8:829-838.

82. Dawson H: A congenital deformity of the forearm and its operative treatment. Br Med J 1912;2:883.

83. Green W, Mital MA: Congenital radio-ulnar synostosis: surgical treatment. J Bone Joint Surg Am 1979;61:738-743.

84. Castello JR, Garro L, Campo M: Congenital radioulnar synostosis. Surgical correction by derotational osteotomy. Ann Chir Main Memb Super 1996;15:11-17.

85. Sachar K, Akelman E, Ehrlich MG: Radioulnar synostosis. Hand Clin 1994;10:399-404.

86. Yammine K, Salon A, Pouliquen JC: Congenital radioulnar synostosis. Study of a series of 37 children and adolescents. Chir Main 1998;17:300-308.

87. Kelikian H: Congenital Deformities of the Hand and Forearm. Philadelphia, WB Saunders, 1974:939-975.

88. Tachdjian M: Orthopedics. Philadelphia, WB Saunders, 1972.

89. Wood V: Congenital radio-ulnar synostosis. In Buck-Gramcko D, ed: Congenital Malformations of the Hand and Forearm. London, Churchill Livingstone, 1998:509-515.

90. Tajima T, Ogisho N, Kanaya F: Follow-up study of joint mobilizations of proximal radioulnar synostoses. American Society for Surgery of the Hand annual meeting, 1994.

91. Yebe Y: New operative method for congenital radio-ulnar synostosis. Seikeigeka 1971;22:900-903.

92. Jupiter JB, Ring D: Operative treatment of post-traumatic proximal radioulnar synostosis. J Bone Joint Surg Am 1998;80:248-257.

93. Kanaya F, Ibaraki K: Mobilization of a congenital proximal radioulnar synostosis with use of a free vascularized fascio-fat graft. J Bone Joint Surg Am 1998;80:1186-1192.

94. Kanaya F: New approach to congenital radio-ulnar synostosis. In Gupta A, Kay SPJ, Scheker LR, eds: The Growing Hand: Diagnosis and Management of the Upper Extremity in Children. London, Churchill Livingstone, 2000:237-241.

95. Sugimoto M, et al: Treatment of traumatic radioulnar synostosis by excision, with interposition of a posterior interosseous island forearm flap. J Hand Surg Br 1996;21:393-395.

96. Bolano L: Congenital proximal radioulnar synostosis: treatment with the Ilizarov method. J Hand Surg Am 1994;19:977-978.

97. Chevallier A, Kieny M, Mauger A: Limb-somite relationship: origin of limb musculature. J Embryol Exp Morphol 1977;41:245-258.

98. Streeter G: Developmental horizons in human embryos IV. A review of histogenesis of cartilage and bone. Contrib Embryol 1949;33:149-167.

99. Shellswell G, Wolpert L: The pattern in muscle and tendon development in the chick wing. In Ede D, Hinchcliff J, Balls M, eds: Vertebrate Limb and Somite Morphogenesis. Cambridge, Cambridge University Press, 1977.

100. Scott J, Haigh M, Neo GE, Gibson S: The effect of muscle paralysis on the radial growth of collagen fibrils in developing tendon. Clin Sci 1987;72:359-363.

101. Beckham C, Dimond R, Greenlee TK Jr: The role of movement in the development of a digital flexor tendon. Am J Anat 1977;150:443-459.

102. Chiquet M, Fambrough DM: A monoclonal antibody as a marker for tendon and muscle morphogenesis. J Cell Biol 1984;98:1926-1936.

103. Borck C: The development of the myo-tendinous junction in the upper extremity mouse embryos (days 15 p.c.-1 p.p.). Z Mikrosk Anat Forsch 1977;91:229-240.

104. Graham J, et al: Determinants in the morphogenesis of muscle tendon insertions. J Pediatr 1982;101:825-831.

105. Tamplin R: Lecture on the Nature and Treatment of Deficiencies. London, Longman, Brown, Green, Longman and Robert, 1846:256-267.

106. Weckesser E: Congenital flexion-adduction deformity of the thumb (congenital "clasped thumb"). J Bone Joint Surg Am 1955;37:977-984.

107. Dinham J, Meggitt DF: Trigger thumbs in children: a review of the natural history and indications for treatment in 105 patients. J Bone Joint Surg 1974;56:153-155.

108. Miller J: Pollex varus: a report of two cases. Univ Hosp Bull Ann Arbor 1944;10:10-11.

109. Matev I: Surgical treatment of spastic "thumb-in-palm" deformity. J Bone Joint Surg Br 1963;45:703-708.

110. Rayan G, Saccone PG: Treatment of spastic thumb-in-palm deformity: a modified extensor pollicis longus tendon rerouting. J Hand Surg Am 1996;21:834-839.

111. Broadbent T, Woolf R: Flexion-abduction deformity of the thumb—congenital clasped thumb. Plast Reconstr Surg 1964;34:612-616.

112. De Smet L, Keymolen K, Fryns JP: Unilateral longitudinal radial ray deficiency of the hand and metacarpal 4-5 synostosis. Genet Couns 1999;10:369-372.

113. Rodgers W, Waters PM: Incidence of trigger digits in newborns. J Hand Surg 1994;19:364-368.

114. Moon W, Park MJ, Ha CW: Trigger digits in children. J Hand Surg Br 2001;26:11-12.

115. Thomas S, Dodds RD: Bilateral trigger thumbs in identical twins. J Pediatr Orthop 1999;8:59-60.

116. Vyas B, Sarwahi V: Bilateral congenital trigger thumb: role of heredity. Indian J Pediatr 1999;66:949-951.

117. Van Heest A, House J, Krivit W, Walker K: Surgical treatment of carpal tunnel syndrome and trigger digits in children with mucopolysaccharide storage disorders. J Hand Surg Am 1998;23:236-243.

118. Notta A: Recherches sur une affection particuliere des gaines tendineuses de la main, caracterisee par le development d'une nodosite sur le trajet des tendons flechisseurs des doigts et par leurs movements. Arch Gen Med 1850;24:142-161.

119. Hudson H: Snapping thumb in childhood. N Engl J Med 1934;210:854-857.

120. Eyres K, McLaren MI: Trigger thumb in children: results of surgical correction. J R Coll Surg Edinb 1991;36:197.

121. Ger E, Kupcha P, Ger D: The management of trigger thumb in children. J Hand Surg Am 1991;16:944-947.

122. Fahey J, Bollinger JA: Trigger finger in adults and children. J Bone Joint Surg 1954;36:1200-1218.

123. McCarroll H: Clinical manifestations of congenital neurofibromatosis. J Bone Joint Surg Am 1950;32:601-617.

124. Kay S, Lees VP: Anomalies of tendons. In Gupta A, Kay SPJ, Scheker LR, eds: The Growing Hand: Diagnosis and Management of the Upper Extremity in Children. London, Churchill Livingstone, 2000:319-322.

125. Claisse RH: A special form of symphalangism: generalized biphalangia caused by proximal interphalangeal synostosis with brachymetapody of the 1st radius [in French]. Rev Rhum Mal Osteoartic 1965;32:118-125.

126. Van Genechten F: Familial trigger thumb in children. Hand 1982;14:56.

127. White J, Jensen WE: Trigger thumb in infants. Am J Dis Child 1953;85:141.

128. Zadek I: Stenosing tenovaginitis of the thumb in infants. J Bone Joint Surg 1942;14:326.

129. Slakey J, Hennrikus WL: Acquired thumb flexion contracture in children: congenital trigger thumb. J Bone Joint Surg Br 1996;78:481.

130. Tan A, Lam KS, Lee EH: The treatment outcome of trigger thumb in children. J Pediatr Orthop B 2002;11:256-259.

131. Littler J: Personal communication, 1978.

132. Hueston J, Wilson W: Aetiology of trigger finger, explained on the basis of intratendinous architecture. Hand 1972;4:257-260.

133. Herdem M, Bayram H, Toqrul E, Sarpel Y: Clinical analysis of the trigger thumb in childhood. Turk J Pediatr 2003;45:237-239.

134. Dunsmuir R, Sherlock DA: The outcome of treatment of trigger thumb in children. J Bone Joint Surg Br 2000;82:736.

135. Mulpruek P, Prichasuk S: Spontaneous recovery of trigger thumbs in children. J Hand Surg Br 1998;23:255.

136. Nemoto K, Nemoto T, Terada N, et al: Splint therapy for trigger thumb and finger in children. J Hand Surg Br 1996;21:416.

137. Yuichi T, Koichi T, Hidea K: Splint therapy for trigger finger in children. Arch Phys Med Rehabil 1983;64:75.

138. Upton J: Discussion of percutaneous trigger thumb release in children. Plast Reconstr Surg 2005; in press.

139. Wang HC, Lin GT: Percutaneous release for trigger thumb in children under general and local anesthesia. Kaohsiung J Med Sci 2004;20:546-551.

140. Gilberts E, Wereldsma JC: Long-term results of percutaneous and open surgery for trigger fingers and thumbs. Int Surg 2002;87:48-52.

141. Maneerit J, Sriworakun C, Budhraja N, Nagavajara P: Comment on: Trigger thumb: results of a prospective randomised study of percutaneous release with steroid injection versus steroid injection alone. J Bone Joint Surg Am 2004;86:1103.

142. Skov O, Bach A, Hammer A: Trigger thumbs in children: a follow-up study of 37 children treated below 15 years of age. J Hand Surg Br 1990;15:466.

143. Lin G, Chien SH, Hu HT, et al: Percutaneous trigger finger release. J Orthop Surg 1997;14:23.

144. Gilberts E, Beekman WH, Stevens HJ, Wereldsma JC: Prospective randomized trial of open versus percutaneous surgery for trigger digits. J Hand Surg Am 2001;26:497.

145. Eastwood D, Gupta KJ, Johnson DP: Percutaneous release of the trigger finger: an office procedure. J Hand Surg Am 1992;17:114.

146. Nowinski R, Bamberger HB: Midlateral incision for trigger thumb release. Orthopedics 2001;24:334-336.

147. McAdams T, Moneim MS, Omer GE Jr: Long-term follow-up of surgical release of the A(1) pulley in childhood trigger thumb. J Pediatr Orthop 2002;22:41-43.

148. Lin G, Chien SH, Hu HT, et al: Percutaneous trigger finger release. J Orthop Surg 1997;14:23.

149. Weckesser E, Reed J, Heiple K: Congenital clasped thumb (congenital flexion-adduction deformity of the thumb): a syndrome, not a specific entity. J Bone Joint Surg Am 1968;50:1417-1428.

150. Tsuyuguchi Y, Tada K, Kawai HX: Splint therapy for trigger finger in children. Arch Phys Med Rehabil 1983;64:75-76.

151. Loomis L: Congenital clasped thumb. J La State Med Soc 1958;110:23-25.
152. McCarroll H: Congenital flexion deformities of thumb. Hand Clin 1985;1:567-575.
153. McCarroll HJ: Congenital flexion deformities of the thumb. Hand Clin 1985;1:567-575.
154. Neviaser R: Congenital hypoplasia of the thumb with absence of the extrinsic extensors, abductor pollicis longus and thenar muscles. J Hand Surg Am 1979;4:301-303.
155. Kay P, Lees VC: Anomalies of the tendons. In Gupta A, Kay SPJ, Scheker LR, eds: The Growing Hand: Diagnosis and Management of the Upper Extremity in Children. London, Churchill Livingstone, 2000:319-331.
156. Snow J: A method for reconstruction of the central slip of the extensor tendon of a finger. Plast Reconstr Surg 1976;57:455-459.
157. Flatt A: The inadequate thumb. The Care of Congenital Hand Anomalies, 2nd ed. St. Louis, Quality Medical Publishing, 1994.
158. Crawford H, Horton C, Adamson J: Congenital aplasia or hypoplasia of the thumb and finger extensor tendons. Report of six cases. J Bone Joint Surg Am 1966;48:82-91.
159. Tsuyuguchi Y, et al: Congenital clasped thumb: a review of forty-three cases. J Hand Surg Am 1985;10:613-618.
160. Lipskier E, Weizenbluth M: Surgical treatment of the clasped thumb. J Hand Surg Br 1989;14:72-79.
161. Bianchine J, Lewis RC: The MASA syndrome: a new heritable mental retardation syndrome. Clin Genet 1974;5:298-306.
162. Littman A, Yates J, Treger A: Camptodactyly a kindred study. JAMA 1968;206:1565-1567.
163. Engber W, Flatt A: Camptodactyly: an analysis of sixty-six patients and twenty-four operations. J Hand Surg Am 1977;2:216-224.
164. Foucher G, Khouri RK, Medina J, et al: Camptodactyly as a spectrum of congenital deficiencies: a treatment algorithm based on clinical examination. Plast Reconstr Surg, in press.
165. Murphy D: Familial finger contracture and associated familial knee-joint subluxation. JAMA 1926;86:395-397.
166. Welch J, Temtamy S: Hereditary contractures of the fingers (camptodactyly). J Med Genet 1966;3:104-113.
167. Baraitser M, Burn J, Fixsen J: A recessively inherited windmill-vane camptodactyly/ichthyosis syndrome. J Med Genet 1983;20:125-127.
168. Eyler D, Markee J: The anatomy and function of the intrinsic musculature of the fingers. J Bone Joint Surg Am 1954;36:1-9.
169. Mehta H, Gardner W: A study of lumbrical muscles in the human hand. Am J Anat 1961;109:227-238.
170. Montant R, Baumann A: Recherches anatomiques sur le systeme tendineux extenseur des doigts de la main. Ann Anat Pathol 1937;14:311-336.
171. Stack H: A study of muscle function in the fingers. Ann R Coll Surg Engl 1963;33:307-322.
172. Smith R, Kaplan E: Camptodactyly and similar atraumatic flexion deformities of the proximal interphalangeal joints of the fingers. J Bone Joint Surg Am 1968;50:1187-1204.
173. Courtemanche A: Camptodactyly: etiology and management. Plast Reconstr Surg 1969;44:451-454.
174. McFarlane R, Curry G, Evans H: Anomalies of the intrinsic muscles in camptodactyly. J Hand Surg Am 1983;8:531-544.
175. McFarlane R, Classen DA, Porte AM, Botz JS: The anatomy and treatment of camptodactyly of the small finger. J Hand Surg Am 1992;17:35-44.
176. Glicenstein J, Haddad R, Guero S: Surgical treatment of camptodactyly. Ann Chir Main Memb Super 1995;14:264-271.
177. Smith P, Grobbelaar AO: Camptodactyly: a unifying theory and approach to surgical treatment. J Hand Surg Am 1998;23:14-19.
178. Zancolli E, Zancolli ER: Congenital ulnar drift and camptodactyly produced by malformation of the retaining ligaments of the skin. Bull Hosp Jt Dis Orthop Inst 1984;44:558-576.
179. Stoddard S: Nomenclature of hereditary crooked fingers. J Hered 1939;30:511-512.
180. Ogino T, Kato H: Operative findings in camptodactyl of the little finger. J Hand Surg Br 1992;17:661-664.
181. Todd A: Case of hereditary contracture of the little fingers. Lancet 1929;2:1088-1090.
182. Steindler A: Congenital malformations and deformities of the hand. J Orthop Surg 1920;2:639-668.
183. O'Brien J, Hodgson A: Congenital abnormality of the flexor digitorum profundus, a cause of flexion deformity of the long and ring fingers. Clin Orthop 1974;104:206-208.
184. Millesi H: Macrodactyly: a case study. In Littler J, Cramer L, Smith J, eds: Symposium of Reconstructive Hand Surgery. St. Louis, CV Mosby, 1974:173-174.
185. McCash C, Backhouse K: Demonstration of a Representative Series of Congenital Hand Deformities in Children. London, British Club for Surgery of the Hand, 1966.
186. Miura T: Non-traumatic flexion deformity of the proximal interphalangeal joint—its pathogenesis and treatment. Hand 1983;15:25-34.
187. Ochi T, et al: The pathology of the involved tendons in patients with familial arthropathy and congenital camptodactyly. Arthritis Rheum 1983;26:896-900.
188. Koman L, Poehling GG: Congenital flexion deformities of the proximal interphalangeal joint in children: a subgroup of camptodactyly. J Hand Surg Am 1990;15:582-586.
189. Wilhelm A, Kleinschmidt W: Neue ätiologische und therapeutische Gesichtspunkte bei der Kamptodaktylie und Tendovaginitis stenosans. Chir Plast Reconstr 1968;5:62-67.
190. Millesi H: Camptodactyly. In Littler J, Cramer L, Smith J, eds: Symposium on Reconstructive Hand Surgery. St. Louis, CV Mosby, 1974:175-177.
191. Lister G: The Hand: Diagnosis and Indications. New York, Churchill Livingstone, 1984:312-349.
192. Hueston J: Dupuytren's Contracture. Edinburgh, Churchill Livingstone, 1963.
193. Carneiro R: Congenital attenuation of the extensor tendon central slip. J Hand Surg Am 1993;18:1004-1007.
194. Miura T, Nakamura R, Tamura Y: Long-standing extended dynamic splintage and release of an abnormal restraining structure in camptodactyly. J Hand Surg Br 1992;17:665-672.
195. Goffin D, Lenoble E, Marin-Braun F, Foucher G: Camptodactyly: classification and therapeutic results. Apropos of a series of 50 cases. Ann Chir Main Memb Super 1994;13:20-25.
196. Frank U, Krimmer H, Hahn P, Lanz U: Surgical therapy of camptodactyly. Handchir Mikrochir Plast Chir 1997;29:284-290.
197. Maeda M, Matsui T: Camptodactyly caused by an abnormal lumbrical muscle. J Hand Surg Br 1985;10:95.
198. Gupta A, Burke FD: Correction of camptodactyly. Preliminary results of extensor indicis transfer. J Hand Surg Br 1990;15:168-170.
199. Oldfield M: Camptodactyl: flexor contracture of the fingers in young girls. Br J Plast Surg 1956;8:312-317.
200. Siegert J, Cooney WP, Dobyns JH: Management of simple camptodactyly. J Hand Surg Br 1990;15:181-190.
201. Berger A, Millesi H: Late results of surgical treatment of camptodactylia. Handchirurgie 1975;7:75-79.
202. Benson L, Waters PM, Kamil NI, et al: Camptodactyly: classification and results of nonoperative treatment. J Pediatr Orthop 1984;14:814.
203. Hersch A, Demarinis F, Stecher R: On the inheritance and development of clinodactyly. Am J Hum Genet 1953;5:257-268.
204. Fort A: Des difformites congenitales et acquises des doigts et des moyens d'y remedier [these]. Paris, A. Delahaye, 1869.

205. Ashley L: The inheritance of streblomicrodactyly. J Hered 1947;38:93-86.

206. Burke F, Flatt A: Clinodactyly. A review of a series of cases. Hand 1979;11:269-280.

207. Jones KG: Megalodactylism. Case report of a child treated by epiphyseal resection. J Bone Joint Surg Am 1963;45:1704-1708.

208. Jaeger M, Refior H: The congenital triangular deformity of the tubular bones of the hand and foot. Clin Orthop 1971;81:139-150.

209. Theander G, Carstam N: Longitudinally bracketed diaphysis. Ann Radiol 1974;17:355-360.

210. Theander G, Carstam N, Rausing A: Longitudinally bracketed diaphysis in young children: radiologic-histopathologic correlations. Acta Radiol Diagn (Stockh) 1982;23:239-299.

211. Light T, Ogden J: The longitudinal epiphyseal bracket: implications for surgical correction. J Pediatr Orthop 1981;1:299-305.

212. Ogden J, Light T, Conlogue G: Correlative roentgenography and morphology of the longitudinal epiphyseal bracket. Skeletal Radiol 1981;6:109.

213. Watson H, Boyes J: Congenital angular deformity of the digits—delta phalanx. J Bone Joint Surg Am 1967;49:333-338.

214. Blevens A, Light T: Crooked fingers. In Flatt A, ed: The Care of Congenital Hand Anomalies. St. Louis, Quality Medical Publishing, 1994:212-213.

215. Kirner J: Doppelseitige Verkrümmungen des Kleinfingerendgliedes als selbständiges Krankheitsbild. Fortschr Rontgenstr 1927;36:804-806.

216. Thomas A: A new dystrophy of the fifth finger. Lancet 1936;1:1412-1413.

217. Freiberg A, Forrest C: Kirner's deformity: a review of the literature and case presentation. J Hand Surg Am 1986;11:28-32.

218. Flatt A: The fingers. The Care of Congenital Hand Anomalies. St. Louis, Quality Medical Publishing, 1994.

219. Grandis C, Bonanno F: Surgical treatment of Kirner's deformity. Handchir Mikrochir Plast Chir 1982;14:204-209.

220. Carstam N, Eiken O: Kirner's deformity of the little finger. J Bone Joint Surg Am 1970;52:1663-1665.

221. Wood V: Clinodactyly. In Green DP, ed: Operative Hand Surgery. New York, Churchill Livingstone, 1982:352-353.

222. Carstam N, Theander G: Surgical treatment of clinodactyly caused by longitudinally bracketed diaphysis. Scand J Plast Reconstr Surg 1975;9:199-202.

223. Vickers D: Langenskiold's operation (physolysis) for congenital malformations of bone producing Madelung's deformity and clinodactyly. J Bone Joint Surg Br 1984;66:778.

224. Vickers D: Clinodactyly of the little finger: a simple operative technique for reversal of the growth abnormality. J Hand Surg Br 1987;12:335-342.

225. El-Shami I: Congenital partial gigantism. Case report and review of literature. Surgery 1969;65:683-688.

226. Temtamy S, Rogers J: Macrodactyly, hemihypertrophy and connective tissue nevi: report of a new syndrome and review of the literature. J Pediatr 1976;89:924-927.

227. Ruppert V, Friedel R, Mentzel T, Markgraf E: Fibrolipomatous hamartoma of the nerve—a rare etiology of macrodactyly. A case report. Handchir Mikrochir Plast Chir 1999;31:53-56.

228. DeLaurenzi V: Macrodattilia de medio. G Med Mil 1962;112:401-405.

229. Upton J: Congenital anomalies of the hand and forearm. In May JW Jr, Littler JW, eds: The Hand. Philadelphia, WB Saunders, 1990:5340-5341. McCarthy JG, ed: Plastic Surgery; vol 8.

230. Halderman D: Monstrosity of a hand. Med Rec 1883;23:320-321.

231. Klein V: Ausschaltung eines ungewohnlich grossen Fingers aus dem Gelenk. Graefe und von Walther J Chir 1824;6:379-382.

232. Recklinghausen F: Über die multiplen Fibroma der Haut und ihre Beziehung zu den multiplen Neuromen. Berlin, A. Hirshwald, 1882.

233. Wood V: Macrodactyly. J Iowa Med Soc 1969;59:922-928.

234. Dell P: Macrodactyly. Hand Clin 1985;1:511-524.

235. Frykman G, Wood V: Peripheral nerve hamartoma with macrodactyly in the hand: report of three cases and review of the literature. J Hand Surg 1978;3:307-312.

236. Price A, Compson JP, Calonje E: Fibrolipomatous hamartoma of nerve arising in the brachial plexus. J Hand Surg Br 1995;20:16-18.

237. Barsky A: Macrodactyly. J Bone Joint Surg Am 1967;49:1255-1266.

238. Amadio P, Reiman HM, Dobyns JH: Lipofibromatous hamartoma of nerve. J Hand Surg Am 1988;13:67-75.

239. Al-Quattan M: Lipofibromatous hamartoma of the median nerve and its associated conditions. J Hand Surg Br 2001;26:368-372.

240. Hueston J, Millray B: Macrodactyly associated with hamartoma of major peripheral nerves. Aust N Z J Surg 1968;37:394-397.

241. Mirza M, King ET, Reinhart MK: Carpal tunnel syndrome associated with macrodactyly. J Hand Surg Br 1998;23:609-610.

242. Ranawat C, Arora M, Singh R: Neurodystrophia lipomatosa with carpal tunnel syndrome. J Bone Joint Surg Am 1968;50:1242-1244.

243. Tsuge K, Ikuta Y: Macrodactyly and fibrofatty proliferation of the median nerve. Hiroshima J Med Sci 1973;22:83-100.

244. Warhold L, Urban MA, Bora FW, et al: Lipofibromatous hamartomas of the median nerve. J Hand Surg Am 1993;18:1032-1037.

245. Rudolph R, Jaffee S: Painless fibrofatty hamartoma of the median nerve. Br J Plast Surg 1975;28:301-302.

246. Lauschke H: Foot-like macrodactyly with syndactyly of the hand. J Hand Surg Br 1988;13:353-355.

247. Edgerton M, Tuerk D: Macrodactyly (digital gigantism): its nature and treatment. In Littler J, Cramer L, Smith J, eds: Symposium on Reconstructive Hand Surgery. St. Louis, CV Mosby, 1974:157-172.

248. Thorne F, Posch J, Mladick R: Megalodactyl. Plast Reconstr Surg 1968;41:232-239.

249. Appenzeller O, Kornfeld M: Macrodactyly and localized hypertrophic neuropathy. Neurology 1974;24:767-771.

250. Ben-Bassat M, et al: Congenital macrodactyly. A case report with three year follow-up. J Bone Joint Surg Br 1966;48:359-364.

251. Minkowitz S, Minkowitz F: A morphological study of macrodactylism: a case report. J Pathol Bacteriol 1965;90:323-328.

252. Brooks B, Lehman E: The bone changes in Recklinghausen's neurofibromatosis. Surg Gynecol Obstet 1964;38:587-597.

253. McCarroll H: Soft tissue neoplasms associated with congenital neurofibromatosis. J Bone Joint Surg Am 1956;38:717-731.

254. Moore B: Peripheral nerve changes associated with congenital deformities. J Bone Joint Surg Am 1944;26:282-288.

255. Inglis K: Local gigantism manifestation of neurofibromatosis: its relation to general gigantism and to acromegaly; illustrating influence of intrinsic factors in disease when development of body is abnormal. Am J Pathol 1950;26:1059-1085.

256. Streeter G: Focal deficiencies in fetal tissues and their relation to intrauterine amputations. Contrib Embryol 1930;22:1-44.

257. Ogino T: Macrodactyly. In Buck-Gramcko D, ed: Congenital Malformations of the Hand and Forearm. London, Churchill Livingstone, 1998:183-193.

258. Tropet Y, Merle M, Vichard P, Michon J: An unusual form of macrodactyly. Ann Chir Main 1982;1:342-346.

259. Heiple K, Elmer R: Chondromatous hamartomas arising from the volar digital plates. J Bone Joint Surg Am 1972;54:393-398.

260. Johnson R, Bonfiglio M: Lipofibromatous hamartoma of the median nerve. J Bone Joint Surg Am 1969;51:984-990.

261. Posner M, McMahon MS, Desai P: Plexiform schwannoma (neurolemmoma) associated with macrodactyly: a case report. J Hand Surg Am 1996;21:707-710.

262. Holt J, Wright E: The radiologic features of neurofibromatosis. Radiology 1948;51:647-663.

263. Tsuge K: Treatment of macrodactyly. J Hand Surg Am 1985;10:968-969.

264. Hensinger R, Rhyne D: Multiple enchondromatous hamartomas. Report of a case. J Bone Joint Surg Am 1974;56:1068-1070.

265. Schuind F, Merle M, Dap F, et al: Hyperostotic macrodactyly. J Hand Surg Am 1988;13:544-548.

266. Bjorklund S: Hemihypertrophy and Wilms tumor. Acta Paediatr 1955;44:287-292.

267. Fraumeni JF Jr, Miller R: Adrenocortical neoplasms and hemihypertrophy, brain tumors, and other disorders. J Pediatr 1967;70:129-138.

268. Pillukat T, Lanz U: Congenital unilateral muscular hyperplasia of the hand—a rare malformation. Handchir Mikrochir Plast Chir 2004;36:170-178.

269. Lanz U, Hahn P, Varela C: Congenital unilateral muscle hypertrophy of the hand with ulnar deviation of the fingers. J Hand Surg Br 1994;19:683-688.

270. Grunert K, Langer M: Angeborene Windmuhlenflugelstellung der Finger. Diagnostic, Symptomatik und Pathogenese. Chir Praxis 1994;48:249-263.

271. Wiedemann HR: Malformation-retardation syndrome with bilateral absence of the 5th rays in both hands and feet, cleft palate, malformed ears and eyelids, radioulnar synostosis [author's transl; in German]. Klin Padiatr 1973;185:181-186.

272. Barmakian J, Posner MA, Silver L, et al: Proteus syndrome. J Hand Surg Am 1992;17:32-34.

273. Burgio G, Wiedemann HR: Further and new details on the Proteus syndrome [letters to the editor]. Eur J Pediatr 1984;143:71-73.

274. Choi M, Way PD, Borah GL: Pediatric peripheral neuropathy in Proteus syndrome. Ann Plast Surg 1998;40:528-532.

275. Clark R, Donnai D, Rogers J, et al: Proteus syndrome: an expanded phenotype. Am J Med Genet 1987;27:99-117.

276. Biesecker L, Happie R, Mulliken JB, et al: Proteus syndrome: diagnostic criteria, differential diagnosis and patient evaluation. Am J Med Genet 1999;84:389-395.

277. Biesecker L, Peters KF, Darling TN, et al: Clinical differentiation between Proteus syndrome and hemihyperplasia. Am J Med Genet 1998;79:311-318.

278. Buck-Gramcko D: Proteus syndrome. In Buck-Gramcko D, ed: Congenital Malformations of the Hand and Forearm. London, Churchill Livingstone, 1998:194-196.

279. Vaughn R, Selinger AD, Howell CG, et al: Proteus syndrome: diagnosis and surgical management. J Pediatr Surg 1993;28:5-10.

280. Fryns J, DeSmet L: Letters to the Editor. J Hand Surg Br 1995;20:565-566.

281. So Y: An unusual association of the windblown hand with upper limb hypertrophy. J Hand Surg Br 1992;17:113-117.

282. Reardon W, Harding B, Winter RM, Baraitser M: Hemihypertrophy, hemimegalencephaly and polydactyly. Am J Med Genet 1996;66:144-149.

283. Allende B: Macrodactyly with enlarged median nerve associated with carpal tunnel syndrome. Plast Reconstr Surg 1967;39:578-582.

284. McCullough H, Harper J, Pitt MC, et al: Median nerve compression in the Proteus syndrome. Pediatr Surg Int 1998;13:499-500.

285. Mulliken J, Glowacki J: Hemangiomas and vascular malformations in infants and children: a classification based on endothelial characteristics. Plast Reconstr Surg 1982;69:412-420.

286. Upton J, Mulliken J, Murray J: Classification and rationale for management of vascular anomalies in the upper extremity. J Hand Surg Am 1985;10:970-975.

287. Upton J, Coombs CJ, Mulliken JB, et al: Vascular malformations of the upper limb: a review of 270 patients. J Hand Surg Am 1999;24:1019-1035.

288. Boyd J, et al: Skeletal changes associated with vascular malformations. Plast Reconstr Surg 1984;74:789-795.

289. Frykman G, Wood V: Macrodactyly. In Green DP, ed: Operative Hand Surgery. New York, Churchill Livingstone, 1982:410-419.

290. Salon A, Guero A, Glicenstein J: Fibrolipoma of the median nerve. Review of 10 surgically treated cases with a mean recall of 8 years. Ann Chir Main Memb Super 1995;14:284-295.

291. Paletta F, Rybka F: Treatment of hamartomas of the median nerve. Ann Surg 1972;176:217-222.

292. Ishida O, Ikuta Y: Long-term results of surgical treatment for macrodactyly of the hand. Plast Reconstr Surg 1998;102:1586-1590.

293. Kotwal P, Farooque M: Macrodactyly. J Bone Joint Surg Br 1998;80:651-653.

294. Boyes J: Macrodactylism—a review and proposed management. Hand 1977;9:172-181.

295. Kostakoglu N, Kayikciglu A, Safak T, et al: Macrodactyly: report of eight cases of a rare anomaly. Turk J Pediatr 1996;38:73-79.

296. Akinci M, Ay S, Ercetin O: Surgical treatment of macrodactyly in older children and adults. J Hand Surg Am 2004;29:1010-1019.

297. Pho R, Patterson M, Lee Y: Reconstruction and pathology in macrodactyly. J Hand Surg Am 1988;13:78-83.

298. Rosenberg L, Yanai A, Mahler D: A nail island flap for treatment of macrodactyly. Hand 1983;15:167-172.

299. Tsuge K: Macrodactyly. In Boswick J, ed: Complications in Hand Surgery. Philadelphia, WB Saunders, 1986:347-351.

Hypoplastic or Absent Thumb

Joseph Upton III, MD

Before classification and management of the deficient thumb, a careful surgeon must assess its size, position, relation to other fingers of the hand, osseous components, joint integrity and stability, intrinsic and extrinsic musculotendinous units, first web space depth and width, and associated malformations of the hand and elsewhere. A thumb should be considered hypoplastic when there is a deficiency of any one structure or all structures that contribute to the "normal" thumb. In the past, all definitions were restricted to the radiographic appearance alone; however, presently, we understand that other tests and factors contribute to the overall diagnosis.

For the first 3 months of life, the thumb is adducted and flexed within the palm and serves primarily as a pacifier. By 9 months of age, though, this first ray gains its independence and mobility from the palm, and at 1 year, it has become a crucial portion of the hand.[1] In the normal hand, the strength and mobility needed for a wide variety of pinch and grasp functions rapidly develop, and by the time the baby is ambulatory, the thumb is used creatively to manipulate the environment.

As relied on in the past, radiographs are required for a complete evaluation of the osteoarticular column.

Normal primary ossification centers of the phalanges and metacarpal of the thumb appear in the second to fourth fetal months, but abnormalities of the skeleton of the thumb (e.g., triangular bones) may not be seen radiographically until well into the first or second year of life. Secondary ossification centers within the epiphyses of the thumb normally appear between 13 months and 4 years of age.[2] The delayed appearance of both primary and secondary ossification centers in the hypoplastic thumb is highly relevant to the diagnostic process because the development of those centers is often prolonged in proportion to the degree of hypoplasia.

CLASSIFICATION

The varying degrees of differences between hypoplastic thumbs have been classified in a number of ways that have few common characteristics.[3] Flatt[4] stressed function potential and designated the digits as "adequate" or "inadequate." Bayne[5] relied on localized positions or deficiencies, and three generations of German authors referred to the degree of skeletal hypoplasia.[6-8] The last of these three systems recognizes the progressive degree of hypoplasia from a slight size discrepancy, with all normal structures present, to total aplasia of the thumb. In time, this system has been amended by others,[9] who subdivided type III (severe hypoplasia) into two groups, those with an intact carpometacarpal joint and those without, which is important in terms of management. The five designated types of thumb hypoplasia-aplasia (Fig. 208-1) are commonly associated with radial (preaxial) dysplasia, and the majority of hand surgeons consider most types of thumb with a normal radius part of this spectrum. It is well recognized that concomitant soft tissue anomalies accompany the skeletal abnormalities. Because the correlation of soft tissue and skeletal deficiencies has been so well defined, this refined system works well for clinical decision-making.

Hypoplasia of the thumb is associated with many other congenital differences, specifically central and transverse deficiencies. Because the anatomic makeup of the thumb does not always allow easy categorization under the current system, five additional categories[10] include the constriction ring syndrome, central deficiencies, radial duplication, the five-fingered hand, and short skeletal rays. In these conditions, the thumb ray usually has characteristic deficiencies that fall into the German type II and type III hypoplasia categories, and the anatomic abnormalities relevant to clinical decision-making are presented here.

INCIDENCE

The true incidence is difficult to determine because of the large number of congenital malformations within which a hypoplastic thumb is a component part. All reported reviews are subject to study of the genetic composition of the population of patients as well as any discrepancies of nomenclature and sampling. Entin[11,12] reported a 16% incidence of thumb hypoplasia in his Canadian patients, whereas Flatt[4] published an 11.2% incidence of thumb abnormalities and a 3.6% incidence of thumb hypoplasia or aplasia. We have seen a 37% incidence within our entire registry, which includes many additional categories.[10] The majority of the children treated surgically are those with radial dysplasia—with and without a partial or complete absence of the radius. We have also seen a large incidence in syndromic patients, such as those with the Apert syndrome, who are commonly referred to large children's hospitals for treatment of their multiple malformations.

ETIOLOGY

Because radial or preaxial longitudinal deficiencies occur in many conditions with a wide variety of causes, the etiology of these malformations spans the entire spectrum of genetic, environmental, teratogenic, and other factors (Table 208-1). Therefore, consultation with a genetic specialist is strongly recommended, and referral to standard genetic textbooks or the OMIM Web site is a must for any responsible hand surgeon.

ASSOCIATED MALFORMATIONS

The many potential associations with thumb and radial hypoplasias and aplasia may involve any organ system within the body (see Table 208-1). Most significant are those of the cardiothoracic, gastrointestinal, and genitourinary systems. Associated hematologic problems, specifically Fanconi anemias, can be detected at birth but usually become clinically apparent later in childhood.

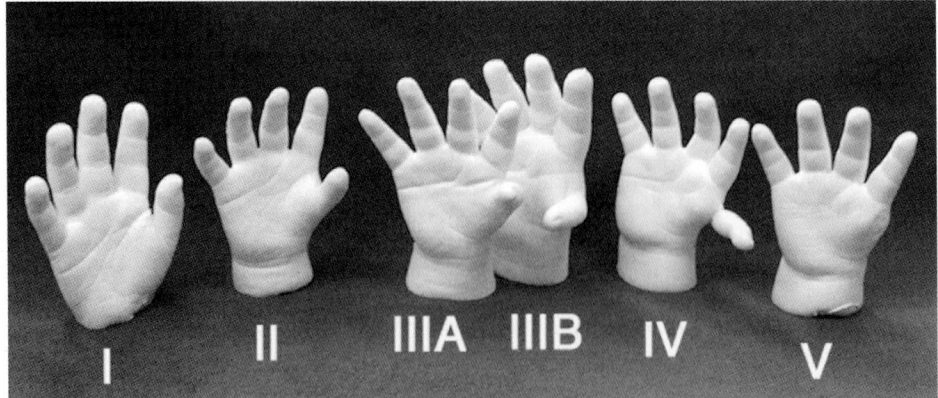

FIGURE 208-1. Thumb hypoplasia. Molds of the right hands of six children with the five classic types of thumb hypoplasia are displayed. Type III has been subclassified into two categories, one with (IIIA) and one without (IIIB) an intact CMC joint. Type IV is often called pouce flottant or floating thumb.

TABLE 208-1 ✦ THUMB AND RADIAL HYPOPLASIA-APLASIA ASSOCIATIONS

Thumb* and Radial† Hypoplasia-Aplasia

Frequent in

Aase syndrome*,†
Baller-Gerold syndrome*,†
Facial-auricular-vertebral spectrum*
Fanconi syndrome*,†
Holt-Oram syndrome*,†
Levy-Hollister syndrome*,†
Nager syndrome*
Radial aplasia-thrombocytopenia (TAR) syndrome*,†
Roberts-SC phocomelia syndrome*,†
Rothmund-Thomson syndrome*
Townes syndrome*
VACTERL association*,†
13q– syndrome*
EEC syndrome

Occasional in

Cat-eye syndrome†
de Lange syndrome*,†
Fetal aminopterin effects*
Fetal valproate effects*
Fibrodysplasia ossificans progressiva*
MURCS association*
Nager syndrome†
Seckel syndrome†
Trisomy 13 syndrome†
Trisomy 18 syndrome†

Metacarpal Hypoplasia: first‡, all§

Frequent in

CHILD syndrome§
Coffin-Siris syndrome§

Cohen syndrome§
Diastrophic dysplasia†
Dyggve-Melchior-Clausen syndrome‡
Grebe syndrome§
Otopalatodigital syndrome, type II§
Partial trisomy 10q syndrome‡
Poland anomaly§
Ruvalcaba syndrome§
Short rib-polydactyly, Majewski type§
Short rib-polydactyly, non-Majewski type§
Trichorhinophalangeal syndrome§
Trisomy 9p syndrome§
5p– syndrome§
18q– syndrome§

Occasional in

de Lange syndrome‡
Larsen syndrome§
Robinow syndrome§
Triploidy syndrome‡

Broad Thumb

Frequent in

Apert syndrome
Carpenter syndrome
Pfeiffer syndrome
Rubinstein-Taybi syndrome
Saethre-Chotzen syndrome

Occasional in

Robinow syndrome
Trisomy 13 syndrome

Modified from Jones KL: Smith's Recognizable Patterns of Human Malformations, 5th ed. Philadelphia, WB Saunders, 1997.

VACTERL

These children may have a wide spectrum of anomalies, including vertebral malformations, anal atresia or hypoplasias, cardiac anomalies, all degrees of tracheoesophageal fistula, renal malformations, and limb abnormalities—which in the upper extremity involve all degrees of radial dysplasia. Not every category on this list needs to be fulfilled for a diagnosis of VACTERL to be considered.

Fanconi Anemia and Other Hematologic Abnormalities[13]

Children with Fanconi anemia develop all degrees of a pancytopenia, which can be life-threatening.[14,15] Most are small with slow growth. Although many other organ systems may be abnormal, deficiencies of the thumb and, to a lesser extent, the entire radial ray are the most common and are present at birth in more than half of these patients. Although children with Fanconi anemia were in the past rarely diagnosed early in life, this condition can now be diagnosed at birth with a DEB (diepoxybutane) test.[14,16] However, because this test involves an unstable gas, butane, it is not available in all medical centers. Other types of treatable childhood anemias, such as the Blackfan type, may occur in the later childhood years and are easily distinguished by routine hematologic tests including the DEB test.[15] Treatment of children with Fanconi anemia by oxymetholone and prednisone therapy has a 70% response rate, and nonresponders can be treated with bone marrow transplantation.[14]

Holt-Oram Syndrome

Two pediatricians, Holt in Philadelphia and Oram in London, independently described the association of congenital heart disease and radial longitudinal defects of the upper limb, and their names have subsequently been associated with all degrees of congenital cardiovascular malformations and radial dysplasias. Interestingly, there is no correlation of the severity of the anatomic deficiency in one system relative to the other. Common to the upper limbs are a stiff hypoplastic thumb joined to a stiff index digit by a complete simple syndactyly, radial deficiencies, and proximal radioulnar synostoses. Hypoplasia of the glenohumeral joint is often not diagnosed until adolescence when shoulder abduction is diminished.

Thrombocytopenia–Absent Radius Syndrome

This unique group of children may be born with normal hematologic parameters, but they usually have a low platelet count, which may decrease rapidly during the first year of life. They are easily distinguished from other types of radial dysplasia by the presence of a thumb despite all degrees of radial deficiencies. The thumb is hypoplastic, and extrinsic flexion and extension vary tremendously. Thenar intrinsic muscles are usually present and provide some palmar abduction by the age of 2 years. The low platelet count commonly reaches normal levels by the age of 4 to 5 years, and the clinical results from centralization are among the best.

CLINICAL PRESENTATION (RADIAL DYSPLASIA TYPES)

In the past, routine radiography was the sole tool used for diagnosis of the hypoplastic thumb. However, this mode of assessment did not reveal any detail about the normal and abnormal soft tissue structures of individual hands. Therefore, surgeons today use a more complete analysis of intrinsic muscles, web space size, extrinsic tendons, and joint stability—all of which have a direct impact on treatment (Figs. 208-2 and 208-3; see also Fig. 208-1).

Type I: Mild Hypoplasia

In this mildest type of hypoplasia, the thumb is slender and slightly shorter than a normally configured first ray (Fig. 208-4). The phalanges and metacarpal can be slightly thinner than usual, but the trapezium and scaphoid are present and the distal radius and styloid process are not affected. The interphalangeal (IP), metacarpophalangeal (MP), and carpometacarpal (CMC) joints are stable and exhibit normal passive and active motion. Whereas there may be a slight hypoplasia and weakness of the abductor pollicis brevis, opponens pollicis, and lateral head of the flexor pollicis brevis muscles, all intrinsic muscles are present.[17] The joints, ligaments and capsules, tendons, nerves, and vascular structures are all normal, and there may be minimal narrowing of the first web space.

Type II: Moderate Hypoplasia

The metacarpal and phalanges are all present but small, and the trapezium, trapezoid, scaphoid, and—to a lesser extent—lunate may be hypoplastic. The first web space is short with the thumb adducted, the ulnar collateral ligament at the MP joint is lax, and the median-innervated thenar muscles are underdeveloped or occasionally absent (Fig. 208-5).[18] The flexor pollicis brevis and opponens pollicis are normally innervated by the median nerve, but the flexor pollicis brevis varies and is reported to be 40% median, 48% ulnar, and 12% both median and ulnar.[19] The ulnar-innervated intrinsics, particularly the adductor pollicis, pull the metacarpal into adduction and narrow the first web space, which on surgical exploration has tight fibrous bands between muscle groups. Type II thumbs contain two neurovascular bundles, and the recurrent motor branch of the median nerve is consistently found.

Many different muscle and tendon anomalies seen on the radial side of the hand have been identified in conjunction with the type II and type IIIA thumbs. In fact, the clinical designation of a given thumb may vary greatly because of this large spectrum of soft tissue abnormalities. Obviously, the absence of IP or MP flexion or extension creases in a slender thumb is the best clinical indicator of flexor and extensor abnormalities. Within this designation, many variations of the long flexor to the thumb may be found. Both the tendon and the muscle belly of the flexor pollicis longus may be abnormal,[20] may have proximal duplications,[21-25] and may have a more radial distal insertion.[23] In some patients, one can observe this muscle originating from the index profundus tendon,[22] the transverse carpal ligament, or the fascia of the thenar intrinsics and inserting into the flexor sheath[21] or the extensor mechanism.[26] In other cases, this muscle may be absent entirely.[27-32] Some of these anomalies may represent abnormal radial wrist extensors or short thumb abductors instead of malformed or malpositioned terminal thumb flexors.[33] On occasion, a small abnormal "musculus lumbricalis pollicis" may extend from the thumb origin across the first web space and attach to the flexor system of the index finger.[34] I have seen this peculiar (atavistic) muscle extending across the first web space in children with the Freeman-Sheldon syndrome and in complex thumb duplications at the metacarpal level.

Normal

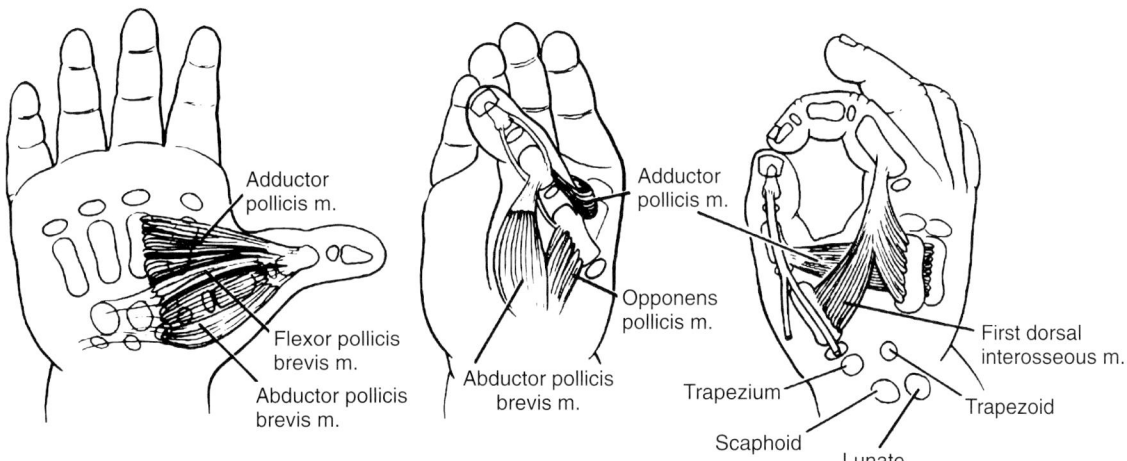

FIGURE 208-2. Normal anatomy. The normal intrinsic muscle anatomy is shown in three views. The median-innervated muscles to the thumb include flexor pollicis brevis (lateral head), abductor pollicis brevis, and opponens pollicis. The ulnar-innervated muscles include adductor pollicis, flexor pollicis brevis (medial head), and first dorsal interosseous. In the normal hand, the extensor pollicis longus tendon attaches to the dorsal lip of the distal phalanx and the extensor pollicis brevis to the dorsal lip of the proximal phalanx. With normal intrinsic muscles, the thenar eminence is full and there is no dorsal depression between the first and second metacarpals.

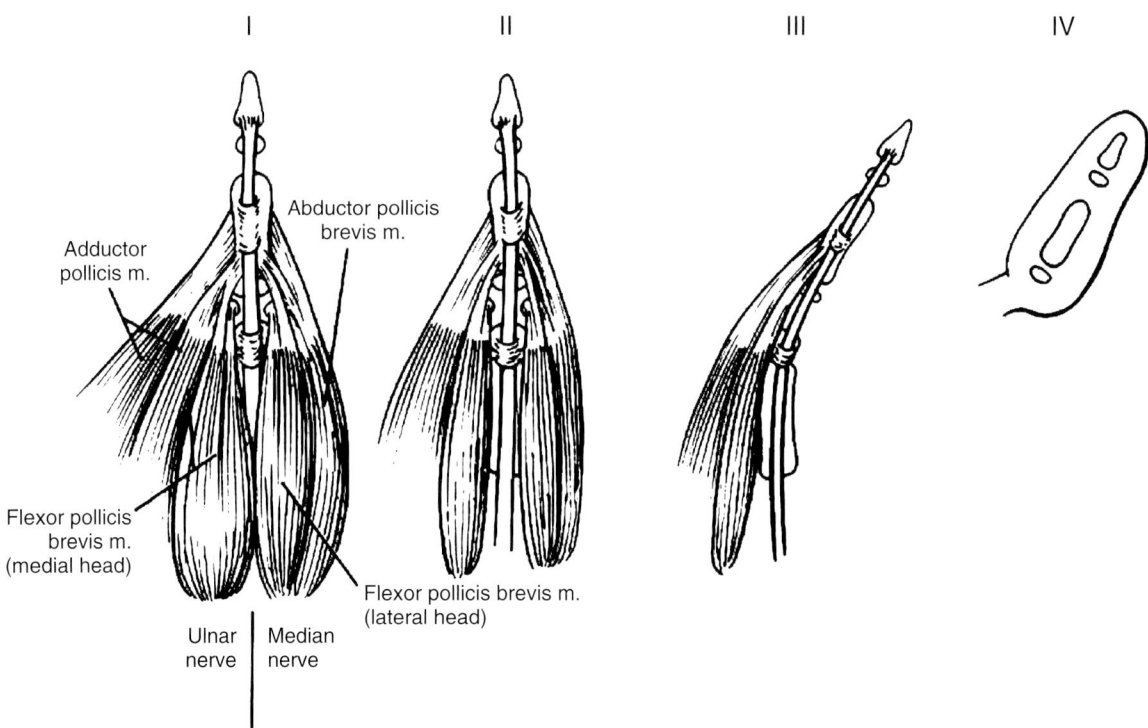

FIGURE 208-3. Thumb hypoplasia. The normal median-innervated intrinsic muscles (abductor pollicis brevis; flexor pollicis brevis, lateral head; and opponens pollicis) and ulnar-innervated intrinsic muscles (adductor pollicis; first dorsal interosseous; and flexor pollicis brevis, medial head) to a right thumb are illustrated. Within the spectrum of thumb deficiencies seen with radial dysplasias,[8,17,135] the intrinsic muscles are all present in type I thumbs but are severely hypoplastic or absent in type III thumbs. Only the ulnar-innervated adductor pollicis and flexor pollicis brevis medial head are present and functional in these hypoplastic type III thumbs. Rudimentary muscles may be present in the type IV floating thumbs. The first dorsal interosseous (also called the abductor indicis muscle) with its second metacarpal origin is found only when the index digit is present.

A. Type I

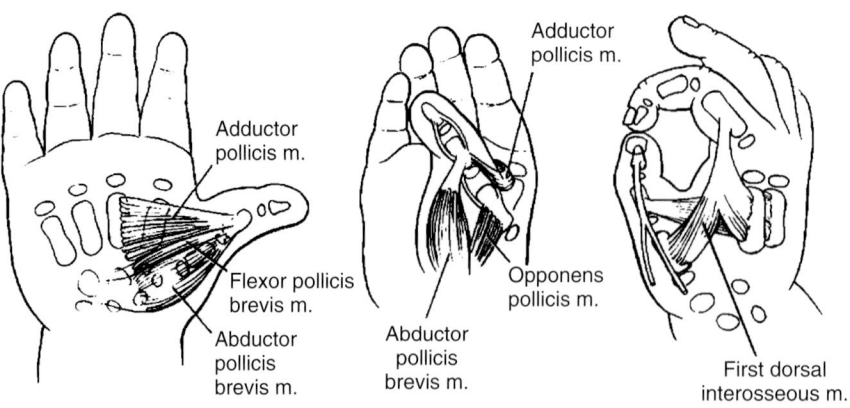

B.

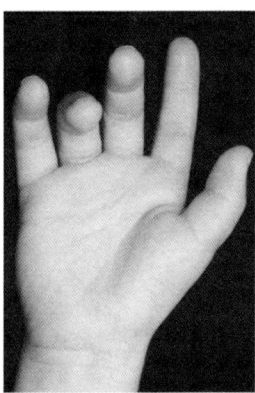
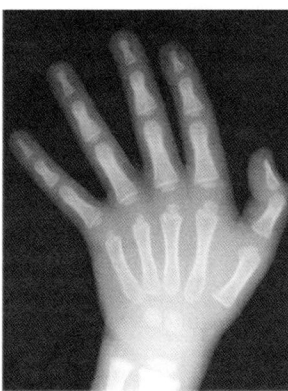

FIGURE 208-4. Type I thumb hypoplasia—mild. *A,* The skeletal ray is well segmented and may be short. All intrinsic muscles and extrinsic tendons are intact. First web space narrowing is minimal to moderate. *B,* Clinical appearance and radiograph of a child who did not require any surgical correction. Although his thenar muscles are weak, there were no significant functional problems.

In addition, the extrinsic extensors may have abnormal insertions,[35,36] extend over the MP joint in a noncentralized position, and reveal abnormal connections with the extrinsic flexor.[24,26,34,37] These abnormal insertions of both flexors and extensors, combined with their deviated course, conspire to make both tendons act primarily as radial deviators and not primary flexors or extensors. In addition, the lax ulnar collateral ligament at the MP joint results in an abduction of the phalangeal portion of the thumb. Tupper[37] has called this pollex abductus and noted that when these muscles contract, there is no IP flexion or extension, only abduction or radial deviation of the thumb. Many anatomic variations of this structure exist, but the functional result is the same (Fig. 208-6). A paper by Graham[24] has summarized the large list of muscle and tendon abnormalities, which often originate in the forearm. Although type II thumbs may present with

these intratendinous connections, the abducted posture and wide degree of muscle and tendon anomalies are primarily seen with type IIIA thumbs (see Fig. 208-6). When followed proximally to the wrist and forearm level, many of these tendons have abnormal origins and long muscle bellies that extend well beyond the wrist into the metacarpal region.

Type III: Severe Hypoplasia

In these cases, the degree of skeletal shortening and narrowing is much more pronounced, particularly at the metacarpal level (Figs. 208-7 and 208-8). The hand and wrist may be radially deviated because of hypoplastic or aplastic carpal bones. The trapezium is usually very small, and the scaphoid is frequently absent. The distal radius is smaller and the styloid process absent, giving the radius a blunted appearance.[38] The extreme

A. Type II

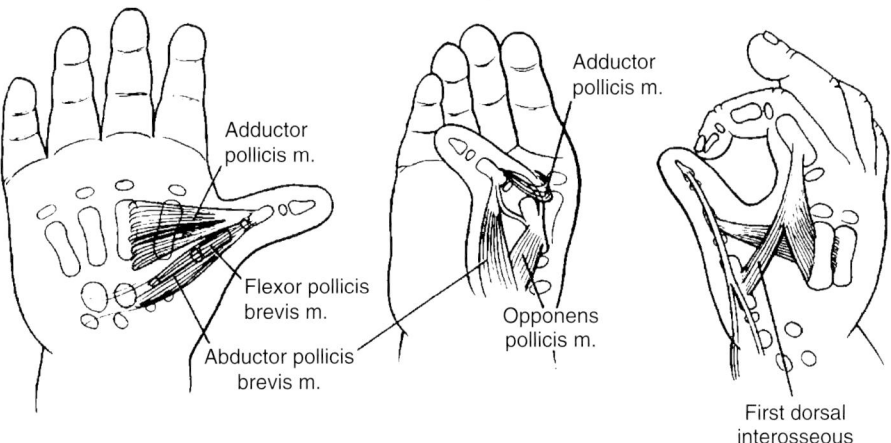

B.

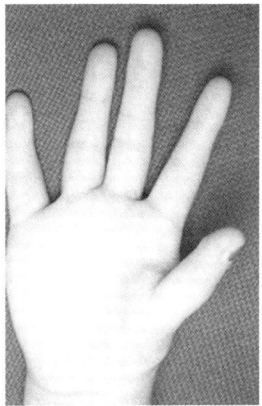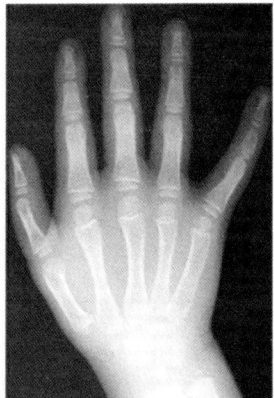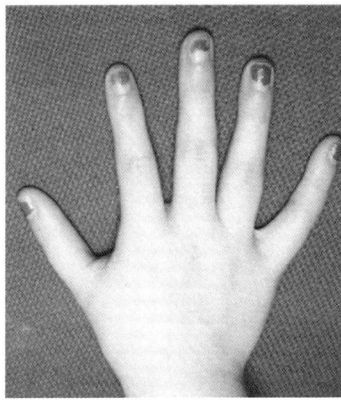

FIGURE 208-5. Type II thumb hypoplasia—moderate. *A,* There is minimal to moderate shortening of the skeletal ray. All bones are present, and ligaments at the MP joint may be lax. The ulnar-innervated intrinsic muscles, adductor pollicis and first dorsal interosseous (second metacarpal origin), are strong, and the median-innervated intrinsics are weak. Anomalous anatomy is common. Adduction contractures from fibrous structures and MP joint instability accompany a deficient first web space. *B,* Clinical appearance and radiograph of a child with a type II hypoplasia of the right hand. The thenar intrinsic muscles are hypoplastic, the first web space is tight, and the thumb is much narrower than normal. Key pinch was weak, and the patient could not hold heavy objects between the thumb and digits. In addition, the ulnar collateral ligament was weak at the MP joint.

amount of anatomic variation within this group prompted Manske et al[39] to subdivide it into type IIIA, with a full-length metacarpal and an intact CMC joint, and type IIIB, with a tapered first metacarpal and no CMC joint. Buck-Gramcko[40] has included an additional variation, called the type IIIC thumb, that possesses only the metacarpal. There are no tendons or muscles in this variant, and the skin bridge is much wider than that seen in type IV (see Fig. 208-1). In the B and C variants, a fibrous band may connect the hypoplastic metacarpal to a cartilaginous nubbin that

represents either a trapezium or metacarpal base. A small abductor pollicis tendon often attaches to this remnant.

Median-innervated intrinsic muscles are either severely hypoplastic or absent entirely; however, if they are present, they may actively flex the MP joint. The ulnar-innervated adductor pollicis pulls the metacarpal medially. The MP joint is lax on both radial and ulnar sides, and anatomically either collateral ligament and the volar plate may be severely hypoplastic or missing. The small thumb with a short web space is abducted

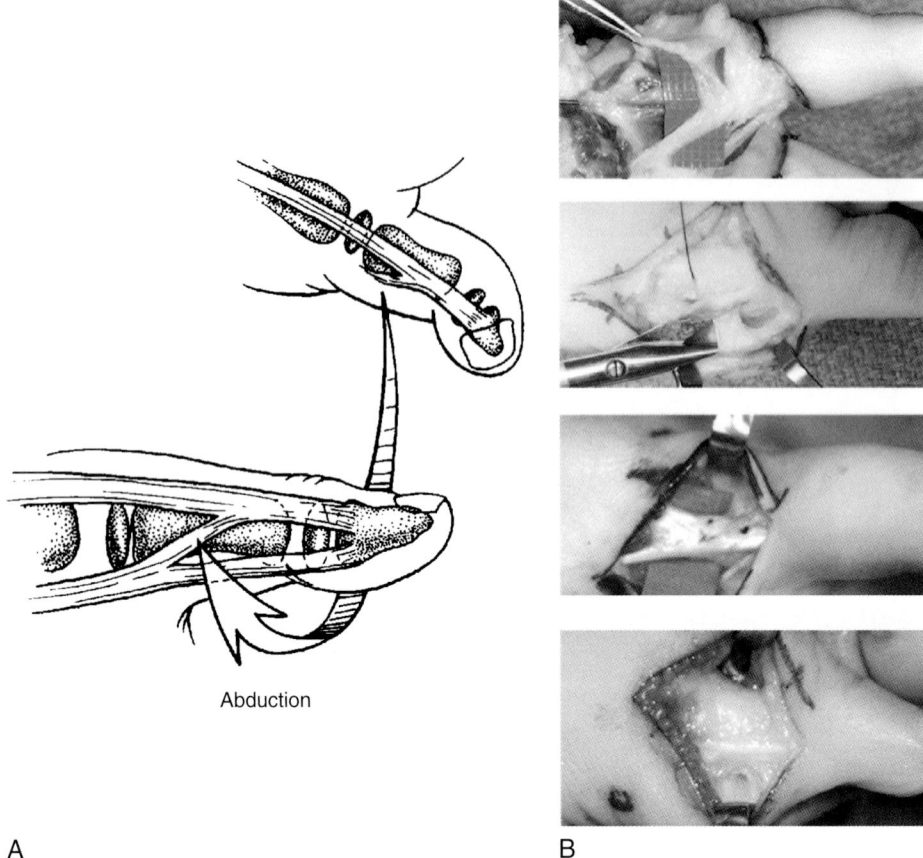

A   B

FIGURE 208-6. Pollex abductus. *A,* In severe type II and many type III thumbs, there may be little if any IP joint flexion, and there may be a radial deviation of the thumb at the MP joint. This is due to the abduction force created by the combined action of the extrinsic flexor and extensor tendons joined by intertendinous connections, the pollex abductus. *B,* Within type II and type III thumb hypoplasias (and proximal thumb duplications), intratendinous connections may vary from a wide, loose, almost areolar band *(top)* to a complete coalition of the flexor and extensor into a single tendon. With excursion from either the flexor or extensor side, the resultant movement in all these thumbs is abduction of the MP joint.

at the MP joint because of the frequent pollex abductus deformity. The radial origin of the first dorsal interosseous from the thumb metacarpal is more severely affected than that from the index metacarpal. The radial head is usually hypoplastic and commonly subluxed, occasionally dislocated.

Abnormal anatomy is the rule. The many intrinsic and extrinsic anatomic variations described within the type II group may exist with greater degrees of hypoplasia. The extrinsic flexor and extensor are usually present and weak, but they may be missing in some cases.[27,32,35] The flexor retinaculum is poorly developed with either attenuation or absence of the major pulleys. In some patients, the motor branch of the median nerve is absent, and there may be only one neurovascular bundle.[22] The radial origin of the first dorsal interosseous to the index finger is severely hypoplastic, and the first web space is severely restricted. Pollex abductus anomalies are common and must be recognized if IP flexion is to be achieved.

Type IV: Floating Thumb (Pouce Flottant, Pendeldaumen)

These thumbs arise distally from the palm and usually lie along the radial midaxial border (Fig. 208-9). They are attached only by a soft tissue pedicle, which has been described by Littler[41] as "nature's own neurovascular pedicle" because of the presence of a digital artery, two venae comitantes, and one or two nerves within the skin bridge. There may be anomalous vascular or neural rings involving neurovascular structures[1,6] that could affect the outcome of a pollicization. There is no metacarpal, and two small

A. Type IIIA

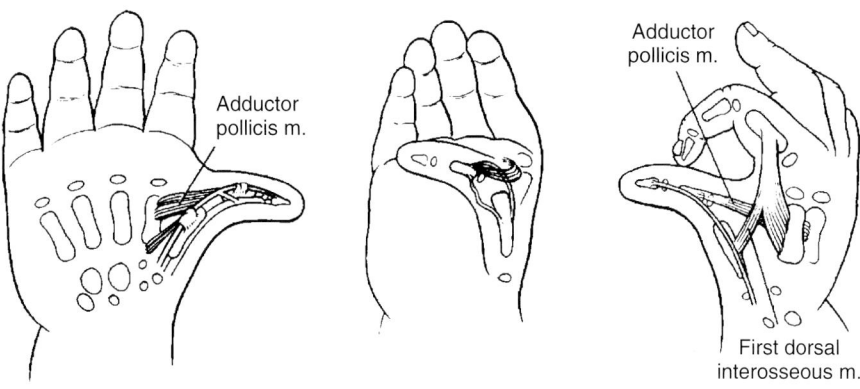

B.

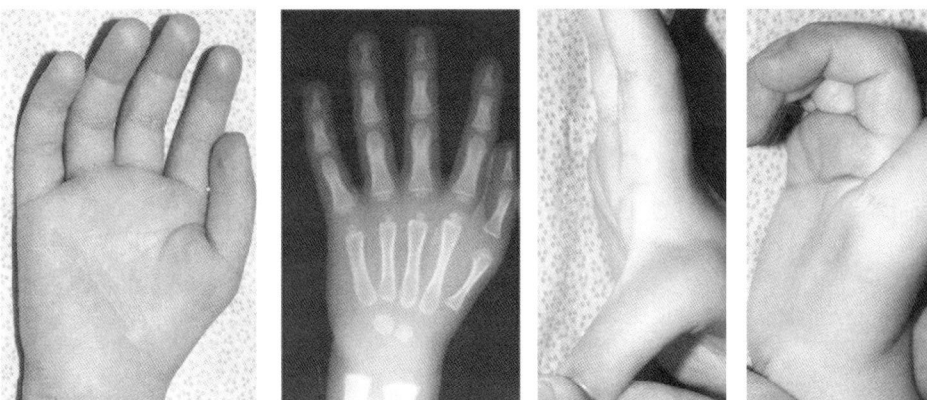

FIGURE 208-7. Type IIIA thumb hypoplasia—severe. *A,* These thumbs exhibit more severe skeletal hypoplasia, including of the carpal bones. Median nerve-innervated thumb intrinsic muscles are severely hypoplastic or absent, and the ulnar-innervated muscles are present but weak. Extrinsic tendons are abnormal, the pollex abductus deformity is frequent, the first web space is small, and the MP joint is unstable (more on the ulnar than the radial side). The CMC joint and thumb metacarpal are intact in IIIA thumbs. *B,* The clinical appearance and radiograph show the short and slender metacarpal, intact CMC joint, severe hypoplasia of the thenar eminence, and lax MP joint. The absent IP flexion crease is indicative of a deficient or absent flexor pollicis longus.

phalanges tend to be present within the soft tissue envelope, which contains a nail. A diminutive nail represents the presence of a distal phalanx. Intrinsic muscles do not insert onto these bones. A first dorsal interosseous muscle (abductor indicis) may be detected by abduction of the index finger. At the carpal level, the trapezium and less often the scaphoid are missing. The radial styloid may be absent, but the distal end of the radius is normal in most of these children.

Type V: Aplasia

The thumb is completely absent in this category (Fig. 208-10). In half of the author's patients[42] and half of those described by Flatt,[43] there is an associated

deficiency of the radius. When the radius is normal, the index digit is normal and has strong abduction at the MP joint owing to the presence of a strong first dorsal interosseous muscle (e.g., abductor indicis). Many of these children with a normal radius will demonstrate "autopollicization." The pulp of the index finger widens and the digit pronates and sits in a more abducted position, resulting in a widening of the intermetacarpal space and attenuation of the intermetacarpal ligament. At best, this posture is a poor substitute for normal key pinch. In the case of a deficient radius, the index ray is stiffer, shorter, and often joined by a simple syndactyly to the long digit. There is a direct correlation between the degree of radial hypoplasia and the index finger deficiencies; the

A. Type IIIB

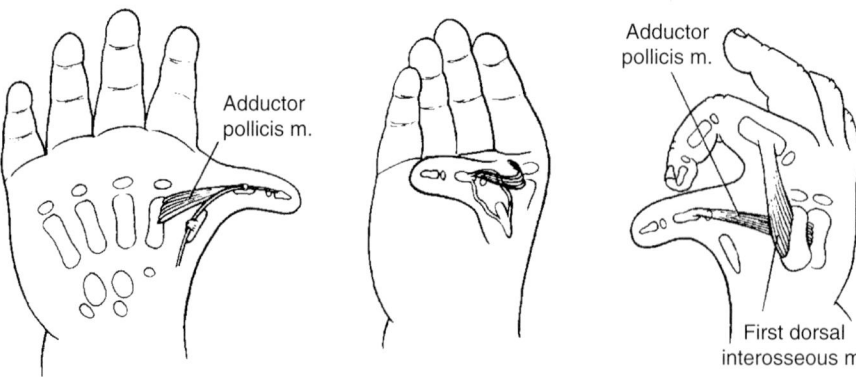

B.

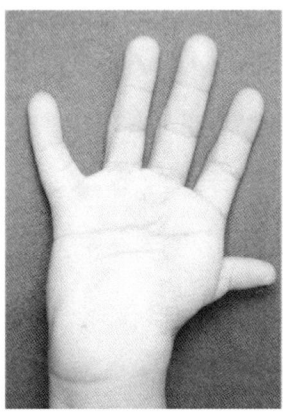 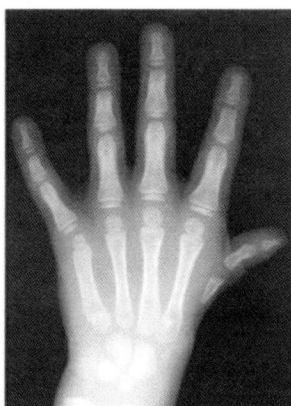 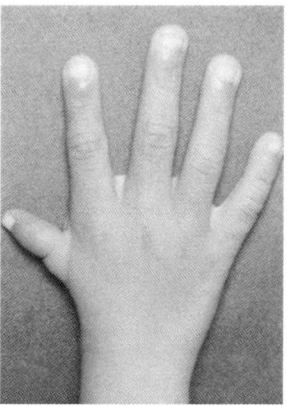

FIGURE 208-8. Type IIIB thumb hypoplasia—severe. *A,* The median-innervated thenar intrinsic muscles are absent entirely. There is severe hypoplasia of the adductor pollicis, the flexor pollicis brevis (lateral head), and the ulnar origin of the first dorsal interosseous. The CMC joint articulation of the proximal metacarpal is absent. The MP joint is lax or absent on both radial and ulnar sides. Flexor and extensor extrinsic tendons are severely hypoplastic or absent. *B,* Clinical appearance and radiograph of a 4-year-old patient with a well-formed but functionless floppy thumb. There is no skeletal stability or extrinsic flexion or extension. Small flexor or extensor tendons may be present and can result in some movement.

index ray is never normal when there are significant associated radial deficiencies. In these hands, the degree of stiffness decreases from the radial to the ulnar digits, and the fifth finger is always the best on the hand.

TREATMENT

Principles

Children with thumb hypoplasia may present many unique problems with both pinch (precision, pulp, key) and grasp (precision, span, power) despite their ability to adapt remarkably to their deficiency.[3] The general ideal prerequisites for construction of a functional thumb include[44]

1. a mobile, stable CMC joint with an intact metacarpal;
2. a scar-free first web space of adequate width and depth lined with full-thickness skin;
3. mobility in at least two of its three joints (CMC, MP, IP);
4. MP joint stability, particularly of the ulnar collateral ligament;
5. adequate motors for strong MP or IP flexion and extension; and
6. capacity to be placed in a palmar abducted (i.e., opposition) position for pinch and grasp maneuvers.

All six of these components should be considered in any detailed analysis of the thumb.

A. Type IV   B.

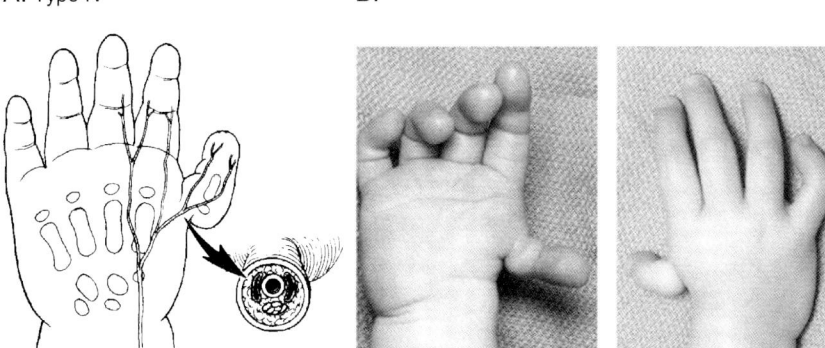

FIGURE 208-9. Type IV thumb hypoplasia—floating thumb. *A*, The hypoplastic thumb is attached to the hand only by a soft tissue bridge, which contains neurovascular structures and rarely hypoplastic tendons and fascia. There is no skeletal connection. *B*, The attached thumb is small with diminutive phalanges and a nail. There is no active flexion or extension. The radial deviation of the wrist and hand is due to hypoplasia of the trapezium, scaphoid, and lunate.

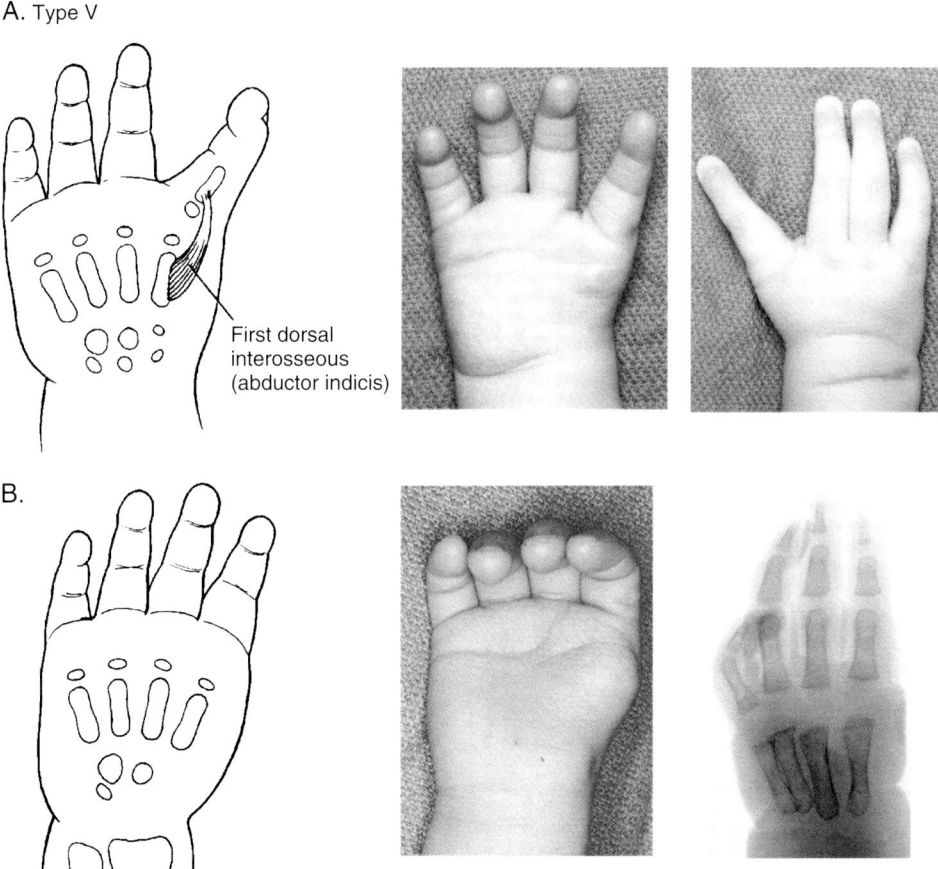

FIGURE 208-10. Type V thumb hypoplasia-aplasia. *A,* With complete aplasia, no thumb structures are present. In approximately half of these patients, the radius is normal. The trapezium, trapezoid, and scaphoid are often hypoplastic, and a strong first dorsal interosseous (abductor indicis) pulls the index digit in abduction and in as much pronation as the intermetacarpal ligament will allow. *B,* Index digits that are not abducted are often stiff at the IP joints and are commonly associated with some degree of radial hypoplasia or aplasia. The amount of stiffness decreases from radial to ulnar digits. Accordingly, the ring and small fingers are always the most functional components of these hands.

Timing

As researchers and clinicians struggle with the possibilities of fetal surgery, many surgeons wonder whether they should wait rather than performing reconstructive procedures of the congenitally different hand as soon as possible (Fig. 208-11). Early reconstruction of the hypoplastic or absent thumb is certainly attractive in an effort to allow the infant to adapt more rapidly with optimal cortical representation. This ideal needs to be tempered with the knowledge that a congenital hand difference is, in itself, not a life-threatening condition (but may be associated with one), and the surgeon can use time to allow the affected part to grow, to observe development, and to assess functional needs. The construction of the thumb with a stable osteoarticular column of adequate length, mobile joints, growth potential, scar-free first web, and gliding muscle-tendon units is not easily accomplished in very small hands despite our refined microvascular instruments, microscopes, and skills. Many other factors need to be considered.

However, the arguments that are forwarded by the proponents of the early surgery persist. The most powerful points include anatomic, cognitive, and psychological factors. Anatomically, the release of tethered musculotendinous units and joint contractures will allow unrestricted growth, and physiologic adaptation of the reconstructed thumb will occur secondary to growth and functional use.[44] On a cognitive level, early surgery will allow the development of the child with a reconstructed thumb to occur before thumb

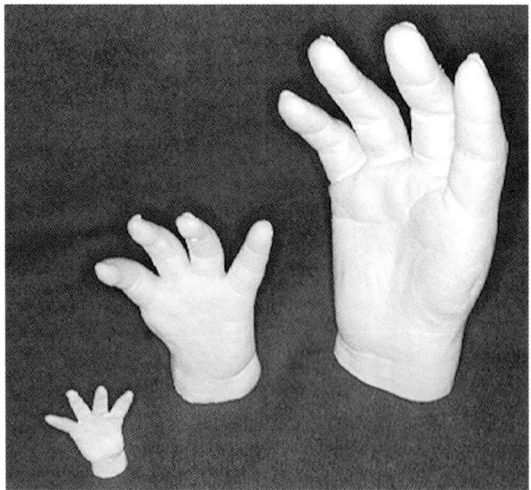

FIGURE 208-11. Timing. Plaster molds of patients with type V hypoplasia made at 32 weeks of gestation and at 12 months and 8 years of age *(left to right)* demonstrate the tremendous growth difference. Despite their discrepant sizes, the anatomy of these hands was remarkably similar with normal index active and passive range of motion. Any surgery on the hand on the left would be quite challenging.

corticalization, which takes place at around 18 months of age. Psychologically, correction will alleviate anxiety in the parents and therefore in the child.

Of course, the advantages of early surgery need to be weighed against those of delayed procedures, which consider growth-related complications, functional need assessment, and cooperation of the patient. In slightly older patients, the affected thumb is larger, so potential problems with osteotomies, alteration of growth, skeletal fixation, joint reconstruction, and potential for compromise of blood supply are reduced. Also with an older patient, the surgeon is better able to accurately assess the functional needs of the child according to his or her interests, current adaptations, and lifestyle. Finally, and perhaps most important, an older child is potentially a more cooperative patient.

In the absence of other organ system complications, I try to reconstruct these problems when the child is between 10 and 18 months of age (see Fig. 208-10). Pollicization at 1 year is often preceded by centralization of the hand and wrist between 5 and 8 months of age. In children with radial deficiencies and thumb aplasia of one upper limb and a less severe thumb hypoplasia on the opposite limb, surgeons should treat the stronger side, with hypoplastic thumb, before attempting pollicization on the more deficient side. Because this hypoplastic thumb will be the child's best thumb, it behooves everyone to strengthen and improve it as soon as possible. However, parents often prefer to have the pollicization performed first and to have nothing done on the more complete side.

The timing for correction of type IIIB deformities may be problematic. Although pollicization is the procedure of choice, some parents and families simply will not allow it. I agree with other surgeons that the alternatives involve difficult reconstructions, often including one or more stages, and are wisely deferred until the child is 4 to 5 years old, when the hand is larger and the patient may be more cooperative with the postoperative therapy regimen.[3,6,24] Surgically speaking, the worst time to approach these youngsters is between the ages of 18 months and 3 years, the "terrible twos."

Surgical correction of the hypoplastic or absent thumb must be individualized. Because these children may have other congenital anomalies, an early assessment of the upper limb deficiencies and a coordinated management plan can be formulated and instituted. Perhaps the most important and least emphasized variables are the confidence, surgical skill, and experience of the surgeon and his or her team. Beware of the young dynamo ready to perform a pollicization without having assisted on many such procedures.

Type I: Mild Hypoplasia

These children are not usually functionally impaired (see Fig. 208-4). In fact, many patients with type I thumb hypoplasia, along with their parents, do not recognize anything abnormal about these hands. These thumbs are commonly found in patients who have a more severe radial dysplasia in the opposite upper limb. However, in this stronger limb, they have little or no difficulty with key pinch, pulp to pulp pinch, opposition, and grasping activities. Because functional problems are rare, surgical correction is not often needed. On occasion, a child with a type I hypoplastic thumb will require release of a mildly contracted web (see type II management). All web releases involve more than simple skin incisions. Careful attention must be directed to tight fascial bands within the web space, anomalous tendon and muscle anatomy, and joint ankylosis.[45] Of all the methods available, the four-flap Z-plasty provides the best contour and appearance (Fig. 208-12). Dorsal transposition flaps from the index finger[27] and rotation flaps[45,46] are effective but require skin

grafting on the visible dorsal surface of the hand. Of course, any method must be carefully individualized to the patient.

OUTCOMES. There are no difficulties with key pulp or nail pinch, grasp, or precision pinch that requires palmar abduction of the thumb. However, the recorded strengths may not reach normal levels. The motion depends on the preoperative condition of the joints, and strength of key pinch and chuck pinch are directly related to the existing thenar musculature.

Type II: Moderate Hypoplasia

Specific problems in the type II thumb that must be addressed individually are narrowed first web space, instability of the MP joint, poor palmar abduction (opposition) for pinching and grasping, lack of IP joint

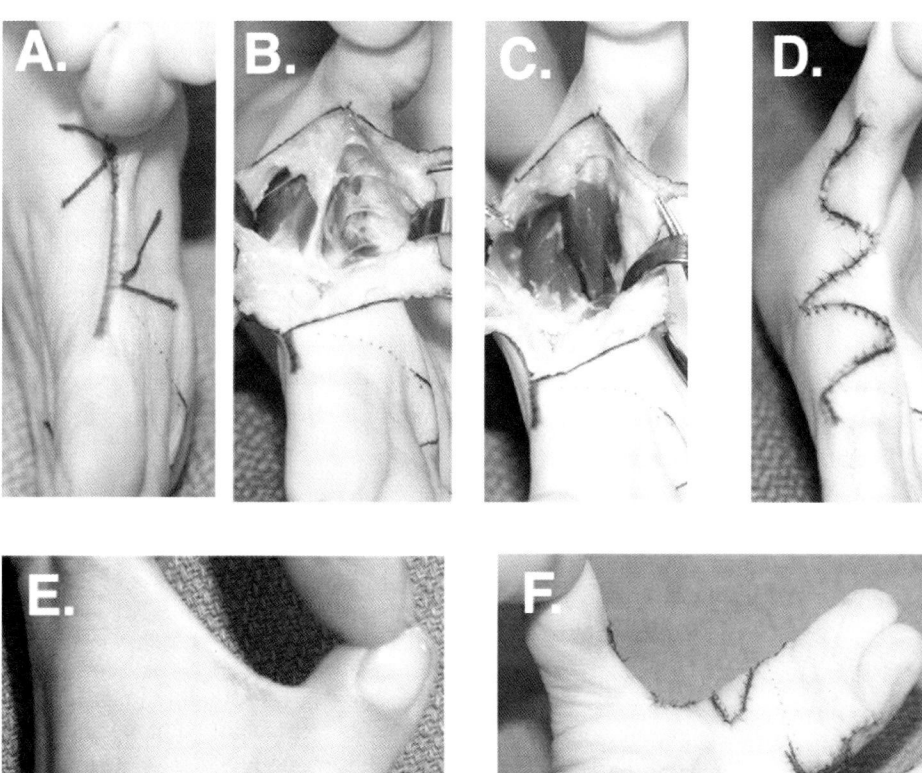

FIGURE 208-12. First web space release. *A,* The skin markings have been made for a four-flap Z-plasty, which includes two 90-degree incisions perpendicular to the tight web between the thumb and index finger. Each is then bisected at a 45-degree angle. *B,* After the four separate flaps have been mobilized, reflected dense septal bands may be identified between the skin and muscle fascia, and larger fascial bands between the intrinsic muscle groups. *C,* Incision and excision of these bands may require dissection to the CMC joint level. *D,* Trimming and minor flap adjustments are always needed with the proper inset of the more mobile dorsal flaps with the more rigid palmar flaps. A skin redundancy on the radial side of the index finger has been eliminated with a straight extension. *E,* The preoperative appearance with a dorsal view. *F,* The postoperative contour is shown from the palmar surface. This technique provides the best contour of all available methods of first web release.

flexion, and abduction posturing of the thumb (pollex abductus) (see Fig. 208-5). Usually all that is needed to correct these thumbs is release of the first web space and stabilization of the MP joint, with or without a transfer for palmar abduction or opposition. When a pollex abductus deformity is encountered, the surgeon should next look for abnormalities of the flexor pollicis longus muscle. A more detailed description is presented in the section on clinical problems and treatment options.

OUTCOMES. Although these are not normal thumbs, functional restoration after early surgery is good.[6,24,28,47] Although motion of the MP joint is decreased after ligament stabilization or chondrodesis, good mobility of the CMC and IP joints will provide excellent function. Attempts to stabilize through chondrodesis often result in a nonunion. In these thumbs, flexion at the IP joint level is diminished and pinch strength reduced not because of a poor adductor pollicis muscle but because of the weak flexor pollicis longus, which is usually malformed. Precision and power grasp between the thumb and three opposing digits is much less than normal. The amount and degree of loss are proportional to the anatomic variations encountered, including the pollex abductus abnormality, the deficient flexor muscle mass, and the amount of surgery required for correction. Stiff thumbs with poor mobility are much more common when there is partial or complete loss of the radius in the same forearm.

Type IIIA: Severe Hypoplasia

Most hand surgeons agree that this variation should be reconstructed surgically (see Fig. 208-7). The individual problems to be addressed are the same as those listed for type II; the options and preferred solutions are listed later. Most authors opt to complete all necessary procedures including widening of the first web space, stabilization of the MP joint, and some type of opposition transfer at one time. The major variable becomes the status of the flexor mechanism, which may require a staged approach. After 25 years of experience, my preference is to replace the anomalous flexor mechanism with a tendon transfer in the presence of at least one good pulley at the level of the metacarpal head. The treatment of the more deficient type IIIB and type IIIC varieties constitutes one of the more interesting ongoing controversies in hand surgery.

OUTCOMES. The type IIIA reconstructed thumbs are short, slender, and less mobile than the type II thumbs, and functional use is highly individual. The only certainty is that these thumbs are never normal. Many studies have correlated the outcome with the degree of anatomic abnormality and the amount of

surgery required.[24,47,48] After MP joint stabilization, motion is diminished; after web release, the first ray is much more mobile and grasp is markedly improved; and after opposition transfers, palmar abduction is maintained if the muscle or tendon transfer is functional.[49] Chondrodesis in young children frequently needs to be repeated as arthrodesis when they are older. Thumb IP joint flexion is rarely normal, and in fact the chance of obtaining good functional flexion in a child born without a flexion crease is poor despite one optimistic report.[24] With a pollex abductus anomaly and a lax or flail MP joint, both MP and IP joint motion will be significantly reduced after reconstruction. The average IP motion in Lister's series[47] was 21 degrees after one- or two-stage reconstruction of the flexor mechanism in the presence of multiple musculotendinous anomalies. Children receiving flexor reconstruction also require joint stabilization at either the MP or IP joint. Efforts to release anomalous flexor tendons, interconnections, or muscles and to use these parts to salvage IP joint motion can be frustrating, particularly if one watches these children grow beyond adolescence.

Type IIIB and Type IIIC: Severe Hypoplasia

For most hand surgeons in Europe, North America, and South America, pollicization is the treatment of choice because a well-performed pollicization provides a much better outcome than any alternative type of staged reconstruction (see Fig. 208-8). However, cultural and parental beliefs may demand one of two alternatives—staged reconstructions with[50-53] and without[54] a microvascular joint transfer, which have both become popular in the eastern Asian countries. Osteoplastic thumb reconstruction has a long history.[7,55-57] The osteoarticular column is connected with an intercalated bone graft between the index and hypoplastic thumb metacarpal (Fig. 208-13). Multiple stages are then needed, first to stabilize MP and IP joints and to construct pulleys. At that point, tendon transfers are performed for opposition as well as IP flexion and extension. The major disadvantages of this procedure include the lack of CMC joint mobility, lack of growth, poor motion, and multiple stages required. Insensate abdominal pedicle flaps have been used to provide tissue for an adequate first web space.

Another alternative is to transfer either the second[54,58-61] or third[62] or first metatarsophalangeal joint in a hyperextended position to make a new CMC joint and proximal metacarpal. This composite joint must be harvested with a large dorsalis pedis pedicle, which provides venous drainage and adds bulk to the deficient thenar region. Tendon transfers are then performed to provide motion at either the MP or IP joint.

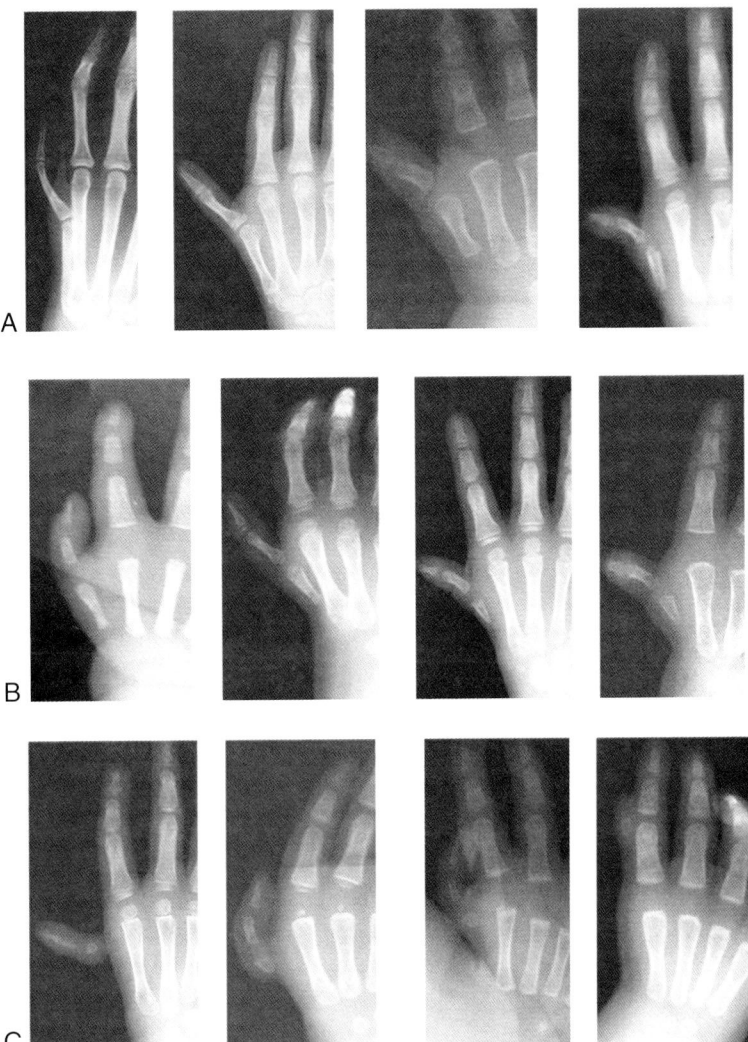

FIGURE 208-13. Spectrum of metacarpal hypoplasia. *A,* There is no arbitrary distinction between specific categories of thumb hypoplasia based on the skeletal appearance alone. These thumbs, which show varying degrees of hypoplasia with a presumably intact CMC joint, are classified as type IIIA. *B,* The smaller metacarpals in these examples signify type IIIB thumbs. *C,* These thumbs, with no skeletal connection, are classified as floating thumbs, type IV. When a tight syndactyly exists between the thumb and index digit, an associated congenital heart defect (the Holt-Oram syndrome) may be present.

The management of these thumbs remains controversial. Without exception, experienced hand surgeons prefer a well-performed pollicization over a staged reconstruction to salvage these deficient thumbs. Any reconstruction will require stabilization of the thumb metacarpal with first web release, MP joint stabilization and opponensplasty, and staged extrinsic tendon transfers—ring flexor digitorum superficialis to flexor pollicis longus for thumb flexion and extensor indicis proprius to extensor pollicis longus for thumb extension. Additional transfers for adduction may also be required. The size of these thumbs at birth makes reconstruction appear attractive to many parents who are often reluctant to consider any other option. Observation of the child at play will usually direct the surgeon and family toward the best course of management. For instance, a child who bypasses the hypoplastic thumb before reconstruction will usually continue to do so after reconstruction. Most undecided parents usually make up their minds after observing other patients with their new pollicized thumbs.

OUTCOMES. Outcome studies[63] indicate that these reconstructed thumbs are short, slender, and relatively immobile. Some surgeons think that the functional pinch and appearance are well worth the effort involved in such complicated microvascular reconstructions.[59,60,64,65] However, lack of growth and immobility are major deterrents.[1,7,57,66-69]

The clinical outcomes after pollicization and alternative staged reconstructions are not controversial and are discussed with the type V thumbs. Staged reconstructions after intercalated bone graft or tendon graft stabilization are predictable. The web space remains deficient. The thumbs are rigid with poor MP or IP joint motion, and the collateral ligament reconstruction at the MP joint level becomes lax with time. There is no metacarpal growth, and as teenagers these children often express dissatisfaction with the thumb "they do not use." However, long-term follow-up interviews with a number of these children, now adults, reveal that some of these patients and their families are attached to and enthusiastic about their small and stiff thumbs.

The advantage of the microvascular procedures to stabilize the metacarpal base and to augment soft tissue is that of growth and restoration of an adequate first web space. The functional results of a number of small series[54,58-60,62,64,70] verify that stability can be achieved but motion is severely impaired. These thumbs are small and have a rudimentary nail complex and scarred web space, which is generally less aesthetically acceptable than a well-executed index pollicization (Fig. 208-14). The technical difficulties and risks of any free tissue transfer in young children may also be significant.

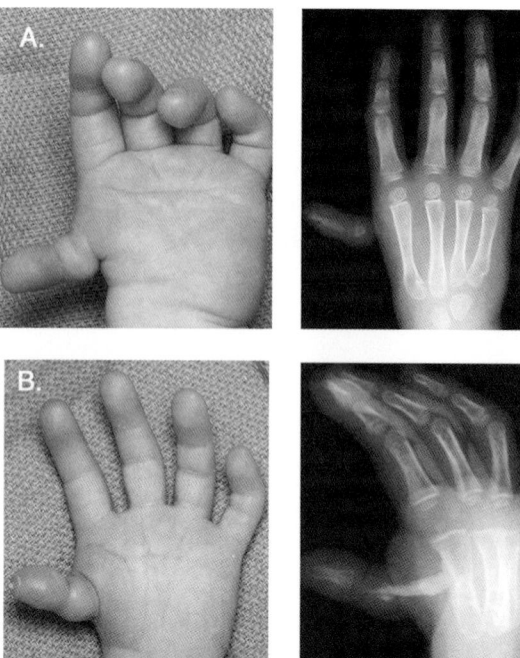

FIGURE 208-15. Type IIIB staged reconstruction. *A,* The preoperative radiograph and clinical appearance of a type IV thumb in a child whose parents insisted on saving it. *B,* A bridging iliac corticocancellous bone graft was used to stabilize the thumb, which became an immobile post and did not grow commensurately with the child. At age 14 years, the same child came to our clinic and asked when I would give her a "normal" thumb.

Type IV: Floating Thumb

Index finger pollicization is the treatment of choice (see Fig. 208-9). If there are too many cultural or parental concerns, consideration is given to the alternative staged reconstructions.

OUTCOMES. The outcomes for pollicization are discussed in the next section. When a staged reconstruction for the floating thumb is chosen, the first ray is smaller and narrow and shows limited motion, depending on the tendons transferred. The thumb does not grow at the metacarpal level if a bone graft has been used (Fig. 208-15), but it will grow and have some CMC joint mobility if a vascularized joint has been transferred. Under the cultural influence of not losing any digits, most of these transfers have been reported from eastern Asia. The results are not very successful compared with an index pollicization.[63,71]

Type V: Absence

Index finger pollicization is the treatment of choice (see Fig. 208-10). Osteoplastic reconstructions and microvascular transfers are not. The technique is described in detail later.

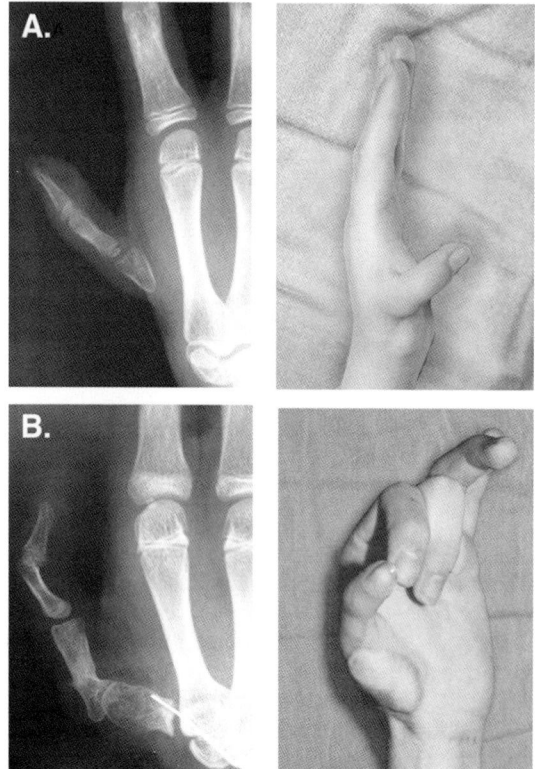

FIGURE 208-14. Type IIIB microvascular reconstruction. *A,* The radiograph and clinical picture show a type IIIB thumb hypoplasia in which there is no proximal metacarpal or CMC joint. This thumb has no skeletal attachment to the rest of the hand. *B,* A second-toe metatarsophalangeal joint, with a covering soft tissue flap, has been transferred to provide the skeletal connection and stability. The clinical picture shown here is at skeletal maturity. Tendon transfers were needed to provide extrinsic flexion and extension to the thumb, and the skin flap helped build up the thenar region. (Case provided by G. Fouchet, MD.)

OUTCOMES

Pollicization. The adequacy of the functional and aesthetic postoperative result depends on the preoperative condition of the index finger. A child with normal skin, bones, joints, tendons, and muscles will achieve an excellent outcome from a *properly performed* pollicization. A youngster with a stiff, partially mobile digit associated with a radial clubhand due to a radial absence will have a less functional outcome. In such a hand, it is important to accurately position the new thumb in greater opposition to the other digits for avoidance of too much CMC joint extension, which would position the thumb in a vulnerable posture. Although assessment of these procedures is difficult, there is no paucity of outcome reports.[9,38,72-82] Most corroborate that preoperative condition determines postoperative result. The most thorough report is that of Manske et al.[9]

Secondary Procedures. Additional procedures have been unusual in my experience. The most common has been opposition transfers for patients with a partial or complete absence of the radius and inadequate median-innervated thenar muscles. In all of these patients, this procedure was discussed as part of the initial "game plan" before pollicization. In 8 of 213 patients (256 pollicizations), an osteotomy was necessary to correct the CMC joint hyperextension, and in 7 patients (treated early in the series), it was necessary to stop persistent growth of the metacarpal.[83] Eleven children have come back as adults to have symptomatic bone spicules from retained periosteum removed. Extensor tendon tenolysis or shortening was necessary in only 10 hands. It is expected that the revision rate would be higher if the patients were less mobile and diligent about long-term follow-up.

Many revisions have been performed on patients whose pollicization was performed by another surgeon. The most common problems were poor position of the skeletal ray, excessive scarring from initial skin loss, adherent extensor tendons, and lack of palmar abduction (opposition). Ten patients have come back as adults, five to have a carpal tunnel release and five to have a painful, dysplastic carpal bone removed. Symptoms were related to repetitive activities at work or pregnancy, and all patients were between 20 and 35 years of age.

Clinical Problems and Treatment Options

DEFICIENT FIRST WEB SPACE

The most effective single procedure performed for congenital hand differences is the correction and widening of the first web space. A scar-free web line, created by full-thickness flaps, is essential for thumb mobility and growth. The many options include local transposition flaps,[84-86] local rotational or sliding flaps with or without skin grafts,[27,46,87] regional vascular island flaps,[88] free fasciocutaneous tissue transfer,[89] distant pedicled flaps,[17,55,90] and use of skin expansion.[10,44] Most are illustrated in Chapter 204.

For all type II situations, local flaps are all that is necessary. Each of the techniques uses the same principle, lengthening the contractual limb of the Z-plasty by transposing tissue perpendicular to it. In general, the four-flap Z-plasty is preferred because it provides the most predictable contour and release (see Fig. 208-12). The five-flap ("jumping man") technique is equally effective but usually involves small flaps with vulnerable tips. A simple Z-plasty, on the other hand, does not give the proper contour and usually creates a central depression at the base of the web space.[91] The surgeon should learn and refine one technique. Local flaps with skin grafts, either on the dorsum of the hand or on the index ray, are popular[27,46] but not preferred because of the conspicuous appearance of the dorsal grafts and the associated contracture when they are harvested along the radial side of the index finger. If the hand requires repeated operations, such as those needed in the Apert hand, dorsal advancement or sliding flaps may be effective because with each procedure, the dorsal tissue is readvanced to make a broader web space.[44,92] The most frequent error in the treatment of these hands is the tendency to use local tissue when the deficit requires more tissue to be moved into the web space.

Additional methods must be considered with more severe narrowing of the first web space seen with type II and type IIIA thumbs. Distally based radial artery or dorsal interosseous arterial flaps can provide more than enough tissue to line the first web space and allow primary closure of the donor site.[44,88] The preferred donor is the radial artery. Preoperative Allen testing must demonstrate an intact palmar arch. I do not hesitate to obtain either a magnetic resonance angiogram or a direct puncture angiogram if there is any question. Predictably, the dorsal interosseous flaps are nourished by the abundant rete network of the carpal region. I would not use an ulnar artery distally based flap unless this artery, the major conduit to the hand, is revascularized with a reversed vein graft. Free groin flaps are effective with minimal donor site morbidity. The major disadvantages are the anomalous vascular anatomy and the specialized training necessary for pediatric microsurgery. Distant pedicle flaps are not indicated and should be considered only under special circumstances.

Technique of First Web Release with Four-Flap Z-Plasty

The contractual limb of the Z-plasty is marked first along the leading edge of the web with the thumb and index finger abducted as much as possible (see

Fig. 208-12). The length of this limb determines the lengths of each of the four flaps. At each end of this line, two lines of the same length are drawn at right angles (90 degrees), with the most radial line passing along the dorsal side of the web (parallel to the thumb metacarpal) and the most ulnar border passing on the palmar side of the web, which is usually close to the thenar flexion crease. These two right angles are then bisected, making four flaps (two palmar, two dorsal), each with a tip angle of 45 degrees. The less mobile glabrous skin on the palmar surface is incised first because minor adjustments are often necessary and more easily accomplished with the mobile dorsal skin. Dorsal veins and nerves are protected with spreading dissection, and all four flaps are retracted as the web space is inspected. The radial neurovascular bundle to the index finger is protected. An arborization of the ulnar digital artery on the thumb side often runs along the distal edge of the adductor pollicis muscle.

Skin incisions alone are usually inadequate for a full release of this web space. Tight fascial investments of the thenar muscles and intermetacarpal bands must be excised before a dramatic release is obtained (see Fig. 208-12*B* and *C*). If necessary, these explorations extend to the level of the CMC joint, where branches of the princeps pollicis artery should be protected. The origin of the first dorsal interosseous on the thumb metacarpal is next inspected and partially recessed if necessary. Release of the adductor pollicis from the third metacarpal carries a potential loss of important pinch strength. Although the first dorsal interosseous and adductor pollicis rarely require release with type II thumbs, they are frequently the tightest deforming force in severe contractures associated with type IIIA thumbs. When myotomies are performed as part of the web release, a 0.35-mm C wire is passed between the thumb and index metacarpals to hold this position for 3 weeks postoperatively. If the radial digital artery (arteria radialis indicis) to the index finger remains as the tightest structure, it can be ligated with impunity when there is a common digital artery to the second web space.

Occasionally in type II thumbs, anomalous muscles acting as adductors may be encountered passing from the flexor surface of the thumb to the extensor surface of the index finger.[34] These muscles are excised. Additional MP joint stabilization procedures or tendon transfers are performed before the flaps are closed with 6-0 mild chromic sutures. When the correct incisions have been made, these flaps will naturally fall into place.

MP JOINT INSTABILITY

The release of a moderate or severe first web space contracture will often unmask a lax ulnar collateral ligament at the MP joint level. Stabilization of this lax joint in type II and type IIIA thumbs can be accom-

plished with a number of procedures: tightening of the existing ligament and capsule,[24] free tendon graft reconstruction,[93] arthrodesis or chondrodesis,[28] and ligament reconstruction with the end of a tendon used to improve palmar abduction (opposition).[3] In the growing child, all must be performed without injury to the epiphysis.[35] Simple imbrication of the attenuated collateral ligament on one or both sides of the MP joint is advocated by some[24] for type II and type IIIA thumbs but has not been permanent in my series. Reefing of the attenuated ulnar collateral ligament and joint capsule can be addressed by either plication or incision and closure of the lax structures with a "pants over vest" repair. The extensor mechanism, with its attenuated shroud fibers, is usually displaced radially and needs to be identified and mobilized from the dorsal joint capsule. A free palmaris or extensor digiti quinti tendon graft passed either through subperiosteal tunnels in the young child or through drill holes in the older youngster is more predictable. One portion of the graft must be palmar enough to reconstruct the volar accessory portion of the ligament. Both radial and ulnar sides of the joint require reconstruction in most type IIIA thumbs. When a flexor digitorum superficialis is used simultaneously for palmar abduction (opposition), one slip is passed through the metacarpal to be used on the ulnar side and the other slip for the radial side of the joint (see Fig. 208-6). Excess tendon on either side may be used for pulley reconstruction if needed.[47]

In type IIIA thumbs with flail joints and poor or absent extrinsic motors, stability of the MP joint is much more critical than motion. Here, a chondrodesis in the young child or arthrodesis in the adolescent is indicated. In the young child, the metacarpal head can be shaved without injury to the growth plate and then fused to the epiphysis of the proximal phalanx.[28,35] Thumbs that have grown in an abducted position and have an asymmetric joint can be stabilized only by fusion.[44] These stabilization procedures must be held with small C wires with the joint in slight flexion (20 degrees). Unless held rigidly, these thumbs can easily drift into hyperextension with minimal cast motion.

Technique of Tendon Graft Stabilization

A palmaris or another common tendon donor is harvested and the MP joint adequately exposed. An extension of the most radial limb of a four-flap Z-plasty provides good exposure for both sides of the joint (Fig. 208-16). After inspection of the extrinsic flexor and extensor tendons with or without intratendinous fibrous connections, joint capsule and collateral ligaments are inspected and imbricated if present. A subperiosteal vertical tunnel is made distal to the growth plate along the metaphysis of the proximal phalanx, and a transverse gauge hole proximal to the metacarpal head will provide the bone fixation for the graft. The

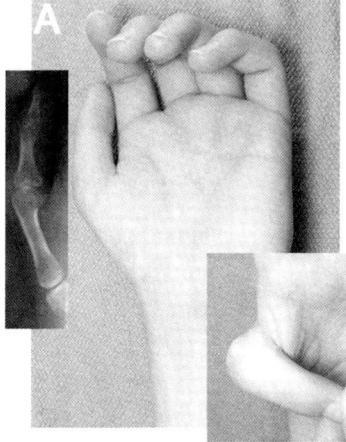
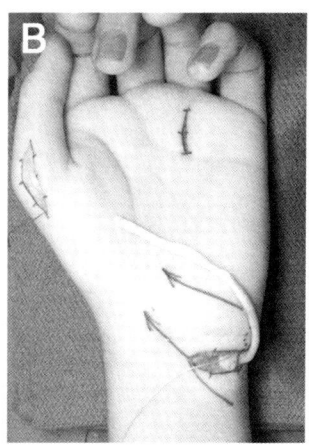
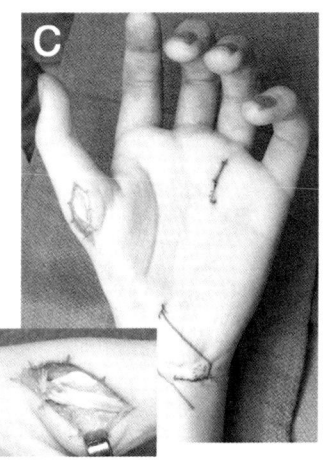
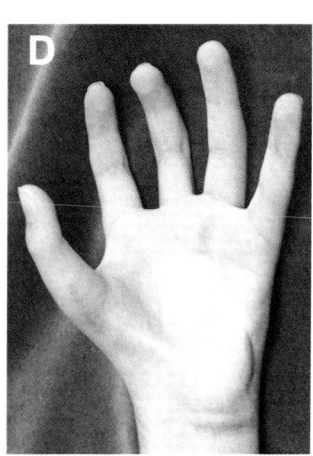

FIGURE 208-16. Type IIIA thumb—joint instability. *A,* The total absence of median-innervated thenar muscles and an unstable MP joint are characteristic of a type IIIA hypoplastic thumb. *B,* The superficial flexor tendon to the ring finger has been looped around the flexor carpi ulnaris and passed through Guyon canal toward the thumb. *C,* The transfer is secured tightly, and both free ends are used to reconstruct the absent collateral ligaments. The inset shows the upper (cord) and lower (volar accessory) portions of the new radial collateral ligament. *D,* Three months postoperatively, the transfer is strong and the MP joint stable on both ulnar and radial sides.

tendon is then passed from the metacarpal fixation point, beneath the extensor shroud, through the periosteal tunnel from dorsal to palmar. It is then passed below the adductor aponeurosis and shroud to the metacarpal. At this point, it is important that the upper portion of this graft mimic the cord (upper) portion of the collateral ligament and that the lower portion provide stability similar to that of the volar accessory portion of the collateral ligament. If this lower portion is fixed at or dorsal to the axis of joint rotation, an MP joint extension contracture will predictably result. The graft is tightened with nonabsorbable sutures in 10 to 15 degrees of flexion and in neutral between radial and ulnar deviation. Pin fixation should not be necessary.

When the ring flexor digitorum superficialis transfer is performed for palmar abduction (opposition), either bifurcation of the tendon is of adequate length for radial and ulnar collateral ligament reconstructions. Most type IIIA and some type II thumbs need both sides of the joint stabilized. In the past, many surgeons have neglected a lax radial side of the joint in their enthusiasm to correct the obviously deficient ulnar

collateral ligament responsible for the abduction of the floppy thumb.

POOR OR ABSENT PALMAR ABDUCTION (OPPOSITION)

The degree of first web space contracture is a good clinical indication of the degree of hypoplasia of thumb abductors, and the need for opposition transfers can be determined both by thenar muscle examination and by assessment of the thumb position during play activities. The child often tends to use key pinching maneuvers because he or she cannot abduct the thumb adequately to obtain a pulp to pulp pinch or grasp and will use a two-handed grasp for holding larger objects. Substitution for the missing or hypoplastic thenar intrinsic muscles is not effective without a mobile CMC joint, adequate first web space, and stabile MP joint. Most commonly, adequate palmar abduction (opposition) of the thumb is obtained by transfer of either the abductor digiti quinti minimi[49,94-96] or the flexor digitorum superficialis of the long or ring finger (Fig. 208-17; see also Fig. 208-16).[43,69,18,97]

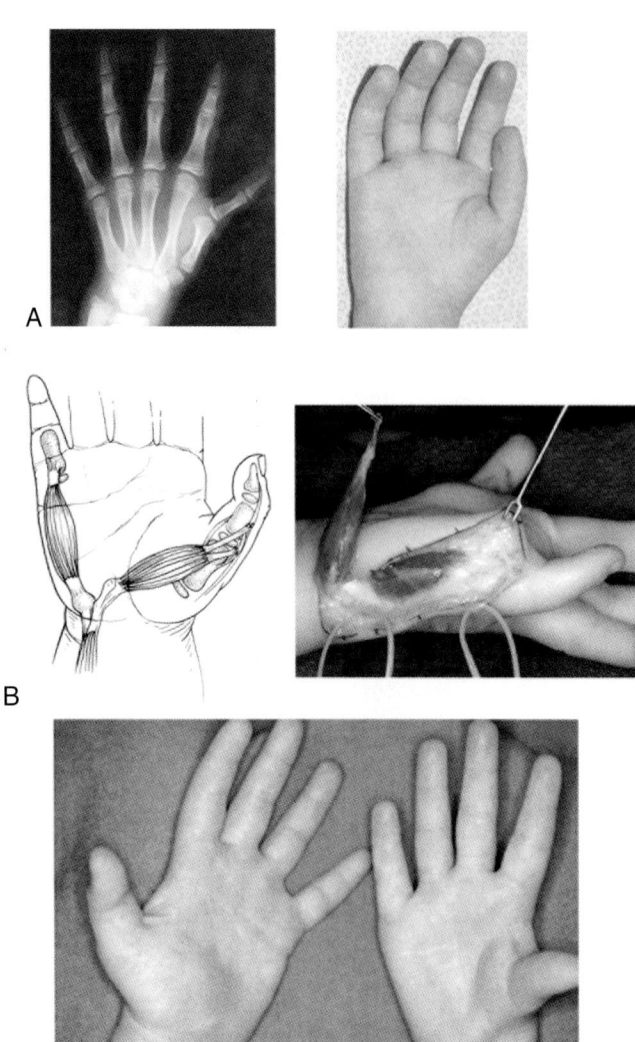

A

B

C

FIGURE 208-17. Abductor digiti quinti minimi transfer for opposition. *A,* The radiograph of this type IIIA thumb shows a small web space and tightly adducted first metacarpal. The clinical photograph shows a marked deficiency of the median-innervated thenar muscles. The radial and ulnar collateral ligaments are stable. *B,* The abductor digiti quinti muscle is isolated on its origin from the pisiform and passed through a subcutaneous tunnel above the palmar fascia to the radial side of the thumb. If two distal tendons can be dissected, separate insertions into the thumb are performed. If one tendon is present, the preferred insertion is into the radial collateral ligament region. When a proximal dissection of the muscle is performed, its neurovascular bundle must be preserved. *C,* The patient shown in *A* is seen 16 years later with functional palmar abduction from the muscle transfer.

Technique of Abductor Digiti Quinti Minimi Transfer

The muscle is raised from an incision extending from the pisiform proximally to the midaxial line of the proximal phalanx (see Fig. 208-17). A skin island can be taken with the muscle, which is then detached from its distal extensor and bone insertions. If there are difficulties separating the abductor digiti quinti minimi muscle from the flexor digiti quinti minimi muscle, both muscles must be raised as a single unit.[49] A distal nutrient artery from the ulnar digital artery to the fifth finger must be ligated if it is present.[98] Additional length can be obtained with detachment from the pisiform[94] and retention on the flexor carpi ulnaris tendon. During this extra mobilization, the proximal axial pedicle to the muscle must be inspected carefully. The muscle is passed through a generous subcutaneous tunnel made between the skin and palmar fascia and then attached to the metacarpal, the radial collateral ligament at the MP joint, or the abductor aponeurosis. Insertion to the proximal phalanx or extensor mechanism should not be performed with any laxity of the ulnar collateral ligament.

Technique of Flexor Digitorum Superficialis Transfer

Harvest of the flexor digitorum superficialis tendon to the ring finger is done through a longitudinal incision at the base of the ring finger. The A1 pulley is released, the finger is flexed, and both slips of the flexor digitorum superficialis are pulled into the wound and cut as far distally as possible. The tendon is then delivered through an incision over the flexor carpi ulnaris and passed through a subcutaneous tunnel to the radial side of the thumb, where the insertion options are the same as for the abductor digiti quinti. The pivot point for the transfer is either through Guyon canal[44] or around the flexor carpi ulnaris. Note that I no longer make a loop from a slip of the flexor carpi ulnaris through which the tendon pivots. The thumb is placed in 45 degrees of palmar abduction and held with a transverse C wire through the thumb and index metacarpals. One slip of the flexor digitorum superficialis tendon is passed through a transverse drill hole near the metacarpal neck and secured. The two slips of the ring flexor digitorum superficialis are then used for reconstruction of the radial and ulnar collateral ligaments as described (see Fig. 208-16). At the same time, the existing ligament and capsule are tightened.

LACK OF IP JOINT MOTION

The most difficult function to reconstruct in type II and type IIIA thumbs is IP joint motion. Dorsal capsulotomy and tendon recentralization will improve the minimal deformities. In the pollex abductus anomaly, flexors and extensors with good proximal excursion need to be centralized with pulley construction. In cases of poor motion, tendon transfers are needed as a second stage. An available ring flexor digitorum superficialis is the most appropriate for IP flexion and an extensor indicis proprius for IP joint extension. Secondary transfers for extension include brachioradialis or extensor carpi radialis longus plus a tendon graft to the extensor pollicis longus.[42]

Pollex Abductus

The clinical presentation of thumb abduction with limited IP motion is indicative of this anomaly (see Fig. 208-6).[34,99] Both the flexor and extensor tendons are exposed through a radial incision or the retracted flap of the web space release. Exploration and traction on the extrinsic tendons will give an estimation of distal IP motion and proximal muscle belly excursion. The interconnecting bands are divided and excised along the radial side of the MP joint and proximal phalanx.[34] The reconstruction here depends on the degree of anomalous anatomy. Absence of both the short and long thumb flexors (flexor pollicis brevis and longus) will severely impair both pinch and grip functions. In those without a pollex abductus, the flexor pollicis longus is usually satisfactory and the pulley system can be strengthened by a slip of tendon—usually taken from the end of a flexor digitorum superficialis transfer. A piece of extensor retinaculum will also make a good pulley.[100] The flexor pollicis longus in the pollex abductus has a poor proximal excursion and can be transferred to the base of the thumb to act as an abductor pollicis longus. Transfer of these abnormal aberrant tendons into a normal position as IP motors is not effective.

After release of the extrinsic tendons and excision of anomalous muscles, a difficult decision must be made with regard to construction of the terminal flexor and at least one strategic pulley. IP joint flexion can be obtained by transfer of an unscarred flexor digitorum superficialis tendon (ring or long) at the same time that palmar abduction (opposition) is restored by an abductor digiti quinti minimi (Huber) transfer.

Technique of Pollicization

Working independently in Europe, Gosset[101] and Hilgenfeldt[102] developed the procedure of digital transposition for post-traumatic thumb losses. In the decades after World War II, Bunnell[103] described similar digital transpositions. Littler[88,104] also refined their techniques and applied them to congenital differences. After the thalidomide crisis in Europe, Buck-Gramcko[68] amassed a large clinical experience and set present-day standards.

Even though pollicization greatly enhances the function of these hands, the index finger is only placed in a more strategic position to simulate a thumb. The newly constructed CMC joint was the index MP joint and therefore does not have the same degree of freedom as the normal CMC joint of the thumb (Figs. 208-18 and 208-19). Because the normal cone of thenar intrinsic muscles is absent, the strength and stability of these thumbs in both pinch and grasp maneuvers do not approach normal.

PRINCIPLES

The principles of this procedure, the most elegant in hand surgery, include transposition of the index digit as a vascular island, rotation and recession shortening of the ray, rebalancing of muscles and tendons, and incisions to construct a normal first web. The operation itself is divided into a number of steps.

INCISIONS AND PLAN

A number of different incisions have been used during the past 3 decades (see Fig. 208-19).[1,68,82,88,105-109] Although the markings of Buck-Gramcko[68] are used most frequently, I prefer a modification of the Littler incisions, which permit much greater flexibility for construction of a broad thumb-index web space.[42,83] A racquet-shaped incision is made around the base of the index ray along the MP flexion crease and extends down the radial border of the hand. The site of the new thenar flexion crease is marked in the palm, and the distal portion of the incision is connected to the incision around the index ray. It is best to plan these incisions as though no thumb or thumb remnant is present and to incorporate this extra tissue into the flap designs only if it is appropriate. If a type IIIB, type IIIC, or type IV thumb is present, the skeleton is

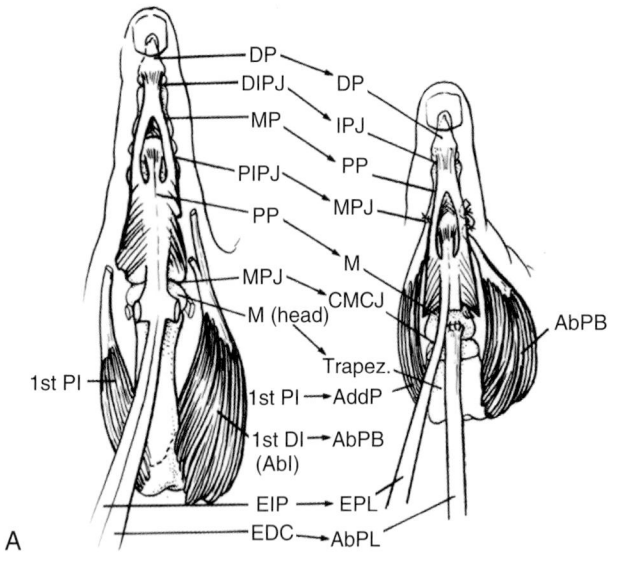

A

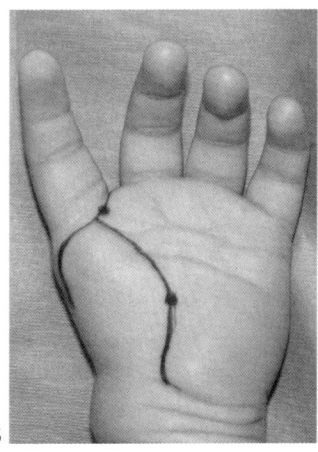

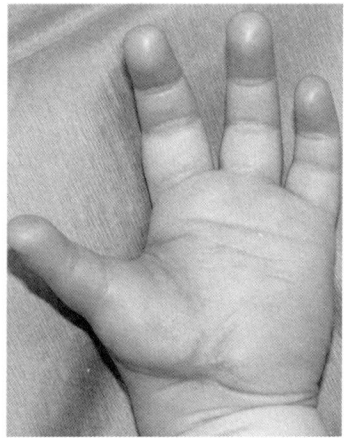

B

FIGURE 208-18. Pollicization. *A,* Rebalancing of the extrinsic and intrinsic muscles from a left index finger to the new left thumb (right). DP, distal phalanx; DIPJ, distal interphalangeal joint; IPJ, interphalangeal joint; MP, middle phalanx; PP, proximal phalanx; PIPJ, proximal interphalangeal joint; MPJ, metacarpophalangeal joint; M, metacarpal; CMCJ, carpometacarpal joint; 1st PI, first palmar interosseous (ulnar interosseous) muscle; 1st DI, first dorsal interosseous (also termel radial interosseous or abductor indicis); EDC, extensor digitorum communis tendon; EIP, extensor indicis proprius tendon; EPL, extensor pollicis longus; AbPB, abductor pollicis brevis muscle; AddP, adductor pollicis muscle; AbPL, abductor pollicis longus tendon. *B,* The preoperative markings are compared with the clinical appearance 6 months after pollicization. The dot in the midpalmar aspect of the index finger is relocated to the midportion of the thenar flexion crease in the postoperative state.

filleted from its soft tissue envelope, and intrinsic muscles are transferred to the new thumb. It is not necessary to isolate and use this skin to augment the web space.

DISSECTION AND EXPOSURE

The dorsal flap is raised in the subcutaneous fat plane above the large dorsal veins, nerves, and lymphatics—all of which are preserved in a single layer of fat and areolar tissue above the extensor mechanism. One large vein is usually present on either side of the dorsum of the digit. The neurovascular structures are dissected, and the palmar flap is raised above the level of the palmar aponeurosis, exposing the superficial palmar arch. The common digital bundle to the index-long web space and the floating thumb (if present) are exposed but individually dissected. Arterial loops around the nerve are present in less than 10% of cases;

however, neural loops around the artery are more common and are opened by spreading the nerve back to the level of the superficial arch. I have not seen the arterial anomalies previously described[110] and do not think that preoperative angiography is necessary. The radial bundle to the index digit is usually hypoplastic but rarely absent. In the presence of a thumb, a common bundle gives one artery to the thumb and one to the index ray. With clear retraction of the neurovascular structures and skeletal and extensor origins of the volar interosseous, first dorsal interosseous and adductor pollicis (if a thumb is present) are detached and the muscles dissected back to their periosteal origin. The index extrinsic flexors are not altered and the lumbrical is left intact. Then the A1 pulley is decompressed. On the dorsal side, the extrinsic extensor digitorum communis and extrinsic indicis proprius to the index are isolated and divided at the level of the MP joint. The lateral bands are gently separated from

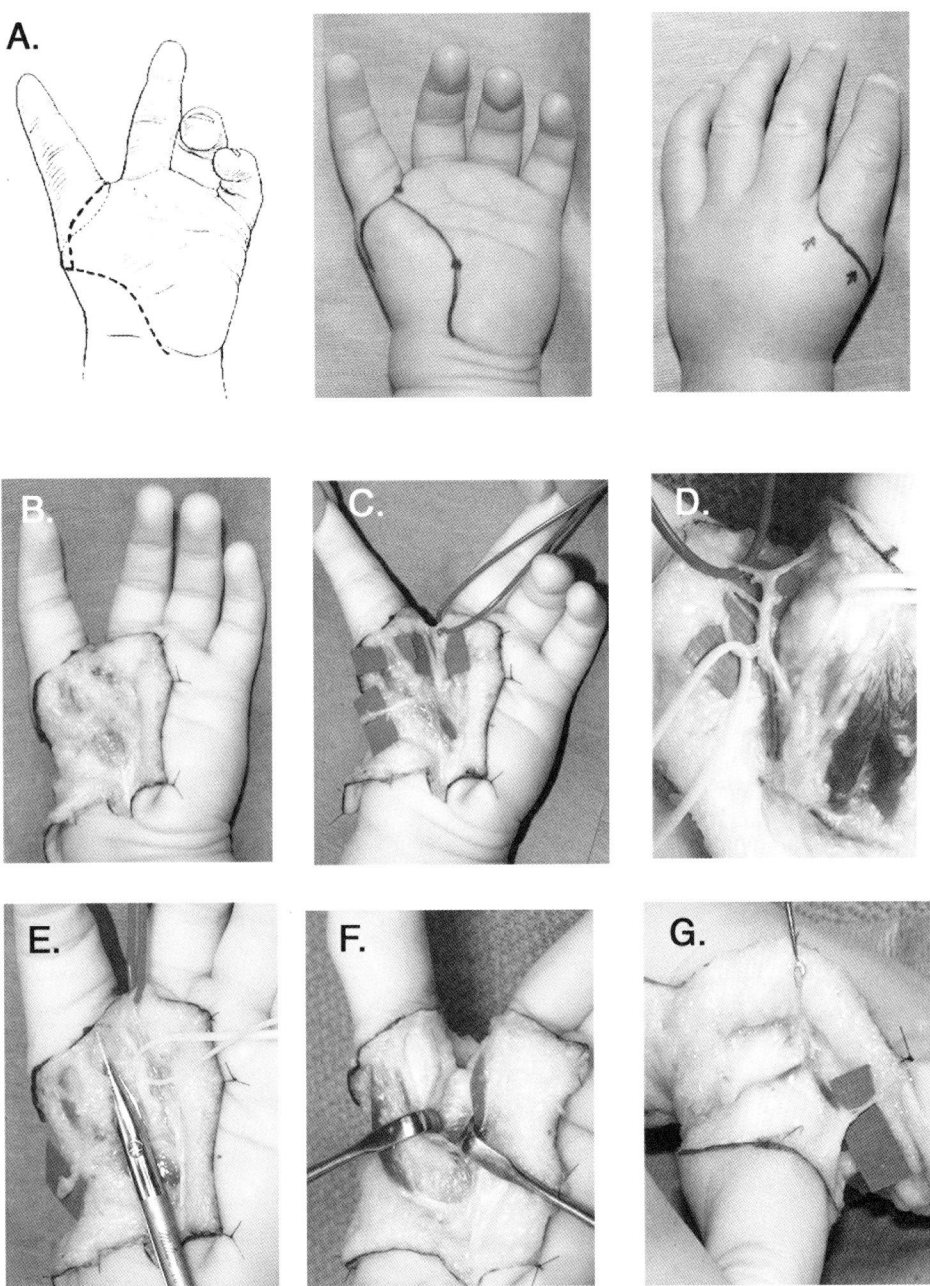

FIGURE 208-19. Pollicization technique. *A,* The illustration and palmar view show the site of the incisions. The most important marking is the location of the future thenar flexion crease within the palm. The volar base of the index finger will be the midportion of this flexion crease. The dorsal marking is made, and the visible dorsal draining veins are marked by arrows. *B,* The palmar flaps are elevated above the palmar aponeurosis. *C,* The common digital bundle to the index-long web space is isolated. The arborization to the radial side of the long finger (dark loop) will be ligated. Note the neuroma in the dissected sensory nerve to the floating thumb, which was ligated in the newborn nursery. *D,* A neural loop around the common vessels to the web space must be carefully teased apart back to the level of the palmar arch. *E,* A full release of the first (A1) annular pulley is completed. *F,* The transverse metacarpal ligament is exposed before its transection, which then provides increased mobility of the ray for the intrinsic muscle dissection. *G,* The dorsal venous system is easily exposed by scissor dissection between the two layers of dorsal fat and areolar tissue.   *Continued*

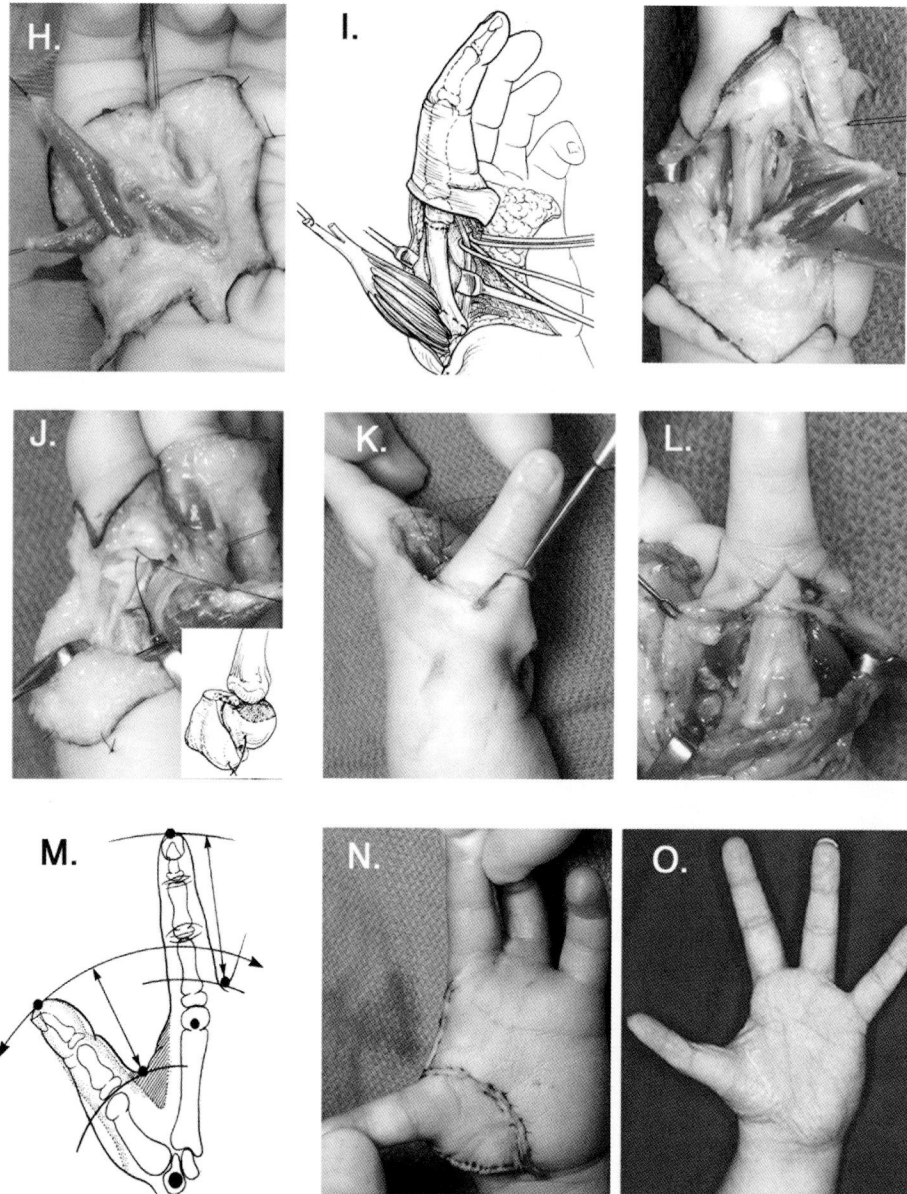

FIGURE 208-19, cont'd. *H,* The first dorsal interosseous (abductor indicis) muscle has been detached from its distal bone and extensor insertions. Two distinct muscles are often found. *I,* The illustration and clinical picture show that the muscles are attached to their periosteal origin, which has been elevated off the metacarpal. The distal osteotomy is through the epiphysis, and the proximal cut leaves the dorsal cortex of the metacarpal base. *J,* The metacarpal head becomes the new thumb trapezium and is placed in a hyperextended position in front of the metacarpal base *(inset).* Interosseous suture fixation is preferred to C wires, which can cause problems in young children. *K,* With the thumb in its new position, the available skin is then draped over the dorsal surface before the cutback incision is made. This maneuver makes maximal use of all the available tissue. *L,* The extrinsic tendons have been shortened and reattached, and the intrinsic muscles have been attached distally either to bone or to the extensor mechanism by the lateral bands. *M,* The normal-appearing first web space is a gentle curve between the MP joint of the thumb and that of the long finger. The shaded area represents the area covered by the additional flaps rotated to form this web. *N,* After closure, a broad web allowing maximal abduction should be present. *O,* The same hand is seen 21 years later.

the common extensor over the proximal phalanx, which will soon become the new thumb metacarpal.

SKELETAL SHORTENING

From both dorsal and palmar approaches, a subperiosteal dissection of the metacarpal is completed, and osteotomy sites are marked (Fig. 208-19I). The intrinsic muscle origins are carefully protected during this dissection, which extends anterior to the index metacarpal to the level of the CMC joint. The proximal osteotomy site is marked and an oblique cut made through the metacarpal, leaving a small post of dorsal cortex to which the metacarpal head will be attached. Here, I have left the entire shaft intact and fixed the metacarpal head to the anterior cortex. The distal metacarpal osteotomy is made through the epiphysis to arrest the growth of the metacarpal head, which becomes the new thumb trapezium. The index finger is now "recessed and rotated"[111] and secured anterior to the base of the index metacarpal with one or more interosseous sutures.[42,100,112] In this position, the MP joint must be in a hyperextended position[68,113] of more than 60 and less than 80 degrees, a position that permits only a few degrees of additional extension of the new CMC joint. Nonabsorbable sutures are preferred to C wires, which can become problematic in young children. This difficult fixation is facilitated by optimal assistance and retraction. At this point in the operation, the tourniquet is deflated for a minimum of 30 minutes.

TENDON AND INTRINSIC MUSCLE REBALANCING

The dorsal flap is first draped over the repositioned index finger, which is held in 45 degrees of palmar abduction, and the dorsal cutback incision is made (Fig. 208-19L). This incision is intentionally delayed because optimal use of all available skin can be crucial for construction of a broad web space. Once it is made, wide exposure to the new thumb is provided. The extensor digitorum communis tendon is advanced and sutured to the ulnar base of the index proximal phalanx (now the thumb metacarpal) so that it provides both extension and pronation. The independent extensor indicis proprius is advanced, and a portion is resected and sutured side by side to the extensor hood with the new thumb held in no more than 10 degrees of MP and IP flexion. Recently, I have accomplished this by simple plication.[104] In rare instances when there is only one extensor on the index finger, this should be used as the extensor pollicis longus.[78]

The intrinsic muscle rebalancing is critical to the resting posture of the thumb. The small first volar interosseous, which becomes the new adductor pollicis, is attached either to the ulnar collateral ligament at the MP joint or into the wing tendon of the extensor mechanism.[104,114] Preferably, the much larger first dorsal interosseous (or abductor indicis), which becomes the new abductor pollicis brevis, is inserted into the radial collateral ligament or the radial base of the new proximal phalanx. When two separate muscles are dissected, one is inserted into bone and the other into the wing tendon on the radial side of the extensor mechanism. Nothing is done with the lumbrical attached to the index flexor digitorum profundus. Additional muscles may be found and used when a hypoplastic thumb is present[88,104] to increase the bulk of the thenar portion of the hand. In those cases in which the first dorsal interosseous (abductor indicis) is absent,[38,111,115] the extensor digitorum communis tendon can be transferred to the palmar surface of the new thumb metacarpal (formerly index proximal phalanx).

The final position of the new thumb is in extension (not hyperextension), which will be properly balanced within 3 to 5 months when the extrinsic flexors tighten. Primary shortening of the new extrinsic flexor can be performed initially, especially with the stiff index finger.[81]

SKIN CLOSURE AND WEB CONSTRUCTION

After skeletal rotation and recession and reattachment of all available musculotendinous parts, one of the most challenging portions of this procedure, tension-free closure, begins (Fig. 208-19M and N). Each hand has a different amount of tissue with which to construct a normal-appearing, broad thumb-index web space. First, the new thumb thenar flexion crease is sutured with the thumb in the appropriate amount of pronation in the palmar abducted position. In this position, the dorsal flap of the hand is advanced over the new thumb, and the dorsoradial flap of the index finger is advanced toward the MP joint of the long finger to construct a normal-appearing web space.[48] This may require additional mobilization and trimming of flaps. As a rule, I try to avoid a straight-line closure dorsally. Finally, the flaps on the radial side of the thumb are trimmed and closed. This skin closure provides a remarkable amount of stability to the new thumb's position. Whereas many different incisions have been proposed,[6,68,82,88,106,116] this particular one is a modification of the Littler and Buck-Gramcko approaches.[44,88] The major differences are that the position of the new thenar crease is the most important point to be determined and the cutback incision into the index is delayed until the available skin can be draped over the index.

POSTOPERATIVE MANAGEMENT

During the 3 weeks of immobilization in a long-arm cast, the tip of the thumb is allowed to move. For the next 6 to 8 weeks, the hand is wrapped in Coban at night to reduce swelling. Ideally, the child works with the parents in special play activities, during which time the long and ring digits are buddy taped to encourage key pinch and grasp with use of the new thumb. It comes as no surprise that there is a positive correlation between good functional results and involved, attentive parents. Other than monthly evaluations by an occupational therapist, no additional therapy is necessary. While the child is outside of the house or in play groups, the thumb is protected with an Orthoplast splint, and within 3 to 6 months, a patient has actively integrated his or her new thumb into the activities of daily living.

COMPLICATIONS

My experience with more than 200 pollicization procedures is similar to that of Buck-Gramcko, who has performed more than three times this number.[78,113] The major learning curve relates to the incisions, muscle rebalancing, and construction of a normal first web space. Devascularization secondary to trauma to the neurovascular pedicle can occur, particularly in patients with clubbed hands and no radial digital artery. This potential problem is avoided by microvascular repair and vein grafting if needed. Invariably, flap losses and their resulting contractures and disfigurement are related to technical problems during surgery. I have never seen a venous compromise in my practice, but this could occur with excessive dissection of the dorsal veins, kinking, or tight dressings. Injury to the innervation of intrinsic muscles may go unrecognized during dissection and can be reconstructed with later transfers. To avoid this problem, these muscles are left attached to their periosteum and are not dissected proximal to the level of the palmar arch. Adduction contractures of the new thumb are the result of either poor positioning and immobilization of the skeletal ray or tight adductor pollicis muscle pull. Aseptic necrosis of the new trapezium (formerly the metacarpal head) has not been a problem in my cases but has been seen. A fibrous union will function well as the new CMC joint. Ossification of the periosteal tissue is common because of periosteum left behind with the intrinsic muscles. Symptomatic spicules are simply excised.

OUTCOMES

The new thumb will never be normal. The adequacy of the functional and aesthetic postoperative result depends, of course, on the preoperative condition of the index finger. Outcomes are predictably divided into two general groups; for specifics, see the section on results of treatment of type V absence. The most thorough study of this is the report of Manske et al.[39] When patients are considered as a single group, total active range of motion averaged 50% of normal, standard grip strength 21%, lateral pinch 22%, and use in normal activities 84%. Interestingly, these results are not significantly altered by the age of the patient at the time of operation.[9] Despite these minor drawbacks, the pollicized index digit is still the best substitute for the congenitally deficient thumb.

The appearance of a pollicized digit is much more difficult to determine because of the subjective interpretation required. Some have tried to quantify appearance by measuring the length of the digit relative to the proximal interphalangeal flexion crease, the resting posture of the new thumb, and the rotation relative to the other digits.[73,80] Meanwhile, others have emphasized the construction of a web across the first web space, which avoids the appearance of a finger positioned on the side of the hand.[39,83] I have observed that the parents and grandparents are almost uniformly pleased with the postoperative appearance of pollicization and that the young patients do not express much of an opinion until they are teenagers, at which time many will let you know whether they like their thumbs or not. Just ask!

The influence of the age at the time of pollicization is always debated. As stated earlier, many surgeons postulate that under ideal circumstances, this operation should be completed within the first year of life[68,80,97] to improve an earlier cortical awareness of the new "thumb." Developmentalists have demonstrated that the child is aware of the thumb as a radial post by 1 year of age.[117] Some argue that because there is no thumb, the index digit is the radial substitute and that pollicization represents a repositioning of the radial post. Manske's data[39] do not support early pollicization for functional reasons. I believe that the size of the hand and the experience, knowledge, and confidence of the surgeon are more important considerations because the surgeon has only one chance to get a pollicization right!

THE INADEQUATE INDEX FINGER

CLINICAL PRESENTATION. In many clinical cases, a less than normal (i.e., stiff) index finger is available for potential pollicization. These include the following:

1. a syndactylized index ray in a child with the Holt-Oram syndrome;
2. an index joined to the long finger with a complete simple syndactyly (i.e., typical cleft hand, index-long syndactyly with absent or hypoplastic thumb);
3. a stiff index finger associated with a complete or partial absence of the radius;
4. a stiff index ray with a fixed proximal interphalangeal (PIP) joint flexion contracture with or

without a complete or partial absence of the radius;

5. the mirror hand (ulnar dimelia); and
6. the five-fingered hand.

In all of these cases, the clinical deficiencies of the index ray are obvious on physical examination, and the major question is whether anything can be accomplished surgically to improve either the clinical function or appearance of the hand (Fig. 208-20). The absence of flexion creases indicates that there has been little if any motion in utero and that there are deficient joints, muscles, and tendinous structures. At surgery, fibrous bands are present between the phalanges, which may not appear joined on radiographs. Flexion contractures (camptodactyly) may be present in the index or all digits with decreasing degrees of severity from the radial to the ulnar digits. These clinical situations do not present frequently but occur more often than anticipated. In my experience with 256 pollicizations performed during the past 25 years, one of

these clinical scenarios is present at least 15% of the time.[83]

TREATMENT. There are no standard guidelines for treatment in the literature, and surgical recommendations depend more on a given surgeon's experience than on practical reasoning. Most recommendations have been overwhelmingly conservative.[9,39,74,75,78,80,83,113,118-125] Options for reconstruction include no surgical treatment, rotation-recession osteotomy of the index ray,[126] formal pollicization of the index ray, and pollicization of the fifth finger.[87]

The determination of what to do and how to do it can be made much easier by an analysis of larger series of pollicizations.[9,39,74,78,113,118-122] Logically, the quality of the result depends predominantly on the preoperative condition of the index ray.

For those with syndromic associations, which include major central neurologic deficits, no surgical treatment is indicated. Pollicization alone for the stiff index digit is considered by some for aesthetic reasons.

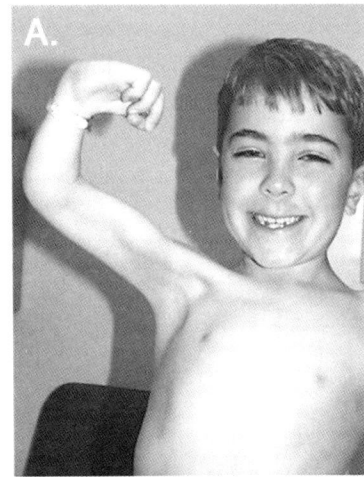
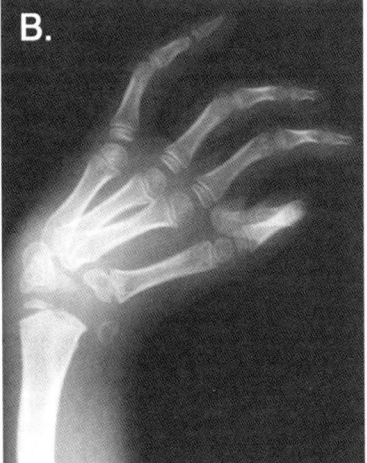
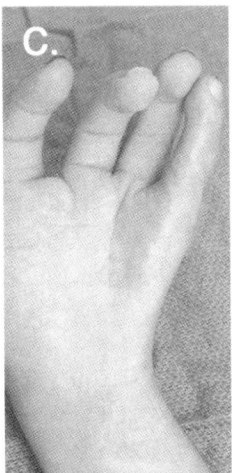
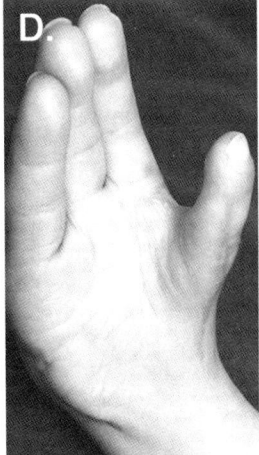
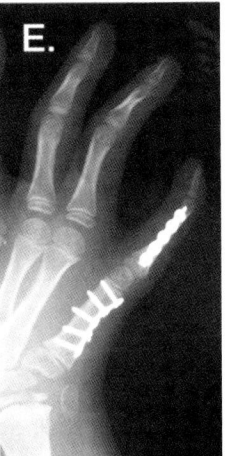

FIGURE 208-20. Inadequate index finger. *A,* This 7-year-old boy with bilateral absence of the radius shows his pectoralis major muscle transfer, which is now working as an elbow flexor. After preliminary distraction, the hand and wrist were then centralized over the distal ulna. *B,* The characteristic widening of the distal ulna is seen. From ulnar to radial, the PIP joints of the digits had an increasing amount of fixed flexion contractures to the extent that the index digit was flexed 100 degrees and was useless. After he had recovered from a successful pollicization on his opposite hand, the patient asked if anything could be done on his right hand. *C,* First, the proximal and middle phalanges were shortened, and an arthrodesis was performed at the PIP joint level. *D,* Next, a rotation-recession osteotomy placed the new thumb in enough palmar abduction to allow pulp to pulp pinch with the long finger and grasping of small objects. This position purposely keeps the thumb from becoming caught in pants pockets and other objects. *E,* Internal plate and screw fixation was used. Motion is present only at the MP joint. Within weeks of the first operation, he began to use this previously ignored digit.

Often, a more mobile index has been moved to the thumb position on the opposite hand. It is important to place the stiffer thumb in a more adducted position. Proper length and the construction of a normal web that extends to the index PIP joint in the thumb position are both crucial to a good appearance.

One alternative rarely chosen for these patients is the rotation-recession osteotomy in lieu of a formal pollicization.[126] I have preferred this procedure in older children, teenagers, and adults with a stiff and flexed index finger, those with scarring from previous procedures, mirror hands, the five-fingered hand, and the stiff index ray associated with a radial clubhand. The principles of treatment are the same, but the ray is not shortened to the full extent of a formal pollicization. Any intrinsic muscles that are present are reattached, and the extrinsic flexors and extensor tendons are shortened as appropriate. The position of the new thumb must be carefully chosen for optimal pinch. Many radial clubhand patients are born with a camptodactyly involving all PIP joints, which progressively becomes more severe in the most radial index and long digits. In these contracted digits, I also perform full releases with Z-plasties or full-thickness skin grafts if needed. Then I consider a rotation-recession osteotomy instead of a classic pollicization as previously described.

The possible combination of deformities with congenital hand differences is almost infinite, and there are many instances in which it is possible to pollicize an index digit after a number of previous procedures involving this ray have been completed. Most examples involve either a syndactylized index finger within a mitten hand or a typical cleft hand in which the index and long fingers are joined within a simple syndactyly.[127] In either case, the syndactyly is released before formal repositioning of the index digit.

OUTCOMES. Optimal results are predictable after a well-performed operation on an index finger with normal active and passive range of motion and a full complement of thenar intrinsic muscles. The radius is usually normal in these children. With less optimal conditions—such as the radial clubhand, the mirror hand, the Holt-Oram syndrome with a syndactylized hypoplastic thumb, or after a syndactyly release—the index and long digits have a diminished range of motion (i.e., stiffness). Meanwhile, the ring and small fingers are the most flexible. The position of the pollicized index finger is crucial for a pinch to the long finger and a grasp to the fifth finger (see Fig. 208-20).[78,113] The new thumb will usually have diminished extrinsic motion, particularly in extension, because the muscles originating on the radial side of the forearm are either abnormal or absent. It is most important that this thumb be positioned for good opposition to the fifth finger, a posture that places it in less

abduction than normal. If it is placed in too much palmar abduction and extension, this immobile post will become caught on objects or within pockets.

ADDITIONAL TYPES OF THUMB HYPOPLASIA

Type VI: Central Deficiencies

CLEFT HAND (TYPICAL)

CLINICAL PRESENTATION. Cleft hand is characterized by hypoplasia or aplasia of the central rays of the hand, thus forming a V- or funnel-shaped cleft (Fig. 208-21). All degrees of simple syndactyly of the first web are seen, resulting in moderate to severe deficiencies of the first web space. In addition, all degrees of hypoplasia, extending to aplasia of the central two rays, may exist.[28] The ulnar two digits in the ring and fifth positions are commonly webbed with simple syndactylies. The thumb in the cleft hand anomaly is usually slightly small with all components of the osteoarticular skeleton present. A Blauth type II thumb classification would be appropriate for the strict constructionist.[17] The wrist and forearm bones are normal, and the median-innervated thenar intrinsics are present. The major deficiency of the thumb in this form of hypoplasia is that the ulnar-innervated intrinsic muscles are severely hypoplastic or absent. In particular, the ulnar-innervated adductor pollicis is usually severely hypoplastic or absent, and the first dorsal interosseous is moderately hypoplastic and contracted. The presence or absence of the third metacarpal is often an excellent indicator of the status of the adductor pollicis muscle. Finally, the extrinsic flexor and extensor musculotendinous units to the thumb tend to be unaffected.

In another variation of typical cleft hand, thumb duplications at all levels may be observed. The more distal type I and II duplications[128] are often associated with the absence of index phalanges that have an intact metacarpal. Super digits and transversely oriented tubular bones at the distal metacarpal level with complete absence of the index (and long) digits are often seen in this variation.[129] With more proximal type III, IV, and V duplications, the central (third) ray is often severely hypoplastic or absent.[130,131] Triphalangeal rays may also be encountered with the proximal duplications at the metacarpal level.

TREATMENT. In treating a patient with the cleft hand anomaly, the following principles should be followed:

- Release the first web syndactyly and contracture.
- Maintain maximal thumb mobility.
- Complete ulnar transposition of the index digit.
- Preserve the adductor pollicis, if present.
- Rotate full-thickness skin flaps into the first web space.

A. VI A Typical cleft hand thumb

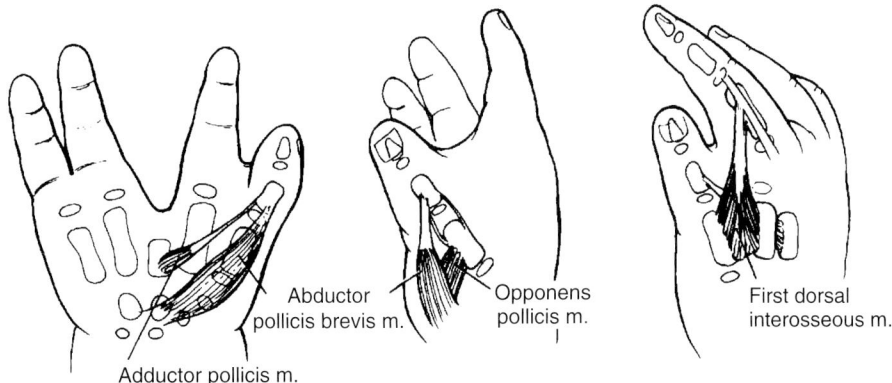

Abductor
pollicis brevis m.

Opponens
pollicis m.

First dorsal
interosseous m.

Adductor pollicis m.

B.

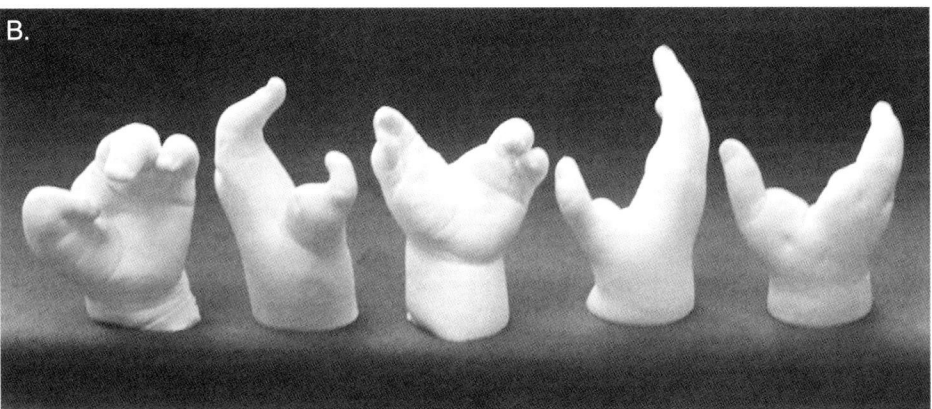

FIGURE 208-21. Thumb in typical cleft hand. *A*, Three layers of median-innervated intrinsic muscles are present in most typical cleft hands. Commonly, the index ray is joined to the thumb by a simple syndactyly. All degrees of absence of the long rays may present. The first dorsal interosseous is present and tight, and the degree of adductor pollicis hypoplasia is proportional to the amount of the third metacarpal present. A very small adductor pollicis is illustrated here. *B*, A sampling of molds shows the wide variation in the size and depth of the central clefting. The thumbs are smaller than normal, and the longer thumbs with flexion contractures are triphalangeal.

- Release any syndactyly involving the two ulnar digits.
- Construct an intermetacarpal ligament between index and ring.
- Treat the thumb duplication in a standard fashion. (See Chapter 206.)

Several procedures and modifications have been described to accomplish these principles for the management of this condition.[21,84,130,132-136] Flaps of the cleft skin based on either the volar or dorsal surface have been used. Unfortunately, both of these designs suffer from the same anatomic problem: the skin flap from the cleft is a random-pattern flap, and the viability of the distal portion of the flap can be suspect. More recently, Tajima has described closure of the newly constructed first web with a dorsal sliding flap.

Undoubtedly, this design poses less risk to the blood supply of the skin flap.

The preferred method of thumb correction uses incisions much like those designed for a pollicization. An incision is made on the ulnar side of the index ray, which is then transposed as a vascular island to the long position. The metacarpal is usually disarticulated and transposed at the CMC joint level. Dorsal and palmar flaps are raised and sutured directly to the skin flaps made by incision of the ulnar side of the cleft. Simple or complex Z-plasties can then be performed on either side of the thumb-index web space as deemed necessary for contour improvement (Fig. 208-22).

When these thumbs are triphalangeal, one of two options is preferred. A stable, well-aligned, mobile but long thumb is usually left uncorrected, and these longer

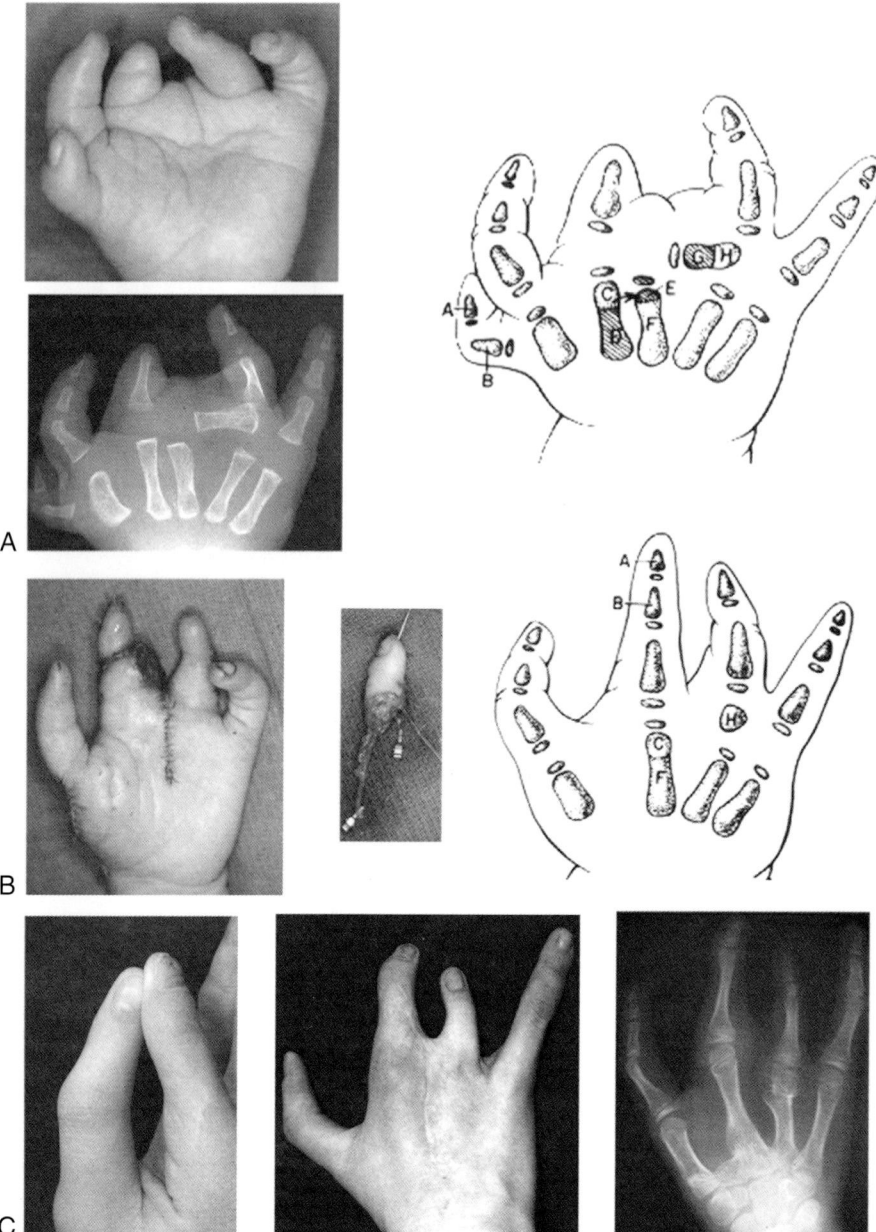

FIGURE 208-22. Cleft (typical) hand thumb. *A,* The left hand and radiograph of a young child with an unusual cleft hand show a triphalangeal thumb, a duplication at the metacarpal level, a short index ray with no distal two phalanges, and a transverse bone connecting the long and ring metacarpals at the MP joint level. The schematic illustration shows the proposed reconstruction. *B,* In a first stage, the index ray (C) was transposed on top of the long metacarpal (F). Only the ulnar portion of the transverse bone (H) was saved because it articulated with the ring proximal phalanx. At the second stage, shown here, the thumb duplication (A, B) was transferred on top of the index ray to make a longer and more complete digit. Nerves and tendons were all joined. *C,* The patient developed a functional pinch between the long (and untouched) triphalangeal thumb and the index finger. At skeletal maturity, her hand and radiograph are seen. The patient has become a confident young lady and, in fact, has won regional New England piano competitions.

thumbs function well. However, with even longer, flexed triphalangeal thumbs, treatment is similar to that described in Chapter 206. The phalangeal components are shortened and fused on one side of the extra phalanx, and the extrinsic tendon insertions are realigned if necessary.

A number of autosomal dominant cleft hand and foot syndromes exist. In these patients, a transverse failure of formation of the thumb may be present at the metacarpal or phalangeal level. When no phalangeal segments are present, vascularized toe to thumb transfer with use of the distal portion of the great toe (if present) is preferred for thumb reconstruction. Distraction lengthening is another alternative.[42,137,138] Motion in these thumbs is poor, but sensation is good, and function is gratifying because the deformities are always bilateral. Secondary procedures for correction of intrinsic joint laxity or deviation are common.

Outcomes. Because most of these thumbs fall into the Blauth type I or type II categories, the results are similar. The major considerations for function relate to the adequacy of the web space construction and the integrity of the first dorsal interosseous and adductor pollicis muscles that are so important in all types of pinch. Strength will be lost from the thumb when the first dorsal interosseous is either recessed or detached during the index transposition. Every effort should be made to preserve what adductor pollicis muscle is present and its periosteal origin. When the index is transposed into the long position, this periosteum is reattached to the index metacarpal. Grip strength is dependent more on the ulnar three digits and not on the thumb.

SYMBRACHYDACTYLY THUMB

Clinical Presentation. The recent change in classification and nomenclature is covered in Chapter 202. For the present, these atypical cleft hands are referred to as symbrachydactyly (Figs. 208-23 and 208-24). This form of deficiency is always unilateral, with

VI B Symbrachydactyly thumb

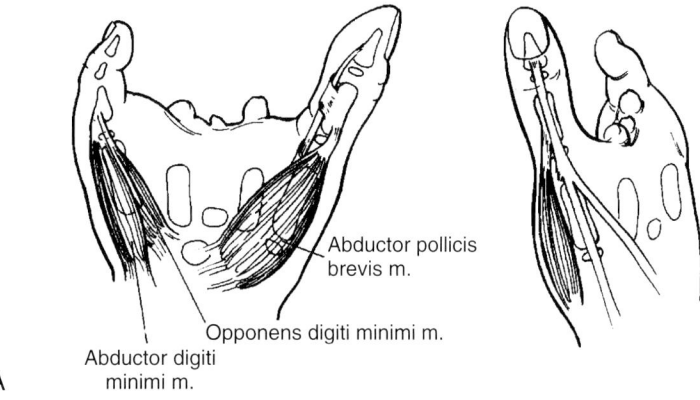

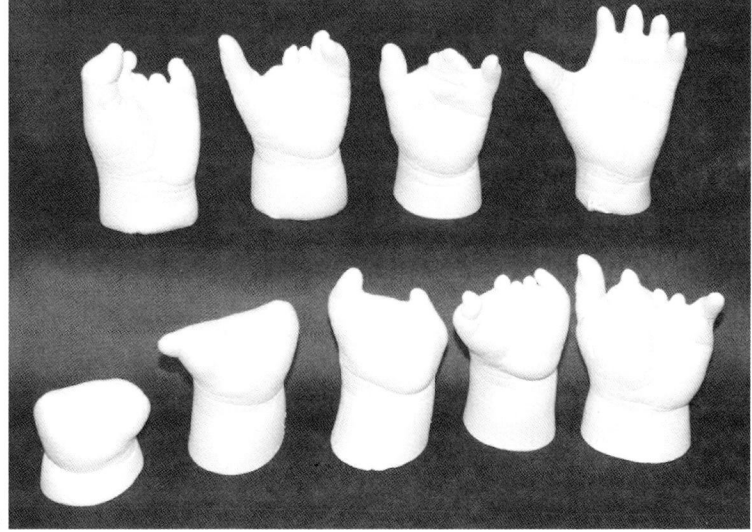

FIGURE 208-23. Symbrachydactyly thumb (atypical cleft). *A,* The border thumb and fifth rays are the most complete in the hand. Thenar and hypothenar muscles are present and often small. Central digits are represented by hypoplastic nubbins. There are all degrees of metacarpal hypoplasia within the central three rays of the hand. Extrinsic flexors and extensors are present but abnormal. *B,* A wide range of variation is present in these hands.

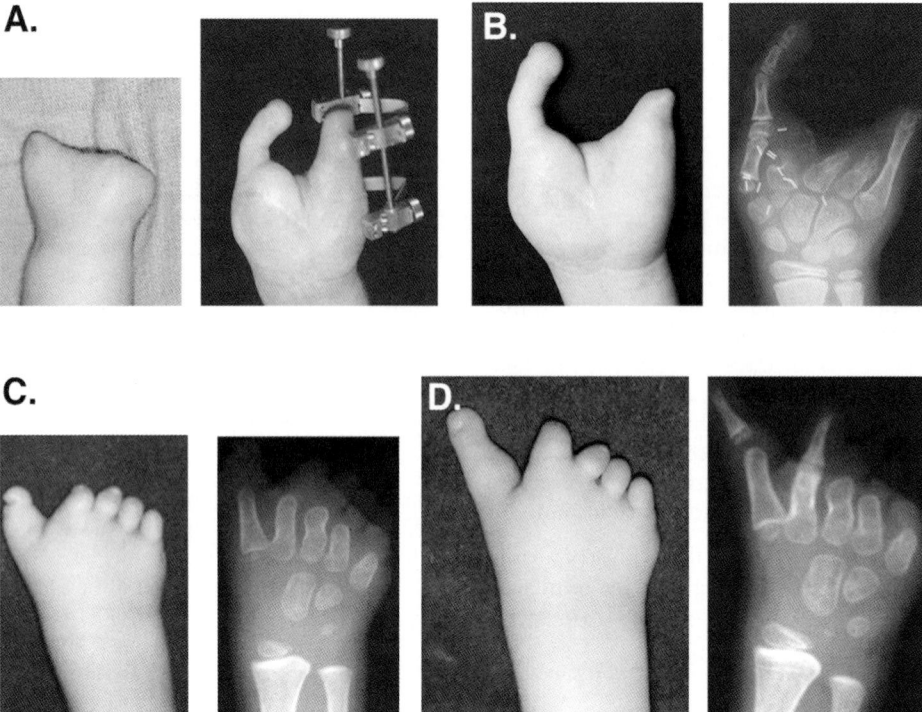

FIGURE 208-24. Symbrachydactyly (atypical cleft) thumbs. *A,* The left hand of this child with the Möbius syndrome was reconstructed with a second-toe transfer at age 18 months and is seen on the right at age 5 years during the distraction lengthening of the fifth metacarpal. The distraction was done in two stages: (1) osteotomy and application of distractor and (2) bone grafting. *B,* Ten years later, the second-toe transfer continued to grow in comparison to the ulnar metacarpal post. *C,* The left hand and radiograph of another patient with generous soft tissue nubbins, which represent the thumb and digits. *D,* He was an ideal candidate for nonvascularized toe phalangeal transfer to the thumb and index rays. The first web space was also deepened and widened with local flaps. Despite the limited mobility of the hand, he had functional use of this hand as a helper hand.

varying degrees of hypoplasia of the central three rays of the hand. Nubbins with minute nail complexes may be present on the distal border of the palm, representing the index, long, and ring fingers, but commonly these central three digits are completely absent with varying degrees of hypoplasia of the central three metacarpals.

All degrees of variation exist, and no two hands are identical. The thumb in this condition is invariably smaller with severe hypoplasia or aplasia of the phalangeal components. On occasion, a metacarpal and distal phalanx are present with a flail thumb at the MP joint level. With an intact third metacarpal, a functional adductor pollicis muscle is often present. Most of these thumbs have weak adduction power. The median-innervated thenar intrinsic muscles are usually intact and range from small to normal in size. The thumb CMC joint is well segmented and mobile, and the IP joint of the thumb may exhibit decreased passive and active motion because of weak extrinsic flexor and extensors. On exploration, the flexor pollicis longus tendon often courses to a hypoplastic or absent muscle

belly in the distal forearm. In the severely hypoplastic thumb, there is marked limitation of MP motion, an absent IP flexion crease, and only a rudimentary flexor pollicis longus tendon. The anomalies seen with the extrinsic flexors and extensors are similar to those described for the types II and IIIA hypoplastic thumbs. The fifth ray is usually the best in the hand with intact intrinsic and extrinsic musculotendinous units. This digit frequently has a radial clinodactyly and a completely unstable MP joint, and the entire hand is hypoplastic. Radius and ulna are present and of equal length but may be small in comparison to the opposite limb.

TREATMENT. Observation of these children at play will provide insight into the need for any thumb reconstruction. Children with symbrachydactyly tend to be among the most functional; virtually all can oppose (not touch) the thumb to the small finger. They all have the components of a basic hand: a mobile radial ray, a cleft, and an additional ray or post on the opposite side of the hand for pinching and grasping functions. Even those with no phalangeal components can effectively grasp or pinch using only their metacarpal motion. Consequently, most of these children will not require any operative intervention, and to do so may be meddlesome. A hypoplastic thumb with good MP motion, stable joints, and present thenar intrinsics should be left alone.

Excision of nonfunctional nubbins will improve the shape of the cleft and provide a deeper web space for grip. Some patients with this anomaly have a thumb deficient in length and unable to oppose to the highly mobile ulnar border digit. Distraction lengthening can improve both function and appearance. These patients may also lack pulp to pulp pinch because of poor pronation of the thumb during pinch maneuvers. Rotational osteotomies at the metacarpal level will resolve this problem by placing the digits in a more favorable position. The severely hypoplastic thumb with an absent or diminutive proximal phalanx and a flail MP joint is best treated with a nonvascularized toe phalangeal transfer into the proximal phalangeal level (see Fig. 208-24). Although motion is not restored, the thumb becomes a more stable, functional post. These transfers are more likely to grow if they are performed before 1 year of age. Ablation of the small distal phalanx with second-toe microvascular transfer is an option best performed between 2 and 4 years of age.

The ulnar digit in symbrachydactyly will often have an unstable MP joint and radial clinodactyly due to its asymmetric proximal phalanx. The flexor tendons are usually strong and the extensors present but unbalanced. Stabilizations of MP joints with chondrodesis, bone grafts, and nonvascularized toe phalanges have been performed with varying degrees of success. Positioned as stable posts, these fifth rays function well for hooking and balancing maneuvers. With time and growth, most of these fifth rays are lengthened with distraction techniques.

OUTCOMES. This thumb is universally smaller than the normal thumb on the contralateral hand. Once stabilized, it provides a mobile radial ray for the rest of the hand, and IP joint motion is either diminished or absent. When the IP flexion crease is absent at birth, results of attempts to restore motion with joint releases and extrinsic tendon reconstructions are dismal. Flexor tendon grafts are also disappointing because of the malformed motors in the forearm; if they are attempted, wrist flexors or extensors should be used.

Type VII: Constriction Ring Syndrome (Amniotic Band Sequence)

CLINICAL PRESENTATION. Amniotic band sequence (constriction ring syndrome, Streeter dysplasia) is a condition that can affect one limb or all limbs and less commonly the face. As defined by Patterson,[139] limb involvement can result in any of the following deformities: simple constriction rings, which may be partial or circumferential; constriction rings with distal deformity, with or without concomitant lymphedema; acrosyndactyly (distal fusion, fenestrated syndactyly); or amputations (Figs. 208-25 to 208-28).

Hypoplasia of the thumb is seen in this condition when there is a deficiency in the length of the thumb, which may have a transverse failure of formation at any level. On occasion, the existing skeletal and soft tissue components of the first ray may be hypoplastic. The hallmark of the amniotic band sequence is that the anatomy proximal to the level of amputation or level of congenital amputation is normal. Either superficial or deep constriction rings around the thumb can be associated with hypoplasia or lymphedema of the distal segment of the digit with hypoplastic nail remnants and slender, truncated phalanges present. Acrosyndactyly is usually seen to involve the central three rays of the hand but can also involve the thumb and fifth finger (see Chapter 204). Amputation of the thumb in this condition is the major cause of partial aplasia of the thumb and can occur at any position along its length. The most practical way to analyze the amputation is to place it at one of three levels: (1) distal to IP joint, (2) proximal phalanx, and (3) metacarpal (see Fig. 208-25). Motion of the IP joint is usually severely affected—even with amputations or deep constriction rings distal to it.

TREATMENT. The following principles apply to the management of these thumbs:

- Immediate treatment of emergency conditions, such as vascular compromise and progressive lymphedema.
- Early liberation of the thumb ray from an acrosyndactylous complex.
- Release of adduction contractures within the first web space when present and resurfacing with full-thickness tissue if needed before any augmentation of thumb length.

After release of the first ray, the functional requirements of the patient need to be accurately determined and the tissues available carefully assessed. In those with distal amputations at the phalangeal level at or beyond the IP joint, no operative intervention may be the best course of action. Often all that needs to be corrected is a proximal constriction ring. Although the nail and palmar pulp may be atrophic, these thumbs are functional. Instability at the IP joint is easily corrected with a collateral ligament reconstruction with either a tendon graft or local tissues (see Chapter 205). Thumb length can be augmented by one of three methods: distraction lengthening at the metacarpal

A. VII Constriction ring thumbs

B.

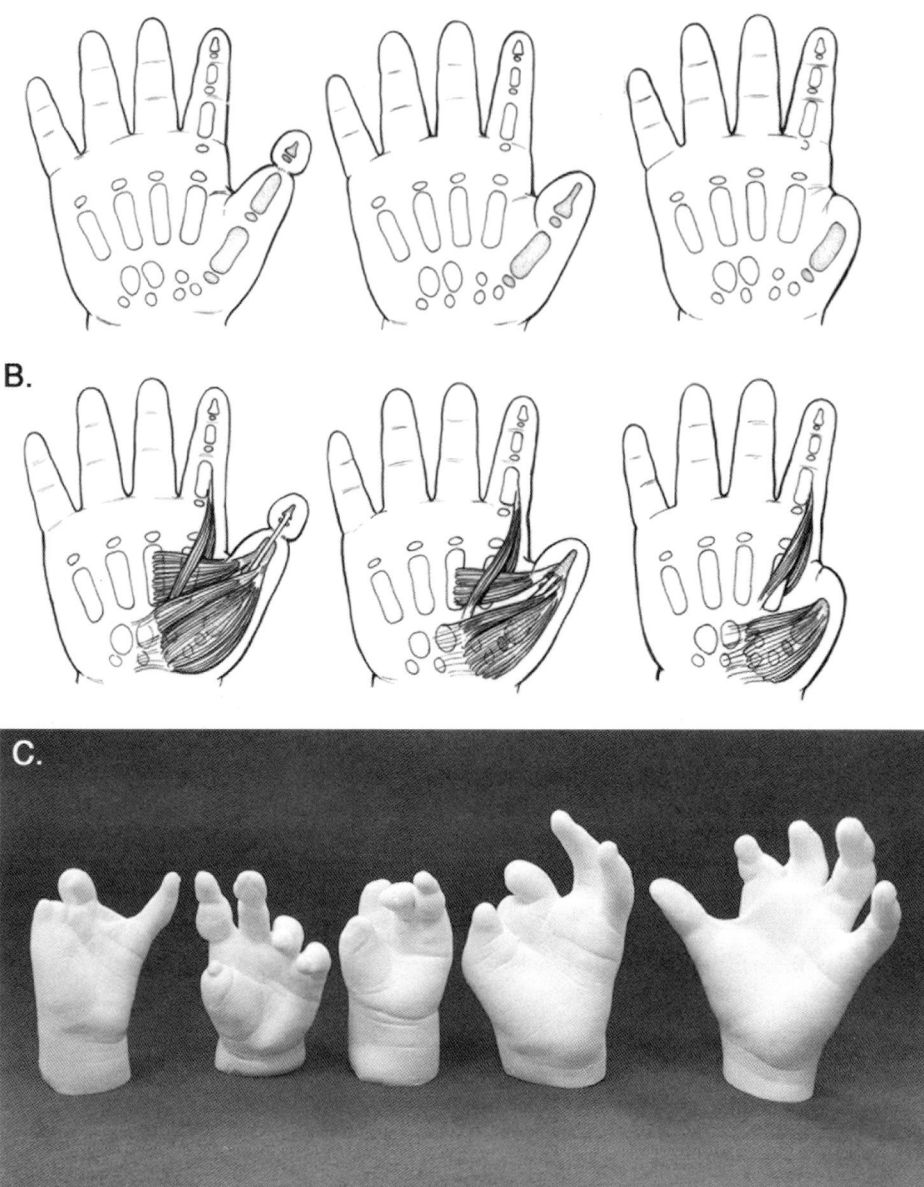

FIGURE 208-25. Constriction ring syndrome thumbs. *A,* The thumb in these hands may present with a shallow or deep constriction ring or an amputation at any level along the skeletal ray. The phalanges at the level of loss are characteristically narrow and taper to the distal stump. *B,* The intrinsic muscles are all present up to the level of the amputation. The proximal anatomy in this condition is normal. *C,* The thumb is absent on the left and shows increasing length in these molds. No two hands are identical. There is great variation in the depth and location of constriction rings along the digits.

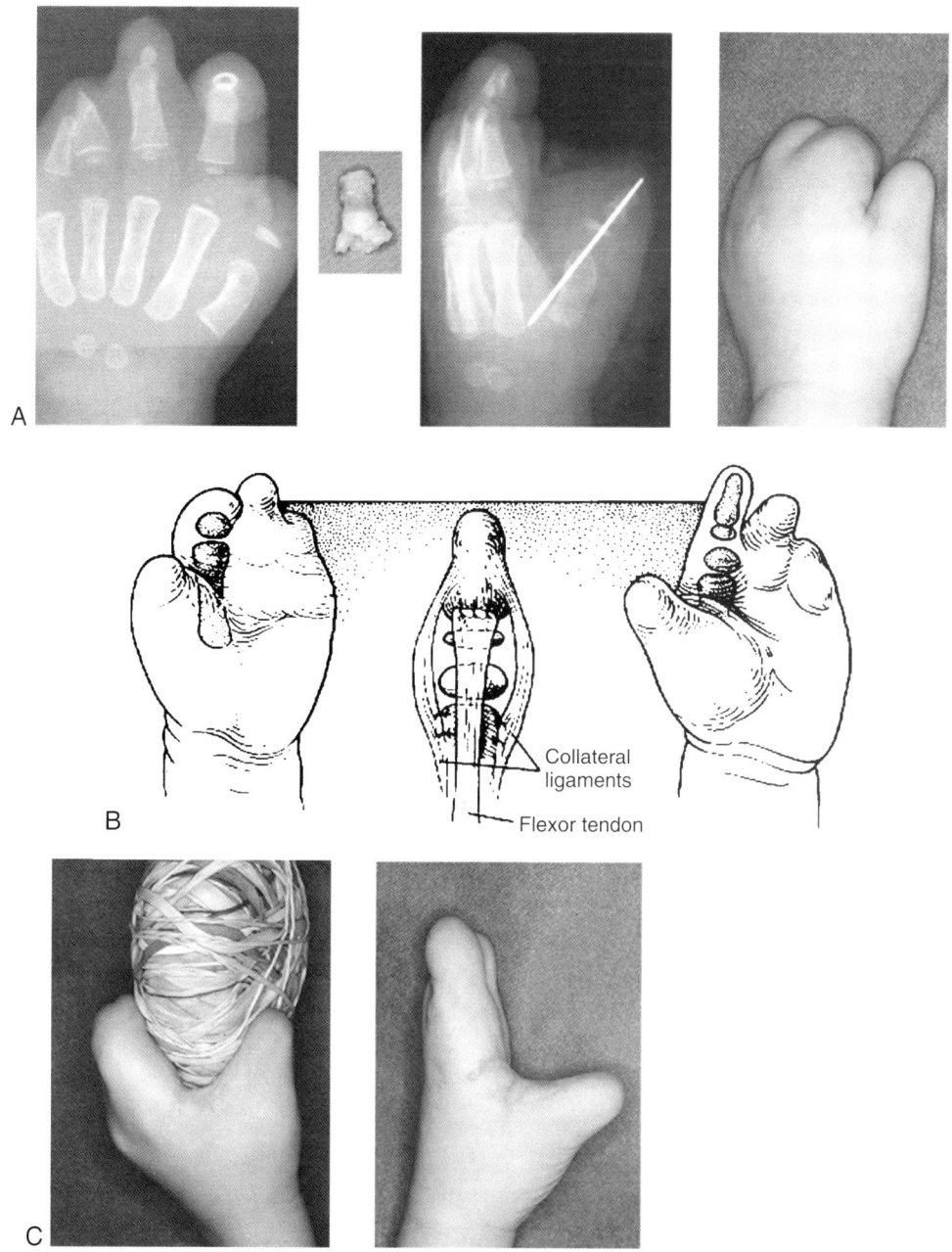

FIGURE 208-26. Constriction ring syndrome thumb treated with toe phalanx. *A,* This child with constriction ring syndrome acrosyndactyly had the fibrous connections holding all fingertips released in the newborn nursery. The thumb ends at the metaphysis of the proximal phalanx and the index finger at the middle phalanx. Nonvascularized toe phalanges from the third and fourth toes were transferred on top of the index and thumb. *B,* The periosteum is intact, and the collateral ligaments and volar plate are attached to the skeletal part at the amputation stump. Joint motion was preserved in this child. *C,* A four-flap Z-plasty deepened the first web space and improved her grasping ability. She is now 20 years old and has had normal growth of the transferred phalanges. No further reconstruction has been performed.

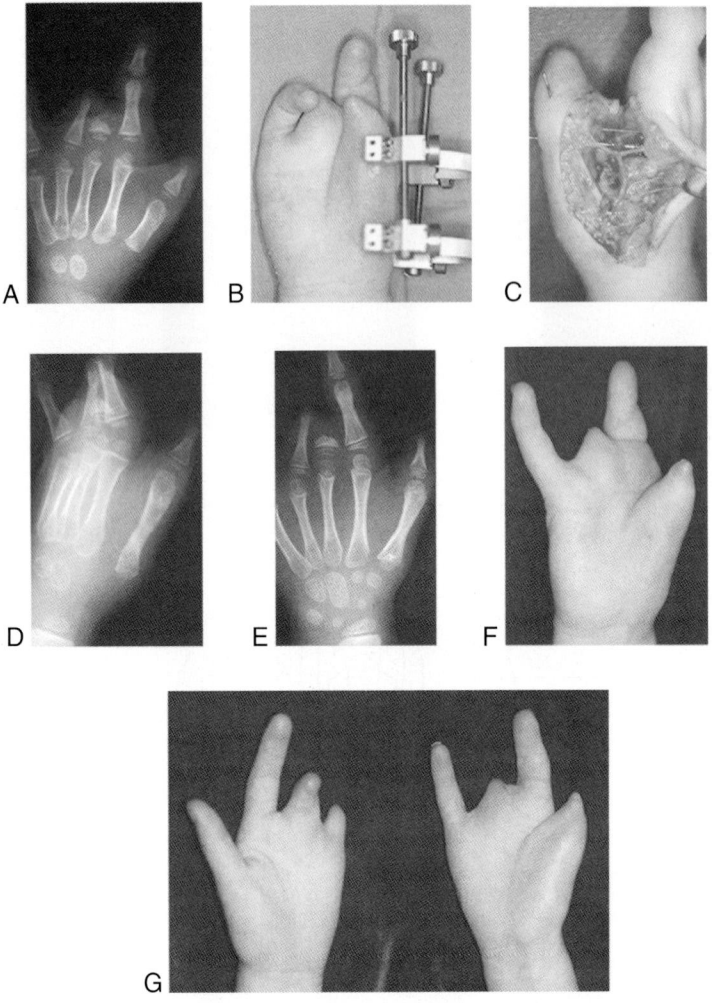

FIGURE 208-27. Constriction ring syndrome thumb treated with distraction lengthening. *A,* The radiograph of a young girl with a congenital amputation at the thumb IP joint level with a tight first web space. Note the tapered appearance of the proximal phalanx. *B,* A distraction apparatus in place is pulling each end of the metacarpal away from the osteotomy site at middiaphyseal level. One clockwise turn of the screw equaled a 1.0-mm gain. *C,* The new bone regenerate (callotasis) advances toward the midportion of the gap created. The stretching injury to soft tissue is impressive! All vessels, nerves, and tendons are intact. *D,* This thumb metacarpal is now as long as the index. *E,* Five years later, both metacarpals are growing, but the index is now longer. *F,* The first web space was deepened to increase the thumb's mobility and span. *G,* Although shorter than normal, this thumb has functioned well on her dominant hand.

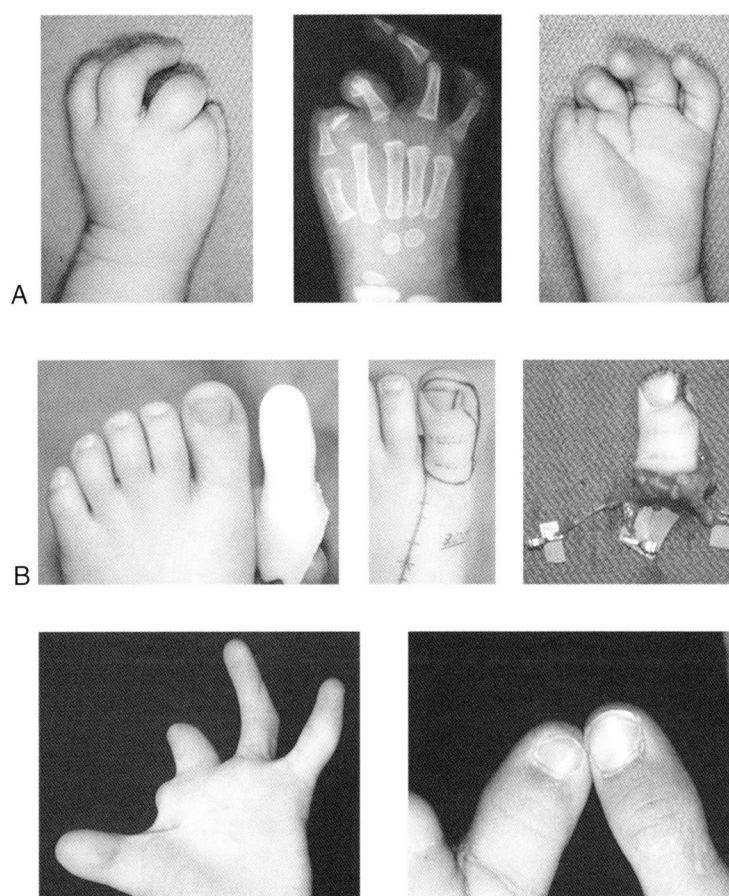

FIGURE 208-28. Constriction ring syndrome thumb treated with microvascular toe transfer. *A,* This boy, born with acrosyndactyly, demonstrated thumb loss at the IP joint level, no first web space, and congenital amputations of the index and long digits at the phalangeal level. Connecting bands present at birth were released in the newborn nursery. His first surgery was a distally based radial forearm fasciocutaneous flap to the first web space and release of the camptodactyly of the ring finger. *B,* Thumb length was augmented with a modified great-toe transfer. A methyl methacrylate mold of the opposite normal thumb is used to measure and contour the larger great toe at the time of operation. The incision markings are shown on the ipsilateral great toe, and the specimen is seen in transit to the recipient left thumb. *C,* The thumb is seen 4 years later. Sensation is normal, and motion measures 30 degrees at the IP joint and 50 degrees at the MP joint. The contour has been excellent. No revisions have been performed.

level, nonvascularized toe phalangeal transfer, and composite vascularized toe to thumb transfer.

Distraction lengthening[42,137,138] is best performed at the metacarpal level when satisfactory bone stock is present. The metacarpal can be easily—but slowly—lengthened up to 100% of its length as a two-staged procedure that includes application of distraction apparatus and osteotomy followed by bone grafting of the intercalated gap and internal fixation (see Fig. 208-27). Lengthening of deficient, terminal, and narrowed phalanges in this condition is not as predictable, and the resulting digits are often stiff and thin. Distal nonunions and exposure of phalanges or hardware used for internal fixation are common complications. Therefore, second-toe composite vascularized transfers are preferred to distraction at the phalangeal level.

Transfer of nonvascularized toe phalanges[140-142] is an excellent way to provide length and growth potential to an empty, redundant soft tissue envelope occasionally seen distal to the level of amputation in this condition. Extraperiosteal harvest and transfer of the third or fourth toe proximal phalanx will result in survival and growth of the phalanx in 90% of patients younger than 2 years (see Fig. 208-26).[140] My experience has not been as successful because only 70% of these phalanges transferred early in life have retained normal growth potential. Survival and growth will occur in patients older than 2 years but at a less predictable rate. The second toe is spared so that the entire toe is available for vascularized composite transfer if required. Secondary distraction lengthening of the transferred phalanx can be performed if further length is required.

In patients with a congenital amputation through the proximal phalanx or metacarpal, composite microvascular transfer of a second toe has been the procedure of choice. The great toe can be transferred as either a complete or a modified unit (see Fig. 208-28), but this option has been reserved for uncorrected thumb deformities, which present later in childhood. Because there is normal anatomy proximal to the level of amputation or band and there is an intact CMC joint, an excellent functional and aesthetic result of the "toe" can be obtained. The presence of functional thenar intrinsics will also enhance the result (see Fig. 208-28). In several children, I have first lengthened a deficient metacarpal with an intact CMC joint to provide a good foundation for second-toe transfer. The keys to the distraction procedure are to proceed slowly, to minimize soft tissue dissection, and to avoid injury to growth centers. The major problem with any toe transfer is the availability of toes, which—like the fingers—may be hypoplastic or aplastic in the constriction ring syndrome.

Various types of on-top-plasties have been described in the hand literature, and most consist of transfer and distal advancement of composite soft tissue and bone segments from adjacent fingers. I prefer free transfers to these local transfers, which tend to require extensive dissection and secondary contractures within the first web space. However, local ray transfers as pollicization procedures can be effective, especially when the index ray is transferred to augment the thumb. A careful surgeon should avoid injury to the median- and ulnar-innervated thenar intrinsic muscles, including the adductor pollicis and its origin from the third metacarpal.

Outcomes. The functional outcome of a thumb with a congenital amputation at the IP joint level is excellent, provided there is a broad, unscarred web space between the thumb and the next digit. Thumbs lengthened with nonvascularized toe phalangeal transfers have the advantage of increased length with little mobility at the MP joint level. Thumbs lengthened with vascularized toe transfers have the advantages of normal length and normal sensation if the transfer is performed in young children and the disadvantage of less than normal motion.[89] The functional results of these transfers in this group are superior because of the normal anatomic motors in the forearm.

Type VIII: Five-Fingered Hand

Clinical Presentation. In this type of hypoplasia, the thumb is smaller in width and longer and has the characteristics of a finger. As the radial border digit, it lies in the same plane as the ulnar four digits and is nonopposable. It is usually the same length as the adjacent index finger. The digit is slender and may be joined to the index finger in an incomplete simple syndactyly. The first web is often severely deficient or nonexistent, and some type of transverse metacarpal ligament is also present. The skeletal anatomy is similar to that of the index ray: a metacarpal with a distal growth center and three phalanges with proximal growth centers. The scaphoid is usually absent or hypoplastic. The thenar muscles (abductor pollicis brevis, flexor

pollicis brevis, opponens pollicis) are also absent, as is the adductor pollicis. Instead, the usual digital intrinsics are present, namely, a lumbrical, palmar interosseous, and dorsal interosseous (Fig. 208-29). The extrinsic flexors and extensors mimic those of the normal fingers. Because the radial digit lies in the same plane as the other fingers in the hand, manipulation of objects is usually performed by using lateral scissoring between the first two digits—or between the second and third if a first web syndactyly is present. Left untreated, those patients without a first web syndactyly tend to attenuate the transverse metacarpal ligament and "autopollicize" into an abducted and slightly pronated posture.

Treatment. The optimal management of these patients is to pollicize the radial digit. The technique employed is similar to that for thumb aplasia (type V). Rebalancing of the intrinsic musculature is paramount to the success of the procedure. In the five-fingered hand anomaly, the dorsal interosseous to the radial digit is only unipennate, and secondary opponensplasty with an abductor digiti quinti minimi or ring flexor digitorum superficialis transfer is occasionally necessary. The most important procedure is the construction of a broad first web space with unscarred flap tissue.

In childhood or during adolescence, two other options are available: (1) the construction of a first web space with a forearm flap plus arthrodesis of the PIP joint or (2) a rotational recession osteotomy of the first metacarpal with pollicization and intrinsic rebalancing (Fig. 208-30). This condition should not be confused with a triphalangeal thumb, in which the thumb is somewhat shorter than the other digits. Although an extra phalanx is present by definition, extrinsic and intrinsic muscle anatomy mimics a thumb more than a finger. The extra phalanx is often angulated and is commonly associated with radial polydactyly.

Outcomes. The results are similar to those described for index pollicization without radial dysplasia. Similar outcomes have been achieved in those who had forearm flaps followed by rotation-recession osteotomies at the metacarpal level. These thumbs are all well positioned in palmar abduction but lack forceful adduction, power pinch, and grasp. The thumbs are long and slender and do not have normal or close to normal key pinch and thumb to index grasping strength.

Type IX: Radial Polydactyly

Clinical Presentation. Despite the level of duplication, each partner thumb is hypoplastic to varying degrees, with the radial duplicate usually being the most

VIII Five-fingered hand

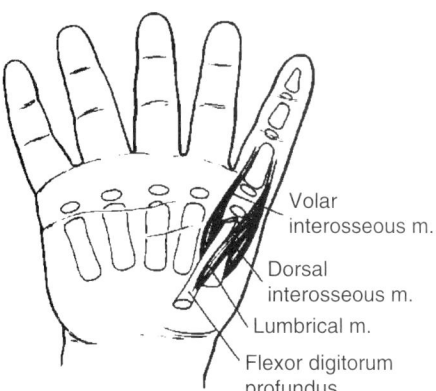

Volar
interosseous m.

Dorsal
interosseous m.

Lumbrical m.

Flexor digitorum
profundus

A

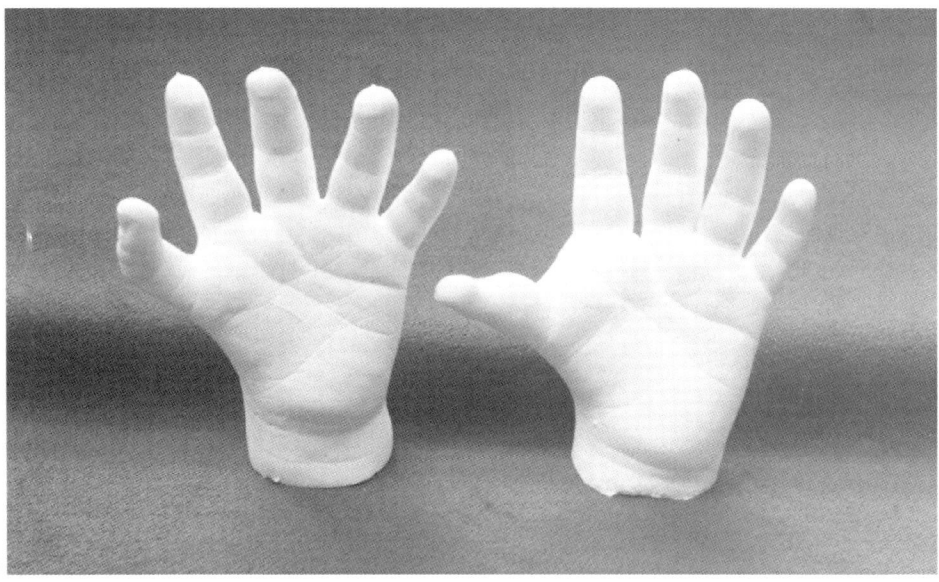

B

FIGURE 208-29. Five-fingered hand. *A,* In the five-fingered hand, the normal complement of median-innervated thenar intrinsic muscles is absent. First dorsal interosseous, volar interosseous, and lumbrical muscles are present in this ray, which anatomically is a digit, not a thumb. *B,* The clinical appearance (preoperative) on the left shows that the patient has tried to flex and autopronate this ray to become a thumb.

severely affected (see Chapter 206). The complexity of the deformity and therefore of the surgical correction increases as the level of the duplication progresses proximally. Associated triphalangia of the ulnar partner further complicates any surgical reconstruction. Specific abnormalities in each duplicate are seen in the nail plate, the osteoarticular column, and both the intrinsic and extrinsic musculotendinous units of each thumb. The nail plate of each duplicate is always narrower than that of the unaffected thumb, and the entire skeletal ray is hypoplastic in duplications proximal to the MP joint.

Musculotendinous abnormalities are common, with the extrinsic extensor almost universally shared.

Indeed, nearly half of the patients described in papers on pollex abductus have duplicate thumbs.[34,37] Deviation of the partners toward each other indicates abnormal insertions of the extrinsic tendons into the distal phalanges, and connections between the extrinsic flexors and extensors are not unusual. These tendinous interconnections will limit function and cause digital angulations. The first web is usually unaffected in duplications involving the distal phalanx, but as the level of duplication lies more proximally, the first web space becomes increasingly deficient.

Treatment. The management of patients with duplications of the thumb varies according to the level

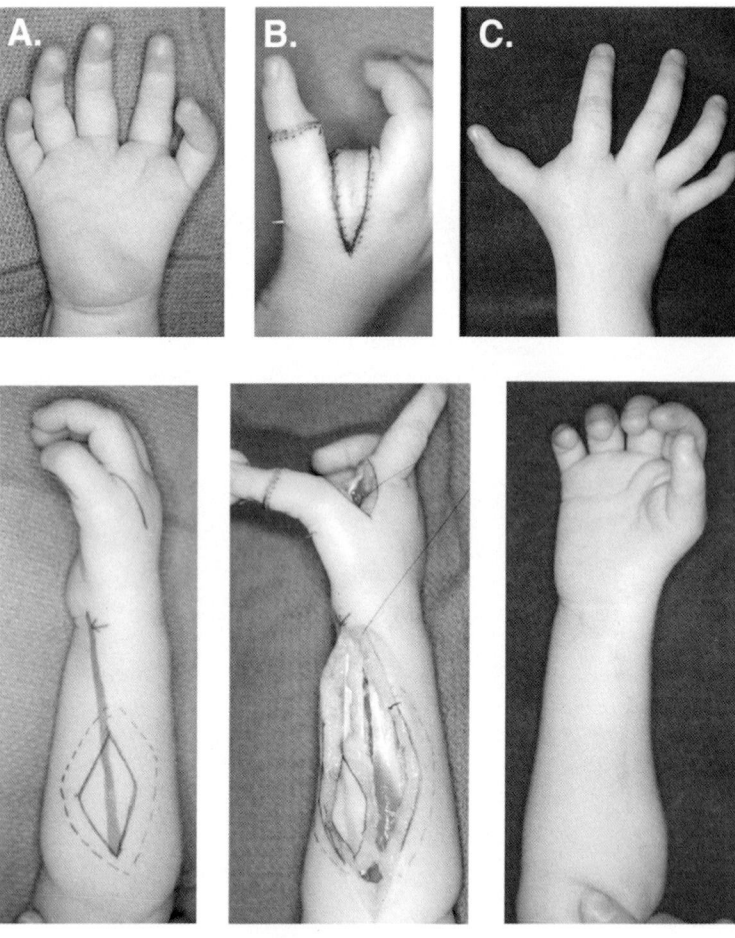

Radial forearm fasciocutaneous flap

FIGURE 208-30. Five-fingered hand. *A,* The right hand of a child with bilateral five-fingered hands is shown. She has autorotated the most radial digit into a pseudothumb position in an effort to function more effectively. *B,* In one procedure, the thumb was shortened and fused at the PIP joint and a first web space constructed with a radial forearm fasciocutaneous flap; below, it is seen before, during, and 5 years after the procedure. A superficial flexor tendon was transferred to improve palmar abduction (opposition). *C,* There has been no contracture or diminution of this web space, which was lined with full-thickness flap tissue.

of duplication and is discussed in more detail in Chapter 206. In general, the surgeon should use the best parts of each thumb to construct the finest thumb possible. Distal duplications (types I and II) are usually managed by preservation of the ulnar duplicate, with extra soft tissue provided from the radial thumb. The resulting nail is smaller than the one on the normal side. The Bilhaut-Cloquet procedure is avoided if possible because of the predictable problems of nail ridging and diminished IP joint motion. The results can, however, be excellent with the more distal level duplications. In addition, duplications at the proximal phalangeal level (types III and IV) are commonly managed with ablation of the radial partner and closure with tissue from this thumb. Musculotendinous abnormalities need to be addressed with the division of interconnections and centralization of insertions. Advancement of the detached thenar intrinsics into the retained extensor mechanism is mandatory, and collateral ligament preservation and

reattachment are key to providing a stable MP joint. The metacarpal head will be broad in these patients and requires trimming on the redundant radial side. Closing wedge osteotomy of the metacarpal may also be required to realign the newly constructed thumb. Appropriate trimming of excess skin should result in wound closure, which should be positioned in the high midaxial position. Duplication in the metacarpal shaft (type V) can often be managed by simple ablation of the radial partner and concomitant four-flap Z-plasty for any first web deficiency. Duplications at the CMC joint level (type VI) and triphalangeal varieties need to be dealt with on their merit. Digital transposition of the ulnar thumb onto the retained base of the radial partner is not unusual. Skeletal realignment, tendon repositioning, and first web releases can usually be completed in a single stage.

OUTCOMES. The results are presented in Chapter 206.

Type X: Syndromic Short Skeletal Thumb Ray

APERT AND PFEIFFER SYNDROMES

CLINICAL PRESENTATION. Deficiencies of the osteoarticular column of the thumb may result in a short, hypoplastic thumb (Figs. 208-31 and 208-32). Bone abnormalities can occur in isolated bone (brachymetacarpia, brachyphalangia); to all bones in combination; or as part of a generalized syndrome, such as the acrocephalosyndactyly (e.g., Apert, Pfeiffer, Carpenter) syndromes or the Rubinstein-Taybi syndrome. Joint function is usually impaired on either side of the abnormal bones. In patients with anomalies of a single bone, brachymetacarpia or brachyphalangia, the remaining components of the thumb tend to be unaffected; in patients with generalized syndromes, other abnormalities of the thumb components are common. In the acrocephalosyndactyly syndromes, delta phalanges are common. They usually involve the proximal phalanx with a longitudinal epiphyseal bracket on the radial side. This abnormal growth plate checks growth on the radial side and results in a radial clinodactyly of the thumb, which becomes more severe over time. The metacarpal is usually short, and the distal phalanx is short and broad. Incidentally, many believe that the abnormal proximal phalanx and broad distal phalanx are variations of a duplication. Musculotendinous anomalies are associated with poor joint function but are not as common as those with type IIIA thumbs. Deficiencies of the first web are most common, occurring along a spectrum of mild

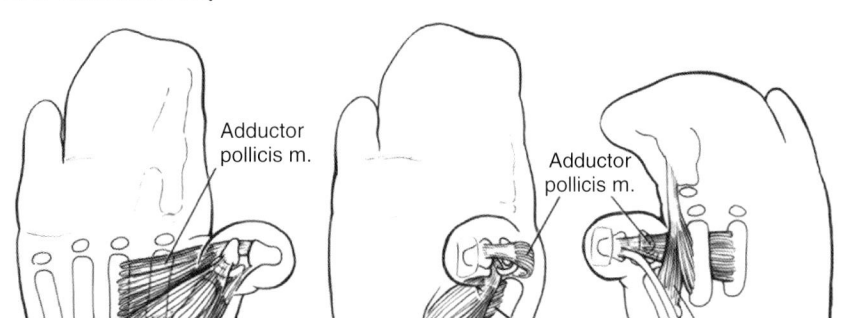

A. X Short skeletal ray

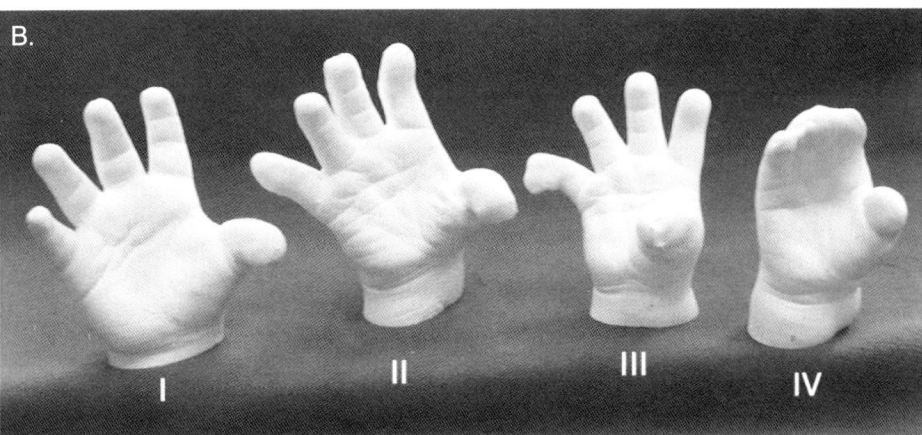

FIGURE 208-31. Type X, short skeletal ray. *A,* A short thumb with or without radial clinodactyly is seen in many syndromes. The primary osseous abnormalities are usually seen at the proximal phalangeal joint level. The median- and ulnar-innervated intrinsic muscles are all present and hypertrophied. Extrinsic and intrinsic flexors and extensors are normal up to the phalangeal level. *B,* The left thumbs of children with four different syndromes all look similar. I, Rubinstein-Taybi; II, Pfeiffer; III, Greig cephalopolysyndactyly; and IV, Apert acrocephalosyndactyly.

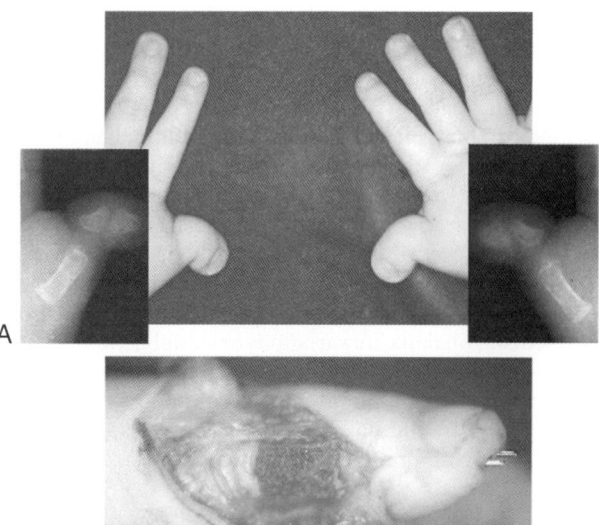

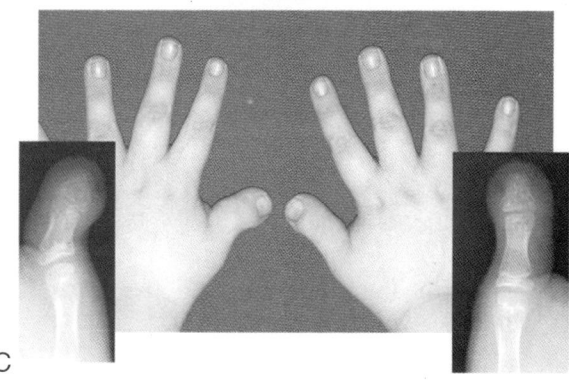

FIGURE 208-32. Type X, short skeletal ray. *A,* The preoperative appearance and thumb radiographs of a young boy with bilateral radial clinodactyly of the thumbs ("hitchhiker thumbs") associated with the Rubenstein-Taybi syndrome. *B,* The soft tissue was lengthened on the radial side with a large Z-plasty, and a composite graft and the bone seen lengthened here with an opening wedge osteotomy and corticocancellous bone graft were held with two C wires. *C,* The same thumbs are seen 7 years later. The right side has grown normally, and on the left side, the deformity has recurred because of the premature closure of the most radial border of the physis.

adduction contracture to complex syndactyly involving the first two rays.

The whole spectrum of metabolic bone diseases, skeletal dysplasias, benign skeletal tumors, and many syndromes may include thumb hypoplasia. In general, little surgical correction is required for these youngsters. The need for surgical improvement is determined by critical observation of these children at play.

TREATMENT. Many patients with short thumbs that are not associated with generalized conditions do not require any treatment because the length deficiency is mild. In those who do have an obvious length deficiency, distraction lengthening with a secondary bone graft to the subsequent bone defect at the metacarpal level is possible.

Patients with generalized syndromes require a multidisciplinary approach to their management, and hand procedures can be coordinated with other required treatments. Children with complex hand anomalies, such as those with Apert syndrome, require special attention so that the function of these thumbs and hands can be optimized.

First web syndactylies need to be managed in the first 3 to 6 months of life so that the child can develop with his or her thumb released before the development of prehension. The options for treatment are the same as those outlined in a previous section. The deficiency of the first web in the majority of the children with craniosynostoses can be adequately treated with a four-flap Z-plasty. In the more complex type II and type III hand anomalies[42] in Apert syndrome, in which there is complete syndactyly of the first web, tissue expansion of the first web is a satisfactory means of producing a long-lasting release of the first web.[44] The deficiencies of length and angulation in these complex anomalies are best managed by a later osteotomy and an iliac crest bone graft. Because these bones are quite small, this procedure is usually delayed until 4 or 5 years of age.

OUTCOMES. Results must be individualized to the specific thumb condition. For those with the Apert syndrome, the thumb is longer, motion is present at the MP and CMC joints, and the degree of independent function depends more on the quality of the first web space.

Thumbs that have been lengthened with distraction techniques are longer, thinner at the phalangeal level, and stiffer at joints distal to the distraction. If distraction is performed slowly, at approximately 0.5 mm/day, damage to the intrinsic muscles is minimized.

REFERENCES

1. Edgerton M, Snyder G, Webb W: Surgical treatment of congenital thumb deformities (including impact of correction). J Bone Joint Surg Am 1965;47:1453-1474.
2. Caffey J: Pediatric X-ray Diagnosis: A Textbook for Students and Practitioners of Pediatrics, Surgery and Radiology, 7th ed. Chicago, Year Book, 1978.
3. Lister G: Absent tendons excluding thumb deficiencies. In Buck-Gramcko D, ed: Congenital Malformations of the Hand and Forearm. London, Churchill Livingstone, 1998:327-330.
4. Flatt A: The Care of Congenital Hand Anomalies. St. Louis, CV Mosby, 1977:55-79.
5. Bayne LG, Klug MS: Long-term review of the surgical treatment of radial deficiencies. J Hand Surg Am 1987;12:169-179.
6. Buck-Gramcko U, Buck-Gramcko D: Free toe transplantation in congenital hand defects. Handchir Mikrochir Plast Chir 1995;27:181-188.
7. Blauth W: The hypoplastic thumb [in German]. Arch Orthop Unfallchir 1967;62:225-246.
8. Müller W: Die angeborenen Fehlbildungen der menschlichen Hand. Leipzig, Germany, Thieme, 1937.
9. Manske PR, McCarroll HR Jr: Reconstruction of the congenitally deficient thumb. Hand Clin 1992;8:177-196.
10. Coombs C, Upton J: The hypoplastic and absent thumb. In Bentz M, ed: Pediatric Plastic Surgery. Stamford, Conn, Appleton & Lange, 1997:907-957.
11. Entin M: Congenital anomalies of the upper extremity. Surg Clin North Am 1960;40:497.
12. Entin M: Reconstruction of congenital anomalies of the upper extremities. J Bone Joint Surg Am 1959;41:681-701.
13. Fanconi G: Familiare infantile perniziosaartige anamie. Jahrbuch Kinder 1927;117:257.
14. Auerbach AD, Rogatko A, Schroeder-Kurth TM: International Fanconi Anemia Registry: relation of clinical symptoms to diepoxybutane sensitivity. Blood 1989;73:391-396.
15. Alter BP: Fanconi's anemia: current concepts. Am J Pediatr Hematol Oncol 1992;145:170-176.
16. Giampietro PF, Adler-Brecher B, Verlander PC, et al: The need for a more accurate and timely diagnosis in Fanconi anemia: a report of the International Fanconi Anemia Registry. Pediatrics 1993;91:1116-1120.
17. Blauth W, Schneider-Sickert F: Congenital Deformities of the Hand: An Atlas of Their Surgical Treatment. Berlin, Springer-Verlag, 1981:10-72.
18. Su C, Hoopes JE, Daniel R: Congenital absence of the thenar muscles innervated by the median nerve: report of a case. J Bone Joint Surg Am 1972;54:1087-1090.
19. O'Rahilly R: Morphological patterns in limb deficiencies and duplications. Am J Anat 1951;89:135-194.
20. Lane W: Abnormal muscle of the hand. J Anat Phys 1887;21:674.
21. Miura T, Komada T: Single method for reconstruction of the cleft hand with an adducted thumb. Plast Reconstr Surg 1979;64:65-67.
22. Blair W, Buckwalter JA: Congenital malposition of the flexor pollicis longus—an anatomy note. J Hand Surg Am 1983;8:93-94.
23. Blair W, Omer GE Jr: Anomalous insertion of the flexor pollicis. J Hand Surg 1981;6:241-244.
24. Graham T, Cleveland OH, Louis DS: A comprehensive approach to surgical management of the type IIIA hypoplastic thumb. J Hand Surg Am 1998;23:3-13.
25. Dellon A, Rayan G: Congenital absence of the thenar muscles: report of two cases. J Bone Joint Surg Am 1981;63:1014-1015.
26. Fitch RD, Urbaniak JR, Ruderman RJ: Conjoined flexor and extensor pollicis longus tendons in the hypoplastic thumb. J Hand Surg Am 1984;9:417-419.
27. Strauch B: Dorsal thumb flap for release of adduction contracture of the first web space. Bull Hosp Joint Dis 1975;36:34-39.
28. Manske PR, McCarroll HR Jr, James M: Type III-A hypoplastic thumb. J Hand Surg Am 1995;20:246-253.
29. Miura T: An appropriate treatment for postoperative Z-formed deformity of the duplicated thumb. J Hand Surg Am 1977;2:380-386.
30. Koster G: Isolated aplasia of the flexor pollicis longus: a case report. J Hand Surg Am 1984;9:870-871.
31. Tsuchida Y, Kasai S, Kojima T: Congenital absence of the flexor pollicis longus and brevis: a case report. Hand 1976;8:294-297.
32. Arminio J: Congenital anomaly of the thumb: absent flexor pollicis longus tendon. J Hand Surg 1979;4:487-488.
33. Chase R: Discussion of pollex abductus due to congenital malposition of the flexor pollicis longus. J Bone Joint Surg Am 1969;51:1290.
34. Lister G: Pollex abductus in hypoplasia and duplication of the thumb. J Hand Surg Am 1991;16:626-633.
35. Neviaser R: Congenital hypoplasia of the thumb with absence of the extrinsic extensors, abductor pollicis longus and thenar muscles. J Hand Surg 1979;4:301-303.
36. Kobayashi A, Ohmiya K, Iwakuma T, Mitsuyasu M: Unusual congenital anomalies of the thumb extensors: report of two cases. Hand 1976;8:17-21.
37. Tupper J: Pollex abductus due to congenital malposition of the flexor pollicis longus. J Bone Joint Surg Am 1969;51:1285-1290.
38. Kleinman WB: Management of thumb hypoplasia. Hand Clin 1990;6:617-641.
39. Manske PR, Rotman MB, Dailey LA: Long-term functional results after pollicization for the congenitally deficient thumb. J Hand Surg Am 1992;17:1064-1072.
40. Buck-Gramcko D: Congenital malformations. In Lister G, ed: Hand Surgery. Stuttgart, Thieme, 1988:12.1-12.114.
41. Littler J: Reconstruction of the thumb. The Monks Lecture. 1977.
42. Upton J: Treatment of congenital forearm and hand anomalies. In May JW Jr, Littler JW, eds: The Hand. Philadelphia, WB Saunders, 1990:5352-5356. McCarthy J, ed: Plastic Surgery; vol 8.
43. Flatt A: The Absent Thumb in Congenital Hand Anomalies, 2nd ed. St. Louis, Quality Medical Publishing, 1994:96-119.
44. Coombs CJ, Mutimer KL: Tissue expansion for the treatment of complete syndactyly of the first web. J Hand Surg Am 1994;19:968-972.
45. Caroli A, Zanasi S: First web-space reconstruction by Caroli's technique in congenital hand deformities with severe thumb ray adduction. Br J Plast Surg 1989;42:653-659.
46. Friedman R, Wood VE: The dorsal transposition flap for congenital contractures of the first web space: a 20 year experience. J Hand Surg Am 1997;22:664-670.
47. Lister G: The choice of procedure following thumb amputation. Clin Orthop 1985;195:45-51.
48. Manske PR, McCaroll HR Jr: Index finger pollicization for a congenitally absent or nonfunctioning thumb. J Hand Surg Am 1985;10:606-613.

49. Manske PR, McCaroll HR Jr: Abductor digiti minimi opponensplasty in congenital radial dysplasia. J Hand Surg Am 1978;3:552-559.

50. Foucher G, Greant P, Merle M, Michon J: Congenital abnormalities of the thumb. Contribution of microsurgical technics [in French]. Chirurgie 1988;114:60-66.

51. Foucher G, Navarro R, Medina J, Allieu Y: Pollicization, remains of the past or current operation [in French]. Bull Acad Natl Med 2000;184:1241-1253.

52. Cooney WP 3rd, Wood MB: Microvascular reconstruction of congenital anomalies and post-traumatic lesions in children. Hand Clin 1992;8:131-146.

53. Reichert B, Berger A: Microsurgical tissue transplantation for correction of hand abnormalities [in German]. Handchir Mikrochir Plast Chir 1994;26:200-205, discussion 206.

54. Nishijima N, Matsumoto T, Yamamuro T: Two-stage reconstruction for the hypoplastic thumb. J Hand Surg Am 1995;20:415-419.

55. Barsky A: Congenital Anomalies of the Hand and Their Surgical Treatment. Springfield, Ill, Charles C Thomas, 1958:114-121.

56. Barsky A: Congenital anomalies of the thumb. Clin Orthop 1959;15:96-110.

57. Matthews D: Congenital absence of functioning thumb. Plast Reconstr Surg 1960;26:487-493.

58. Yamauchi Y, Fujimaki A, Yanagihara Y, Yoshizaki K: Reconstruction of floating thumb—especially on the use of vascularized metatarsophalangeal joint grafting. Seikeigeka Mook 1979;30:1645-1648.

59. Ono H, Yajima H, Tamai S, Mizomoto S: Vascularized toe joint transfer for floating thumb. J Jpn Soc Surg Hand 1979;8:510-514.

60. Foucher G, Medina J, Navarro R: Microsurgical reconstruction of the hypoplastic thumb, type IIIB. J Reconstr Microsurg 2001;17:9-15.

61. Fujimaki A, Yamauchi Y: Application of microsurgery in congenital anomaly of the hand. Seikeigeka Mook 1984;35:142-150.

62. Kanaya F, Tokeshi M, Annri H, et al: Transposition of the third metatarsus for the reconstruction of Blauth type III hypoplastic thumb. J Jpn Soc Surg Hand 1996;12:776-780.

63. Horii E, Nakamura R, Innoye G, et al: Functional assessment for thumb hypoplasia by questionnaire. J Jpn Soc Surg Hand 1996;12:772-775.

64. Tajima T, ed: Reconstruction of the floating thumb. In Buck-Gramcko D, ed: Congenital Malformations of the Hand and Forearm. London, Churchill Livingstone, 1998:369-373.

65. Tsai TM, Lim BH: Free vascularized transfer of the metatarsophalangeal and proximal interphalangeal joints of the second toe for reconstruction of the metacarpophalangeal joints of the thumb and index finger using a single vascular pedicle. Plast Reconstr Surg 1996;98:1080-1086.

66. Barsky A: Cleft hand: classification, incidence and treatment. Review of the literature and report of nineteen cases. J Bone Joint Surg Am 1964;46:1707-1720.

67. Blauth W: Indication and technics of the index-finger thumb in thumb aplasia [in German]. Handchirurgie 1969;1:28-33.

68. Buck-Gramcko D: Pollicization of the index in case of aplasia and hypoplasia of the thumb. Methods and results [in French]. Rev Chir Orthop Reparatrice Appar Mot 1971;57:35-48.

69. Tajima T: Classification of thumb hypoplasia. Hand Clin 1985;1:577-594.

70. Shabata M, Yoshizu T, Seki T, et al: Reconstruction of hypoplastic thumb using toe transfer. In Yastamaki M, ed: Current Trends in Hand Surgery. Amsterdam, Elsevier, 1995:467-471.

71. Tajima T, Watanabe Y, Uchiyama J: Treatment and study of the hypoplastic thumb [in Japanese]. Keisei Geka 1967;10:227-234.

72. Gilbert A: Current treatment of malformations of the hand [in French]. Chirurgie 1990;116:180-183.

73. Percival NJ, Sykes PJ, Chandraprakasam T: A method of assessment of pollicisation. J Hand Surg Br 1991;16:141-143.

74. Roper BA, Turnbull TJ: Functional assessment after pollicisation. J Hand Surg Br 1986;11:399-403.

75. Sekiguchi J, Ohmori K, Kobayashi S, et al: Functional results after pollicization in congenital cases. J Jpn Soc Surg Hand 1994;10:890-894.

76. Harrison SH: Pollicization for congenital deformities of the hand. Proc R Soc Med 1973;66:634-637.

77. Kozin SH, Weiss AA, Webber JB, et al: Index finger pollicization for congenital aplasia or hypoplasia of the thumb. J Hand Surg Am 1992;17:880-884.

78. Buck-Gramcko D: Pollicization in congenital malformations of the hand and forearm. In Buck-Gramcko D, ed: Congenital Malformations of the Hand and Forearm. London, Churchill Livingstone, 1998:379-402.

79. Langlais F, Malek R: Pollicizations in congenital malformations of the thumb. Indications, technical problems, results, apropos of 30 cases [in French]. Ann Chir 1973;27:1217-1223.

80. Sykes PJ, Chandraprakasam T, Percival NJ: Pollicization of the index finger in congenital anomalies. J Hand Surg Br 1991;16:144-147.

81. Bartlett GR, Coombs CJ, Johnstone BR: Primary shortening of the pollicized long flexor tendon in congenital pollicization. J Hand Surg Am 2001;26:595-598.

82. Egloff DV, Verdan C: Pollicization of the index finger for reconstruction of the congenitally hypoplastic or absent thumb. J Hand Surg Am 1983;8:839-848.

83. Upton J: Pollicization for the aplastic thumb. In Marsh J, ed: Current Therapy in Plastic and Reconstructive Surgery: Trunk and Extremities. Philadelphia, BC Decker, 1989:232-236.

84. Sandzen SJ: Classification and functional management of congenital central defect of the hand. Hand Clin 1985;1:483-498.

85. Woolf R, Broadbent T: The four-flap Z-plasty. Plast Reconstr Surg 1972;49:48-51.

86. Hirshowitz B, Karev A, Rousso M: Combined double Z-plasty and Y-V advancement for thumb web contracture. Hand 1975;7:291.

87. Flatt A: The Care of Congenital Hand Anomalies, 2nd ed. St. Louis, Quality Medical Publishing, 1994:292-314.

88. Upton J, Havlik RJ, Coombs CJ: Use of forearm flaps for the severely contracted first web space in children with congenital malformations. J Hand Surg Am 1996;21:470-477.

89. Kay SE, Wiberg M, Bellew M, Webb F: Toe to hand transfer in children. Part 2. Functional and psychological aspects. J Hand Surg Br 1996;21:735-745.

90. Bunnell S: Surgery of the Hand, 3rd ed. Philadelphia, JB Lippincott, 1956:81-91.

91. Furnas D, Fischer G: The Z-plasty: biomechanics and mathematics. Br J Plast Surg 1971;24:144-160.

92. Fereshetian S, Upton J: The anatomy and management of the thumb in Apert syndrome. Clin Plast Surg 1991;18:365-380.

93. Brown D, Upton J, Khouri R: Free flap coverage of the hand. Clin Plast Surg 1997;24:57-62.

94. Littler J, Cooley S: Opposition of the thumb and its restoration by abductor digiti quinti transfer. J Bone Joint Surg Am 1963;45:1389-1396.

95. Ogino T, Minami A, Fukuda K: Abductor digiti minimi opponensplasty in hypoplastic thumb. J Hand Surg Br 1986;11:372-377.

96. Huber E: Hilssoperation bei Medianuslahung. Dtsch Z Chir 1921;162:271-275.

97. Lister G: The choice of procedure following thumb amputations. Clin Orthop 1985;195:45-51.

98. Oberlin C, Gilbert A: Transfer of the abductor digiti minimi (quinti) in radial deformities of the hand in children. Ann Chir Main 1984;3:215-220.

99. Lister G: Pollex abductus. Presented at the Symposium on Congenital Deformities of the Upper Limb, Paris, 1988.
100. Lister G: Intraosseous wiring of the digital skeleton. J Hand Surg Am 1978;3:427-435.
101. Gosset J: La pollicisation de l'index. (Technique chirurgicale.) J Chir (Paris) 1949;65:403-413.
102. Hilgenfeldt O: Operativer Daumenersatz und Beseitigung von Greifstorungen bei Fingerverlusten. Stuttgart, Ferdinand Enke Verlag, 1950.
103. Bunnell S: Digit transfer by neurovascular pedicle. J Bone Joint Surg Am 1952;34:772-774.
104. Littler J: The neurovascular pedicle method of digital transposition for reconstruction of the thumb. Plast Reconstr Surg 1953;12:303-319.
105. Harrison SH: Pollicisation in children. Hand 1971;3:204-210.
106. Malek R, Grossman JA: The skin incision in pollicization. J Hand Surg Am 1985;10:305-306.
107. White W: Fundamental priorities in pollicisation. J Bone Joint Surg Br 1970;52:438-443.
108. Zancolli E: Transplantation of the index finger in the absence of the thumb. J Bone Joint Surg Am 1960;42:658-660.
109. Carroll R: Pollicization. In Green D, ed: Operative Hand Surgery. New York, Churchill Livingstone, 1988:2263-2280.
110. Huffstadt A, Broker F: Arterial patterns of the hand and pollicisation. Handchirurgie 1978;10:31-35.
111. Littler J: Digital transposition. Curr Pract Orthop Surg 1966;3:157-172.
112. Dobyns J, Bayne L, Wood V: Congenital hand deformities. In Green D, ed: Operative Hand Surgery. New York, Churchill Livingstone, 1982:277-281.
113. Buck-Gramcko D: Complications and bad results in pollicization of the index finger (in congenital cases). Ann Chir Main Memb Super 1991;10:506-512.
114. Riordan D: Technique of pollicization. In Crenshaw AH, ed: Campbell's Operative Orthopedics. St. Louis, CV Mosby, 1971:278-280.
115. Hentz VR, Littler JW: Abduction-pronation and recession of second (index) metacarpal in thumb agenesis. J Hand Surg Am 1977;2:113-117.
116. Blauth W: Principles of pollicisation with special emphasis on new incision methods [in German]. Handchirurgie 1970;2:117-121.
117. Erhardt R: Sequential levels in the development of prehension. Am J Occup Ther 1974;28:592-596.
118. Flatt A: The absent thumb. In Flatt A: The Care of Congenital Hand Anomalies, 2nd ed. St. Louis, Quality Medical Publishing, 1994:96-119.
119. Harrison H: Upper limb anomalies: pollicization for congenital deformities of the hand. Proc R Soc Med 1973;66:634-638.
120. Michon J, Merle J, Bouchon Y, Foucher G: Functional comparison between pollicization and toe-to-hand transfer for thumb reconstruction. J Reconstr Microsurg 1984;1:103-112.
121. Ward J, Pensler JM, Parry SW: Pollicization for thumb reconstruction in severe pediatric hand burns. Plast Reconstr Surg 1985;76:927-932.
122. Egloff D, Verdan CL: Pollicization of the index finger for reconstruction of the congenitally hypoplastic or absent thumb. J Hand Surg Am 1983;8:839-848.
123. Dijkstra R, Bos KE: Functional results of thumb reconstruction. Hand 1982;14:120-128.
124. Lister G: Reconstruction of the hypoplastic thumb. Clin Orthop 1985;195:52-65.
125. Harrison S: Pollicisation in cases of radial club hand. Br J Plast Surg 1970;3:192-200.
126. Hentz VR, Littler JW: The surgical management of congenital hand anomalies. In Littler JW, ed: The Hand and Upper Extremity. Philadelphia, WB Saunders, 1977:3306-3349. Converse JM, ed: Reconstructive Plastic Surgery; vol 6.
127. Eaton C, Lister GD: Syndactyly. Hand Clin 1990;6:555-575.
128. Wassel H: The results of surgery for polydactyly of the thumb. Clin Orthop 1969;64:175-193.
129. Wood V: "Super digit." Hand Clin 1990;6:673-684.
130. Barsky J: Cleft hand: classification, incidence and treatments. J Bone Joint Surg Am 1964;46:1707.
131. Ogino T: Cleft hand. Hand Clin 1990;6:661.
132. Snow J, Littler J: Surgical treatment of the cleft hand. Transactions of the 4th International Congress of Plastic and Reconstructive Surgery, Rome, 1967. Amsterdam, Excerpta Medica, 1969:888-893.
133. Ueba Y: Plastic surgery for the cleft hand. J Hand Surg Am 1981;6:557-560.
134. Tada K, Kurisaki E, Yonenobu K, et al: Central polydactyly—a review of 12 cases and their surgical treatment. J Hand Surg Am 1982;7:460-465.
135. Buck-Gramcko D: Cleft hands: classification and treatment. Hand Clin 1985;1:467-473.
136. Nutt J, Flatt A: Congenital central hand deficit. Hand Surg 1981;6:48-60.
137. Matev I: Congenital absence of the thumb [in German]. Z Orthop Ihre Grenzgeb 1966;102:166-169.
138. Kessler I, Baruch A, Hecht O: Experience with distraction lengthening of digital rays in congenital anomalies. J Hand Surg Am 1977;2:394-401.
139. Patterson T: Congenital ring constrictions. Br J Plast Surg 1961;14:1-31.
140. Goldberg N, Watson H: Composite toe (phalanx with epiphysis) transplants in the reconstruction of the aphalangic hand. J Hand Surg Am 1982;7:454-459.
141. Carroll R: Insertion of toe phalangeal grafts in hypoplastic digits. In Flatt A, ed: The Care Congenital Hand Anomalies. St. Louis, CV Mosby, 1977:143-144.
142. Buck-Gramcko D: The role of non-vascularized toe phalanx transplantation. Hand Clin 1990;6:643-659.

Vascular Anomalies of the Upper Extremity

JOSEPH UPTON III, MD ✦ JENNIFER J. MARLER, MD

The diagnosis and management of vascular tumors and malformations in the upper extremity remain a daunting and sometimes frustrating experience for surgeons who focus on disorders of the upper limb. These are not impossible problems and, in most cases, are treatable with predictable outcomes.[1] This review focuses on the entire spectrum of benign and malignant vascular lesions in the upper extremity. Primary emphasis is placed on the classification, diagnostic work-up, treatment algorithm, complications, and outcomes for each group of lesions. Principles of treatment are emphasized, instead of the many possible methods of reconstruction.

CLASSIFICATION

The etiology of vascular birthmarks has long stimulated the fertile imagination of man. At any point in time, classification systems have reflected a balance between folklore and science. Well into the 19th century, the doctrine of maternal impressions dictated that a gravid mother's craving for strawberries, sight of an accident, or emotional longing could imprint a vascular blemish, a naevus maternus, on her unborn child.[2] With the development of histopathology, Virchow and others introduced the term *angioma,* containing the Greek suffix -oma, meaning swelling or tumor.[3,4] Present-day use of this term denotes a tumor with cellular proliferation. During the past 100 years, the literature on this subject has been confused by a

potpourri of descriptive histologic, embryologic, and biologic classification systems. In most hand surgery textbooks, all vascular anomalies have been mistakenly labeled hemangiomas.[3]

In 1982, a biologic classification of vascular anomalies was proposed that separates vascular tumors from vascular malformations (Table 209-1).[5] It is based on cellular characteristics and correlates with both physical examination findings and natural history of the two types of lesions. Vascular tumors are characterized by endothelial cell proliferation, whereas vascular malformations do not exhibit cellular proliferation. Hemangiomas are the most common vascular tumor but are not the only proliferative vascular lesions seen by the hand surgeon. There are a small group of tumors (2%) that do not involute. Their biologic growth incorporates a benign to malignant spectrum, ranging from a slowly proliferating hemangioendothelioma to a rapidly expanding angiosarcoma.

Malformations represent those lesions that do not involute. These biologically quiescent lesions are classified by their predominant channel type and can be rheologically subdivided into slow- and fast-flow lesions. Change in size can be affected by mechanical factors and cellular changes with aging and hormonal modulation. They may be associated with skeletal overgrowth and fast-flow lesions, in particular, and can cause challenging, occasionally life-threatening clinical problems.

TABLE 209-1 ✦ OVERVIEW OF VASCULAR ANOMALIES

Vascular Tumors

Hemangiomas
  Congenital
    Rapidly involuting congenital hemangioma
    Noninvoluting congenital hemangioma
  Infantile
  Hemangiomatosis
Pyogenic granuloma
Kaposiform hemangioendothelioma
Rare tumors
  Hemangiopericytoma
  Hemangioendothelioma
  Giant cell angioblastoma
  Angiosarcoma

Vascular Malformations

Telangiectasias
  Cutis marmorata telangiectasia congenita
  Hereditary hemorrhagic telangiectasia
Capillary malformations
Venous malformations
  Blue rubber bleb nevus syndrome
Lymphatic malformations
  Lymphangiomatosis
Arteriovenous malformations
Combined (eponymous) slow-flow malformations
  Capillary-lymphatic-venous malformation (Klippel-Trénaunay syndrome)
  Proteus syndrome
  Maffucci syndrome
  Bannayan-Riley-Ruvalcaba syndrome
Combined (eponymous) fast-flow malformations
  Capillary-arteriovenous malformation (Parkes Weber syndrome)

This review discusses the spectrum of vascular anomalies that affect the upper extremity. Vascular tumors and vascular malformations are considered in separate sections.

VASCULAR TUMORS

Hemangioma

PATHOGENESIS

The term *angiogenesis*, introduced by Folkman et al[6] in the early 1970s, refers to blood vessel development but is also associated with the recruitment of new blood vessels by a tumor. The hemangioma is a tumor of vascular endothelial cells and represents a pure model of angiogenesis. Elegant experiments have demonstrated that many cancers are angiogenesis dependent, with vessel recruitment controlled by a complicated balance of both angiogenesis stimulators (up-regulating blood vessel formation) and angiogenesis inhibitors (down-regulating blood vessel formation). In the treatment section, we shall see how the growth of these tumors can be suppressed by angiogenic inhibitors.

Most hemangiomas are solitary. One fifth of affected infants have more than one lesion. The female-to-male ratio varies between 3:1 and 5:1 and is reported to be higher in association with other vascular anomalies[7] or pediatric tumors. The incidence is up to 10 times higher in children whose mothers have had chorionic villus sampling.[8] The effect of hormonal modulation on blood vessel recruitment, especially during pregnancy, is not understood.

The natural history of a hemangioma has been well defined by both light microscopy and immunohistochemistry into three phases: the proliferating phase (0 to 1 year), the involuting phase (1 to 7 years), and the involuted phase (>7 years).[9] Proliferation occurs during the first year of life and is characterized by rapid growth of plump endothelial cells that form tightly packed sinusoids. A number of endothelial markers are present, including CD31, von Willebrand factor, and E-selectin, among others.[9-11] The concentration of two well-known angiogenic peptides, vascular endothelial growth factor and basic fibroblast growth factor, is up-regulated during this phase.[9,12] The clinical course can be monitored by urine levels of basic fibroblast growth factor, which peak during this phase.[13] Endothelial cells from hemangiomas isolated in culture rapidly form vascular loops and channels.[14]

The involuting phase occurs between 1 and 7 years of age and is characterized by a flattening of endothelial cells, dilatation of vascular channels, and ingrowth of fibrous tissue.[15] Mast cells and macrophages are more prominent; mast cells are thought to produce proteins that down-regulate endothelial turnover. Metalloproteinases, proteins known to inhibit angiogenesis, are present in higher concentration.[9] After 2 months of age, apoptosis begins and reaches its peak at 2 years of age, at which time at least one third of the dying cells are endothelial.[11] In situ hybridization studies have shown that the skin overlying a hemangioma is not normal and lacks the normal development of the outer keratin layer. Within this hyperplastic skin are high levels of basic fibroblast growth factor and low levels of interferon-β.[16] During the involuting phase, these levels reverse, and keratin production occurs with normal interferon-β levels. During the involuted phase, the regression of blood vessels is completed. Some small feeding vessels, some large draining veins, and an admixture of fibrofatty and loose connective tissue are all that remain. The multilaminated basement membranes around residual capillaries are the only remnant of the proliferating phase.[15]

CLINICAL FEATURES

Hemangiomas are the most common tumor of infancy and childhood. The incidence is between 4% and 10% in white infants,[17] lower in dark-skinned babies, and as high as 23% in low-weight premature infants.[18] Girls are more commonly affected than are boys (Table 209-2). Eighty percent are solitary, and 20% are multiple; in the latter group, involvement of internal organs is likely, including the central nervous system. The head and neck (60%) and trunk (25%) are more commonly involved than the upper and lower extremity (15%).[19] Between one third and one half of hemangiomas are not present at birth. In retrospect, most of these have a premonitory red blush or spot that appeared to be an ecchymosis.[2]

Severe life-endangering problems occur in children with hemangiomas around the airway, liver hemangiomas, or "hemangiomatosis" (multiple cutaneous and internal organ hemangiomas). These children present with liver failure, anemia, congestive heart failure, and respiratory failure, which are rarely seen with isolated upper extremity lesions.

PROLIFERATING PHASE. During the early proliferating phase, the skin is raised with a bright crimson-red color. The evolving mass is warm and firm, and most have the appearance of strawberries (Fig. 209-1). These lesions can develop deep to the subcutaneous fatty layers, even deep to muscle in the forearm or upper arm without any dermal or epidermal component. On initial examination, it is impossible to accurately predict the onset of involution; it usually occurs by 12 months of age. Frequent observation and reassurance of parents are best.

INVOLUTING PHASE. After 1 year of age, the exponential growth subsides and the tumor decreases in size relative to the growth of the child. The mass becomes less tense, the color fades, and size decreases (Fig. 209-2). Small gray areas called herald spots appear on the surface of the lesion, representing regions of necrosis and healing. The involution process extends from 1 to 8 years. The rate of regression is not related to the initial size or location of the lesion or the gender of the patient. Involution is complete in 50% of patients by the age of 5 years, in 70% by 7 years, and in 100% by 10 to 12 years.[20] At complete regression, the skin is almost normal histologically. If the tumor was large, there may be redundant folds of loose skin with residual underlying fibrofatty tissue, typically on the dorsum of the hand or forearm. Deep lesions often regress without a visible cutaneous trace. Hemangiomas do not involve skeletal structures and are not related to skeletal overgrowth.[21] Even with the most extensive hemangiomas of the upper extremity, we have not documented increased growth.

CONGENITAL HEMANGIOMAS

There are at least two subsets of hemangioma that demonstrate different patterns of histologic and biologic behavior compared with typical infantile hemangiomas (Fig. 209-3). These are both "congenital" hemangiomas that form during prenatal life and are fully developed at birth.

One type involutes rapidly during the first few weeks or months of life.[22] These have a characteristic red-violaceous color and coarse telangiectasias, often with a peripheral or central area of pallor. Their distribution more commonly involves the trunk and extremities. Rapidly involuting congenital hemangioma is the term proposed for this distinct group.

A second, less common subset of congenital hemangioma persists into later childhood. Noninvoluting congenital hemangioma is the term proposed for this type.[23]

RADIOLOGIC CHARACTERISTICS

Ultrasonography

An ultrasound examination is usually the only study needed for accurate diagnosis of a solitary, well-localized hemangioma. A proliferating hemangioma is characteristically a dense, homogeneous lesion with fast flow. There is decreased arterial resistance and increased venous flow velocity within a discrete mass.[24,25] As involution progresses, there is more diffuse infiltrating soft tissue mass and less vessel flow.[26] An experienced ultrasonographer has no difficulty with

TABLE 209-2 ◆ COMPARISON OF TYPICAL INFANTILE HEMANGIOMAS AND VASCULAR MALFORMATIONS

	Hemangioma	Vascular Malformation
Present at birth	70% of cases—no 30% of cases—premonitory spot	Yes (may not be clinically evident)
Growth characteristics	Rapid growth during first year of life followed by spontaneous involution	Growth commensurate with child Subject to extrinsic modulation by hormonal and other factors
Female-to-male ratio	3:1	1:1

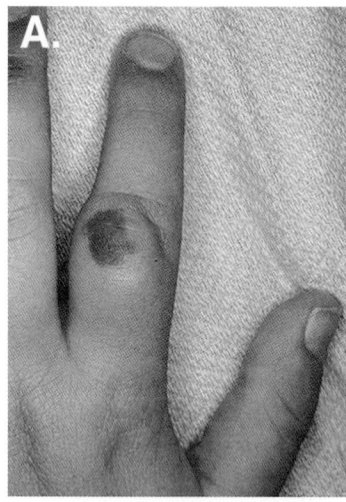

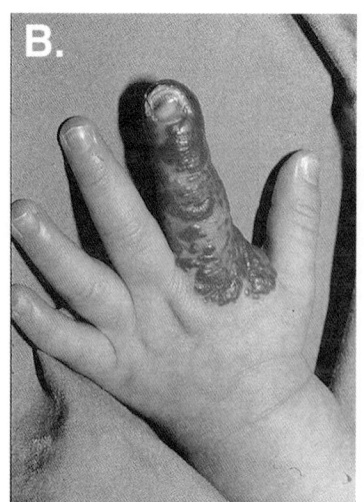

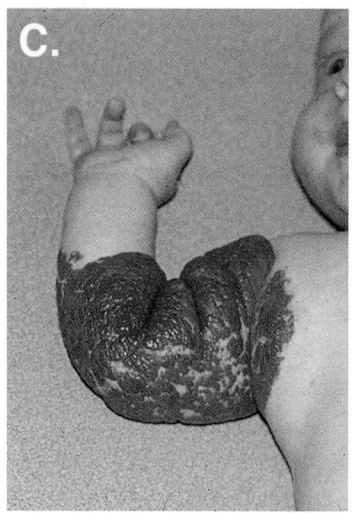

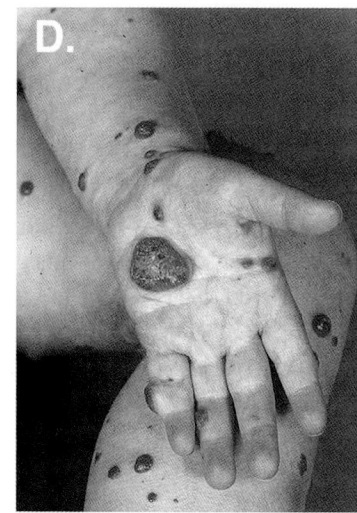

FIGURE 209-1. Diverse presentations of upper limb hemangioma. *A,* A subcutaneous lesion with an overlying capillary stain. *B,* A rapidly enlarging index lesion with an associated paronychial infection that was aggravated by finger sucking in a 6-month-old baby. *C,* A circumferential lesion of the axilla, arm, and elbow region demonstrating involvement of the superficial and deep dermis. *D,* Multiple raised, sessile lesions of all four limbs, trunk, and abdomen are known as hemangiomatosis; internal organ involvement must be ruled out.

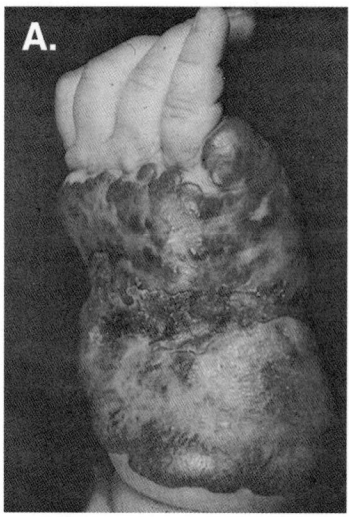

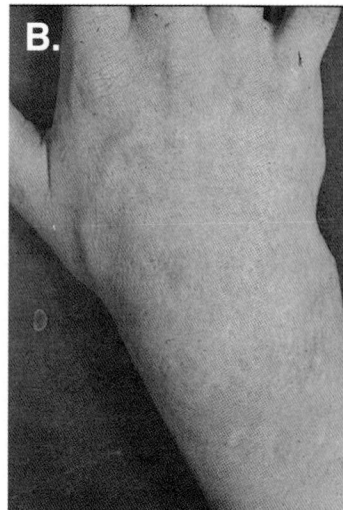

FIGURE 209-2. Hemangioma, spontaneous resolution. *A,* A soft, raised red lesion at 1 year of age at the start of involution. *B,* Same wrist and hand 10 years later. No surgery has been performed.

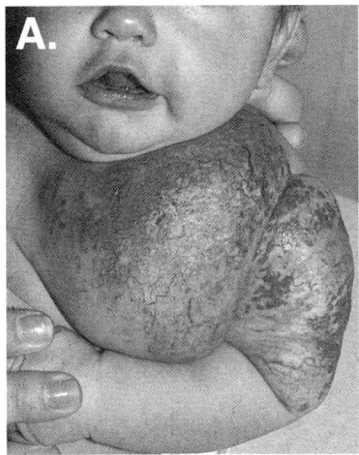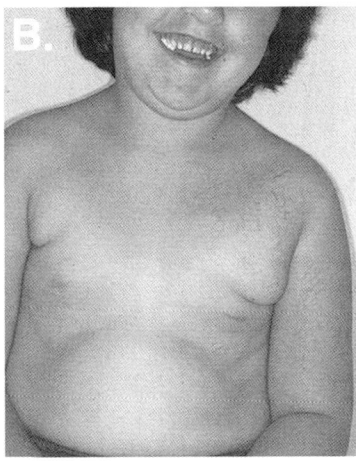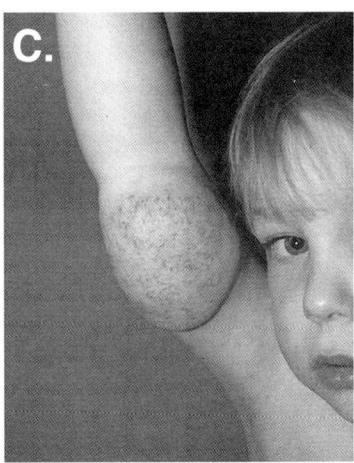

FIGURE 209-3. Two types of congenital hemangioma. *A* and *B,* Rapidly involuting congenital hemangioma. This extensive lesion involving the left arm, axilla, and chest wall was fully formed at birth and involuted by 6 months of age. At 3 years of age, there is little fibrofatty residuum. *C,* Noninvoluting congenital hemangioma. There has been no obvious involution of this congenital lesion seen in a 4-year-old boy.

the differentiation of arteriovenous malformations, venous malformations, and malignant tumors from hemangiomas. The stages of involution and responses to pharmacologic therapy are often documented with ultrasonography as well as by urine levels of basic fibroblast growth factor.

Magnetic Resonance Imaging

Magnetic resonance imaging (MRI) of proliferating hemangiomas shows a solid tissue of intermediate intensity on T1-weighted sequences and moderate hyperintensity on T2-weighted spin echo images (Fig. 209-4). Flow voids are indicative of the rapid flow between feeding arteries and large draining veins. Gradient-recalled sequences confirm the presence of high-flow vessels within and around the soft tissue mass. As involution progresses, these flow voids disappear; T1-weighted images show high signals indicative of fat; T2 images show decreased signals, also indicative of fat; and the lobularity of the lesion becomes more obvious.[27,28]

Nuclear Scanning

Radionuclear scanning with technetium-tagged erythrocytes is not useful in the upper extremity. It is occasionally used to detect deep hemangiomas within the central nervous system and gastrointestinal system.[29]

Angiography

Invasive angiography is not used for initial diagnosis but may document both the diagnosis and embolic treatment course of large lesions involving the arms, axilla, and chest wall. An early arterial blush with large feeding arteries and draining veins is characteristic of the proliferating lesion. After regression, these lesions are avascular.

ASSOCIATED MALFORMATIONS

Although geneticists list hemangiomas as a part of many syndromes, these lesions are usually malformations.[30] Mulliken[31] has noted that because hemangiomas are so frequent in infants and young children, their occurrence with other anomalies may be coincidental; to be designated a true association, there must be at least a 10% frequency with another defect. True hemangiomas do coexist rarely with carotid and great vessel anomalies[26] and central nervous system malformations.[32,33] These are easily distinguished by ultrasonography and MRI scanning. In general, upper extremity vascular anomalies that are part of syndromes are malformations (usually venous malformations, lymphatic malformations, or combined lesions).

DIFFERENTIAL DIAGNOSIS

Most hemangiomas are evident by their strawberry appearance and proliferative growth during the first year of life. However, not all lesions with a strawberry appearance are hemangiomas.[34] Pyogenic granulomas within the digits and forearm are not as large and have a sessile base.[35] Deep expanding lesions may represent other childhood tumors, such as infantile fibrosarcoma,[36] hemangiopericytoma,[37] and tufted angioma, also called angioblastoma of Nakagawa.[38]

Typical hemangiomas should not, by definition, result in coagulopathy. Massive hemangiomas in the arm, axilla, and chest wall with thrombocytopenia and coagulopathy should be considered to be kaposiform

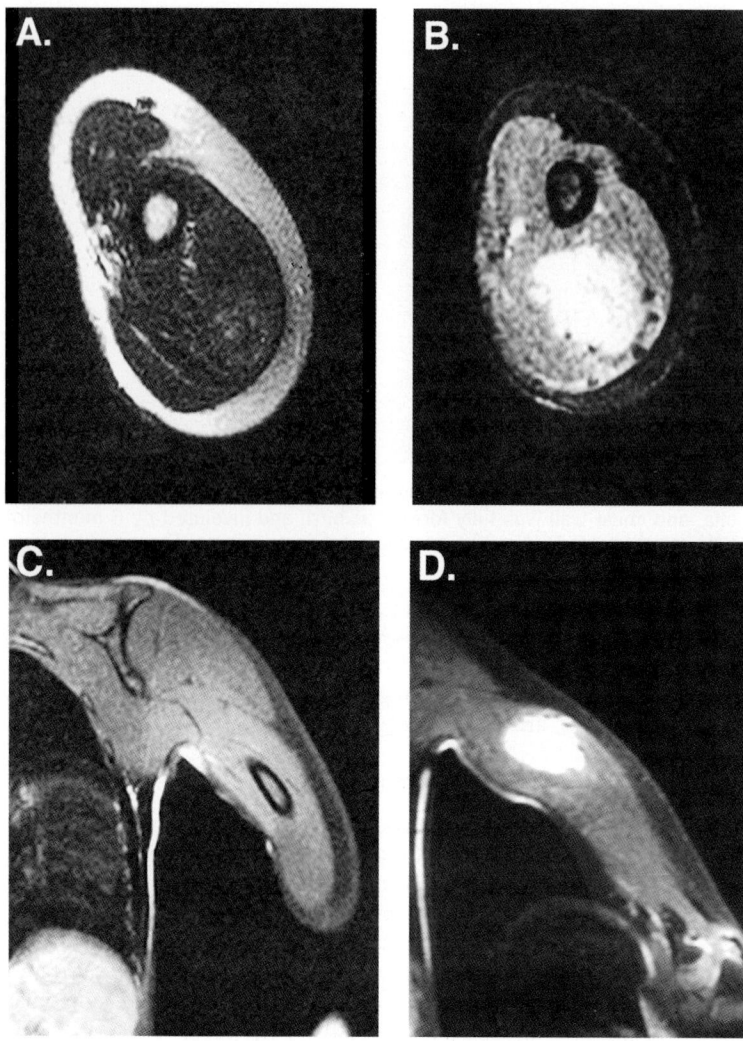

FIGURE 209-4. Hemangioma, MRI characteristics. *A* and *B,* Transverse T2-weighted *(A)* and T1-weighted *(B)* sequences with and without gadolinium enhancement demonstrate an intramuscular triceps hemangioma of the upper arm. *C* and *D,* The same sequences on sagittal view.

hemangioendothelioma, a vascular tumor associated with platelet trapping (discussed later), unless it is proved otherwise. Although MRI will usually direct the correct diagnosis, tissue biopsy is mandatory if there is any question about the diagnosis.

TREATMENT

Observation

After surfing the Internet, computer-savvy parents will arrive at the consultant's offices with a wrong diagnosis. These people often obtain information that is neither from peer-reviewed publications nor accurate. It is important to gain their confidence by making the correct diagnosis and providing a thorough explanation of the natural history of their child's hemangioma. Frequent office visits for serial photographs and reassurance may be necessary. Although lesions in the head

and neck regions cause most distress to parents, those involving the upper limb, particularly large diffuse lesions, can become the focus of an entire family. This is one clinical situation in which the surgeon, trained to operate, expends maximal time and energy urging the parents to do nothing.

Most hemangiomas in the upper extremity are solitary and cause no functional problems. Rapidly growing lesions in the arm, axilla, elbow, or forearm must be watched for ulceration, maceration, crusting, or bleeding, which may occur in up to 10% of extremity lesions (Fig. 209-5).[39] Lesions of the fingertips, of the paronychial folds, and within the interdigital web spaces break down much more frequently and are irritated by the child's scratching or sucking. Local cleaning and wound care with application of dressings to open ulcers will promote spontaneous epithelialization. The first layer of any dressing should contain a

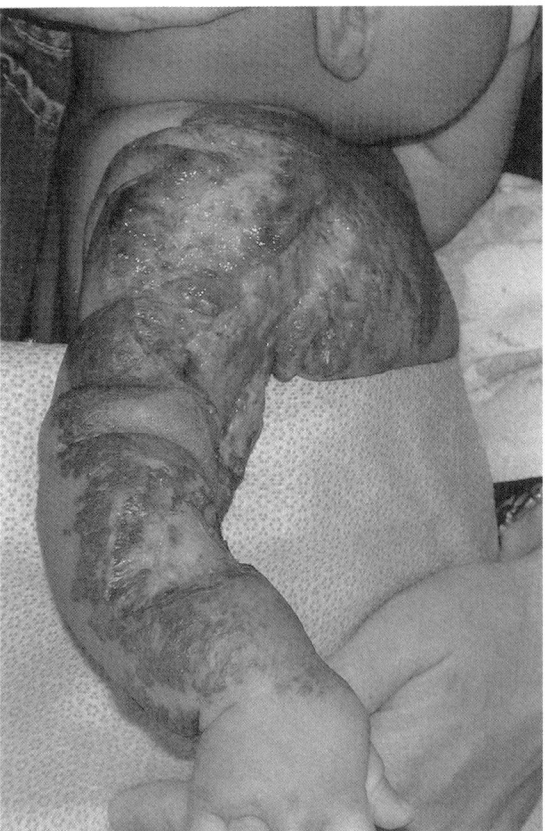

FIGURE 209-5. Hemangioma ulceration. Small areas of necrosis heralded massive axillary, upper arm, and forearm ulceration in this 5-month-old girl. Topical treatment with hydrogel dressings resulted in nearly complete wound closure. An axillary skin graft was required, although this is unusual; skin grafts are almost never needed with careful wound care.

petrolatum base so that removal of the gauze will not prompt brisk bleeding from the fragile epithelial surface. Rigid welcome sleeves used in patients with cleft lip and palate will help keep the child's hands out of his or her mouth. Topical antibiotics effectively reduce surface bacterial counts. Parenteral antibiotics are reserved for clinical cellulitis. Superficial ulcerations and infections should heal within 10 to 14 days. Full-thickness loss will take several weeks, depending on the extent of the lesion.

Because hemangiomas will naturally completely regress, the urge to operate should be avoided. Parents often ask what the surgeon would do if this were his or her child. The answer is to wait patiently. They may be frightened by persistent oozing or bleeding. All bleeding from hemangiomas of the upper limb can be controlled with application of a pressure dressing and elevation. In rare lesions, suture ligature of a bleeder may be required.

Medical Therapy

The incidence of life-endangering problems caused by hemangiomas is unknown but has been conservatively estimated to be not higher than 10%.[40] Almost all involve lesions within or around the cervicofacial region, gastrointestinal tract, eyes, or airways. Those lesions involving the upper limb are usually large with extension into the axilla and ipsilateral chest wall. There are effective pharmacologic treatments, which include the following.

Intralesional Corticosteroid Injection. Triamcinolone (10 mg/mL, 25 mg/mL) is injected slowly through a 25-gauge needle while the periphery of the lesion is compressed with a pressure ring. Dosage should not exceed 3 to 5 mg/kg per injection. Complications include subcutaneous tissue atrophy and hypopigmentation. The response rate is equal to that for intravenous corticosteroid administration.[41]

Systemic Corticosteroid Therapy. Oral or intravenous administration of equivalent doses of prednisone or prednisolone at 2 to 3 mg/kg per day for 2 weeks is used for acute situations. Within 7 to 10 days after initiation of the drug, decreased growth rate, lightening of color, and softening of the tumor are indicative of a response. If there is a response, the steroid is slowly tapered every 2 to 4 weeks.[31] The drug should be discontinued by the age of 1 year. Outcome studies show accelerated regression in 30%, stabilization of growth in 40%, and minimal or no response in up to 30%. At our institution, the response rate has been as high as 80% to 90%. Others have reported similar results with dosages as high as 5 mg/kg per day.[42] The well-known untoward effects of this therapy include cushingoid facies, weight gain, and decreased growth in virtually all of these children. By 24 months of age, these children return to the normal height and weight for their ages.[43] Myopathy and infections may occur in those receiving larger doses for prolonged periods.

Interferon Alfa-2a or Alfa-2b. Recombinant interferon alfa-2a or alfa-2b is our second-line drug for the treatment of problematic hemangiomas, although some have used it as a primary agent.[44-47] There is no evidence that it is synergistic with corticosteroids.[48] Our indications for use include failure to respond to corticosteroids, complications from corticosteroid use, and parental refusal of corticosteroid use.

Interferon is given at a dose of 2 to 3 million units/m^2 administered by subcutaneous injection daily. Because the response rate is much slower and less dramatic than with corticosteroids, treatment must last for 6 to 12 months. Interferon has been successful for 80% of children treated, a group that includes the 30% who did not respond to systemic corticosteroids.[31] Most children have a low-grade fever during the first 1 to 2 weeks of treatment. This is effectively treated with aceta-minophen. Transient elevation in transaminase enzymes, neutropenia, and anemia are reversed with discontinuation of the drug. The most serious side effect is a spastic diplegia, which is reported in up to 10% of children receiving long-term interferon therapy.[49,50] In our experience, the incidence is higher, on the order of 25% of infants who were younger than 12 months when they received interferon. These children should be monitored by a pediatric neurologist during treatment; the drug should be discontinued if signs of spastic diplegia develop.

ANGIOGENIC INHIBITORS. Whereas it is anticipated that angiogenesis inhibitors will play a role in the medical treatment of hemangiomas, no short-term outcome studies have been reported.

Interventional Radiology

Embolization is effectively used in rapidly growing lesions causing congestive heart failure, in patients whose pharmacologic treatment has failed, or in patients who are moribund. This generally occurs in the setting of large pelvic, hepatic, or lower extremity hemangiomas. Indications in the upper limb are rare. Sclerotherapy is not used for extremity hemangiomas.

Surgery

Surgical resection for proliferating or involuting hemangiomas in the upper extremity is rarely needed because these lesions predictably involute. Problematic ulcers with persistent bleeding or chronic infection may be more appropriately resected surgically. Lesions within intertriginous regions and periungual spaces can be difficult in babies and young children. We have successfully treated large ulcerated lesions in the extremities by closed suction with the vacuum-assisted closure device. Surgery in childhood is indicated if it is obvious that it will be needed after involution, if the resulting scar does not cause new contractures, and if no normal tissue is lost during the excision. It is often best to postpone excision until regression is complete in the young, active mobile child.

Pyogenic Granuloma

CLINICAL FEATURES

Pyogenic granulomas are rare before 6 months of age and cannot be considered a congenital birthmark. They appear without a history of trauma or cutaneous rash. They frequently arise within a cutaneous capillary malformation. They occur more commonly on the face or within the mouth than on the arm, hand, or fingertips. These sessile lesions arise from a distinct pedicle, rarely exceed 1.0 cm in width, and persistently crust and bleed (Fig. 209-6).[43] Multiple calls and visits to the

frustrated pediatrician for bleeding usually result in referral to the hand specialist or plastic surgeon.

DIAGNOSIS

Although the diagnosis is obvious from the sessile pedunculated morphology, these lesions can be confused with cutaneous hemangiomas, retained foreign bodies in the glabrous skin of the hand, and undetected Salter II injuries of the distal phalanges. MRI scans and ultrasonography are not necessary. Histologic examination shows a dense fibrous stromal network surrounding lobules of plump, compact endothelial cells. Tritiated thymidine uptake studies show high indices (indicative of cellular proliferation) in both the epidermis and endothelial cells.[2]

TREATMENT

A wide variety of local treatments include curettage, shave excision, excision and laser photocoagulation,[51] and full-thickness skin excision.[2] Our preferred treatment is either thorough curettage and cauterization of small lesions or full-thickness excision and direct closure of larger lesions.

Kaposiform Hemangioendothelioma

PATHOGENESIS

Kaposiform hemangioendothelioma is an invasive vascular tumor of infancy that has a natural history more consistent with a low-grade malignant neoplasm. It is also called a tufted angioma.[52-54] Thrombocytopenia and coagulopathy can be profound in these large lesions. This has become known as the Kasabach-Merritt phenomenon, in recognition of the authors of a single case report in 1940 describing a patient with thrombocytopenia and bleeding within a large truncal lesion.[55] Mistakenly, this term has been applied to the coagulopathies that may occur with slow-flow venous malformations and lymphatic-venous malformations. The mechanism for trapping of platelets and other clotting factors is not known.

CLINICAL FEATURES

Both sexes are affected equally. Lesions are usually present at birth and involve large areas of the body. The upper extremity is involved when this vascular tumor invades the chest, shoulder, axilla, and arm. The skin has a deep purple color and is tense and edematous (Fig. 209-7). Petechiae and ecchymosis are often present on the surface of this coagulopathic tumor. Hematologic studies show thrombocytopenia (usually less than 10,000 platelets/mm^3) with low fibrinogen and increased fibrin split products. Biopsy is rarely indicated because the clinical picture is pathognomonic.

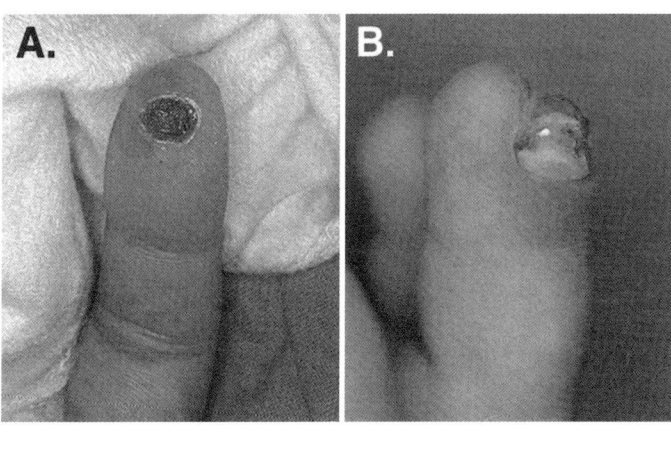

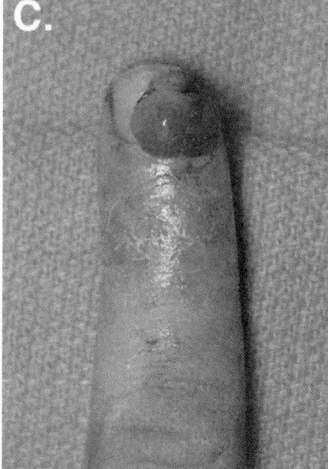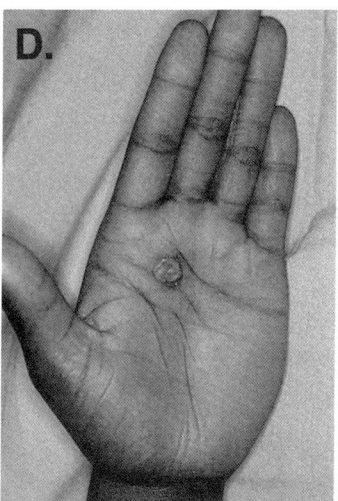

FIGURE 209-6. Diverse presentations of pyogenic granuloma. These granulomas are vascular tumors that are frequently seen in the digits and hand. Most are initially diagnosed as retained foreign bodies, although a history of trauma is lacking. Granulomas arising beneath the eponychial fold may also represent untreated epiphyseal dislocations of the distal phalanx.

DIAGNOSIS

MRI distinguishes kaposiform hemangioendothelioma from hemangioma. Kaposiform hemangioendothelioma is not well delineated as it crosses tissue boundaries and has poorly defined margins. Soft tissues are thickened on T1-weighted images, with diffuse enhancement on contrast-enhanced sequences and stranding of subcutaneous tissues similar to that seen in lymphatic obstruction on T2-weighted images. The signal voids are not flow voids but represent spaces filled with hemosiderin or other blood products.[54] Osteolysis may be present adjacent to the tumor.

Histologic examination shows aggressive patterns that contain sheets of endothelial cells lining narrow vascular channels filled with blood and hemosiderin. Also present are dilated lymphatic channels.

TREATMENT

Treatment of kaposiform hemangioendothelioma is medical, not surgical, and similar to the treatment of hemangiomas (see earlier). The primary drug is interferon alfa, which is successful in 50% of children with kaposiform hemangioendothelioma and bleeding.[44] Vincristine has also been used. Mortality rates are still in the 20% to 30% range. Drug therapy is successful in shrinking the tumor and controlling the coagulopathy. However, many of these kaposiform hemangioendotheliomas do not completely regress and remain as a much smaller asymptomatic tumor later in life.[56]

Glomus Tumor

The reader is referred to most hand surgery textbooks and atlases, in which the nature and management of this common periungual mass are discussed.

Rare Tumors

HEMANGIOPERICYTOMAS

Hemangiopericytomas are rare subcutaneous tumors arising from pericytes. They bear histologic similarity

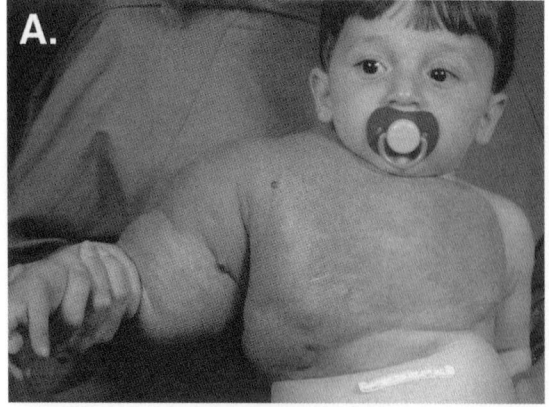

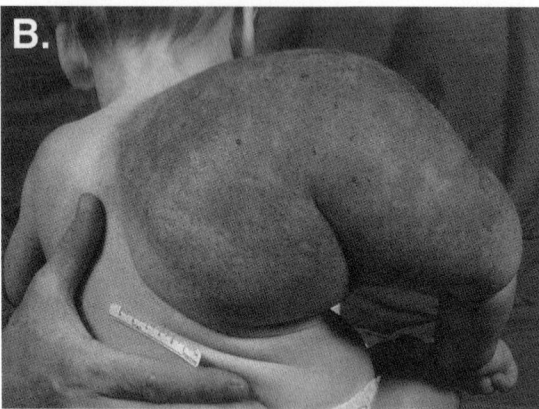

FIGURE 209-7. Kaposiform hemangioendothelioma. The large lesion shown here in frontal *(A)* and dorsal *(B)* views developed on the arm and chest wall of this infant. Additional findings included thrombocytopenia (<5000/mm³), hypofibrinogenemia, and increased fibrin split products. Ecchymosis and petechiae may be evident in these children. A deep red-purple color and tense nature are characteristic of the lesion.

to glomus tumors but are more locally invasive.[57] They are more common in adults; only 5% to 10% of cases occur in children.[58] Children younger than 1 year have a better prognosis than do older children or adults. Treatment options include resection and neoadjuvant chemotherapy.[57-59]

HEMANGIOENDOTHELIOMA

Hemangioendothelioma is a rare vascular tumor that can affect the upper extremity. There are conflicting reports concerning its histologic definition, malignant potential, and optimal therapy. It can be congenital[60] and may present during infancy,[61] childhood, or later life.[62] It has been reported in association with underlying bone tumors.[63] It may be benign or malignant[64] and, in certain histologic forms, has been reported to share similarity with a low-grade angiosarcoma (Fig. 209-8).

GIANT CELL ANGIOBLASTOMA

Giant cell angioblastoma is a rare destructive pediatric tumor that can affect the upper extremity.[65-67] Whereas amputation was the only reported treatment,[65] we successfully treated a neonate with a congenital hand lesion by use of an antiangiogenic regimen of interferon alfa (Fig. 209-9).[67] Without this pharmacologic therapy, hand amputation would have been mandated.

ANGIOSARCOMA

We have not seen this rare tumor develop de novo in the upper extremity but have documented its occurrence in the axillary region in two female patients. In both women, it developed many years after extensive radiation therapy for breast carcinoma.

VASCULAR MALFORMATIONS
Pathogenesis

Vascular malformations are believed to arise from errors in embryogenesis.[2] Clinical classification is based on the particular type of vascular channel within the malformation.[14] Research designed to clarify the mechanisms of normal blood vessel formation is beginning to provide insight into the pathogenesis of abnormal blood vessel formation. *Vasculogenesis* refers to the process of primitive blood vessel or channel formation; *angiogenesis* refers to the formation of new vessels from this preexisting vasculature.[68-70] Embryonic endothelial cells can be identified as precursors for either arteries or veins; arteries express the ligand ephrin-B2 and veins ephrin-B4.[69] The genetic imprint of an endothelial cell can now be determined before its differentiation.

The field of molecular genetics is also providing insight into the possible mechanisms of malformation. Osler-Rendu-Weber syndrome, known as hereditary hemorrhagic telangiectasia, involves capillary malformations in skin and mucous membranes. These patients also have more serious lung, liver, and central nervous system anomalies, including arteriovenous malformations. Genes on chromosomes 9q and 12q have defined three different clinical patterns of this disease (hereditary hemorrhagic telangiectasia types 1 to 3).[71]

Telangiectasias: Cutis Marmorata Telangiectasia Congenita

Cutis marmorata telangiectasia congenita is a distinct pathologic entity first described by van Lohuizen.[72] This rare vascular anomaly manifests as congenital livid

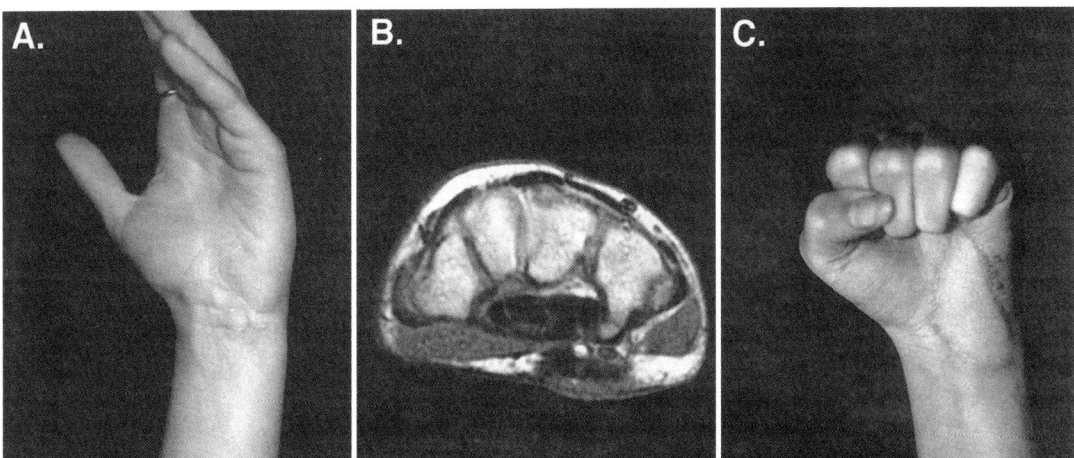

FIGURE 209-8. Hemangioendothelioma. *A,* Several hard, immobile cutaneous nodules of the volar wrist in an adolescent with ulnar paresthesias. These recurrent lesions followed three previous resections, including a neurolysis of the ulnar nerve within Guyon canal and resection of the ulnar artery at age 7 years. *B,* A T2-weighted sequence on MRI documents the loss of the normal fat signal and replacement by scar and recurrent tumor. *C,* Result 5 years after resection of the involved skin and resurfacing with a thin radial forearm free flap from the opposite forearm as a flow-through revascularization. The affected ulnar nerve was resected and replaced with sural nerve grafts. Intrinsic muscle function is normal at this follow-up evaluation, and two-point sensory discrimination is 5.0 mm.

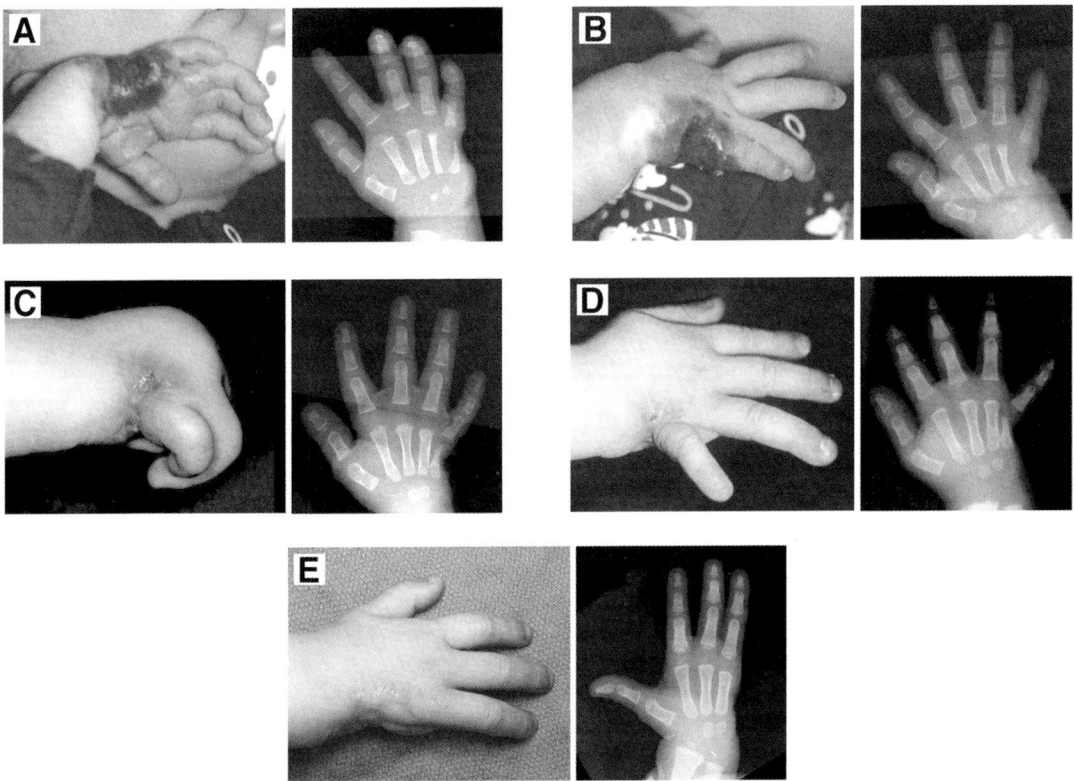

FIGURE 209-9. Giant cell angioblastoma. *A,* The clinical appearance and radiograph of an infant born with an ulcerated erythematous lesion over the hypothenar eminence. *B,* Within 3 months, the ulcer progressed and skeletal erosion worsened. Biopsy was consistent with giant cell angioblastoma. The baby was prescribed interferon alfa, an angiogenesis inhibitor, at a dosage of 3 million units m^2/day injected subcutaneously. *C,* Near closure of the open ulcer after 4 months of therapy. *D,* Wound contraction and fifth metacarpal remineralization after 1 year of treatment. *E,* Result after definitive resection of all residual tumor, the ulnar artery and nerve, and the fifth ray of the hand. Nerve grafts were used for ulnar motor and sensory reconstruction.

cutaneous marbling, even at normal temperatures, that becomes more pronounced with lower temperatures or with crying. The involved skin is depressed in a serpiginous, reticulated pattern and has a distinctive deep purple color (Fig. 209-10). Ulceration may be present. It occurs in a localized, segmental, or generalized distribution, more frequently involving the trunk and extremities than the face or scalp. In one reported series, cutis marmorata telangiectasia congenita was unilateral in 65% of patients and involved a lower extremity in 69% of patients.[73] The affected extremity is often hypoplastic compared with its nonaffected counterpart.[74,75]

Differential diagnoses include cutis marmorata (or livedo reticularis) and a telangiectatic variant of hemangioma. Cutis marmorata is merely an accentuated pattern of normal cutaneous vascularity. It is seen as a transient mottling pattern when the child is placed in a low-temperature environment but disappears on warming. Telangiectatic hemangioma, most often seen on an extremity, has a fine, variegated pattern. It is not associated with depression of the involved skin and regresses, as do the other forms of hemangioma.[34]

Almost all affected infants with cutis marmorata telangiectasia congenita show improvement of the skin

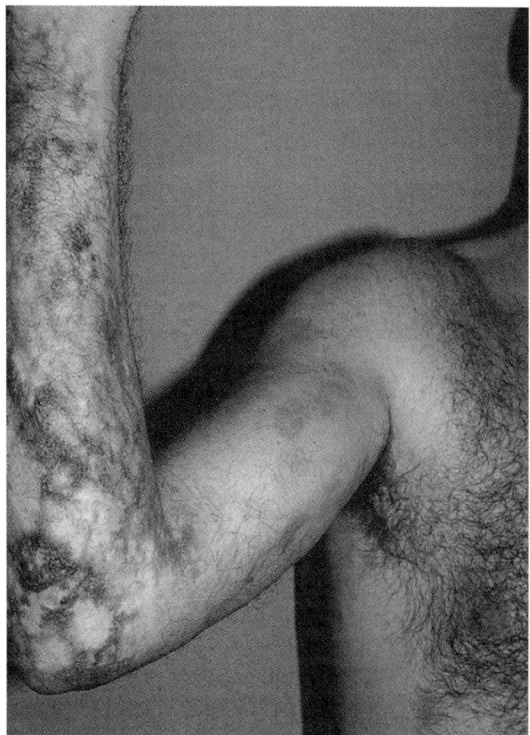

FIGURE 209-10. Cutis marmorata telangiectasia congenita. The characteristic features include a reticulated, marble-like appearance with a typical deep purple color. Involved limbs may have both soft tissue and skeletal atrophy.

changes during the first year of life, continuing into adolescence.[2,76] However, atrophy and pigmentation often persist into adulthood in association with ectasia of the superficial veins in the involved limb (see Fig. 209-10).

Capillary Malformations

CLINICAL FEATURES

Capillary malformations are capillary- to venule-sized vessels within the superficial and deep dermal layers of skin. Their red color is from circulating erythrocytes. They have also been referred to as port-wine stains. Immunohistochemical studies have shown that these dilated vessels lack the normal smooth muscle layer within their walls and vasa nervorum.[77] These are often confused with the most common birthmark of infancy (known as the angel kiss on the forehead, nose, or lip and the stork bite on the back of the neck) that represents a "transient dilatation" of dermal vessels and fades within months.

Capillary malformations in the upper extremity have varied appearances (Fig. 209-11). Mulliken and others have noted that the extremity and trunk lesions do not become as dark and nodular as those lesions in the head and neck region with aging. Extensive cutaneous capillary malformations often may be associated with hypertrophy (circumferential and axial) of both soft tissue and bone. There is no predictable pattern.

Upper extremity capillary malformations are often associated with a deeper venous or lymphatic malformation.[1] A patient with the Sturge-Weber syndrome may have extremity capillary malformations on one or both upper limbs and in one or all of the trigeminal nerve distributions on the face with other intracranial and ocular vascular anomalies. Those with staining in the V1 distribution are at greatest risk. All need MRI evaluation of the head and thorough neurologic and ophthalmologic examinations.[78]

TREATMENT

Although no treatment is usually elected for extremity capillary malformations, the tunable pulsed-dye laser can effectively decrease the color of the cutaneous blush. Some believe that the results are better during infancy,[79] whereas others have recorded no significant difference in the timing of laser treatment.[80] In general, there is a marked decrease in the color of the capillary malformation. More dramatic results are obtained on the face and neck than on the trunk and extremities.[48]

The soft tissue debulking and skeletal procedures required with overgrowth are particular to the associated venous, lymphatic, or lymphatic-venous malformations and are described in those sections.

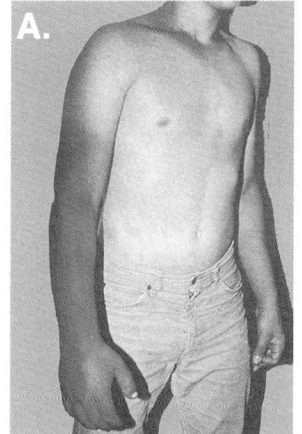

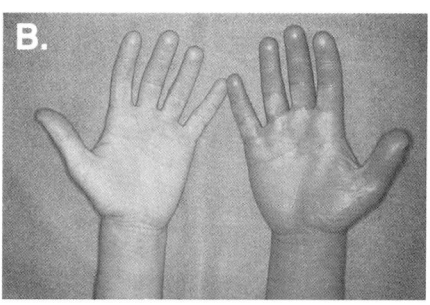

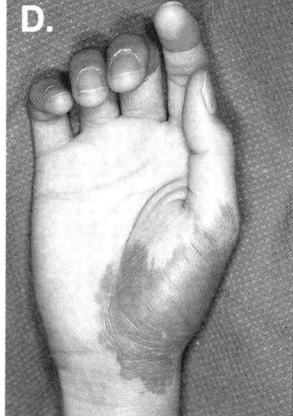

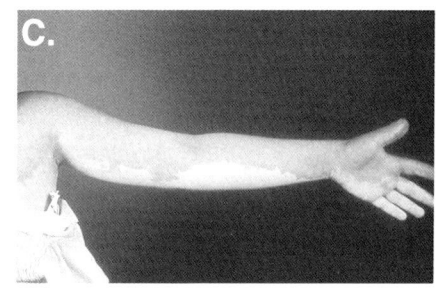

FIGURE 209-11. Diverse presentations of capillary malformation. Capillary malformations can involve any portion of the upper extremity and do not necessarily follow a segmental or dermatologic pattern. *A,* An extensive circumferential lesion of the arm, forearm, and hand. Note the less intense capillary malformation of the ipsilateral chest and abdomen. *B,* Diffuse enlargement of the hand is noted in the patient shown in *A. C,* Capillary malformation involving the C3-5 distribution of the upper limb. *D,* Capillary malformation involving the thenar eminence.

Venous Malformations

PATHOGENESIS

The knowledge of the molecular genetics of venous malformations (VMs) is just beginning. Most VMs are sporadic, but there are families with an autosomal dominant pattern and mutation that maps to chromosome 9.[81] A type of VM called glomangioma maps to chromosome 1p,[82] and a type of cerebral VM (cavernous) prevalent in Mexican American populations maps to chromosome 7q. These studies suggest a genetic pattern of or susceptibility for certain types of VM.

CLINICAL FEATURES

Although VMs of the upper extremity are all present at birth, not all are obvious. Within the first 5 to 6 years of life, all but the smallest or deepest lesions will become clinically evident. Less than 10% are clinically indolent until adolescence.[1] They grow commensurately with the child and slowly expand during the adolescent growth spurt.

The most common presenting symptoms are a mass, swelling, and cutaneous discoloration. These are slow-flow malformations that engorge with the limb in a dependent position and decompress with the limb held above the level of the heart. Most VMs are in the subcutaneous tissue planes external to the muscular fascia in the axilla, arm, and forearm (Fig. 209-12).

Most VMs are solitary but many are multiple. A small number of patients have extensive lesions that may extend into the axilla and ipsilateral chest wall. Large VMs without a lymphatic component do not characteristically penetrate the pulmonary cavities or mediastinum.

Symptoms of pain and paresthesias with VMs are usually the result of local inflammation around intralesional thrombi or nerve compression at the usual levels.[1] Areas with phlebothrombosis become swollen, firm, and painful, especially when compression garments are applied. Most symptoms are aggravated after exercise in which repetitive movements such as lifting, gripping, or pinching are involved.

Not all lesions are superficial. Intramuscular VMs occur with equal frequency in the extensor muscles and in the flexor-pronator groups of the forearm. Within the hand, the dorsal interossei and thenar and hypothenar intrinsic muscles are affected much more commonly than the lumbricals and palmar interossei. The skin overlying affected muscles usually has a VM within the subcutaneous space. We have noted a subgroup of deep VMs that run along either side of the interosseous membrane and spread along fascial planes between muscle groups. Although these lesions are not as dense as subcutaneous or intramuscular VMs, calcified phleboliths found anywhere between the wrist and shoulder make these some of the most symptomatic. In the absence of phleboliths, nerve

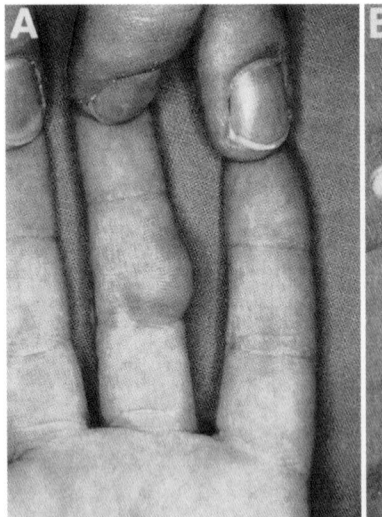
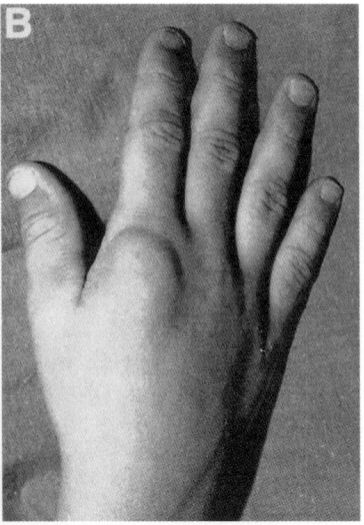
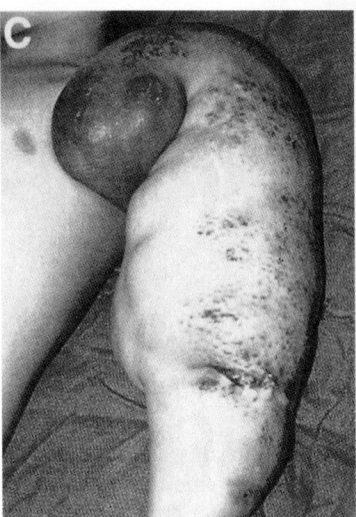
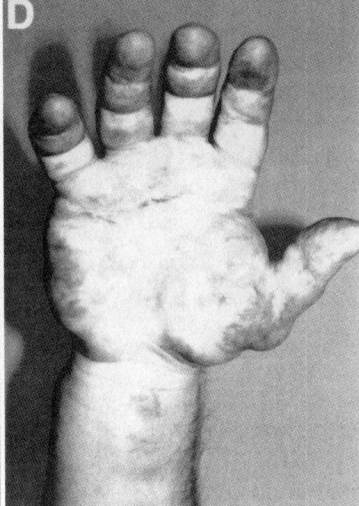

FIGURE 209-12. Diverse presentations of venous malformation. *A,* An isolated venous malformation along the palmar surface of a digit will be symptomatic if intralesional thrombi compress digital nerves. *B,* This dorsal lesion is soft and compressible and symptomatic. *C,* Extensive venous malformations may involve the entire extremity and chest wall. This patient is septic from an infected phlebothrombosis in the anterior axillary region. *D,* This diffuse venous malformation involves every soft tissue structure of the hand and distal forearm. Surgery is indicated only for symptomatic regions.

compression, or intralesional bleeding, most VMs are asymptomatic. Subtle deficiencies in grip and pinch strength may be measured with extensive intramuscular involvement; however, these generally seem minimal in comparison to the extent of involvement on MRI scans.

VMs do occasionally involve skeletal structures. Radiographs of these limbs show cortical lucencies where vessels penetrate the medullary canals. Large areas of osteolysis are not present. However, pathologic fractures can occur with significant stress loading of upper limbs with large diffuse lesions. Both overgrowth and undergrowth of limbs with large VMs have been documented.[21] Synovial VMs in the wrist and elbow may cause hemarthrosis and arthritis from hemosiderin deposits. These problems are not as common in the upper as in the lower extremity.

VMs do not progress from a slow-flow to a high-flow state. All grow commensurately with the child (Fig. 209-13). Enlargement after partial resection represents redirection of flow into adjacent anomalous channels. There is a hormonal modulation in women with medium-sized and large VMs and lymphatic-venous malformations, which may increase in size during adolescence, during menses, with oral contraceptives, and during pregnancies. In women who experienced exacerbations of their symptoms during pregnancy, there was no improvement (reversal of size and flow) after pregnancy.[1]

Large VMs can be coagulopathic. A thorough coagulation profile should be obtained in all patients with extensive VMs, with or without capillary or lymphatic components, particularly if there is any history of bleeding or ecchymosis. In contrast to the Kasabach-Merritt

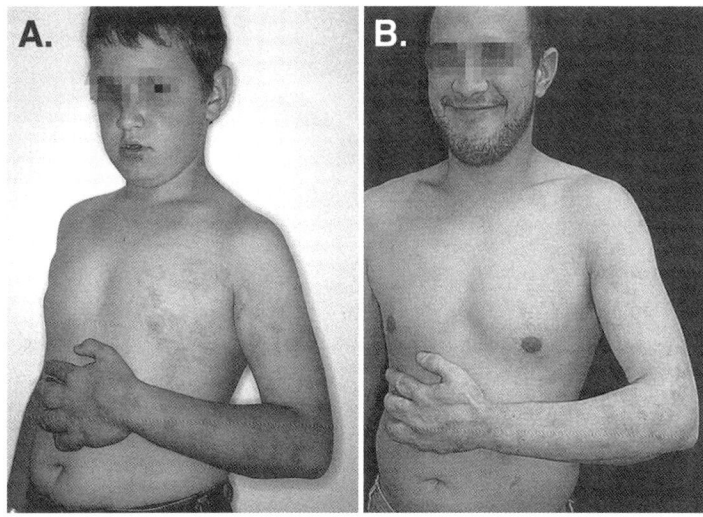

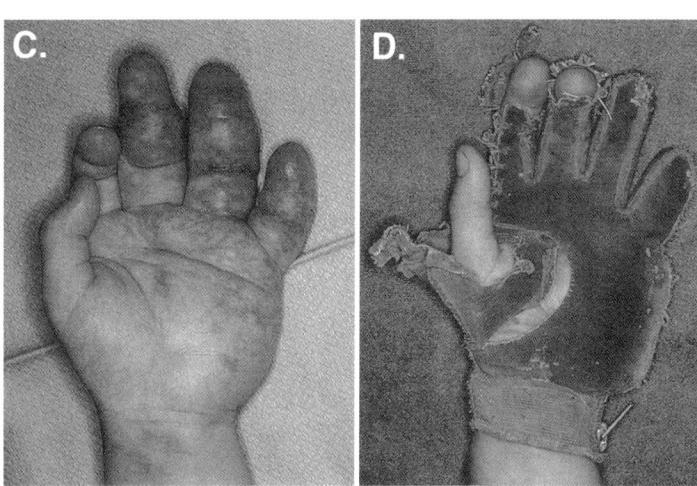

FIGURE 209-13. Extensive venous malformation. *A*, An extensive venous malformation in a 9-year-old boy involving the entire hand and extending up the forearm and arm onto the ipsilateral chest wall. Surgery is reserved for isolated regions of pain or phlebothrombosis. *B*, The same patient is seen 22 years later, demonstrating a stable clinical picture. *C* and *D*, All tissues of the hand are involved. For the first 9 years of this boy's life, a compression glove was sufficient to control his symptoms. The well-worn appearance of the glove attests to this young man's compliance.

phenomenon associated with thrombocytopenia, patients with coagulopathic VMs have platelet counts in the 100,000 to 150,000/mm³ range. Prothrombin time may be increased, with normal activated partial thromboplastin time, low fibrinogen levels (150 to 200 mg/dL), and increased fibrin split products.

RADIOLOGIC CHARACTERISTICS

Ultrasonography

Ultrasound examination is useful only to confirm what is known on physical examination: slow flow in a compressible lesion.

Magnetic Resonance Imaging

MRI scans provide the "gold standard" for the evaluation of VMs (Fig. 209-14). These lesions have no characteristic size and can involve all tissue layers. On T1-weighted sequences, these lesions are isointense;

gradient-weighted images show diffuse, inhomogeneous enhancement. T2-weighted images show septation within the soft tissue mass and signal voids characteristic of phleboliths. Flow-sensitive gradient-weighted sequences show no evidence of high flow but signal voids (phleboliths) that are not flow voids. Magnetic resonance venography is helpful for evaluation of large VMs anywhere in the upper limb.

Phlebography

Direct puncture phlebography can be used to obtain a more detailed evaluation of the intrinsic anatomy of a VM and to visualize the extrinsic drainage of the limb. It is usually performed before sclerotherapy.

Angiography

Arterial anatomy is normal in limbs with VMs, lymphatic-venous malformations, and capillary-lymphatic-venous malformations, although there may

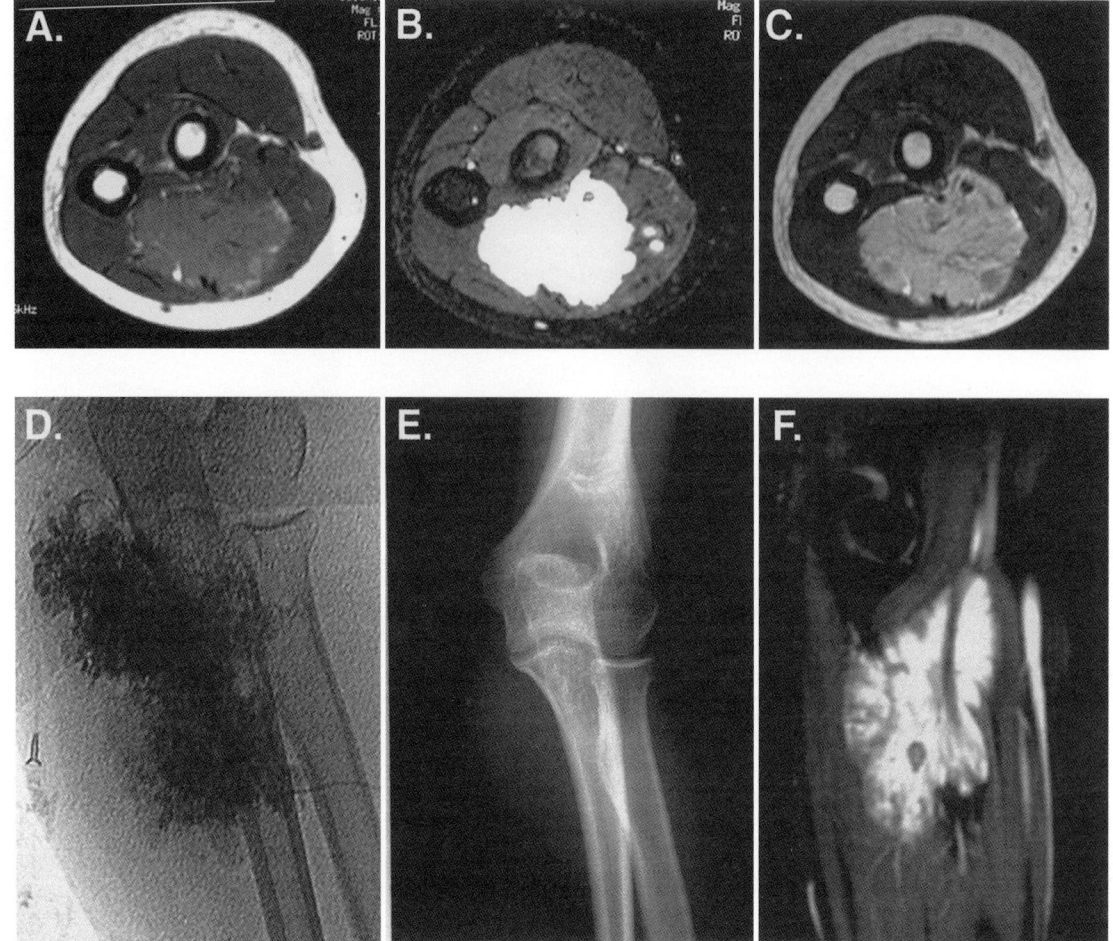

FIGURE 209-14. Imaging of a venous malformation in an adult patient with a forearm lesion. *A to C,* Transverse MRI sequences of the forearm, which are differently weighted, highlight characteristic findings of a venous malformation. On a T1-weighted sequence *(A),* the venous malformation is isointense to adjacent skeletal muscle. On a T1-weighted sequence with gadolinium administration *(B),* there is diffuse enhancement of the venous malformation. On a T2-weighted sequence *(C),* there is a high signal with signal voids within the venous malformation that represent phleboliths. *D,* Intravenous injection of contrast material at the time of sclerotherapy reveals an abnormal collection of saccular venous structures. *E,* Phleboliths are seen in soft tissues on a lateral plain radiograph. *F,* T2-weighted sagittal MRI sequence.

be some distortion on the basis of mass effect, particularly within the hand. Abnormalities on the venous side show puddling of contrast material and delayed flow out of the VM. Angiograms are helpful in the preoperative evaluation of large VMs or of lesions in difficult areas for dissection, such as the brachial plexus, antecubital fossa, and palmar spaces of the hand.

TREATMENT

An algorithm for treatment of VMs is outlined in Figure 209-15.

Observation

The initial treatment of all VMs is conservative. Most large and small lesions are asymptomatic. A carefully tailored compression garment is helpful to control the enlargement of the VM during or after exercise and to control the bulk and weight of the distended lesion (see Fig. 209-13). Pain associated with phlebothrombosis may be aggravated by garment wear. Low-dose aspirin therapy is helpful to reduce thrombus formation. We encourage and continue conservative measures unless functional symptoms or aesthetic considerations become significant.

Sclerotherapy

Our second line of treatment is provided by the interventional radiologist for all but the small well-localized lesions in the upper limb that are most expeditiously removed with surgical resection.

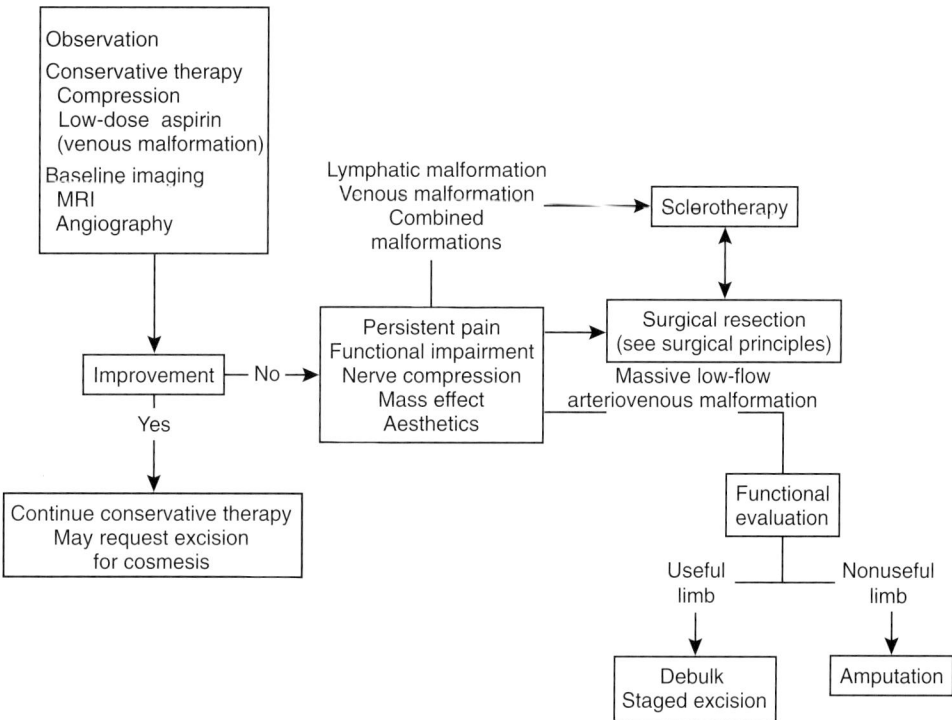

FIGURE 209-15. Treatment algorithm for slow-flow vascular malformations.

Sclerotherapy is used for functional or aesthetic considerations and is most successful in lesions with large saccular channels. Absolute alcohol (100%) is the preferred sclerosant in the United States[83]; Ethibloc,* a mixture of zein (a corn protein), alcohol, and contrast medium, is used outside of this country.[84]

The passage of sclerosant into the general circulation can be potentially dangerous if a proximal tourniquet is not used. Direct injections adjacent to neurovascular structures anywhere in the limb, especially around the brachial plexus, into the antecubital fossa, or in the volar wrist crease region, and directly into the palm of the hand are performed with great caution, if at all. Our radiologists prefer to treat specific areas at multiple bimonthly intervals[83] and have the best outcomes with large VMs in the arm and proximal forearm (Fig. 209-16). Although sclerotherapy has been performed on the dorsal surface of the hand, direct injections into the hand are avoided.

Complications extend from ecchymosis, blistering, and occasionally full-thickness loss of overlying skin to damage of adjacent soft tissue structures (Fig. 209-17). Extensive hemolysis may lead to renal toxicity. Excessive intravenous sclerosant may cause cardiac compromise.[83]

Careful pretreatment planning is necessary whenever sclerotherapy is used before a single or staged surgical resection. The inflammatory reaction and scar formation after this modality are significant and will cross tissue planes. The surgeon must be available when the interventional radiologist plans to treat extensive VMs. With smaller lesions, we often go directly to surgical resection, which leaves adjacent structures less traumatized. Embolization from the arterial side is not used with VMs.

Surgery

The indications for surgical treatment are primarily functional but can be aesthetic.[1,85] Technical details and principles of treatment are summarized in Table 209-3. Judicious resections of VMs are both safe and predictable. Small well-localized lesions anywhere in the subcutaneous tissue planes, on the dorsum of the hand, or along the sides of a digit or thumb are easily removed. Larger diffuse lesions may be more of a problem, depending on regional anatomy. Any resection involving the neurovascular structures in the antecubital fossa, pronator tunnel, and deep palmar spaces of the hand requires careful planning and an experienced surgeon. Single or staged debulking on the dorsum of the hand may extend through the intermetacarpal spaces into the deep palmar spaces, a difficult area in which to control bleeding. Loupe

*Ethicon, Hamburg, Germany.

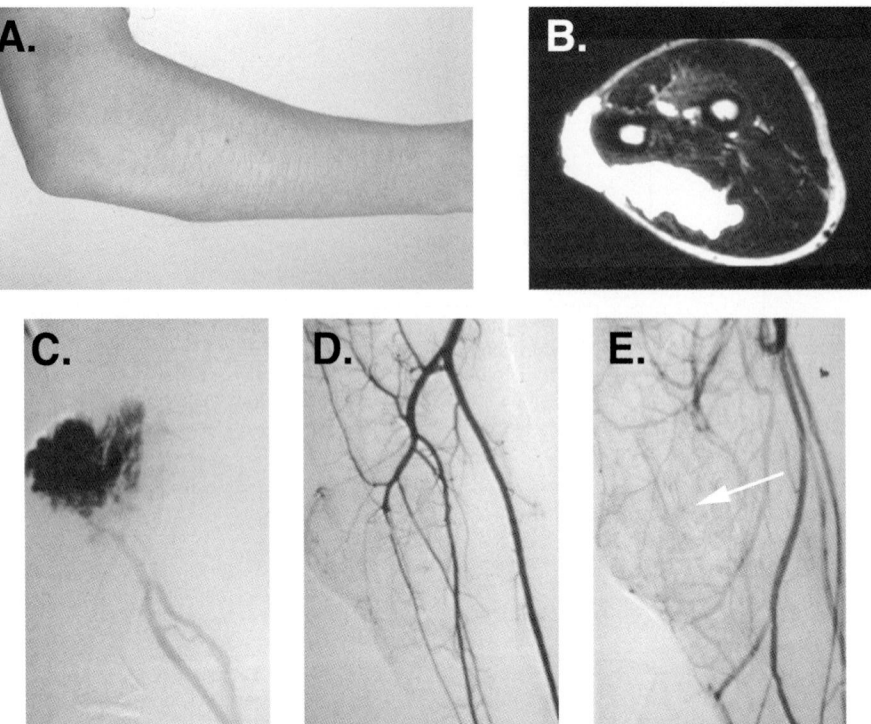

FIGURE 209-16. Sclerotherapy of an upper extremity venous malformation. *A,* Venous malformation involving the superficial flexor and extensor compartments of the forearm. *B,* T1-weighted MRI sequence demonstrates the extent of involvement. Physical examination alone may be deceiving. *C,* Injection of contrast material at the time of sclerotherapy demonstrates the abnormal venous vessels. *D,* Arterial-phase angiogram after sclerotherapy demonstrates a normal arterial circulation. *E,* Venous-phase angiogram after sclerotherapy shows lack of contrast material at the site of the sclerosed venous malformation *(arrow).*

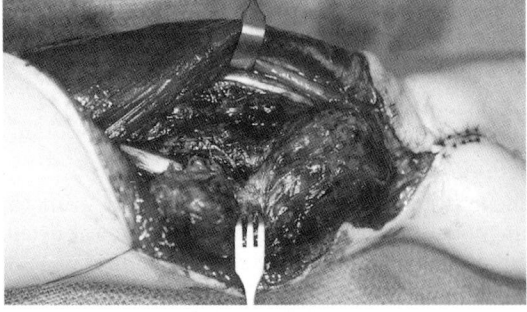

FIGURE 209-17. Sclerotherapy complication. An acute compartment syndrome developed within hours after this venous malformation was injected. The lesion extended along the interosseous membrane, involving all four superficial flexor muscle bellies and the terminal flexor to the thumb. Clots and thrombi are seen during the fasciotomy. Involved portions of muscles were excised. The only residuum 4 years later was a weak thumb flexor.

TABLE 209-3 ✦ OPERATIVE PRINCIPLES FOR RESECTION OF UPPER EXTREMITY VASCULAR MALFORMATIONS

Maintain absolute hemostasis under tourniquet control.
Carefully plan dissection within a well-defined region.
Preserve nerves, arteries, and joint cavities. Avoid intraneural dissection.
Avoid reoperation in a previously scarred region by performing a thorough initial dissection.
Avoid dorsal and palmar dissections.
Use separate procedures for debulking of digit, hand, forearm, and arm. Debulk axilla and chest wall together.
Perform joint synovectomies and tendon dissections within the digital sheath sparingly.

magnification is used at all times, and we do not hesitate to use the operating microscope in dissection of peripheral nerves or within the palm or along digits.

We avoid intramuscular dissections unless symptoms in that particular area are due to phlebothrombosis and are always surprised by the perioperative function of an extensively infiltrated muscle. Within the arm or forearm, it is often better to resect the affected muscle completely and to restore its function, if needed, with a transfer or replacement. In the patient with a large, extensive VM with localized areas of pain, we will resect that specific region, which invariably contains inflamed varices with thromboses (Fig. 209-18).

It is impossible to completely excise large, diffuse lesions with and without muscle involvement. Symptomatic, enlarged digits can be debulked in two stages with the incision placed in the midlateral line. Microscopic preservation of digital arteries, including individual vincular branches and nerves, is important (Fig. 209-19). In dorsal digital debulking, it is unwise to proceed beyond Cleland ligaments on the opposite side of the digit. Forearm debulkings are completed in the same two-staged fashion (Fig. 209-20). Fortunately, extensive VMs rarely extend through the brachial plexus, a structure that precludes dissection with the aid of a tourniquet. These resections should be avoided in asymptomatic patients with normal distal radial, ulnar, and median nerve function.

Large VMs extending along the entire arm into the axilla and ipsilateral chest wall are challenging, especially when the patient may be septic from localized phlebothrombosis. Coagulopathies are often present. When the mass is primarily extramuscular, a total resection is often best (see Fig. 209-12). Surgical aids include catheters in the subclavian artery and vein, Cell Saver, hypotensive anesthesia, pneumatic tourniquet for the most distal portion of the VM, and experienced

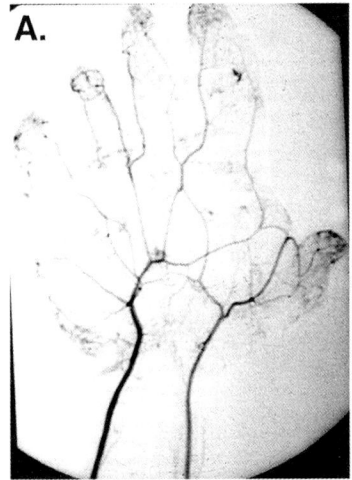
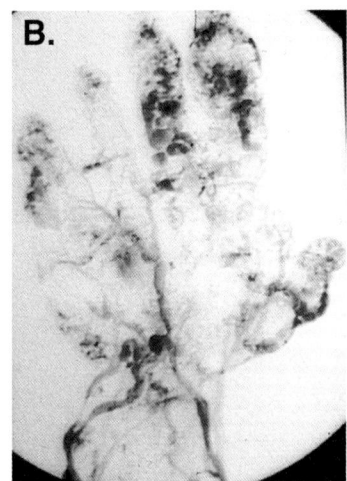
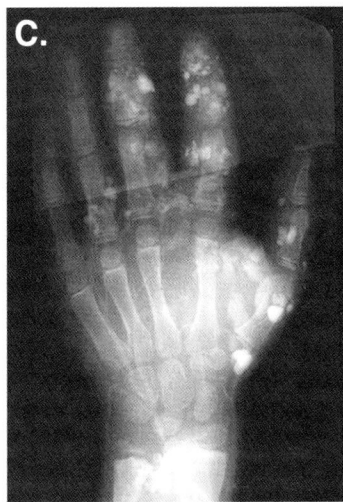
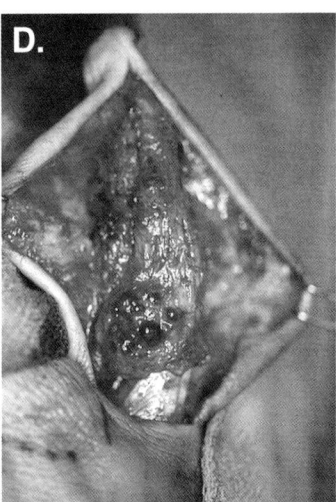

FIGURE 209-18. Venous malformation. *A,* The arterial phase on this angiogram shows normal arterial anatomy. *B,* Saccular venous lakes, tortuous veins, and pooling are clearly demonstrated on venous-phase angiography. *C,* Plain radiography of the same patient demonstrates many calcified phleboliths. *D,* The thrombi and phleboliths within the venous malformation, shown here at digital surgical resection, may cause direct compression and irritation of both dorsal and palmar digital nerves.

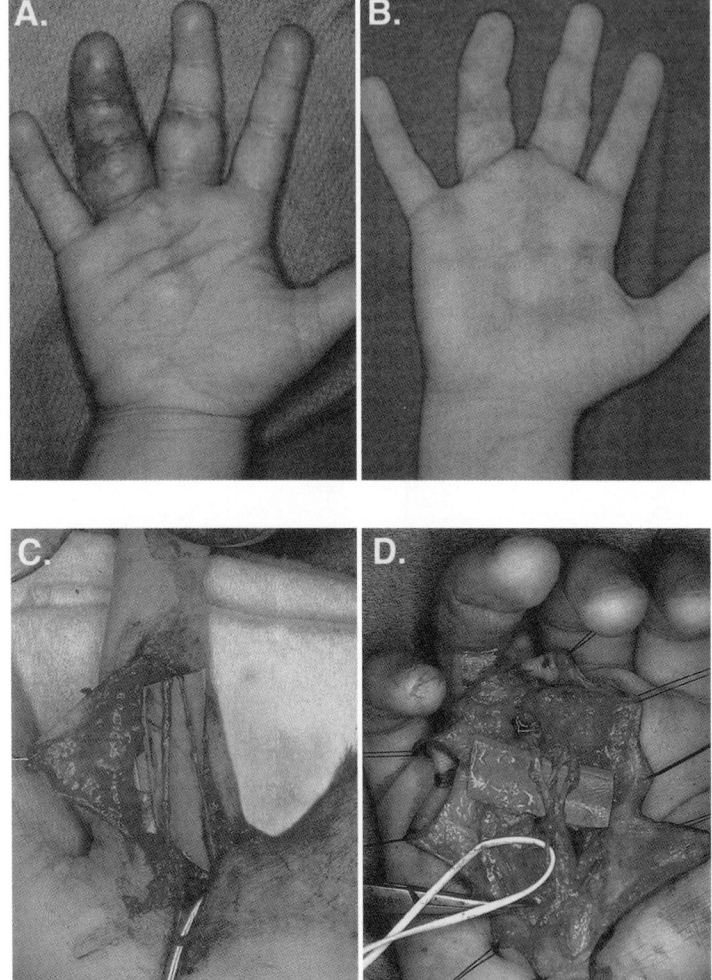

FIGURE 209-19. Surgical resection of a venous malformation involving the palm and long and ring digits. *A*, Preoperative appearance. The extent of involvement is always much greater than is estimated on physical examination. *B*, The first of multiple staged procedures consisted of debulking half of each of the long and ring fingers. Microscopic dissection is invaluable for preservation of neurovascular structures. *C*, The radial digital nerve and artery are seen after microscopic dissection. *D*, All neurovascular structures (except the venae comitantes) are preserved during a full palmar dissection.

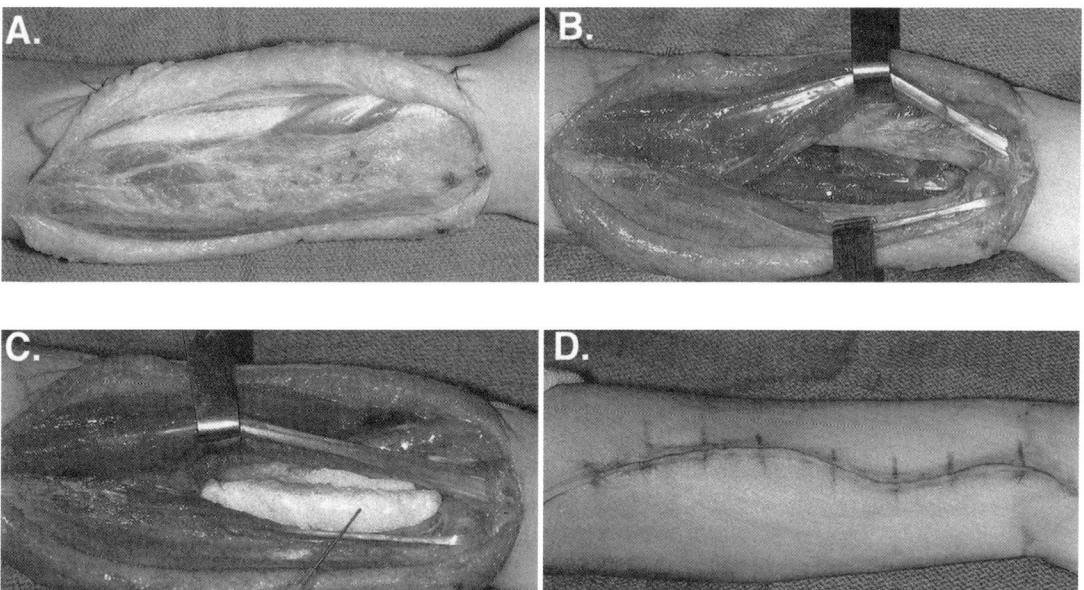

FIGURE 209-20. Persistent venous malformation after surgical resection. *A,* A 9-year-old boy presented after an unsuccessful excision of a symptomatic venous malformation at another institution, during which the surgeons found themselves operating "in an ink well." At the time of reoperation at our institution, the skin flaps have been reflected, and the scarred muscular fascia has been exposed. *B,* Excision included the interosseous membrane and all involved soft tissue as well as several distal muscle bellies. *C,* Before closure, Gelfoam has been placed within the dead space along with drainage catheters. *D,* An intradermal subcutaneous closure should always be performed on the exposed dorsal surface of the forearm.

assistants who can compress the lesion while the primary surgeon dissects it off the muscular fascia. One unit of fresh frozen plasma must be replaced with every three units of blood. We try to limit total blood replacement to one blood volume in these children.

The complication rate after partial or complete removal of slow-flow VMs is less than 10%. Patients with complications usually had more than one problem, directly proportional to the size and specific location of the VM.[1] Because postoperative hematomas are common, we have used delayed primary closures at 24 to 72 hours after resection of large VMs. In contrast to the head and neck and truncal regions, hematomas can be avoided in the upper limb with elevation and a good compression dressing. One should not rely on drains alone. The most common long-term problems have been neuromas in continuity, loss of function, contracture after intramuscular resections, and soft tissue losses.[1] All can be difficult problems to treat.

BLUE RUBBER BLEB NEVUS SYNDROME

Blue rubber bleb nevus syndrome is a rare, sporadic disorder consisting of cutaneous and gastrointestinal VMs. This is the most common vascular anomaly responsible for chronic gastrointestinal hemorrhage. Autosomal dominant inheritance has been reported,

but no genetic locus has yet been identified.[86] The cutaneous lesions are soft and dome shaped or nodular; they have a predilection for occurrence on the trunk, palms, and soles (Fig. 209-21).[86] The lesions increase in size and number with age. Orthopedic dysfunction may result.[87] The gastrointestinal lesions are widely distributed, most commonly in the small bowel, ranging in number from a few to several hundred per patient. In addition to bleeding, these lesions may lead to intussusception and volvulus.[88] Lesions are frequently present in the liver, gallbladder, mesentery, and retroperitoneum.

Lymphatic Malformations

PATHOGENESIS

Since Sabin's classic proposal[89] that lymphatics develop in a centrifugal fashion from existing veins, there has been great controversy. Some have reasoned that these endothelial channels develop independently (centripetal) before connecting to veins. Studies by Kaipainen[90] and Wigle[91] support the centrifugal hypothesis. Studies of the molecular genetics of lymphatics have shown that lymphatic endothelial cells express vascular endothelial growth factor receptor 3 (VEGFR3).[90] When this gene is eliminated in knockout mice, these animals die with major venous

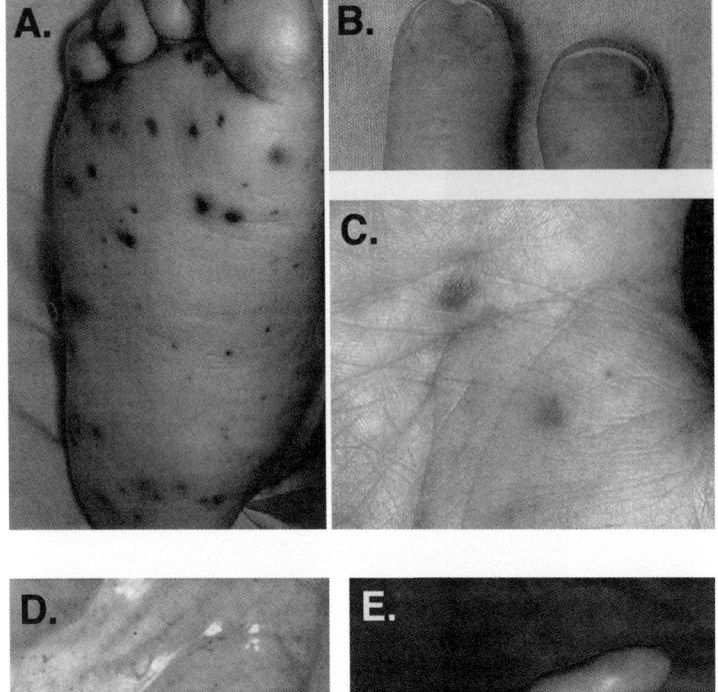

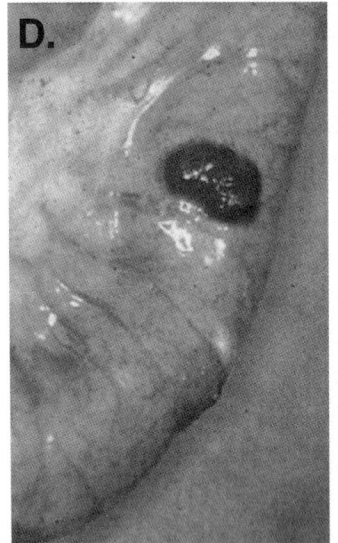

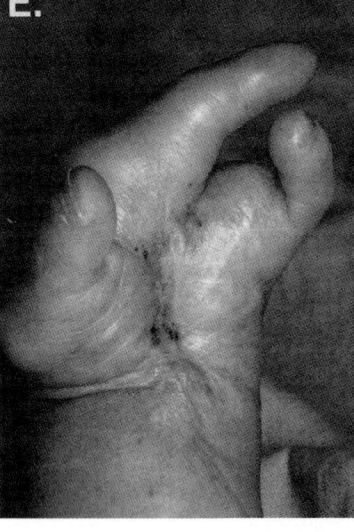

FIGURE 209-21. Blue rubber bleb nevus syndrome. *A* to *C,* Multiple small localized nodular venous malformations are seen on the plantar surface of the foot, in subungual locations, and beneath the glabrous surfaces of the palm. *D,* The gastrointestinal tract is commonly involved. Anemia caused by mucosal ulcerations is the major clinical problem. Several hundred lesions may be present. *E,* Appearance of the patient's hand after multiple ray resections during childhood done as a result of venous malformations.

anomalies and no lymphatics.[92] Transgenic mice who overexpress VEGFR3 ligand VEGF-C develop abnormal, distended lymphatic channels.

Milroy disease is a type of hereditary lymphedema that has been localized to loci on chromosomes 5q and 16q.[93-96] This type of lymphedema is the result of a lymphatic anomaly.

CLINICAL FEATURES

Lymphatic anomalies are usually present at birth. Smaller lesions in less conspicuous regions, such as the interdigital web spaces, axilla, buttock, and perineum, become evident by 4 years of age. In contrast to VMs, lymphatic malformations (LMs) have a rubbery consistency and do not decompress with elevation or direct pressure. Boys and girls are affected equally. LMs are most commonly found in the cervicofacial region, where large lesions are often detected by prenatal ultrasound examination. The arm-axilla, retroperitoneum, mediastinum, buttock, and anorectal regions are also involved. Although thoracic duct anomalies can occur, they are rarely seen with isolated upper extremity and chest wall LMs.

LM is best described macroscopically as a sponge with large (macroscopic), small (microscopic), or combined spaces. Using now outdated terminology, previous authors used the terms lymphangioma for microscopic LMs and cystic hygroma for macroscopic lesions in the cervicofacial region. In the upper limb, either solitary or diffuse lesions in the arm, axilla, and chest wall have both macroscopic and microscopic channels. Distal to the elbow, almost all LMs are predominantly microscopic, a characteristic that makes them less amenable to sclerotherapy. Diffuse lesions involving the dorsum of the hand, wrist, and forearm usually contain microcystic spaces with large amounts of adjacent adipose tissue. On histologic examination, the walls of lymphatic spaces contain both smooth and skeletal muscle cells and are of variable thickness. The lumens and cystic spaces are filled with protein-rich fluid. Lymphocytes and small germinal centers may be present.[31] In all upper extremity locations, LMs are accompanied by large amounts of fat within the subcutaneous tissue plane.

LMs in the upper limb have many forms (Fig. 209-22). A dermal capillary malformation is often present in large lesions. The skin may have a bluish discoloration. With dermal involvement, the skin is thick and may have deep cutaneous puckering (Fig. 209-23),[31] much like the peau d'orange skin seen in acquired types of lymphedema. LMs in the superficial layers present as single or coalesced vesicles that often weep and provide a portal of entry for bacterial flora. Dark blue or red nodules represent vesicles filled with blood. Skin involvement does not follow any neurologic patterns and is usually patchy in the presence of extensive deep LMs. One variant of LM has a venous component, termed lymphatic-venous malformation (LVM).

Lymphatic anomalies in the upper limb are most commonly isolated to a specific region in a digit, hand, forearm, or arm. Axillary LMs typically extend onto the ipsilateral chest wall and into the supraclavicular space and neck. Extensions into the mediastinum are appreciated only after an MRI scan has been obtained. There is no characteristic pattern of anatomic involvement. Fortunately, most LMs are confined to the subcutaneous tissue planes and skin. LMs do not penetrate the intermuscular fascia into muscle but can spread along these fascial planes. With small LMs, hand,

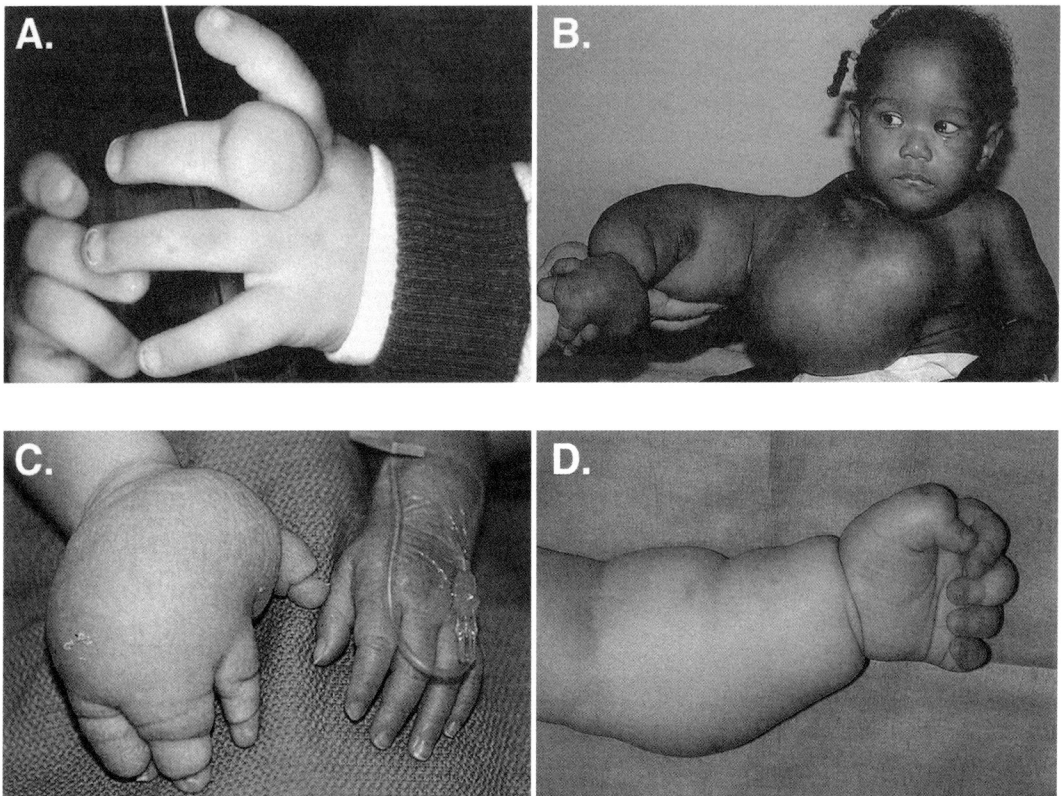

FIGURE 209-22. Diverse presentations of lymphatic malformations. *A,* Hard, rubbery semimobile mass on the dorsum of the ring finger in an 18-month-old boy. *B,* Gross involvement of the upper limb, ipsilateral chest, mediastinum, and neck in a 2-year-old girl. *C,* Lymphatic malformation involving the right hand and wrist of a neonate who had an erroneous diagnosis of amniotic band syndrome on prenatal ultrasound examination, resulting in unnecessary fetal surgery at another institution. The tissue is rubbery and minimally compressible. *D,* A common presentation of more extensive lymphatic malformations is on the forearm and dorsum of the hand and digits.

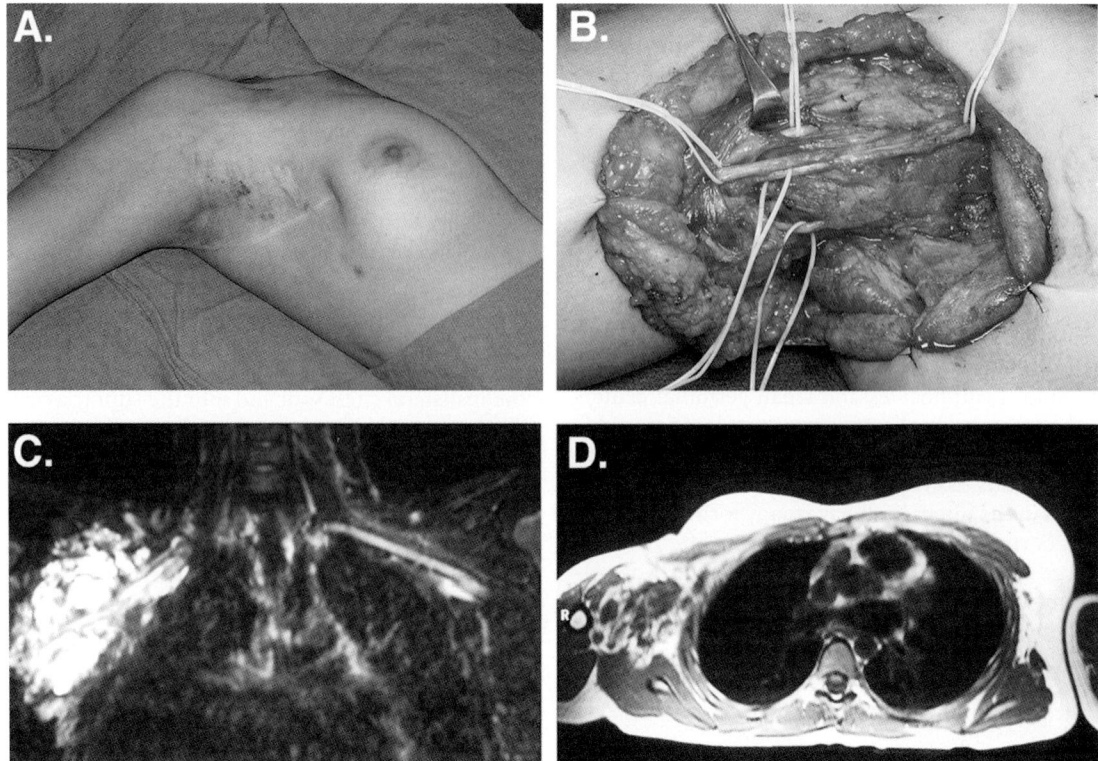

FIGURE 209-23. Lymphatic malformation, axilla. *A,* Deep dermal lymphatic malformation and cutaneous vesicles have been a source of bleeding, drainage, and recurrent cellulitis in this teenager who had an axillary lymphatic malformation partially resected during the first month of life. Surgical removal is the only method that will eliminate these symptoms. Appropriate breast augmentation is planned when the patient reaches maturity. *B,* The medial and lateral cords of the brachial plexus have been identified during a dissection, which must be meticulous. Only the symptomatic portions of the plexus need to be dissected. All of these axillary lesions extend deep to the chest wall. *C* and *D,* Axillary and chest wall extension is well demonstrated on these MRI sequences after gadolinium administration. The three-dimensional breast deficiency is also seen.

forearm, and arm function is normal. Most symptoms in larger lesions are related to the size, weight, and noncompressibility of the lesion or the weeping, maceration, and ulcers of infected regions. In contrast to pure VMs, nerve compression and phlebothrombosis are uncommon.

LM in the upper and lower extremity can be associated with both skeletal and soft tissue overgrowth that in varying degrees progresses to gigantism. In most of these limbs, there is an accompanying adipose overgrowth. Bones and joints are not characteristically invaded by the lymphatic channels.

Lymphangiomatosis refers to a condition of unique patients who have evidence of disseminated LM. This constellation typically includes diffuse thoracic duct anomalies with recurrent pleural effusions together with pathognomonic osteolytic bone lesions. These bone lesions were originally described as Gorham-Stout syndrome, disappearing bone disease, or phantom bone disease.[97] Whereas bone lesions alone have been reported in isolated patients, they are much more frequently seen in the setting of intrathoracic disease.

RADIOLOGIC CHARACTERISTICS

Ultrasonography

Ultrasound examination is useful only to document the existence of large and small fluid-filled soft tissue spaces with or without fibrous septations.

Magnetic Resonance Imaging

T1-weighted images are hypointense, and secondary to the high water content, T2-weighted sequences are hyperintense (Fig. 209-24). Large macrocysts may have fluid levels from protein or blood. Administration of contrast material may reveal absent or slight rim enhancement, and gradient-weighted sequences show no evidence of high-flow voids.[26] Large venous channels may also be present with LMs and are more frequently dispersed within combined LVMs.[26]

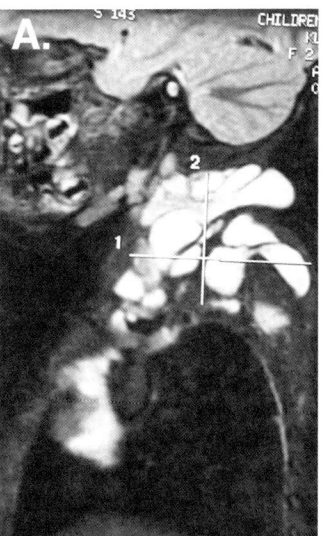
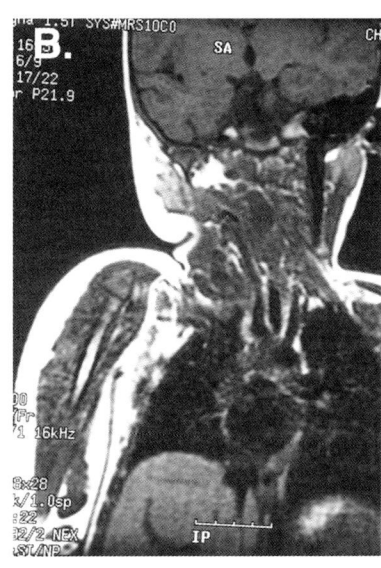
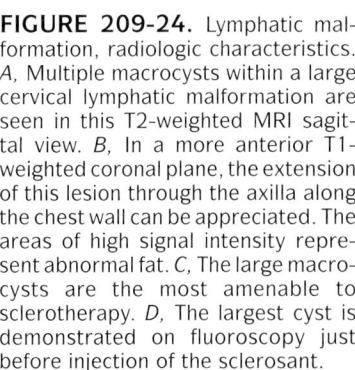
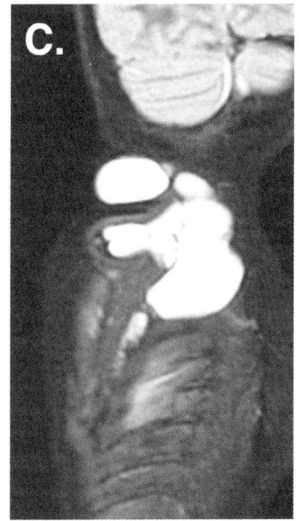
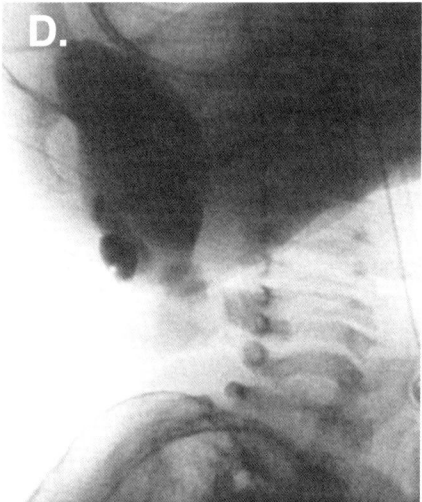

FIGURE 209-24. Lymphatic malformation, radiologic characteristics. *A,* Multiple macrocysts within a large cervical lymphatic malformation are seen in this T2-weighted MRI sagittal view. *B,* In a more anterior T1-weighted coronal plane, the extension of this lesion through the axilla along the chest wall can be appreciated. The areas of high signal intensity represent abnormal fat. *C,* The large macrocysts are the most amenable to sclerotherapy. *D,* The largest cyst is demonstrated on fluoroscopy just before injection of the sclerosant.

TREATMENT

Observation

As with VMs, there are three treatment options for LMs: conservative measures, sclerotherapy, and surgical resection (see Fig. 209-15). Small lesions and involved areas of skin are easily observed and treated with local wound care. The two major problems with LMs are infection and intralesional bleeding. Bleeding within a pure LM is not necessarily indicative of a coagulopathy, but a hematologic work-up is advised with all large LMs or combined lesions. Bleeding causes the LM to enlarge and to become bluish and sometimes painful. Cold compression, elevation, rest, and empirical antibiotic therapy provide effective treatment.

Infection is a more serious problem. Bacteria from a systemic infection may seed channels within an LM. The mechanism may be due to altered lymphatic flow or lymphocyte function in the wall of anomalous channels.[31] A rapidly progressing cellulitis in children is usually secondary to an upper respiratory infection. Beta-streptococcal organisms are the major pathogens and respond to the prompt administration of penicillin or a broad-spectrum antibiotic. These wildfire infections usually resolve as rapidly as they progress. Parents must be warned to start the oral administration as soon as the signs of infection become evident.

Simple aspiration of large cysts provides only temporary relief. Sustained intermittent compression of large lesions in the upper extremity adequately decompresses one region, displacing fluid into adjacent portions of the LM. Without continuous wear of an elastic garment, the fluid will eventually reaccumulate.

Sclerotherapy

The second line of treatment is sclerotherapy by direct injection into the cystic cavities (see Fig. 209-24). Macrocystic LMs respond much more favorably than microcystic lesions do, and for this reason, sclerosants are rarely used around the wrist, hand, or digits. Pure ethanol, sodium tetradecyl sulfate, and doxycycline are the most frequently used sclerosants.[26] A new agent, OK-432, derived from group A *Streptococcus pyogenes*, has been used for LMs[98,99] and, in one report, improved osteolysis.

Surgery

Surgical resection is the most predictable way to control or "cure" LMs. It is elected more frequently for LMs than for VMs. Operative indications for both LMs and LVMs include pain; intralesional thrombi (venous component present); episodic bleeding; recurrent infection; chronic ulceration and maceration; and functional problems specific to the size, weight, and bulk of extensive lesions. Local resections in the arm, axilla, and chest wall are often necessary to control excessive drainage.

Expertise and knowledge of neural and vascular anatomy are essential for dissections of the brachial plexus, antecubital fossa, and palmar spaces of the hand (including the carpal and ulnar tunnels) and along the digits and thumb. We have noted most difficulty with extensive lesions within the antecubital fossa and the pronator tunnel, where the multiple motor branches of the ulnar and median nerves must be preserved. Within the palm of the hand, both superficial and deep palmar arches must be preserved with the common digital vessels and all motor branches to intrinsic muscles; these dissections should not be performed unless there is a compelling reason to do so.

The general principles are reviewed in Table 209-3. Additional caveats exist for each specific location in the upper limb. The digits and thumb should be approached through midaxial incisions. Zigzag incisions in the glabrous skin hypertrophy and should be avoided. One neurovascular bundle should be left untouched during each of two staged debulkings of a massively enlarged digit (Fig. 209-25). Cleland ligaments (which are typically stretched or attenuated) represent important landmarks during dissection. Dorsal debulking should not extend beyond this ligament to the opposite side of the digit. The adventitia around digital arteries and the epineurium of digital nerves can help indicate the location of neurovascular structures in these often distorted digits. Despite

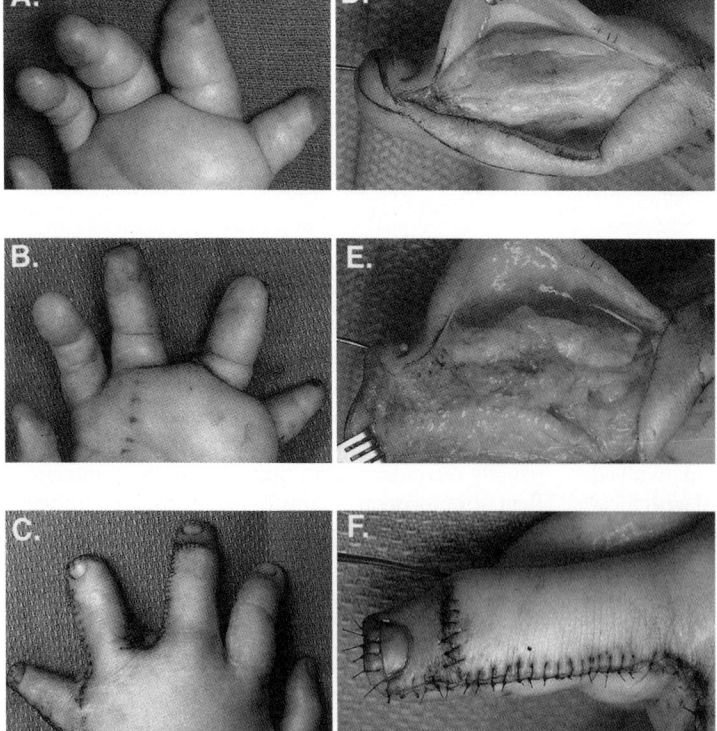

FIGURE 209-25. Lymphatic malformation, digital resection. *A,* The digital and palmar dissections of this lymphatic malformation are performed separately. One side of the digit will be debulked at a time. *B,* Postoperative appearance of palmar surface. *C,* Dorsal surface closure. *D,* Flaps are raised through a high midaxial incision. Estimated regions of skin excision include a large portion of the pulp tissue. There is significant scar tissue from a previous excision. *E,* The radial neurovascular bundle, including vincular branches of the artery, has been preserved. An excess amount of fat is admixed with the microcystic lymphatic malformation. The ulnar neurovascular bundle is untouched. *F,* Excess skin is excised through dorsal skin creases. A 2-mm skin bridge is preserved on the distal fingertip for suturing of the palmar flap.

resection of large amounts of both glabrous and dorsal skin, all closures must be tension free. Early use of Coban wrapping and continuous passive motion machines will decrease postoperative swelling and the residual scar that often develops postoperatively.

The dorsal surfaces of the hand and wrist should be debulked in stages with incisions along the borders of the hand or through a single incision parallel to the third metacarpal (Fig. 209-26). When this skin contains deep dermal LM and epidermal vesicles, consider total excision and replacement with either a full-thickness skin graft or a thin fasciocutaneous flap. The tissue over the thumb and thenar muscles and that over the hypothenar muscles are easy to debulk. In contrast, a thorough dissection of LM within the palm is one of the most difficult procedures in all of hand surgery.

The forearm is ideally approached through a straight medial incision, extending from wrist to elbow. Each stage can extend no more than 200 degrees around the circumference of the forearm. The elbow and arm are best approached medially, and extensive LMs or LVMs are removed in two or more stages. The use of continual compression garments and com-pression pumps preoperatively and postoperatively makes a tremendous difference in achieving a satisfactory result. Although fluid collection can be partially controlled with compression, most resections proximal to the elbow will drain for weeks postoperatively.

After performing separate resections of the chest wall and axilla for many years, we now perform this in a single stage during which all neurovascular structures can be clearly identified (Fig. 209-27). These are long, meticulous operations during which blood loss can be insidious and assistants can become fatigued. A thorough preoperative preparation of the entire surgical and anesthesiology teams is essential. Difficult decisions must be made in regard to replacement of involved skin (lymphangioma circumscriptum). Hypothermic-hypotensive anesthesia and a Cell Saver may help limit blood loss. After one complete blood volume has been replaced, fresh frozen plasma should be available.

The principle of performing as thorough a resection as possible is more important in the resection of an LM than with any other vascular anomaly. The inflammation and angiogenesis of these healing

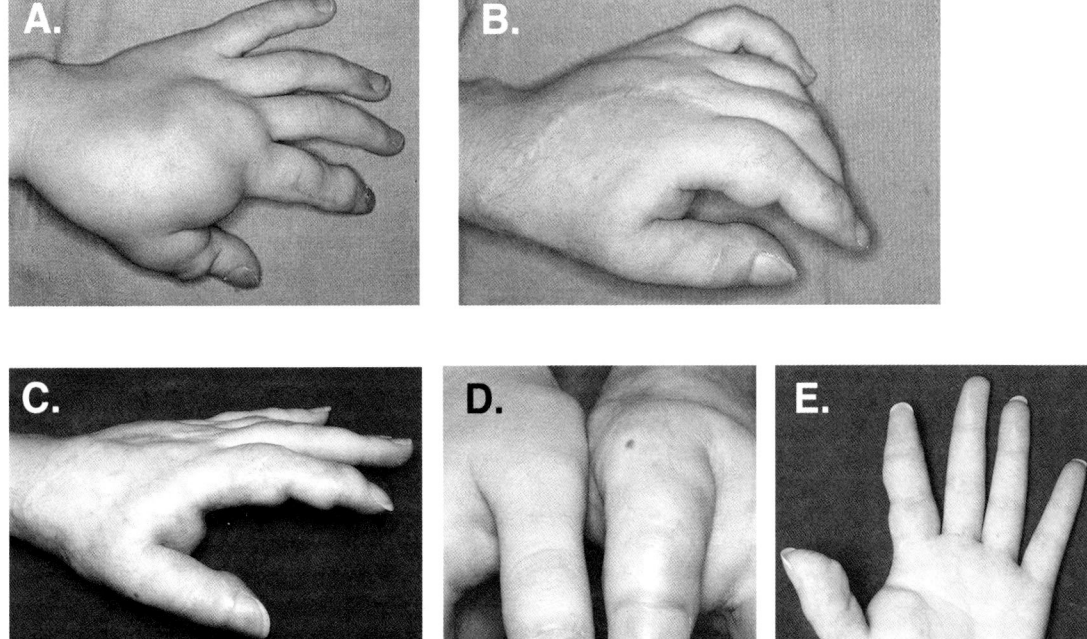

FIGURE 209-26. Lymphatic malformation, dorsal hand resection. *A,* This young girl is seen at age 6 years after debulking of the index and long digits. Resection of the dorsum of the hand and thumb is planned in two additional procedures. *B,* Postoperative result, 24 years later. *C,* Result 30 years after resection. *D* and *E,* Regions over the radial side of the index finger and the palmar pulp of the thumb continue to be swollen and hyperhidrotic as a result of the intradermal lymphatic malformation.

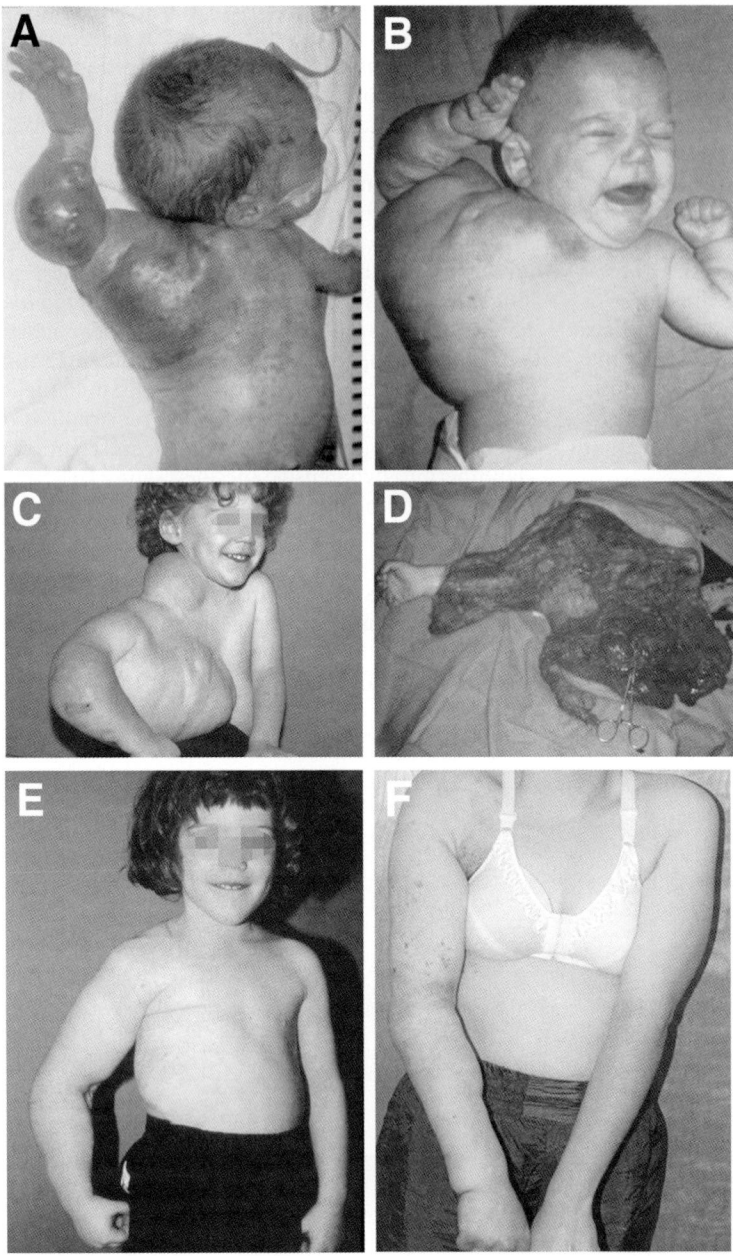

FIGURE 209-27. Extensive lymphatic malformation, natural history and resection. *A,* At birth, this baby had a rubbery mass with peau d'orange skin and a bluish hue within the arm and axilla. The diagnosis of lymphatic malformation can be made on physical examination alone. *B,* During the next 3 months, the mass enlarged and was not compressible. *C,* By 20 months of life, the size and weight of the lesion had become problematic. *D,* The lesion along chest wall, axilla including brachial plexus, and arm was dissected and resected during one procedure. *E,* The chest and arm with residual malformation have been well controlled with compression wrapping at age 5 years. *F,* Despite three additional debulkings of the forearm and arm, it has been difficult to control swelling in this region. Bleeding and maceration from direct dermal involvement within the axilla have necessitated antibiotic treatment for an average of 3 months per year.

wounds can be profound. Hypertrophic scars are common. Swelling may be difficult to control, particularly within the palm of the hand, which cannot be effectively wrapped circumferentially. The bleeding and fibrosis encountered on re-entry of these previously dissected regions are unique and profound. Dissect these areas in such a way that re-entry will not be necessary. Compression pumps augment circumferential wrapping of the wrist, forearm, and axillary regions. With extensive LMs or LVMs, these modalities will displace fluid into the mediastinal LM. Thick skin with dermal involvement (either with or without vesicles)

contains lymphatic channels and will invariably fissure, ulcerate, or become infected; it invariably requires surgical replacement.

The outcomes of aggressive surgery are satisfactory, with a complication rate of 22%.[85] Scar revisions, resection of neuromas, and replacement of drains for persistent drainage in the proximal portions of the limb and chest wall were the most common complications in our reported series.[85] Amputation is often elected for massively enlarged digits, hands, or portions of the arm or after unsuccessful limb salvage attempts. During the past 3 years, we have effectively used continuous passive motion machines to maintain motion in released joints at all levels from fingertip to glenohumeral joint.

Arteriovenous Malformations

PATHOPHYSIOLOGY

The pathogenesis of arteriovenous malformations (AVMs) is not understood. They are believed to result from errors of vascular development between the fourth and sixth weeks of embryonic gestation. One hypothesis holds that they result from failure of arteriovenous channels in the primitive retiform plexus to regress.[100]

Tissue from the epicenter of an AVM, termed the nidus, demonstrates close juxtaposition of medium-sized arteries, veins, and vessels. It is difficult, by light microscopy, to determine whether any particular abnormal vascular channel is part of the original (primary) malformation or secondarily altered by increased flow and pressure. In time, the veins become "arterialized" and exhibit intimal thickening, increased smooth muscle within the media, and dilatation of the vasa vasorum.[101] There is also progressive dilatation of the proximal arteries, with fibrosis, thinning of the media, and diminished elastic tissue.[101]

Several mechanisms have been proposed to account for the tendency of AVMs to expand to involve previously quiescent adjacent tissue. Reid[101] believed that the thin-walled arteries and veins could rupture into one another secondary to increased pressure and flow, forming new fistulous connections, an explanation for the rapid enlargement of arteriovenous anomalies that occurs after trauma or during pregnancy. Other authors have proposed that local ischemia plays a role in the pathogenesis. Local ischemia can result from the steal phenomenon, producing both pain and ulceration. It is well known that an AVM can enlarge rapidly after proximal ligation.[102-104] In a complementary way, Hurwitz[105] proposed that the failure of enlargement of residual malformation after microvascular tissue transfer may be a result of enhanced vascularity of the reconstructed field. Finally, an intrinsic cellular abnormality has been implicated. Cells cultured from surgical AVM specimens demonstrate a higher proliferation rate, are less responsive to cytokines, and express a c-*ets*-1 proto-oncogene, suggesting defective regulation of proliferation possibly resulting in reduced apoptosis.[106]

CLINICAL FEATURES

Fast-flow malformations are usually present at birth but visible only as a red blush that may be mistaken for a port-wine stain. During childhood, a thrill or bruit and a mass that does not respond to elevation develop. The adolescent growth spurt stimulates growth and expansion by an unknown mechanism; thrills, bruits, and warmth beneath the cutaneous stain become clinically obvious. The pain does not always respond to elevation, especially after exercise, and may be accompanied by hyperhidrosis. In female patients, the lesion's size increases during the adolescent growth spurt and with menses, oral contraceptive use, and pregnancy; it does not regress to its previous size after delivery. The mechanism of hormonal modulation is not known. Symptoms of distal ischemia and discoloration of digits progressing to ulceration may develop with increased shunting through proximal arteriovenous fistulas (AVFs). Children with large lesions with extensive AVFs may go into congestive heart failure. These AVMs are occasionally localized to the hand and wrist but usually extend through the arm and forearm into the axilla.

CLASSIFICATION

A clinical staging system of AVMs in all anatomic regions has been introduced by Schobinger (Table 209-4).[107] Not all lesions predictably progress through stages II and IV, particularly in the upper extremity.

We have subclassified upper limb lesions into three separate groups that correlated well with treatment (Fig. 209-28). In each group, the physical findings correlated well with the anatomic findings on angiography.[1]

TYPE A. These fast-flow anomalies include single or multiple AVFs, aneurysms, or ectasias on the arterial side of the circulation. They primarily involve either the radial or ulnar system with or without shunting to the interosseous system. Symptoms occur only with exercise.

TYPE B. Type B consists of more extensive AVMs localized primarily to one axial arterial system in the forearm, hand, or digit. These fast-flow AVMs have stable flow characteristics and provoke minimal or no distal symptoms. A steal phenomenon can develop after exercise early in life and progress with time.

TABLE 209-4 ✦ CLINICAL STAGING SYSTEM FOR ARTERIOVENOUS MALFORMATIONS

Stage	Description
I Quiescence	Pink-blue stain, increased warmth, arteriovenous shunting detectable on 20-MHz Doppler study
II Expansion	Stage I plus enlargement, pulsations, thrill and bruits, tortuous-tense veins
III Destruction	Stage II plus dystrophic skin changes, ulceration, bleeding, persistent pain, soft tissue necrosis
IV Decompensation	Stage III plus cardiac failure

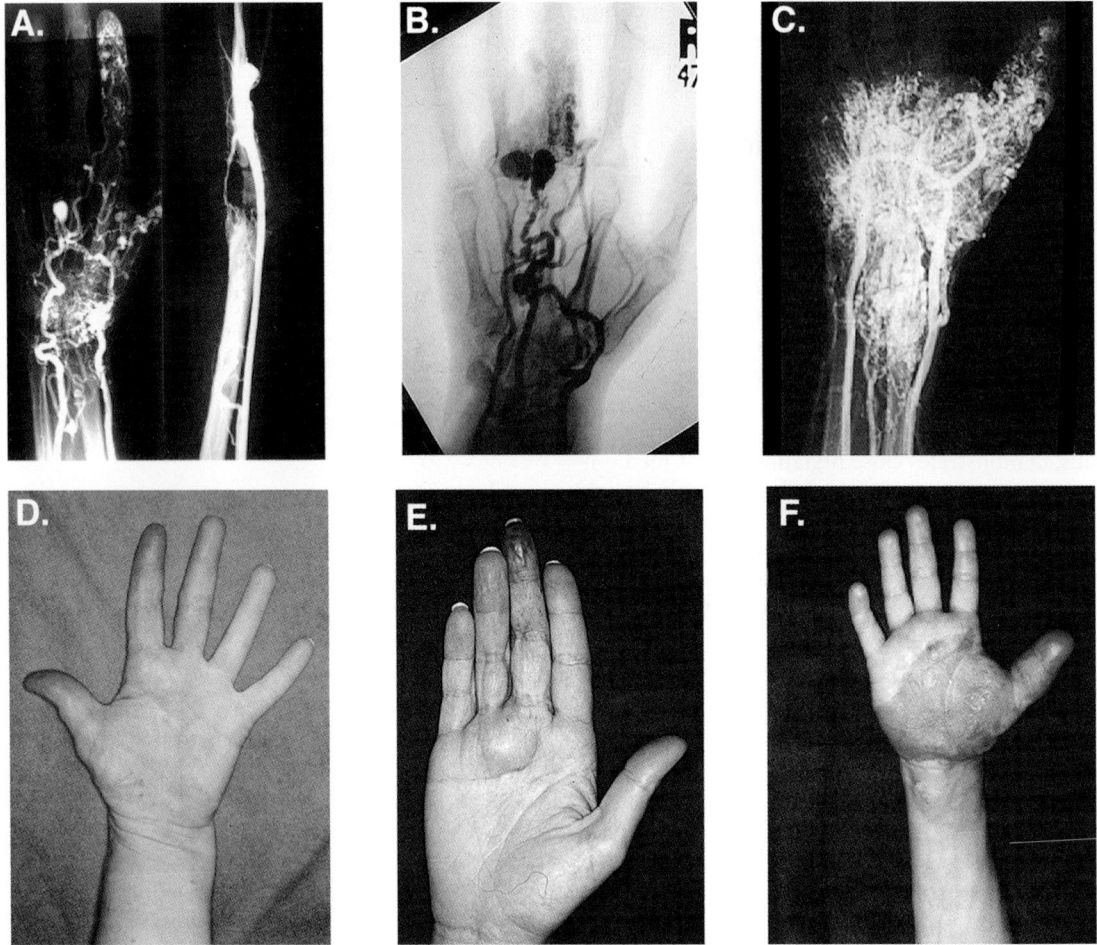

FIGURE 209-28. Types of fast-flow AVMs. *A* and *D,* Type A consists of single or multiple AVFs, aneurysms on the arterial side of the circulation. *B* and *E,* Type B lesions are more extensive but localized primarily to one or two of the three axial systems on the arterial side (radial, interosseous, or ulnar). The discoloration of the tip of the long finger is secondary to the steal phenomenon. *C* and *F,* Type C malformations are extensive, involve all three systems, and are symptomatic. The many micro-AVFs involve all tissues of the wrist and hand.

TYPE C. These malformations are more diffuse, involving at least two of the three axial systems, with microfistulous and macrofistulous AVMs involving all tissue of the extremity. They are usually evident at an early age and expand into previously uninvolved areas of the hand. Increased warmth, pain, hyperhidrosis, and progressive distal steal phenomenon are present.

RADIOLOGIC CHARACTERISTICS

Ultrasonography

The clinical diagnosis and presence of fast flow are confirmed by ultrasonography and color Doppler studies. Ultrasound examination of large lesions shows high-flow voids with a low arterial resistance. Arteriovenous shunts are well demonstrated. Type A and type B lesions can easily be observed with yearly ultrasound examinations. More invasive studies are deferred until the time of treatment.

Magnetic Resonance Imaging

MRI scans are obtained to gain a baseline with large lesions or lesions involving the palmar spaces of the hand (Fig. 209-29). Scans are not obtained for AVMs isolated to a single digit. Soft tissue thickening and flow voids are easily detected by T1- and gradient-weighted sequences. Magnetic resonance angiography obtained synchronously will demonstrate the location and caliber of feeding vessels and shunts (AVFs).

Angiography

Angiography is the best way to demonstrate the specific abnormal anatomy of the malformation. Superselective angiography is not used until interventional or

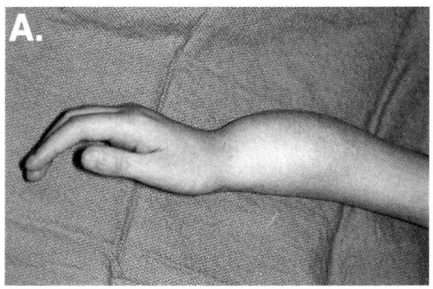
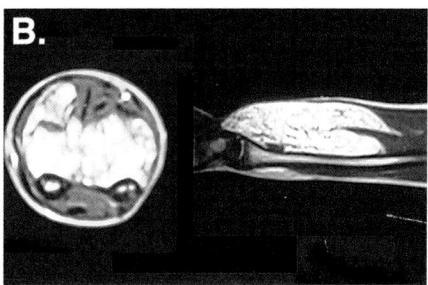
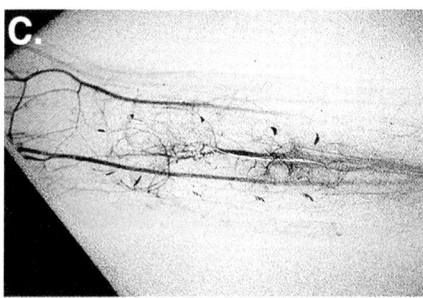
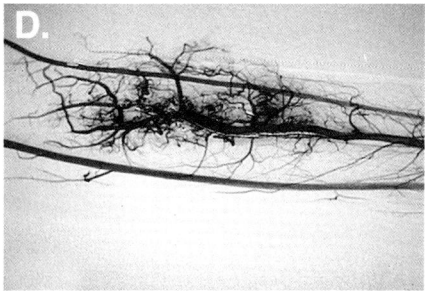
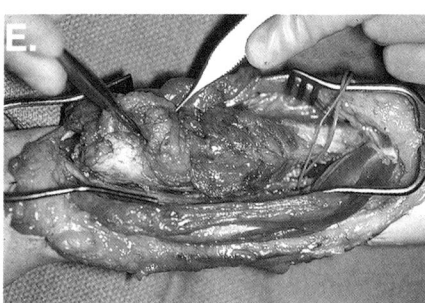
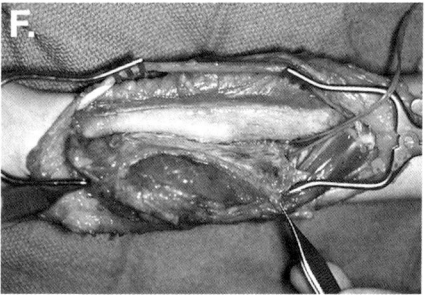

FIGURE 209-29. Type B fast flow. *A,* An 8-year-old girl presented with a persistent mass with thrills and bruits over the distal third of the right forearm. *B,* T1-weighted MRI sequences show flow voids and a mass involving all soft tissue structures dorsal to the interosseous membrane of the forearm. *C,* Early views during angiography demonstrate the many microshunts and AVFs along the interosseous system. *D,* The nidus of the AVM remains along the interosseous membrane with diffuse extension into the adjacent soft tissue mass. *E,* After preoperative embolization, the mass is well visualized. *F,* Resection included the interosseous membrane and involved periosteum of both the radius and ulna. Normal digital and thumb extension was restored postoperatively.

surgical treatment is planned. Sequential images demonstrate the size and location of the feeding arteries, the AVM nidus, and the early opacification of draining veins (see Fig. 209-29). Magnified subtraction images are used in the planning of all resections.

TREATMENT

An algorithm for treatment is outlined in Figure 209-30.

Observation

Early in life, observation and compression garments are the mainstays of treatment. Asymptomatic patients

are not considered surgical candidates despite the presence of well-localized type A and type B lesions. We have treated one 67-year-old man conservatively with compression wraps for a type C macrofistulous AVM with multiple AVFs (Fig. 209-31). Most patients with type B and type C lesions develop pain as a result of distention of the lesion and progression of a distal steal phenomenon.

Sclerotherapy

Sclerotherapy can be used to obliterate large tortuous arteries if ligated feeding arteries prevent passage of an embolization catheter. Local arterial and venous

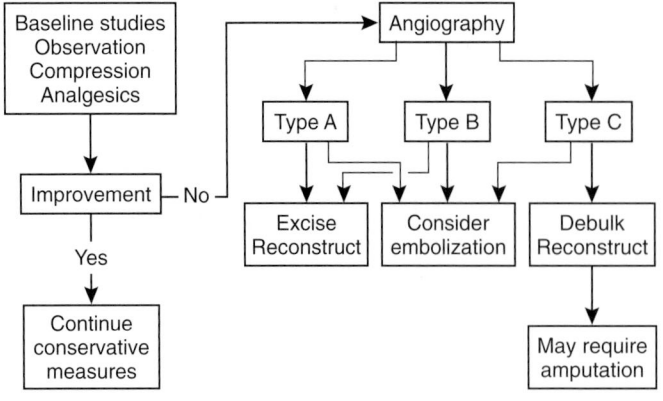

FIGURE 209-30. Treatment algorithm for fast-flow malformations.

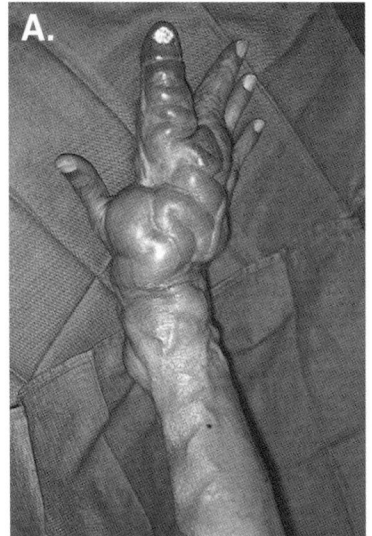

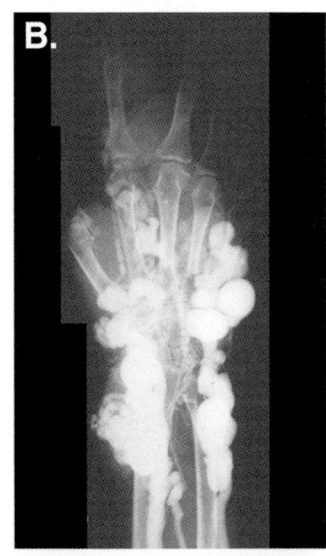

FIGURE 209-31. AVM type C, fast flow. *A,* This 67-year-old executive noted a gradual swelling and pulsation in his hand since his teenage years. Earlier in life, surgical removal of symptomatic regions was aborted because of bleeding that could be controlled only with elevation and pressure. *B,* Early angiographic sequences show macrofistulous shunts involving the radial and ulnar arteries and both palmar arches. With aging, these vascular channels have dilated and become tortuous. He experiences a persistent steal phenomenon in the long and index fingers, and the mass within the palm partially obstructs a functional grasp unless he wears his compression glove. *C* and *D,* Extrinsic flexion and extension have remained normal. The distorted nail matrix of the index finger has been the source of a chronic paronychia.

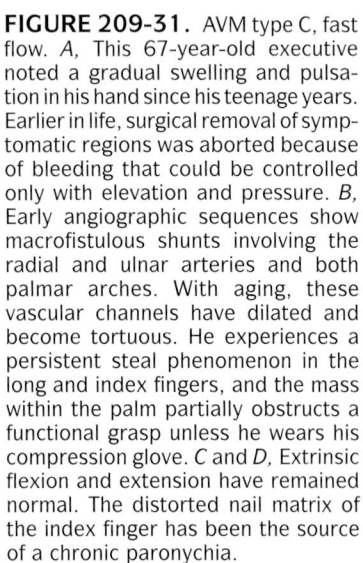

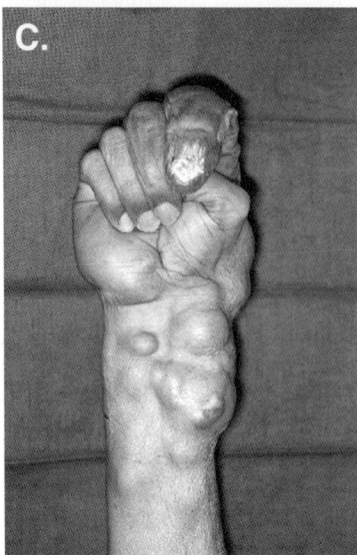

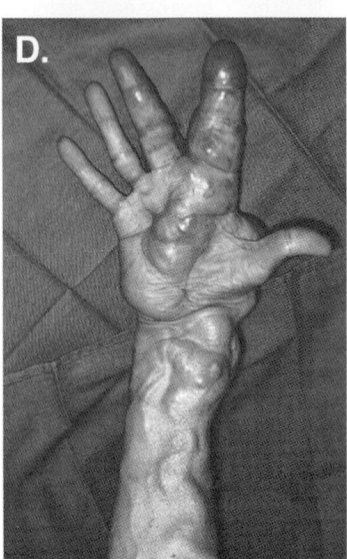

occlusion is necessary to prevent spread of the sclerosant solution beyond the injected nidus. Some well-localized AVMs have been successfully treated with a combination of embolization followed by sclerotherapy.[108] Most of these have been for head and neck and lower extremity lesions. The risks and morbidity after this combined approach are high.[107] We have not used this combination in the treatment of upper limb AVMs.

Embolization

The decision to use embolization with or without surgery is made jointly by the surgeon and the interventional radiologist. For minimally to moderately symptomatic type A or type B AVMs, embolization is the less traumatic procedure (Fig. 209-32). Indications include rapid growth of the AVM with increased flow of AVFs, pain, distal discoloration and ulceration, cardiac overload or congestive heart failure, and failure to thrive. This progression is illustrated in Figure 209-33. The most common symptoms are well localized to specific areas of microfistulous or macrofistulous shunting; these are best controlled with superselective embolization by use of various types of particles, coils, Gelfoam packs, and the like. For type C lesions and those in the Schobinger III and IV groups, palliative embolization is often used before surgery (Figs. 209-34 and 209-35).

Surgery

The old technique of deafferentation or ligation of feeding vessels to an AVM is no longer used for two reasons: it blocks later passage of an embolization catheter, and it stimulates the rapid recruitment of adjacent vessels toward the nidus of the AVM. In all but the least complicated resections, angiography and superselective embolization precede surgical resection by 24 to 72 hours. Under pneumatic tourniquet control, the embolized regions are easy to find and provide excellent landmarks for the surgeon. With large lesions, embolization alone can be palliative for difficult problems such as congestive heart failure, continued bleeding, and localized pain. Surgery is mandated for uncontrolled intralesional bleeding, compartment syndromes, nerve compressions, chronic ulceration, and gangrene. Wound dehiscence, bleeding, and infection are common early sequelae, and neuroma-related pain, sympathetic dystrophies, and contracture often follow the unsuccessful resection. Partial resections of type B and type C AVMs are doomed to fail. All dissections must be as thorough as possible. The need for microvascular revascularization of the hand or individual digits must be addressed. Most of the preoperative pain in these patients is steal phenomenon related. The creative reconstructive surgeon should be aggressive with both the resection and methods of reconstruction. Regional and distant tissue transfers have increased our ability to cover and reconstruct these wounds successfully (Fig. 209-36).

Both the young tyros and experienced surgical veterans agree that the most difficult aspect of these resections is defining the limits of the malformation, which characteristically cross tissue planes. Our approach has been to perform preoperative angiography and embolization of the symptomatic portion of the AVM to define the resection margins anatomically before an incision is made. Even in the ideal bloodless field afforded by the tourniquet, the surgeon may not have

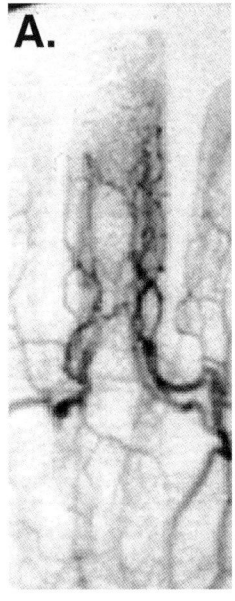 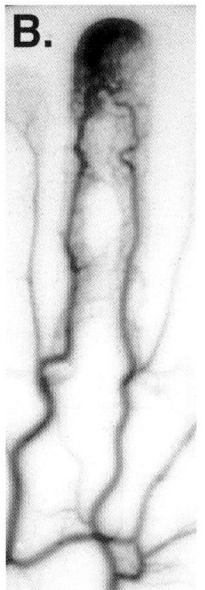 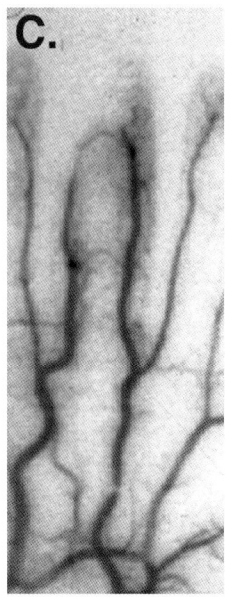

FIGURE 209-32. AVM type B, fast flow. *A,* The angiogram of a 6-month-old child with a swollen, red, tense fingertip. Localized thrills were consistent with a microfistulous AVM involving only the pulp tissue. *B,* Superselective embolization was performed through a catheter that was passed into the ulnar digital artery of this small child. *C,* Follow-up angiography demonstrates complete obliteration of the mass.

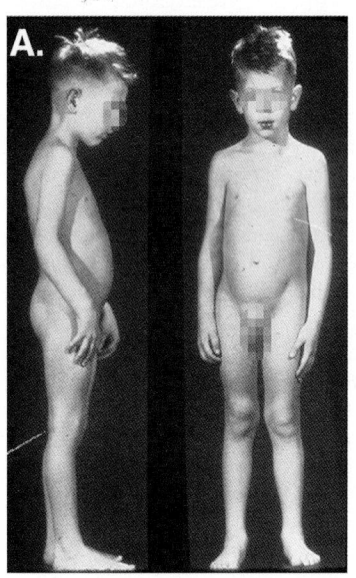
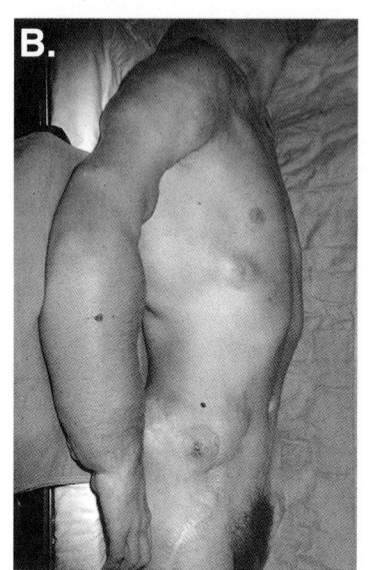
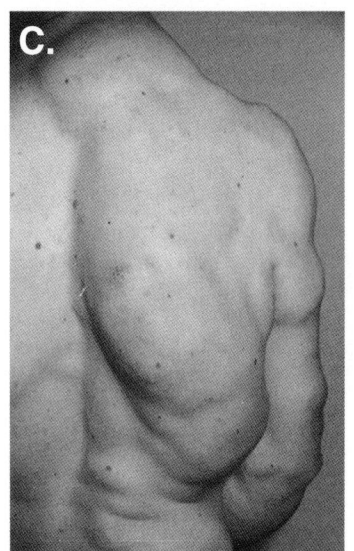
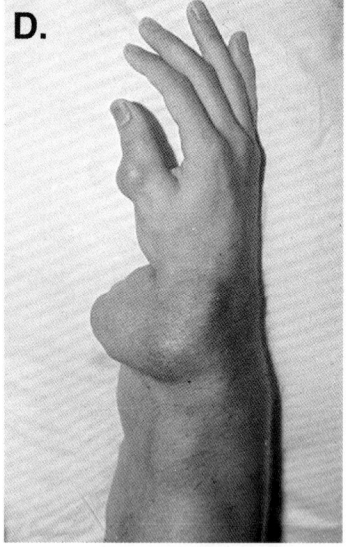

FIGURE 209-33. AVM type C, progressive compartment syndrome. *A,* At age 5 years, this youngster presented with a painful right elbow, wrist, and hand. Localized thrills were also noted along the ipsilateral chest wall. *B,* Twenty-five years later, these masses are still painful after exercise and swollen in spite of futile attempts to ligate feeding vessels (deafferentation). *C,* The untreated chest wall and trunk have become progressively larger. *D,* Compression garments only aggravated his forearm and hand pain. A ligation procedure resulted in an acute forearm compression syndrome. The bulk and weight of the malformation have interfered with hand function. A below-elbow amputation was necessary.

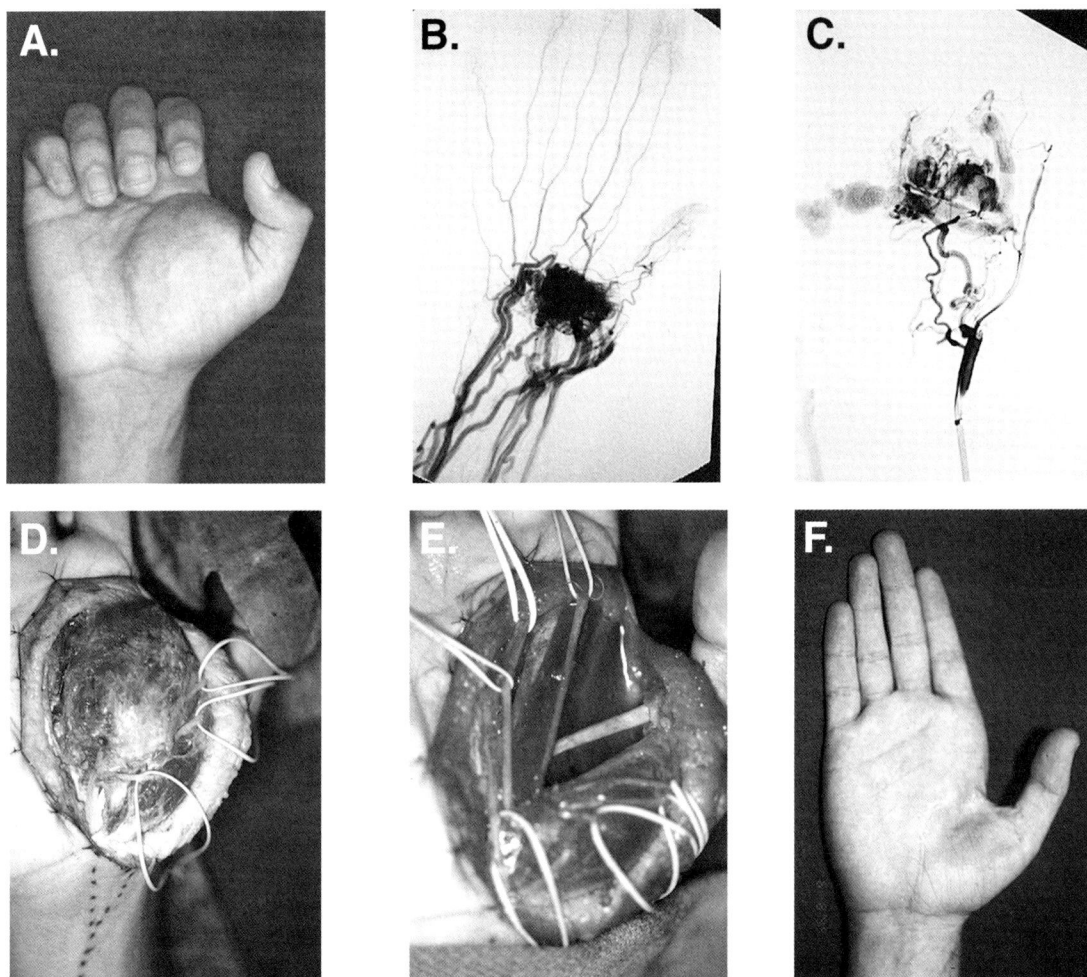

FIGURE 209-34. AVM type B, embolization and surgery. *A*, This professional wrestler presented with a painful mass within the thenar muscles. A thrill was first noted during adolescence. There was no history of trauma. *B*, The nidus of the AVM was demonstrated at the level of the superficial palmar arch, supplied by radial, interosseous, and ulnar vessels. Distal digital and thumb arterial architecture was shown to be normal. *C*, The postembolization study showed obliteration of most of the AVM with large draining veins. *D*, Two days later, the mass was explored surgically. Vessel loops mark the recurrent motor branch and sensory branches of the median nerve. *E*, All nerves and flexor tendons were preserved during surgical resection. *F*, Five years later, he continues to demonstrate good function. Palmar abduction is present through the abductor pollicis, but key pinch is weak because of the resection of the adductor pollicis muscle.

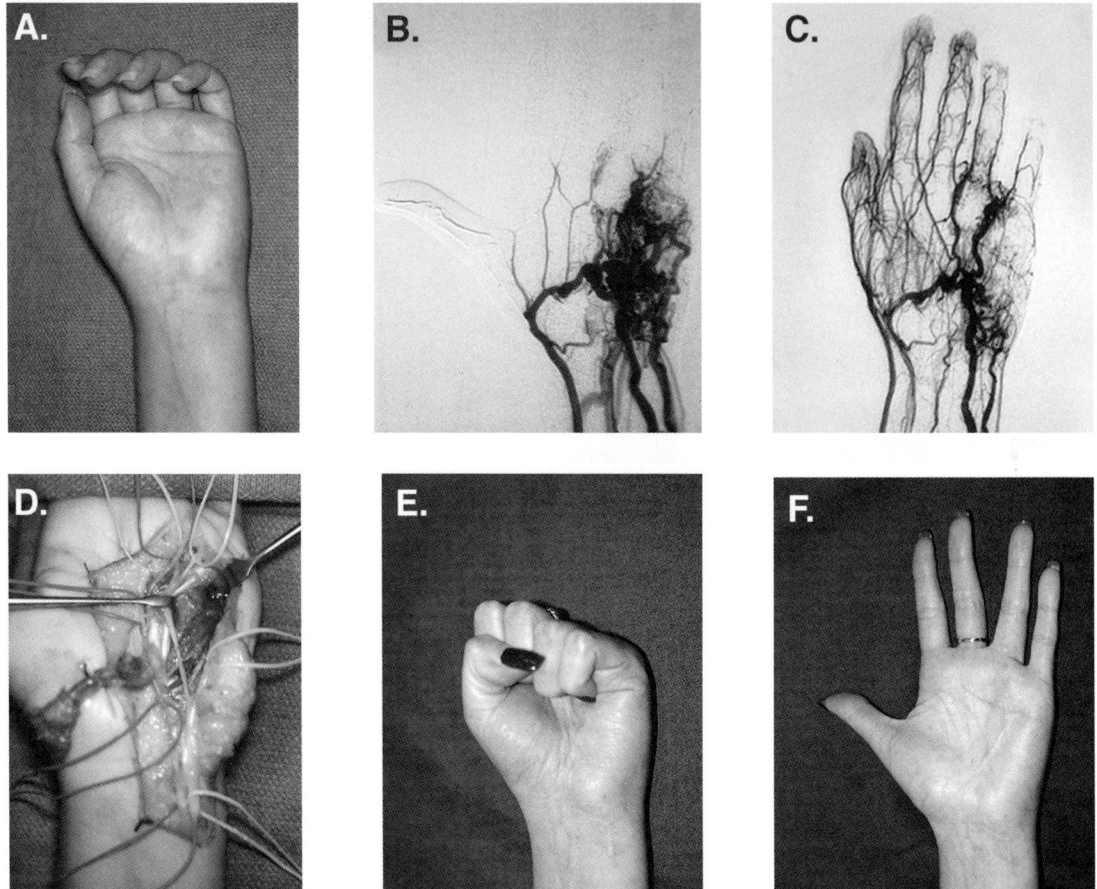

FIGURE 209-35. AVM type B, embolization, surgery, and repeated embolization. *A,* A pulsatile mass within the hypothenar eminence of this young woman became larger and painful when she started antiovulant medication. *B,* Early angiographic sequences showed a macrofistulous AVM in Guyon canal fed by both ulnar and interosseous vessels. *C,* A postembolization sequence showed persistence of many shunts. Note the lack of perfusion of the pulp tissue of both ring and long digits, which were most symptomatic. The caliber of the ulnar artery was twice normal. *D,* Surgical excision included removal of ulnar artery and common digital vessel to the fourth web space. Sensory and motor nerves and flexor tendons were preserved, and revascularization to the ulnar side of the ring finger and both sides of the fifth digit was performed with autogenous vein grafts. *E,* Normal flexion and extension without claw posturing was noted 2 years postoperatively. *F,* Five years later, she presented with a painful mass at the base of the ring finger. This represented some residual AVM at the margin of the previous resection within the intermetacarpal space and was easily embolized without the need for more surgery.

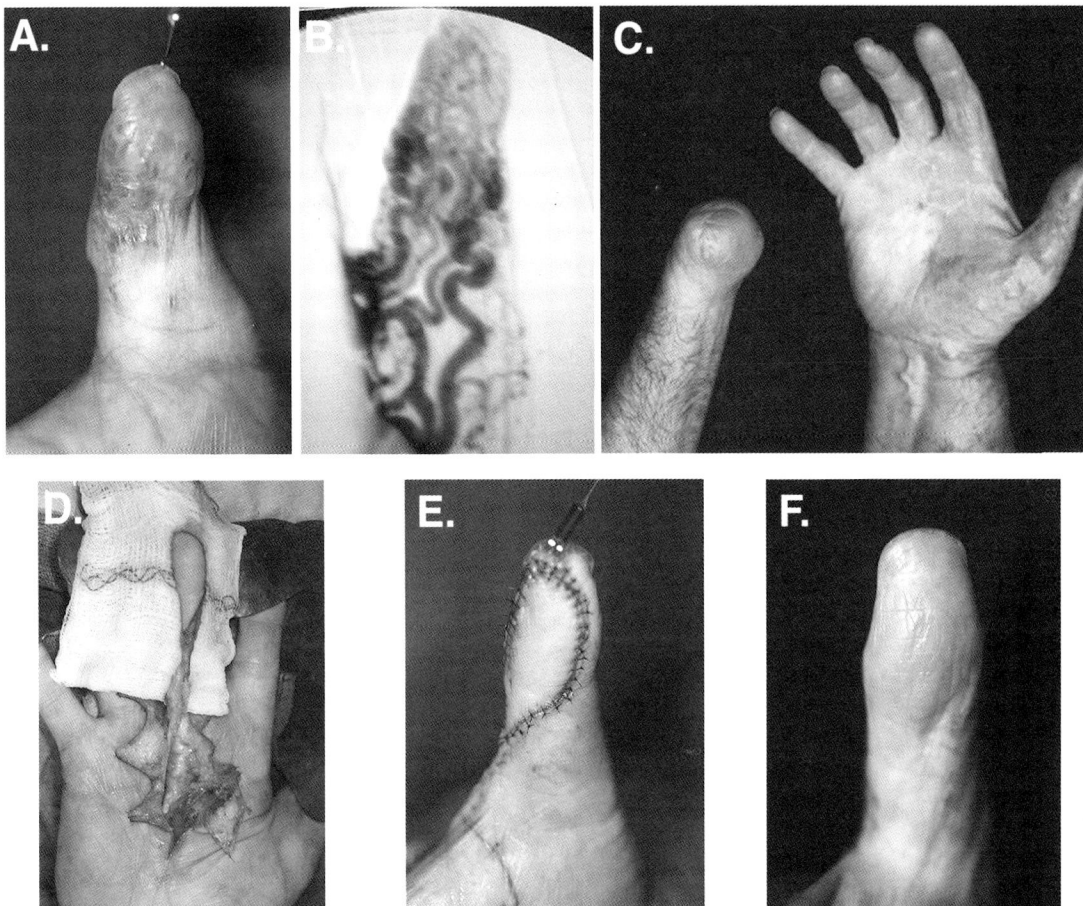

FIGURE 209-36. AVM type C, neurovascular island flap. *A,* The pulsatile bleeding from excoriated regions of this 60-year-old man's right thumb had become the focus for a severe depression. *B,* An angiogram showed an extensive type C macrofistulous AVM involving the radial side of his dominant hand. *C,* The congenital absence of his left hand made him completely dependent on the function of his right side. *D,* After surgical resection of the scarred and unstable pulp surface and debulking of the entire thumb, resurfacing was accomplished with a neurovascular island flap from the ulnar side of the long finger. *E,* The flap extended to the nail plate distally and included the entire working pulp surface of the thumb. *F,* A grateful patient has a stable thumb that he still perceives is on the ulnar side of the ring finger.

a clear delineation of small anomalous vessel malformation margins.[1]

Long-term outcome for patients with type B and type C AVMs (Schobinger II-IV) after upper extremity resections or amputations is not available. Our preliminary experience with approximately 45 patients is that most show expansion of residual malformations somewhere near the periphery of the resection within 10 years. The majority observed beyond this time became symptomatic in those areas within 10 years. The spread of the malformation into previously uninvolved portions of the extremity has been much greater for microfistulous AVMs and macrofistulous lesions (Fig. 209-37).

It is difficult for the surgeon to know when not to operate. Some will categorically refuse to consider any

surgical approach after witnessing colleagues trying to operate "in an inkwell" after uncontrolled hemorrhage from macrofistulas. For upper extremity lesions, tourniquets, embolization, careful planning, good surgical technique, and aggressive resections and reconstructions together provide opportunities that are not readily available in other anatomic regions, such as the head and neck, trunk, pelvis, and peritoneum. These dilemmas are not necessarily impossible surgical problems but should be approached with great caution. Symptomatic type A and type B lesions are the most amenable to surgery.

The recommendation to amputate is both difficult for the surgeon and exasperating for the parents, who in desperation often seek multiple additional opinions. Unfortunately, few experts are available

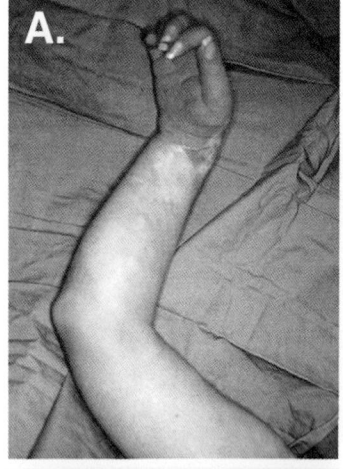

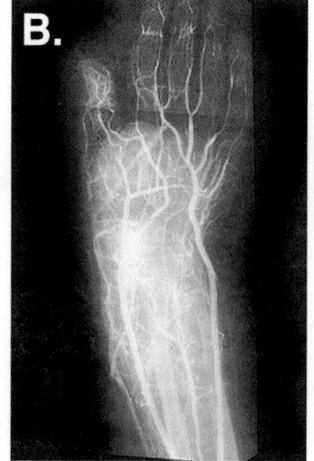

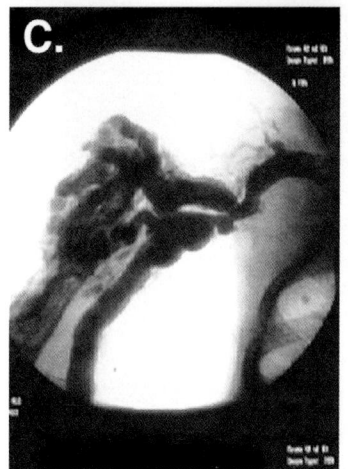

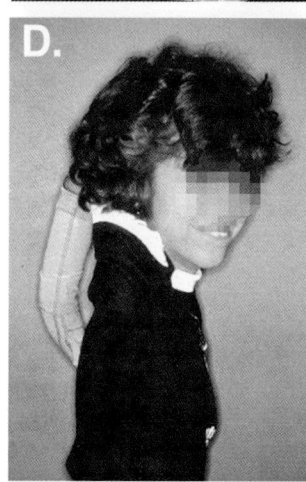

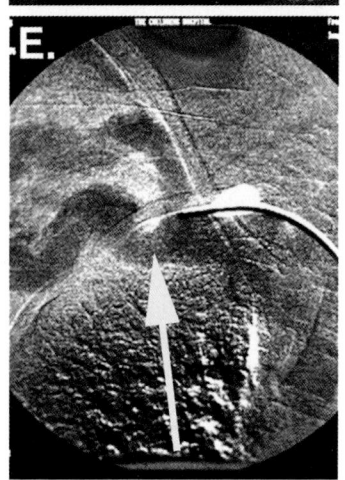

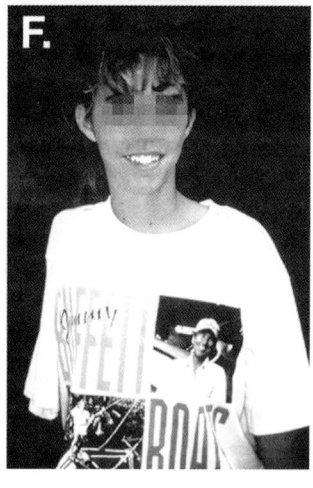

FIGURE 209-37. AVM type C, microfistulous, progressive. *A,* At age 1 year, this child presented with a capillary malformation of the hand and pulsatile mass of the distal forearm. The diagnosis of Parkes Weber syndrome was made, and she was treated with compression garments. *B,* An angiogram at age 6 years showed a progressive microfistulous, painful AVM of the distal forearm. By the time she was 12 years old, she was in continual pain. *C,* Massively enlarged subclavian and axillary arteries were demonstrated, and at the same time, she showed early signs of cardiac compromise. *D,* She learned to control her pain by dislocating her glenohumeral joint and compressing her axillary artery, a position in which she often slept. *E,* Intra-arterial balloon catheters were helpful at the time of shoulder disarticulation for removal of her parasitic and extremely painful limb. *F,* Preservation of the scapula helps drape clothing and makes the appearance of these patients less conspicuous. Within 6 months, she gained 20 pounds, became less morose, and excelled in school and cross-country running.

worldwide. If the patient is requesting amputation, he or she is usually right, and the request should not be denied by the surgeon. Pain, impending gangrene, symptoms secondary to severe steal, early cardiac compromise, and failure of young children and adolescents to maintain normal growth parameters are all indications for selective amputation (Figs. 209-38 and 209-39). Our outcome study of patients with type C AVM (Schobinger IV) showed an amputation rate of more than 90% during a 30-year period. In retrospect, with 9 of 17 patients eventually requiring amputation at the forearm, arm, or shoulder level, we prolonged the inevitable amputation for a number of reasons. The recovery after ablation of the parasitic part and elimination of the chronic pain is both remarkable and predictable. Rapid weight gain, improved disposition, and increased level of activity are all notable.

These problems await a pharmacologic cure! Promising results have been obtained in one patient, a 3-year-old girl with multiple soft tissue and skeletal AVMs and AVFs of the upper extremity, treated with marimastat (unpublished data). This matrix metalloproteinase inhibitor acts by an antiangiogenic mechanism. Such preliminary results await long-term confirmation. Multiple clinical phase I studies evaluating angiogenic inhibitors are in progress.

Combined (Eponymous) Malformations

Combined malformations contain more than one vascular element (capillary, arterial, venous, and lymphatic) and are named accordingly: capillary-lymphatic malformation, capillary-venous malformation,

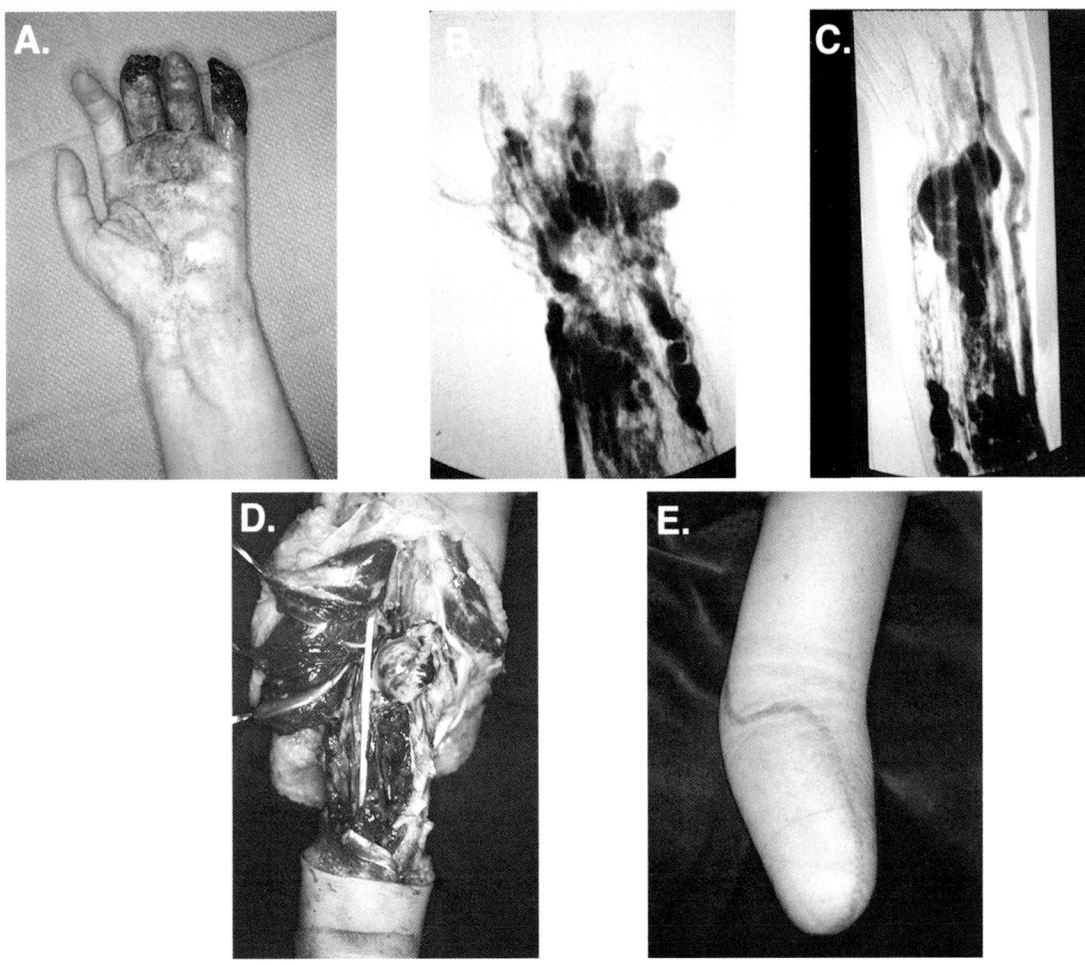

FIGURE 209-38. AVM type C, below-elbow amputation. *A,* A 25-year-old secretary with a known type C AVM presented after embolization of a massive lesion involving the entire forearm and hand. *B,* An angiogram showed macrofistulous shunting involving all three arterial systems of the hand. The digital vessels to the ulnar three digits were not visualized at any stage of the study. *C,* The shunts and fistulas with the forearm appeared to be massive. *D,* Appearance during amputation. *E,* With a well-healed, nonpainful below-elbow amputation stump, she functioned well with and without a myoelectric prosthesis. She regretted that she did not have this procedure performed much earlier in life.

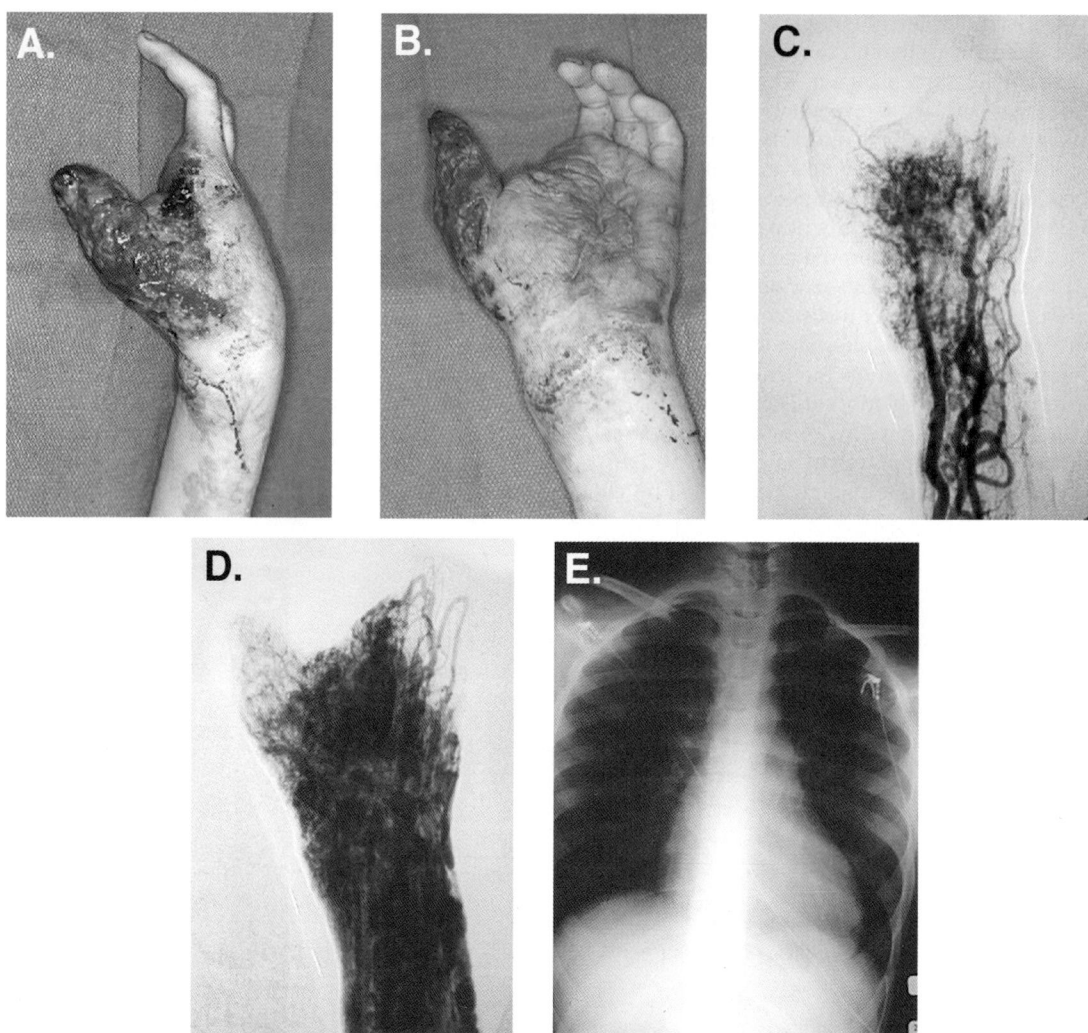

FIGURE 209-39. Type C, microfistulous and macrofistulous shunting, congestive heart failure, below-elbow amputation. *A* and *B,* Both this teenager with a type C AVM and his parents wanted to save this hand. The index ray had been resected for uncontrollable pulsatile bleeding. The thumb then became ulcerated and congested, and the patient became suicidal because of the unrelenting pain. *C,* Angiography showed massively tortuous and enlarged axial vessels feeding microfistulous shunts within the forearm and hand. *D,* A later sequence demonstrated the extent of the shunting and lack of distal digital perfusion. *E,* Chest radiograph and electrocardiogram were consistent with congestive heart failure. A below-elbow amputation was followed by a predictable recovery and normal adolescent growth spurt.

capillary-lymphatic-venous malformation (also known as Klippel-Trénaunay syndrome), arteriovenous malformation, and so on. In addition, they can be subdivided by rheology. If an arterial component is present, they are fast flow (arteriovenous malformation, capillary-arteriovenous malformation); otherwise, they are slow flow (capillary-lymphatic malformation, capillary-venous malformation, capillary-lymphatic-venous malformation). These combined and often complex malformations can involve any part of the upper extremity and indeed any anatomic region of the body. Many are associated with skeletal overgrowth.[21] The treatment corresponds

to whether slow-flow or fast-flow components are present.

SLOW-FLOW EPONYMOUS COMBINED MALFORMATIONS

Capillary-Lymphatic-Venous Malformation (Klippel-Trénaunay Syndrome)

Capillary-lymphatic-venous malformation (CLVM) is associated with skeletal and soft tissue overgrowth.[1,109-112] Klippel-Trénaunay syndrome is a well-known eponym for this anomaly. CLVM is often confused with the Parkes Weber syndrome (capillary-arteriovenous malformation; see Fig. 209-37) or, in fact, any condition that is associated with limb hypertrophy.

In this sporadic anomaly, boys and girls are equally affected. In 80%, only the lower limb is involved. The upper limb alone is affected in 5%, and both upper and lower limbs are involved in 15% of patients. Eighty-five percent of cases are unilateral, and one arm and the contralateral leg are occasionally affected. In a few cases, the entire trunk is part of the malformation. Upper extremity lesions can extend into the mediastinum and retropleural space but rarely evoke symptoms. Venous hypoplasias and anomalies may be present. Lymphatic hypoplasia is present in more than half of the patients, and generalized lymphedema is common in these extremities. Upper extremity CLVM presents with skeletal overgrowth of the arm, forearm, or hand (Figs. 209-40 and 209-41). However, undergrowth can occur. Pulmonary embolism may occur in up to 25% of patients.

Proteus Syndrome

Proteus syndrome refers to a sporadic, progressive vascular, skeletal, and soft tissue condition that truly lies at the interface of vascular anomalies and overgrowth syndromes. Its name is not eponymous but reflects an elusive understanding of this disorder; Proteus, the Greek god, was able to assume any shape or form to elude capture.

In response to the protean manifestations of this disorder, a consensus workshop was held at the National Institutes of Health in 1998 to recommend diagnostic criteria, differential diagnoses, and guidelines for the evaluation of patients. The diagnostic criteria include three mandatory general criteria, which are (1) mosaic or asymmetric distribution of lesions, (2) progressive course, and (3) sporadic occurrence.[113] In addition, some number of "category signs" must be present. These include verrucous (linear) nevus, lipomas and lipomatosis, macrocephaly (calvarial hyperostoses), asymmetric limbs with partial gigantism of the hands or feet, and curious cerebriform plantar thickening ("moccasin" feet). As a rule, Proteus syndrome is not present at birth. These features suggest that this syndrome may be the result of a dominant lethal gene that survives by somatic mosaicism.[113]

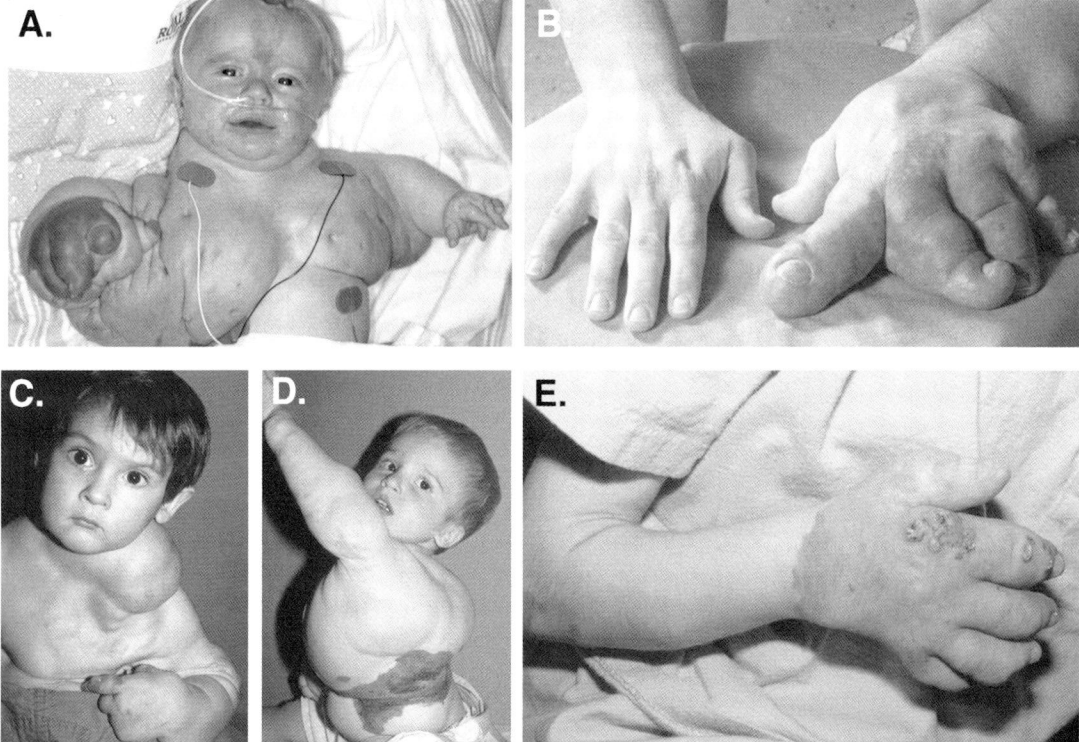

FIGURE 209-40. CLVM, Klippel-Trénaunay syndrome. *A,* This CLVM involves all portions of both upper extremities and the entire thorax with intrathoracic extension into the mediastinum and pleural cavities. Debulking of the pleural cavities and heart was necessary to relieve cardiac failure. *B,* Overgrowth of skeletal and soft tissue structures is commonly seen in the hand. *C,* Macrocystic lymphatic components are common in the neck in these combined lesions. *D,* Extension into the abdomen and pelvis may occur. *E,* Epidermal lymphatic vesicles often become the source of a rapidly spreading cellulitis.

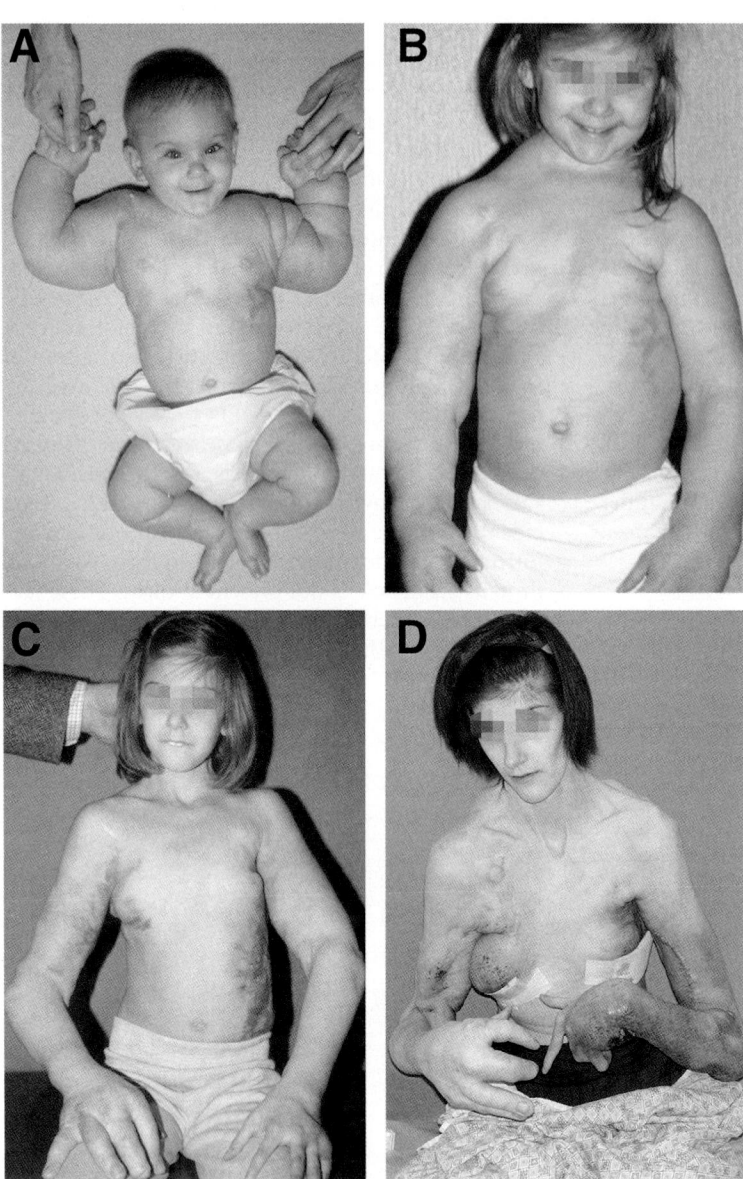

FIGURE 209-41. CLVM progression. *A to D,* The progression of a combined CLVM is seen at the ages of 6 months and 3, 12, and 28 years. Manifestations of upper limb involvement included skeletal and soft tissue overgrowth, macrodactyly, development of extensive lymphatic vesicles, and worsening of joint contractures after multiple operations at another institution. At the age of 22 years, she delivered a normal infant, and 6 years later, she died of a suspected pulmonary embolus.

Maffucci Syndrome

Maffucci syndrome denotes the coexistence of exophytic VMs with bone exostoses and enchondromas.[114] This extremely rare condition typically presents in late childhood. The osseous lesions appear first, most often in the hands, feet, long bones of the extremity, ribs, pelvis, and cranium.[115] There may be a history of recurrent fractures secondary to enchondromatous weakening of bone diaphyses; this occurs before the development of cutaneous vascular lesions.

The VMs involve the subcutaneous tissues and bones and are generally distributed in the extremities; they may be unilateral or bilateral (Figs. 209-42 and

209-43). Their distribution does not necessarily correlate with that of the enchondromas. They are most commonly located on the hands and feet, reported to be 57.1% and 41%, respectively.[116] They may occur anywhere, however, and have been reported in the leptomeninges, eyes, and lungs and throughout the gastrointestinal tract from mouth to anus.[117-123]

These patients often develop spindle cell hemangioendotheliomas within the VMs. These are a reactive vascular proliferation rather than a true tumor.[124] Malignant transformation, usually chondrosarcoma, occurs in 20% to 30% of patients.[116,125] Chondrosarcomas arise from sites of enchondromas and have been reported at a variety of anatomic sites, including the

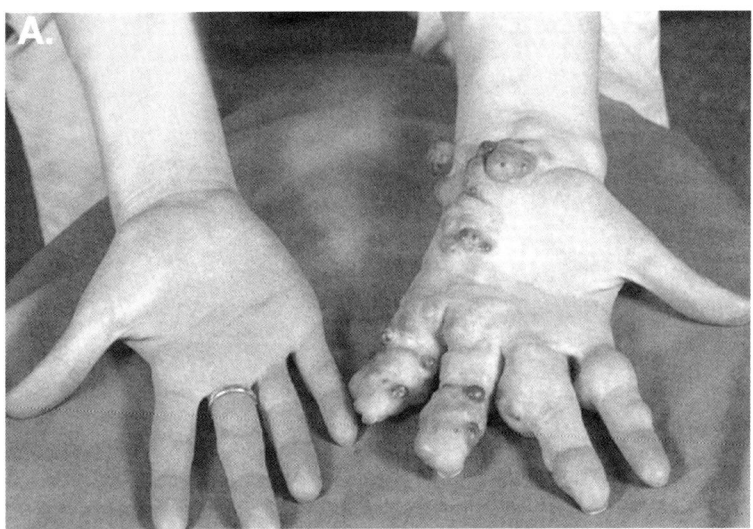

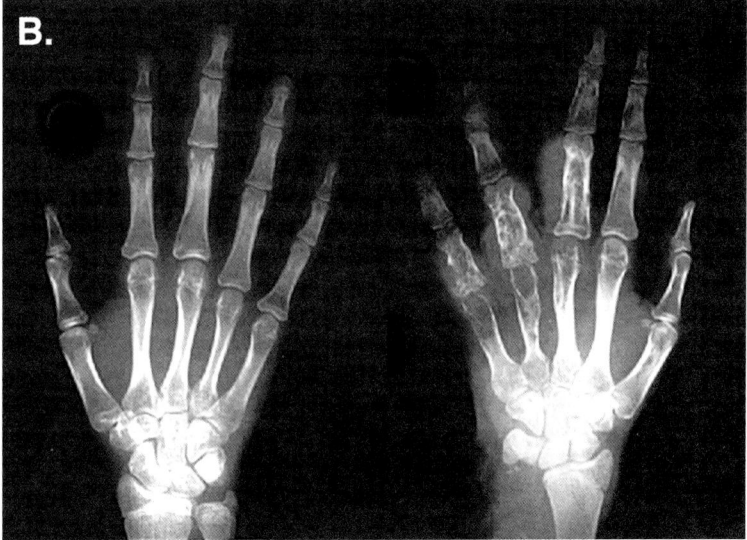

FIGURE 209-42. Maffucci syndrome. *A,* The unilateral hand of a girl with the Maffucci syndrome shows the characteristic sessile, pedunculated venous malformations. *B,* Radiographs demonstrate multiple phalangeal and metacarpal lucencies secondary to enchondromas. Her right distal ulna has been previously resected.

skull.[126] The average age at development of chondrosarcomas is 40 years, but it has ranged from 13 to 69 years in reported cases.[115,116,125] A majority of the chondrosarcomas are of histologically low grade and can often be cured with surgical resection.[127,128]

Bannayan-Riley-Ruvalcaba Syndrome

Three syndromes, Riley-Smith, Bannayan-Zonana, and Ruvalcaba-Myhre-Smith, once considered distinct entities, have been integrated as Bannayan-Riley-Ruvalcaba syndrome to reflect their overlapping clinical features.[129] The characteristic clinical features of Bannayan-Riley-Ruvalcaba syndrome are macrocephaly with normal ventricular size, multiple subcutaneous or visceral lipomas (encapsulated or diffusely infiltrating), vascular anomalies, and skeletal abnormalities.[130] At least half of the patients have central nervous system abnormalities, such as hypotonia, minor to moderate mental retardation, and seizures.[130] Additional features may include hamartomatous polyps of the distal ileum and colon,[131] Hashimoto thyroiditis, and retinal abnormalities.[132] The cutaneous vascular lesions, reported to be capillary, venous, and possibly arteriovenous, are usually a minor component of the syndrome. Other cutaneous lesions include, in decreasing frequency, lentigines of the penis, facial verrucae, acanthosis nigricans, and multiple acrochordons. This autosomal dominant disorder is caused by germline mutations in *PTEN*, a tumor suppressor gene that maps to 10q23.[133]

Clinical features pertinent to the upper limb surgeon include hypotonia and mild to moderate delay in motor skills in two thirds of patients. Lipomas in any subcutaneous location are more common than

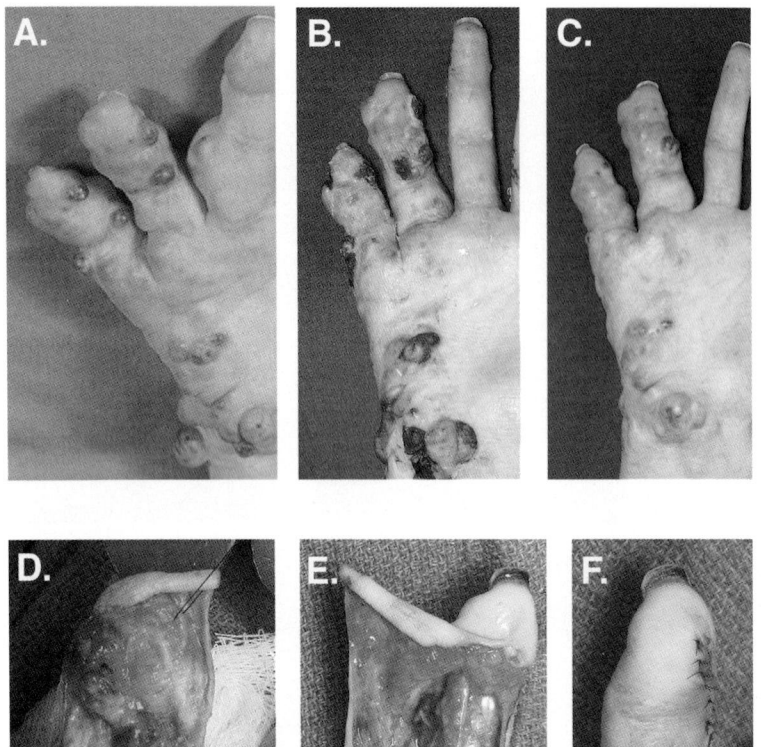

FIGURE 209-43. Maffucci syndrome. *A,* Preoperative appearance of multiple lesions on the ulnar side of the hand. *B,* Sclerosis is noted in multiple regions 5 days after sclerotherapy. *C,* The same hand 6 months later. *D,* Multiple sessile, thrombosed lesions cover the flexor tendons. The arrow marks the ulnar digital nerve of the fifth digit. *E,* Both digital arteries and nerves, including dorsal sensory branches, have been dissected and preserved microscopically. *F,* Appearance after skin resection and closure.

VMs, which we have seen in the forearm and dorsum of the hand. Treatment consists of excision of problematic lipomas, VMs, or the occasional LM as previously outlined.

FAST-FLOW EPONYMOUS SYNDROMES

Parkes Weber Syndrome (Capillary-Arteriovenous Malformation)

CLINICAL FEATURES. This syndrome is much less prevalent than CLVM but is seen more commonly than CLVM in the upper extremity. The capillary malformation is usually more diffuse and pink (see Fig. 209-37). The major difference is the presence of the AVM with AVFs, which all present early in childhood. These lesions become progressively worse and carry a poor long-term prognosis. With time, the involved regions of the arm and forearm form large macrofistulous shunts. CLVM (Klippel-Trénaunay

syndrome) and capillary-arteriovenous malformation (Parkes Weber syndrome) are distinctly different but frequently confused malformations. Some physicians have erroneously labeled patients as having "Klippel-Trénaunay-Weber syndrome," which does not exist. A clear comparison of these two syndromes is provided in Table 209-5.

TREATMENT. Surgical treatment is helpful only for well-localized symptomatic shunts, compartment syndromes, or compression syndromes. Because many of these upper extremity lesions are so diffuse, surgical resection is unrealistic. Attempted surgical resections often lead to wound dehiscence, bleeding, full-thickness skin loss, and chronic infection. Embolization has been the mainstay of treatment. Complications of this treatment include localized soft tissue necrosis, migration of embolized particles outside the limb, and distal gangrene leading to amputation.

TABLE 209-5 ✦ COMPARISON OF KLIPPEL-TRÉNAUNAY AND PARKES WEBER SYNDROMES

	Klippel-Trénaunay (CLVM)	Parkes Weber (CAVM)
Capillary stain	Present, typically deep purple	Present, pink
Lymphatic vesicles	Often present	Absent
Arteriovenous fistulas	Absent	Present
Deep venous anomalies	Common	Absent
Lateral venous anomaly	Common	Absent
Limb hypertrophy	Moderate	Major
Gigantism	Disproportionate	Proportionate
Lymphatics	Hypoplastic	Hyperplastic
Associated anomalies	Common	Uncommon
Prognosis	Stable clinical course	Often progressive deterioration

CLVM, capillary-lymphatic-venous malformation; CAVM, capillary-arteriovenous malformation.

All of these upper extremity lesions are in the type C category, in which 60% lead to amputation.[1] After amputation, these children and adults must be observed carefully for cardiac compromise. These malformations can involve areas of the limb proximal to the amputation. We presently observe several asymptomatic adolescent below-knee amputees who are active in sports yet show early signs of cardiac compromise and presence of a Branham sign.

REFERENCES

1. Upton J, Coombs CJ, Mulliken JB, et al: Vascular malformations of the upper limb: a review of 270 patients. J Hand Surg Am 1999;24:1019-1035.
2. Mulliken J, Young A: Vascular Birthmarks: Hemangiomas and Malformations. Philadelphia, WB Saunders, 1988.
3. Virchow R: Angioma in die krankhaften Geschwulste, vol 3. Berlin, Hirschwald, 1863:306-425.
4. Wegener G: Über Lymphangiome. Arch Klin Chir 1877;20:641-707.
5. Mulliken JB, Glowacki J: Hemangiomas and vascular malformations in infants and children: a classification based on endothelial characteristics. Plast Reconstr Surg 1982;69:412-422.
6. Folkman J, Mulliken J, Ezekowitz R: Angiogenesis and hemangiomas. In Oldham K, Colombani P, Foglio R, eds: Surgery of Infants and Children: Scientific Principles and Practice. Philadelphia, Lippincott-Raven, 1997:569-579.
7. Gorlin RJ, Kantaputra P, Aughton DJ, Mulliken JB: Marked female predilection in some syndromes associated with facial hemangiomas. Am J Med Genet 1994;52:130-135.
8. Burton BK, Schulz CJ, Angle B, Burd LI: An increased incidence of haemangiomas in infants born following chorionic villus sampling (CVS). Prenat Diagn 1995;15:209-214.
9. Takahashi K, Mulliken JB, Kozakewich HP, et al: Cellular markers that distinguish the phases of hemangioma during infancy and childhood. J Clin Invest 1994;93:2357-2364.
10. Martin-Padura I, De Castellarnau C, Uccini S, et al: Expression of VE (vascular endothelial)–cadherin and other endothelial-specific markers in haemangiomas. J Pathol 1995;175:51-57.
11. Kraling BM, Razon MJ, Boon LM, et al: E-selectin is present in proliferating endothelial cells in human hemangiomas. Am J Pathol 1996;148:1181-1191.
12. Chang J, Most D, Bresnick S, et al: Proliferative hemangiomas: analysis of cytokine gene expression and angiogenesis. Plast Reconstr Surg 1999;103:1-9, discussion 10.
13. Chang E, Boyd A, Nelson CC, et al: Successful treatment of infantile hemangiomas with interferon-alpha-2b. J Pediatr Hematol Oncol 1997;19:237-244.
14. Mulliken JB, Zetter BR, Folkman J: In vitro characteristics of endothelium from hemangiomas and vascular malformations. Surgery 1982;92:348-353.
15. Dethlefsen SM, Mulliken JB, Glowacki J: An ultrastructural study of mast cell interactions in hemangiomas. Ultrastruct Pathol 1986;10:175-183.
16. Bielenberg DR, Bucana CD, Sanchez R, et al: Progressive growth of infantile cutaneous hemangiomas is directly correlated with hyperplasia and angiogenesis of adjacent epidermis and inversely correlated with expression of the endogenous angiogenesis inhibitor, IFN-beta. Int J Oncol 1999;14:401-408.
17. Holmdahl K: Cutaneous hemangiomas in premature and mature infants. Acta Pediatr Scand 1955;44:70-79.
18. Amir J, Metzker A, Krikler R, Reisner SH: Strawberry hemangioma in preterm infants. Pediatr Dermatol 1986;3:331-332.
19. Finn MC, Glowacki J, Mulliken JB: Congenital vascular lesions: clinical application of a new classification. J Pediatr Surg 1983;18:894-900.
20. Bowers R, Graham E, Tomlinson K: The natural history of the strawberry nevus. Arch Dermatol 1960;82:667-680.
21. Boyd JB, Mulliken JB, Kaban LB, et al: Skeletal changes associated with vascular malformations. Plast Reconstr Surg 1984;74:789-797.
22. Boon LM, Enjolras O, Mulliken JB: Congenital hemangioma: evidence of accelerated involution. J Pediatr 1996;128:329-335.
23. Enjolras O, Mulliken J, Boon L, et al: Noninvoluting congenital hemangioma: a rare cutaneous vascular anomaly. Plast Reconstr Surg 2001;107:1647-1654.
24. Dubois J, Garel L, Grignon A, et al: Imaging of hemangiomas and vascular malformations in children. Acad Radiol 1998;5:390-400.
25. Paltiel HJ, Burrows PE, Kozakewich HP, et al: Soft-tissue vascular anomalies: utility of US for diagnosis. Radiology 2000;214:747-754.
26. Burrows PE, Laor T, Paltiel H, Robertson RL: Diagnostic imaging in the evaluation of vascular birthmarks. Dermatol Clin 1998;16:455-488.
27. Meyer JS, Hoffer FA, Barnes PD, Mulliken JB: Biological classification of soft-tissue vascular anomalies: MR correlation. AJR Am J Roentgenol 1991;157:559-564.
28. Huston J 3rd, Forbes GS, Ruefenacht DA, et al: Magnetic resonance imaging of facial vascular anomalies [see comments]. Mayo Clin Proc 1992;67:739-747.

29. Barton DJ, Miller JH, Allwright SJ, Sloan GM: Distinguishing soft-tissue hemangiomas from vascular malformations using technetium-labeled red blood cell scintigraphy. Plast Reconstr Surg 1992;89:46-52, discussion 53-55.

30. Burns A, Kaplan L, Mulliken J: Is there an association between hemangiomas and syndromes with dysmorphic features? Pediatrics 1991;88:1257-1267.

31. Mulliken J, Fishman S, Burrows P: Vascular anomalies. Curr Probl Surg 2000;37:517-584.

32. Goldberg NS, Hebert AA, Esterly NB: Sacral hemangiomas and multiple congenital abnormalities. Arch Dermatol 1986;122:684-687.

33. Albright AL, Gartner JC, Wiener ES: Lumbar cutaneous hemangiomas as indicators of tethered spinal cords. Pediatrics 1989;83:977-980.

34. Martinez-Perez D, Fein NA, Boon LM, Mulliken JB: Not all hemangiomas look like strawberries: uncommon presentations of the most common tumor of infancy. Pediatr Dermatol 1995;12:1-6.

35. Patrice SJ, Wiss K, Mulliken JB: Pyogenic granuloma (lobular capillary hemangioma): a clinicopathologic study of 178 cases. Pediatr Dermatol 1991;8:267-276.

36. Boon LM, Fishman SJ, Lund DP, Mulliken JB: Congenital fibrosarcoma masquerading as congenital hemangioma: report of two cases. J Pediatr Surg 1995;30:1378-1381.

37. Chung KC, Weiss SW, Kuzon WM Jr: Multifocal congenital hemangiopericytoma associated with Kasabach-Merritt syndrome. Br J Plast Surg 1995;48:240-242.

38. Jones EW, Orkin M: Tufted angioma (angioblastoma). A benign progressive angioma, not to be confused with Kaposi's sarcoma or low-grade angiosarcoma. J Am Acad Dermatol 1989;20:214-225.

39. Margileth AM, Museles M: Cutaneous hemangiomas in children. Diagnosis and conservative management. JAMA 1965;194:523-526.

40. Enjolras O, Gelbert F: Superficial hemangiomas: associations and management [see comments]. Pediatr Dermatol 1997;14:173-179.

41. Sloan GM, Reinisch JF, Nichter LS, et al: Intralesional corticosteroid therapy for infantile hemangiomas. Plast Reconstr Surg 1989;83:459-467.

42. Sadan N, Wolach B: Treatment of hemangiomas of infants with high doses of prednisone [see comments]. J Pediatr 1996;128:141-146.

43. Boon LM, MacDonald DM, Mulliken JB: Complications of systemic corticosteroid therapy for problematic hemangioma. Plast Reconstr Surg 1999;104:1616-1623.

44. Ezekowitz RA, Mulliken JB, Folkman J: Interferon alfa-2a therapy for life-threatening hemangiomas of infancy [see comments] [published errata appear in N Engl J Med 1994;330:300 and 1995;333:595-596]. N Engl J Med 1992;326:1456-1463.

45. Ricketts RR, Hatley RM, Corden BJ, et al: Interferon-alpha-2a for the treatment of complex hemangiomas of infancy and childhood. Ann Surg 1994;219:605-612, discussion 612-614.

46. Soumekh B, Adams G, Shapiro R: Treatment of head and neck hemangiomas with recombinant interferon alpha-2B. Ann Rhinol Laryngol 1994;105:201-206.

47. Greinwald JH Jr, Burke DK, Bonthius DJ, et al: An update on the treatment of hemangiomas in children with interferon alfa-2a. Arch Otolaryngol Head Neck Surg 1999;125:21-27.

48. Mulliken J, Boon L, Takahashi K: Pharmacologic therapy for endangering hemangiomas. Curr Opin Dermatol 1995;2:109-113.

49. Barlow CF, Priebe CJ, Mulliken JB, et al: Spastic diplegia as a complication of interferon alfa-2a treatment of hemangiomas of infancy [see comments]. J Pediatr 1998;132:527-530.

50. Dubois J, Hershon L, Carmant L, et al: Toxicity profile of interferon alfa-2b in children: a prospective evaluation. J Pediatr 1999;135:782-785.

51. Kirschner RE, Low DW: Treatment of pyogenic granuloma by shave excision and laser photocoagulation. Plast Reconstr Surg 1999;104:1346-1349.

52. Zukerberg LR, Nickoloff BJ, Weiss SW: Kaposiform hemangioendothelioma of infancy and childhood. An aggressive neoplasm associated with Kasabach-Merritt syndrome and lymphangiomatosis. Am J Surg Pathol 1993;17:321-328.

53. Enjolras O, Wassef M, Mazoyer E, et al: Infants with Kasabach-Merritt syndrome do not have "true" hemangiomas. J Pediatr 1997;130:631-640.

54. Sarkar M, Mulliken JB, Kozakewich HP, et al: Thrombocytopenic coagulopathy (Kasabach-Merritt phenomenon) is associated with kaposiform hemangioendothelioma and not with common infantile hemangioma. Plast Reconstr Surg 1997;100:1377-1386.

55. Kasabach H, Merritt K: Capillary hemangioma with extensive purpura: report of a case. Am J Dis Child 1940;59:1063-1070.

56. Enjolras O, Mulliken JB, Wassef M, et al: Residual lesions after Kasabach-Merritt phenomenon in 41 patients. J Am Acad Dermatol 2000;42:225-235.

57. Lim JK, Teston L, Pennington DG, May J: Hemangiopericytoma of the hand: a literature review and case study. J Hand Surg Am 1992;17:1051-1055.

58. Rodriguez-Galindo C, Ramsey K, Jenkins JJ, et al: Hemangiopericytoma in children and infants. Cancer 2000;88:198-204.

59. Templeton PA, Gordon DJ, O'Hara MD: Infantile haemangiopericytoma of the hand. J Hand Surg Br 1996;21:121-123.

60. Moss LA, Stueber K, Hafiz MA: Congenital hemangioendothelioma of the hand—case report. J Hand Surg Am 1982;7:53-56.

61. Chia J, Teh M, Pho RW: Haemangioendothelioma in an infant's wrist. J Hand Surg Br 1997;22:119-121.

62. Acharya G, Merritt WH, Theogaraj SD: Hemangioendotheliomas of the hand: case reports. J Hand Surg Am 1980;5:181-182.

63. Quante M, Patel NK, Hill S, et al: Epithelioid hemangioendothelioma presenting in the skin: a clinicopathologic study of eight cases. Am J Dermatopathol 1998;20:541-546.

64. Patel MR, Srinivasan KC, Pearlman HS: Malignant hemangioendothelioma in the hand: a case report. J Hand Surg Am 1978;3:585-588.

65. Gonzalez-Crussi F, Chou P, Crawford SE: Congenital, infiltrating giant-cell angioblastoma. A new entity? Am J Surg Pathol 1991;15:175-183.

66. Vargas SO, Perez-Atayde AR, Gonzalez-Crussi F, Kozakewich HP: Giant cell angioblastoma: three additional occurrences of a distinct pathologic entity. Am J Surg Pathol 2001;25:185-196.

67. Marler J, Rubin J, Trede N, et al: Successful antiangiogenic therapy of giant cell angioblastoma with interferon alfa-2b: report of two cases. Pediatrics 2002;109:E37.

68. Risau W, Sariola H, Zerwes HG, et al: Vasculogenesis and angiogenesis in embryonic-stem-cell-derived embryoid bodies. Development 1988;102:471-478.

69. Wang HU, Chen ZF, Anderson DJ: Molecular distinction and angiogenic interaction between embryonic arteries and veins revealed by ephrin-B2 and its receptor Eph-B4. Cell 1998;93:741-753.

70. Vikkula M, Boon L, Mulliken J, Olsen B: Molecular basis of vascular anomalies. Trends Cardiovasc Med 1998;8:281-292.

71. Guttmacher AE, Marchuk DA, White RI: Hereditary hemorrhagic telangiectasia. N Engl J Med 1995;333:918-924.

72. van Lohuizen C: Über eine seltene angeborene Hautanomalie (cutis marmorata telangiectatica congenita). Acta Derm Venereol 1922;3:202.

73. Amitai DB, Fichman S, Merlob P, et al: Cutis marmorata telangiectatica congenita: clinical findings in 85 patients. Pediatr Dermatol 2000;17:100-104.

74. Fitzsimmons JS, Starks M: Cutis marmorata telangiectatica congenita or congenital generalized phlebectasia. Arch Dis Child 1970;45:724-726.

75. Dutkowsky JP, Kasser JR, Kaplan LC: Leg length discrepancy associated with vivid cutis marmorata [see comments]. J Pediatr Orthop 1993;13:456-458.

76. Devillers AC, de Waard-van der Spek FB, Oranje AP: Cutis marmorata telangiectatica congenita: clinical features in 35 cases. Arch Dermatol 1999;135:34-38.

77. Smoller BR, Rosen S: Port-wine stains. A disease of altered neural modulation of blood vessels? Arch Dermatol 1986; 122:177-179.

78. Enjolras O, Riche MC, Merland JJ: Facial port-wine stains and Sturge-Weber syndrome. Pediatrics 1985;76:48-51.

79. Tan OT, Sherwood K, Gilchrest BA: Treatment of children with port-wine stains using the flashlamp-pulsed tunable dye laser [see comments]. N Engl J Med 1989;320:416-421.

80. van der Horst CM, Koster PH, de Borgie CA, et al: Effect of the timing of treatment of port-wine stains with the flash-lamp-pumped pulsed-dye laser [see comments]. N Engl J Med 1998;338:1028-1033.

81. Boon LM, Mulliken JB, Vikkula M, et al: Assignment of a locus for dominantly inherited venous malformations to chromosome 9p. Hum Mol Genet 1994;3:1583-1587.

82. Boon LM, Brouillard P, Irrthum A, et al: A gene for inherited cutaneous venous anomalies ("glomangiomas") localizes to chromosome 1p21-22. Am J Hum Genet 1999;65:125-133.

83. Berenguer B, Burrows PE, Zurakowski D, Mulliken JB: Sclerotherapy of craniofacial venous malformations: complications and results. Plast Reconstr Surg 1999;104:1-11, discussion 12-15.

84. Dubois JM, Sebag GH, De Prost Y, et al: Soft-tissue venous malformations in children: percutaneous sclerotherapy with Ethibloc. Radiology 1991;180:195-198.

85. Upton J, Mulliken JB, Murray JE: Classification and rationale for management of vascular anomalies in the upper extremity. J Hand Surg Am 1985;10:970-975.

86. Oranje AP: Blue rubber bleb nevus syndrome. Pediatr Dermatol 1986;3:304-310.

87. McCarthy JC, Goldberg MJ, Zimbler S: Orthopaedic dysfunction in the blue rubber-bleb nevus syndrome. J Bone Joint Surg Am 1982;64:280-283.

88. Tyrrel RT, Baumgartner BR, Montemayor KA: Blue rubber bleb nevus syndrome: CT diagnosis of intussusception. AJR Am J Roentgenol 1990;154:105-106.

89. Sabin F: On the origin of the lymphatic system from the veins and the development of the lymph hearts and thoracic duct in the pig. Am J Anat 1905;1:367.

90. Kaipainen A, Korhonen J, Mustonen T, et al: Expression of the fms-like tyrosine kinase 4 gene becomes restricted to lymphatic endothelium during development. Proc Natl Acad Sci USA 1995;92:3566-3570.

91. Wigle JT, Oliver G: Prox1 function is required for the development of the murine lymphatic system. Cell 1999;98:769-778.

92. Dumont DJ, Fong GH, Puri MC, et al: Vascularization of the mouse embryo: a study of flk-1, tek, tie, and vascular endothelial growth factor expression during development. Dev Dyn 1995;203:80-92.

93. Ferrell RE, Levinson KL, Esman JH, et al: Hereditary lymphedema: evidence for linkage and genetic heterogeneity. Hum Mol Genet 1998;7:2073-2078.

94. Evans AL, Brice G, Sotirova V, et al: Mapping of primary congenital lymphedema to the 5q35.3 region. Am J Hum Genet 1999;64:547-555.

95. Mangion J, Rahman N, Mansour S, et al: A gene for lymphedema-distichiasis maps to 16q24.3. Am J Hum Genet 1999;65:427-432.

96. Kimak M, Karkkainen M, Alitalo K, et al: Mutations in the vascular endothelial growth factor receptor (VEGF-3;Flt 4) cause hereditary lymphedema [abstract]. J Hum Genet 1999;65:253.

97. Gorham L, Stout A: Massive osteolysis (acute spontaneous absorption of bone, phantom bone, disappearing bone): its relation to hemangiomatosis. J Bone Joint Surg 1955;37:986-1004.

98. Ogita S, Tsuto T, Tokiwa K, Takahashi T: Intracystic injection of OK-432: a new sclerosing therapy for cystic hygroma in children. Br J Surg 1987;74:690-691.

99. Ogita S, Tsuto T, Nakamura K, et al: OK-432 therapy in 64 patients with lymphangioma. J Pediatr Surg 1994;29:784-785.

100. Halsted W: Congenital arteriovenous and lymphaticovenous fistulae: unique clinical and experimental observations. Trans Am Surg Assoc 1919;37:262.

101. Reid M: Abnormal arteriovenous communications, acquired and congenital. II. The origin and nature of arteriovenous aneurysms, cirsoid aneurysms and simple angiomas. Arch Surg 1925;10:601.

102. Reinhoff WJ: Congenital arteriovenous fistula: an embryological study with report of a case. Bull Johns Hopkins Hosp 1924;35:271.

103. Braverman I, Keh A, Jacobson B: Ultrastructure and three-dimensional organization of the telangiectases of hereditary hemorrhagic telangiectasia. J Invest Dermatol 1990;95:422.

104. Coleman CJ: Diagnosis and treatment of congenital arteriovenous fistulas of the head and neck. Am J Surg 1973;47:354.

105. Hurwitz D, Kerber C: Hemodynamic considerations in the treatment of arteriovenous malformations of the face and scalp. Plast Reconstr Surg 1981;67:421.

106. Wautier MP, Boval B, Chappey O, et al: Cultured endothelial cells from human arteriovenous malformations have defective growth regulation. Blood 1999;94:2020-2028.

107. Kohout MP, Hansen M, Pribaz JJ, Mulliken JB: Arteriovenous malformations of the head and neck: natural history and management. Plast Reconstr Surg 1998;102:643-654.

108. Yakes WF, Rossi P, Odink H: How I do it. Arteriovenous malformation management. Cardiovasc Intervent Radiol 1996;19:65-71.

109. Baskerville PA, Ackroyd JS, Lea Thomas M, Browse NL: The Klippel-Trénaunay syndrome: clinical, radiological and haemodynamic features and management. Br J Surg 1985;72:232-236.

110. Gloviczki P, Stanson AW, Stickler GB, et al: Klippel-Trénaunay syndrome: the risks and benefits of vascular interventions. Surgery 1991;110:469-479.

111. Samuel M, Spitz L: Klippel-Trénaunay syndrome: clinical features, complications and management in children. Br J Surg 1995;82:757-761.

112. Jacob AG, Driscoll DJ, Shaughnessy WJ, et al: Klippel-Trénaunay syndrome: spectrum and management. Mayo Clin Proc 1998;73:28-36.

113. Biesecker LG, Happle R, Mulliken JB, et al: Proteus syndrome: diagnostic criteria, differential diagnosis, and patient evaluation. Am J Med Genet 1999;84:389-395.

114. Maffucci A: Di un caso di encondroma ed angioma multiplo contribuzione al a genesi embrionale dei tumor. Movimento Med Chir (Naples) 1881;3:399.

115. Lewis R, Ketcham A: Maffucci's syndrome: functional and neoplastic significance. J Bone Joint Surg Am 1979;55:1469.

116. Kaplan RP, Wang JT, Amron DM, Kaplan L: Maffucci's syndrome: two case reports with a literature review. J Am Acad Dermatol 1993;29:894-899.

117. Bean W: Dyschondroplasia and hemangiomata. Arch Intern Med 1955;95:767.

118. Cameron A, McMillan D: Lipomatosis of skeletal muscle in Maffucci's syndrome. J Bone Joint Surg Br 1956;38:692.

119. Kennedy J: Dyschondroplasia and hemangiomata (Maffucci's syndrome): report of a case with oral and intracranial lesions. Br J Dent 1973;135:18.

120. Loewinger R, Lichtenstein J, Dodson W, et al: Maffucci's syndrome: a mesenchymal dysplasia with multiple tumor syndrome. Br J Dermatol 1977;96:317.

121. Lowell S, Mathey R: Head and neck manifestations of Maffucci's syndrome. Arch Otolaryngol 1979;105:427.

122. Moorthy A: Oral manifestations in Maffucci's syndrome. Br Dent J 1983;155:160.

123. Johnson TE, Nasr AM, Nalbandian RM, Cappelen-Smith J: Enchondromatosis and hemangioma (Maffucci's syndrome) with orbital involvement. Am J Ophthalmol 1990;110:153-159.

124. Perkins P, Weiss SW: Spindle cell hemangioendothelioma. An analysis of 78 cases with reassessment of its pathogenesis and biologic behavior. Am J Surg Pathol 1996;20:1196-1204.

125. Sun TC, Swee RG, Shives TC, Unni KK: Chondrosarcoma in Maffucci's syndrome. J Bone Joint Surg Am 1985;67:1214-1219.

126. Dahlin D, Henderson E: Chondrosarcoma. A surgical and pathological problem. Review of 212 cases. J Bone Joint Surg Am 1956;38:1025.

127. Coley B, Higinbotham N: Secondary chondrosarcoma. Ann Surg 1954;139:1954.

128. Cook P, Evans P: Chondrosarcoma of the skull in Maffucci's syndrome. Br J Radiol 1977;50:833.

129. Cohen MM Jr: Bannayan-Riley-Ruvalcaba syndrome: renaming three formerly recognized syndromes as one etiologic entity [letter]. Am J Med Genet 1990;35:291-292.

130. Fargnoli MC, Orlow SJ, Semel-Concepcion J, Bolognia JL: Clinicopathologic findings in the Bannayan-Riley-Ruvalcaba syndrome. Arch Dermatol 1996;132:1214-1218.

131. Gorlin RJ, Cohen MM Jr, Condon LM, Burke BA: Bannayan-Riley-Ruvalcaba syndrome. Am J Med Genet 1992;44:307-314.

132. DiLiberti J, D'Agostino A, Ruvalcaba R, Schimschock J: A new lipid storage myopathy observed in individuals with Ruvalcaba-Myhre-Smith syndrome. Am J Med Genet 1984;18:163-167.

133. Marsh DJ, Dahia PL, Zheng Z, et al: Germline mutations in PTEN are present in Bannayan-Zonana syndrome [letter]. Nat Genet 1997;16:333-334.

Pediatric Upper Extremity Trauma

EDWARD J. HARVEY, MD ✦ L. SCOTT LEVIN, MD

CRITICAL AND EMERGENCY CARE

Treatment of the pediatric upper extremity injury has many pitfalls that do not present themselves in the adult injury. Evaluation and diagnosis are difficult, particularly in an age group in which communication is sometimes nearly impossible. The physical examination and observation of the extremity in question relative to the physical and mental state of the patient are often the only things that the surgeon has to determine a diagnosis. In a patient with incomplete ossification, interpretation of normal results of diagnostic studies such as radiography is difficult at times. The surgeon must not hesitate to perform more invasive tests, such as arteriography, arthrography, and examination under anesthesia, to maximize outcome in this group of patients.

Initial treatment of an open upper extremity injury in the emergency department uses not only a rigid splint but also early application of a biologic dressing, which includes saline dressings and antibiotic cream, to prevent further desiccation and damage to the wound. The open hand injury should receive the same tetanus and antibiotic coverage that any open fracture would receive.[1,2] Knowledge of the mechanism of injury will delineate the zone of injury and tissue death to be expected. Thermal injury from machinery may involve fractures, but the zone of death will often include the intrinsic muscles and deeper tissues. Débridement of the wound will better

indicate the tissue replacement that is needed. Any underlying skeletal fixation must be coordinated with the soft tissue plan, which takes precedence. A single examination (one supervising physician) of the hand under adequate sedation should take place (Table 210-1).

The outcome of a simple wound of the hand is rarely complicated if there is timely treatment. Dressings with antibiotic ointment and gauze bandage are changed at 48 hours after the injury. Adjustment in treatment depends on the individual case. This dressing is usually protected with an above-elbow cast for the 2 to 4 days that it is needed. Casts should not be used if there is extensive soft tissue loss, swelling, or suspicion that there will be inadequate follow-up.

Because of the proximity of any wound in the hand to major neurovascular structures, great care must be taken in the examination of the patient. The clinical picture is usually apparent regardless of the amount of pain or lack of cooperation demonstrated by the child. The unconscious patient with tendon lacerations holds the hand in an unmistakable attitude. Patients with tendon injuries will not demonstrate the normal cascade of the hand. Examination should include the digital Allen test and two-point discrimination, when appropriate, for every laceration on both the volar and dorsal hand. All clean wounds without neurovascular damage can be closed primarily and protected in a splint for 3 to 4 days. A decision on individual digital nerve or artery lacerations must be made

TABLE 210-1 ✦ MEDICATIONS MOST COMMONLY USED FOR SEDATION IN PEDIATRIC FRACTURE REDUCTION[8]

Medication	Dosage	Comments
Midazolam	0.05-0.2 mg/kg IV	Rapid onset, brief duration of action
Diazepam	0.04-0.3 mg/kg IV	Good muscle relaxant
Morphine	0.1-0.2 mg/kg IV	Long duration of action
Meperidine	1.0-2.0 mg/kg IV	Long duration of action
Fentanyl	1.0-5.0 mg/kg IV	Potent, rapid onset of action, titrates slowly
Ketamine	1.0-2.0 mg/kg IV	Manage emergence reactions with small
	3.0-4.0 mg/kg IM	doses of midazolam
Naloxone	1.0-2.0 mg/kg IV	Narcotic reversal agent
Flumazenil	5.0-10.0 μg/kg IV (maximum, 0.2 mg)	Benzodiazepine reversal agent
Atropine	0.01 mg/kg IV or IM (maximum, 0.5 mg)	Antisialagogue
Glycopyrrolate	4.0-10.0 μg/kg IV or IM (maximum, 0.25 mg)	Antisialagogue

IM, intramuscular; IV, intravenous.

by the surgeon and the patient. Wounds are dressed with antibiotic ointment and a bulky dressing. All sutures placed in the hand should be 5-0 or 6-0 in size. Wounds in small children should be closed with subcutaneous sutures if wound cleanliness is adequate. Sutures are removed at 1 week, and range-of-motion exercises are encouraged.

MUTILATING HAND INJURIES: ASSESSMENT AND GENERAL MANAGEMENT PRINCIPLES

Examination of the extensive hand injury usually occurs in the operating room because of difficulty with examination of the child without adequate anesthesia (Fig. 210-1). The ultimate function of the hand should be determined before the planning of any operation, and this may require excusing yourself from the operating room to discuss prognosis and plan with the patient's family (see Fig. 210-1). Remaining elements of the hand must be examined for assessment of ultimate function. A viable hand must be treated aggressively with fracture fixation and soft tissue replacement for motion to be retained. A plan for stabilization that includes the replacement of as many tissues as possible early in the course is the preferred treatment plan. The desire for total reconstruction must be tempered with the realization that extensive surgery may do as much to impede the patient's recovery as it does to promote the rehabilitation. Multiple procedures on both the volar and dorsal hand should be staged so that the more important procedures for recovery are accomplished primarily. Débridement always results in the loss of tissue volume. In an area such as the hand, a small amount of tissue loss can result in the exposure of vital structures. The surgeon must be prepared to accept the fact that nonviable tissues cannot be used to cover wounds while waiting

for granulation to occur. Marginal tissue left in the wound is only a nidus for infection. Waiting for an open hand wound to declare itself will only result in increased fibrosis and decreased ultimate function because of the attendant immobilization and more difficult rehabilitation. Critical neurovascular structures can be cleaned. Neurovascular structures should be stripped of dirt but not sacrificed to remove all contaminant. Tendons can be trimmed or shortened to remove foreign bodies. These structures are then covered promptly with tissue transfer, which will retain their viability.[3]

Primary débridement is accomplished with the limb exsanguinated and the tourniquet inflated. Vital structures are easily differentiated from dead tissue with the aid of loupe magnification. Secondary débridement is carried out immediately afterward with the tourniquet deflated to further trim any remaining devitalized tissue. This gives the benefit of minimizing blood loss while allowing primary débridement in a clear wound. Careful attention should be paid to the soft tissue envelope after release of the tourniquet. Simple trauma will allow débridement to bleeding dermal edges; however, with torsion, avulsion, and thermal or electrical injuries, there will be skip lesions of devitalized tissue, which will compromise results if they are allowed to remain. In these cases, knowledge of anatomic planes and the location of the perforating blood supply to the tissue envelope is useful. The avascular skin may be débrided while leaving a vascularized dermal layer in some avulsion or torsion injuries. Laser Doppler flowmetry of the margins is a reliable method of evaluating viable soft tissue and dermal remnants. If there is any question as to the viability of the envelope and it does not overlie a vital structure, it should be sacrificed and the area should be reconstructed with tissue reconstruction techniques.

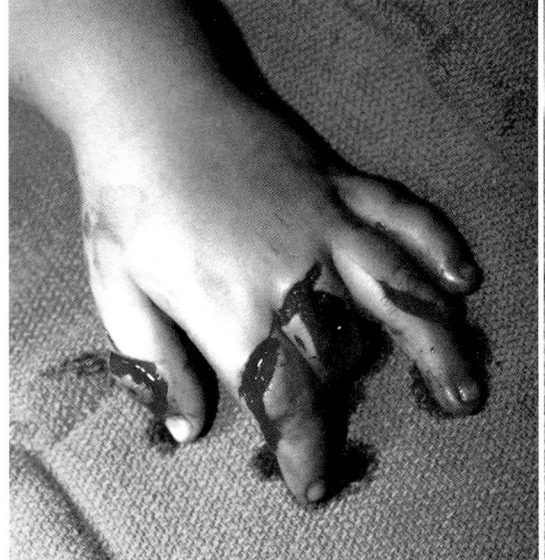

A

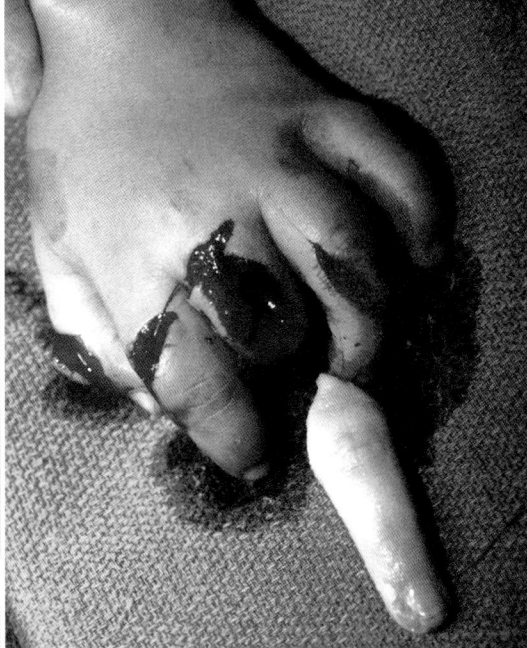

B

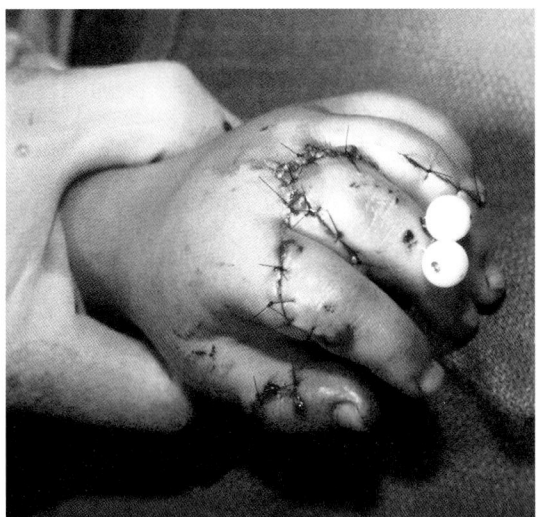

C

FIGURE 210-1. Lawn mower injury of the hand. *A,* A young patient sustained a lawn mower injury to four digits of the left hand, with sparing of the little finger. The initial examination was made after adequate general anesthesia, which allowed full cleaning of the wound, including the amputated third digit. *B,* The third digit examined under the microscope shows adequate vascular elements out of the zone of injury to allow replantation. Other wounds were shown to be repairable as well with minimal tissue loss. This permitted the physician time to obtain more information in a controlled atmosphere and a better understanding of the problem. At this time, discussion with the family was accomplished with better information exchange. Even though this necessitated some time out of the operating room, the plan of treatment was clarified for both the family and the surgeon. *C,* Postoperatively, the wounds are closed, and the replantation has been accomplished.

Débridement is initiated at the skin surface and carried toward the depths of the wound. Any extensive wound in the palm should be extended to decompress the median nerve by incision of the transverse carpal ligament (Fig. 210-2). This extension into non-traumatized anatomy allows a reference to the planes of the palm. Wounds on the extensor surface can be débrided because of the lack of vital structures and greater elasticity of the skin. Denuded tendon, nerve, and vessels can be cleaned and retained. Frayed tendon should be débrided at least partially. Contused nerves are retained, but avulsed nerves are trimmed back to normal fascicles. Nerve grafting is carried out primarily if possible. Vessels with intimal hemorrhage are resected and grafted. Any bone fragments that are maintained on a soft tissue pedicle should be retained if they are not grossly contaminated.

After débridement, thorough scrubbing with solution containing bacitracin is carried out. New drapes are used for the definitive procedures. If soft tissue reconstruction cannot be performed, repeated débridement at 24 to 48 hours will allow inspection of marginal areas.[4]

The timing of the reconstruction of combined injuries depends on several factors. Primary repair of all injured structures is desired therapy; however, enthusiasm must be tempered in certain cases. Segmental gaps in the skeleton can be maintained with

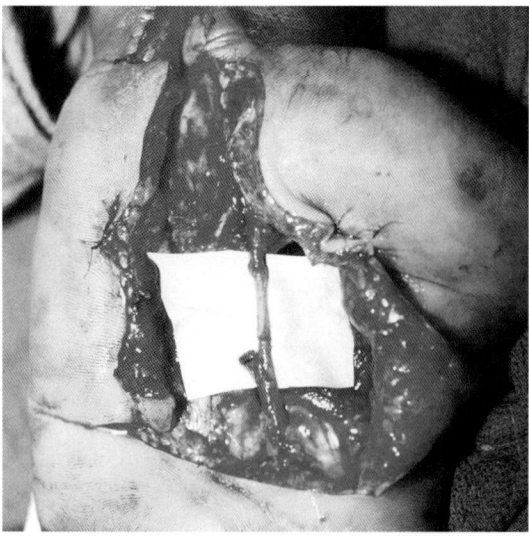

FIGURE 210-2. Gunshot wound to the midpalm of a 10-year-old boy. Decompression and débridement to viable tissue have been carried out. Release of the carpal tunnel is obvious at the superior portion of the image. To maximize viable tissue and peripheral circulation, a vein bypass for the individual digits has been performed. Soft tissue coverage is paramount for successful repair in these injuries.

methyl methacrylate or silicone spacers while soft tissue reconstruction is carried out. If tendons are irreparable with a poor soft tissue envelope, silicone tendon spacers or pediatric feeding tubes can be substituted for flexor or extensor tendons, and they can be grafted later when the soft tissue envelope is stable. Spare parts from amputated areas can be used to decrease donor site morbidity and to increase the reconstruction options. Amputated fingers can be used as fillet grafts to improve coverage of the hand. Neurovascular structures for grafts to other areas of the hand can be useful. Proximal interphalangeal joints or wraparound grafts can be used for other digits to maximize function. The cleanliness of the wound should not dissuade the surgeon from early reconstruction. Early microvascular reconstruction will decrease bacterial counts and avoid chronic infections.[5] A consideration of the final function of the hand may dictate early arthrodesis or emergent flap coverage to rehabilitate the hand to the maximum potential. Amputation of part of the hand as a primary procedure should be considered an option in the severely traumatized hand.[6] Secondary heterotopic tissue transplantation should be planned in these cases. However, it is generally agreed that the indication for replantation in children can be broader than in adults.[7] A single-digit amputation is considered for replantation in children, even for an isolated amputation of a second or fifth finger (Fig. 210-3).

SPECIAL CONSIDERATIONS IN CHILDREN'S FRACTURES

Anesthesia

In most centers, including ours, a large proportion of fractures are treated outside the operating room, which requires the treating physician to administer anesthesia.[8] The American Academy of Pediatrics has established strict guidelines for conscious sedation. Many surgeons do not keep up with these recommendations. A survey indicated that as many as one third of orthopedic surgeons were not in compliance with these guidelines.[9] Options include quick reduction without anesthesia, hematoma or intravenous regional block, axillary block, intravenous sedation, self-administered nitrous oxide (50:50 ratio of nitrous oxide and oxygen) with or without adjuvant block, and general anesthesia.

Intravenous sedation and regional block have traditionally been the most widely used. Varela et al[10] reported on the use of meperidine and midazolam for this purpose. The target doses were 2 mg/kg of body weight and 0.1 mg/kg, respectively. Half of the recommended dose was infused during a period of 1 to 3 minutes. After an additional 3 to 5 minutes of observation, the remainder was titrated to achieve adequate sedation. Regional intravenous blocks have the advantages of rapid onset of effect, simple administration, and good muscle relaxation. Disadvantages include pain when the injured limb is exsanguinated by wrapping or elevation. Premature cuff deflation may lead to major neurologic and cardiac complications when high doses are used.

Self-administered nitrous oxide anesthesia is relatively safe[11] and has the advantage of having more rapid onset and effect with greater satisfaction of patients. Nitrous oxide is contraindicated for patients with middle ear infections or effusions. Hennrikus et al[11] demonstrated 97% successful analgesia with self-administered nitrous oxide and oxygen plus hematoma block. Use of general anesthesia avoids the burden of providing anesthesia. In addition, if several reduction attempts are required or surgery is decided on, general anesthesia provides total relaxation with minimal constraints. A synopsis of the different agents and their effects is provided in Table 210-1.

FRACTURES OF THE FOREARM BONES

Pediatric forearm and distal radius fractures are common injuries. Resultant deformities are usually a product of indirect trauma involving angular loading combined with rotational displacement. Fractures are classified by location, completeness, angular and rotational deformities, and fragment displacement. Successful outcomes are based on restoration of adequate

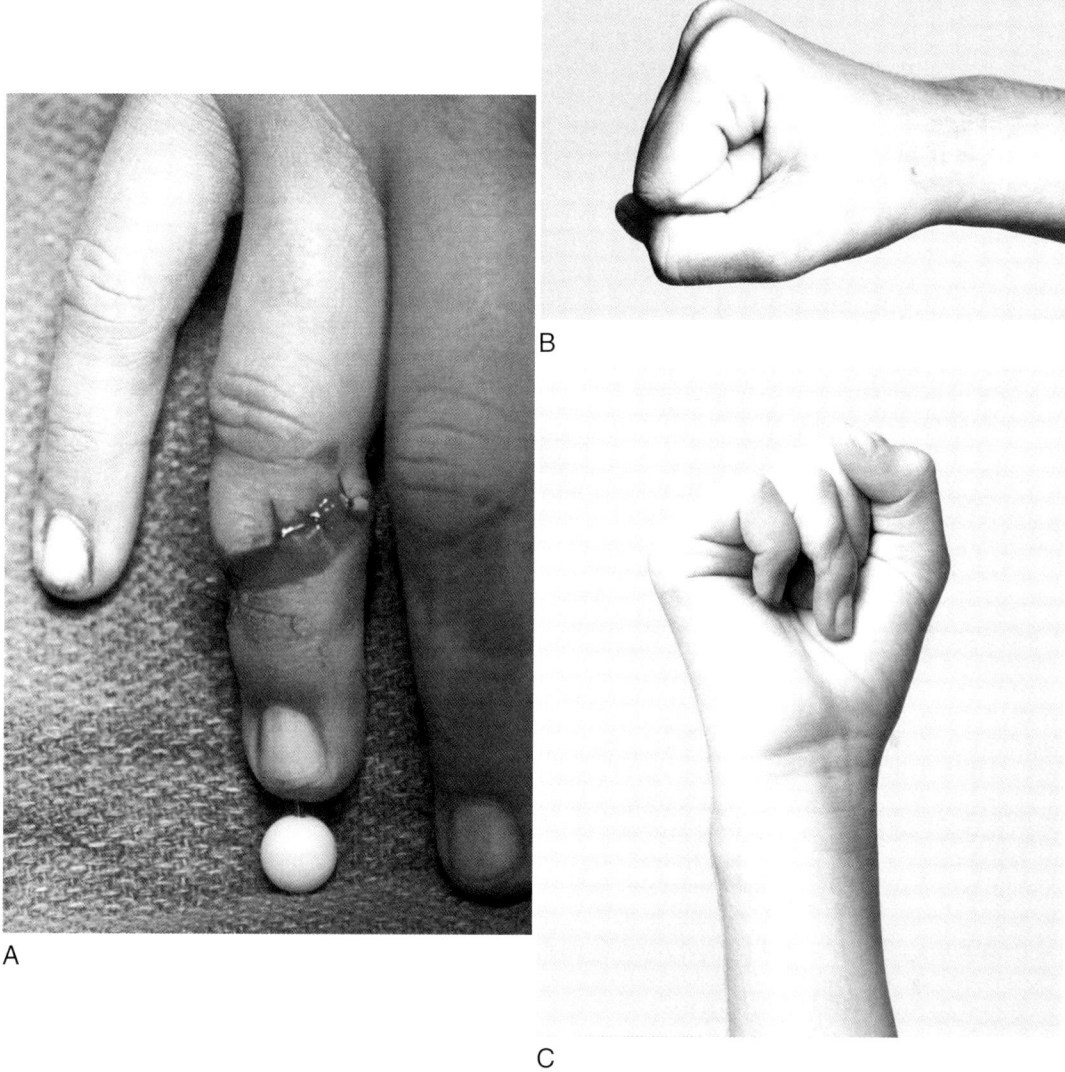

FIGURE 210-3. Single-digit replantation. *A,* Sharp laceration amputation involving the middle phalanx of the third digit. Replantation in this young patient was carried out successfully. This surgery may not have been attempted in some adult patients. *B,* One year postoperatively, there is good recovery of function in the hand. *C,* Full flexion of the digit has not been achieved, but the patient has neurologic recovery and does not complain of any limitation in the digit.

pronation and supination and, to a lesser degree, acceptable cosmesis. When several important concepts are kept in mind, these goals are usually met with conservative treatment by reduction and immobilization. Rotating the forearm such that the palm is directed toward the fracture apex reduces greenstick fractures. Complete fractures are manipulated and reduced with traction and rotation; extremities are then immobilized in well-molded plaster casts until healing, which usually takes about 6 weeks. Radiographs should be obtained between 1 and 2 weeks after initial reduction to detect early angulation. The predominant

motions affected by malunion are pronation and supination, which are a function of skeletal length and axial and rotational alignment. Normal supination from neutral is 80 to 120 degrees; normal pronation from neutral is 50 to 80 degrees. Common activities of daily living require 100 degrees of forearm rotation, equally split between pronation and supination. In fractures at any level in children younger than 9 years, complete displacement, 15 degrees of angulation, and 45 degrees of malrotation are acceptable. In children 9 years of age and older, 30 degrees of malrotation is acceptable, with 10 degrees of angulation for proximal fractures and 15 degrees for more distal fractures. Complete bayonet apposition is acceptable, especially for distal radius fractures, as long as angulation does not exceed 20 degrees and 2 years of growth remains.[8] Vittas et al[12] have reviewed the ability of the forearm to remodel. Thirty-six children treated for angulated midshaft forearm fractures were re-examined by radiography after a median time of 4 years (range, 2 to 5.8 years). In children younger than 11 years, there was a significant correlation between fracture correction and change in epiphyseal plate angulation, with the highest degree of correction being 13 degrees. In children older than 11 years, no correlation was found, and the degree of fracture correction was unpredictable.

The indications for surgical intervention in pediatric forearm fractures include open fractures; fractures shortly before skeletal maturity; irreducible fractures, with or without soft tissue interposition; unstable fractures after reduction; and Monteggia fractures with an unstable radial head and residual ulnar angulation. Traditional therapy for forearm fractures has been closed treatment and casting. Although recent authors have tried to determine indications for operative therapy for this problem, the "gold standard" for fractures in the skeletally immature patient is closed therapy. Jones and Weiner[13] reviewed their experience with closed therapy. A retrospective review was undertaken to evaluate the efficacy of primary nonoperative treatment (closed reduction and long-arm casting) along with pins and plaster as a salvage technique for those reduction failures. A total of 730 closed fractures were compiled. Of the 300 fractures requiring closed reductions, 22 went on to require remanipu-lations, and 12 required the use of pins and plaster technique for satisfactory reduction to be obtained or maintained. Complications in the group treated in this manner included two superficial pin infections treated with antibiotics and two forearms with moderate loss of pronation-supination not requiring treatment. They concluded that closed reduction of pediatric forearm fractures remains the accepted standard and that the technique of pins and plaster should be considered a reliable alternative for the unstable injuries.

Despite this, there has been a movement toward open reduction and internal fixation in pediatric fractures—particularly with minimally invasive fixation techniques. Elastic intramedullary nailing represents one of the more dynamic and topical surgical concepts in the treatment of upper extremity fractures in children (Fig. 210-4). Several publications have examined the use of these fixation devices. Cullen et al[14] looked at the complication rate with this technique. Their retrospective review of 20 children with forearm fractures treated with intramedullary fixation noted several complications. Intramedullary fixation of both bones was performed in eight cases, of the ulna alone in nine, and of the isolated radius in three. A limited open approach to one or both bones was necessary for insertion of the intramedullary rod in 15 of 20 cases, including the eight open fractures. Eighteen complications occurred in 10 of 20 patients, including hardware migration, infection, loss of reduction, reoperation, nerve injury, significantly decreased range of motion, synostosis, muscle entrapment, and delayed union. Despite the complications, 17 patients had excellent outcomes and 2 had good outcomes.

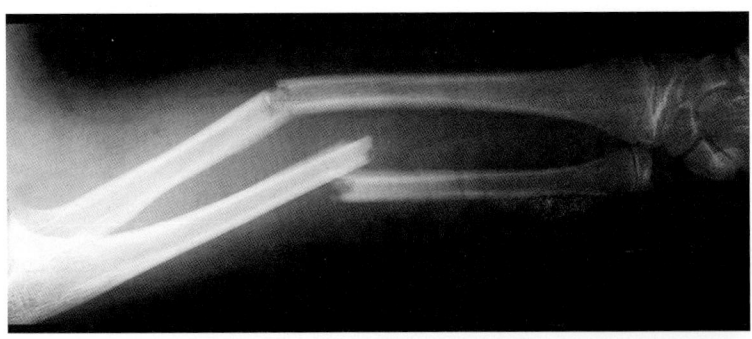

A

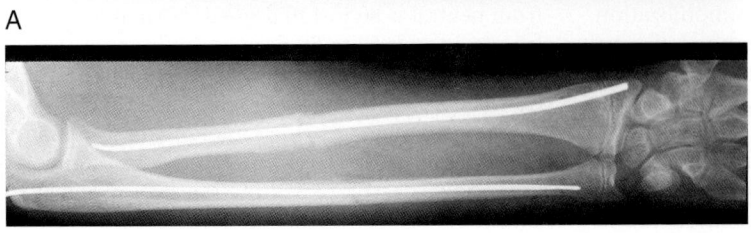

B

FIGURE 210-4. Intramedullary fixation of the forearm. *A,* Open midshaft fracture in a 12-year-old patient. *B,* Intramedullary fixation with titanium flexible nails was accomplished with minimal stripping of the already damaged fracture site. Irrigation and débridement were carried out per protocol before fixation at the same operative session. Healing at 6 weeks allowed removal of fixation devices.

Lascombes et al[15] reviewed 85 forearm fractures in which single curved nails were inserted into each forearm bone with closed reduction. Immediate mobilization was allowed postoperatively. In a 3.5-year follow-up of 76 patients, 92% had excellent results with a full range of movement. There were neither nonunions nor infections.

Griffet et al[16] reported on nailing used 67 times for a displaced fracture, 3 times for a recurrent fracture, 3 times after a secondary displacement, and 7 times in patients with multiple injuries. Sound union was achieved in 78 patients and normal motion in 79. The seven skin complications (three in the ulnar fractures and four in the radial fractures) consisted of three major local infections, one radial osteomyelitis, and three minor skin breakdowns. One patient had limited thumb extension, and two patients fell a second time. Most authors reporting on intramedullary flexible nails for forearm fractures have declared an advantage because plaster casts are avoided, allowing children to go back to school early. Sound union is achieved as quickly as with orthopedic treatment, and recovery is excellent. Although excellent clinical results can be expected with intramedullary fixation, complications related to the surgical technique can be expected.

Recent literature has examined whether there is a need for fixation of both bones in the forearm.[17] Bhaskar and Roberts[18] thought that if reduction and fixation of the fracture of the ulna alone restore acceptable alignment of the radius in unstable fractures of the forearm, operation on the radius can be avoided. Kirkos et al[19] believed that fixation of the radius is sufficient. They retrospectively reviewed the results of 50 children who had unstable diaphyseal forearm fractures of both bones for which closed reduction had been unsuccessful and so were treated with open reduction and internal fixation of the radius only. In this series, the functional and the anatomic results in all children at a mean follow-up of 4 years were excellent. Flynn and Waters[20] thought that fixation of one bone was adequate and that an intramedullary device would be sufficient.

The authors think that the ideal fixation is intramedullary fixation of at least one bone and then closed treatment or intramedullary fixation of the other bone, depending on the fracture. If there is any comminution at either bone, plating must be used on at least one bone—with closed reduction or intramedullary fixation or possibly plating of the other bone. If there is any limitation to motion, particularly pronation and supination, plating after anatomic reduction should be carried out. Prebending of the intramedullary device is sometimes needed to ensure maintenance of the anatomic bow of the forearm bones. Removal of plates from the radius is associated with a high complication rate and should be avoided at all costs.

CARPAL INJURIES

Carpal injuries are uncommon in children. The ability to arrive at a correct diagnosis has been facilitated by improvements in imaging, including wrist arthroscopy. Because the carpus of the infant is entirely cartilaginous, it is relatively immune to injury. As the carpus begins to ossify, it becomes more vulnerable to fracture and ligamentous injury (Fig. 210-5). By adolescence, the nearly completely ossified carpus demonstrates injury patterns similar to those of adults.[21] The diagnosis of intercarpal ligamentous injuries is complicated by the normal sequence of ossification of carpal bones. Partial carpal ossification makes it more difficult to establish the true axis of partially ossified carpal bones and to detect carpal malalignment. The distance between adjacent carpal ossific nuclei narrows as the wrist matures, confusing diagnosis of intercarpal diastasis.[22]

The scaphoid is the most frequently fractured bone in children, as in adults. The scaphoid ossifies eccentrically, with the distal pole ossifying before the proximal pole. The distance between the ossified scaphoid and the ossified lunate decreases as the child grows.

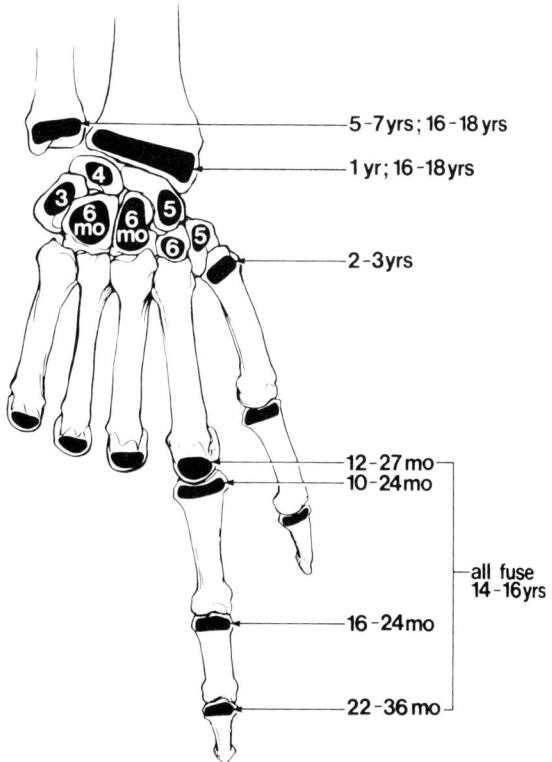

FIGURE 210-5. Ossification centers of the wrist. Knowledge of the timeline of ossification (as well as bilateral radiographs) is important in planning treatment. (From Rockwood CA, Wilkins KE, King RE: Fractures in Children, vol 3. Philadelphia, JB Lippincott, 1984:230.)

The median distance between ossific regions of the two bones varies from an average of 9 mm in 7-year-old children to 3 mm in 15-year-old children.[23] The radiographic gap is filled by unossified and articular cartilage and is often misinterpreted as scapholunate dissociation. Comparative films of the contralateral wrist may prove helpful, remembering that carpal ossification is not perfectly symmetric.

The patterns of fractures are different in children, with far more distal third fractures in children than in adults. Avulsion of the distal, radial aspect of the scaphoid is an injury seen in young children. Many of these fractures are not apparent on initial films but are seen on films repeated 1 to 2 weeks after injury. These injuries heal with 4 or 5 weeks of simple immobilization, with minimal long-term sequelae. Many pediatric scaphoid fractures are incomplete, disrupting only a single cortex. Most pediatric scaphoid fractures are nondisplaced and heal with 4 to 6 weeks of immobilization. When scaphoid fractures are displaced in children, open reduction is indicated to prevent the development of nonunion. Nonunions are also treated with open reduction and internal fixation.[24,25]

Fractures of the lunate and most other bones are extremely uncommon. The triquetrum is more susceptible to injury. The majority of these injuries occur between 11 and 13 years. Typically, the injury results from hyperextension of the wrist in which the ulnarly deviated carpus impinges on the distal ulna. A flake of the triquetrum is split off by the injury. Diagnosis is suggested by localized tenderness over the dorsum of the triquetrum. Small avulsion fracture fragments are best seen on oblique radiographic views. All injuries heal with immobilization in a short-arm cast for 3 weeks.[21]

FRACTURES AND DISLOCATIONS IN THE CHILD'S HAND

Hand fractures are frequent in children[26,27] and often follow a predictable, uneventful course. Joint involvement is an adverse prognosis that is mentioned by some authors[28,29] dealing specifically with articular fractures and in most general series of hand fractures in children, in particular if the fracture is displaced initially. The Salter classification of injuries has done much for the understanding of pediatric fractures and is applicable to fractures about the hand as well (Fig. 210-6). A review[30] (58 articular fractures of the hand in 55 children) demonstrated that the results were far from normal in a number of cases, with a complication rate as high as 50% when the fracture was displaced initially. A number of these fractures are initially overlooked, especially in small children, because of examination difficulties. This often delays the diagnosis by many days, sometimes even until the stage of altered function. Remodeling of bone malunion occurs

only in the sagittal plane (posteroanterior angulation), very little in the frontal plane (lateral angulation), and never in rotational deformities. Remodeling is most important in the metaphyseal area, much less so in the epiphyseal area. The older the child, the less remodeling of bone takes place. Remodeling of the articular cartilage can be expected only in young children (before 2 years).[27]

Fractures through the neck of the proximal and middle phalanges in children are relatively uncommon and represent approximately 1% of fractures in children's hands.[31,32] In young children, the condyles of the phalanges are not fully ossified, and the distal fragment in these fractures therefore has also been called the cartilaginous cap. The ossified portion (which is seen on the radiograph) is actually within this cartilaginous cap. Cartilaginous cap fractures may be displaced or undisplaced. In most cases, the injury occurs when the digit is entrapped in a closing door. It is thought that displacement of the distal fragment occurs as the child violently attempts to withdraw the trapped digit. This withdrawal reaction opens the fracture site enough for rotation of the distal fragment to occur. The lack of tendon attachments to the cartilaginous cap allows rotation, which is usually in a dorsal direction.[33] The best method of diagnosis and assessment of the degree of displacement is a true lateral radiograph. Undisplaced fractures can be treated conservatively, with splinting alone. Displaced fractures are usually unstable and require reduction and Kirschner wire fixation. The surgical approach to open reduction is through a dorsal or midlateral incision. Reduction of the fracture is best done under intraoperative radiographic control. In one author's experience, only 10% of displaced cap fractures could be reduced adequately by closed reduction, and open reduction is often necessary.[33] Furthermore, maintenance of reduction without the use of internal fixation is difficult in these unstable fractures. Cartilaginous cap fractures occur at the neck of the phalanx (where there is no epiphysis), and the fractures therefore show little remodeling in either plane.

TENDON INJURIES

Controversy about timing of tendon repair is focused mainly on the flexors. As a general rule, direct early repair, at all levels of injury, is agreed on,[34] provided wound conditions permit. This is even more pertinent in the youngest age group, those younger than 4 to 6 years, in whom flexor tendon grafting is particularly difficult. Tendon repairs should be carried out at the same time as replantation regardless of level. When injury to the flexors is diagnosed, surgical repair of both tendons, if possible, is carried out at all levels (with the possible exception of the zone IV carpal

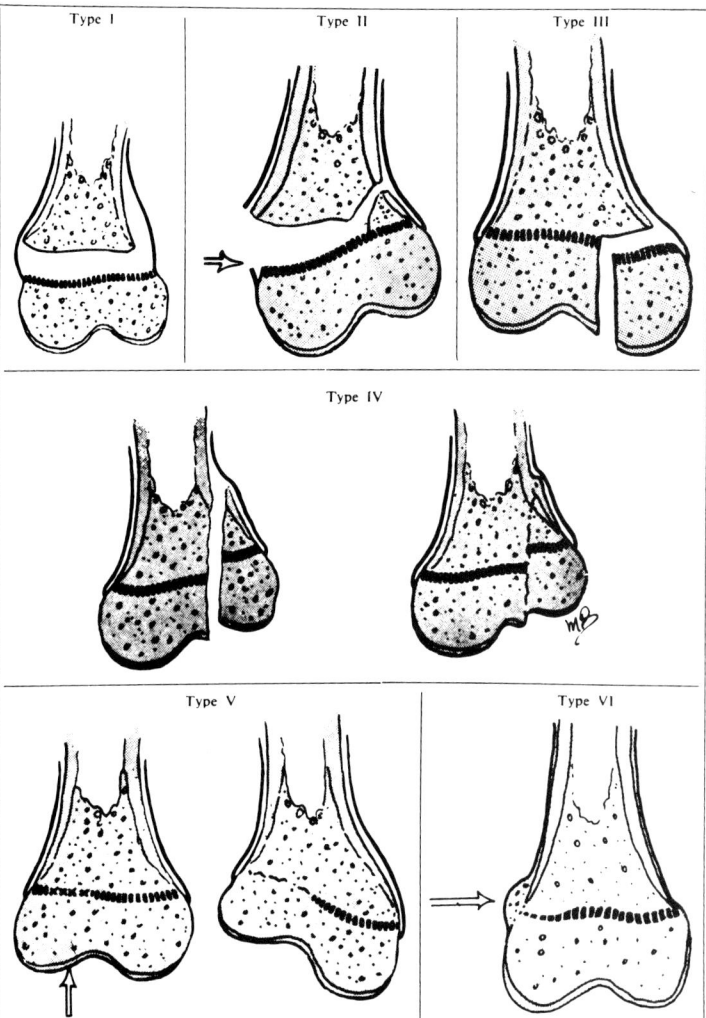

FIGURE 210-6. Salter classification of pediatric fractures. Well-known injury patterns for pediatric fractures apply to those fractures in the hand. Type I fractures are epiphyseal separation. Displacement may occur, but growth can be normal. Type II fractures are physeal fractures that exit through a small portion of the metaphysis. This makes the fracture easier to recognize and to reduce but may cause asymmetric growth after fracture. Intra-articular fractures of the epiphysis are type III fractures. These are associated with a higher incidence of growth arrest, may be difficult to recognize, and usually need to be operated on. Type IV fractures are also epiphyseal splitting fractures that exit the metaphysis rather than through the physis. Migration usually occurs unless the fragment is stabilized. Type V is a crushing injury and is rarely recognized but almost always results in some growth arrest. Type VI was added to the classification and is a peripheral injury that through healing results in a bone bridge and possible growth abnormality. (From Rockwood CA, Wilkins KE, King RE: Fractures in Children, vol 3. Philadelphia, JB Lippincott, 1984:121.)

tunnel level, where it may be better to repair only the flexor profundus).[35] The appropriate time to perform a flexor tendon graft in children has been debated. Some authors believe that age is no contraindication to grafting, although others have hesitated to perform flexor tendon grafts in children. The latter cite technical difficulties because of the small size of the tendons and the inability of children to cooperate in postoperative care and rehabilitation. Conventional free tendon grafts are indicated if there is no extensive scarring in the digit, the pulley is intact, and joints are capable of complete passive mobility. Two-staged flexor reconstruction is a complicated surgical technique but represents a salvage procedure in severely scarred digits, with incompetent pulley and joint contracture.[36,37]

The technique in children is essentially the same as that in adults, except that the distal juncture is not placed in the distal phalangeal bone. If possible, it should be placed into the distal profundus stump. If there is no distal stump, the graft should be sutured directly into bone with nonabsorbable sutures through drill holes placed distal to the epiphysis. If tendon grafting is to be performed, the preferred graft material is the palmaris longus or the flexor superficialis of the injured finger. The plantaris in children is often too thin to hold sutures.[35] The flexor tendon graft, if successful, may grow along with the child's hand. Hage and Dupuis[38] could not prove this. They did report that despite good function, the involved finger did lag slightly in growth and remained minimally smaller than the uninjured fingers. For staged procedures, Valenti and Gilbert[37] described a technique that they have used for 26 children. The effect of age on the results was also assessed, and it was a significant factor in the percentage of total active motion: older children (10 to 15 years, five cases) had a mean result of 81.5%; younger children (1 to 3 years, nine cases) had a mean result of 53%. The total active motion of the finger increased with the age.

The procedure is described as follows. A Brunner palmar incision is used to expose the scarred tendon sheath. A lateral digital incision is preferred to prevent secondary skin necrosis. The digital neurovascular bundle has to be identified and protected. The scarred tendons and damaged pulley elements are excised. All the undamaged segments are spared. A stump of flexor digitorum profundus is left to allow good distal fixation. A distally based tail of the flexor digitorum superficialis is preserved to prevent a proximal interphalangeal hyperextension deformity and to facilitate reconstruction of the pulley. After complete exposure of the digital canal, the incision is carried on the palm to expose the proximal part of the flexor tendons. The proximal stump of the flexor digitorum profundus is transected at the level of the lumbrical muscle. It is also possible to harvest the palmaris longus and approximate this to the proximal stump of the flexor digitorum profundus. If, after resection of scarred tendons and fibrous tissue, there is a contracture of the joint (proximal interphalangeal or metacarpophalangeal), release of the checkrein ligament and a capsulotomy of the volar plate may be necessary. The transverse arterial branches (from the collateral digital arteries) that supply the epiphysis plate must be preserved to avoid disturbance of digital growth. In most cases, the remaining tissue at the level of the old pulley is sufficient for reconstruction of the A2 and A4 pulleys. If it is not sufficient, these authors[37] used a tendon graft such as the palmaris longus or the rest of the flexor digitorum superficialis, fixing this to the periosteum. The authors believe that attachments around or through the bone are aggressive for the child. A remaining tail of the flexor superficialis tendon, left attached at its insertion, can be used for reconstruction of the A3 pulley. The implant is secured to the profundus stump at the distal phalanx; the authors use a U stitch with 9-0 nonabsorbable suture material. The adequacy of the pulley system is checked by traction on the proximal tip of the tendon implant. The proximal tip of the implant is introduced into the carpal tunnel until the distal forearm, where the area is free of scar. Before closure, it is important to check for good gliding of the implant at the level of the digital canal (quality of the pulley reconstruction) and in the distal forearm. It is important to detect a kinking of the tendon implant when the finger is flexed and a buckling if the tendon implant is too big. The results were better when the proximal tendon juncture was performed in the palm (68%, 13 cases) than in the distal forearm (56%, 10 cases).[37]

Passive joint rehabilitation is begun after 10 days and continued until stage 2 surgery. Stage 2 surgery is undertaken after 2 months of rehabilitation and if the skin is soft and passive motion of the joint is complete. At stage 2, the tendon implant is removed and a graft is inserted. Two small incisions are performed—a fingertip approach on the palmar aspect of the distal interphalangeal joint and a proximal approach in the palm or in the distal part of the forearm. The tendon graft is sutured to the distal stump of the flexor digitorum profundus. The tendon graft is passed through the pulp under the nail plate and then tensioned and fixed with nonabsorbable sutures (4-0). The tension of the graft is correct if the attitude of the finger is in slightly more flexion than the other digits.

FINGERTIP AND NAIL INJURIES

In the pediatric population, the most frequent level of digital amputation is through the distal phalanx. Advances in microsurgery allow replantation of distal amputation even in young children and infants, and such a procedure is no longer a technical challenge. When successful, replantation at this level leads to good functional and cosmetic results, superior to what is achieved by local or pedicled flaps. The overall success rate of replantation has been reported to be adequate in some studies.[39,40] Dautel uses a zone classification to determine replantation procedures. In zone 1, the amputated part does not include any bone fragment. Examination under magnification usually fails to demonstrate any vessel suitable for anastomosis. In young children, when the amputated part is available, it should be replaced as a composite graft. In zone 2, amputation goes through the nail bed, preserving at least half of the nail bed and sterile matrix. The central artery of the pulp can be retrieved and used for revascularization. No dorsal vein is available at this level. Venous drainage of the replanted part is achieved by repair of a palmar vein or by controlled bleeding. Technical problems are similar in zone 3 (at or near the nail fold), but because the remaining nail bed is shorter, a hooked nail deformity is likely to occur if the replantation fails or if the distal remnant is pulled tightly to meet the pulp and the nail matrix. This necessitates repair procedures that are much more extensive than the original surgery (Fig. 210-7).[41] In zone 4, proximal to the proximal nail fold, a dorsal vein can usually be dissected and repaired to ensure venous drainage of the replanted part.[40]

Nail bed injuries should be repaired. Ardouin et al[42] looked at medium-term outcome in 241 cases of distal finger trauma. Nail deformities were found in 42%, and 40% had sensory disturbances. Fourteen nail beds were sutured, leading to 12 normal nails (86%), whereas unsutured nail beds led to 52% normal nails. Small resorbable suture repair of the matrix after nail removal is the best way to ensure good functional and aesthetic outcome.

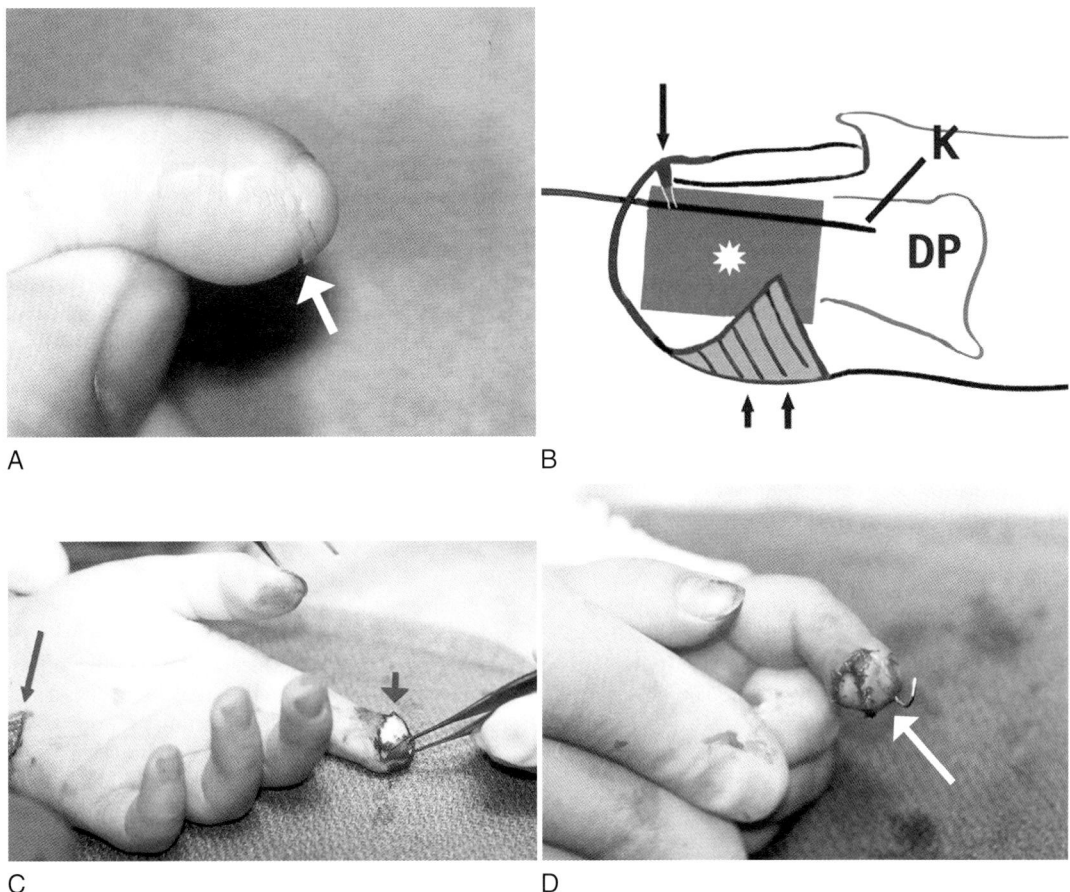

FIGURE 210-7. Hook nail in a 5-year-old after distal pulp avulsion. *A,* Overzealous attempt at lengthening of the volar flap to permit closure has resulted in tension on the dorsal surface including the nail matrix. This results in the classic hook nail deformity. The arrowhead shows the position of the end of the hook nail. *B,* Schematic representing operative plan for reconstruction. DP, distal phalanx; K, fixation wire that can hold bone block (white star) for increased length and also supports nail bed—one or two wires can be used for support; single arrow, trimmed nail bed with pulp transposed superiorly to meet the bed after relaxing incision is made in the volar finger; double arrows, full-thickness skin graft placed in the defect after transposition. *C,* Intraoperative picture of volar skin graft *(arrowhead)* being positioned in the defect as pulp is transposed distally. The arrow shows full-thickness skin graft donor site. *D,* Postoperative picture shows good repositioning of both sensory pulp and nail bed in more anatomic positions. Wire fixation is left for 4 weeks. The arrow indicates sensate pulp position. Secondary healing or less rigorous attempts to close the finger will often have better outcome.

PERIPHERAL NERVE INJURIES

There is a general impression that all nerve injuries can be treated with surgical repair and the surgeon can expect a favorable outcome. Functional remodeling does occur in the pediatric central nervous system. Remarkable levels of recovery of sensory function recorded by quantitative measurement of pressure sense, heat and cold threshold, sweating, and localization have been demonstrated in children in whom the skin of the hand was reinnervated from inappropriate spinal nerves or by the intercostal nerve.[43] There is some evidence that motor plasticity exists as well. The other positive factor relating to the recovery of

nerves in children is the relative rarity of pain. Injury to peripheral nerves is not always accompanied or followed by pain; many cases of complete division are painless. Incomplete lesions can be accompanied by pain of varying duration and severity. Certain of these pain states, which cause definite difficulties when they are present in the adult, are scarcely ever seen in the child (i.e., causalgia, reflex sympathetic dystrophy, and central pain). On the other hand, pain is associated with a nerve entrapped within fractures or dislocations, and pain occurs when nerve injuries are associated with an arterial lesion, provoking ischemia. The observation of better outcome after nerve repair in children may have as much to do with events within the central nervous system as it does with regeneration across the suture line and better reconnection with the target organs.[43]

There are many pitfalls in the diagnosis of injuries to peripheral nerves, especially in children. The goal must be to recognize the injury as soon as possible after the event and determine whether the nerves are affected, the level of injury, and the extent and depth of the lesions. The early symptoms of acute nerve injury are abnormal sensations, alteration or loss of sensibility, weakness, motor paralysis, impairment of function, and sometimes pain. The patient may be aware of warming or dryness of the skin. Pain is an important symptom. Its occurrence after injury often suggests that the cause is continuing, such as when a nerve is stretched over a bone projection or compressed by a hard object, constricted by a suture, or involved in an expanding hematoma.[43] In the young child, the anesthetic hand or digits may be wholly excluded from function, and the posture of the part hints at nerve injury. One sign is present in the first 48 hours after deep injury of a nerve with a cutaneous sensory component. Because the small as well as the large fibers are affected, the skin in the distribution of the affected nerve is warm and dry.[44]

Electrophysiologic examination is an aid to diagnosis. Perhaps the most important role of electrophysiologic examination is to distinguish between degenerative and nondegenerative lesions. If axons are damaged (degenerative lesion), stimulation of the nerve below the level of the lesion 6 days after injury will not elicit a motor response.[45] If the axons are intact (conduction block), stimulation will evoke a motor response. A firm diagnosis of neurapraxia should never be made unless stimulation of the nerve below the level of the lesion produces a motor response 1 week after the injury.

There is a relatively high incidence of lesions involving children's nerves caused by or associated with damage to the adjacent skeleton. The nerves may be damaged by traction from displacement, laceration by a fragment of bone, entrapment within the dislocated joint or fracture, or late entrapment and compression by callus. On the whole, dislocations are more damaging. Seigal and Gelberman[46] reviewed these nerve injuries in both adults and children. They found that 85% of nerve palsies from closed fractures recovered, and about 65% to 70% did so after open fractures. Of the nerves that recovered, 90% had done so by 4 months. Their recommendations for intervention were the fractures needing internal fixation, the presence of an associated vascular injury, the need for wound exploration of an open fracture, and a fracture or dislocation that is irreducible. The elbow is an area of difficulty in treatment of nerve injuries in children because of the proximity of all three major nerves to the bone and because of the constant risk of damage

to the brachial artery and compartment syndrome in the flexor muscles of the forearm. Ottolenghi[47] reported 830 cases of supracondylar fractures in children and recognized three patterns of injury to the median nerve and brachial artery: they were tented over the spike of the proximal fracture, the nerve was entrapped within the fracture, or both were entrapped in the fracture. Thirty-nine of these cases required treatment of vascular complications. Wilkins[48] found an 11% incidence of nerve palsy in 285 children with fractures and fracture-dislocations in the elbow region; only one failed to recover spontaneously. Dutkovsky and Kasser[49] reviewed nerves injured by fractures in children and commented that an irreducible supracondylar fracture with associated nerve damage represents an indication for open reduction and exploration. They cautioned against the percutaneous approach for insertion of the medial pin in fixation.

The prognosis for recovery after repair is determined by the severity of the original injury. The worst results are seen in complete lesions of the supraclavicular brachial plexus and in high-velocity injuries, in which penetrating missiles destroyed the proximal humerus and the adjacent nerves.[43] One of the most significant variables in determining prognosis is delay to repair. Skillful primary repair, however, may be followed by recovery to nearly normal levels, even in complex cases. Adequate follow-up is essential for detection and treatment of progressive deformity, especially at the ankle and foot.[43]

UPPER EXTREMITY VASCULAR INJURIES

Studies of upper extremity vascular injuries do not exist and we must extrapolate from other reviews. Gross and Yau[50] issued a strong warning against accepting a diagnosis of spasm. In the treatment of trauma, any persistent ischemia should be considered arterial injury and not caused by spasm; if distal ischemia persists after reduction of the fracture or dislocation, it should be assumed that arterial occlusion is the result of vessel damage or thrombosis rather than spasm.

Reichard et al[51] reviewed the cases of 87 children treated for penetrating extremity trauma during a 5-year period to define the usefulness of arteriography. The ages ranged from 2 to 16 years. Arteriography was performed for 24 children; 12 exhibited physical signs of vascular injury (diminished pulse, distal ischemia, expanding hematoma, and bruits or thrills over the wound), and 12 were asymptomatic with wounds in proximity to major vessels. Two other patients with ongoing hemorrhage were taken directly to the operating room. Of the 12 arteriograms obtained for abnormal physical signs, 8 (67%) showed vascular injuries. None of the studies performed for proximity alone had abnormal results. All patients with vascular injuries had abnormal physical findings, whereas only 4 of 77 patients without vascular injuries had abnormal findings (sensitivity 100%, specificity 95%). No missed injuries or complications were found. Timely diagnosis with repair is the cornerstone for successful management of vascular injuries. These authors found that arteriography is an important adjunct for patients who have abnormal physical findings. Proximity to major vessels alone fails to identify patients at risk for significant injuries. With these data, angiography may not be warranted in patients with penetrating trauma whose physical examination results are normal. Noninvasive modalities such as B-mode ultrasonography and Doppler study may have future application in the evaluation of these cases. Early and aggressive surgical intervention and repair are warranted to prevent long-term sequelae. The authors think that all vessels should be repaired (see Fig. 210-2).

CONCLUSIONS

The pediatric upper extremity injury is associated with many difficulties in evaluation and diagnosis, particularly in an age group in which communication is sometimes nearly impossible. The authors stress the difficulty in relying on normal diagnostic test results in a patient with incomplete ossification. The surgeon must not hesitate to perform more invasive tests, such as arteriography, arthrography, and examination under anesthesia, to maximize outcome in this group of patients. Long-term follow-up is essential to ensure early treatment of any sequelae.

REFERENCES

1. Freeland A, Jabaley M: Stabilization of fractures in the hand and wrist with traumatic soft tissue and bone loss. Hand Clin 1988;4:425-436.
2. Patzakis M, Wilkins J: Factors influencing infection rate in open fracture wounds. Clin Orthop 1989;243:36-40.
3. Rockwell W, Lister G: Coverage of hand injuries. Orthop Clin 1993;24:411-423.
4. Breidenbach W: Emergency free tissue transfer for reconstruction of acute upper extremity wounds. Clin Plast Surg 1989; 16:505-514.
5. Chen S, Wei F, Chen H, et al: Emergency free-flap transfer for reconstruction of acute complex extremity wounds. Plast Reconstr Surg 1992;89:882-888.
6. Kleinert H, Jablon M, Tsai T: An overview of replantation and results of 347 replants in 245 patients. J Trauma 1980;20:390-397.
7. Saies A, Urbaniak J, Nunley J, et al: Results after replantation and revascularization in the upper extremity in children. J Bone Joint Surg Am 1994;76:1766-1776.
8. Noonan K, Price C: Forearm and distal radius fractures in children. J Am Acad Orthop Surg 1998;6:146-156.
9. Price C, Choy J: Current practice of sedation and pain management in the reduction of pediatric forearm fractures: a survey. Orthop Trans 1995;19:42.
10. Varela C, Lorfing K, Schmidt T: Intravenous sedation for the closed reduction of fractures in children. J Bone Joint Surg Am 1995;77:340-345.
11. Hennrikus W, Shin A, Klingelberger C: Self-administered nitrous oxide and a hematoma block for analgesia in the outpatient reduction of fractures in children. J Bone Joint Surg Am 1995;77:335-339.
12. Vittas D, Larsen E, Torp-Pedersen S: Angular remodeling of midshaft forearm fractures in children. Clin Orthop 1991;265:261-264.
13. Jones K, Weiner D: The management of forearm fractures in children: a plea for conservatism. J Pediatr Orthop 1999;19:811-815.
14. Cullen M, Roy D, Giza E, Crawford A: Complications of intramedullary fixation of pediatric forearm fractures. J Pediatr Orthop 1998;18:14-21.
15. Lascombes P, Prevot J, Ligier J, et al: Elastic stable intramedullary nailing in forearm shaft fractures in children: 85 cases. J Pediatr Orthop 1990;10:167-171.
16. Griffet J, el Hayek T, Baby M: Intramedullary nailing of forearm fractures in children. J Pediatr Orthop B 1999;8:88-89.
17. Till H, Huttl B, Knorr P, Dietz H: Elastic stable intramedullary nailing (ESIN) provides good long-term results in pediatric long-bone fractures. Eur J Pediatr Surg 2000;10:319-322.
18. Bhaskar A, Roberts J: Treatment of unstable fractures of the forearm in children. Is plating of a single bone adequate? J Bone Joint Surg Br 2001;83:253-258.
19. Kirkos J, Beslikas T, Kapras E, Papavasiliou V: Surgical treatment of unstable diaphyseal both-bone forearm fractures in children with single fixation of the radius. Injury 2000;31:591-596.
20. Flynn J, Waters P: Single-bone fixation of both-bone forearm fractures. J Pediatr Orthop 1996;16:655-659.
21. Light T: Carpal injuries in children. Hand Clin 2000;16:513-522.
22. Light T: Injury to the immature carpus. Hand Clin 1988;4:415-424.
23. Leicht P, Mikkelsen J, Larsen C: Scapholunate distance in children. Acta Radiol 1996;37:625-626.
24. Caputo A, Watson H, Nissen C: Scaphoid nonunion in a child: a case report. J Hand Surg Am 1995;20:243-245.
25. Onuba O, Ireland J: Two cases of nonunion of fractures of the scaphoid in children. Injury 1984;15:109-112.
26. Landin L: Fracture patterns in children. Analysis of 8682 fractures with special reference to incidence, etiology and secular changes in a Swedish urban population. Acta Orthop Scand 1983;202:1-109.
27. Leclercq C, Korn W: Articular fractures of the fingers in children. Hand Clin 2000;16:523-534.
28. Fischer M, McElfresh E: Physeal and periphyseal injuries of the hand. Hand Clin 1994;10:287-301.
29. Torre B: Epiphyseal injuries in the small joints of the hand. Hand Clin 1988;4:113-121.
30. Leclercq C: Articular fracture in children (acute and chronic). In Bruser P, Gilbert A, eds: Finger, Bone and Joint Injuries. London, Dunitz, 1999:365-371.
31. Fischer M, McElfresh E: Physeal and periphyseal injuries of the hand. Hand Clin 1994;10:287-301.
32. Beatty E, Light T, Belsole R, Ogden J: Wrist and hand skeletal injuries in children. Hand Clin 1990;6:723-738.
33. Al-Qattan M: The cartilaginous cap fracture. Hand Clin 2000;16:535-540.
34. Herndon J: Treatment of tendon injuries in children. Orthop Clin North Am 1976;7:717-731.
35. Schneider L: Flexor tendons—late reconstruction. In Green DP, Hotchkiss RN, Pederson WC, eds: Green's Operative Hand Surgery. Philadelphia, Churchill Livingstone, 1999:1898-1949.

36. Hunter J, Salisbury R: Use of the gliding artificial implants to produce tendon sheaths: techniques and results in children. Plast Reconstr Surg 1970;45:564-572.

37. Valenti P, Gilbert A: Two-stage flexor tendon grafting in children. Hand Clin 2000;16:573-578.

38. Hage J, Dupuis C: The intriguing fate of tendon grafts in small children's hands and their results. Br J Plast Surg 1965;18:341-349.

39. Dautel G, Ferreira A, Corcella D: Replantations digitales distales. A propos d'une série de 61 cas. La Main 1997;2:329-335.

40. Dautel G: Fingertip replantation in children. Hand Clin 2000;16:541-546.

41. Atasoy E, Godfrey A, Kalisman M: The "antenna" procedure for the "hook-nail" deformity. J Hand Surg Am 1983;8:55-58.

42. Ardouin T, Poirier P, Rogez J: Fingertips and nailbed injuries in children. Apropos of 241 cases. Rev Chir Orthop Reparatrice Appar Mot 1997;83:330-334.

43. Birch R, Achan P: Peripheral nerve repairs and their results in children. Hand Clin 2000;16:579-595.

44. Birch R, Bonney G, Dowell J, Hollingdale J: Iatrogenic injuries of peripheral nerves. J Bone Joint Surg Br 1991;73:280-282.

45. Landau W: The duration of neuromuscular function after nerve section. Neurosurgery 1953;10:64-68.

46. Seigel D, Gelberman R: Peripheral nerve injuries associated with fractures and dislocations. In Gelberman RH, ed: Operative Nerve Repair and Reconstruction. Philadelphia, JB Lippincott, 1991:619-633.

47. Ottolenghi C: Prophylaxie du syndrome de Volkmann dans les fractures supra-condyliennes du coude chez l'enfant. Rev Chir Orthop 1971;57:517-525.

48. Wilkins K: Fractures and dislocations of the elbow region. In Rockwood CA Wilkins K, King RE, eds: Fractures in Children. Philadelphia, JB Lippincott, 1991:363-577.

49. Dutkovsky J, Kasser J: Nerve injury associated with fractures in children. In Gelberman RH, ed: Operative Nerve Repair and Reconstruction. Philadelphia, JB Lippincott, 1991:635-653.

50. Gross W, Yao J: Vascular problems. In Wadsworth TG: The Elbow. Edinburgh, Churchill Livingstone, 1982:223-241.

51. Reichard K, Hall J, Meller J, et al: Arteriography in the evaluation of penetrating pediatric extremity injuries. J Pediatr Surg 1994;29:19-22.

Hand Management for Patients with Epidermolysis Bullosa

AMY L. LADD, MD ✦ JOHN M. EGGLESTON III, MD

Mechanobullous diseases impart epithelial fragility, causing cutaneous breakdown after minimal trauma to the skin. When the skin of the hands is involved, it becomes susceptible to blistering and subsequent scarring. Even with proper care, severe manual crippling with profound physical and emotional impact can ensue. Epidermolysis bullosa (EB) describes a cluster of genetically determined mechanobullous disorders with varied modes of inheritance, mechanisms of action, pathologic processes, and management needs.

Although more than 25 subtypes have been described,[1] EB can best be classified into the following three groups according to microscopic level of pathologic change:

1. EB simplex: a defective formation of basal keratin that causes intraepidermal blistering.[2,3] It is transferred in an autosomal dominant and rarely autosomal recessive pattern. The hands generally heal without significant scarring.[4]
2. Junctional EB: abnormal production of hemidesmosomes (a structure for cellular adhesion) and their associated subbasal dense plate.[5-7] It causes blistering at the lamina lucida of the dermal-epidermal junction and heals with skin attenuation but rarely scarring.[4]
3. Dystrophic EB: linked to multiple different mutations on chromosome 3p21 of the COL7A1 gene that codes for type VII collagen.[8] Type VII collagen composes the building blocks of anchoring fibril proteins of the epidermal basement membrane. Deficiency or abnormality of fibrils causes blistering of the skin below the lamina densa, and severe scarring can result on healing. Autosomal recessive forms of this disorder are quantitatively more severe than are dominant forms and typically yield more clinically morbid blistering.[9,10]

The severe blistering seen in patients with recessive dystrophic epidermolysis bullosa (RDEB) affects the epithelium of multiple organ systems. Hair, skin, and nails are among the most visible. Dental caries are prevalent and may reflect dental enamel defects.[11] Ocular changes include symblepharon (restriction of the opening between eyelids) and corneal opacification. Oral and perioral blistering can lead to ankyloglossia and microstomia; esophageal manifestations can lead to severe circumferential stricture of the lumen. Perianal blistering and fissuring are common and can lead to stenosis and, secondarily, to fecal retention. Seventy-seven percent of children (86% of adults) with RDEB suffer from malnutrition.[12] Serum vitamin and mineral counts are generally low, and an anemia of chronic disease is typically refractory to iron supplementation. Immune function is reduced because of decreased natural killer cell activity[13] and impaired immunoglobulin secretion.[14] As a result, patients demonstrate developmental delay and short stature.[15]

Blistered skin of the hand heals with sheets of scar. Subsequent cicatricial contraction leads insidiously to

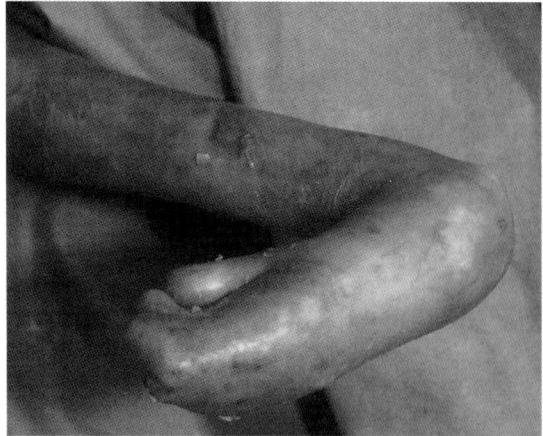

FIGURE 211-1. A preoperative view of the hand of a patient with RDEB. Notice wrist flexion, adduction of thumb, loss of web spaces, and mitten-like deformity called pseudosyndactyly.

marked obliteration of the first web space with progressive adduction of the thumb into the palm. The remaining digits, the palm, and the wrist are similarly drawn into severe flexion. As the blistered extremity heals, a "mitten" of normal and necrotic keratinocytes beneath a thickened stratum corneum covers the hand. The deep surface of this mitten forms at the usual level of blistering: just deep to the lamina densa of the basement membrane. Few dermal structures and no anchoring fibrils are seen on microscopic section.[16] As the web spaces of these hypoplastic hands are lost, distinction between the digits is lessened, a process called pseudosyndactylization. Although the deformity results uniquely from soft tissue contracture, secondary articular fibrosis and both tendon shortening and adhesion ensue (Fig. 211-1).

DIAGNOSIS

Most patients with RDEB requiring surgery of the hand will have been diagnosed before referral to the surgeon. Prenatal testing and diagnosis have been available for more than 2 decades for select scenarios.[17-20] Owing to the recessive nature of RDEB, however, parents' carrier status is often unknown, and such testing is rarely performed. The undiagnosed patient in whom EB is suspected should be referred to a dermatologist for work-up, specific diagnosis, and early presurgical management. A preliminary diagnosis of EB is made largely on the basis of clinical history and examination and sometimes family history. Because many other skin diseases may obscure the diagnosis, particularly in the neonate, microscopic and laboratory studies are warranted. Electron microscopic evaluation of a skin biopsy specimen is the standard for evaluating the level

of blistering and other diagnostic ultrastructural characteristics.[21,22] Skin biopsy specimens for this study must be harvested according to a special protocol to avoid tissue disruption in the sample. Specimens should also be harvested for specific antibody probes[23] and possible antigen mapping with indirect immunohistochemical staining.[24] Obtaining a specific diagnosis is critical to provide genetic and family counseling, to direct therapy, and to allow prediction of disease course and prognosis.

PROGNOSIS

Patients with most forms of inherited EB, with the exception of recessive dystrophic, have normal life spans. Certain phenotypically more severe forms (herpetiformis subtype of EB simplex, Herlitz subtype of junctional EB, and Hallopeau-Siemens subtype of RDEB) are more often associated with death in infancy or childhood. With improved medical and surgical management, patients with most variants of dystrophic EB are living longer than ever before, many reaching middle age or beyond. Improved longevity has evoked ongoing research into reproductive medicine,[25] associated oncology,[26,27] and general care for older patients.

GENERAL TREATMENT

Whereas corrective surgical and nonsurgical treatment modalities represent a promising area of research, the mainstays of management are prevention of cutaneous trauma and meticulous health and hygiene practices. Preventive and therapeutic treatment of this multisystemic disease is best managed by a team approach. Referral to regional EB centers initiates coordinated management by a dermatologist, dentist, gastroenterologist, nutritionist, occupational and physical therapists, pediatrician or internist, and surgeon.[28] The dermatologist, with whom maintenance visits are recommended every 6 months, generally orchestrates treatment.

Prevention of cutaneous trauma entails avoidance of excessive heat and blunt or shearing trauma. Protective pads at bone prominences, articulations, and vulnerable skin are necessary during activities. Meticulous care of blistered skin with antibiotic ointments, nonadherent dressings, and tape-free bandaging with circumferential wraps or elastic tubular nets should be supervised by a dermatologist. Some authors[29] advocate drainage of intact blisters by a sterile needle to prevent the extension of tissue separation.

In addition to general skin care, the dermatologist treats episodic infection of the skin (usually *Staphylococcus aureus*) with topical agents, dressings, and occasional incision and drainage. Chronic wounds require diligent monitoring for the development of squamous cell carcinoma. These lesions appear most frequently in the third and fourth decades[30] and pose a significant threat of metastasis and death (up to one in three).[31,32] Most appear over bone prominences at the limbs,[33] and thus the dermatologist or hand surgeon should perform biopsy of suspicious lesions seen on examination. Excision with skin graft is standard, although free tissue transfer with donor site coverage by use of tissue expansion has been documented.[34]

Virtually all patients with RDEB suffer from gastrointestinal manifestations of their disease.[35,36] Ankyloglossia, microstomia, reflux of gastric content, and esophageal or anal strictures may require reconstructive surgery or balloon dilatation by a gastroenterologist. Blistering gums, caries, and dental enamel defects[37] add to mechanical challenges to proper nutrition intake. Thus, both meticulous dental care and close outpatient management by a nutritionist are important.

Not only is total calorie *intake* generally reduced in severe EB patients, nutritive *uptake* is often poor across affected mucosal tissue of the gut. Both external and internal weeping wounds create sumps on protein stores. Accordingly, patients with dystrophic EB typically possess slight stature and fall as low as the third percentile for height and weight.[38] Patients require supplementation including iron, zinc, and total protein[39] among other elements. Many benefit from placement of a percutaneous gastrostomy feeding tube.[40] Despite repletion of iron stores, chronic blood loss from weeping wounds is common, and an anemia of chronic disease persists. Although patients can tolerate a hemoglobin level as low as 8 g/dL without symptoms, concentrations may fall well below this. Preoperative evaluation of protein and blood counts is important. Nutritional supplementation and agents such as erythropoietin have been advocated in the hematologic literature.[41]

Seventy-five percent of patients with RDEB suffer ophthalmologic sequelae. Blistering of the periocular skin and conjunctiva[42] as well as corneal abrasions[43] lead to scarring. Resultant cicatrices can lead to lid ectropion, symblepharon, and restriction of the lacrimal ducts, thus desiccating the eye surface. Vigilant monitoring and prompt management of ocular or eyelid disease require ophthalmologic and plastic surgical specialists.

Severe EB is psychologically challenging for both the patient and the primary caretakers or family. Whereas psychologists are inconstant components of an EB team, their contribution to the welfare of a patient with EB and compliance with the care plans may be significant. Support groups are helpful for many patients and families.

HAND-SPECIFIC TREATMENT

Numerous proposals have been published for surgical management of the hand in patients with EB.[44-51]

Approaches to treatment vary, but surgeons generally concur that the ongoing deformation cannot be arrested but is temporarily reversed and significantly slowed by surgical release of the contracted digits and extensive preoperative and postoperative splinting and therapy.

Nonoperative Management

In dystrophic EB, progressive hand deformity is virtually the rule. Although scar formation after cutaneous trauma appears to be the primary cause, a multifactorial pathophysiologic mechanism is suggested in one study[52] by the involvement of both hands with inconsistent regard to hand dominance or history of blistering trauma. Crippling flexion and adduction have been found to commence at the ulnar aspect of the hand and to progress radially. Subtle frictional damage from simple digital posturing has been proposed in explanation. Minimizing gross trauma and meticulous skin care must be paired with ongoing hand evaluation for treatment of the inevitable deformation.

Patients require examination by a hand therapist once a year for maintenance or more often when problems arise. Stretching exercises, protective and web-retaining gloves, and splinting are generally beneficial while patients are still in early childhood. Detailed education of a patient's caretaker promotes improved understanding and thus better compliance with treatment and lessens anxiety about future hurdles. An ongoing relationship with an occupational or hand therapist provides not only preoperative and perioperative therapy but encourages practices that facilitate independence in daily living and scholastic and professional pursuits. With the current level of management, many patients with RDEB attend university and pursue gainful employment.

Operative Management

Patients with dystrophic EB frequently require multiple surgeries on each hand during the course of a lifetime. The first surgery may be required in the first year of life or may not be indicated or possible until teenage years. The average age at initial surgery is around 6 years.[28] Indications for operation include rapid progression of hand contractures and loss of hand function. Treatment of deformities when they are still mild to moderate is preferred, although patients usually present only after severe contractures have developed. Finally, patients and their families must be willing and able to perform the demanding postoperative regimen before consideration is given to scheduling. Intensive counseling from the surgeon and therapist is essential to clarify a patient's predictable postoperative needs. Patients generally undergo surgery on one hand at a time to maintain maximum independent function, although simultaneous surgery on both hands may be appropriate for the infant or very debilitated patient.

Anesthesia

Anesthesia is induced according to the preferred method of the pediatric anesthesiologist. Intravenous sedation is generally preferred over endotracheal intubation to minimize oropharyngeal trauma.[53] Mask general anesthesia may also be used with special attention to skin protection and lubrication beneath the mask. Adjunctive regional nerve block anesthesia is also well tolerated and provides intraoperative and postoperative pain relief.[50,51,54] When airway control or length of operation is in question, intubation has been documented and advocated by multiple authors for up to 12 hours.[55-57]

The demands of managing patients with EB require specific education of the nursing teams. All pressure points must be well padded; adhesives are avoided. Electrocardiographic leads can be applied with conductive gel and a light nonadhesive overlay and tubular elastic fishnet. A bipolar cautery obviates the need for a grounding pad. A blood pressure cuff may be applied over cotton padding, but the authors do not routinely use a tourniquet because the bleeding is minimal. After anesthesia has been induced, an intravenous catheter is placed and wrapped with Coban. Instead of scrubbing, the extremity is washed by pouring dilute chlorhexidine soap over the surgical sites.

Surgery

Perioperative antibiotic therapy consists of only three weight-appropriate doses of intravenous cefazolin, a deviation from the long-term courses documented in older sources.[58,59] Despite its traditional use,[60,61] the tourniquet is unnecessary and is a source of potential trauma. Blood loss is both easily controlled and minimal. Hemostatic collagen (Avitene) or thrombin-soaked cellulose may be applied to wounds to promote clotting. After mitten degloving, serous oozing slicks the surface of the hand, posing a larger technical problem than does bleeding and causing fluid losses that warrant monitoring.

After provision of a wrist block with 0.25% bupivacaine, the hand and fingers are "de-cocooned" of their epidermal mitten. The keratinocytic mitten is scored along the volar surface at the level of the wrist, where contracture release is often necessary. Dorsally, the mitten is separated only as far proximally as the perceived level of blistering, a deviation from earlier techniques in which circumferential incision was made at the wrist.[61] Care must be taken to score only the keratinocytic mitten, which is quite thin, and not the

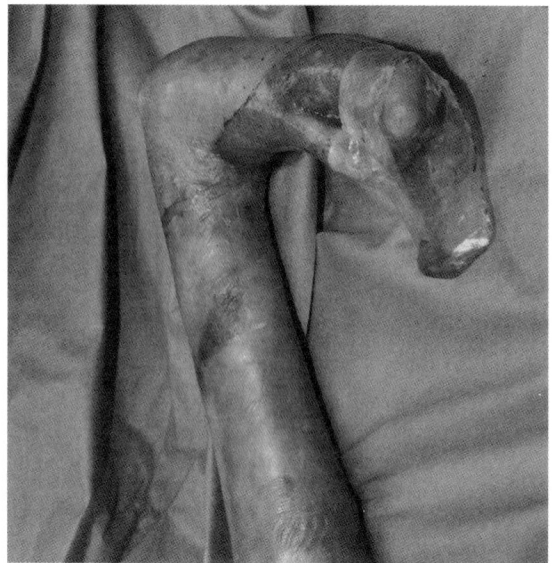

FIGURE 211-2. Removal of keratinocytic mitten. Composed primarily of necrotic keratinocytes and devoid of intact basement membrane, it is inadequate for use as skin graft.

underlying dermis. The line of dissection is extended with careful progression by use of fine scissors. The mitten is gently removed with a Freer elevator or forceps with manual traction (Fig. 211-2). Degloving alone has been demonstrated to be ineffective treatment,[62] and the lack of an intact basement membrane and prevalence of necrotic keratinocytes in the mitten render it useless as autograft stock.[63]

The adducted thumb and first web space are released with gentle but firm manipulation aided by a small scissors or scalpel. Because a true syndactyly involving the adductor fascia is often present, fascial division may be necessary to liberate the thumb. Release of the adductor or first dorsal interosseous muscles has been reported[61,62] but is not routinely necessary. Mild traction in abduction will indicate areas in need of sharp release. The rigid, maneuverable 6700 Beaver blade is well suited for this function. Care to avoid damage to the neurovascular bundles must be practiced because the dermal defects leave them vulnerable. The remaining fingers are similarly separated along their obliterated web spaces and are extended with moderate force, aided by dermal scoring along lines of tension. The distal interphalangeal joint may not be amenable to complete extension, and a certain extensor lag may be accepted.

Because of the unpredictable thickness of the stratum corneum of potential skin graft donor sites and the inherently greater potential for secondary contraction of split-thickness compared with full-thickness graft, full-thickness skin grafts are used for

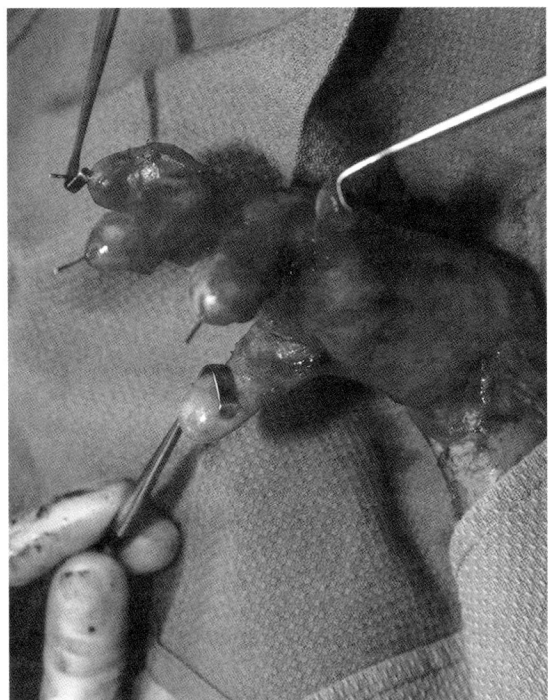

FIGURE 211-3. Lateral view after interphalangeal joint pinning and tissue release. Observe re-creation of web spaces. Pins to the proximal phalanx facilitate digital extension for 2 weeks.

coat of mupirocin antibiotic ointment (Bactroban) is applied to all wounds, which are then wrapped in petrolatum gauze. Bulky mineral oil-soaked cotton inserts are secured in the web spaces before casting. A well-padded long-arm cast is used for small children, whereas a short-arm cast is preferred for older children and adults. The cast completely envelops the hand. The wrist is secured in neutral or slightly extended position, the fingers are extended, and the thumb is maximally abducted. The axillary portion of the cast may be lined externally with sheepskin to protect the trunk from abrasive trauma. This system obviates the traction bow described by Greider and Flatt,[61] the external frame described by Zarem et al,[64] and the prolonged hospital stays and dressing changes required by those techniques (Fig. 211-5).

POSTOPERATIVE CARE

Hand surgery for the patient with EB is largely an outpatient procedure, but occasionally a patient may require overnight admission for pain control. At 10 to 14 days, the cast and pins are removed under intravenous and mask anesthesia. To facilitate removal, dressings may require soaking with normal saline or, when significant dried blood is present, with dilute hydrogen peroxide. One dose of antibiotics (cefazolin) is given preoperatively. Minimal débridement is generally needed, and new blisters, should they be present,

coverage of dermal defects. Split-thickness grafts have been advocated by some authors to conserve donor sites[58,60-62]; others[47] argue that adequate quantities of unblistered full-thickness skin are available for harvest, most often from the abdomen or inguinal fold. The epidermal layer may slough from the harvested tissue, but excellent dermal graft "take" is typical. Graft width greater than 2 cm is rarely needed. Given the inelastic nature of affected skin, flexion of the hip may be beneficial to decrease tension at the donor site during closure. The donor defect is best closed with *absorbable* interrupted deep dermal and epidermal sutures. Permanent sutures should be avoided because wounds heal quickly, often incorporating and burying sutures within their scar. The donor incision is dressed with a nonadhesive bandage, gauze, and a tubular fishnet rather than adhesive tape.

K-wires are then passed from the fingertips across the interphalangeal joints to preserve digital extension (Figs. 211-3 and 211-4). The abducted thumb is maintained in position by large bolster padding and generally does not require pinning.[47] Skin graft is sutured in place with 6-0 ophthalmic chromic gut. This filament is preferred because of its spatula-tip needle and the ease with which the coated suture glides through skin rendered "sticky" by serous ooze. A liberal

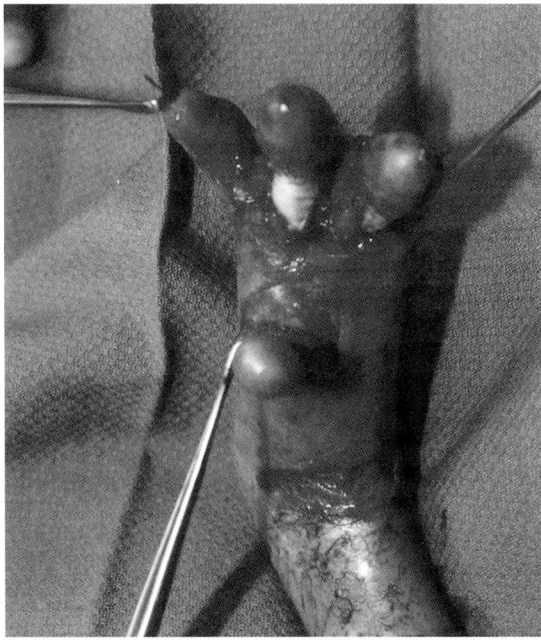

FIGURE 211-4. Volar view. Small full-thickness skin grafts are anchored with 6-0 ophthalmic chromic gut suture.

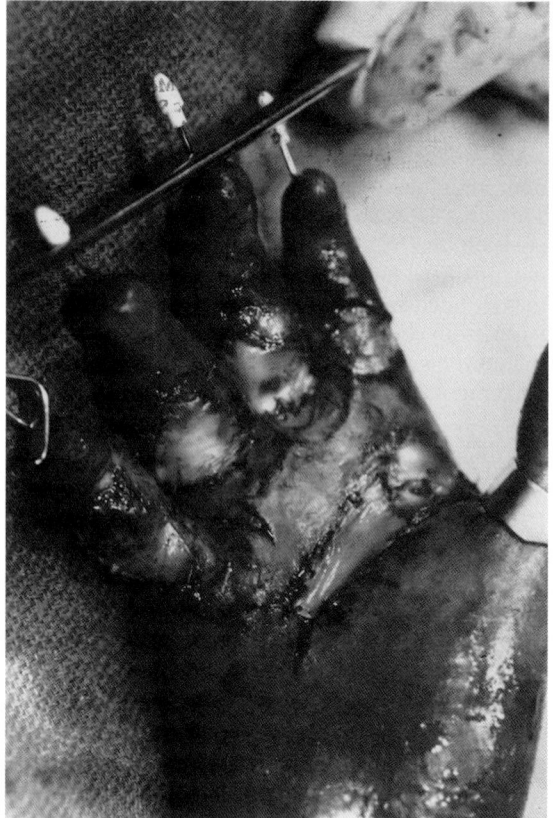

FIGURE 211-5. A postoperative view of a hand requiring five grafts for complete release and coverage.

are treated. Wounds and grafts are dressed in antibiotic ointment, and a hand therapy specialist fits the patient for a temporary thermoplastic splint and measures for a well-padded thermoplastic splint with web-retaining partitions augmented with silicone putty, which will be used after several weeks (Fig. 211-6). Patients rarely require overnight admission postoperatively, although patient and family assistance facilities (like the Ronald McDonald House) are often ideal. Patients may require 1 to 5 days' stay in proximity to the medical center for extensive splinting and ranging of the extremity. A longer stay is necessary when the family and local therapist are new to the procedure. Sedation is often needed for the first several days of this regimen.

After discharge, the patient wears a splint at all times, except during dressing changes and ranging exercises, until all wounds and grafts have healed, typically 4 to 6 weeks postoperatively. Thereafter, the splint is worn by night, and a custom-made, web-retaining elastic compression glove* is used by day (Fig. 211-7). Some

---

*For example, Barton-Carey Medical Products, Perrysburg, Ohio.

patients prefer wrapping with dressings to wearing gloves. A local hand therapist performs frequent monitoring of extremity progress, compliance of the patient, and glove and splint maintenance.

Whereas this procedure never improves manual dexterity and range of motion to the level of unaffected hands, it readily delivers functional hands from cocooned "clubs." Residual flexion deformities of 15 to 30 degrees at the interphalangeal joints and a total range of as little as 45 degrees at the metacarpophalangeal joints often constitute acceptable results. Because the disease process is ongoing, recurrence of pseudosyndactylization is the rule. Repeated surgeries are necessary from months to years (on average 2 years) after release.[28,51,59,60] Prolongation of the interval between procedures relies on the patient's compliance, the interaction of and intervention by the therapist, and the patient's nutritional status. The patient's phenotypic expression also plays a major role in the rate of recurrence. In our experience, compliance was found to be worst in young patients with uninformed care providers and in adolescents and young adults with poor motivation.

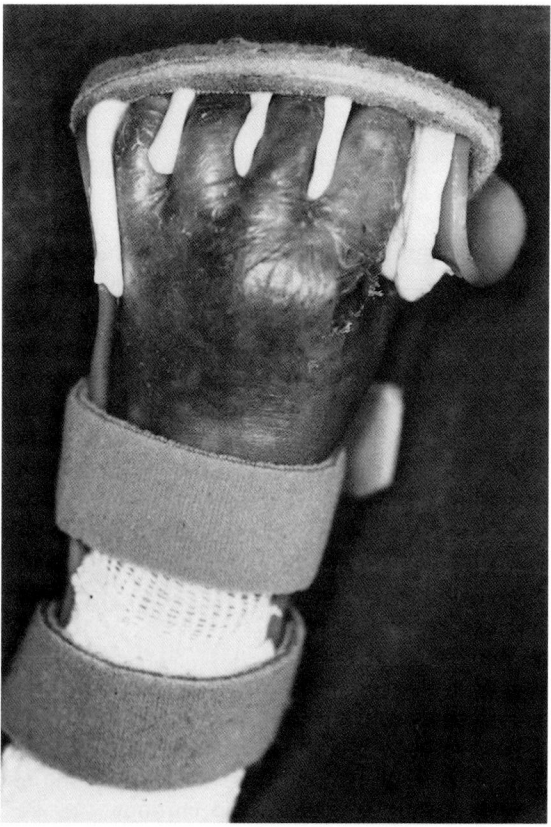

FIGURE 211-6. Splint in wrist extension, metacarpophalangeal flexion, and interphalangeal extension. Web space retainers are augmented with silicone putty.

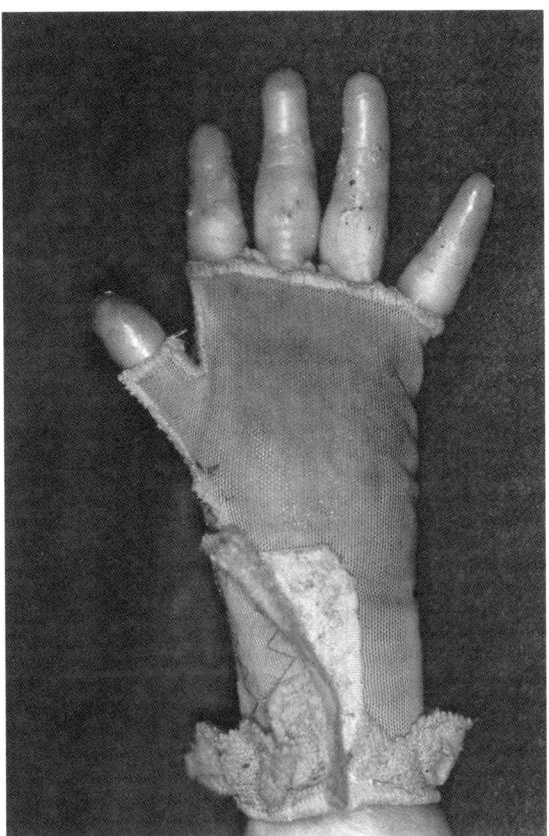

FIGURE 211-7. Success in maintaining web spaces and functional hand posture largely depends on compliance with maintenance splinting and custom-made elastic compression gloves or other web-retaining dressings.

FUTURE TREATMENT MODALITIES

Although the efforts described in this chapter compose the current management for patients with RDEB with manual pathologic changes, they address only the physical manifestations of EB and do nothing to reverse the underlying process of faulty collagen production. Genetic engineering for the molecular treatment of EB is currently an active area of research and may provide a systemic cure for EB in the future. A spontaneously occurring phase-shifting mutation has been studied[65] that reduces the phenotypic severity of RDEB, but in vivo therapeutic interventions have not yet induced such amelioration. Phenotypic reversion has been genetically achieved in some patients with junctional, but not yet dystrophic, EB. This has been implemented by use of retroviral vectors for transduction of cultured skin cells with curative cDNA and delivery of the resultant product at both the molecular and functional planes.[66] Until a cure at the cellular level is obtained for dystrophic EB, rigorous surgical, rehabilitational, and medical interventions remain the best hope for providing an active and long life to patients with dystrophic EB.

REFERENCES

1. Fine J-D, Bauer EA, Briggaman RA, et al: Revised clinical and laboratory criteria for subtypes of inherited epidermolysis bullosa. J Am Acad Dermatol 1991;24:119-135.
2. Leigh IM, Lane EB: Mutations in genes for epidermal keratins in epidermolysis bullosa and epidermolytic hyperkeratosis. Arch Dermatol 1993;129:1571-1577.
3. Corden LD, McLean WH: Human keratin diseases: hereditary fragility of specific epithelial tissues. Exp Dermatol 1996;5:297-307.
4. Lin AN, Carter DM: Epidermolysis bullosa simplex: a clinical overview. In Lin AN, Carter DM, eds: Epidermolysis Bullosa: Basic and Clinical Aspects. New York, Springer, 1992:89-117.
5. Eady RAJ, McGrath JA, McMillan JR: Ultrastructural clues to genetic disorders of skin: the dermal-epidermal junction. J Invest Dermatol 1994;103:13s-18s.
6. Christiano AM, Uitto J: Molecular complexity of the basement membrane zone. Exp Dermatol 1996;5:1-11.
7. Tidman MJ, Eady RAJ: Hemidesmosome heterogeneity in junctional epidermolysis bullosa revealed by morphometric analysis. J Invest Dermatol 1986;86:51-56.
8. Parente MG, Chung LC, Ryynanen J, et al: Human type VII collagen: cDNA cloning and chromosomal mapping of the gene. Proc Natl Acad Sci USA 1991;88:6931-6935.
9. Leigh IM, Eady RAJ, Heagerty AHM, et al: Type VII collagen is a normal component of epidermal basement membrane, which shows altered expression in recessive dystrophic epidermolysis bullosa. J Invest Dermatol 1988;90:639-642.
10. McGrath JA, Ishida-Yamamoto A, O'Grady A, et al: Structural variations in anchoring fibrils in dystrophic epidermolysis bullosa: correlation with type VII collagen expression. J Invest Dermatol 1993;100:366-372.
11. Wright J, Capps J, Fine JD: Dental caries variation in the different epidermolysis bullosa diseases. J Dent Res 1989;68:416.
12. Birge K: Nutrition management of patients with epidermolysis bullosa. J Am Diet Assoc 1995;95:575-579.
13. Trying SK, Chopra V, Johnson L, et al: Natural killer cell activity is reduced in patients with severe forms of epidermolysis bullosa. Arch Dermatol 1989;125:797-800.
14. Sweet SP, Ballsdon AE, Harris JC, et al: Impaired secretory immunity in dystrophic epidermolysis bullosa. Oral Microbiol Immunol 1999;14:316-320.
15. Wojnarowska F, Eady RAJ, Burge SM: Bullous eruptions. In Champion RH, Burton JL, Burns DA, Breathnach SM, eds: Rook/Wilkinson/Ebling Textbook of Dermatology, 6th ed. Oxford, Blackwell Science, 1998:1817-1844.
16. McGrath JA, O'Grady A, Mayou BJ, Eady RA: Mitten deformity in severe generalized recessive dystrophic epidermolysis bullosa: histological, immunofluorescence, and ultrastructural study. J Cutan Pathol 1992;19:385-389.
17. Christiano AM, Uitto J: Molecular complexity of the basement membrane zone. Exp Dermatol 1996;5:1-11.
18. Shimizu H, Suzumori K, Nishikawa T: Heterogeneous reactivity with LH7.2 and the first prenatal diagnosis of generalized recessive dystrophic epidermolysis bullosa among Japanese patients. Dermatology 1996;192:203-207.
19. Rodeck CH, Eady RAJ, Gosden CM: Prenatal diagnosis of epidermolysis bullosa letalis. Lancet 1980;1:949-952.
20. Klingberg S, Mortimore R, Parkes J, et al: Prenatal diagnosis of dominant dystrophic epidermolysis bullosa, by COL7A1 molecular analysis. Prenat Diagn 2000;20:618-622.
21. Eady RAJ, Tidman MJ: Diagnosing epidermolysis bullosa. Br J Dermatol 1983;108:621-626.
22. Hanna W, Silverman F, Boxall L, Krafchik BR: Ultrastructural features of epidermolysis bullosa. Ultrastruct Pathol 1983;5:29-36.

23. Heagerty AH, Kennedy AR, Leigh IM, et al: Identification of an epidermal basement membrane defect in recessive forms of dystrophic epidermolysis bullosa by LH 7.2 monoclonal antibody: use in diagnosis. Br J Dermatol 1986;115:125-131.

24. Hintner H, Stingl G, Schuler G, et al: Immunofluorescence mapping of antigenic determinants within the dermal-epidermal junction in the mechanobullous diseases. J Invest Dermatol 1981;76:113-118.

25. Buscher U, Wessel J, Anton-Lamprecht I, Dudenhausen JW: Pregnancy and delivery in a patient with mutilating dystrophic epidermolysis bullosa (Hallopeau-Siemens type). Obstet Gynecol 1997;89(pt 2):817-820.

26. Hoss DM, McNutt NS, Carter DM: Atypical melanocytic lesions in epidermolysis bullosa. J Cutan Pathol 1994;21:164-169.

27. McGrath JA, Schofield OMV, Mayou BJ: Metastatic squamous cell carcinoma resembling angiosarcoma complicating dystrophic epidermolysis bullosa. Dermatologica 1991;182:235-238.

28. Eggleston J, Ladd A: Hand management for patients with recessive dystrophic epidermolysis bullosa: a multidisciplinary approach. Adrian E. Flatt Residents and Fellows Conference in Hand Surgery (American Society for Surgery of the Hand), Boston, September 1999.

29. Dunnill MGS, Eady RAJ: The management of dystrophic epidermolysis bullosa. Clin Exp Dermatol 1995;20:179-188.

30. McGrath JA, Schofield OMV, Mayou BJ: Epidermolysis bullosa complicated by squamous cell carcinoma: a report of 10 cases. J Cutan Pathol 1992;19:116-123.

31. Keefe M, Wakeel RA: Death from metastatic, cutaneous squamous cell carcinoma in autosomal recessive dystrophic epidermolysis bullosa despite permanent inpatient care. Dermatologica 1988;177:180-184.

32. Bosch RJ, Gallardo MA, Ruiz del Portal G, et al: Squamous cell carcinoma secondary to recessive dystrophic epidermolysis bullosa: report of eight tumours in four patients. J Eur Acad Dermatol Venereol 1999;13:198-204.

33. Newman C, Wagner RF, Tyring SK, Spigel T: Squamous cell carcinoma secondary to recessive dystrophic epidermolysis bullosa. J Dermatol Surg Oncol 1992;18:301-305.

34. Whitney TM, Ramasastry S, Futrell JW: Combined tissue expansion and free tissue transfer for reconstruction of the hand in epidermolysis bullosa-associated malignancy. Ann Plast Surg 1993;31:552-555.

35. Ergun GA, Lin AN, Dannenberg AJ, Carter DM: Gastrointestinal manifestations of epidermolysis bullosa. A study of 101 patients. Medicine (Baltimore) 1992;71:121-127.

36. Travis SPL, McGrath JA, Turnbull AJ, et al: Oral and gastrointestinal manifestations of epidermolysis bullosa. Lancet 1992;340:1505-1506.

37. Wright JT, Fine J-D, Johnson L: Hereditary epidermolysis bullosa: oral manifestations and dental management. Pediatr Dent 1993;15:242-247.

38. Allman S, Haynes H, MacKinnon P, et al: Nutrition in dystrophic epidermolysis bullosa. Pediatr Dermatol 1992;9:231-238.

39. Fine J-D, Tamura T, Johnson L: Blood vitamin and trace metal levels in epidermolysis bullosa. Arch Dermatol 1989;125:374-379.

40. Haynes L: Epidermolysis bullosa. In Shaw V, Lawsib M, eds: Clinical Pediatric Dietetics, Oxford, Blackwell, 1994:295-302.

41. Fridge JL, Vichinski EP: Correction of the anemia of epidermolysis bullosa with intravenous iron and erythropoietin. J Pediatr 1998;132:871-873.

42. Iwamoto M, Haik BG, Iwamoto T, et al: The ultrastructural defect in conjunctiva from a case of recessive dystrophic epidermolysis bullosa. Arch Ophthalmol 1991;109:1382-1386.

43. Gans LA: Eye lesions of epidermolysis bullosa. Arch Dermatol 1988;124:762-764.

44. Marin-Bertolin S, Valero JVA, Giménez CN, et al: Surgical management of hand contractures and pseudosyndactyly in dystrophic epidermolysis bullosa. Ann Plast Surg 1999;43:555-559.

45. Witt P, Cheng C, Mallory S, et al: Surgical treatment of pseudosyndactyly of the hand in epidermolysis bullosa: histological analysis of an acellular allograft dermal matrix. Ann Plast Surg 1999;43:379-385.

46. Mullett F: A review of management of the hand in dystrophic epidermolysis bullosa. J Hand Ther 1998;11:261-265.

47. Ladd AL, Kibele A, Gibbons S: Surgical treatment and postoperative splinting of recessive dystrophic epidermolysis bullosa. J Hand Surg Am 1996;21:888-897.

48. Eisenberg M, Llewelyn D: Surgical management of hands in children with recessive dystrophic epidermolysis bullosa: use of allogeneic composite cultured skin grafts. Br J Plast Surg 1998;51:608-613.

49. Campiglio GL, Pajardi G, Rafanelli G: A new protocol for treatment of hand deformities in recessive dystrophic epidermolysis bullosa (13 cases). Ann Chir Main Memb Super 1997;16:91-100.

50. Ikeda S, Yaguchi H, Ogawa H: Successful surgical management and long-term follow-up of epidermolysis bullosa. Int J Dermatol 1994;33:442-445.

51. Le Touze A, Viau D, Martin L, et al: Recessive dystrophic epidermolysis bullosa: management of hand deformities. Eur J Pediatr Surg 1993;3:352-355.

52. Mullett F, Wade A, Smith P: A survey of predisposing factors and the development of the hand deformity in children with dystrophic epidermolysis bullosa. Br J Hand Ther 1996;2:18-21.

53. Schaffer S: Head and neck manifestations of epidermolysis bullosa. Clin Pediatr 1992;31:81-88.

54. Boughton R, Crawford MR, Vonwiller JB: Epidermolysis bullosa: a review of 15 years' experience, including experience with combined general and regional anaesthetic techniques. Anaesth Intensive Care 1988;16:260-264.

55. Yonker-Sell AE, Connolly LA: Twelve hour anaesthesia in a patient with epidermolysis bullosa. Can J Anaesth 1995;42:735-739.

56. James I, Wark MB: Airway management during anesthesia in patients with epidermolysis bullosa dystrophica. Anesthesiology 1982;56:323-326.

57. Griffin RP, Mayou BJ: The anaesthetic management of patients with dystrophic epidermolysis bullosa: a review of 44 patients over a 10 year period. Anaesthesia 1993;48:810-815.

58. Swinyard CA, Swenson JR, Rees TD: Rehabilitation of hand deformities in epidermolysis bullosa. Arch Phys Med Rehabil 1968;49:138-144.

59. Vozdvizhensky SI, Albanova VI: Surgical treatment of contracture and syndactyly of children with epidermolysis bullosa. Br J Plast Surg 1993;46:314-316.

60. Terrill PJ, Mayou BJ, Pemberton J: Experience in the surgical management of the hand in dystrophic epidermolysis bullosa. Br J Plast Surg 1992;45:435-442.

61. Greider JL, Flatt AE: Care of the hand in recessive dystrophic epidermolysis bullosa. Plast Reconstr Surg 1983;72:222-228.

62. Horner RL, Wiedel JD, Bralliar F: Involvement of the hand in epidermolysis bullosa. J Bone Joint Surg Am 1971;53:1347-1356.

63. McGrath JA, O'Grady A, Mayou BJ, et al: Mitten deformity in severe generalized recessive dystrophic epidermolysis bullosa: histological, immunofluorescence, and ultrastructural study. J Cutan Pathol 1992;19:385-389.

64. Zarem HA, Pearson RW, Leaf N: Surgical management of hand deformities in recessive dystrophic epidermolysis bullosa. Br J Plast Surg 1974;27:176-181.

65. McGrath JA, Ashton GH, Mellerio JE, et al: Moderation of phenotypic severity in dystrophic and junctional forms of epidermolysis bullosa through in-frame skipping of exons containing non-sense or frameshift mutations. J Invest Dermatol 1999;113:314-321.

66. Spirito F, Meneguzzi G, Danos O, Mezzina M: Cutaneous gene transfer and therapy: the present and the future. J Gene Med 2001;3:21-31.

Effect of Growth on Pediatric Hand Reconstruction

ALAIN GILBERT, MD

Growth has usually been considered a positive factor in the assessment of long-term results after surgery done at a young age. Most authors have even suggested that surgical reconstruction be performed as early as possible to give more chances of improving the results.[1] This is largely true, but in several instances, growth may have a deleterious effect. If some persisting anomalies are improved, others can be aggravated. The surgeon should keep a few basic principles of growth in mind in deciding the age at treatment and the type of procedure to use.

THE POSITIVE EFFECTS OF GROWTH

Correction of Axial Deformities

In younger children, axial deviation may be corrected spontaneously if the deviation is anteroposterior (in the flexion-extension plane). Of course, the deviation will be corrected only if it is due to a malposition of the fragments but not if the growth plate is involved. Lateral deviations are rarely corrected completely, and rotation deformities will not improve.[2] The closer the deformity to the growth plate, and the younger the patient, the better the correction. It is then necessary in finger fractures to precisely reduce any rotational deformity or lateral deviation. The commonly accepted idea that finger fracture treatment in children is usually successful is true, provided these principles are respected.

In congenital deformities, there may be a spontaneous improvement after treatment of syndactylies with distal fusion or bone grafting[1]; but there are many deformities, such as distal bone fusion, that will not improve. The clinodactyly (lateral deviation) and rotation may even increase with time. This is why distal bone fusion (e.g., in acrosyndactyly) should be separated very early so the resulting lateral deviation may be minimized.

Improvement in Joint Surface Anomalies

In cases of articular fractures, slight anomalies will certainly provoke arthritis in adults. In children, provided the deformity is not too severe, the joint may reconstruct with time, and although mobility may be affected, the new joint may function well for many years.[3] However, if the deformity is too severe, there is no hope of any functional improvement. Improvement is limited; in some types of synchondrosis, there is still a joint space, but it has two flat joint surfaces. All attempts to carve these surfaces and to reconstruct a moving joint will fail. After an initial period of mobility, the joint will become stiff again in a few weeks. In radial clubhand after centralization or radialization, the head of the ulna will enlarge and progressively cover the carpus like a new radius.

Muscle and Tendon Adaptation

Growth is important for adaptation of the length of the muscles and tendons after various procedures, particularly after pollicization. The adequate rebalancing of tension between the agonist and antagonist muscles may take 6 to 12 months after the operation. The abductor digiti minimi transferred to the thumb will hypertrophy and give the shape of a real thenar eminence.

Function and Cosmesis

Other than the reconstructed thumb, which will become more cosmetic when it is more efficient, all parts of the hand that are nonfunctioning or poorly functioning will improve in appearance with time when they are used in everyday life. This is true for fingers after separation, reconstruction of tendons, and restoration of sensation.

THE NEGATIVE EFFECTS OF GROWTH

Unfortunately, negative aspects of growth are common and not always predictable. They may be due to several factors outlined in the following section.

Injury to the Growth Plate (Fig. 212-1)

One of the most well known consequences of growth plate involvement occurs after centralization of the ulna

in radial clubhand (Figs. 212-2 to 212-5). There is a natural shortening due to the malformation, but it is often severely augmented by the surgical procedure. Centralization, in particular, has been accused of destroying a large part of the blood supply of the lower ulna epiphysis. This was one of the reasons that led Buck-Gramcko to propose a radialization to put less pressure on the epiphysis.[1]

Another specific influence can be observed after traumatic amputation and replantation at the level of the growth plate of the proximal or middle phalanges of the fingers (Fig. 212-6). In this instance, an immediate success may ultimately fail because of progressive relative shortening of the finger. The uninjured fingers grow to their full potential while the injured finger lags farther behind as the child ages. Destruction of one or two growth plates in a young child may be a contraindication for replantation. More limited but still deleterious functional consequences can be seen with the partial destruction of the growth plate in epiphyseal fractures. The reduction may be perfect, but with time, a partial epiphysiodesis may occur and be responsible for severe deviation (Fig. 212-7).

Passing a Kirschner wire across the growth plate may result in a partial epiphysiodesis. In the author's experience, it is very rare. In looking retrospectively at

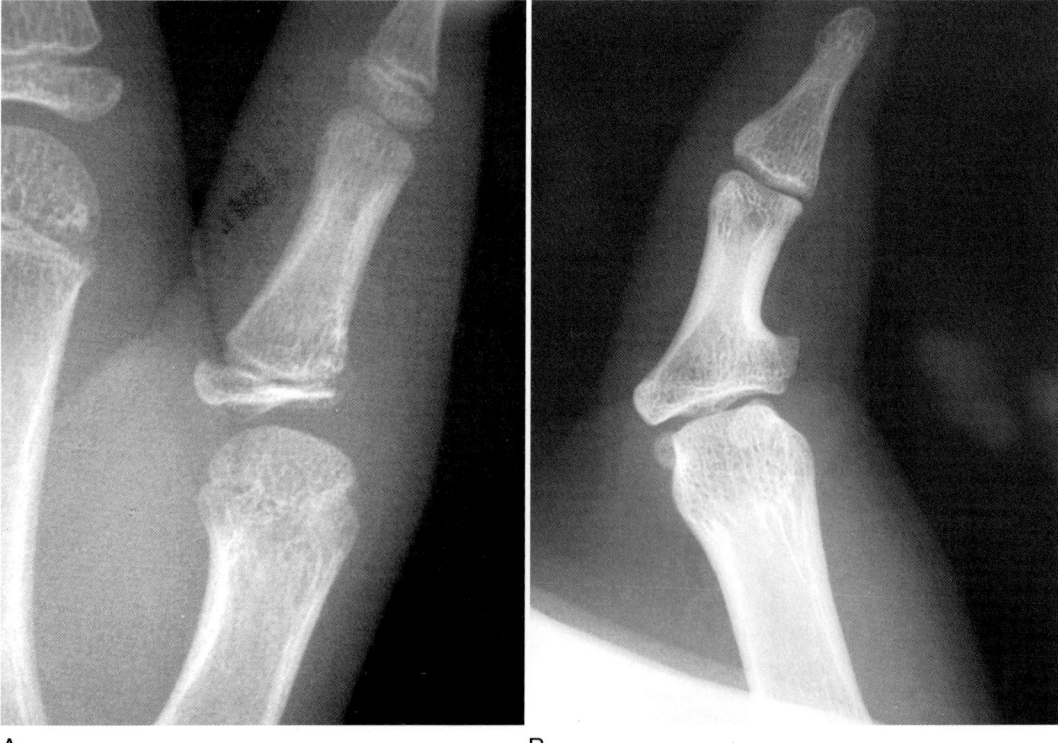

A   B

FIGURE 212-1. *A,* Trauma to the growth plate with lateral deviation. *B,* At the end of growth, deviation is not corrected.

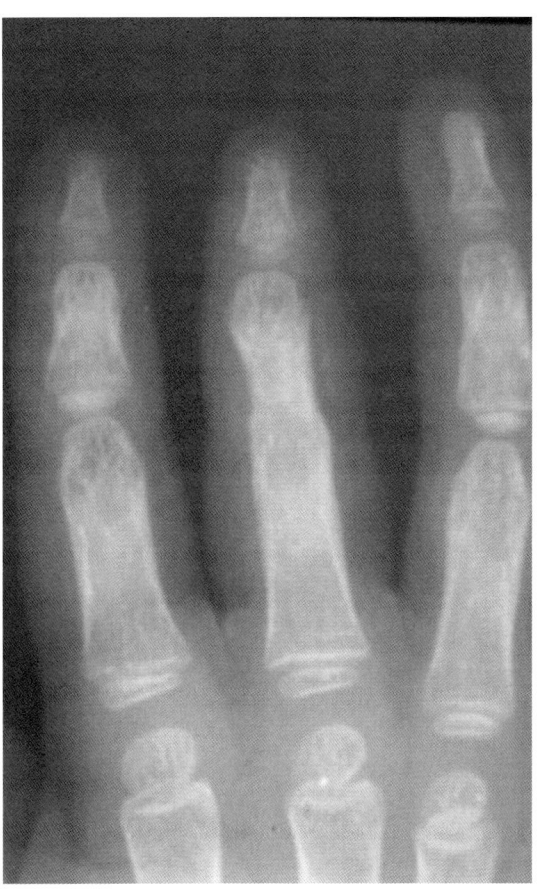

FIGURE 212-2. The radiograph shows fusion of the proximal interphalangeal joint and destruction of the growth plate.

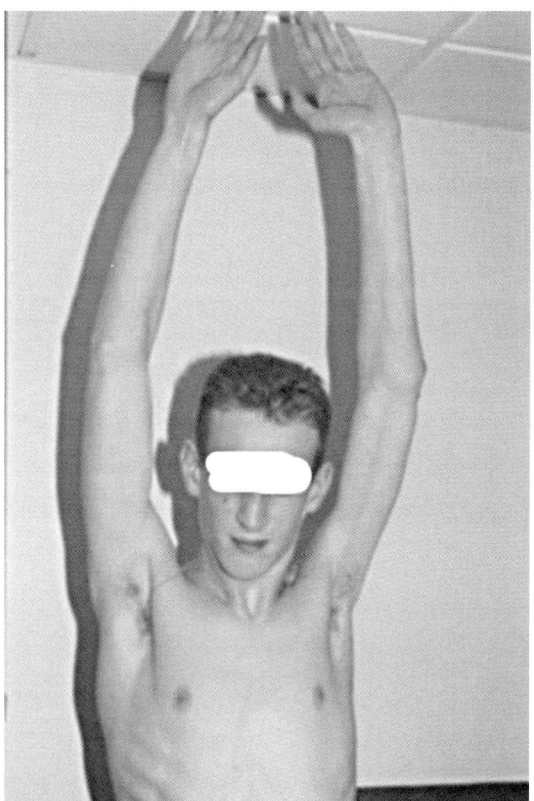

FIGURE 212-3. In this instance, there is little shortening.

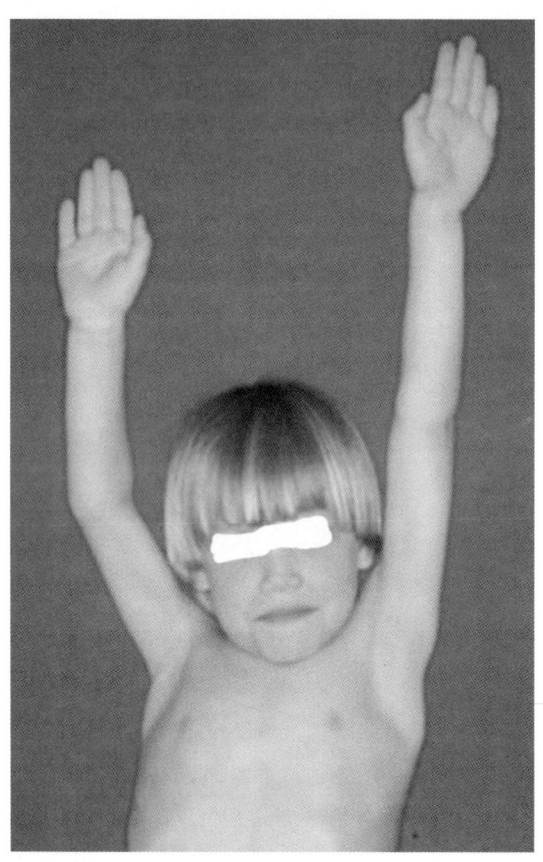

FIGURE 212-4. Despite a good recovery, the shortening is severe.

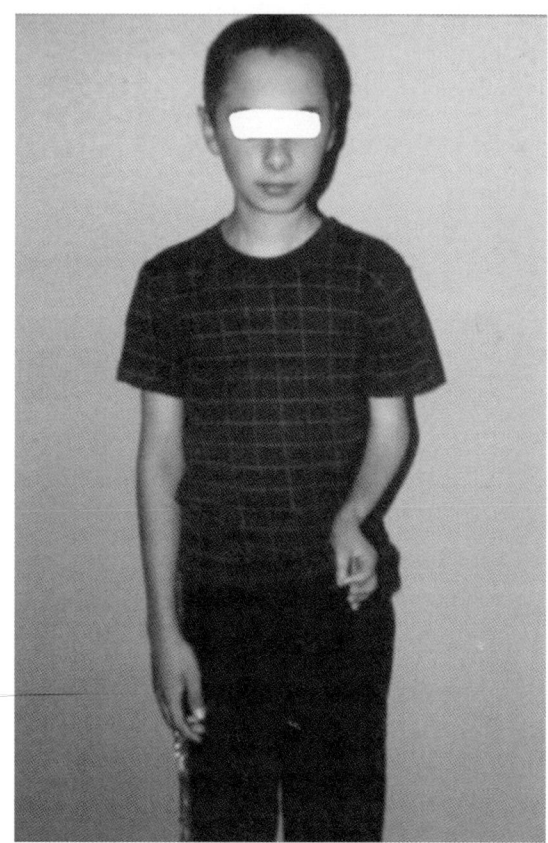

FIGURE 212-5. After complete paralysis, there is maximum shortening.

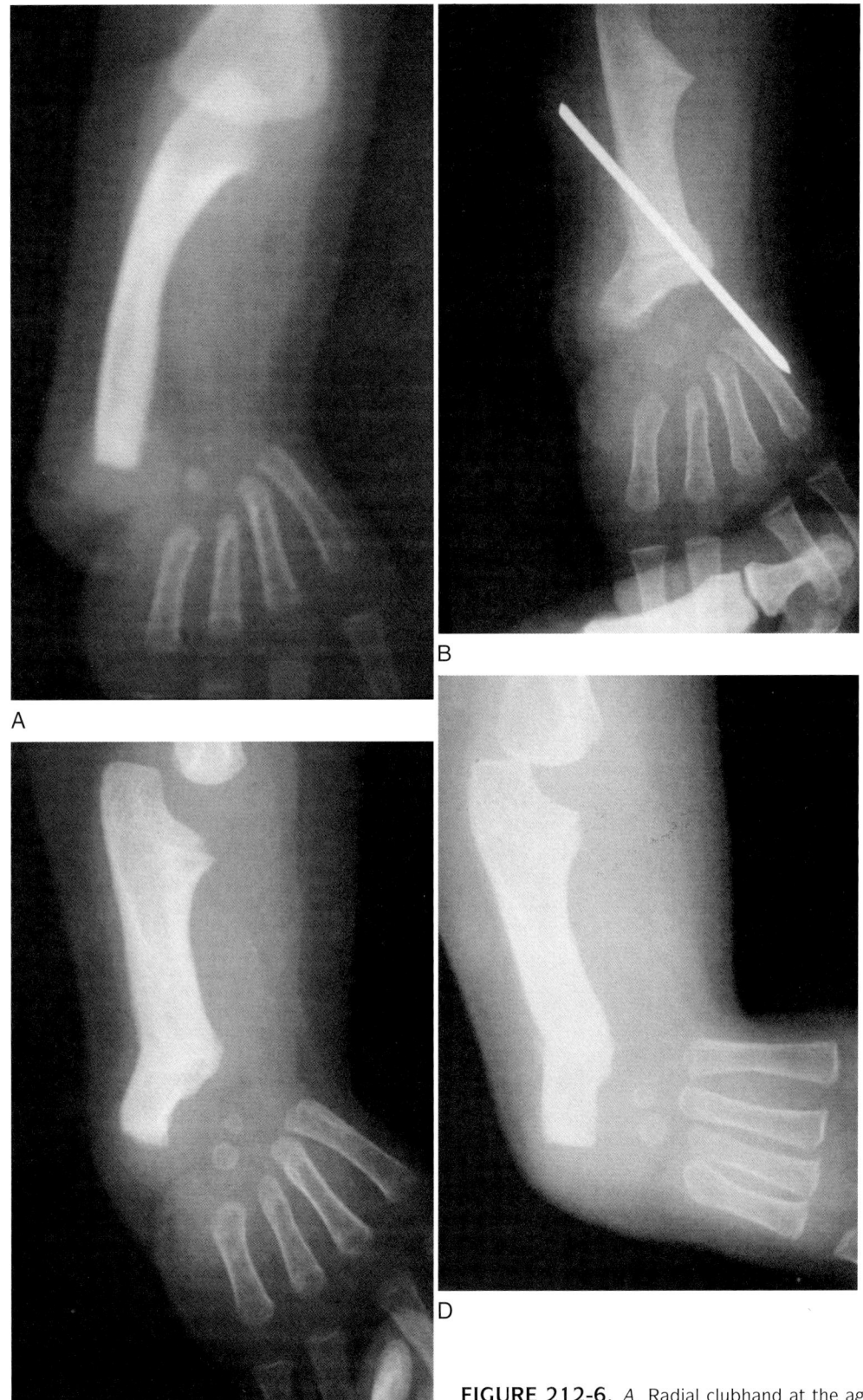

FIGURE 212-6. *A,* Radial clubhand at the age of 10 months. *B,* Rotation osteotomy of the lower epiphysis. *C,* After 8 months, recurrence has started. *D,* Two years later, recurrence is complete.

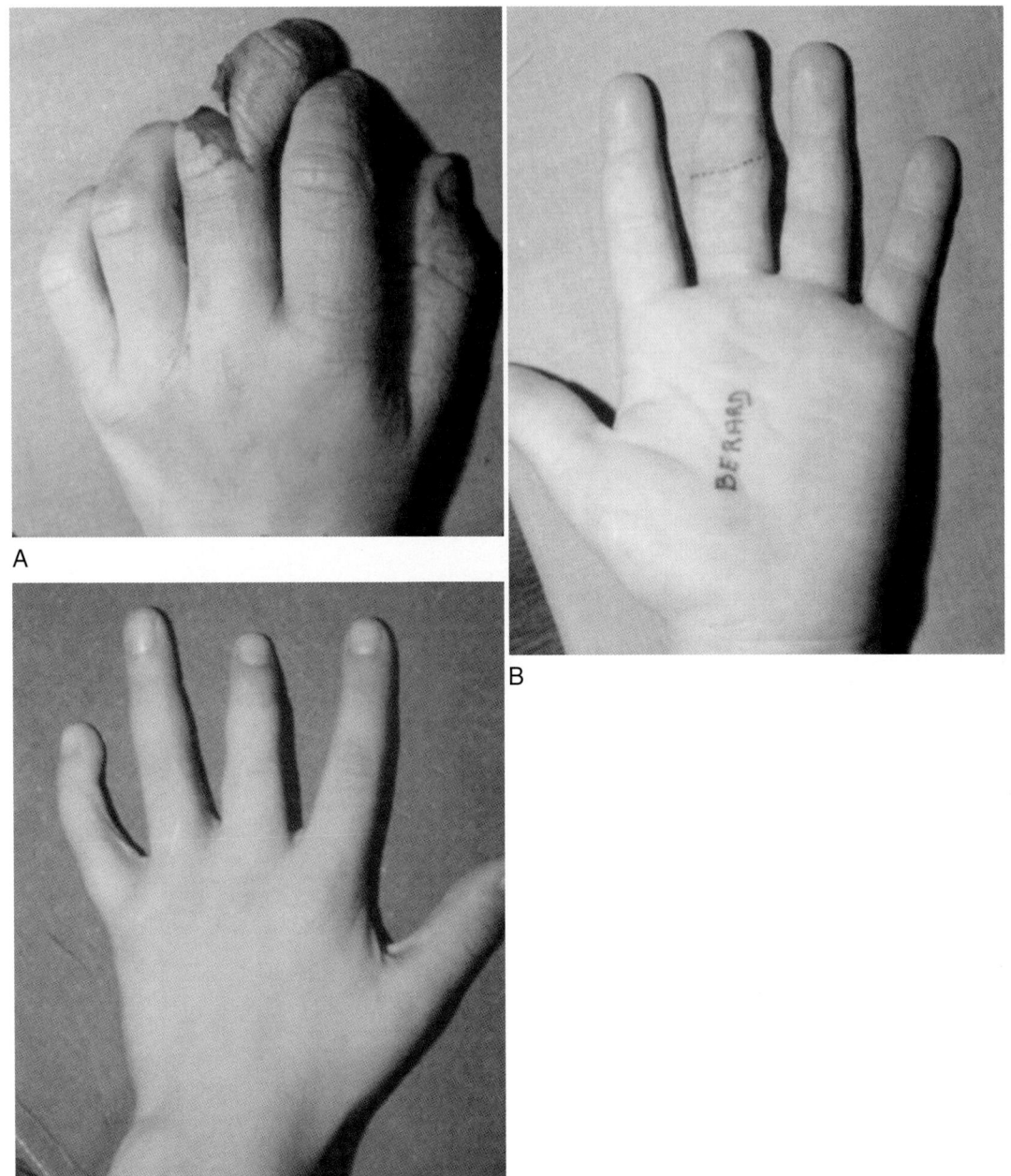

A

B

C

FIGURE 212-7. *A,* Nearly complete amputation of middle finger at the level of the proximal interphalangeal joint. *B,* After replantation. *C,* Six years after replantation, severe shortening of the finger.

a large series of toe transfers, there was no explanation for particular growth defects, and no relation was found with pinning.

In some osseous syndactylies or for the treatment of duplications, it is necessary to cut through the epiphysis. This procedure may induce lateral epiphysiodesis. This type of complication is rare when the osteotomy is done on a nonossified epiphysis.

Limitation of Growth due to Paralysis and Absence of Movements

Long-standing, extensive paralysis will impair growth and eventually result in a severe size discrepancy between the upper extremities. The best example is represented by the consequences of obstetric brachial palsy (Figs. 212-8 and 212-9). The length discrepancy starts early and is aggravated over time. It is more severe in extensive paralysis than in partial lesions. At the completion of growth, the difference in size (length discrepancy) may be up to 8 to 10 cm. An early repair of the plexus may limit the shortening of the arm but never results in completely equal limb lengths. The basis of this discrepancy is not clear. There is the influence of nerve lesion, as can be found in other proximal nerve injuries; however, the dominant factor is probably disuse. It seems that the earlier and more extensively the arm is reintegrated into the voluntary brain scheme, the less difference in length there will be with the other arm.

Absence of repair of the flexor tendons is also a cause of shortening of the finger as growth occurs. Sometimes the tendon is not repaired for several years, and there is time for the growth discrepancy to appear. After repair or grafting, the finger grows again normally but will not overcome the established shortening.

Poor Planning of Reconstruction

Many problems are due to poor planning of reconstruction. In a congenital absence of fingers, reconstruction may involve lengthening the first and

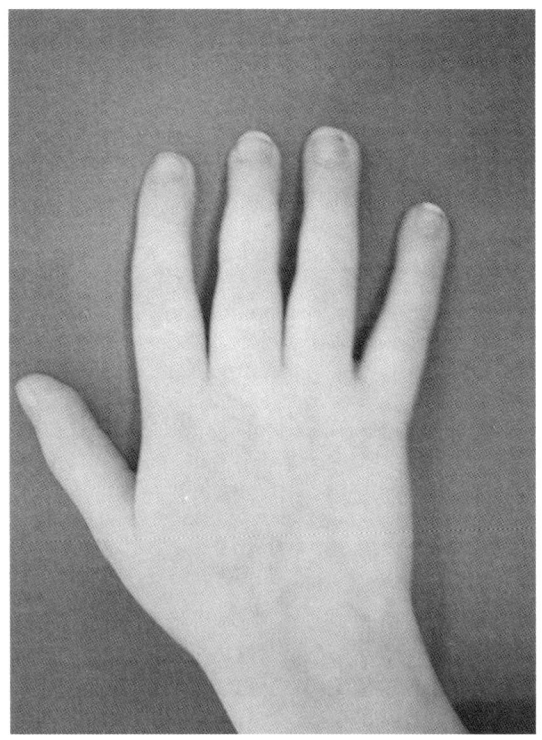

FIGURE 212-8. After several years, there is a growth defect due to an unrepaired flexor tendon to the third finger.

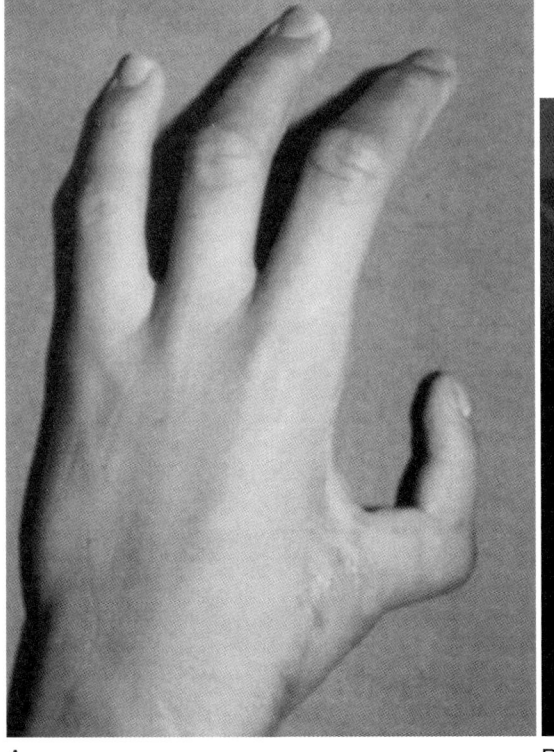

A

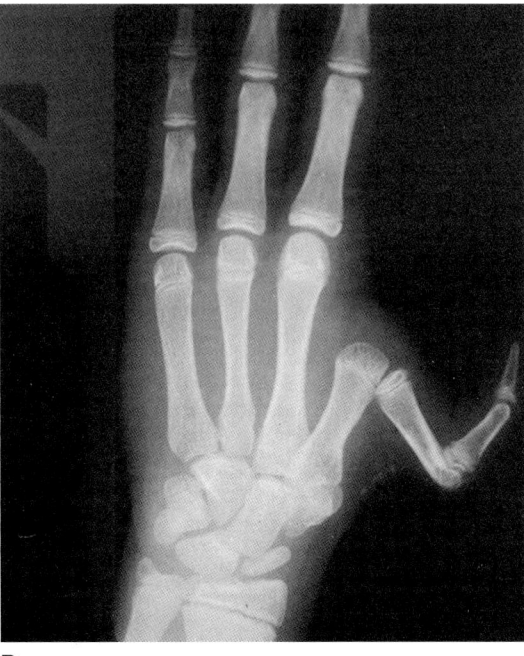

B

FIGURE 212-9. *A,* Fourteen years after successful pollicization. The initial result was excellent. *B,* The progressive deterioration is due to continued growth of the second metacarpal.

fifth ray by toe transfers. The toe will grow, but sometimes only one of the metacarpals will grow normally; with time, the two reconstructed fingers will be of such different sizes that there will soon be no more possibility for prehension (pinch) between the two reconstructed digits. This transformation of an early satisfactory procedure into a poor long-term result is one of the most frustrating events in reconstructive pediatric hand surgery (see Fig. 212-7B and C).

Lateral deviation may be due to external factors, such as that seen in syndactyly of fingers of different sizes or after scars and contractures. Early release will probably allow development without deformity. If the pathologic factor is not suppressed, the scar not treated, or the syndactyly not released, the apparent bone deviation will become permanent. In patients in whom the growth is impaired by soft tissue contractures, the treatment must be early. If the situation is not corrected, growth may cause severe deviations.

MANAGING GROWTH ANOMALIES

Prevention

In many cases, growth anomalies can be prevented by early treatment (syndactyly), but in other cases, it will be preferable to wait a few years. The delta phalanx can be treated in the first months or years of life, but the high incidence of recurrences has led many authors to wait at least 3 or 4 years before any attempt is made to correct the deviation.

In growth disturbance due to paralysis, an early repair of the nerve may avoid a great part of the length disturbance. However, even an early repair with excellent results will eventually have some length discrepancy. In obstetric paralysis, the extent of the paralysis is also an important factor. The prevention of shortening is one of the arguments for an early decision and operation of the plexus.

Treatment

Lengthening is the most common way to treat lack of growth. In the hand, this procedure is difficult to perform in a very young child because the result is always a percentage of the original size (up to 150% or 200%). If the bone is very small, the gain will be limited and quickly lost by growth of the other structures. There are few indications for lengthening in young infants, mostly when the growth disturbance prevents pinch and function. In these instances, the family should be aware that further lengthening might be needed in the future.

In older children, lengthening is done as a final corrective procedure (e.g., brachymetacarpal, radial

clubhand) by use of a progressive technique and external fixation. In the hand, bone grafting is usually not necessary between the distracted bone ends because spontaneous callus will heal the defect in 1 or 2 months. In the forearm, spontaneous healing, although possible, is not the best choice because it is a long process (4 to 6 months) and results in poor quality of bone. For forearm reconstruction in the adolescent, it is preferable to use a vascularized fibular graft that will heal in 6 to 8 weeks.

In the treatment of partial closure of the growth plate, the techniques of desepiphysiodesis can be used (Fig. 212-10). This procedure is mostly recommended after traumatic disturbance. Although rare, post-traumatic epiphysiodesis can provoke serious deviations. The procedure has also been used for the treatment of congenital delta phalanx or Madelung deformity.[4] This procedure can produce interesting results, but it is quite unpredictable. When the procedure fails, it is sometimes better to complete the epiphysiodesis of the growth plate and later complete a lengthening operation.

In complete premature closure of the growth plate, the length discrepancy may become a severe problem, and the only solution in the young child is growth plate transplantation. These transplantations have also been used in congenital disorders such as radial clubhand and thumb aplasia. The most common donor site is the upper fibular epiphysis, with its nutrient vessels,[5] but the iliac crest can also be used. The results of these transplantations seem better in the lower than in the upper limb.[5-7]

On the contrary, hypergrowth is also a possibility, and its treatment is not always satisfactory. The main treatment of hypergrowth is therapeutic epiphysiodesis. It is a difficult operation because destruction of the growth plate without disturbing the stability of the phalanx is not easy to perform. It is mainly done for macrodactyly, but the procedure is not always predictable. It is sometimes necessary to perform a secondary procedure (Fig. 212-11).

CONCLUSIONS

The influence of growth in pediatric hand surgery is crucial and should always be taken into account in deciding which procedure will be optimal for a child. Growth can sometimes be a positive factor; however, in many cases, it is the cause of late failure of surgical repairs. Good knowledge of the growth potential of the finger or hand, atraumatic technique, and adequate follow-up are necessary. It is sometimes better to postpone an operation when the risks of growth interference are too high. In other patients, an early operation may re-establish a normal growth pattern.

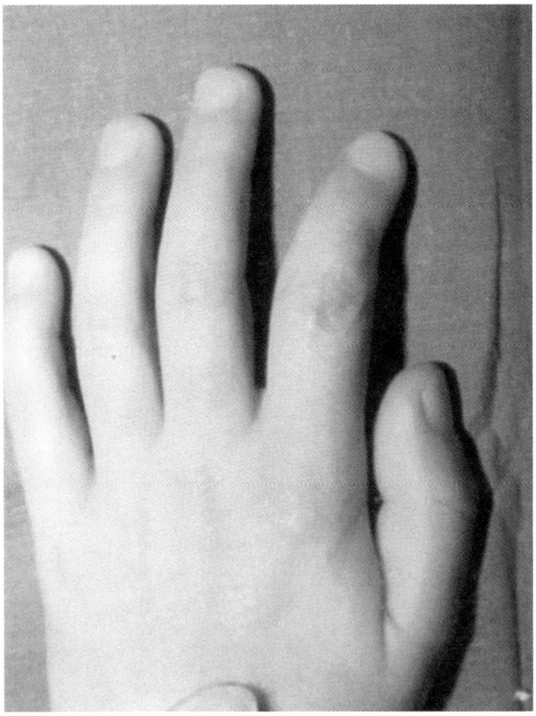

A

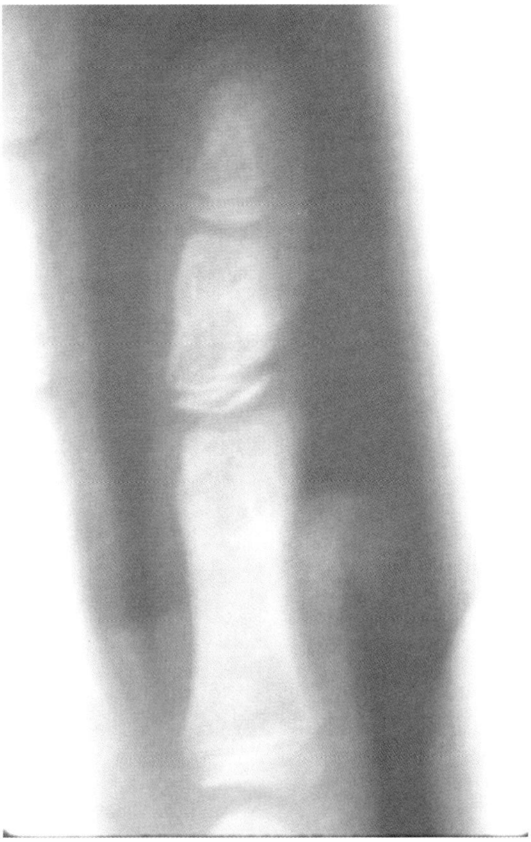

B

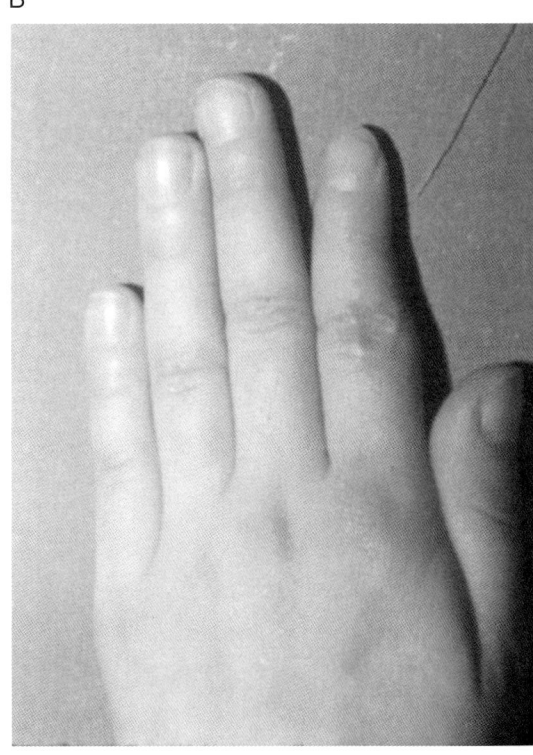

FIGURE 212-10. *A*, Deviation after electrical burn. There is a lateral epiphysiodesis. *B*, Desepiphysiodesis is done with fat inclusion. *C*, Progressive reduction of the deformity.

C

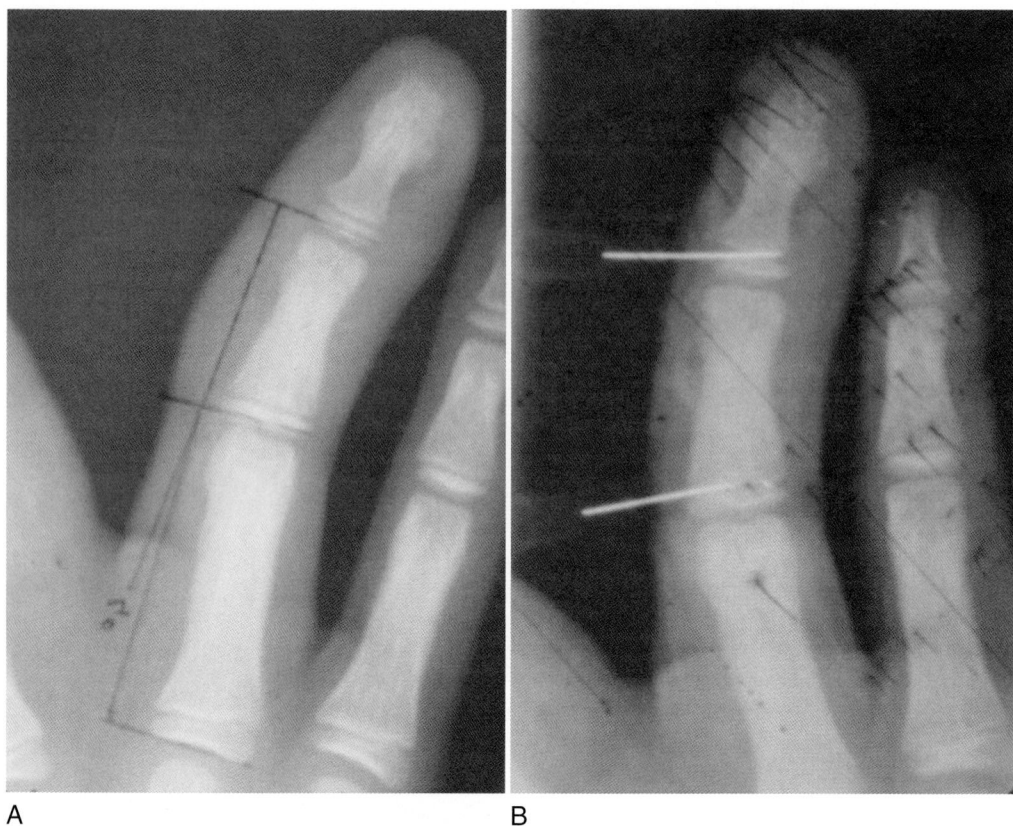

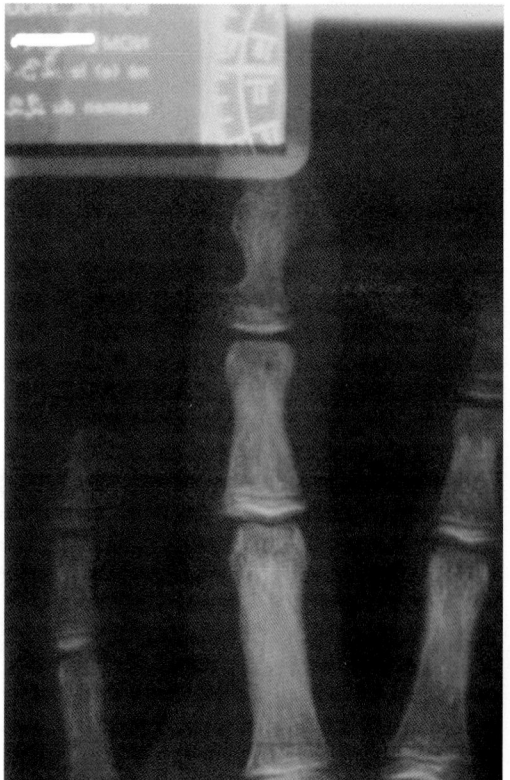

FIGURE 212-11. *A,* Deviation associated with a macrodactyly. *B,* Epiphysiodesis of two growth plates. *C,* Result after 4 years.

REFERENCES

1. Buck-Gramcko D: Influence of growth and altered function on bones and muscles. In Tubiana R, ed: The Hand. Philadelphia, WB Saunders, 1999:737.
2. Gilbert A: Fractures of the fingers in children. In Bruser P, Gilbert A, eds: Finger Bone and Joint Injuries. London, Dunitz, 1999:359-364.
3. Leclercq C, Korn W: Articular fractures of the fingers in children. Hand Clin 2000;16:523-534.
4. Vickers D: Madelung deformity: surgical prophylaxis. J Hand Surg Br 1992;17:401-407.
5. Wood M, Gilbert A: Microvascular Bone Reconstruction. London, Dunitz, 1997.
6. Tsai TM, Lowing G, Tonkin M: Vascularized fibular epiphyseal transfer. Clin Orthop 1986;210:228-234.
7. Vilkki SL: Distraction and microvascular epiphysis transfer for radial club hand. J Hand Surg Br 1998;23:445-452.

Paralytic Disorders

Tendon Transfers in the Upper Limb

Neil F. Jones, MD, FRCS ◆ Kayvan T. Khiabani, MD, MSc, FRCS(C), FACS

Tendon transfers are reconstructive techniques that restore motion or balance to the hand lost secondary to impaired or absent function of the extrinsic or intrinsic muscle-tendon units of the forearm and hand. In a typical tendon transfer, the tendon of insertion of a functioning muscle is detached, mobilized, and then reattached to another tendon or bone to substitute for the action of a nonfunctioning muscle-tendon unit. On occasion, both the tendon of origin and the tendon of insertion are detached and then reattached at different locations. Unlike a tendon graft, the transferred donor tendon remains attached to its parent muscle. A tendon transfer also differs from a microsurgical free muscle transfer in that the neurovascular pedicle to the muscle of the transferred tendon remains intact.

There are three general indications for tendon transfers in the upper extremity: to restore function to a paralyzed muscle because of injuries of the peripheral nerves, the brachial plexus, or the spinal cord; to restore function after closed tendon ruptures or open injuries to the tendons or muscles; and to restore balance to a hand deformed by various neurologic diseases. Tendon transfers are best conceptualized as a means to restore a lost "function" rather than as a means to substitute for a specific muscle (e.g., restoration of strong pinch as opposed to restoration of function of the flexor pollicis longus). Tendon transfers are performed predominantly after peripheral nerve injuries and therefore are discussed according to a specific nerve palsy. However, the general principles described in this chapter apply to all transfers (Table 213-1).

TABLE 213-1 ◆ BASIC PRINCIPLES OF TENDON TRANSFERS

Soft tissue equilibrium
Full passive range of motion of involved joints
Adequate amplitude of donor muscle
Direct line of pull
Single function for each transferred tendon
Synergy of transfer

GENERAL PRINCIPLES

Bone and Soft Tissue Healing

Steindler[1] first suggested that tendon transfers cannot glide through edematous or scarred soft tissues, nor can they flex or extend stiff metacarpophalangeal (MCP) and proximal interphalangeal (PIP) joints. He therefore advocated that tendon transfers be delayed until "tissue equilibrium" has been restored.[1]

Before a tendon transfer is performed, all fractures should be healed or rigidly fixed by internal fixation. Chronic scarred skin and subcutaneous tissues or skin grafts in the projected line of pull of a tendon transfer should be excised; the defect should be resurfaced with a flap that itself is allowed to heal and the new scars become mature. If secondary tendon transfers are likely to be necessary, initial split-thickness skin grafting of soft tissue defects of the hand and forearm, simply to achieve a healed wound, should be avoided if possible. Instead, consideration should be given to a pliable flap, ideally of skin and subcutaneous tissues, as a delayed primary coverage by use of pedicled flaps (such as the groin flap and reverse radial forearm flap) or free flaps (such as the lateral arm flap, contralateral radial forearm flap, scapular flap, and latissimus dorsi flap). On occasion, silicone rods can be placed at the time of flap coverage, either beneath or through the subcutaneous fat of a transferred flap to make a smooth tunnel through which a tendon transfer may later be passed.

The span of the thumb–index finger web space should be maintained by splinting, especially after median nerve injuries. If a secondary adduction contracture has developed, this should be released by a Z-plasty, skin grafting, or transposition flap and release of the adductor pollicis, if needed, before any opposition tendon transfer. Full passive range of motion of the MCP and PIP joints should be achieved by physical therapy and dynamic splinting before any tendon transfer. Preliminary capsulotomies of the MCP and PIP joints or tenolysis of adherent flexor or extensor tendons may occasionally be required if dynamic splinting fails to achieve adequate joint mobility.

Selection of Donor Muscle-Tendon

EXPENDABILITY

The muscle-tendon unit selected as a potential donor for transfer must be expendable. Its sacrifice must not create an important new deficit. For example, the ring finger flexor digitorum superficialis (FDS) tendon may be used to correct MCP hyperextension (claw deformity) in patients with a low ulnar nerve palsy, but it is not expendable in patients with a high ulnar nerve palsy who have no functioning flexor digitorum profundus (FDP) tendon to the ring finger. The selection of a muscle-tendon unit as a tendon transfer may also be influenced by the patient's occupation. For example, the flexor carpi radialis (FCR) may be a more appropriate transfer to provide finger extension in a working man rather than the more conventional flexor carpi ulnaris (FCU) transfer because the FCU provides the important function of flexion and ulnar deviation of the wrist needed in work activities such as hammering. More important, if multiple tendon transfers are required, a minimum of one wrist flexor, one wrist extensor, and one extrinsic flexor and extensor tendon to each digit should always be retained.

STRENGTH AND AMPLITUDE

In selecting the most appropriate donor muscle-tendon, the surgeon must consider not only the strength of the muscle to be transferred but also the native strength of the now paralyzed muscle or muscles and the strength of the antagonist muscle. Brand[2,3] has emphasized that the maximum potential force of a muscle is directly proportional to its physiologic cross-sectional area. It has been calculated that a muscle can produce a force of 3.65 kg per square centimeter of its cross-sectional area. This potential force is maximal when the muscle is at its resting length, which is defined as the position midway between the length when it is fully stretched passively and the length when it is fully contracted.

The potential amplitude or excursion of a donor muscle-tendon unit must also be sufficient to restore the specific lost function. The finger flexors have an amplitude of 70 mm; the finger extensors, 50 mm; and the wrist flexors and extensors, 33 mm. The tenodesis effect of wrist flexion or extension may also increase the effective amplitude of a tendon transfer by 25 mm. Excursion of a donor muscle may also be increased by extensive release of its surrounding fascia and is best exemplified by transfer of the brachioradialis muscle. The distal portion and tendon of the brachioradialis muscle are surrounded by dense fascia. Division of these fascial attachments will add an additional 2 to 3 cm of passive excursion.

DIRECTION OF TRANSFER AND INTEGRITY

A tendon transfer should pass in a direct line from the origin of the donor muscle to its new insertion. Unless early tendon transfers are being performed, when there is still a chance of reinnervation after nerve repair, the recipient tendons should be divided proximal to the site of the tendon juncture to create a more direct line of pull (end-to-end) rather than producing a Y- shaped end-to-side juncture. Tendon transfers should act only across one joint and perform only one single function. This maintains the "integrity" of the muscle. However, a transfer may be inserted into several recipient tendons as long as they each perform the same function in adjacent digits. Finally, the donor muscle selected should preferably be synergistic with the function of the muscle to be restored or at least be potentially retrainable.

The surgeon has to determine the specific functions to be restored, select the appropriate donor muscle-tendon units, and decide on the timing of the tendon transfer. For this selection to be made, every muscle still functioning in the forearm and hand should be tested by manual muscle testing to document which are functioning and to grade their strength. From this list of functioning muscles, only those that are expendable are available as donor transfers. The specific functions of the hand that need to be restored are then listed in order of priority. The final step is to match the available donor muscles with the functions that need to be restored on the basis of force, amplitude, and direction of the various muscles available.

Arthrodesis of a more proximal joint such as the wrist may occasionally need to be considered to release a wrist flexor or extensor tendon for transfer. Transfers that require postoperative immobilization with the wrist in flexion are usually performed at a first stage. Those transfers requiring postoperative immobilization with the wrist in extension are performed at a second stage.

Timing of Tendon Transfers

Timing of tendon transfers may be classified as early, conventional, or late. A conventional tendon transfer is usually performed after reinnervation of the paralyzed muscle fails to occur by 3 months after the expected time of reinnervation based on the rate of nerve regeneration of 1 mm per day. Brand,[3] Omer,[4] and Burkhalter[5] have advocated "early" tendon transfers in certain circumstances, in which a tendon transfer is performed simultaneously with the nerve repair or before the expected time of reinnervation of the muscle. This early tendon transfer therefore serves as a temporary substitute for the paralyzed muscle until reinnervation occurs by acting as an internal splint. If reinnervation is suboptimal, the early tendon transfer

acts as a helper to augment the power of the muscle; and if reinnervation fails to occur, it then acts as a permanent substitute.

Surgical Techniques

The success of any tendon transfer depends entirely on prevention of scarring or adhesions along the path of the transferred tendon. Incisions should be carefully planned before elevation of the tourniquet so that the final tendon junctures lie transversely beneath skin flaps rather than immediately beneath and paralleling the incisions. The donor muscle should be carefully mobilized to prevent damage to its neurovascular bundle, which usually enters in the proximal third of the muscle. The transferred tendon should glide in a tunnel through the subcutaneous tissues and not cross bone devoid of uninjured periosteum or pass through small fascial windows. Only the distal end of the tendon should be grasped with surgical instruments and care taken to prevent desiccation of the tendon or the surrounding tissues. Tendon junctures are performed by a Pulvertaft weave technique when possible. The donor and recipient tendons are sutured under normal tension, and after one or two nonabsorbable sutures have been inserted, the tension of the transfer is checked by observing the flexion and extension of the digit during tenodesis of the wrist. The hand is immobilized postoperatively in the desired position for 3 to 4 weeks, at which time gentle active range-of-motion exercises are started, usually under the supervision of a therapist, but the hand is protected for another 3 weeks in a lightweight protective splint.

RADIAL NERVE PALSY

Indications

The functional motor deficit in radial nerve palsy consists of inability to extend the wrist, inability to extend the fingers at the MCP joints, and inability to extend and radially abduct the thumb (Fig. 213-1). However, the most significant disability is that patients are unable to stabilize the wrist so that transmission of flexor power to the fingers is impaired, resulting in marked weakness of grip strength.

Tendon transfers are therefore required to provide wrist extension, extension of the fingers at the MCP joints, and extension and radial abduction of the thumb. Unlike with the median and ulnar nerves, sensory loss after radial nerve injury is not functionally disabling unless the patient develops a painful neuroma.

Timing of tendon transfers for radial nerve palsy remains controversial. The two options are to perform an early tendon transfer simultaneously with repair of the radial nerve to act as an internal splint to provide

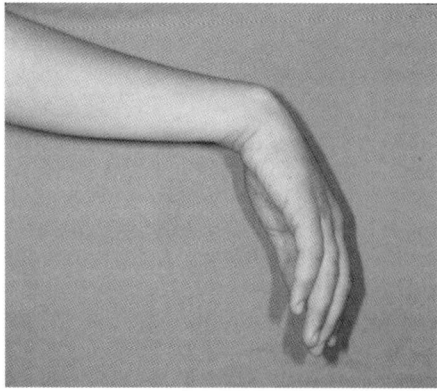

FIGURE 213-1. The typical posture of the hand and wrist of a patient with a high radial nerve palsy. The wrist cannot be extended. The fingers are extended through the tenodesis effect.

immediate restoration of power grip; and more conventionally, to delay any tendon transfers until reinnervation of the most proximal muscles, brachioradialis and extensor carpi radialis longus, fails to occur within the calculated time limit. The more proximal the nerve injury, the less likely that functional muscle reinnervation will occur.[3,5] If the nerve remains in continuity, most surgeons would suggest that observation for 3 months is indicated to await spontaneous recovery in peripheral nerve palsies. Mayer and Mayfield[6] reported 39 cases of posterior interosseous nerve neurorrhaphy with complete recovery in 28 patients and partial recovery in 11 patients. Young et al[7] studied 51 patients with posterior interosseous nerve palsy, of whom only 11 had resolution by 3 months. Of the remaining 40 patients, 20 of the 23 who underwent neurolysis and 10 of the 12 who underwent nerve grafting had excellent or good results. A conflicting study of radial nerve injuries demonstrated useful function in 65%, but only 38% of patients who underwent nerve grafting obtained useful motor function.[8] These studies demonstrate that repair of the radial and posterior interosseous nerves can provide significant return of function and should be considered. With extensive nerve gaps or associated soft tissue injuries and in older patients, the chances of successful reinnervation are much less predictable, and it may therefore be more appropriate for these patients to undergo the full set of tendon transfers early.[9] In a patient awaiting return of nerve function, it is important to maintain supple MCP joints capable of full extension and adequate radial abduction of the thumb with appropriate splinting and therapy.

Operations

Franke[10] provided one of the earliest descriptions of tendon transfers for radial nerve palsy using the FCU

to extensor digitorum communis (EDC) transfer through the interosseous membrane. Capellen in 1899 described the FCR to extensor pollicis longus (EPL) transfer. The pronator teres to extensor carpi radialis longus (ECRL) and extensor carpi radialis brevis (ECRB) transfer for wrist extension was first reported in 1906 by Sir Robert Jones. Zachary[11] emphasized the importance of retaining at least one wrist flexor, preferably the FCR, to facilitate wrist control. Other authors have suggested that the FCU is not an expendable tendon and therefore prefer to use the FCR as the donor tendon to restore finger extension.[12] The advantage of using the FCR is that it preserves the important moment of flexion and ulnar deviation of the wrist that is so important for power grip in a working man. This is particularly true in the patient with a posterior interosseous nerve palsy in which ECRL function is preserved but extensor carpi ulnaris (ECU) activity is lost. This leads to radial deviation of the wrist with attempted wrist extension. Use of the FCU in this setting will increase the radial deviation of the wrist because only radially deviating wrist motors are preserved.

Several different tendon transfers have been reported for radial nerve palsy, but three patterns of transfer have evolved. The use of the pronator teres to provide wrist extension has become universally accepted, the only remaining controversy being whether to insert the pronator teres into the ECRB alone or into both the ECRL and ECRB. The three patterns of tendon transfer differ therefore only in the technique of restoring finger extension and thumb extension and radial abduction (Table 213-2).[11,13-15]

AUTHORS' PREFERRED TRANSFERS

In the patient with a radial nerve palsy, the FCU transfer is the authors' preferred technique; in the patient with a posterior interosseous nerve palsy, the FCR

TABLE 213-2 ✦ TENDON TRANSFERS FOR RADIAL NERVE PALSY

Standard FCU Transfer	FCR Transfer	Boyes Superficialis Transfer
PT to ECRB	PT to ECRB	PT to ECRL + ECRB
FCU to EDC	FCR to EDC	FDS long to EDC long, ring, and small fingers
PL to EPL	PL to EPL	FDS ring to EIP and EPL
		FCR to APL and EPB

APL, abductor pollicis longus; ECRB, extensor carpi radialis brevis; ECRL, extensor carpi radialis longus; EDC, extensor digitorum communis; EIP, extensor indicis proprius; EPB, extensor pollicis brevis; EPL, extensor pollicis longus; FCR, flexor carpi radialis; FCU, flexor carpi ulnaris; FDS, flexor digitorum superficialis; PL, palmaris longus; PT, pronator teres.

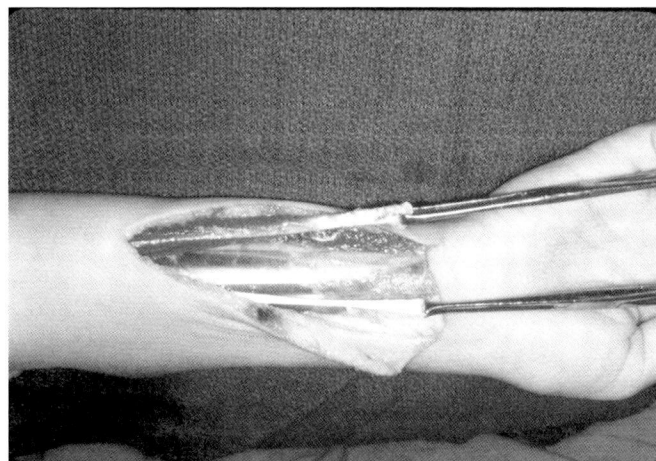

FIGURE 213-2. The FCU tendon and distal muscle are dissected. In this patient, a palmaris longus is present, and its tendon is dissected for later transfer to the EPL.

transfer is preferred. Through an inverted J–shaped incision over the ulnar volar aspect of the distal forearm, the FCU tendon is transected at the wrist crease and released extensively from its fascial attachments up into the proximal third of the forearm, with care taken not to damage the neurovascular pedicle; a second incision is used in the proximal forearm if necessary (Fig. 213-2). Through the same distal incision, the palmaris longus tendon is transected at the wrist crease and the muscle mobilized into the middle third of the forearm (see Fig. 213-2). An S-shaped incision is then made beginning over the volar radial aspect of the middle third of the forearm and passing dorsally and ulnarly over the radial border of the forearm (Fig. 213-3). The tendon of pronator teres is elevated from the radius in continuity with a 2- to 3-cm strip of periosteum (Fig. 213-4). The ECRB is transected at its musculotendinous junction if there is no chance of future reinnervation of the wrist extensors. The pronator teres is then rerouted around the radial border of the forearm superficial to the brachioradialis and ECRL in a straight direction to its insertion into the

ECRB (see Fig. 213-4). The FCU tendon is passed through a subcutaneous tunnel made with a Kelly clamp from the palmar incision around the ulnar border of the forearm into the dorsal incision to lie obliquely across the EDC tendons proximal to the extensor retinaculum. If no return of EDC function is to be expected, the EDC tendons can be transected at their musculotendinous junctions so that a more direct line of pull can be achieved (Fig. 213-5). Otherwise, an end-to-side juncture is performed. The EPL tendon is divided at its musculotendinous junction, removed from the third dorsal extensor tendon compartment, and passed through a subcutaneous tunnel from the base of the thumb metacarpal to the volar wrist incision (Fig. 213-6). If the palmaris longus is not present, the tendon of the EPL is included with the tendons of the EDC and the FCU, which provides for both finger and thumb extension. To prevent a collapse flexion deformity at the carpometacarpal joint of the thumb, tenodesis of the abductor pollicis longus (APL) will be necessary. After transection of the APL tendon in the distal forearm,

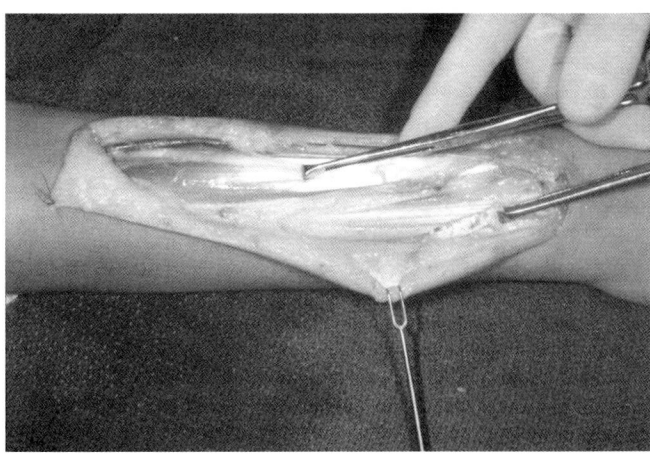

FIGURE 213-3. A dorsal incision exposes the wrist and finger extensors. The FCU tendon has been brought from palmar to dorsal, around the ulna through a large gap made in the intermuscular septum.

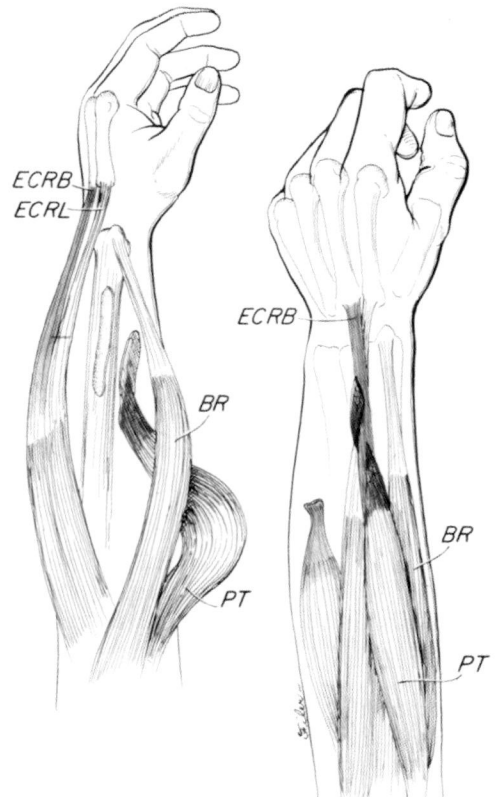

FIGURE 213-4. *Left,* The relatively short tendon of insertion of the pronator teres (PT) can be extended by elevating a strip of periosteum. *Right,* The pronator teres will be woven into the tendon of the extensor carpi radialis brevis (ECRB). BR, brachioradialis; ECRL, extensor carpi radialis longus.

it is looped around the brachioradialis proximal to the radial styloid and sutured to itself with the thumb metacarpal held in extension with the wrist in 30 degrees of extension.

The proper tension in radial nerve tendon transfers should be tight enough to provide full extension of the wrist and digits but without restricting full flexion of the digits when the wrist is fully extended. The pronator teres at resting tension is woven through the ECRB tendon with the wrist in 45 degrees of extension. The distal ends of the four EDC tendons to the index, long, ring, and small fingers are sutured to the FCU tendon proximal to the extensor retinaculum. The extensor digiti minimi (EDM) is usually not included unless there is still an extensor lag when proximal traction is applied to the EDC tendon to the small finger. With the wrist in neutral and the FCU under maximal tension, each individual EDC tendon is sutured to provide full extension at the MCP joint, starting with the index finger and finishing with the small finger. Appropriate tension is then evaluated by checking that all four digits extend synchronously when the wrist is palmar flexed and, most important, that all four digits can be passively flexed into a fist when the wrist is extended. Finally, palmaris longus and EPL are interwoven over the radial volar aspect of the wrist with both tendons under resting tension with the wrist in neutral. The wrist is immobilized in 45 degrees of extension in a volar splint with the MCP joints positioned in slight flexion and the thumb in full extension and abduction.

Active flexion and extension of the fingers and thumb are started at $3^{1}/_{2}$ to 4 weeks; active exercises of the wrist are begun at 5 weeks. Protective splinting is continued until 6 to 8 weeks postoperatively. Results have been uniformly good (Fig. 213-7).

FCR Transfer

The skin incision begins from the radial volar aspect of the midforearm and extends dorsally over the third and fourth extensor tendon compartments. The pronator teres is transferred to the ECRB and the palmaris longus is transferred to the EPL exactly as described in the standard FCU transfer. The FCR is divided at the wrist crease and mobilized approximately to the level of the midforearm and rerouted around the radial border of the forearm. The four EDC tendons and, if necessary, the EDM may be woven through the donor FCR tendon proximal to the extensor retinaculum, but more usually the extensor tendons need to be rerouted superficial to the extensor retinaculum to obtain a straighter line of pull (Fig. 213-8). To prevent a bulky tendon juncture, the small finger EDC and EDM may be sutured side-to-side to the ring finger EDC and the index finger EDC sutured side-to-side to the long finger EDC under appropriate tension. Then only the two EDC tendons to the long and ring fingers require weaving through the FCR tendon. As with the standard FCU transfer, these tendon junctures are performed with the wrist in neutral and the MCP joints in full extension with the FCR tendon under maximal traction. Postoperative management is similar to that for the FCU transfer.

Boyes Superficialis Transfer

Boyes[13] was the first to suggest that neither the FCU nor the FCR has sufficient amplitude (30 mm) to produce full excursion of the digital extensor tendons (50 mm) without the potential increase in amplitude obtained with the tenodesis effect of wrist flexion. He therefore advocated use of the superficialis tendons to the long and ring fingers, which have an amplitude of 70 mm, to act as donor tendons to restore finger extension.[13,14] The advantages of the Boyes transfer are that it will potentially allow simultaneous wrist and finger extension, it may allow independent thumb and index finger extension, and it does not weaken wrist flexion. However, the long and ring fingers are deprived

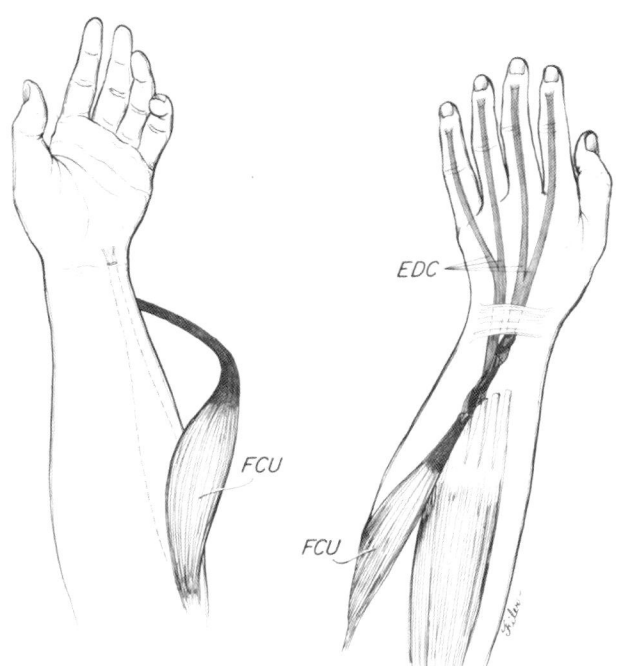

FIGURE 213-5. The FCU is brought around the ulnar border of the forearm. The muscle-tendon junction of the EDC is excised to increase the excursion potential of this transfer, and the FCU is woven into the tendons of the EDC.

of superficialis function, and this may result in weak grip. Harvesting of the superficialis tendons may also lead to the subsequent development of either a "swan-neck" deformity or a flexion contracture at the PIP joint.

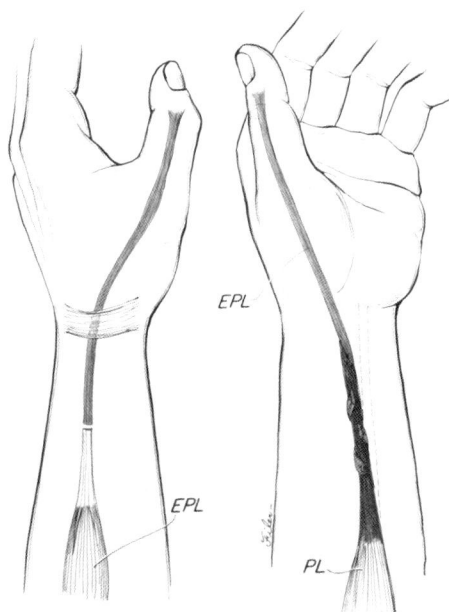

FIGURE 213-6. The palmaris longus (PL), if present, can be attached to the rerouted EPL tendon to provide both thumb extension and some radial abduction.

The superficialis tendons to the long and ring fingers are exposed between the A1 and A2 pulleys through either one transverse incision at the base of the fingers or two separate longitudinal incisions. The superficialis tendons are divided just proximal to their decussation and then withdrawn proximally into a longitudinal incision over the volar aspect of the middle third of the forearm. The tendon of pronator teres can be transected and rerouted through this same incision as described previously. Blunt dissection on either side of the flexor profundus muscles allows a window to be excised in the interosseous membrane just proximal to the pronator quadratus (Fig. 213-9). This window should be made as large as possible, at least 4 cm long and as wide as the interosseous space, so that the muscle bellies of the two superficialis tendons can be passed through this window to minimize the development of adhesions. It is important to pass the superficialis tendons of the ring and long fingers to their respective sides of the median nerve to prevent scissoring over the nerve and compression.

Thompson and Rasmussen[16] prefer to transfer the two superficialis tendons through subcutaneous tunnels around the radial and ulnar borders of the forearm. Through a J-shaped incision passing transversely across the dorsum of the wrist and then extending proximally along the dorsum of the ulna, the extensor tendons are isolated as well as the ECRB. In Boyes' original description, the pronator teres was sutured to both the ECRL and ECRB,[13] but to prevent excessive radial deviation, the pronator teres should

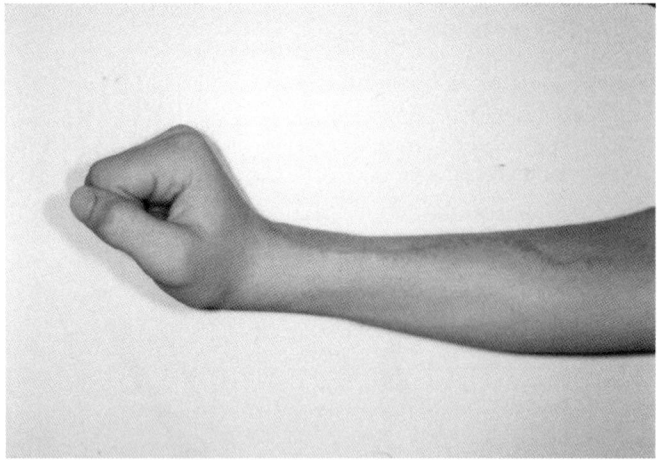

A

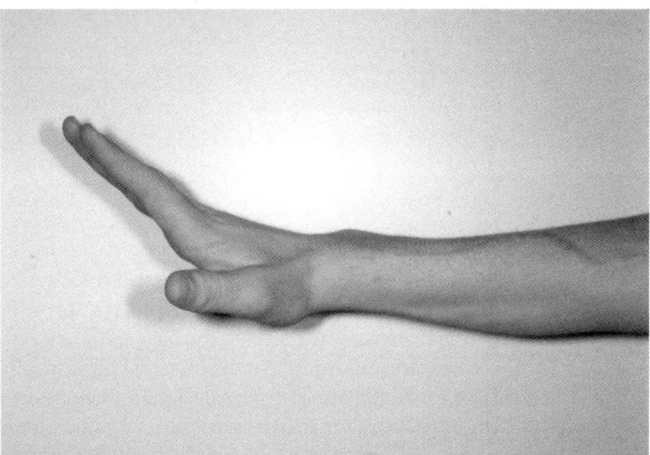

B

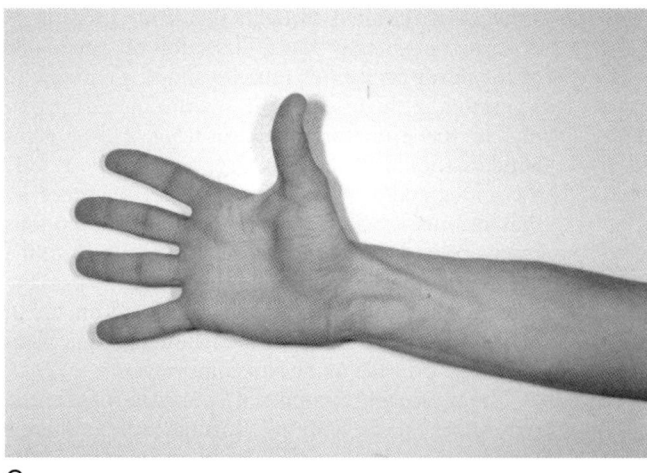

C

FIGURE 213-7. A patient 5 years after pronator teres to ECRB, FCU to EDC, and palmaris longus to EPL transfers. *A,* Wrist extension and finger flexion. *B,* Full finger extension. *C,* Excellent thumb extension and radial abduction.

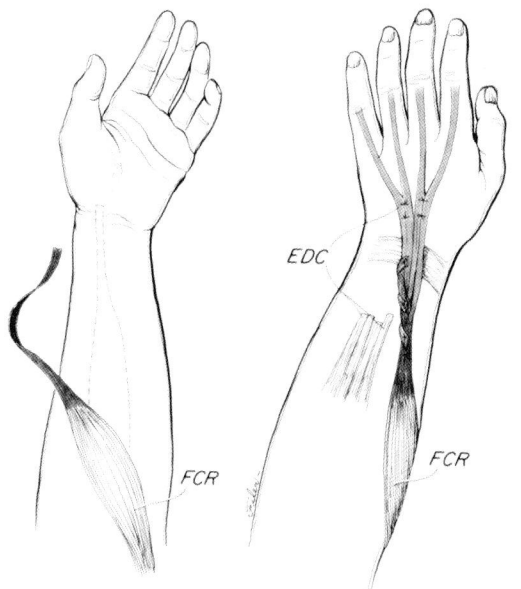

FIGURE 213-8. Transfer of the FCR to the combined tendons of the EDC.

be woven only end-to-end into the ECRB with the wrist in 30 degrees of extension. The long finger superficialis is then passed to the radial side of the profundus muscles and the ring finger superficialis to the ulnar side through the interosseous window into the dorsal incision. After transection of the EPL and extensor indicis proprius (EIP) tendons, they are woven end-to-end into the long finger superficialis tendon. Similarly, the transected EDC tendons to the index, long, ring, and small fingers are woven end-to-end into the ring finger superficialis tendon, although this arrangement can be reversed. The tendon junctures are performed proximal to the extensor retinaculum with resting tension in the donor superficialis tendons and full extension at the MCP joints.

If necessary, the APL is transected at its musculotendinous junction and passed through a subcutaneous tunnel from the base of the thumb into the volar forearm incision. Either the palmaris longus or the FCR is transected at the wrist crease and woven end-to-end with the APL tendon to provide abduction of the thumb and to prevent a collapse deformity of the thumb metacarpal. The tourniquet should be deflated before the closure of the incisions because of the likelihood of bleeding from the anterior or posterior interosseous vessels.

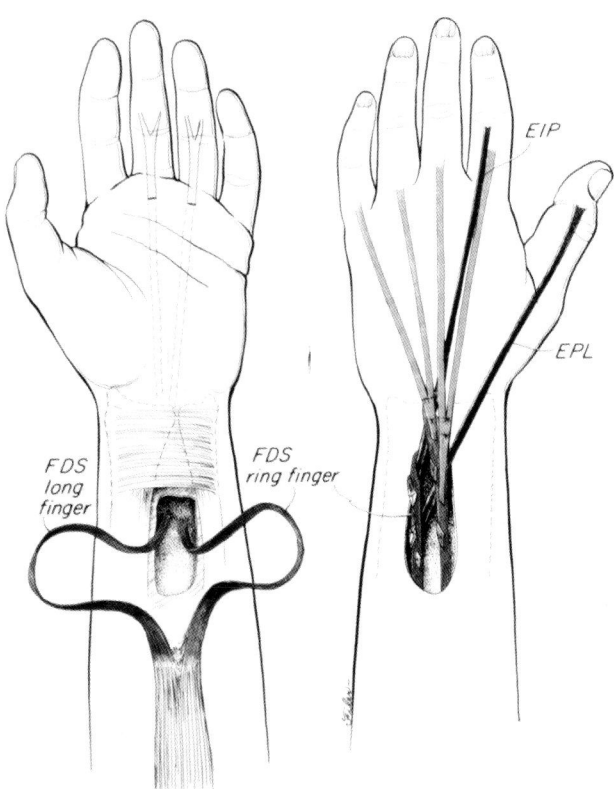

FIGURE 213-9. Transfer of the long and ring finger superficialis tendons (FDS) through a window in the interosseous membrane to restore function to the extensor digitorum communis tendons and extensor indicis proprius (EIP) and extensor pollicis longus (EPL).

Outcomes

Tendon transfers for radial nerve palsy are generally predictable. Tsuge[17] described the evolution of his technique in 69 patients during a 25-year period. Using the FCU transfer and insertion of pronator teres into both ECRL and ECRB in the initial 41 patients, he reported "fairly satisfactory" results but thought that there were three problems: development of radial deviation of the wrist, restriction of wrist flexion, and marginal thumb abduction. Because of these concerns, the pronator teres was transferred only to the ECRB and the FCR was transferred through the interosseous membrane for finger extension, leaving the FCU intact; good results were obtained in 24 of 27 cases. A long-term functional study of the FCU transfer in six patients by Raskin and Wilgis[18] revealed adequate wrist motion and power to perform daily activities; a work simulation protocol showed that patients were able to perform tasks without significant difficulty. Problems of inadequate ulnar deviation, grip strength, and wrist instability were not seen. A subjective outcome study by Riordan[19] also revealed satisfaction with the standard FCU transfer.

Chuinard et al[14] studied 21 patients who had undergone the Boyes superficialis transfers with excellent results in 10, good results in 6, and only fair results in 5 patients. Subjectively, 13 patients thought that they had obtained an excellent result and 8 a good result. Complications requiring a second procedure were reported in 5 patients and included adhesions, dehiscence of the transfer, MCP and wrist extension contractures, and problems with correct tensioning of the transfers. A report of 13 patients with radial nerve palsy and 5 patients with posterior interosseous nerve palsy by Fujiwara[20] documented generally good results with the Boyes transfers. No patient in either of these studies developed postoperative median nerve compression despite the potential for this complication with this transfer.

All three techniques have been reported to yield good results, but there are few quantitative studies to substantiate the reported outcomes and no prospective comparison of the three different techniques. The FCU transfer is perhaps the simplest technique and provides reproducibly good results in patients with radial nerve palsy.

LOW MEDIAN NERVE PALSY

Anatomic Considerations

The functional deficit that follows injury to the median nerve distal to the innervation of the extrinsic forearm flexor muscles consists primarily of loss of opposition of the thumb and absent sensation over the thumb, index and long fingers, and radial half of the ring finger.

Opposition is a composite motion that occurs at all three joints to position the thumb pad opposite the distal phalanx of the partially flexed long finger. Abduction, pronation, and flexion occur at the carpometacarpal joint, abduction and flexion at the MCP joint, and either flexion or extension at the interphalangeal joint. Approximately 40 degrees of abduction of the thumb metacarpal occurs at the carpometacarpal joint, and 20 degrees of abduction of the proximal phalanx occurs at the MCP joint. From a starting position of full extension and adduction, the thumb pronates approximately 90 degrees during opposition to the long finger. Extension of the thumb interphalangeal joint is required for pulp to pulp pinch, whereas slight flexion of the interphalangeal joint allows tip to tip pinch. Of the three intrinsic thenar muscles, the flexor pollicis brevis (FPB) muscle typically, although not always, receives a dual innervation from both the median and ulnar nerves. Because the FPB may remain innervated by the ulnar nerve in approximately 70% of median nerve injuries, patients may not notice any significant functional loss, but careful testing will reveal decreased strength of abduction and lack of pronation.

Before any opposition transfer, patients with median nerve injuries should be instructed to prevent the development of an adduction or supination contracture of the thumb by a program of passive abduction exercises. A static thumb–index finger web space splint may be used at night, but this usually interferes with the already compromised function of the hand if it is used during the day. Care should be taken to ensure that such splints abduct the thumb metacarpal rather than the proximal phalanx; otherwise, the median nerve palsy will be compounded by attenuation of the ulnar collateral ligament of the MCP joint. If patients present with an established adduction or supination contracture of the thumb, release of the thumb–index finger web space skin, fascia over the first dorsal interosseous muscle, or even the first dorsal interosseous and adductor muscles themselves may be required before any opposition tendon transfer.

Bunnell[21] first emphasized that the pull of an opposition tendon transfer should be in an oblique direction from the thumb MCP joint to the region of the pisiform and, second, to produce pronation, that the transfer should be inserted into the dorsal ulnar base of the proximal phalanx. Opposition transfers that are directed along the radial aspect of the palm will produce a greater component of palmar abduction, whereas transfers that pass from the pisiform will produce both abduction and pronation. The more distal the transfer passes across the palm, the greater the power of thumb flexion. Several methods of insertion of opposition transfers have been advocated, including attachment to the dorsal ulnar base of the proximal phalanx[21-23]; insertion into the abductor pollicis brevis (APB) tendon[24]; dual insertion into the APB and continuation distally into the MCP joint capsule and EPL tendon[19]; insertion into the APB, dorsal joint capsule, and adductor pollicis[25]; and use of a distally based extensor pollicis brevis (EPB) tendon.[26] However, a biomechanical study has shown that opposition tendon transfers inserted into the APB tendon alone will produce full abduction and pronation.[27] Therefore, the more complex dual insertions should probably be reserved for combined median and ulnar nerve palsies.

Several factors influence the likelihood of useful motor and sensory return after median nerve injury, including age of the patient, level of injury, length of nerve defect and interposition graft, and period of preoperative delay. The best results are realized in distal injuries in young patients requiring only primary repair. Associated injuries such as vascular damage, tendon injury, and concomitant ulnar nerve transection portend a worse prognosis. The chances of reinnervation of the thenar muscles after group fascicular repair of a distal median nerve laceration should be reasonably optimistic. Therefore, conventional timing of an opposition tendon transfer may be required only in those patients who fail to demonstrate signs of reinnervation within the usual calculated time interval. For older patients or those with poor prognostic comorbid factors, early tendon transfers should be considered.

Careful observation of thumb function after either a low or high median nerve palsy will reveal whether an early tendon transfer for thumb opposition is necessary. The FPB remains innervated by the ulnar nerve in approximately 70% of median nerve injuries so that thumb function may not be significantly compromised. Consequently, an early opposition transfer may not be necessary. Other patients, however, will adapt to their loss of opposition and abduction by substitution of the APL to provide thumb abduction, but this can be achieved only with the hand positioned in pronation. This places patients at an even greater disadvantage in that not only do they have absent sensation in the median nerve distribution, but also, with the forearm in pronation, they cannot even see the palmar surface of the hand to compensate for the loss of sensation. Therefore, if the surgeon or therapist observes the patient attempting to grasp objects by radial abduction of the thumb with the forearm in pronation, an early opposition tendon transfer should be strongly considered. If, however, the patient is able to pick up an object with the forearm in neutral or to grasp an object with the forearm in supination, it is likely that the FPB remains innervated by the ulnar nerve, and consequently the decision for performing an early opposition tendon transfer can be delayed.

Operations

EXTENSOR INDICIS PROPRIUS (BURKHALTER TRANSFER)

The EIP transfer[28] is the authors' preferred technique, except in elderly patients with thenar atrophy secondary to severe carpal tunnel syndrome (Fig. 213-10). The

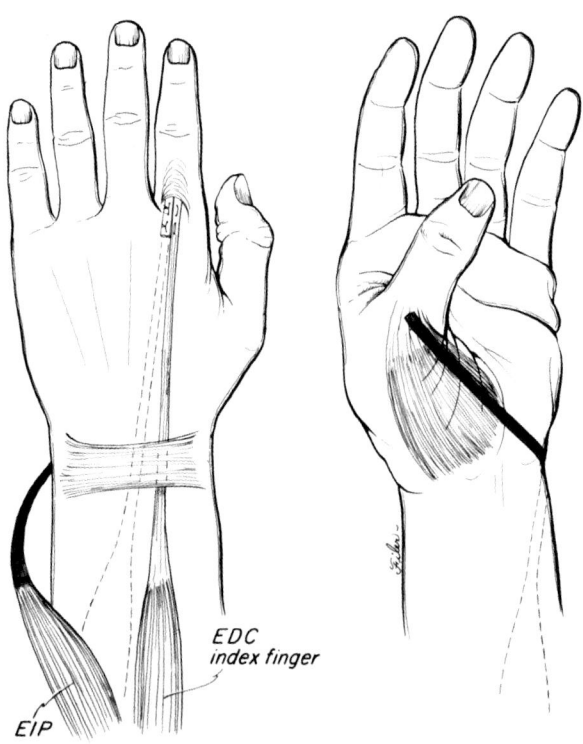

FIGURE 213-10. The EIP transfer to restore opposition is schematically depicted. See text for details. EDC, extensor digitorum communis.

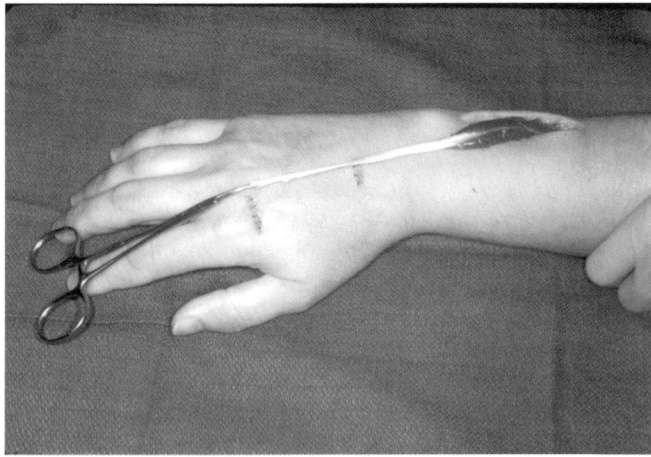

FIGURE 213-11. Incisions for harvesting the EIP.

EIP tendon is transected through a small transverse incision just proximal to the MCP joint of the index finger. The distal stump of the EIP tendon is then repaired to the EDC tendon of the index finger to prevent extensor lag at the MCP joint. The EIP tendon is mobilized through two small transverse incisions, one proximal and one distal to the extensor retinaculum, and the muscle belly is mobilized through a longitudinal incision over the ulnar aspect of the dorsum of the midforearm (Fig. 213-11). A transverse incision is made just proximal to the pisiform bone, and a subcutaneous tunnel is developed to connect this incision to the dorsal forearm incision. The EIP tendon is then passed subcutaneously around the ulnar border of the distal forearm superficial to the ECU tendon into the pisiform incision (Fig. 213-12). The APB tendon is identified through a small incision over the radial aspect of the MCP joint of the thumb, and a subcutaneous tunnel is made connecting this incision with the pisiform incision. The tendon transfer is passed obliquely across the palm and woven into the tendon of the APB under maximum tension with the wrist in neutral position and the thumb in maximal palmar abduction.

The tension of the transfer is then tested by the tenodesis effect of the wrist. Wrist flexion should allow the thumb to be passively adducted. If wrist extension produces excessive flexion or extension of the thumb at the MCP joint, this indicates that the transfer has been inserted either too far volarly or too far dorsally and should be adjusted accordingly.

The thumb is immobilized in full abduction with the wrist in slight palmar flexion for 4 weeks, at which time active abduction and opposition movements are begun with protective splinting for another 3 to 4 weeks. The only potential disadvantage with this tendon transfer is that the EIP tendon is only just long enough to reach the APB tendon. The postoperative results have been predictable (Fig. 213-13).

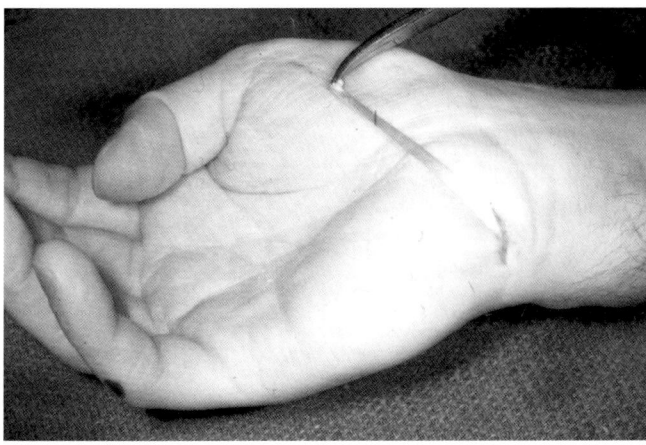

FIGURE 213-12. The palmar incision and the direction of the EIP transfer.

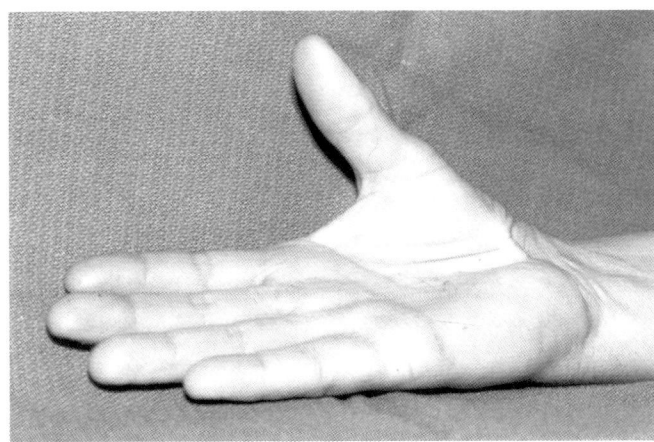

A

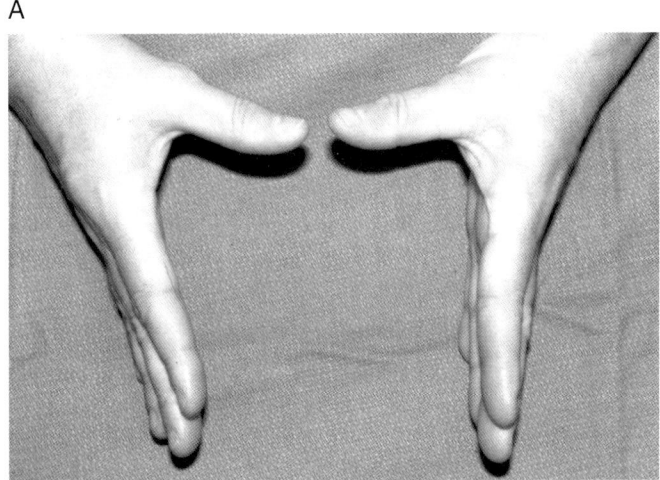

B

FIGURE 213-13. *A* and *B,* The postoperative opposition restored by EIP transfer.

RING FINGER FLEXOR DIGITORUM SUPERFICIALIS (BUNNELL TRANSFER)
(Fig. 213-14)

In the flexor superficialis transfer described originally by Bunnell,[21] the ring finger superficialis tendon is isolated through a small transverse incision just distal to the distal palmar crease. The tendon is transected between the A1 and A2 pulleys and delivered into a proximal incision made over the volar aspect of the distal forearm (Fig. 213-15*A*). The FCU tendon is split longitudinally to make a distal-based strip of the radial half of the tendon. This is then passed through a slit in the FCU tendon just proximal to the pisiform and sutured to itself to make a pulley (Fig. 213-15*B*). The distal end of the ring finger superficialis tendon is passed through the pulley and through an oblique subcutaneous tunnel across the palm into an incision over the radial aspect of the MCP joint of the thumb. All the other incisions are then closed, and the tension

on the tendon transfer is adjusted as described previously.

Simple looping of the ring finger superficialis around the FCU tendon rather than use of a fixed pulley rapidly becomes ineffective, and the transfer becomes converted to a flexor of the MCP joint rather than a true opposition transfer. Other pulleys for the ring finger superficialis transfer are made by passing the tendon through Guyon canal and through a window in the transverse carpal ligament.

Compared with the EIP transfer, the ring finger superficialis is relatively stronger and has greater length. However, the ring finger superficialis is not available as a donor tendon in a high median nerve palsy or in low median nerve injuries in which there have been associated injuries to the flexor tendons. The ring finger superficialis transfer should also not be selected in combined low median and high ulnar nerve palsies because the ring finger superficialis is the only remaining flexor tendon in the ring finger.

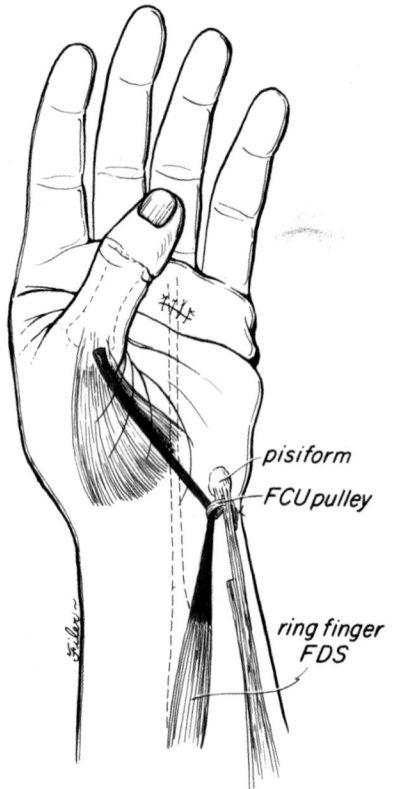

FIGURE 213-14. The FDS to APB transfer to restore thumb opposition is schematically depicted. FCU, flexor carpi ulnaris.

In low median-low ulnar nerve palsies, the ring finger superficialis may be required for correction of clawing. In addition, harvesting of the superficialis tendon may result in either a flexion contracture or a swan-neck deformity of the PIP joint of the donor finger. This is perhaps the strongest of the opposition transfers (Fig. 213-15C and D).

PALMARIS LONGUS (CAMITZ TRANSFER)
(Fig. 213-16)

The palmaris longus tendon Camitz transfer[29-31] is a simple transfer that will provide abduction of the thumb but little pronation or flexion and is particularly indicated in elderly patients with thenar atrophy due to long-standing carpal tunnel syndrome. A strip of palmar fascia is dissected in continuity with the distal palmaris longus tendon through a standard carpal tunnel incision in the palm extending proximally into the distal forearm. A subcutaneous tunnel is developed from the radial aspect of the distal forearm incision along the thenar eminence into a midaxial incision on the radial aspect of the MCP joint of the thumb. The fascial extension of the palmaris longus tendon is passed through the subcutaneous tunnel and sutured to the

APB tendon under maximal tension with the wrist in neutral position (Fig. 213-17).

OTHER OPPOSITION TENDON TRANSFERS

Huber[32] and Nicholaysen[33] described transfer of the abductor digiti minimi, which may occasionally be indicated in patients with a combined median and radial nerve palsy and in children with congenital anomalies affecting the thumb. Because the muscle originates at the pisiform, this transfer provides excellent flexion and pronation of the thumb but little palmar abduction. The tendinous insertion of the abductor digiti minimi is transected from the ulnar lateral band through an ulnar midaxial incision along the proximal phalanx of the small finger. The incision is then extended proximally along the radial aspect of the hypothenar eminence, and the muscle is elevated in a distal to proximal direction; care is taken to protect the neurovascular bundle that enters the muscle just beyond the pisiform. A wide subcutaneous tunnel is dissected between the hypothenar incision and the insertion of the APB at the MCP joint of the thumb. Hemostasis is achieved after release of the tourniquet, and the entire abductor digiti minimi muscle is rotated 180 degrees through the subcutaneous tunnel in the palm and sutured into the APB tendon. This transfer has been compared with turning the page of a book.[32]

Phalen and Miller[26] advocate the use of the EPB tendon activated by the ECU. The EPB is divided at its musculotendinous junction in the distal forearm and retrieved through an incision at the MCP joint of the thumb. This distally based tendon may then be passed through a subcutaneous tunnel obliquely across the palm to the area of the pisiform. The ECU tendon is transected at the base of the fifth metacarpal and routed subcutaneously around the ulnar border of the wrist to be interwoven with the EPB tendon.

Taylor[34] described the use of the EDM as an opposition tendon transfer. This transfer, which was also described by Schneider,[35] reroutes the EDM around the ulnar side of the hand to the thumb MCP joint.

HIGH MEDIAN NERVE PALSY

Indications

The functional deficit after injury to the median nerve proximal to its innervation of the extrinsic forearm flexor muscles consists of inability to flex the index finger at the PIP and distal interphalangeal (DIP) joints and the thumb at the interphalangeal joint in addition to loss of opposition (Fig. 213-18). This is due to paralysis of all four FDS muscles, the FDP tendons to the index and long fingers, and the flexor pollicis longus

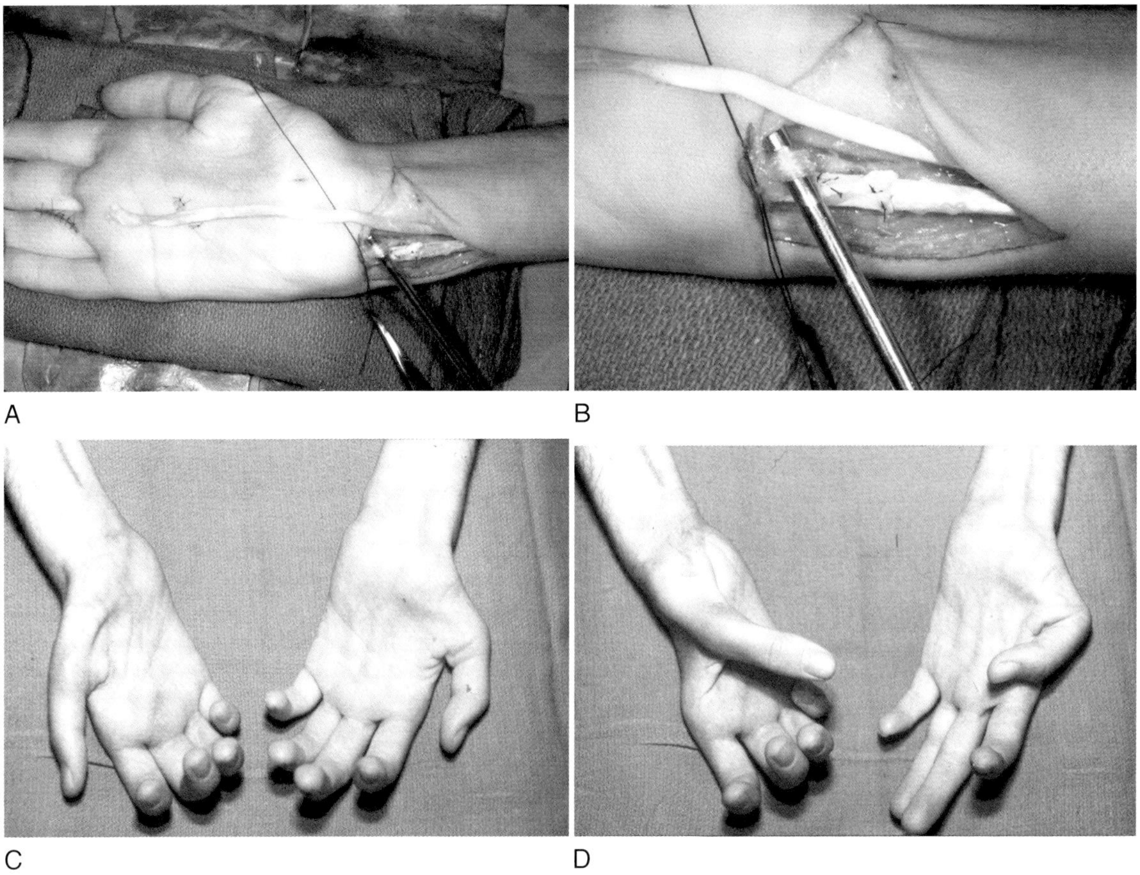

FIGURE 213-15. *A,* Incisions used to obtain the superficialis tendon of the ring finger FDS. *B,* The technique of using half of the FCU sutured to itself as a pulley is demonstrated. *C,* A patient who lacks opposition secondary to Charcot-Marie-Tooth disease, preoperative appearance. *D,* Postoperatively, opposition has been restored to the right hand.

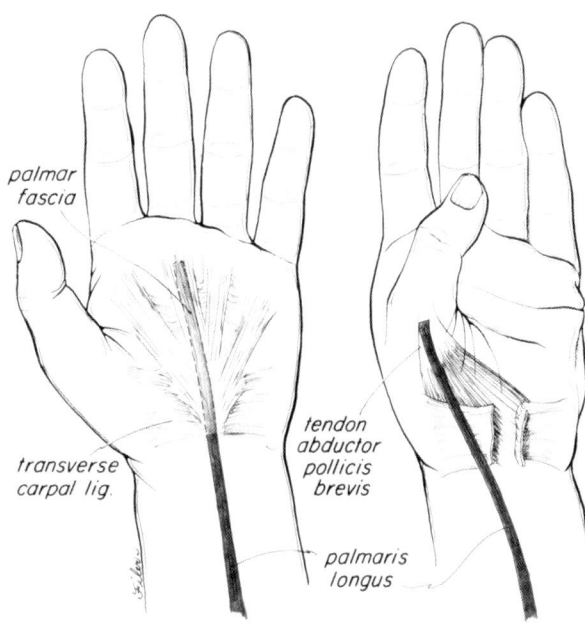

FIGURE 213-16. The Camitz transfer using the palmaris longus with its tendon extended by palmar fascia is schematically depicted.

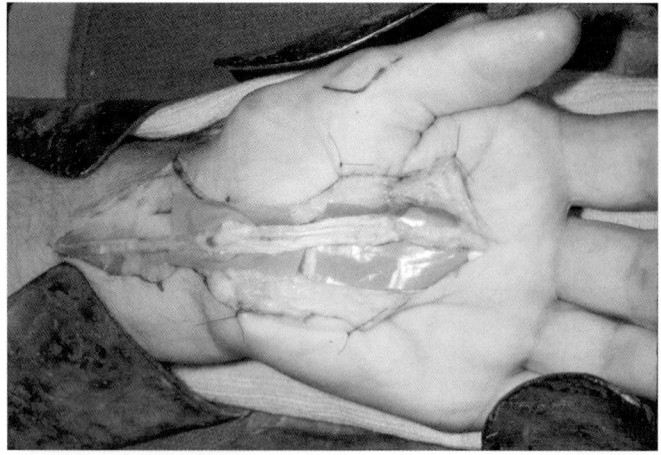

A

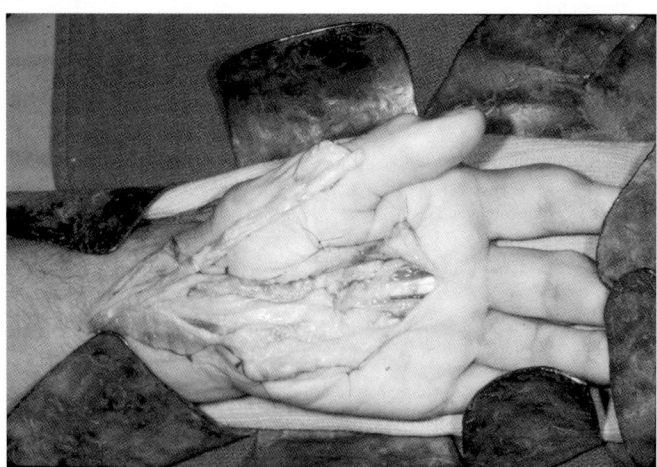

B

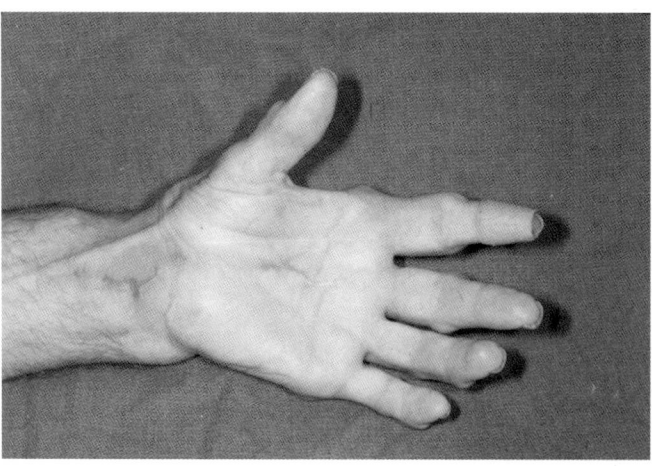

C

FIGURE 213-17. *A,* A wide strip of palmar fascia is dissected in continuity with the tendon of the palmaris longus. *B,* This is directly transferred to be inserted into the tendon of the APB. *C,* A postoperative result of the Camitz transfer.

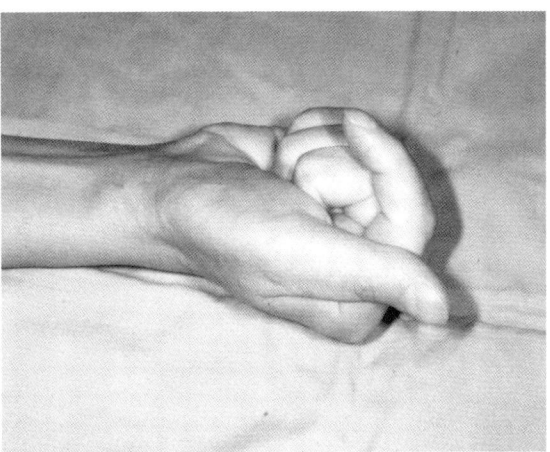

FIGURE 213-18. Inability to flex the interphalangeal joint of the thumb and the distal interphalangeal joint of the index finger as a consequence of high median nerve palsy.

(FPL) muscle. Patients are often still able to flex the long finger because of interconnections between the profundus tendons to the long, ring, and small fingers in the distal forearm. Therefore, the two functions that need to be restored in patients with a high median nerve palsy are flexion at the interphalangeal joint of the thumb and flexion of the PIP and DIP joints of the index and long fingers, together with a conventional opposition tendon transfer.

Operations

Flexion of the interphalangeal joint of the thumb may be restored by transfer of brachioradialis to FPL and flexion of the distal interphalangeal joint of the index and middle fingers by side-to-side tenodesis of the FDP II and III to IV and V (Fig. 213-19). The brachioradialis is divided at its insertion on the radial styloid and extensively mobilized from its investing fascia up into the proximal third of the forearm so that the freed muscle can develop approximately 30 mm of excursion. If reinnervation of the FPL muscle is not expected to occur after repair or grafting of the median nerve, the tendon can be divided at its musculotendinous junction and woven end-to-end into the brachioradialis tendon. However, if there is any possibility of reinnervation of the FPL, the brachioradialis tendon should be woven end-to-side into the FPL tendon, which remains in continuity.

Through the same volar forearm incision, the profundus tendons to the index and long fingers can be sutured side-to-side to the ulnar-innervated profundus tendons to the ring and small fingers (see Fig. 213-19). The results of these two transfers are also relatively predictable (Fig. 213-20).

If power flexion of the index and long fingers is required, formal transfer of the ECRL tendon to the index and long finger profundus tendons may be performed. The ECRL is transected through a small transverse incision at the base of the index finger metacarpal and passed subcutaneously around the radial border of the distal forearm into the volar incision. The profundus tendons to the index and long fingers are woven into the ECRL tendon so that with the wrist in 30 to 45 degrees of extension, the tips of the index and long fingers almost touch the palm. Similarly, with the wrist in full palmar flexion, the fingers will assume an almost fully extended position. Adjusting tension on this transfer by use of the tenodesis effect of the wrist is absolutely critical because the donor ECRL tendon has only 30 mm of amplitude, whereas the profundus tendons normally have 70 mm of excursion. If this transfer is sutured under too much tension, it will result in flexion contractures of these two fingers.

The timing of tendon transfers in a high median nerve palsy remains controversial.[5] If a good primary or delayed primary nerve repair can be performed, there is a reasonable chance of reinnervation of the extrinsic flexor muscles in a young patient. Consequently, early transfer of brachioradialis to FPL or side-to-side repair of the index and long finger profundus tendons to the ring and small finger profundus tendons is not necessary. However, if the patient is seen late and requires secondary nerve grafting of the median nerve, tendon transfers for restoration of

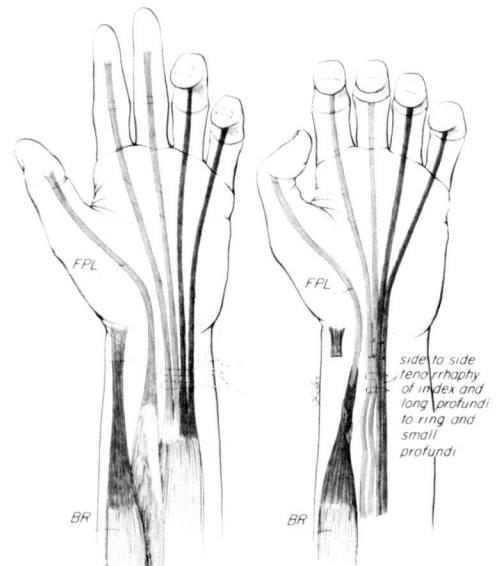

FIGURE 213-19. Transfer of the brachioradialis (BR) to flexor pollicis longus (FPL) and side-to-side FDP tenorrhaphy is schematically depicted.

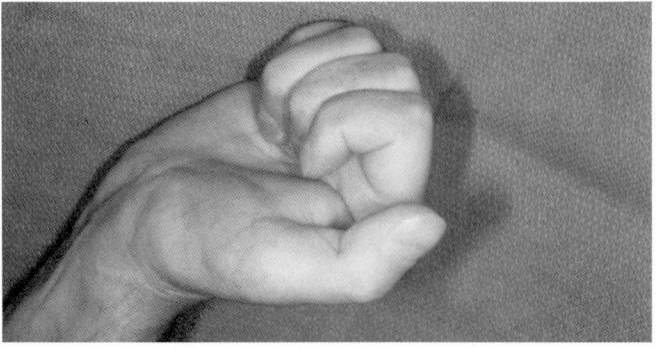

A

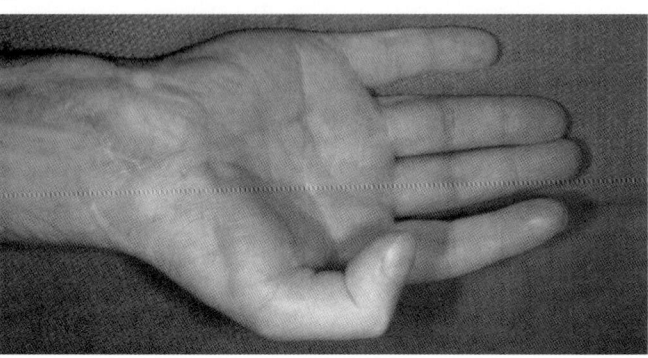

B

FIGURE 213-20. *A,* The finger flexion cascade has been restored by side-to-side tenorrhaphy of the FDP tendons. *B,* Semi-independent flexion of the interphalangeal joint of the thumb after brachioradialis to FPL transfer. Thumb interphalangeal joint flexion independent of finger flexion is not so predictable because the brachioradialis, after transfer, is not an easily retrained muscle in many individuals.

thumb flexion and index and long finger flexion should be performed simultaneously with the nerve graft.

Outcomes

There is no standard measurement of opposition in the literature. Some authors have developed functional scales to rate outcome, whereas others have reported the patient's subjective satisfaction.[36,37] An anatomic and biomechanical study by Cooney et al[27] showed that the FDS of the ring finger and the ECU were the best transfers to replace thenar strength, abduction, and pronation. They calculated that the ECU and FDS transfers restored 60% and 40%, respectively, of required thenar muscle strength. The Camitz transfer provided good abduction but weak flexion and opposition.

Excellent or good results were obtained in approximately 88% after EIP transfer in patients with nerve deficits secondary to leprosy.[38] Similar results have been reported by other authors, but few data documenting thumb range of motion or rigorous functional outcomes exist. There are few publications containing objective data that discuss the long-term functional outcomes of the Bunnell superficialis transfer. Brandsma et al[39] reported 32% excellent and 51% good results. Some of the other patients in this study under-

went FDS transfers for intrinsic function. Of the 158 donor fingers, swan-neck deformities were seen in 15%, DIP flexion contractures in 29%, and PIP flexion contractures in 18%. Groves and Goldner[40] reported 75% success in 16 patients with high median nerve or brachial plexus lesions reconstructed with superficialis opposition transfers.

Whereas Phalen and Miller[26] reported good results with the ECU transfer, another study described the development of significant radial deviation in one third of cases.[41] These authors cautioned that the FCU must have normal strength to maintain proper wrist balance after ECU transfer.

Terrono et al[42] retrospectively reviewed their experience with 33 Camitz transfers for severe median nerve compression in patients with a mean age of 65 years. Ninety-four percent of the patients thought that their thumb dexterity and speed were improved by the operation; only two patients were unhappy with the results. Braun[29] reported similar good results in 28 patients who underwent the Camitz transfer. No objective biomechanical data are available for this transfer.

Success is often defined differently in clinical studies, and thus a cohesive evaluation and enlightened recommendations are difficult to make (Table 213-3). Data on high median nerve palsy reconstruction are even more scarce.

TABLE 213-3 ◆ OPPOSITION TRANSFERS

Opposition Technique	Etiology	Reported Author	Success
Huber	Trauma Neurologic disease	Wissinger, 1977	80%
Camitz	Nerve compression	Terrono, 1993 Foucher, 1991	94% 91%
Extensor indicis proprius	Mixed trauma	Anderson, 1991 Burkhalter, 1973	88% 88%
Bunnell	Leprosy Leprosy Trauma Trauma	Brandsma, 1992 Palande, 1975 Kirkland, 1948 Groves, 1975	83% 94% 85% 75%
Extensor digiti quinti	Trauma	Schneider, 1969	80%

LOW ULNAR NERVE PALSY

Indications

Injury to the ulnar nerve distal to the innervation of the ring and small finger FDP and FCU muscles produces a functional deficit consisting of paralysis of all seven interossei, the ulnar two lumbricals, three hypothenar muscles and the adductor pollicis, and part of the FPB muscles. This results in an imbalance of the flexor and extensor forces at the MCP, PIP, and DIP joints of the fingers. Because the interossei are the main flexors of the MCP joints, extension of the proximal phalanges by the extrinsic extensor tendons is unopposed and MCP joint hyperextension occurs to the extent allowed by the volar plates. Because the extrinsic extensor tendons concentrate their extension at the MCP joints and the interossei are unable to actively extend at the PIP and DIP joints, the increased tension in the flexor tendons that occurs as the MCP joints begin to hyperextend will be unopposed at the PIP and DIP joints. This therefore produces the typical claw hand with hyperextension at the MCP joints and reciprocal flexion at the PIP and DIP joints (Fig. 213-21A). Imbalance between the extrinsic extensor and flexor tendons leads to weak grip strength and asynchronous flexion of the fingers. The MCP joints do not flex until after the interphalangeal joints have become completely flexed, resulting in curling of the tips of the fingers into the palm with loss of ability to grasp large objects (Fig. 213-21B and C). In a low ulnar nerve palsy, the clawing and loss of integrated MCP and interphalangeal joint flexion are confined to the ring and small fingers and to a lesser extent to the long finger because the lumbricals to the index and long fingers remain innervated by the median nerve. However, with a combined median and ulnar nerve palsy, all four fingers are affected. Fowler[43] has shown that the PIP joints can be extended by the extrinsic extensor tendons provided the MCP joints are stabilized against hyperextension. Both the claw deformity and the asynchronous flexion may therefore be improved either by static procedures to prevent hyperextension at the MCP joints or by dynamic tendon transfers either to produce MCP joint flexion alone or to provide both MCP joint flexion and interphalangeal joint extension.

The other significant impairment in patients with low ulnar nerve palsy is weak thumb–index finger pinch, which may be only 30% of normal because of paralysis of the adductor pollicis, half of the FPB, and the first dorsal interosseous muscles. However, in 58% of ulnar nerve injuries, there is dual innervation of the FPB muscle, which can to some extent provide thumb MCP joint flexion and key pinch to the index finger. Loss of key pinch is usually manifested by compensatory activation of the FPL, producing excessive flexion at the interphalangeal joint (Froment sign) (Fig. 213-22) and occasionally hyperextension at the MCP joint (Jeanne sign) as the patient attempts forceful pinch. In such patients with weak pinch, tendon transfers will be required to restore adduction of the thumb and abduction of the index finger.

Patients may also develop an irritating ulnar deviation of the small finger in addition to clawing at the MCP joint of the small finger (Wartenberg sign) caused by the unopposed action of the EDM tendon due to paralysis of the third palmar interosseous muscle. A tendon transfer may occasionally be required to correct this ulnar deviation of the small finger.

Timing

Timing of tendon transfers for ulnar nerve palsy is primarily dependent on two factors, the probability of motor recovery and the severity of the functional deficit. Primary microsurgical repair of the ulnar nerve at the

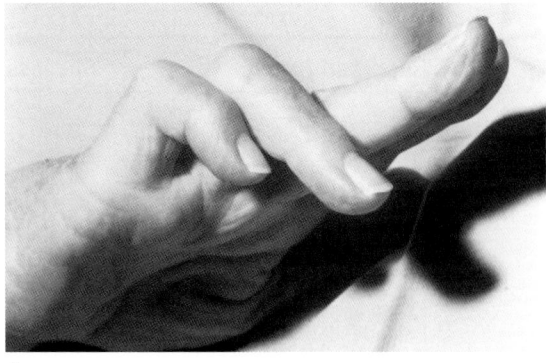

A

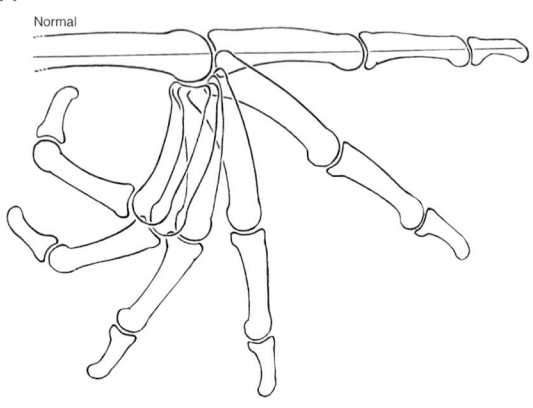

Normal

B

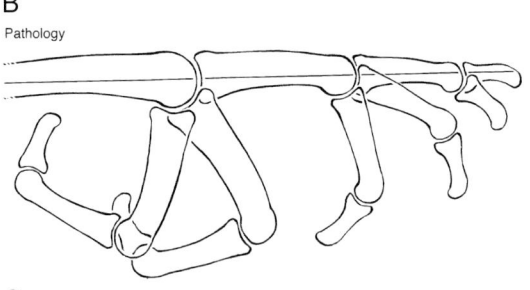

Pathology

C

FIGURE 213-21. *A,* The typical posture of the ulnar "claw" hand characterized by MCP hyperextension and reciprocal PIP and DIP flexion. *B,* The normal flexion arc is initiated at the MCP joints, and the pulp of the fingertip ascribes an equiangular curve as it moves from full extension to full flexion. This allows the normal finger to grasp equally well an object the size of a basketball or the size of a pencil. *C,* As the intrinsic minus fingers flex around an object, the fingers "roll up" with flexion initiated at the DIP and PIP joints, rather than beginning at the MCP joints. (From Hentz V, Chase R: Hand Surgery: A Clinical Atlas. Philadelphia, WB Saunders, 2001:402, 420.)

wrist can be expected to yield useful results in about 75% of patients. Secondary nerve grafting has been reported to provide some functional motor recovery in approximately 40% to 75% of cases, with a somewhat worse prognosis for sensory recovery. As in other peripheral nerve injuries, younger patients, those

with shorter nerve defects, and those without other significant associated injuries have a better chance of obtaining useful results from ulnar nerve repair.

Early tendon transfers should be considered for those with a debilitating claw deformity. Whereas clawing should be treated proactively with a lumbrical block splint, some patients may benefit from early static transfers to prevent MCP hyperextension and clawing. Trevett et al[44] studied the functional results after both high and low ulnar nerve repairs to better define the indications for tendon transfers. They demonstrated continued improvement in intrinsic muscle power, grip strength, and sensation for at least 2 years in high and 3 years in low ulnar nerve repairs. The significant conclusion from this study was that early tendon transfers should be performed only in manual laborers who complain of poor grip or key pinch.

CLAWING OF THE FINGERS

Static procedures to prevent hyperextension of the proximal phalanges at their MCP joints include capsulodesis and various tenodeses. Volar plate capsulodesis of the MCP joint, described by Zancolli,[45] is a simple technique in which the volar plate is advanced proximally and attached to the metacarpal neck to maintain the MCP joint in approximately 20 degrees of flexion. Parkes[46] has described an effective tenodesis both to prevent hyperextension at the MCP joints and to provide extension at the interphalangeal joints by use of a tendon graft sutured to the transverse carpal ligament and passed volar to the deep transverse intermetacarpal (intervolar plate) ligaments to insert into the radial lateral band of each finger. Fowler attached tendon grafts to the radial lateral bands, passed them volar to the deep transverse intermetacarpal ligaments, routed them dorsally through the intermetacarpal spaces, and then attached the grafts to the dorsal carpal ligament.[19] The Riordan tenodesis employs a similar dorsal route using two distally based strips of the ECRL and ECU tendons.[19]

The various dynamic tendon transfers that have been described to correct clawing differ primarily in whether they provide only MCP joint flexion or both MCP joint flexion and interphalangeal joint extension. The surgeon can determine which general type of transfer is most appropriate by preoperative testing of PIP and DIP joint extension with the MCP joints held passively flexed. If the extrinsic extensor tendons can produce full extension at the PIP and DIP joints with the MCP joint flexed (Fig. 213-23), the transfer may need to produce only strong MCP joint flexion by insertion of the transfer into the A1 pulley[45] (Fig. 213-24), into the A2 pulley,[47] or through a drill hole in the proximal phalanx.[48] However, with long-standing flexion deformities of the PIP joints, the central slip of the extensor mechanism may become attenuated.

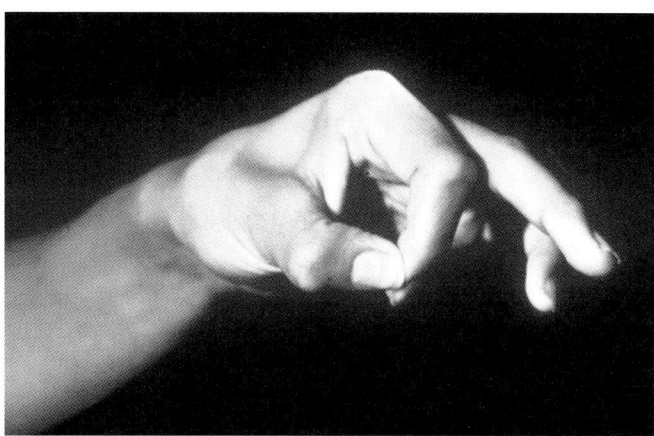

FIGURE 213-22. The thumb in ulnar nerve palsy. In the absence of the adductor pollicis and FPB, the FPL must provide all the power of thumb flexion. As the prime flexor of the interphalangeal joint, it preferentially flexes this joint, leading to interphalangeal hyperextension as greater activation occurs. This leads to a less stable pinch posture between the tip of the thumb and index finger as opposed to a more stable normal pinch between the broad pulp surface of the thumb and the digit. (From Hentz V, Chase R: Hand Surgery: A Clinical Atlas. Philadelphia, WB Saunders, 2001:436.)

Consequently, with passive flexion of the MCP joints, the patient cannot actively extend the PIP joints using the extrinsic extensor tendons. In these circumstances, the transfer should be inserted into one of the lateral

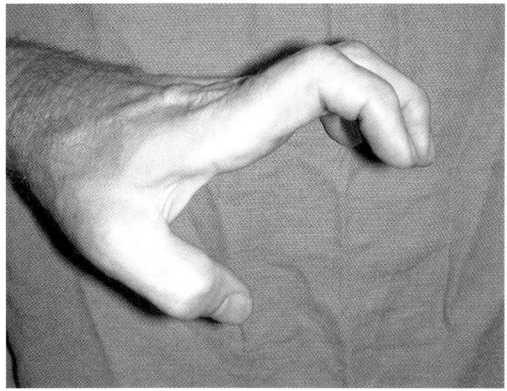

A

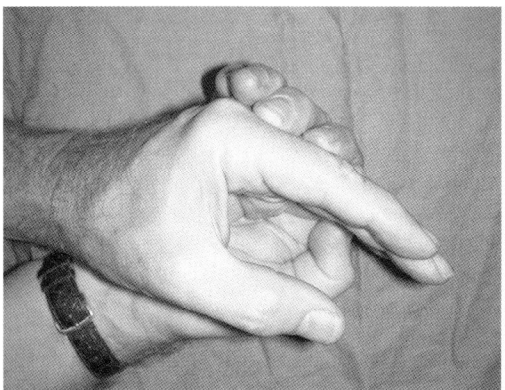

B

FIGURE 213-23. *A*, Fingers claw with unsupported MCP joints. *B*, However, when the MCP joints are held flexed, the patient is able to fully extend the PIP and DIP joints through the action of the still-innervated extrinsic extensors.

bands or into the dorsal base of the middle phalanx so that both MCP joint flexion and PIP joint extension can potentially be restored.

If one of the superficialis tendons is used as a donor tendon to produce either MCP joint flexion alone or both MCP joint flexion and interphalangeal joint extension, it does not produce any increase in power grip. Adding an extra muscle-tendon unit from outside the hand to activate these transfers, such as a wrist flexor or extensor tendon, will potentially lead to increased grip strength.

TENDON TRANSFERS TO PROVIDE MCP JOINT FLEXION ALONE

"Lasso" Transfers

In the Zancolli lasso procedure, the FDS tendons to the ring and small fingers are divided distal to the A1 pulley through a distal palmar crease incision. Each tendon is withdrawn from the flexor sheath between the A1 and A2 pulleys, looped around the A1 pulley, and sutured to itself. In patients with a high ulnar palsy, the ring and small finger superficialis tendons cannot be used; therefore, the long finger superficialis tendon is divided into two slips, and each slip is passed under the A1 pulleys of the ring and small fingers and sutured to itself (see Fig. 213-24).

In a combined high median-ulnar nerve palsy, all the superficialis tendons are paralyzed and consequently an indirect lasso procedure is required. After the superficialis tendons are passed around the A1 pulleys, the proximal ends of the superficialis tendons are activated by either the ECRL or FCR. Brooks and Jones[47] have described a variant of this transfer in which the ECRL or FCR is elongated with plantaris or toe extensor tendon grafts passed through the carpal tunnel and inserted more distally into the A2 pulley.

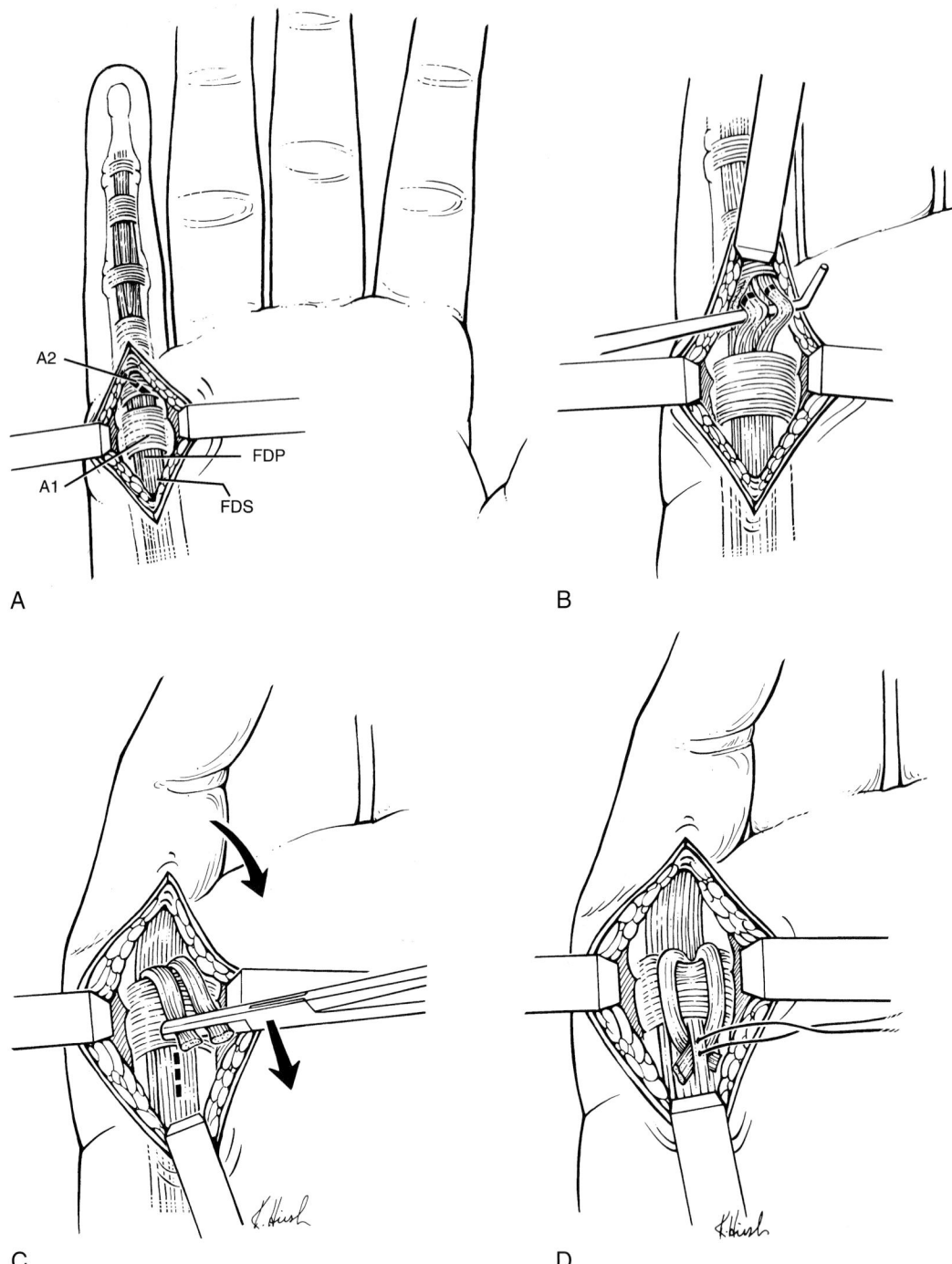

FIGURE 213-24. Illustration of the Zancolli lasso. *A,* The flexor digitorum superficialis (FDS) is isolated and divided distally. *B,* The FDS tendon is looped around the A1 pulley. *C* and *D,* The tendon is sutured to itself under tension. FDP, flexor digitorum profundus. (From Hentz V, Chase R: Hand Surgery, A Clinical Atlas. Philadelphia, WB Saunders, 2001:424.)

Burkhalter and Strait[48] have also used the same donor tendons, the ring finger superficialis and ECRL, but with insertion through a transverse drill hole in the middle third of the proximal phalanx. The ring finger superficialis is divided at the level of the PIP joint, withdrawn into the palm, and divided into two slips. Each slip is then passed down the lumbrical canal and drawn into a transverse drill hole on the radial aspect of the middle third of the proximal phalanx of the ring and small fingers. In patients with a high ulnar nerve palsy or a combined high median-ulnar nerve palsy, the ECRL can be extended with either two or four tendon grafts. The grafts are then passed through the intermetacarpal spaces and down the lumbrical canals volar to the deep transverse intermetacarpal ligaments and again attached into a drill hole on the radial aspect of the middle third of the proximal phalanges of all four digits. All these transfers will produce MCP joint flexion alone. Only those powered by a wrist flexor or extensor tendon will lead to increased power grip.

TENDON TRANSFERS TO PROVIDE SIMULTANEOUS MCP JOINT FLEXION AND INTERPHALANGEAL EXTENSION

Modified Stiles-Bunnell Transfer

In the modified Stiles-Bunnell transfer,[49] for patients with an isolated low ulnar nerve palsy, the ring finger superficialis tendon is divided just proximal to the PIP joint, withdrawn through a transverse distal palmar crease incision, and split longitudinally into two slips. In a high ulnar nerve palsy, the long finger FDS tendon is used. The radial lateral bands of the ring and small fingers are exposed through radial midaxial incisions, and each slip of the superficialis tendon is passed down the lumbrical canals of the ring and small fingers. With the wrist in neutral, each slip is sutured under good tension to the radial lateral band with the MCP joints in 45 degrees of flexion and the interphalangeal joints fully extended (Fig. 213-25). Tension is tested by the tenodesis effect of the wrist; with wrist extension, the fingers should assume the "intrinsic plus" position. The hand is immobilized in a dorsal block splint with the wrist in slight flexion and the MCP joints flexed 70 degrees for $3\frac{1}{2}$ to 4 weeks.

On occasion, the long or ring finger superficialis may be split into three slips should the long, ring, and small fingers need correction. With a total intrinsic palsy, the superficialis tendons to the long and ring fingers are each divided into two slips and passed down the lumbrical canals to the radial lateral bands of the index, long, ring, and small fingers. Brand advocates insertion of the slip to the index finger into the ulnar lateral band to provide improved three-point pinch. However, this may result in scissoring of the index and long fingers.

One of the disadvantages of the modified Stiles-Bunnell transfer is that the ring finger superficialis is

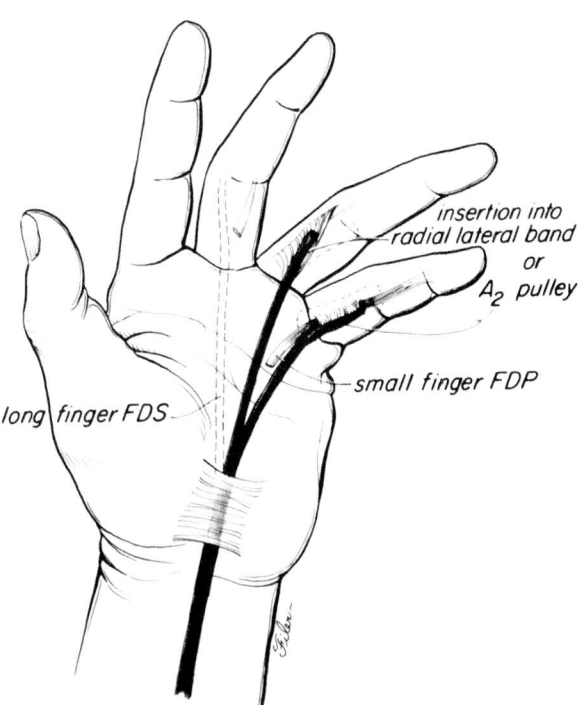

FIGURE 213-25. Transfer of the long finger flexor digitorum superficialis (FDS) to the radial lateral band of the ring finger or the A$_2$ pulley of the small finger is schematically illustrated. FDP, flexor digitorum profundus.

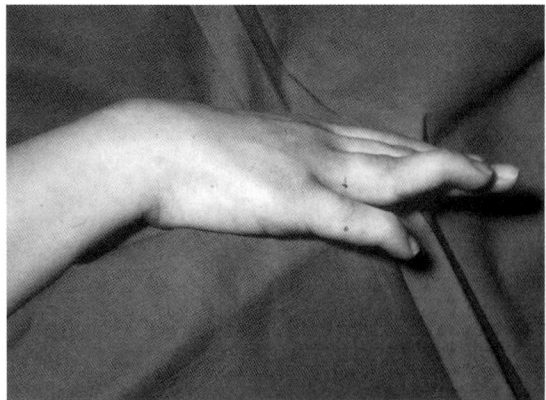

FIGURE 213-26. Attachment of the transfer into the lateral band may lead to a swan-neck deformity, particularly in a patient with inherent PIP volar plate laxity.

not expendable in a high ulnar nerve palsy or in a combined high median-ulnar nerve palsy. Second, the transfer may result in progressive overcorrection of the claw deformity, eventually resulting in a swan-neck hyperextension deformity at the PIP joints (Fig. 213-26). The modified Stiles-Bunnell transfer should therefore be used only in patients with mild PIP joint flexion contractures or stable fingers without passive hyperextension at the PIP joints.

Brand ECRL and ECRB Transfers

From his extensive experience with intrinsic transfers in patients with leprosy, Brand[2,50] has convincingly documented increased grip strength resulting from transfer of the ECRL with four plantaris tendon grafts passed through the lumbrical canals to the radial lateral bands of the long, ring, and small fingers and to the ulnar lateral band of the index finger (Brand II) in patients with a combined intrinsic palsy of leprosy (Fig. 213-27). In an isolated ulnar nerve palsy, this transfer is attached to the radial lateral bands of the ring and little fingers (Fig. 213-28).

In Brand's transfer for combined palsy, two short transverse incisions are made over the second dorsal extensor tendon compartment and over the radial aspect of the midforearm to allow transection of the ECRL tendon, which is withdrawn into the midforearm. The tendon is then passed around the radial border of the forearm into a transverse volar forearm incision approximately 2 to 3 inches proximal to the wrist crease. Each half of a folded plantaris tendon graft is then split longitudinally to make four slips and its proximal end sutured to the ECRL tendon projecting through the volar forearm incision. Through a 3-cm-long incision just to the ulnar side of the thenar crease, a tendon tunneling forceps is passed along the floor of the carpal tunnel to exit on the ulnar side of the

volar forearm incision. The four tendon grafts are then pulled distally through the carpal tunnel into the palmar incision. The proximal tendon juncture therefore lies distal to the volar forearm incision but proximal to the transverse carpal ligament. Through radial midaxial incisions over the proximal phalanges of the ring and small fingers (and the long finger if necessary), the tunneling forceps are passed volar to the deep transverse intermetacarpal ligaments through the lumbrical canals into the palmar incision, and the three tendon slips are brought into each midaxial incision. The tendon slip to the index finger may be tunneled through the first dorsal interosseous muscle to the radial lateral band or passed through the second intermetacarpal space to the ulnar lateral band as advocated by Brand. This will produce supination of the index finger and may provide better three-point pinch. The hand is positioned with the wrist extended 40 degrees, the MCP joints flexed 70 degrees, and the

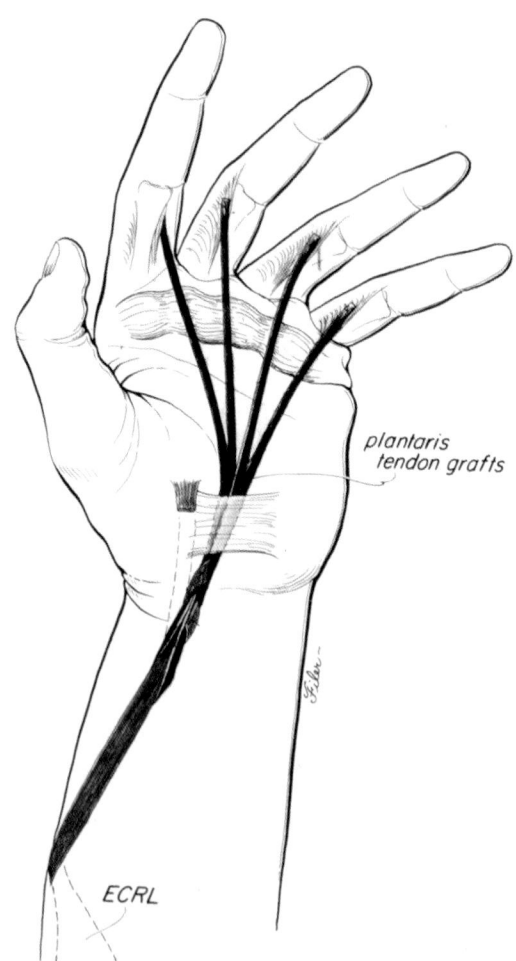

plantaris tendon grafts

ECRL

FIGURE 213-27. Brand II extensor carpi radialis longus (ECRL) transfer into all four lateral bands in a patient with combined low median and ulnar nerve palsy.

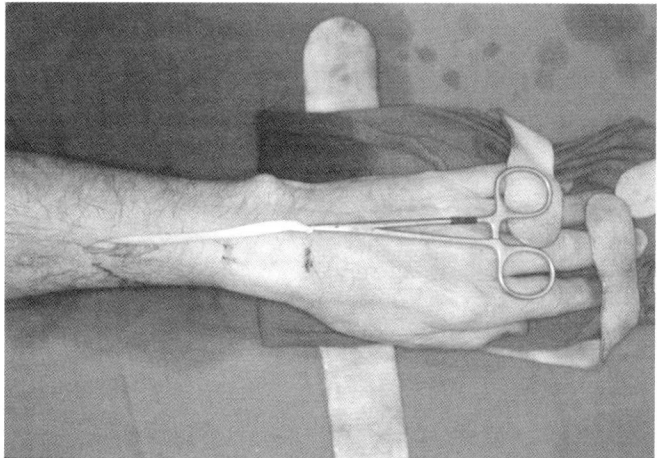

A

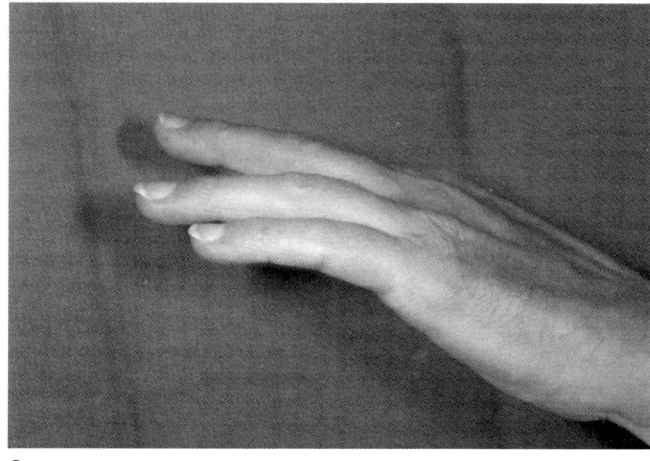

B

C

FIGURE 213-28. *A,* The ECRL is detached from its insertion into the base of the second metacarpal. *B,* A palmaris longus graft is attached to the ECRL, which has been brought volarly around the radial side of the forearm. *C,* Postoperatively, this has corrected the preoperative claw deformity of the fourth and fifth fingers.

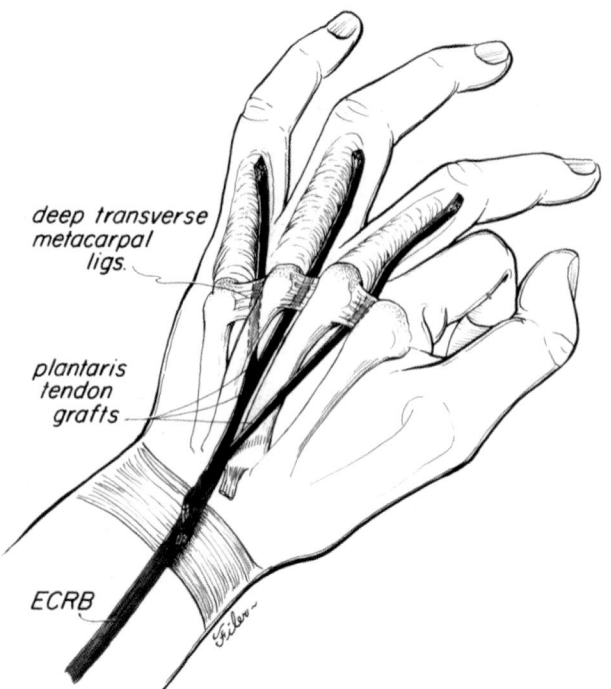

deep transverse
metacarpal
ligs.

plantaris
tendon
grafts

ECRB

FIGURE 213-29. Brand I extensor carpi radialis brevis (ECRB) transfer into the three ulnar fingers may be needed if the middle finger claws.

interphalangeal joints fully extended. After all the slack is taken up in the four plantaris grafts, they are sutured to the lateral bands just proximal to the PIP joints, and the hand is immobilized in this position for 3 weeks.

Brand originally described this intrinsic transfer as a dorsal transfer using the ECRB to activate a four-tailed plantaris graft passed from dorsal to volar through the intermetacarpal spaces (Brand I) (Fig. 213-29). However, during wrist extension, the ECRB and tendon grafts relax, which is a relative disadvantage of this dorsal routing of the original Brand I transfer. Riordan[19] has described a similar transfer using FCR transferred dorsally around the radial border of the forearm and elongated with tendon grafts passed through the intermetacarpal spaces volar to the deep transverse intermetacarpal ligaments to the radial lateral bands. This transfer is mutually beneficial if there is an associated flexion contracture of the wrist. The dorsal route also forms the basis for the Fowler transfer in which the EIP and EDM tendons are each split longitudinally and passed through the intermetacarpal spaces to the radial lateral bands of the fingers.[51] The EIP tendon controls the index and long fingers, and the EDM tendon controls the ring and small fingers. In a modification of this Fowler transfer, Riordan has described splitting only the EIP tendon into two slips and passing them through the third and fourth intermetacarpal spaces to insert into the radial lateral bands to correct clawing of the ring and small fingers.[51]

TENDON TRANSFER TO CORRECT ULNAR DEVIATION OF THE SMALL FINGER

A variant of the Fowler transfer has been advocated by Blacker et al[52] to correct the ulnar deviation deformity of the small finger (Wartenberg sign). The ulnar half of the EDM is detached, passed volar to the deep transverse intermetacarpal ligament, and sutured into the insertion of the radial collateral ligament of the MCP joint on the base of the proximal phalanx; or if there is associated clawing of the small finger, it is looped under the A2 pulley and sutured back to itself (Brooks insertion).

TENDON TRANSFERS TO PROVIDE FLEXION-ADDUCTION OF THE THUMB

The most successful tendon transfers to restore adduction of the thumb have a transverse direction of pull across the palm deep to the flexor tendons and insert into the tendon of the adductor pollicis. Littler[24] has advocated transfer of the ring finger superficialis deep to the flexor tendons of the index and long fingers and parallel to the transverse fibers of the adductor pollicis, where it is inserted into a drill hole just distal to the adductor insertion; he has been able to document an increase in pinch strength to 71% of the opposite hand. Smith[53] described use of the ECRB extended by a free tendon graft passed through the second intermetacarpal space and tunneled deep to the adductor pollicis to its insertion. Other tendon transfers for restoration of adduction of the thumb have included either the brachioradialis[63] or ECRL[13] elongated with a tendon graft and passed through the third intermetacarpal space to the thumb MCP joint and the EIP passed through the second intermetacarpal space.[50] Combined transfers to provide both thumb adduction and index finger abduction have been described by splitting the extensor indicis[63] or EDM.[58] On occasion, arthrodesis of the interphalangeal joint or MCP joint of the thumb may be a simpler alternative to tendon transfers to provide strong key pinch.

Ring Finger Flexor Digitorum Superficialis Transfer

The ring finger FDS tendon is transected between the A1 and A2 pulleys through a short incision at the base of the ring finger.[24] The superficialis tendon is then passed transversely across the palm deep to the index and long finger flexor tendons to the ulnar aspect of the thumb MCP joint, if necessary by a short incision just to the ulnar side of the thenar crease. The transfer is either sutured into the adductor pollicis tendon or passed into a drill hole through the proximal phalanx just distal to the adductor insertion and tied over a button. Tension is set with the wrist in neutral and the thumb adducted against the index finger with the superficialis tendon at its resting length. Appropriate tension is confirmed by tenodesis of the wrist; with wrist flexion, the thumb should be able to be passively abducted. Edgerton and Brand[25] have described a variation of this transfer in which the ring finger superficialis is brought through a window in the palmar fascia and then passed subcutaneously to the adductor insertion. Obviously, the ring finger superficialis cannot be used as an adductor transfer in patients with a high ulnar nerve palsy because this would deprive the ring finger of its only remaining flexor tendon.

Extensor Carpi Radialis Brevis Transfer

The ECRB is transected through a short transverse incision over the second dorsal extensor compartment just distal to the extensor retinaculum and withdrawn through a second transverse incision just proximal to the extensor retinaculum.[53] A small flap is then elevated over the ulnar aspect of the MCP joint of the thumb, and a palmaris or plantaris tendon graft is sutured to the tendon of the adductor pollicis. Through a short transverse incision overlying the proximal third of the second intermetacarpal space, a tendon passer is used to tunnel the tendon graft deep to the adductor pollicis and then to withdraw it dorsally through

the second intermetacarpal space. After the tendon graft is passed subcutaneously to the most proximal incision, it is woven into the ECRB tendon with the wrist in neutral and the thumb adducted (Fig. 213-30). Tension is then checked by tenodesis of the wrist; with palmar flexion, the thumb should become strongly adducted, whereas wrist extension should allow easy passive abduction of the thumb. The thumb is immobilized postoperatively for 3 weeks midway between full abduction and full adduction with the wrist in 20 to 30 degrees of dorsiflexion.

TENDON TRANSFERS TO PROVIDE INDEX FINGER ABDUCTION

Restoration of strong abduction of the index finger is the second component required for powerful pinch. Bunnell[49] described the transfer of extensor indicis extended with a short tendon graft and inserted into the first dorsal interosseous tendon. Bruner[68] divided the EPB tendon over the dorsum of the MCP joint of the thumb and tunneled it subcutaneously beneath the EPL tendon into the first dorsal interosseous tendon. However, one of the accessory tendons of the APL extended with a free tendon graft or attached to the rerouted EDC tendon of the index finger may be the best choice to restore abduction of the index finger.

Accessory Abductor Pollicis Longus and Free Tendon Graft

Neviaser et al[54] described an accessory APL tendon elongated with a palmaris or plantaris tendon graft transferred to the insertion of the first dorsal interosseous tendon (see Fig. 213-30). A small flap is elevated over the radial aspect of the proximal phalanx of the index finger, and a tendon graft is sutured to the first dorsal interosseous tendon just distal to the MCP joint. The proximal end of the tendon graft is then passed subcutaneously to a transverse incision over the first dorsal extensor compartment. After the compartment is opened, one of the accessory APL tendons is transected and interwoven with the tendon graft with the wrist in neutral position and the index finger radially abducted.

HIGH ULNAR NERVE PALSY

Indications and Operations

Many surgeons fail to realize the significant functional deficit in a high ulnar nerve palsy associated with paralysis of the FCU and profundus tendons to the ring and small fingers. The only remaining tendons on the ulnar side of the hand are the superficialis tendon to the ring finger and the usually diminutive superficialis tendon

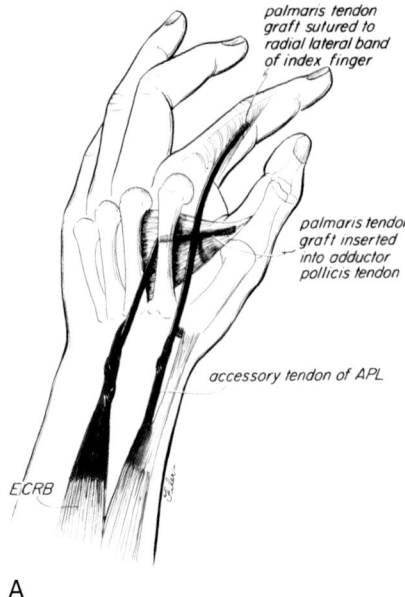

A

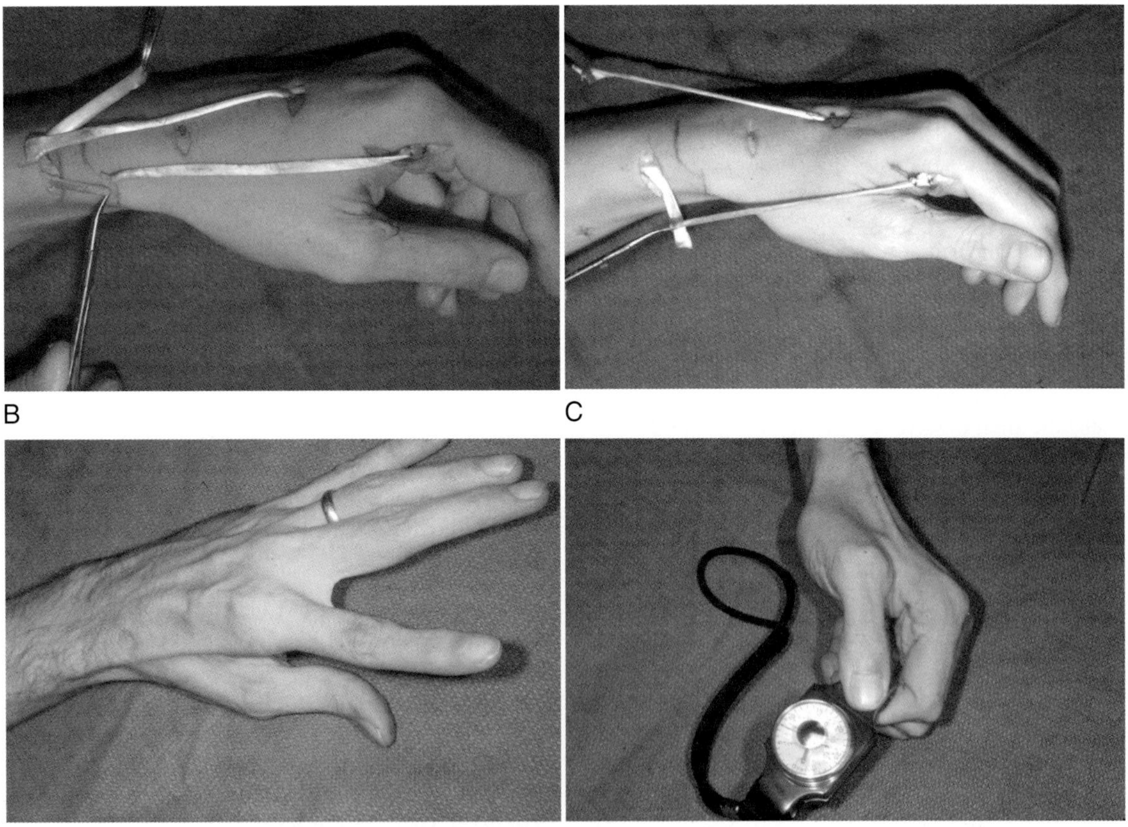

FIGURE 213-30. *A,* Transfers to restore thumb flexion-adduction and abduction of the index finger are schematically illustrated. *B,* A tendon graft has been anchored to the tendon of the adductor pollicis. It is passed dorsal to the flexor tendons and neurovascular bundles and then from palmar to dorsal through the second intermetacarpal space. A tendon graft has been sutured into the tendon of the first dorsal interosseous. *C,* Tension on these two grafts flexes and adducts the thumb and abducts the index finger at its MCP joint. *D,* Postoperative function after these two transfers. *E,* Pinch force is significantly improved. APL, abductor pollicis longus; ECRB, extensor carpi radialis longus.

to the small finger. However, paralysis of the profundus tendons to the ring and small fingers will often be masked by interconnections between these two tendons and the long finger profundus tendon in the distal forearm. If there is significant weakness of flexion of the ring and small fingers, power grip can be restored by side-to-side tenorrhaphy of the ring and small finger profundus tendons to the median-innervated long finger profundus tendon. To restore independent flexion of the ring and small fingers, the superficialis tendon of the long finger may be used as a donor tendon to activate the profundus tendons to the ring and small fingers. Patients requiring strong ulnar deviation and flexion of the wrist may also need to be considered for transfer of the FCR tendon to FCU.

Outcomes

There are few reports to substantiate the relative effectiveness of the various transfers to restore synchronous MCP flexion and interphalangeal extension of the fingers and thumb-index finger pinch. Hastings and Davidson[55] compared four techniques—Zancolli lasso, Stiles-Bunnell, Brand, and Riordan and Fowler transfers—for correction of the claw deformity in 12 patients with high, 14 patients with low, and 3 patients with mixed high and low ulnar nerve palsy. Successful outcomes were seen in the majority of cases. Most failures occurred in the small finger, and transfers using the superficialis tendons were found to further weaken the hand. Only transfers using wrist flexors or extensors have been shown to increase grip strength. A later report examining the effectiveness of the FDS lasso procedure showed similar results, with correction of clawing in 19 of 23 digits but no significant improvement in grip strength.[56] Brandsma et al[39] reported good (57%) or excellent (21%) results with use of the superficialis transfer to restore intrinsic function.

Quantitative measures of pinch strength have been shown to double after ECRB adductorplasty.[57] Hastings and Davidson[55] also showed an approximate doubling of pinch strength in hands treated with the ECRB transfer, although it is interesting that only 18 of the 34 patients in this study thought that pinch strength was compromised enough to warrant a tendon transfer. Robinson et al[58] evaluated the combination of the ulnar slip of EDM to provide thumb adduction and the EIP to restore index finger abduction in six patients and demonstrated an average improvement in pinch strength from 5% to 40% to 50% of the normal side.

TENDON TRANSFERS FOR COMBINED NERVE INJURIES

It is much more difficult to reconstruct the upper extremity affected by multiple nerve injuries. The majority of these patients require multiple reconstructive procedures and tendon transfers. The choice of tendon transfers and the timing of the surgery should be well planned, designed and individualized to address the patient's specific functional needs. It is unwise to adopt a "cookbook" approach for reconstruction of the patient with combined nerve injuries. Basic principles of tendon transfers, such as soft tissue equilibrium, full passive range of motion of involved joints, selection of the appropriate donor muscle, and direction of transfer as outlined earlier, should be carefully considered in preoperative planning.

Before any operation is performed, the patient should be educated about the goals and risks of the procedure and the fact that the injured extremity will never be normal. As a general rule, the results of tendon transfers for combined nerve injuries are inferior to those for a single nerve injury.[59,60]

Adding to the complexity of these problems, the number of donor tendons is limited, more joints need to be mobilized, there is a more profound sensory loss, and the soft tissues may be more scarred in this population of patients. Multiple nerve repairs or nerve grafting should be done as soon as clinically appropriate, but return of motor function rarely extends beyond two major joints distal to the injury.[60] Reinnervated muscles, however, should not be used or should be used only with great caution as donors for tendon transfers.

Dynamic tenodesis is an important concept in reconstruction of these combined nerve injuries. Wrist flexion or extension can be used to augment the excursion of any tendon transfer that crosses the wrist. For example, if a wrist flexor such as the FCR is used to activate the FDP, flexion of the fingers will be enhanced if the patient extends the wrist using the ECRL or ECRB simultaneously with contraction of the FCR transfer. Therefore, if the excursion of a tendon transfer is less than optimal to produce a specific function, increased range of motion can be achieved through wrist tenodesis.[61]

Low Median-Low Ulnar Nerve Palsy

A low median and low ulnar nerve palsy is the most common combined nerve injury in the upper extremity and is usually the result of a "spaghetti-wrist" laceration.[62] This leads to complete loss of sensation on the palmar surface of the hand and a complete intrinsic motor paralysis that results in a claw hand deformity. The hallmark of this injury is a flat transverse metacarpal arch with hyperextension at the MCP joints and hyperflexion of the PIP joints accompanied by an abducted small finger. It is especially important to prevent an adduction contracture of the thumb-index web space.[63] The surgeon should repair or graft the median and ulnar nerves before any tendon transfers are performed to restore some protective sensibility to the hand. The goals of reconstruction in a low median-low ulnar nerve palsy are to restore thumb adduction, thumb abduction and opposition, and abduction of the index finger and to improve extension of the PIP joints of the fingers.

Thumb adduction for key pinch can be restored by transfer of the ECRB extended by a tendon graft through the second intermetacarpal space and inserted into the adductor tubercle of the thumb metacarpal or, alternatively, by transfer of the superficialis tendon from the ring finger to the adductor insertion. The best option for reconstruction of thumb opposition is the EIP transfer rerouted around the ulnar border of the hand and inserted into the APB tendon.[28,49,64] This transfer can be combined with arthrodesis of the MCP joint of the thumb to allow maximum stability.[65] Index finger abduction for strong pinch can be restored by transfer of one of the APL tendon slips extended by a tendon graft to the first dorsal interosseous insertion. Finally, clawing of the fingers can be corrected by use of the ECRL or ECRB or brachioradialis extended by four tendon grafts and inserted into either the A2 pulleys or the radial lateral bands as previously discussed. Alternatively, if the patient has developed a flexion contracture of the wrist, by involuntarily trying to prevent clawing by flexing the wrist, the FCR tendon may be used to motor the four tendon grafts.[19]

If the patient still has poor palmar sensibility despite nerve repair or nerve grafting, consideration should be given to transfer of a superficial radial nerve-innervated flap to the thumb or nerve transfer of the superficial radial nerve to the distal median nerve.

High Median-High Ulnar Nerve Palsy

This is a severe injury in which there is no active flexion of the fingers and thumb and loss of thumb opposition and key pinch in addition to the loss of palmar sensibility. Initially, the fingers may be fully extended even at the interphalangeal joints despite the intrinsic paralysis. However, once tendon transfers are completed to provide active finger flexion, the fingers gradually assume a claw posture. Tendon transfers for reconstruction of a high median-high ulnar nerve palsy have to be performed in two or three stages. The goals are to restore finger and thumb flexion, thumb-index finger pinch, and abduction and opposition of the thumb; and to correct the later development of clawing of the fingers.

Thumb adduction and key pinch can be achieved by transfer of the ECRB with a free tendon graft through the second intermetacarpal space to the

adductor pollicis insertion.[53,66] Finger flexion can be restored by transfer of the ECRL to the four FDP tendons.[67] This can be combined with tenodesis of the DIP joints of the three ulnar fingers.[62] Flexion of the thumb can be restored by transfer of the brachioradialis to the FPL through the same palmar incision.[67] The brachioradialis muscle must be mobilized and elevated off the radius into the proximal third of the forearm. A Pulvertaft tendon weave is then performed between the brachioradialis and FPL in the distal third of the forearm.[59,62] As in a low median-low ulnar nerve palsy, the most reliable procedure for thumb opposition is transfer of the EIP to the APB insertion. If the interphalangeal joint of the thumb tends to assume a flexed position, the EIP transfer should be inserted both into the APB insertion and then into the EPL tendon just proximal to the interphalangeal joint.[19] If thumb pinch remains unstable with MCP extension and interphalangeal joint flexion, arthrodesis of the MCP joint should be considered. A useful procedure that avoids the need to fuse the interphalangeal joint of the thumb involves longitudinal splitting of the FPL tendon, detachment of the radial half from its insertion into the distal phalanx, and transfer of this tendon slip dorsally where it is attached into the EPL tendon proximal to the interphalangeal joint of the thumb. This results in a dynamic stabilization of the interphalangeal joint when the transfer pulls through the FPL.

If the fingers begin to adopt a clawed position after finger flexion has been restored, there are no expendable wrist extensors (ECRL and ECRB) remaining to provide integration of MCP flexion and interphalangeal joint extension; static tenodesis techniques may be necessary. Free tendon grafts can be placed from the deep transverse metacarpal ligaments to the lateral bands[46] or from the dorsal carpal ligament to the lateral bands.[19] Alternatively, hyperextension can be prevented by Zancolli capsulodeses, or arthrodesis of the PIP joints can be performed. Finally, abduction of the index finger for pinch can be restored by an accessory APL tendon extended with a free tendon graft to the first dorsal interosseous or alternatively by use of the EPB.[68]

The importance of restoring sensibility to the radial side of the hand in a high median-high ulnar nerve palsy, by either secondary nerve repair or nerve grafting, cannot be overstated. A sensate hand is the prerequisite for performing the tendon transfers mentioned. If sensation cannot be restored, Omer[59] has advocated a fillet flap of the index finger to resurface the thumb-long finger web space with dorsal skin innervated by the superficial radial nerve. Alternatively, a first dorsal metacarpal artery flap innervated by the superficial branch of the radial nerve can be transferred to the palmar surface of the thumb, or the superficial radial nerve itself can be transferred to the distal median nerve as a "nerve-transfer" technique.

TENDON TRANSFERS FOR RECONSTRUCTION AFTER TRAUMA

Tendon transfers are an excellent method of restoring active motion to the hand and wrist after traumatic injuries of the muscles and tendons of the forearm, wrist, and hand. If there has been segmental loss of tendon, a tendon graft is often used instead of a tendon transfer. With more severe trauma (industrial or motor vehicle accidents, blast, missile and explosion injuries), associated damage to the soft tissues will leave a scarred bed that is unsuitable for tendon grafts; a tendon graft is more likely to become adherent to the scarred surrounding tissue than is a tendon transfer. If a forearm muscle itself has been severely damaged, a tendon graft will be unable to restore active motion, and a tendon transfer will be necessary.

Time is another important consideration in reconstruction of the post-traumatic upper extremity. The unavoidable fate of injured muscle is myostatic contracture and atrophy if there has been a long delay between the traumatic event and the reconstructive procedure, again making a tendon transfer a more suitable option for reconstruction.

Restoration of Thumb Extension

Rupture of the EPL tendon occurs in approximately 1 in 200 distal radius fractures, classically at Lister tubercle, and it may happen at any time from several weeks to several months after the fracture. Ischemia of the tendon due to swelling and edema of the tenosynovium and attrition over the roughened dorsal radial cortex have been postulated to cause this tendon rupture.[69-72] Patients present with weak extension or loss of extension at the interphalangeal joint or paradoxically with incomplete extension at the MCP joint as well as inability to raise the thumb dorsal to the plane of the hand (Fig. 213-31).

The optimal choice for restoration of thumb extension is the EIP to EPL transfer, which can be performed under local anesthesia (see Fig. 213-31). The EIP tendon is harvested through a short transverse incision just proximal to the index finger MCP joint, and its distal stump is then sutured end-to-side to the EDC tendon of the index finger to prevent extensor lag of this finger. The EIP is retrieved through a second transverse incision just distal to the transverse carpal ligament. A third incision is made over the distal third of the thumb metacarpal, and the EIP is channeled subcutaneously to this incision. The distal end of the EIP is sutured to the distal end of the EPL with the wrist held in neutral and the thumb fully extended and parallel or just volar to the plane of the palm.[73] The tension of the transfer can be checked by tenodesis of the wrist. With wrist flexion, the thumb should move dorsal to

the plane of the palm; with wrist extension, the thumb should be able to be placed in full passive abduction and opposition. The patient is even able to use the transferred EIP and extend the thumb on the operating table. The wrist is immobilized postoperatively in 40 degrees of extension with the thumb in abduction and extension for 3 to 4 weeks. A removable splint is used for an additional 3 or 4 weeks, and there is usually no need for retraining.

Restoration of Finger Extension

Restoration of finger extension after trauma can be accomplished by tendon transfers similar to those used for radial nerve palsy. These transfers, which are discussed in detail earlier in this chapter, include transfer of either of the wrist flexors FCU or FCR to the EDC and the Boyes transfer of the FDS of the long and ring fingers to the EDC.

Restoration of Thumb Flexion

Acute lacerations or ruptures of the FPL tendon can be treated by primary or delayed primary repair or tendon grafting. However, with missed diagnosis, the muscle fibers undergo significant shortening, atrophy, and fibrosis within 6 months to a year from injury. In these situations, it is preferable to restore thumb flexion with a tendon transfer, usually the FDS of the ring finger.

The ring finger superficialis is harvested through a transverse incision at the base of the proximal phalanx and retrieved through a second incision in the proximal palm. It is then passed through the FPL sheath to the base of the distal phalanx through an open incision or attached to a fine rubber catheter or feeding tube and withdrawn distally through the sheath. The ring finger FDS to FPL tendon transfer can be performed in one stage or in two stages if the bed is scarred and poor with initial placement of a Silastic tendon rod (Fig. 213-32).[74] If necessary, a pulley can be reconstructed with the old FPL tendon remnant or with a palmaris longus graft.[66] The tendon is sutured to the distal phalanx of the thumb with a pull-out suture fixed over a button. The tension of the transfer can be checked by wrist tenodesis. With the wrist in full flexion, the thumb should extend completely; with wrist extension, the thumb tip should overlie the ring finger MCP joint.

Restoration of Finger Flexion

Patients may occasionally present with severe crushing or avulsion injuries involving the forearm flexor muscles. The options for secondary reconstruction of finger flexion are a tendon transfer of the ECRL to all four FDP tendons or a functioning free gracilis muscle transfer.

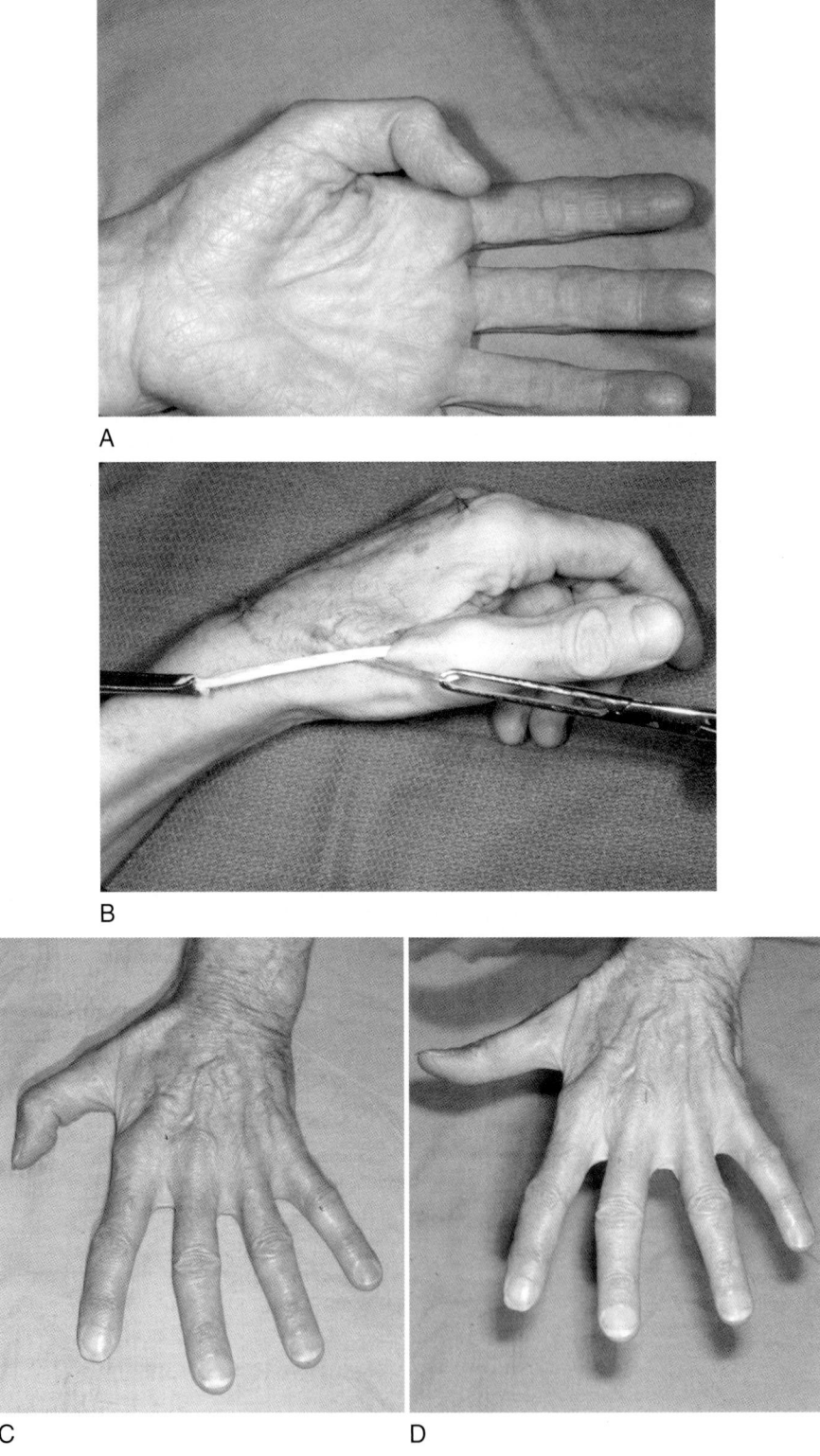

FIGURE 213-31. *A,* Rupture of the EPL. *B,* Transfer of the EIP to the EPL. *C,* Preoperative thumb extension. *D,* Postoperative thumb extension.

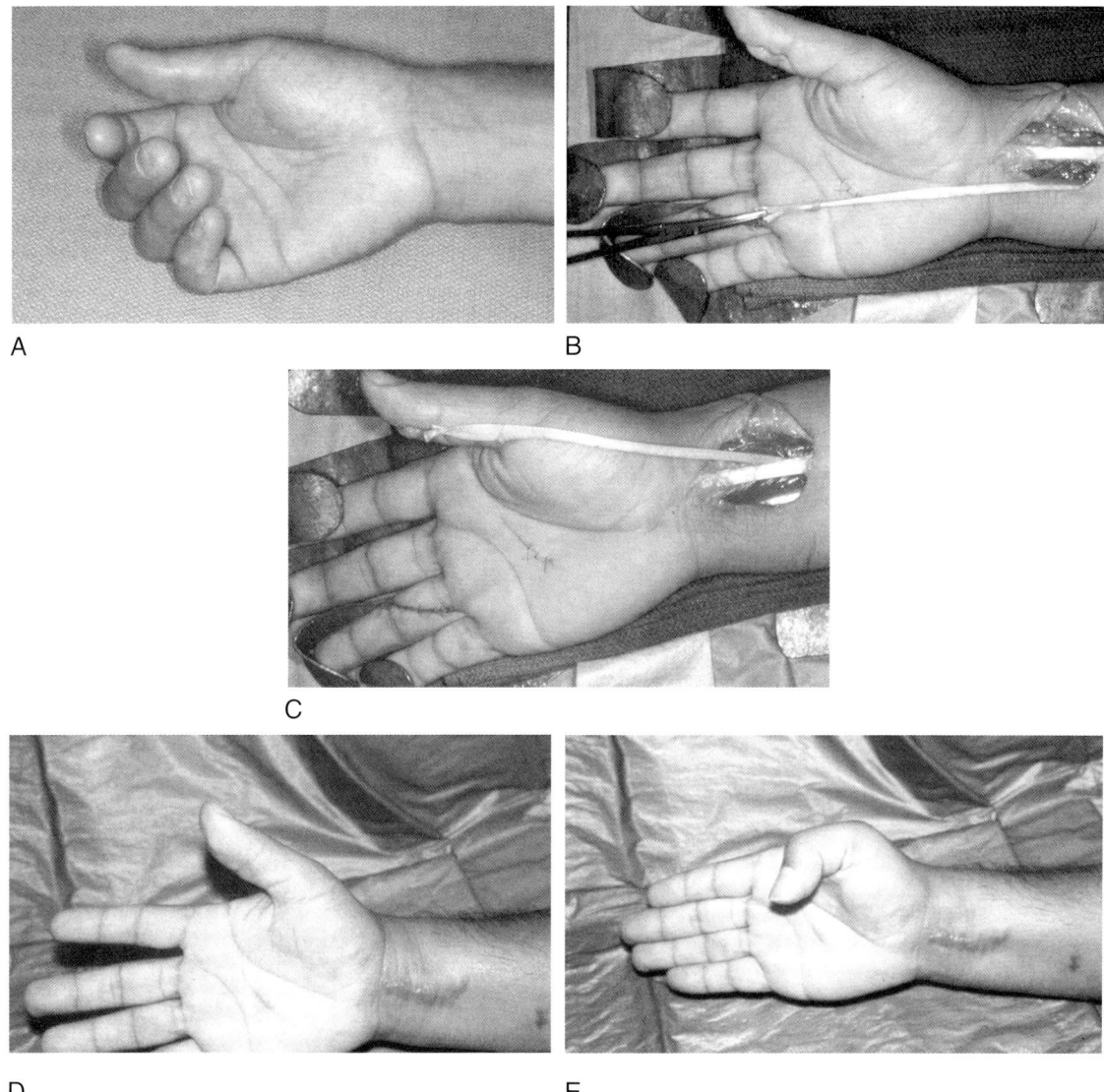

FIGURE 213-32. *A*, Missed laceration of the FPL tendon. *B*, After a first stage insertion of a Silastic rod permits the development of a smooth gliding bed for the transfer of the ring finger FDS tendon. *C*, The FDS tendon is prepared for passage into its new sheath. *D*, Postoperative extension. *E*, Postoperative flexion.

The ECRL is transected at the base of the index finger metacarpal and mobilized through a longitudinal incision on the dorsum of the forearm. It is then tunneled subcutaneously around the radial border of the forearm to a palmar incision over the distal forearm. Great care has to be exercised in adjusting the tension when the ECRL is sutured to all four FDP tendons because the ECRL has only 30 mm of amplitude, and the FDP tendons require 70 mm of excursion for full finger flexion. Insertion of the transfer too tightly will prevent full finger extension. The wrist tenodesis effect is vitally important in this transfer. Wrist extension should cause the fingers to flex down to the palm, whereas wrist flexion should allow the fingers to come out to full extension. If the FPL is also nonfunctioning, thumb flexion can be restored by transferring the brachioradialis to the FPL through the same palmar incision.

SUMMARY

Tendon transfers, if carefully selected and performed meticulously, will provide a gratifying functional improvement to the hand affected by radial, median, ulnar, or combined nerve palsies as well as by severe trauma of the extrinsic flexor and extensor muscles and tendons. Quantitative outcome data are lacking for many of the tendon transfers described, but surgeons and patients can attest to the significant benefits derived from them. Comparative studies must be designed in the future to document the effectiveness of the various transfers and their ultimate impact on hand function and return to work.

REFERENCES

1. Steindler A: Tendon transplantation in the upper extremity. Am J Surg 1939;44:260.
2. Brand PW: Clinical Mechanics of the Hand. St. Louis, CV Mosby, 1985.
3. Brand PW, Beach RB, Thompson DE: Relative tension and potential excursion of muscles in the forearm and hand. J Hand Surg Am 1981;6:209-219.
4. Omer JE: The technique and timing of tendon transfers. Orthop Clin North Am 1974;4:243.
5. Burkhalter WE: Early tendon transfer in upper extremity peripheral nerve injury. Clin Orthop 1974;104:68-79.
6. Mayer JH, Mayfield FH: Surgery of the posterior interosseous branch of the radial nerve: analysis of 58 cases. Surg Gynecol Obstet 1947;84:979.
7. Young C, Hudson A, Richards R: Operative treatment of palsy of the posterior interosseous nerve of the forearm. J Bone Joint Surg Am 1990;72:1215-1219.
8. Kallio PK, Vastamaki M, Solonen KA: The results of secondary microsurgical repair of radial nerve in 33 patients. J Hand Surg Br 1993;18:320-322.
9. Bevin AG: Early tendon transfer for radial nerve transection. Hand 1976;8:134-136.
10. Franke F: Sehnenüberpflanzug. Arch Klin Chir 1896;52:87.
11. Zachary RB: Tendon transplantation for radial paralysis. Br J Surg 1946;23:350.
12. Starr CL: Army experiences with tendon transference. J Bone Joint Surg 1922;4:3.
13. Boyes JH: Tendon transfers for radial palsy. Bull Hosp Joint Dis 1960;21:97.
14. Chuinard RG, Boyes JH, Stark HH, Ashworth CR: Tendon transfers for radial nerve palsy: use of superficialis tendons for digital extension. J Hand Surg Am 1978;3:560-570.
15. Tsuge K, Adachi N: Tendon transfer for extensor palsy of forearm. Hiroshima J Med Sci 1969;18:219-232.
16. Thompson M, Rasmussen KB: Tendon transfers for defective long extensors of the wrist and fingers. Scand J Plast Reconstr Surg 1969;3:71.
17. Tsuge K: Tendon transfers for radial nerve palsy. Aust N Z J Surg 1980;50:267-272.
18. Raskin KB, Wilgis EF: Flexor carpi ulnaris transfer for radial nerve palsy: functional testing of long-term results. J Hand Surg Am 1995;20:737-742.
19. Riordan DC: Tendon transplantations in median nerve and ulnar nerve paralysis. J Bone Joint Surg Am 1953;35:312.
20. Fujiwara A, Ryo F, Kashiwagi D, Fujita H: Evaluation of the Boyes' method in the treatment of radial nerve paralysis [in Japanese]. Seikei Geka 1970;21:954-956.
21. Bunnell S: Opposition of the thumb. J Bone Joint Surg 1938;20:269.
22. Royle ND: An operation for paralysis of the intrinsic muscles of the thumb. JAMA 1938;111:612.
23. Thompson TC: A modified operation for opponens paralysis. J Bone Joint Surg 1942;24:632.
24. Littler JW: Tendon transfers and arthrodeses in combined median and ulnar nerve paralysis. J Bone Joint Surg Am 1949;31:225.
25. Edgerton MT, Brand PW: Restoration of abduction and adduction to the unstable thumb in median and ulnar paralysis. Plast Reconstr Surg 1965;36:150.
26. Phalen GS, Miller RC: The transfer of wrist extensor muscles to restore or reinforce flexion power of the fingers and opposition of the thumb. J Bone Joint Surg 1947;29:993.
27. Cooney WP, Linscheid RL, An KN: Opposition of the thumb: an anatomic and biomechanical study of tendon transfers. J Hand Surg Am 1984;9:777-786.
28. Burkhalter W, Christensen RC, Brown P: Extensor indicis proprius opponensplasty. J Bone Joint Surg Am 1973;55:725-732.
29. Braun RM: Palmaris longus tendon transfer for augmentation of the thenar musculature in low median palsy. J Hand Surg Am 1978;3:488-491.
30. Camitz H: Über die Behandlung der Opposition-Slahmung. Acta Chir Scand 1929;65:77.
31. Littler JW, Li CS: Primary restoration of thumb opposition with median nerve decompression. Plast Reconstr Surg 1967;39:74-75.
32. Huber E: Hilfsoperation bei Medianus Slahmung. Dtsch Z Chir 1921;126:271.
33. Nicolaysen J: Transplantation des m. abductor dig. V bei fehlender Oppositionsfähigkeit des Daumens. Dtsch Z Chir 1922;168:133.
34. Taylor RT: Reconstruction of the hand: a new technique in tenoplasty. Surg Gynecol Obstet 1921;32:237.
35. Schneider LH: Opponensplasty using the extensor digiti minimi. J Bone Joint Surg Am 1969;51:1297-1302.
36. Jensen EG: Restoration of opposition of the thumb. Hand 1978;10:161-167.
37. Kirklin JW, Thomas CG: Opponen transplant: an analysis of the methods employed and results obtained in 75 cases. Surg Gynecol Obstet 1948;86:213.
38. Anderson GA, Lee V, Sundararaj GD: Extensor indicis proprius opponensplasty. J Hand Surg Br 1991;16:334-338.
39. Brandsma JW, Ottenhoff-De Jonge MW: Flexor digitorum superficialis tendon transfer for intrinsic replacement. Long-term results and the effect on donor fingers. J Hand Surg Br 1992;17:625-628.

40. Groves RJ, Goldner JL: Restoration of strong opposition after median-nerve or brachial plexus paralysis. J Bone Joint Surg Am 1975;57:112-115.

41. Wood VE, Adams J: Complications of opponensplasty with transfer of extensor carpi ulnaris to extensor pollicis brevis. J Hand Surg Am 1984;9:699-704.

42. Terrono AL, Rose JH, Mulroy J, Millender LH: Camitz palmaris longus abductorplasty for severe thenar atrophy secondary to carpal tunnel syndrome. J Hand Surg Am 1993;18:204-206.

43. Fowler BS: Extensor apparatus of the digits. J Bone Joint Surg Br 1949;31:477.

44. Trevett MC, Tuson C, de Jager LT, Juon JM: The functional results of ulnar nerve repair. Defining the indications for tendon transfer. J Hand Surg Br 1995;20:444-446.

45. Zancolli EA: Claw hand caused by paralysis of the intrinsic muscles. A simple surgical procedure for its correction. J Bone Joint Surg Am 1957;39:1076.

46. Parkes A: Paralytic claw fingers—a graft tenodesis operation. Hand 1973;5:192-199.

47. Brooks AL, Jones DS: A new intrinsic tendon transfer for the paralytic hand. J Bone Joint Surg Am 1975;57:730.

48. Burkhalter WE, Strait JL: Metacarpophalangeal flexor replacement for intrinsic-muscle paralysis. J Bone Joint Surg Am 1973;55:1667-1676.

49. Bunnell S: Surgery of the intrinsic muscles of the hand other than those producing opposition of the thumb. J Bone Joint Surg 1942;24:1.

50. Brand PW: Tendon grafting illustrated by a new operation for intrinsic paralysis of the fingers. J Bone Joint Surg Br 1961;43:444.

51. Enna CD, Riordan DC: The Fowler procedure for correction of the paralytic claw hand. Plast Reconstr Surg 1973;52:352-360.

52. Blacker GJ, Lister GD, Kleinert HE: The abducted little finger in low ulnar nerve palsy. J Hand Surg Am 1976;1:190-196.

53. Smith RJ: Extensor carpi radialis brevis tendon transfer for thumb adduction—a study of power pinch. J Hand Surg Am 1983;8:4-15.

54. Neviaser RJ, Wilson JN, Gardner MM: Abductor pollicis longus transfer for replacement of first dorsal interosseous. J Hand Surg Am 1980;5:53-57.

55. Hastings H, Davidson S: Tendon transfers for ulnar nerve palsy. Evaluation of results and practical treatment considerations. Hand Clin 1988;4:167-178.

56. Hastings H, McCollam SM: Flexor digitorum superficialis lasso tendon transfer in isolated ulnar nerve palsy: a functional evaluation. J Hand Surg Am 1994;19:275-280.

57. Mannerfelt L: Studies on the hand in ulnar nerve paralysis. A clinical-experimental investigation in normal and anomalous innervation. Acta Orthop Scand Suppl 1966;87:1.

58. Robinson D, Aghasi MK, Halperin N: Restoration of pinch in ulnar nerve palsy by transfer of split extensor digiti minimi and extensor indicis. J Hand Surg Br 1992;17:622-624.

59. Omer GE Jr: Tendon transfers in combined nerve lesions. Orthop Clin North Am 1974;5:377-387.

60. Omer GE Jr: Injuries to nerves of the upper extremity. J Bone Joint Surg Am 1974;56:1615-1624.

61. Eversmann WW Jr: Tendon transfers for combined nerve injuries. Hand Clin 1988;4:187-199.

62. Brand PW: Tendon transfers for median and ulnar nerve paralysis. Orthop Clin North Am 1970;1:447-454.

63. Omer GE Jr: Reconstruction of a balanced thumb through tendon transfers. Clin Orthop 1985;195:104-116.

64. Curtis RM: Opposition of the thumb. Orthop Clin North Am 1974;5:305-321.

65. Williams HW: The leprosy thumb. Br J Plast Surg 1966;19:136-139.

66. Smith RJ. Tendon Transfers of the Hand and Forearm. Boston, Little, Brown, 1987.

67. Omer GE Jr: Evaluation and reconstruction of the forearm and hand after acute traumatic peripheral nerve injuries. J Bone Joint Surg Am 1968;50:1454-1478.

68. Bruner JM: Tendon transfer to restore abduction of the index finger using the extensor pollicis brevis. Plast Reconstr Surg 1948;3:197.

69. Christophe K: Rupture of the extensor pollicis longus tendon following Colles' fracture. J Bone Joint Surg 1953;35:1003.

70. Duplay S: Rupture sous-cutanee du tendon du long extenseur du pouce au niveau dala tabatiere anatomique. Bull Mem Soc Chir 1876;2:788.

71. Schneider LH, Rosenstein RG: Restoration of extensor pollicis longus function by tendon transfer. Plast Reconstr Surg 1983;71:533-537.

72. Strandell G: Post-traumatic rupture of the extensor pollicis longus tendon: pathogenesis and treatment. Acta Chir Scand 1955;109:81.

73. Low CK, Pereira BP, Chao VT: Optimum tensioning position for extensor pollicis longus to extensor pollicis longus transfer. Clin Orthop 2001;388:225-232.

74. Posner MA: Flexor superficialis tendon transfers to the thumb—an alternative to the free tendon graft for treatment of chronic injuries within the digital sheath. J Hand Surg Am 1983;8:876-881.

Free Functioning Muscle Transfers in the Upper Limb

RALPH T. MANKTELOW, MD ◆ RONALD M. ZUKER, MD

THE CLINICAL PROBLEM

Free functioning muscle transfer involves the microneurovascular transfer of a muscle from its donor site to a site in the arm. The objective of the procedure is to reconstruct a major functional deficit in the arm. Viability of the transplanted muscle is obtained by vascular anastomoses between the muscle and the arm. Most critical to the success of the operation is the repair of the muscle's motor nerves to an appropriate motor nerve in the arm.[1]

This is a complex procedure that requires great care in its planning and execution. The indication for this procedure is the reconstruction of a major skeletal muscle deficit. Because this is a complex procedure, if there are simpler methods of carrying out the functional reconstruction, they should be used. In many cases of muscle deficit, tendon transfers are available for reconstruction; for example, for long finger flexors, it is possible to reconstruct finger flexion by transfer of a radial wrist extensor tendon. If a tendon transfer will give an adequate result, it should be used.

The most common mechanisms of muscle loss are direct trauma to the muscle compartment, Volkmann ischemic paralysis, nerve injury, and tumor resection.[2] The procedure of free functioning muscle transfer has been successfully used to replace muscle deficits in the forearm both for finger flexion and extension and for replacement of the biceps, triceps, and anterior deltoid. In other centers where brachial plexus is more commonly treated, free functioning muscle transfer has become a commonly used procedure to replace biceps muscle function.[2-4]

In 1970, Tamai[5] transplanted the rectus femoris in a dog by use of microneurovascular techniques. He presented electrophysiologic and biomechanical evidence of contraction of the muscle and demonstrated useful movement. This paper stimulated many surgeons to consider use of what were at that time the new techniques of microvascular surgery for functioning muscle transfer. In 1973, surgeons at the Sixth Peoples' Hospital in Shanghai transplanted the lateral portion of the pectoralis major for the replacement of forearm flexor musculature. The patient had a Volkmann ischemic contracture of the forearm.[6] One of the authors (R.T.M.) visited Shanghai in 1976 and observed this patient's function, noting a good range of finger flexion and good grip strength. With the stimulation of that observation, functioning muscle transfers have been pursued both for the extremities and for facial paralysis reconstruction. The authors now have experience with more than 400 functioning microneurovascular muscle transfers. The majority of these have been for facial paralysis reconstruction. With subsequent experience, the surgical technique and the indications for muscle transfer in extremity reconstruction have been refined.

BASIC SCIENCE
Critical Muscle Anatomy

For muscle transfer, the critical aspects of muscle anatomy are its tendon or attachment at the origin and insertion; vascular supply; motor nerve; and orientation, length, and cross-sectional area of the muscle fibers. The muscle must have adequate length to fit the recipient site and to provide a suitable tendon for insertion, have vessels at a suitable location for anastomoses to the recipient vessels, and preferably have a single motor nerve. The muscle must be large enough that it will provide sufficient excursion and sufficient strength. Excursion and strength are functions of muscle cross-sectional area and fiber length and are dealt with in the section on functional muscle physiology.

GRACILIS MUSCLE

The gracilis muscle is the preferred muscle for upper extremity reconstruction in children and adults. The advantages of this muscle are that it satisfies all of the requirements for a neurovascular transfer, including good length to fit most recipient sites in the upper extremity, an excellent tendon that can be used for its distal attachment, and good excursion. Furthermore, the muscle is easily harvested from the inner thigh without leaving any functional or aesthetic deficit. The function of more than 100 patients who had this muscle removed was studied, and there were no functional deficits.[7] Thigh adduction is unaffected because the adductor magnus and longus are still present. The resulting scar on the medial upper thigh is reasonably well hidden.

The belly of the gracilis muscle lies just posterior to the adductor longus and sartorius muscles in the medial thigh. It is a superficial muscle and is easily exposed through a longitudinal medial thigh incision. It takes its origin from the body of the pubis and the adjacent ramus of the ischium by a thin fibrous aponeurosis (Fig. 214-1). The muscle fibers insert into a well-defined tendon that attaches to the medial shaft of the tibia just below the tibial tubercle. Although there are often three or more vascular pedicles, the proximal pedicle is the dominant one and reliably perfuses the muscle. The pedicle is 8 to 12 cm distal to the muscle's origin. There is a single artery 1 to 2 mm in diameter and two venae comitantes, each 1 to 4 mm in diameter. The pedicle lies under the adductor longus, taking its origin from the profunda femoris artery (Fig. 214-2). Rarely, the superior pedicle is a double pedicle with two arteries and four venae comitantes. From our injection studies, it appears that the circulation from these double vessels may not be interconnected within the muscle. There is a single constant perforator that usually exits from the superficial surface of the muscle at the same level as the dominant

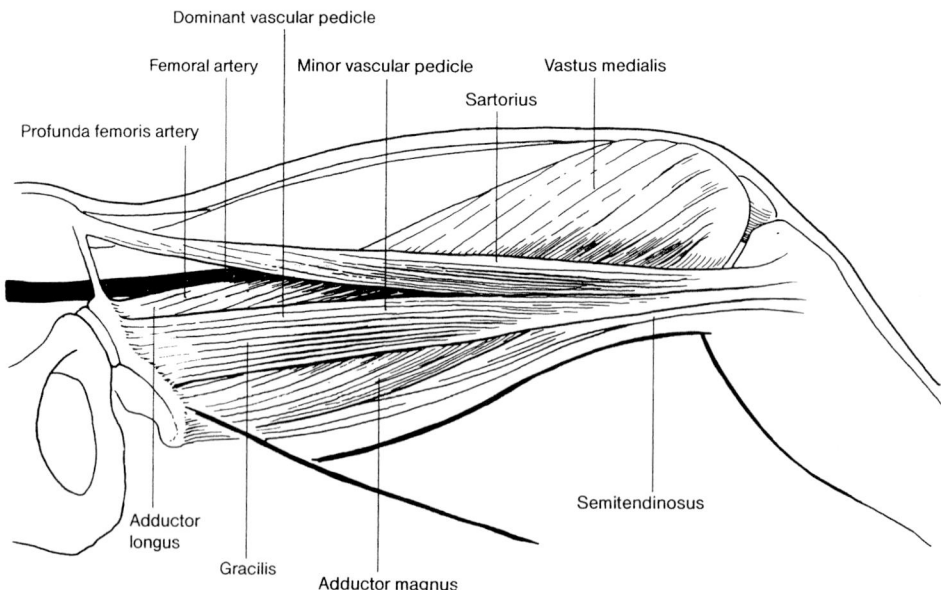

FIGURE 214-1. The anatomic relationship of the gracilis muscle to the surrounding structures. (From Manktelow RT: Microvascular Reconstruction: Anatomy, Applications, and Surgical Technique. New York, Springer-Verlag, 1986:39.)

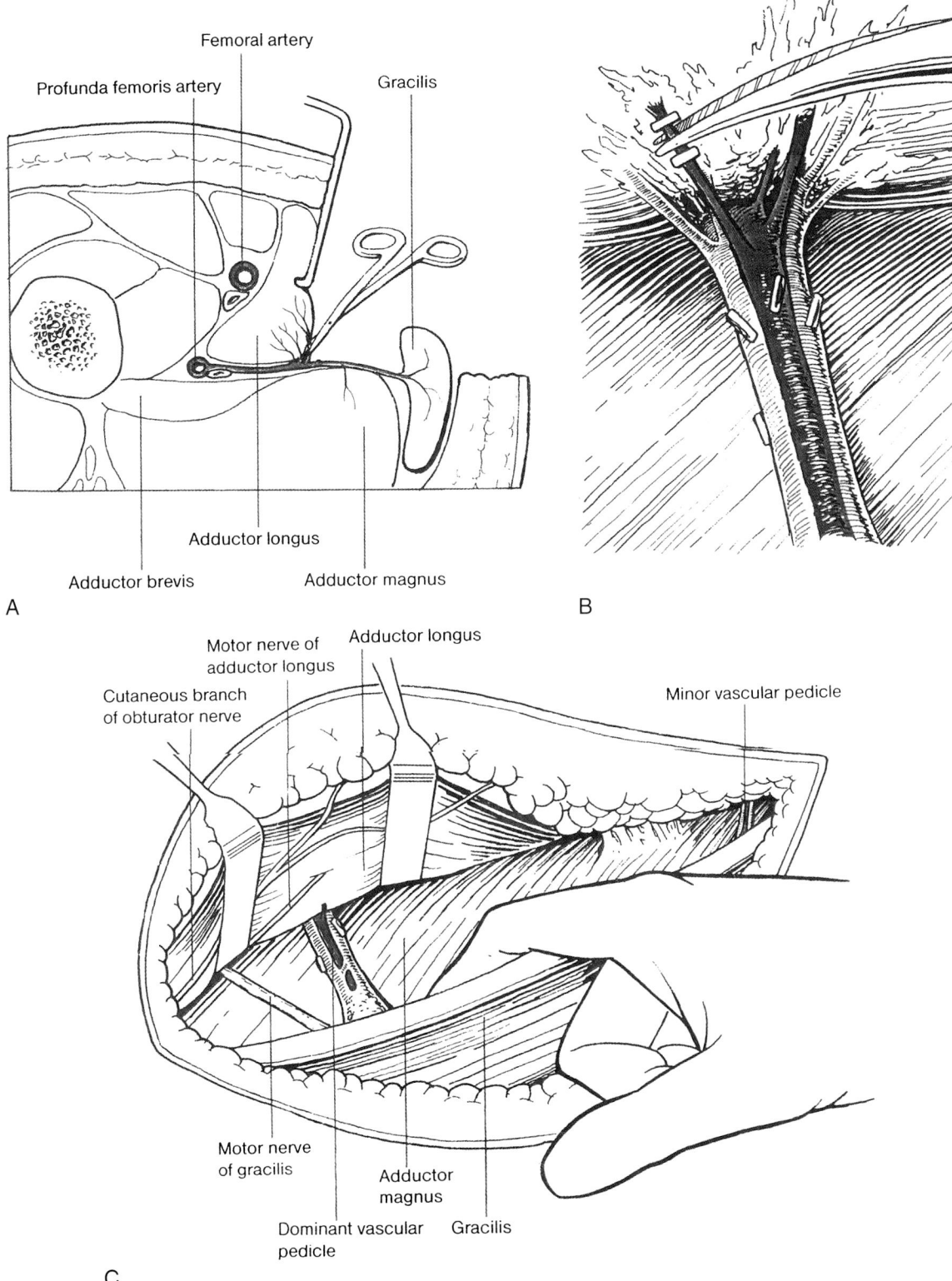

FIGURE 214-2. *A* to *C*, Retraction of the adductor longus allows exposure of the motor nerve and vascular pedicle and division of the vascular branches to the adductor longus. Branches of the pedicle enter the deep surface of the adductor longus and must be divided to obtain the full length of the pedicle. (From Manktelow RT: Microvascular Reconstruction: Anatomy, Applications, and Surgical Technique. New York, Springer-Verlag, 1986:43.)

vascular pedicle. The muscle can be taken with an attached cutaneous flap nourished by this perforator.

Although there are secondary pedicles present, these pedicles are not usually required for nourishment of the muscle. Sometimes, after division of the secondary pedicles, the distal 5 cm of muscle will become dark. This portion can be removed and the raw muscle fibers attached to the tendon so that their functional effect is maintained.

The single motor nerve enters the muscle along with the pedicle on the deep surface of the muscle. It passes into the hilum and then branches into the muscle. There are two to seven fascicles present. However, the nerve can usually be divided into two groups of fascicles. Ninety percent of the time, one of these fascicles will control the anterior 20% to 50% of the muscle, and the remaining fascicle or fascicles will control the posterior portion of the muscle. This is a useful functional separation that may be employed to provide independent thumb and finger motion.

The muscle fiber anatomy appears to have a strap muscle configuration, and this is true in the proximal three fifths of the muscle belly. However, in the distal two fifths, the muscle fibers insert into the tendon that extends up approximately half the length of the muscle. The most posterior muscle fibers are shorter and insert proximally in the tendon, and the longer anterior muscle fibers insert more distally (see Fig. 214-1). The muscle function is primarily to adduct the thigh, to flex and medially rotate it, and to stabilize the hip during flexion and extension.

OTHER MUSCLES THAT HAVE BEEN USED FOR FREE FUNCTIONING MUSCLE TRANSFER

The latissimus dorsi has been used by many for free functioning muscle transfer.[2,8] It has the advantage of having a larger muscle bulk that suggests the potential of a stronger functional transfer. However, although it has an excellent tendon at its origin, it has a diffuse insertion. The superior muscle fibers are short compared with the anterior lateral muscle fibers, and this makes insertion of all of the muscle fibers into the tendons that are to be moved much more complex than if there is a single tendon, as in the gracilis. The pectoralis major has also been used but suffers from a similar disadvantage. The tensor fascia lata is shorter and has a shorter excursion. However, it has an excellent tendon of insertion and origin and suitable neurovascular anatomy.

Functional Muscle Physiology

A muscle is composed of many muscle fibers enclosed in sarcolemma. Each of these muscle fibers is composed of many myofibrils. The functional structure of each myofibril is an arrangement of actin and myosin fibers that lie adjacent to each other. When muscle contraction occurs, it is a process of dynamic sliding of the adjacent actin and myosin fibers over each other into increased fiber overlap. The force of muscle contraction is thought to be proportional to the degree of overlap of the fibers. At maximum extension of the muscle fiber, there is little overlap and thus muscle contraction is particularly weak. With progressive shortening, the overlapping of the fibers becomes greater and the force of contraction stronger. With further shortening, there is crumpling of the myosin fibers with less area of overlap and correspondingly less force of contraction. These events produce the length-tension curve. With muscle fiber contraction, the tension peaks in the midportion of the shortening and decreases with further shortening of the muscle (Fig. 214-3A). In addition to the dynamic force from actin and myosin, an increased force develops as the muscle is extended from the elastic tension of the connective tissue network that surrounds the individual muscle fibers (Fig. 214-3B). These two tensions, dynamic and elastic, are combined to produce the total tension in an intact muscle (Fig. 214-3C).

When a single muscle fiber is stimulated in the laboratory, there is a 57% shortening of the fiber's fully stretched length.[9] However, there is some limitation to the maximum stretch of an intact muscle because of its connective tissue framework, which results in slightly less shortening in the intact muscle. The gracilis is a particularly effective muscle with respect to excursion because it is largely a strap muscle. The authors' clinical experience with stimulating the gracilis muscle in vivo has demonstrated that there is at least 50% shortening of the muscle from its fully stretched length (Fig. 214-4). In adults, the gracilis, when it is maximally stimulated, will shorten more than 12 cm. Because this amount of shortening is more than that required for any functions in the upper extremity, the gracilis provides an excellent excursion for all arm reconstructions. A muscle has decreasing strength after its point of maximum tension, which is developed in the midpoint of the length-tension curve; therefore, it is important to transfer it with sufficient tension such that the muscle's range of excursion is about the midpoint of the curve, the most powerful and dynamic portion of its length-tension curve. Pennate muscles, such as the rectus femoris, have been transferred as free functional muscles.[10] Because a pennate muscle has much shorter muscle fiber units that are attached to a central or lateral tendon, the muscle as a whole has a relatively short excursion. This is because the amount of contraction of the muscle as a whole is proportional to the length of the muscle fibers within the muscle. On the other hand, the pennate muscle generally has more strength of contraction because strength is proportional to the sum of the cross-sectional area of all muscle fibers.

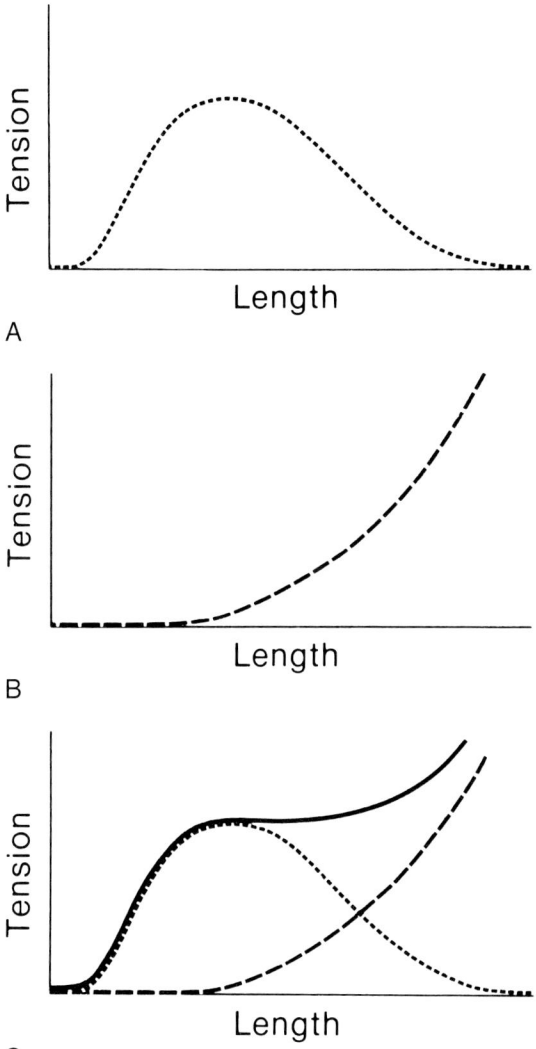

FIGURE 214-3. *A,* Single muscle fiber length-tension curve during active contraction. *B,* Length-tension curve of a whole muscle being passively stretched; with increasing length, there is increasing tension from the connective tissue framework. *C,* The tension developed by a whole muscle under tetanic stimulation is the sum of the forces produced by active contraction and passive stretching (*solid line, A* plus *B*). (From Manktelow RT: Functioning muscle transfer for reconstruction of the hand. In May JW Jr, Littler JW, eds: The Hand. Philadelphia, WB Saunders, 1990:4968. McCarthy JG, ed: Plastic Surgery; vol 8.)

ANALYSIS OF THE CLINICAL PROBLEM

Clinical Assessment of the Extremity

The involved extremity must be evaluated in detail. Particular attention is focused on the specific anatomic structures that will be required at the recipient site.

This includes the recipient vessels, the motor nerve that will reinnervate the transplant, the structures around the tendon repair site that will facilitate tendon gliding, and the range of motion of the joints that will be affected by the transfer. In addition to this, there must be stability and control of the proximal portion of the limb. An adequate history and physical examination will outline the mechanism of injury and offer some insight into whether these structures have been damaged. Surgical débridement of necrotic musculature can lead to extensive scarring and damage to the neurovascular structures. Thus, a thorough history and review of previous operative reports may be valuable. The site of the proposed tendon repairs should be studied carefully. If there is insufficient soft tissue cover in the distal half of the forearm to facilitate tendon gliding, a staged procedure, bringing in either regional or distant soft tissue cover, is required. This should be done well in advance of muscle transplantation to minimize scar formation and to facilitate optimal gliding. Although the gracilis can be transferred with an attached cutaneous skin flap, the flap, coming from the medial thigh, is usually too thick to be aesthetically acceptable and is not reliable over the distal part of the muscle. The proximal half of the muscle can be covered with a skin graft without fear of inhibiting muscle movement and with acceptable appearance.

DIAGNOSTIC STUDIES

To clarify the status of the vascular supply to the limb and specifically to locate vessels that will be used for the transfer, angiography is helpful. For example, it is not uncommon in Volkmann ischemic contracture to see gaps in the brachial artery at the site of the causative supracondylar fracture. These gaps should be reconstructed before muscle transfer. Angiography is also invaluable in locating the site of the artery that will revascularize the transfer. The anterior interosseous artery is often undamaged and available for volar forearm reconstruction. In addition to confirming the availability of the anterior interosseous artery, the angiogram can also give important information about the status of the nerve. If the artery is healthy and pristine in appearance, one can anticipate that the nerve directly adjacent to the artery is also undamaged. This is essential information because the selection of an appropriate undamaged motor nerve is crucial to the success of the procedure. The anterior interosseous nerve is in a deep protected position and thus is usually available. However, if it is not, alternative motor input should be sought. The clinical evaluation can be invaluable in indicating whether the second choice, which is a motor branch of the ulnar nerve going to the flexor digitorum longus nerve, is intact and functioning. Thus, one could potentially use the ulnar nerve input

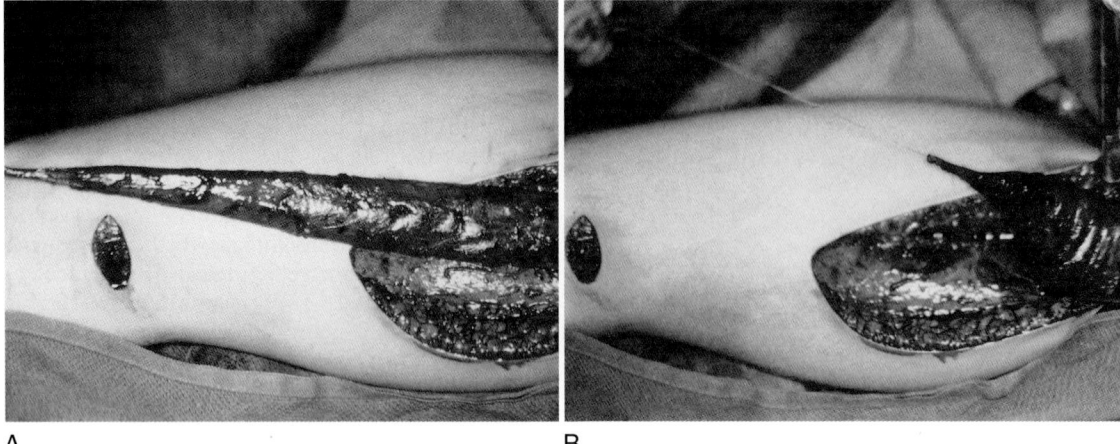

A   B

FIGURE 214-4. *A,* The gracilis muscle has been detached from its insertion and stretched to its fully extended length. *B,* With tetanic stimulation of the gracilis motor nerve, the muscle shortens to less than half of its extended length. (From Manktelow RT: Functioning muscle transfer for reconstruction of the hand. In May JW Jr, Littler JW, eds: The Hand. Philadelphia, WB Saunders, 1990:4969. McCarthy JG, ed: Plastic Surgery; vol 8.)

to the digital flexors to innervate the new muscle transplant.

Another useful tool to evaluate motor nerve function is electromyography of the pronator quadratus muscle. If the pronator quadratus muscle is functioning, there is a high probability that the anterior interosseous nerve will provide normal branches to innervate the functioning muscle transplant. This muscle often has some degree of function in Volkmann ischemic contracture even when the more superficial muscles have become necrotic or damaged. Conversely, if there is loss of function of the pronator quadratus muscle, one should be prepared to look elsewhere for a functioning motor nerve to innervate the transplant. When uncertainty exists, biopsy of the nerve before the date of the intended muscle transfer may be wise to be sure of its capability to innervate the muscle. There may be a nerve injury higher up as well, and this may make it difficult to know for sure that the motor nerve selected will innervate the muscle. In these situations, a biopsy is worthwhile to confirm adequacy of innervation.

Alternatives to Muscle Transfer

Alternative treatments for muscle dysfunction in the extremity are available. For minor degrees of flexion loss, a muscle slide is often all that is necessary. The origin of the flexor mass can be released through an ulnar approach and advanced distally. This releases the contractile elements and allows full digital extension with a functional amount of flexion. In certain situations, tendon transfers may be helpful. Adequate innervation and adequate joint mobility are required for success. Transfers from the extensor aspect of the

extremity to the volar aspect are most effective and may be of value.

TREATMENT GOALS AND REALISTIC EXPECTATIONS

The key factors that affect the outcome of muscle transfer are patient selection, muscle selection, operative technique of muscle transfer, and postoperative management. The goal of surgery is to obtain a well-vascularized and well-innervated muscle that regains a powerful contraction force with good excursion. The most common location for muscle transfer in the authors' experience is for replacement of the forearm long finger flexor musculature. This procedure reconstructs elbow flexion and extension and shoulder flexion.

For good function to be obtained, the recovery of adequate strength must be accompanied by good excursion and tendon gliding. It is important that the surgical technique facilitate these outcomes. Expectations, however, must be realistic. Experimental microneurovascular transplantation of the dog gracilis by McKee and Kuzon[11] produced forces of contraction that varied from 35% to 120% of the control muscle in the opposite normal limb. It was not clear why there was such a range of results. In her study using the rabbit model, Terzis[12] found that the recovery of muscle strength was never as good as in the normal muscle. This decrease in strength was thought to be due to a number of factors, including poor reinnervation and the likelihood that the muscle's origin had become detached, resulting in a tenotomy effect on the muscle's function.

Patient Selection

The patient must have an extremity problem that will be improved in function when a single motor is transferred to it (possibly along with other reconstructive procedures). Particularly in severe trauma, many extremities have lost so many functional components that the addition of a single functioning muscle may not make any difference to the function of the arm as a whole. In reconstructing finger flexion, it is necessary that there be muscles that will balance the transferred muscle, such as the wrist and finger extensor capability, and there should be intact intrinsics and useful hand sensibility. The bed in which the muscle will lie must facilitate good muscle gliding, and the structures that are going to be motored by the muscle must have mobile joints and gliding tendons.

Functioning free muscle transplantation requires considerable cooperation on the part of the patient during the rehabilitative phase. Thus, the psychosocial makeup of the patient is important. If there is a lack of cooperation during the rehabilitation process, success will not be achieved. The patient must be enthusiastic about the reconstruction and understand that considerable time and effort will be required to get the most out of the transplant. If these factors are lacking, it might be best to wait until cooperation can be ensured.

Muscle Selection

Muscle selection is important. The factors to be considered include the anatomic size of the muscle with respect to the recipient site, the availability of tendons for attachment to the origin and insertion, the presence of a suitable neurovascular supply, and a muscle fiber anatomy that will provide sufficient excursion and strength of contraction.

SURGICAL TECHNIQUE

Selection of Appropriate Muscle for Free Functioning Muscle Transfer

There are both donor site and recipient site issues that must be considered in the selection of the appropriate muscle. The important donor site issues are related to the functional capability of the muscle, the ready accessibility of the donor site while a second team is working on the upper extremity, the lack of functional loss after removal of the muscle, and the acceptable location and visibility of the scar.

All muscles for transfer should be readily and reliably transferred on the basis of a single artery and vein repair. Thus, the muscles are limited to type I.[13] There should also be a single motor nerve controlling the muscle. The structure of the muscle should facilitate

its ready attachment in the recipient area. This means that there should be good tissue at the origin and good tissue at the insertion of the muscle for secure attachment to the recipient tissues. It should also be possible to capture all of the muscle fibers in the muscle at the attachment to the insertion. Many muscles, such as the latissimus dorsi and the gracilis, have varying degrees of functional overlap with other adjacent muscles, allowing them to be removed without significant functional loss.

It is helpful if the scars are in a location such as the upper medial thigh for the gracilis because this is easily hidden in most types of clothing. Harvesting of the entire latissimus muscle with an acceptable scar for a female patient requires a fairly small incision and endoscopic techniques.

The recipient needs dictate which muscle is best to use. Excursion is important for all muscle transfers. The muscle must have more excursion in its normal site than it will have in its transferred site because undoubtedly there will be some losses in excursion due to less than perfect tension setting after transfer. The maximum excursion of the finger flexor tendons is 6 cm in an adult man and less in a woman or child. Finger extensors are 4 to 5 cm. Strength is an important feature and is affected by many factors, including the innervation of the muscle, the extent that the patient uses it for resisted activity, and the intrinsic strength of the muscle determined by the cross-sectional area of the muscle fibers.

The anatomic structures of the recipient site dictate how the muscle will have to fit the site (Fig. 214-5). The need for tendons at the insertion of the muscle varies according to the recipient site. For example, a muscle transfer for finger flexion to a forearm that has flexor tendons present in the distal forearm is a much easier insertion than one in which the flexor tendons begin in the midpalm. The location of the recipient vessels is important to minimize the problems of vascular anastomosis. If there are no recipient vessels in the region of the end of the muscle's vascular pedicle, vein grafts will be required. This will decrease the reliability of the vascular transfer. Particularly critical is the location of the selected motor nerve for reinnervation of the transfer. This motor nerve must be located at a site adjacent to the donor muscle so that a tension-free coaptation can be carried out. The innervation strength through a nerve graft is much less than through a direct coaptation.[14] This decrease in innervation strength is markedly apparent when a long cross-facial nerve graft is used to innervate a muscle transfer for lower facial reconstruction.

Skin coverage of the transferred muscle is important because there must be skin and subcutaneous fatty tissues covering the distal half of the muscle and at the site of the tendon attachment to facilitate tendon gliding. In some cases, it will be helpful to carry a

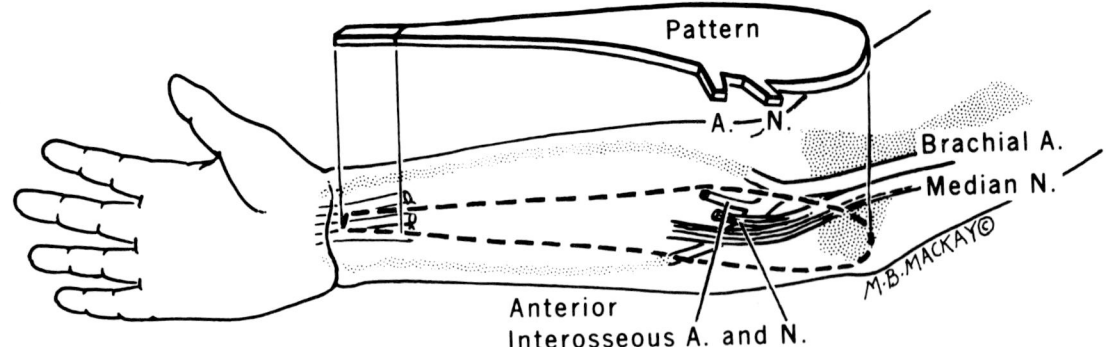

FIGURE 214-5. Preoperative planning identifies the site of the vessels, nerve, and tendons of attachment and allows the design of an anatomic pattern of the muscle to be inserted into the defect. (From Manktelow RT: Functioning muscle transfer for reconstruction of the hand. In May JW Jr, Littler JW, eds: The Hand. Philadelphia, WB Saunders, 1990:4971. McCarthy JG, ed: Plastic Surgery; vol 8.)

cutaneous paddle with the muscle to provide this coverage; in other cases, it may be necessary to design a flap at a preliminary operative sitting.

The authors have had experience in extremity reconstruction with different muscles, including the gracilis, latissimus dorsi, tensor fascia lata, and pectoralis major. However, the most experience has been gained with the gracilis muscle, and it satisfies the donor site requirements for most locations in the upper extremity. Although the muscle may seem to be small, recovery is excellent after transfer. It has provided a remarkably strong contractile force for all locations. The rectus femoris has an even greater strength potential because this is a multipennate muscle; however, the length of the individual muscle fibers is in the range of 5 to 6 cm. This provides a maximum contraction of about 2.5 to 3 cm, which is not enough for most locations. The latissimus dorsi should be used with caution because of the marked difference in muscle fiber length between the shorter posterior-superior fibers and the long anterior-lateral fibers. It is necessary for all fibers to be attached to the tendons of insertion if they are going to be effective for muscle contraction, and this presents a technical difficulty. Some surgeons have reversed this muscle so that its tendon of insertion into the humerus is placed distally and attached to the flexor tendons. This places the neurovascular pedicle in a distal part of the forearm, which may be a problem for neural coaptation. The authors have also had experience with more than 300 microneurovascular muscle transfers to the face. Experience has proved that a piece of muscle centered on the neurovascular hilum and transferred will function well. Most of the authors' experience in the face has been with the gracilis muscle, but the extensor carpi radialis brevis, the pectoralis minor, and the latissimus dorsi have also been used. This approach of custom cutting the muscle to the size of the defect may be suitable for smaller muscle reconstructions, such as transfers for replacement of thenar musculature.

Elevating the Gracilis Muscle

The gracilis is easily harvested through a midline incision in the upper thigh. The incision should be placed in the upper half of the thigh and evenly placed between the front and back of the thigh so that it is minimally visible. This incision always forms a spread scar. Prepare the leg free from above the groin to below the knee. If the hip is positioned in moderate abduction and external rotation with the knee moderately flexed, the medial aspect of the thigh is accessible. Most of the surgery is done with the surgeon on the opposite side of the operating table.

The important surface landmark is the insertion of the adductor longus tendon into the adductor tubercle. Draw a line from this point to the tibial tubercle with the knee flexed at 90 degrees. This marks the upper border of the gracilis muscle. Place the incision posterior to this line in the midline of the thigh, where it is most likely not to be seen from the front or back when the patient is standing.

Carry the incision through the superficial and deep fascia and identify the gracilis muscle by palpating the adductor longus tendon and its muscle. Separate the muscle from the adductor longus and adductor magnus.

Retract the adductor longus with two large right-angled retractors, one on each side of the dominant pedicle. Separate the branches of the dominant pedicle from the adductor longus (see Fig. 214-2). A 6-cm length of pedicle can be developed. There may be one or more small branches from the pedicle going down to the underlying adductor magnus. The motor nerve lies proximal to the pedicle, entering the muscle at the same point as the artery and venae comitantes. By dissection under the adductor longus and separation of the motor nerve from the nerve to the adductor longus, a nerve length of 9 or 10 cm can usually be obtained.

Divide the secondary pedicles. Always divide the muscle's distal tendon before the proximal, or inadvertent stimulation and contraction of the muscle may avulse the pedicle. The tendon is divided through a separate incision proximal to the knee. When the muscle is completely separated from all structures except its dominant pedicle, it should be observed for perfusion. If there is any dark muscle distally, it should be excised and the proximal cut fibers attached to the tendon. After the muscle is removed and transferred to the arm, the recipient area is closed in layers. By closing the deep fascia, one ensures that there will be a symmetrically shaped thigh without any indentation.

Muscle Transfer to the Flexor Aspect of the Forearm

The preoperative examination determines the feasibility of a muscle transfer on the basis of adequate structures. There must be a suitable artery and vein and undamaged motor nerve. The fixation of the muscle origin is usually not a problem; but the insertion may be a problem, and adequate tendons need to be identified. The pathologic process will usually suggest the location of these structures. There must be adequate soft tissue coverage for the muscle except in the proximal half of the forearm. For the proximal half of the forearm, a split-thickness skin graft over the muscle is satisfactory and aesthetically more acceptable than a thick skin paddle taken from the medial thigh. Because the neurovascular pedicle of the muscle is in its proximal third, it will be necessary to have recipient vessels in the forearm in this location. If there is any doubt about the availability of an undamaged motor nerve in the forearm, as may be the case in previous trauma, the arm should be explored as a preliminary procedure. The proposed motor nerve should be identified and biopsy samples taken at the intended site of repair. Because quick section assessment of nerve is difficult, this biopsy is best performed some days before the planned surgery so that careful histologic assessment of the nerve can be carried out. The most suitable nerve for providing long finger flexor musculature is the anterior interosseous nerve. Because this nerve comes off the deep surface of the median nerve, usually a few centimeters distal to the elbow, if the median nerve is intact, the anterior interosseous is usually available in an undamaged condition. Other nerves that may be used are the finger flexor branches of the median nerve to the sublimis and the branches of the ulnar nerve to the flexor digitorum profundus.

It is a good idea to sketch the intended position of the muscle on the forearm, with the expected location of the vessels and nerve and tendons for insertion (see Fig. 214-5). It is then possible to plan an incision that will be appropriate to allow exposure of these structures and provide good coverage of the muscle. It is usually necessary to plan for a skin graft in the proximal portion of the forearm to prevent a tight closure.

After elevation of the skin flaps, the bed is prepared to receive the muscle. Each of the structures that need to be prepared is identified. In a post-traumatic situation, this can be tedious. By identifying arteries, veins, and nerves proximal to the level of injury and dissecting distally, along the structures, one can follow the artery, vein, and nerve into the forearm to the point of the intended repair. If there is any question about the suitability of the nerve, a quick section at this point will at least tell you whether there is a lot of fibrosis. Axon stains are not reliable, and it is difficult to identify nerve structure with a quick section. The appearance of a healthy nerve when it is cut is well known to reconstructive surgeons; there is usually some characteristic pouting of jelly-like tissue after a few minutes. Our experience is that when this is present, the permanent histologic stains also look good. The common flexor origin should be cleaned over the medial epicondyle, preparing whatever fibrous or fascial tissue there is at the common flexor origin. Strong fascia is required for reliable attachment of the muscle proximally. In dissecting the distal forearm, great care must be taken to preserve the median and ulnar nerves and the vasculature to the hand and to identify the flexor tendons. If some adhesions are present between the profundus tendons and the surrounding tissues, they should be removed.

When all of the structures are prepared for attachment to the muscle, the muscle is then detached from the thigh and transferred to the arm. The first step is to tack the muscle loosely in place and identify where the muscle's vessels and nerves are located with respect to the recipient structures to ensure that there is a suitable apposition. The muscle can be moved proximally or distally to accommodate these neurovascular coaptations.

One of the important aspects of the repair is to transfer the muscle with sufficient tension that it can work in the most effective portion of the length-tension curve of muscle function. Before the gracilis is separated from the surrounding muscles in the leg and while it is still attached to its origin and insertion, it should be stretched out to its maximum physiologic extended position by abducting the thigh and extending the knee. When the muscle is so stretched, it is marked at 5-cm intervals. This is best done with small sutures placed in the superficial fibers of the muscle (Fig. 214-6). After transfer of the muscle to the forearm and attachment of the muscle's origin to the common flexor origin of the forearm, the muscle should be stretched distally and allowed to retract within the range of its expected excursion. This allows anticipation of the position of the pedicle and ensures

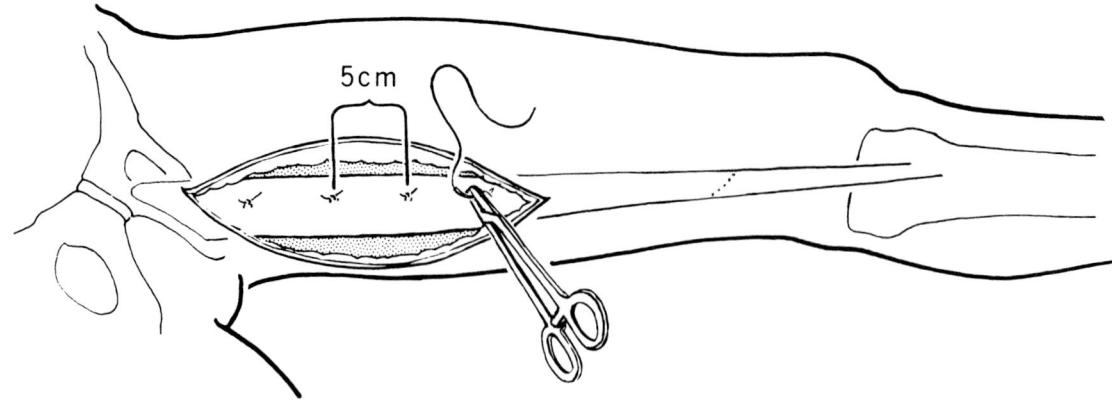

FIGURE 214-6. For optimal strength and excursion in the transplanted muscle, the gracilis must be transferred to the arm at the same tension as it is in the leg. This is accomplished before transfer by placing a suture or other mark every 5 cm on the surface of the muscle. This is done when it is at its fully extended physiologic length, which is with the thigh fully abducted and the knee fully extended. (From Manktelow RT: Functioning muscle transfer for reconstruction of the hand. In May JW Jr, Littler JW, eds: The Hand. Philadelphia, WB Saunders, 1990:4974. McCarthy JG, ed: Plastic Surgery; vol 8.)

that there will be no traction on the pedicle after its repair. The muscle is temporarily fixed in place, and the vascular and nerve repairs are done. On the basis of the laboratory experience of Clarke[15] and our clinical experience, there is no problem with an ischemia time of up to 3 hours after transfer from the leg. Thus, there is no need to rush and possibly compromise the technical quality of the revascularization and nerve repair. This repair should be done right the first time because it is sometimes difficult to revise a vascular thrombosis to muscle without producing damaging ischemia. The nerve repair should be done as close as is reasonable to the muscle to minimize the duration of denervation, but this is really not a major issue. A fascicular repair should be done between the fascicles of the gracilis motor nerve and the anterior interosseous nerve. More than half of the cross section of the gracilis motor nerve is loose areolar and fatty tissue. This should be stripped back so that the individual fascicles themselves can be repaired and there is maximum opportunity for the axons to pass across the nerve coaptation.

When the gracilis muscle is used to provide motor function to all four fingers for a strong grip, it is important that the fingers come down in unison, with the little finger slightly leading the ring and the ring leading the long and the long leading the index. For this cascade to be obtained, the profundus tendons should be sewn side-to-side to each other in such a position that traction on the group of tendons produces a balanced grip with all fingers flexing together in a cascade. This is easily done by an interweaving suture repair; the profundus tendons are woven among themselves with multiple mattress sutures.

The tension is then set by extending the wrist and fingers and pulling on the gracilis tendon until there

is a 5-cm distance between each of the muscle markings that were placed when the muscle was in the thigh. While holding the fingers and wrist in full extension, locate and mark the position of the flexor tendon stumps on the tendon of the stretched gracilis. The gracilis must be sutured to the flexor tendons so that these points are adjacent (Fig. 214-7A). In this position, the muscle will be at its maximum length in which it will be required to function in the arm, which is the same maximum length as was required for it to function in the leg. With the fingers and wrist in flexion, the tension is not excessive for tendon repair (Fig. 214-7B). By weaving of the gracilis tendon through the profundus tendons and with use of multiple mattress sutures, a secure repair can be obtained that allows early mobilization without dehiscence. In tall individuals, the gracilis muscle is usually too long, and muscle extends down into the carpal tunnel. This muscle can be trimmed off and the proximal muscle ends reattached to the gracilis tendon. Loose fibers should not be left free because with contraction, their strength will be dissipated and not available to the fingers.

If the flexor pollicis longus function is being reconstructed as well, the flexor pollicis longus should be inserted into the group of profundus tendons after the gracilis has been attached. The object of the flexor pollicis longus repair is to apply sufficient tension that the thumb will come adjacent to the flexed index finger and produce a key pinch against the middle phalanx of the index finger. If the flexor pollicis longus tendon is inserted too tightly, the thumb will flex into the palm before the fingers come into the palm. This is a dysfunctional position.

If it is desired to produce separate functioning neuromuscular groups, the technique must begin when

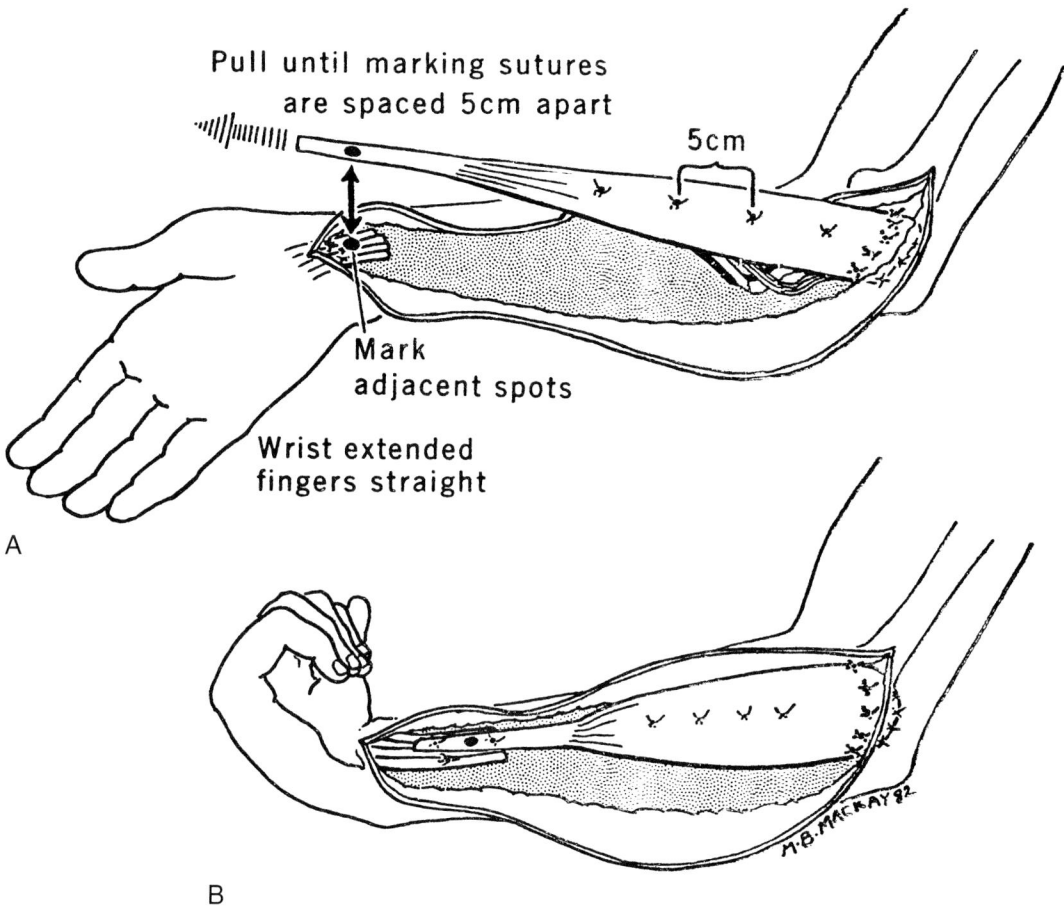

**Pull until marking sutures
are spaced 5cm apart**

5cm

**Mark
adjacent spots**

**Wrist extended
fingers straight**

A

B

FIGURE 214-7. *A,* After transfer of the muscle to the arm and attachment to its new origin, the fingers and wrists are placed in full passive extension and the gracilis is stretched distally. When the suture markers on the muscle are 5 cm apart, marks are placed opposite each other on the profundus tendons and the gracilis tendon. These marks identify the point at which the tendons should be sutured together. This places the muscle in the arm such that its fully extended physiologic length as identified in the leg is now its fully extended physiologic length in the arm. *B,* The interweaving suture repair is done with the wrist and fingers flexed to remove tension from the muscle. (From Manktelow RT: Functioning muscle transfer for reconstruction of the hand. In May JW Jr, Littler JW, eds: The Hand. Philadelphia, WB Saunders, 1990:4974. McCarthy JG, ed: Plastic Surgery; vol 8.)

the muscle is in the thigh. The motor nerve is divided longitudinally into two fascicular groups. There is usually a smaller fascicle that controls the anterior 25% to 50% of the muscle, and the rest of the nerve will control the posterior 50% to 75% of the muscle. By use of a microbipolar nerve stimulator, this separation can easily be identified. The portion of the muscle that is under the control of each fascicle is identified by palpation of the muscle when each fascicle is individually stimulated. The smaller anterior portion of the muscle will be used for thumb flexion and the posterior portion for finger flexion. Because the anterior muscle fibers are in continuity with the anterior tendon fibers, it is possible to split the tendon and the attached muscle fibers. When the muscle is transferred to the forearm, the profundus tendons are woven into the posterior tendon, and the flexor pollicis longus is woven

into the anterior piece of tendon. It is necessary to have independent nerve input that will allow separate control of the thumb and fingers. When the anterior interosseous nerve is identified and traced distally, it is often possible to identify a branch inserting radially into muscle. This is usually the branch to the flexor pollicis longus. There is usually more than one branch inserting toward the ulnar nerve. These branches insert into the flexor digitorum profundus muscle. If it is still present, there will be continuation of the anterior interosseous nerve distally into the pronator quadratus and wrist joint. By selection of nerve fascicles that previously went to the flexors of the thumb and the fingers and attachment of these to the appropriate fascicles of the gracilis muscle, some independent motion can be obtained between the fingers and thumb (Fig. 214-8).

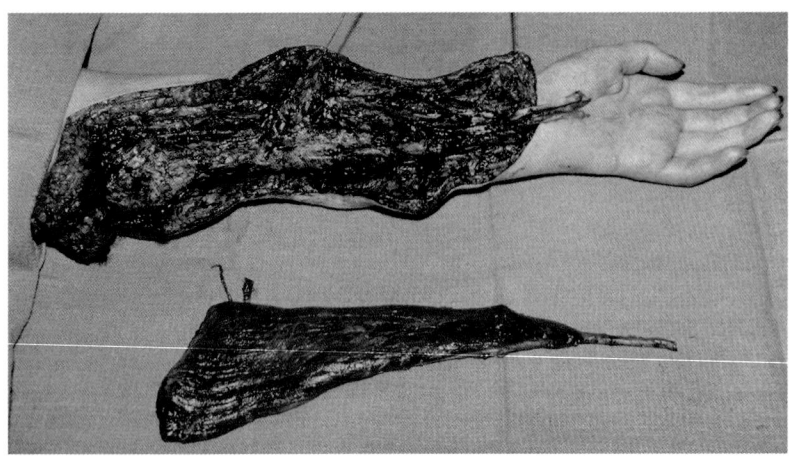

FIGURE 214-8. The flexor aspect of the forearm is prepared to accept the gracilis muscle for reconstruction of finger flexion.

Closure should be obtained securely over the distal half of the muscle with a two-layered firm closure. In the proximal half of the muscle, direct closure will usually be too tight and compress the pedicle. It is preferable to apply a split-thickness skin graft.

The postoperative position of the extremity should be with the hand and wrist in 30 degrees of flexion and the fingers in the position of function. A posterior slab of plaster is used to support the hand in this position. At the split-thickness skin graft in the proximal forearm, a window should be placed in the dressing so that the muscle can be evaluated. A small 1-cm flap of skin graft is folded back on itself to expose the muscle, and a damp gauze is placed on this and removed at half-hour intervals by the nursing staff to observe the color and appearance of the muscle. It is much more difficult to evaluate muscle than skin by its appearance. If the muscle develops venous compromise, it will become dark and blue. If there is arterial insufficiency, the muscle continues to look red, but it gets a somewhat drier granular appearance to it that is quite characteristic; however, this is a relatively subtle change. If there is doubt about the arterial supply to the muscle, a small snip will allow assessment of bleeding.

Muscle Transfer for Finger Extension

The gracilis muscle is an excellent muscle to provide finger and thumb extension because the excursion and strength are more than adequate to straighten the fingers in all wrist positions. The muscle fits well into the extensor aspect of the forearm, and there is a good length of tendon that is useful for attachment to the long finger and thumb extensors. The patient who has a severe extensor forearm muscle loss will also frequently have a severe flexor forearm loss. The authors have had experience with four patients with combined losses who required a microneurovascular muscle transfer for finger flexion and one for finger extension. In this situation, there will usually be a lack of wrist stabilization. The wrist must be held in a stable position during finger flexion or else the wrist will flex with the fingers and the grip will not be useful. Wrist stabilization can be accomplished by tenodesis of the extensor carpi radialis longus and extensor carpi ulnaris tendons through a bone window in the dorsum of the radius. The gracilis muscle, when it is used on the extensor aspect of the arm, will provide finger extension and thumb abduction and extension. If the flexor aspect of the forearm is intact, however, the standard tendon transfers for providing finger, thumb, and wrist extension should be used.

The posterior interosseous nerve is preferred for innervation of the transferred muscle. This nerve may be identified where it passes through the supinator. At this point, the nerve fibers will be supplying finger extension as well as thumb extension and abduction. In addition, there are fibers going to the extensor carpi ulnaris, and these are usually on the most proximal and ulnar aspect of the nerve. Sometimes, there are remnants of finger extensor muscles. This facilitates the identification of the branches of the posterior interosseous that provide finger extension (Fig. 214-9).

The vascular repair requires careful planning because there are frequently no large vessels on the dorsal aspect of the forearm. The pedicle can be attached end-to-side to the radial artery or end-to-end to a radial recurrent branch of the radial artery. The pedicle is best routed under the muscle bellies of the extensor carpi radialis, brevis, and longus and brachioradialis and directly into the radial artery. An adequate tunnel must be designed so that there is no compression of the pedicle. A superficial or deep vein in the forearm is usually available for venous return.

The origin of the muscle is usually the lateral epicondyle and common extensor fascia. The muscle will

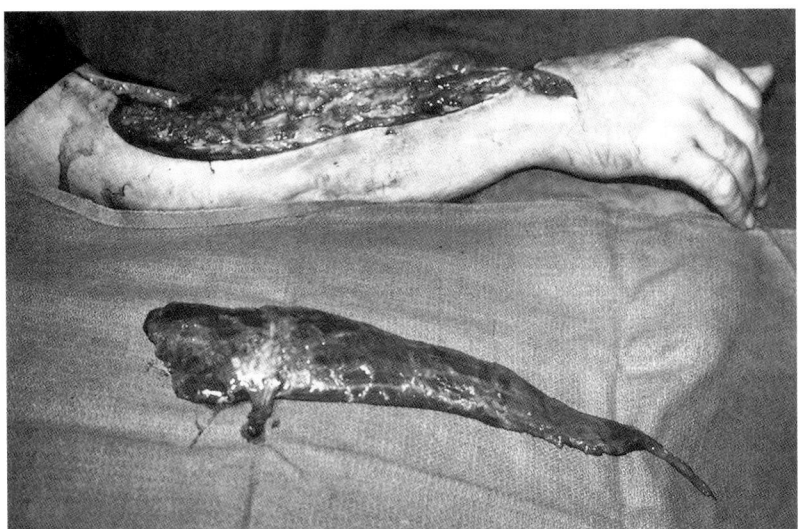

FIGURE 214-9. The extensor aspect of the forearm is prepared to accept the gracilis muscle for reconstruction of finger extension and thumb extension and abduction.

provide finger extension by attachment to the extensor digitorum communis tendons of all four fingers. The four finger tendons should be woven together so that with traction on the tendons, all fingers extend equally and symmetrically. By rerouting of the extensor pollicis longus so that it lies over the extensor pollicis brevis and abductor pollicis brevis, the tendon will both extend and abduct the thumb. This tendon should be inserted into the common extensor tendon mass. The effect of the tendon transfer can be tested by traction on the grouped tendons.

The same technique as described for the finger flexors is used to develop the correct muscle tension. The wrist and fingers are placed in full flexion while the gracilis muscle is stretched to its maximum extended length. Adjacent points on the finger extensor tendons and the gracilis tendon are marked, and this indicates the point of desired tendon repair. When the wrist and fingers are brought back into extension, the tendon repair can easily be done without too much tension. An interweaving repair with multiple mattress sutures will be secure. Good local skin flap coverage must be available to cover the distal half of the gracilis muscle and tendon repair so that good tendon gliding can be obtained. A split-thickness skin graft is appropriate for the proximal half of the muscle.

Postoperative management is similar to that for a flexor muscle repair. The wrist and fingers are splinted in extension for 2 to 3 weeks, and then a passive program of finger and wrist flexion is begun. It is important to get the program going and to be quite vigorous so that joint stiffness and finger and gracilis tendon adhesions are prevented. A resisted exercise program is developed once a useful range of active finger extension has occurred; this usually begins at about 6 months.

Muscle Transfers for Biceps Reconstruction

Local muscle transfers for elbow flexion include the latissimus dorsi and pectoralis major. They should be used if available. They provide an early return of function and are reasonably reliable.

Skin coverage of a muscle transfer in the upper arm is usually not a problem. Skin flaps should be elevated so that with closure, there is flap coverage for at least the distal half of the muscle belly. If necessary, a skin graft can be placed on the proximal half. The humeral circumflex arteries, profunda brachii, and ulnar recurrent artery are available as recipient vessels. There are usually plenty of venae comitantes for venous return. The origin of the muscle will be the acromion and distal end of the clavicle. The gracilis tendon will be inserted into the biceps tendon attachment (Fig. 214-10). The most appropriate nerve for reinnervation is the motor portion of the musculocutaneous nerve. Approximately 50% of the cross section of this mixed nerve is sensory. Because it is more than four times the size of the gracilis nerve, it is possible for the gracilis motor nerve to be attached inadvertently to a part that is only sensory. Identification of the motor component of the musculocutaneous nerve can be done by identification of branches that lead to remnants of the biceps or brachialis muscle. If this is not possible, the technique of awake nerve stimulation or histochemical staining is useful.[16]

The postoperative management involves placement of the arm in flexion at the elbow and the shoulder in neutral. A Velpeau dressing will maintain this position for 2 to 3 weeks. The postoperative management is similar to that previously described; a program of passive stretching is begun at 2 to 3 weeks, and then

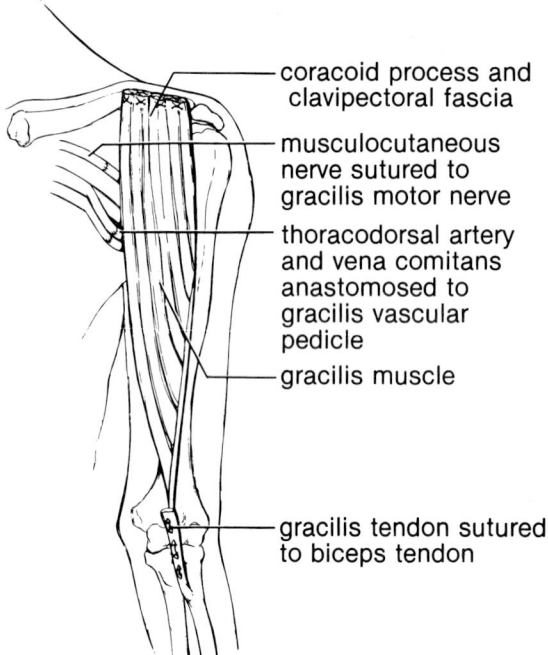

coracoid process and
clavipectoral fascia

musculocutaneous
nerve sutured to
gracilis motor nerve

thoracodorsal artery
and vena comitans
anastomosed to
gracilis vascular
pedicle

gracilis muscle

gracilis tendon sutured
to biceps tendon

FIGURE 214-10. The gracilis muscle is used to reconstruct the biceps and brachialis muscle.

an active exercise program is started once reinnervation has occurred.

Muscle Transfer for Triceps Reconstruction

This transfer is similar to that of the biceps except for the origin, insertion, and innervation. The origin is to the scapula, usually in the region of the glenoid fossa, and the insertion is into the olecranon or the remnants of the triceps tendon. Innervation is with one of the branches of the radial nerve that used to supply the triceps.

Muscle Transfer for Anterior Deltoid Reconstruction

Although the function of the deltoid is shoulder abduction, flexion, and extension, patients who have sustained a complete loss of deltoid function through either axillary nerve injury or deltoid muscle loss will often be able to abduct and flex the shoulder to some extent. This is done by use of the supraspinatus muscle and other shoulder muscles including the pectoralis major, biceps, and coracobrachialis. The ability to do this is variable. Some patients have limited shoulder flexion, which is a major deficit because the patient is then unable to position the hand in front of the body. Deltoid reconstruction, therefore, is done primarily for shoulder flexion and to some extent for abduction. The muscle is placed on the anterior aspect of the shoulder (Fig. 214-11). Soft tissue coverage is usually not a problem. The thoracodorsal artery is most useful because it is a long pedicle and can be brought to the gracilis muscle's artery without difficulty. The venae comitantes of this pedicle will provide venous outflow. Because the axillary nerve is a mixed nerve, it will be necessary to clarify which part is the motor portion (see biceps reconstruction). The acromion and distal end of the clavicle are used for the origin of the muscle. The gracilis tendon is inserted into the anterior portion of the humerus through a drill hole; if there are strong remnants of the deltoid still present,

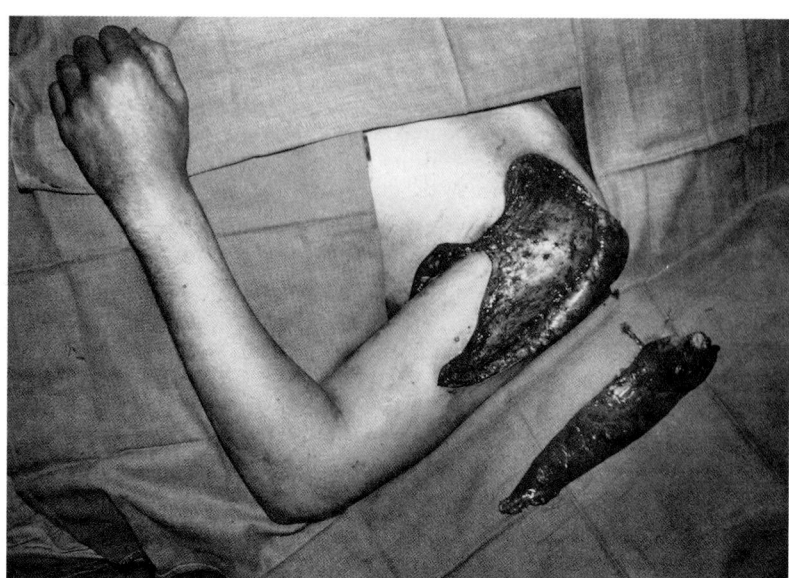

FIGURE 214-11. The gracilis is used to reconstruct the anterolateral deltoid musculature.

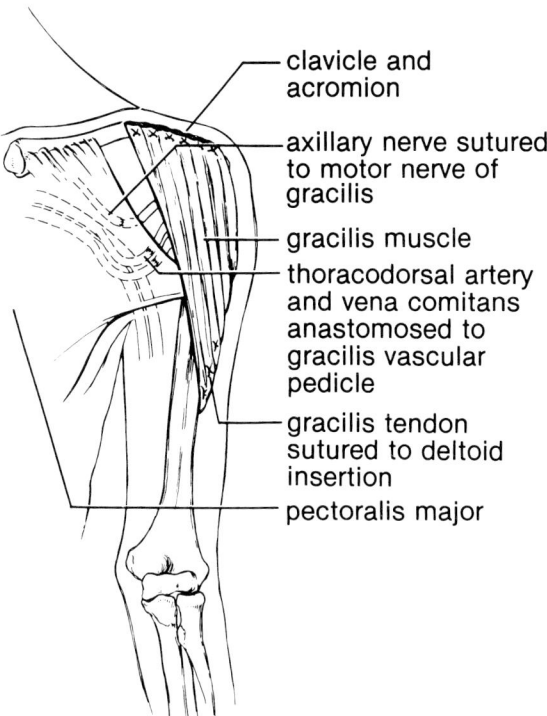

- clavicle and acromion
- axillary nerve sutured to motor nerve of gracilis
- gracilis muscle
- thoracodorsal artery and vena comitans anastomosed to gracilis vascular pedicle
- gracilis tendon sutured to deltoid insertion
- pectoralis major

FIGURE 214-12. Muscle transfer inserted for antero-lateral deltoid reconstruction.

it can be inserted into these (Fig. 214-12). One of the difficult aspects of this surgery may be the identification and exposure of the axillary nerve. If the cause of the paralysis is an axillary nerve avulsion, which may occur in a dislocation of the shoulder, the stump of the nerve may be deeply located. It is possible to identify this either through dissection deep to the intact pectoralis major or, for better exposure, by division of the tendon of the pectoralis major muscle. By identifying the posterior cord of the brachial plexus and tracing it distally, one can find the axillary nerve.

The technique of tension setting is similar to that in other muscle transfers. After attachment of the origin of the muscle, the shoulder is extended and the position of the gracilis muscle is noted on the humerus when the marks on the muscle have been stretched 5 cm apart. A small amount of the distal portion of the muscle will usually need to be removed because the muscle belly is too long. Because the tendon of the gracilis extends to the midpoint of its muscle belly, this is never a problem.

The postoperative care involves a Velpeau dressing in position for 3 weeks. A stretching program is not as critical as in other muscles from the standpoint of muscle and tendon adhesions, but it is important to get the shoulder moving because a stiff shoulder after immobilization will usually take many months of therapy to be overcome. Once the muscle has been reinnervated, a resisted exercise program is developed to build maximum strength.

POSTOPERATIVE MANAGEMENT

The postoperative management is similar for all transfer locations. The initial management involves bed rest for 1 or 2 days and careful observation of the exposed area of muscle. In addition to appropriate positioning of the extremity, it is important to maintain the circulation to the muscle. Thus, maintenance of a high circulating blood volume, adequate urine output, and stable blood pressure and keeping the patient warm are essential to ensure muscle perfusion.

If a thrombosis does occur, its recognition must be immediate. It will be necessary to return the patient to the operating room, revise the anastomosis, and obtain an intact circulation within 3 to 4 hours or severe ischemic damage to the muscle will occur.

Beginning about 3 weeks postoperatively, a program of passive stretching is begun. Because tendon attachments are secure interweaving repairs, early motion is safe, adhesions can be prevented, and the need for a late tenolysis is unusual. The wrist and fingers, elbow, and shoulder are passively mobilized so that the muscle is stretched, and it should be possible to obtain full passive joint motion within a month or so. For example, in the case of a muscle transfer for finger flexion, there should be passive combined finger and wrist extension. The extension will produce distal gliding of the muscle and flexor tendons. If the muscle has been put in with sufficient tension, the mechanical tension of the muscle fibers with passive finger and wrist flexion will produce proximal tendon and muscle gliding. This program of early passive muscle extension is important and will overcome a myotonic muscle contracture, prevent adhesions, and develop a tissue gliding bed at the muscle-tendon junction in preparation for the time when reinnervation occurs and active movement develops.

Reinnervation time varies with the distance between the nerve repair and the muscle belly itself. In general, reinnervation begins at about 2 to 4 months postoperatively. When active contraction begins, the patient is encouraged to contract the muscle frequently throughout the day. One of the most important features of the postoperative program is the application of graduated exercises with increasing resistance as tolerated. This should be commenced as soon as a good range of motion is obtained. A regular exercise program with repetitions to fatigue two or three times per day will stimulate muscle fiber development. This program is similar to a weightlifting program that an athlete would take part in to improve muscle strength.

This important feature of the postoperative program is an often neglected part of therapy after motor nerve repairs in general. A muscle that has undergone atrophy for any reason, the most common being disuse and denervation, will respond by undergoing hypertrophy when it is stressed. This recovery of strength and muscle bulk is an adaptive process that requires forceful contraction against resistance. The exercise program will be beneficial for at least 1 year after the development of a useful range of muscle motion. Eventually, the exercise program will be incorporated into activities of daily living and work-related activities. The development of this program of resistance exercises repeated to fatigue is extremely important for the ultimate development of full strength. A work hardening program can also be introduced and can be extremely effective. The motivation and exercise tolerance of each patient are critically important in obtaining optimum outcomes. In damaged upper extremities, it may be necessary for the therapist to develop innovative solutions involving pulleys, weights, grippers, or elastic strapping to provide resistance exercises.

COMPLICATIONS

Complications from free functioning muscle transplantation to the upper extremity can be broken down into early and late. Vascular insufficiency is the most common and dreaded early complication and needs to be rectified immediately. A warm ischemia period of 5 to 6 hours will lead to muscle necrosis that prevents recovery. Vascular compromise can also occur from inappropriate positioning and a variety of systemic factors leading to reduced circulation.

The late complications are related to the functional issues of the surviving muscle transplant. Inadequate neural input from an inadequate or damaged motor nerve or a disrupted nerve coaptation will lead to poor or negligible function. Even if the muscle is adequately innervated, it may not produce the desired movement because of scarring at the level of the tendon repair or tendon structures. If there is poor tendon gliding, a tenolysis at the junction of the gracilis tendon and digital tendons is indicated. However, one should wait until the muscle is fully innervated so that a program of active exercises can be initiated after the tenolysis. In this way, an effective tendon excursion can take place.

It is uncommon to have a functioning muscle transfer decrease in function after it has reached a plateau. However, a strong blow in the region of the vascular supply could damage the circulation and lead to an ischemic process with loss of function. This rare circumstance has been seen once, and its correction requires another muscle transplantation procedure.

RESULTS OF FREE MUSCLE TRANSFER TO THE UPPER EXTREMITY
Forearm Transfers

The authors have completed long finger flexor reconstruction in 14 adults and 16 children. When there is an extensive muscle loss on the dorsal forearm, there will be instability of the wrist if the wrist extensors are absent. In these instances, an extensor tenodesis should be carried out with use of the wrist extensor tendons fixed to the radius.

The etiology of muscle loss includes Volkmann ischemic contracture and traumatic muscle loss. Although the pectoralis major and the latissimus dorsi were used in three patients with early finger flexor reconstruction, the gracilis was used for all others. Six of the 14 adult patients required secondary procedures. These included tendon length adjustment, capsulotomy, tendon transfer, tenolysis, digital fusion, and metacarpophalangeal capsulodesis.

The results of surgery were very good. All patients thought that the operation was worthwhile. More than half of the finger flexor patients were able to close their fists completely enough to touch their proximal palm (Fig. 214-13). For the adult group, the distal palmar crease to fingertip distance ranged from 0.5 to 4 cm. The average grip strength was 38% compared with the opposite normal extremity. The range was 14% to 81%. The severity of the pretransfer upper extremity injury is a significant factor in determining the functional use of the extremity. The absence of good supination and pronation is a significant detriment to functional use. Incomplete but protective sensation or full sensation was present in all patients. Lack of full sensation did not appear to be a limiting factor to functional use. In all patients who had extensor tendon transfers, close to full finger and thumb extension was obtained.

Biceps Transfer

Although free functioning muscle transfer has been used extensively by others for brachial plexus reconstruction, the authors have little experience in this area. Our experience has been after trauma in which the musculocutaneous nerve was available for innervation of the transfer. Four of five patients with biceps reconstruction had full active elbow flexion and were able to flex their elbows with an average weight of 5 mg held in the hand (Fig. 214-14).

Deltoid Reconstruction

The anterior deltoid has been reconstructed for shoulder flexion in eight patients. The etiology has been muscle loss related to tumor resection and late

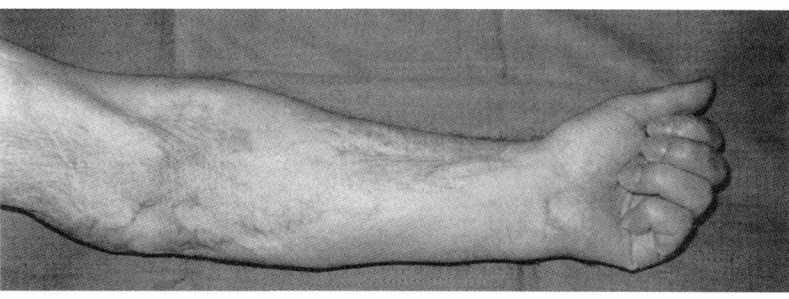

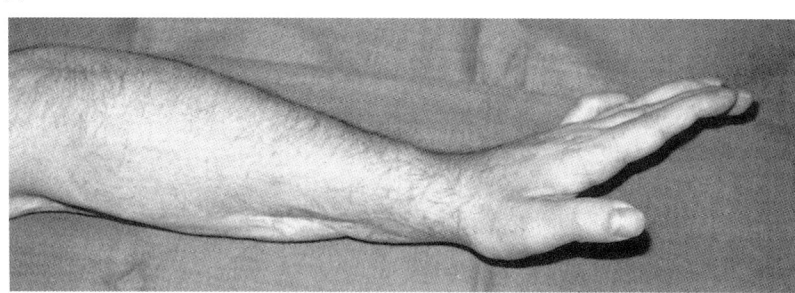

FIGURE 214-13. *A*, After a gracilis muscle transfer to replace finger flexor musculature lost in an industrial accident, a complete fist can be made with active contraction of the muscle. *B*, The muscle will stretch to allow full active wrist and finger extension.

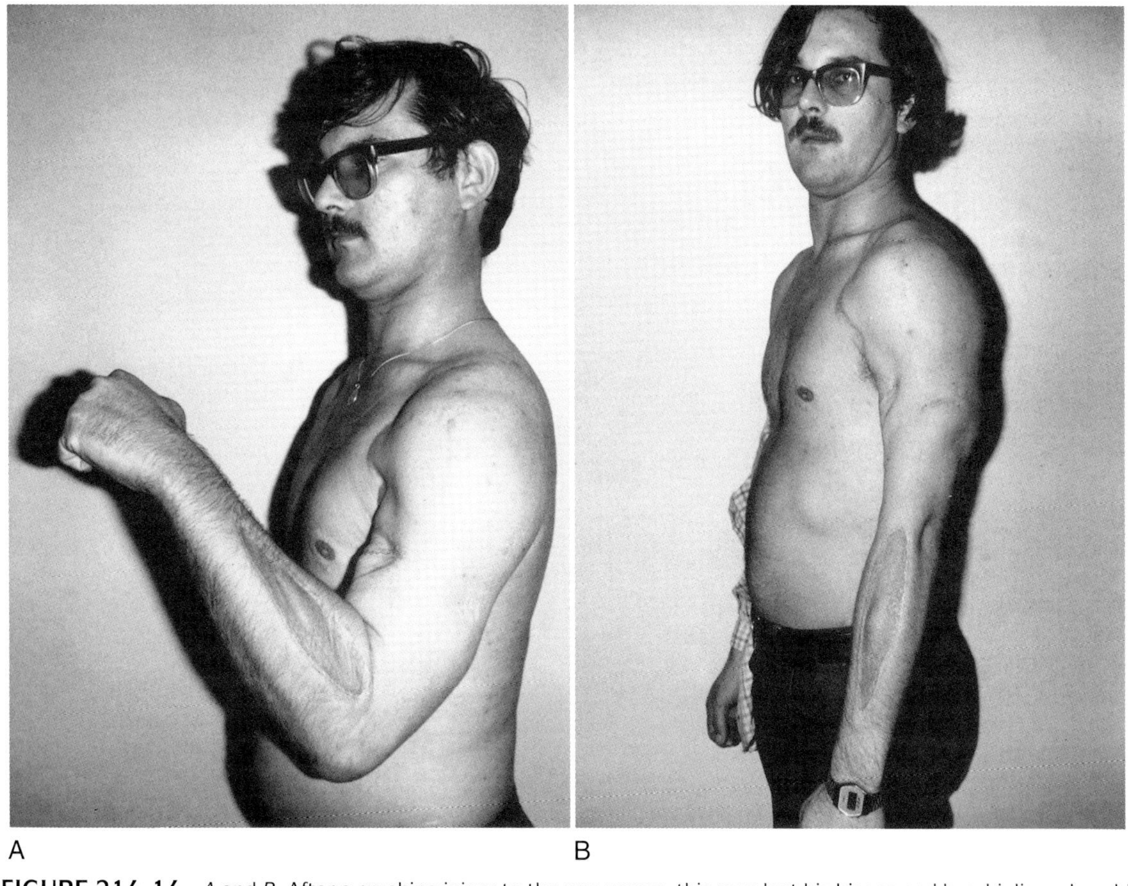

A   B

FIGURE 214-14. *A* and *B*, After a crushing injury to the upper arm, this man lost his biceps and brachialis and could not flex his elbow. He is seen here after a gracilis muscle transfer innervated with the motor component of the musculocutaneous nerve. Note full elbow extension and flexion.

presentation of an axillary nerve avulsion secondary to shoulder dislocation. All patients had weak or no shoulder flexion preoperatively. No patient could flex the shoulder above the horizontal plane, and some were not able to flex it at all. Four of the patients had chronic subluxation of the glenohumeral joint and complained of shoulder pain preoperatively.

One patient did not develop active muscle contraction. Seven patients had useful flexion of the shoulder to 90 to 170 degrees and could fix the humerus in position in front of the body. All four patients with subluxation noted a significant decrease in shoulder pain after muscle transfer.

REFERENCES

1. Manktelow RT, McKee NH: Free muscle transplantation to provide active flexion. J Hand Surg 1978;3:416-426.
2. Zuker RM, Egersaegi EP, Manktelow RT, et al: Volkmann's ischemic contracture in children: the results of free vascularized muscle transplantation. Microsurgery 1991;12:341-345.
3. Chuang DC, Epstein MD, Yeh MC, Wei FC: Functional restoration of elbow flexion in brachial plexus injuries: results in 167 patients (excluding obstetrical brachial plexus injury). J Hand Surg Am 1993;18:285-291.
4. Doi K, Sakai K, Kuwata N, et al: Reconstruction of finger and elbow function after complete avulsion of the brachial plexus. J Hand Surg Am 1991;16:796-803.
5. Tamai S, Komatsu S, Sakamoto H, et al: Free muscle transplants in dogs with microsurgical neurovascular anastomoses. Plast Reconstr Surg 1970;46:219-225.
6. Sixth Peoples' Hospital, Microvascular Service, Shanghai: Free muscle transplantation by microsurgical neurovascular anastomoses. Clin Med J 1976;2:47.
7. Carr MM, Manktelow RT, Zuker RM: Gracilis donor site morbidity. Microsurgery 1995;16:598-600.
8. Manktelow RT, Zuker RM, McKee NH: Functioning free muscle transplantation. J Hand Surg Am 1984;9:32-39.
9. Carlson FD, Wilkie DR: Muscle Physiology. Englewood Cliffs, NJ, Prentice-Hall, 1974.
10. Schenck RR: Rectus femoris muscle and composite skin transplantation by microneurovascular anastomoses for avulsion of forearm muscles: a case report. J Hand Surg Am 1978;3:60-69.
11. McKee NH, Kuzon WM: Functioning free muscle transplantation: making it work? What is known? Ann Plast Surg 1989;23:249-254.
12. Terzis JK, Sweet RD, Dykes RW, Williams HB: Recovery of function in free muscle transplants using microneurovascular anastomosis. J Hand Surg Am 1978;3:37-59.
13. Mathes SJ, Nahai F: Classification of the vascular anatomy of muscles: experiments and clinical correlation. Plast Reconstr Surg 1981;67:177-187.
14. Berger A, Millesi H: Nerve grafting. Clin Orthop 1978;133:49-55.
15. Clarke HM: The Hemodynamics and Viability of Skin and Muscle Flaps [thesis]. Toronto, University of Toronto, 1984:104.
16. Sanger JR, Riley DA, Yousif NJ, et al: Histochemical staining of nerve endings as an aid to free muscle transplantation. Microsurgery 1991;12:361-366.

Restoration of Upper Extremity Function in Tetraplegia

VINCENT R. HENTZ, MD ✦ TIMOTHY R. MCADAMS, MD

With continued improvements in the emergency resuscitation of patients with cervical spinal cord injuries, greater numbers of patients with higher levels of injury are surviving. These patients reach rehabilitation facilities with heightened expectations about recovery and with significant rehabilitative demands.

In addition, because of the increasing acceptance that surgery can play an important role in restoration of function to the paralyzed upper extremity, greater numbers of tetraplegic patients are knowledgeable about upper extremity surgery and inquire about the appropriateness of surgery for their hands and arms. Tetraplegics express a greater desire to have function restored to their hands than, for example, to have sexual function restored.

HISTORICAL PERSPECTIVE

In the minds of both physiatrists and surgeons, the appropriateness of surgical reconstruction for the tetraplegic's upper extremity has waxed and waned in acceptance since the initial reports of Bunnell[1] in the l940s. The many factors that are responsible for the varying attitudes toward surgery are discussed here.

In l949, Bunnell[2] described his results with procedures designed to provide an automatic finger grasp and release and tip-to-tip or so-called opposition pinch

for tetraplegic patients possessing active wrist extension. This was accomplished by tenodeses of multiple extensor and flexor tendons to the radius so that the thumb and fingers would automatically flex with wrist extension and extend with wrist flexion. In addition, with wrist extension, the thumb and the index and middle fingertips were brought together in so-called opposition or three-jawed chuck pinch. Muscle transfers were used occasionally rather than tenodeses, but Bunnell's goal for the thumb remained focused on achieving tip-to-tip pinch because this was thought to represent refined function. In general, Bunnell's patients would be classified at C6 and C7 functional levels according to current standards because they frequently retained active wrist extension and flexion.

Some years later, at Rancho Los Amigos Hospital, Nickel and colleagues[3] attempted to extend hand surgery to tetraplegics with less residual upper extremity function. They devised a complex operation involving fusion of many joints to pre-position the fingers and thumb and multiple tenodeses to achieve an automatic opposition-type or tip-to-tip pinch between the thumb and index and middle fingers. In actuality, it was difficult to achieve the precise digital posture needed for accurate thumb opposition. Some patients were unhappy with the stiff fingers, a consequence of the fusions. Although this surgical procedure fell into

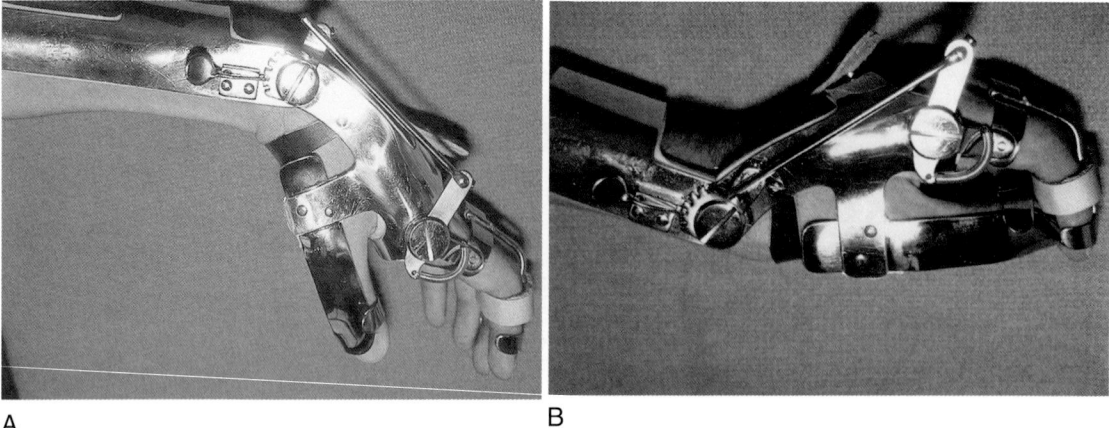

A   B

FIGURE 215-1. In the United States, the wrist-driven flexor hinge splint (*A* and *B*) is the most commonly prescribed dynamic orthosis. It employs a system of rods and levers that reciprocally convert active wrist motion into finger extension and flexion. The device stabilizes all the joints of the thumb so that it becomes a solid post. The interphalangeal joints of the index and middle fingers are similarly stabilized so that motion occurs only at the metacarpophalangeal joints of these two fingers. (From Hentz V, Leclercq C: Surgical Rehabilitation of the Upper Limb in Tetraplegia. London, Harcourt Health Sciences, 2002:3.)

disfavor, its external corollary, a mechanical device or orthosis that holds the fingers and thumbs in the necessary position, became the standard orthosis.[4] In the United States, the Rancho design of the wrist-driven flexor hand splint and various modifications of this splint still remain the standard functional orthosis for the tetraplegic's hand (Fig. 215-1).

During the 1960s and early 1970s, several pioneer reconstructive extremity surgeons, including Lamb[5] in Scotland and Zancolli[6] in Argentina, were reporting good results with use of active muscle-tendon transfers to substitute for missing function. However, during this period, surgery was not held in high regard by physiatrists and rehabilitation specialists because of more than occasional poor results. The results of muscle-tendon transfers were sometimes unpredictable because the transferred muscle was frequently spastic. Patients did not appreciate stiff contracted fingers that could result from transfer of such spastic muscles. Guttmann,[7] in his textbook on spinal cord management, stated in 1976 that less than 5% of tetraplegic patients were candidates for hand surgery.

In 1974,[8] and again in 1975,[9] a Swedish hand surgeon, Erik Moberg, published his philosophy regarding the role of hand surgery in tetraplegia and described his results in reconstructing two important functions missing in the majority of tetraplegic patients, elbow extension and key grasp (Fig. 215-2). Moberg held four strong opinions:

1. Aside from the brain, the hand of the tetraplegic represents the patient's most important residual resource. However, tetraplegic patients use the hands differently from any other patient in that they must "walk" on their hands. Past failure to recognize the functional demands of the tetraplegic's hands led to poorly designed fusions and tenodeses that broke down in response to these demands.

2. As the most important residual resource, the hand has three primary roles: gripping, feeling, and human contact. Moberg believed that supple hands are preferred for human contact and that the stiff clawed hands that followed the multiple joint fusions performed in previous years were unacceptable to the patient.

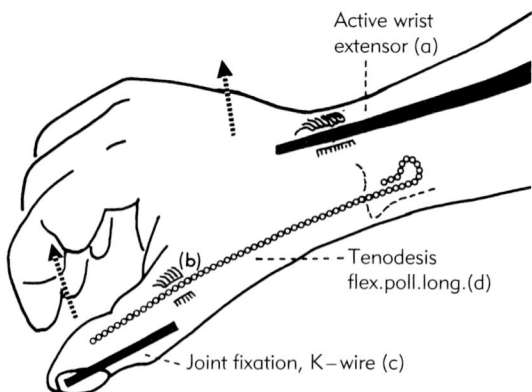

FIGURE 215-2. Moberg's procedures to restore elbow extension and key pinch are illustrated. (From Moberg E: Surgical treatment for absent single-hand grip and elbow extension in quadriplegia. J Bone Joint Surg Am 1975; 57:196-206.)

3. When limited functional resources remain after injury, surgery should represent essentially no risk to these residual resources. Therefore, especially for patients with upper level cervical cord injuries, all surgery should be essentially reversible.

4. Moberg believed that the key grip (i.e., lateral pinch) between the broad pulp of the thumb and the side of the index finger was far more useful for the tetraplegic patient than the opposition-type pinch favored by most predecessors.

Moberg remained a champion of the role of surgery for tetraplegic patients until his death in the spring of 1993. His philosophy has guided the development of our program in surgical reconstruction for tetraplegic patients at the VA Palo Alto Health Care System, Spinal Cord Injury Center, during the past 25 years. We[10-14] have enlarged on Moberg's philosophy as we have gained experience. Tetraplegics with greater numbers of residual motor resources are candidates for the reconstruction of more functional hands than can be achieved by provision of only a key or lateral pinch. Some minimal risk for these patients is acceptable. Still, even after 20 years, we observe Moberg's dicta, especially for the patients who present with little remaining function in the upper limb.

CLASSIFICATION OF THE TETRAPLEGIC UPPER EXTREMITY

An injury to the cervical spinal cord has been classified in many ways, including by the skeletal level of injury and according to the most distal remaining functioning cervical root. However, no two patients, even with injuries at the same skeletal level, are exactly alike, and the same is frequently true of the right and left extremities in the same patient. There may be discrepancies in the motor and sensory distribution of an individual patient's injury. For useful recommendations to be made for treatment, it was necessary to develop a more precise method for classification of the upper limb in the tetraplegic patient. From this need arose the International Classification used today, based not on the spinal level of injury but on the limb's remaining useful motor and sensory resources (Table 215-1). Muscle strength is assessed by the standard Medical Research Council (MRC) of Britain scale of 0 to 5, and the limb is classified according to the residual number of grade 4 or grade 5 muscles under voluntary control distal to the elbow. The grade 4 level was chosen because a grade 4 muscle can be transferred with the expectation that it will be able to perform useful work. A grade 3 muscle loses so much of its power in transfer that it cannot be reliably expected to do useful work after transfer.

Moberg[9,15] encouraged a consideration of remaining sensory resources as well. If sufficient proprioception remains in any part of the hand (typically the thumb and index finger), the patient can control the hand without having to keep it in view. If the hand lacks proprioception, the patient could instead use the eyes for afferent control. However, lack of proprioception limits the patient in performing bimanual activities. Today, static two-point discrimination of less than 12 to 15 mm is acknowledged to indicate the presence of proprioception. The International Classification recognizes the presence or absence of proprioception by including codes to indicate whether afferent control resides in the hands, termed cutaneous or Cu, or only in the eyes of the patient, termed ocular and abbreviated O.

TABLE 215-1 ✦ INTERNATIONAL CLASSIFICATION FOR SURGERY OF THE HAND IN TETRAPLEGIA*

Sensibility O or Cu Group	Motor Characteristics	Description of Function
0	No muscles below elbow suitable for transfer	Flexion-supination of elbow
1	BR	
2	ECRL	Extension of wrist (weak or strong)
3†	ECRB	Extension of wrist
4	PT	Extension and pronation of wrist
5	FCR	Flexion of wrist
6	Finger extensors	Extrinsic extension of fingers, partial or complete
7	Thumb extension	Extrinsic extension of the thumb
8	Partial digital flexors	Extrinsic flexion of the fingers, weak
9	Lacks only intrinsics	Extrinsic flexion of the fingers
X	Exceptions	

*Edinburgh, 1978; modified Giens, France, 1984.
†Caution: it is not possible to determine ECRB strength without surgical exposure.
BR, brachioradialis; ECRL, extensor carpi radialis longus; ECRB, extensor carpi radialis brevis; PT, pronator teres; FCR, flexor carpi radialis.

Later, the International Classification scheme was extended somewhat to include a determination of the presence or absence of active elbow extension. This system was adopted by the International Federation of Hand Surgery Societies,[16] and it is used by essentially all surgeons involved in the care of the upper extremities of these patients.

FORMING A TEAM

Moberg also stressed the need to develop a "critical mass" of like-minded professionals into a team, which should include physiatrists and rehabilitation medicine specialists involved in the rehabilitation and long-term care of tetraplegic patients. Critical to the concept of a team are well-trained therapists, either physical therapists or occupational therapists (preferably both). The hand and upper extremity surgeon, whose primary background may be either orthopedics or plastic and reconstructive surgery, constitutes the remaining professional resource. Others, including social workers and psychologists, may play unique roles. However, the most important part of the team, once identified, is the patient; equally important is the patient's support group, including family, attendant, and others. The role of the professionals in this team seems relatively clear-cut. The physiatrist or rehabilitation medicine specialist assists in determining the appropriateness of surgery for the patient as well as the appropriate timing of surgery relative to overall rehabilitation goals and schedules. The therapist frequently serves as the patient's advocate. He or she knows the patient better than anyone else, particularly the patient's motivation and intelligence and, most important, the patient's expectations, voiced or not.

Upper extremity surgery has perhaps greater emotional impact for the tetraplegic patient than for most other patients. The tetraplegic patient is aware of the somewhat precarious nature of his or her life. Whereas the goal of surgical reconstruction for the upper extremity is greater independence, this can be achieved only at the expense of an occasionally prolonged period of greater dependence. For family and attendants, this greater period of dependence translates into more inconvenience and effort. All the team members must play a role in the decision-making process and must share in the frustrations as well as in the rewards.

EVALUATION AND SELECTION OF THE PATIENT

The hand and upper extremity team should participate in the routine evaluation of even newly injured patients. The cervical cord-injured patient arrives at a rehabilitation facility or spinal cord injury unit usually with fairly supple upper limbs, although with no or only minimal volitional movement. Fortunately today, well-educated therapists involved with the patients in the early days or weeks after injury are aware of the need for protective splinting to avoid the insidious development of pathologic contractures of the shoulders, elbows, wrists, and digits.

Once the patient's vertebral injury has become stabilized and the patient can be up in a wheelchair, an assessment by the upper extremity team takes on new meaning. By the third or fourth month after injury, the eventual functional level is usually clearly established for the majority of patients.[17] At this time, and on the basis of the patient's ability to adapt to adaptive devices for feeding and hygiene, an early determination about the applicability of more complex functional orthoses can be made.[18-20] For some patients, early measurement, fabrication, and fitting of a functional orthosis, such as a wrist-driven flexor hinge splint (see Fig. 215-1), will advance the rate of rehabilitation. For patients with early but weak recovery of wrist extension, the wrist-driven flexor hinge splint represents an excellent exercise therapy directed toward strengthening wrist extensors so that they may eventually actuate a surgically reconstructed pinch or grip.

Hand or upper extremity surgery is rarely indicated during the initial months of rehabilitation after injury. The patient needs time to experience neurologic, psychological, and social stability. From a practical standpoint, there are simply too many more important rehabilitation activities going on. On the other hand, a dogmatic philosophy embracing tired dicta, such as "never operate on a patient before 12 months," has no basis in science. Some patients are clearly candidates for surgery before this calendar date. For example, early surgical intervention to relieve the pathologic effects of a fixed elbow flexion contracture may allow a patient to participate more vigorously in necessary rehabilitation activities.[21] There exists a good rationale for paralyzing for some months a spastic and shortened biceps muscle by botulinum toxin injection in open crush of the musculocutaneous nerve. A good argument can be made for early release of a fixed elbow flexion contracture with simultaneous transfer of the contracted biceps muscle to the triceps. This removes a pathologic or deforming force and reinforces or restores some power to the antagonist.

Once the patient has achieved neurologic and psychological stability, a formal evaluation to establish the appropriateness of upper extremity surgery can be accomplished by the team. The evaluation focuses on both the tangible evidence of recovery by assessment of remaining motor and sensory resources and the important intangibles, such as motivation and intelligence. In addition, the assessment includes an evaluation of the means by which the patient now accomplishes the tasks of daily living, with particular attention to how he or she performs transfers and pushes a wheelchair (Fig. 215-3).

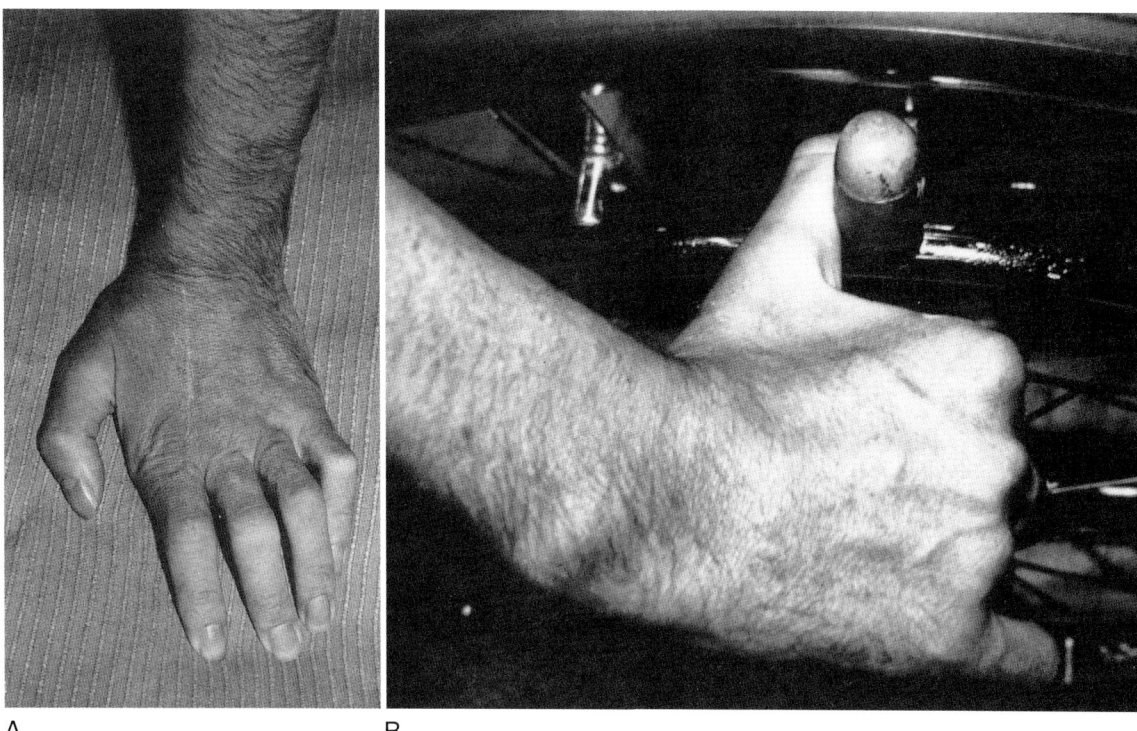

A   B

FIGURE 215-3. Transfers performed on the flattened hand, although stable, will, over time, destroy the collateral ligaments about the thumb and the metacarpophalangeal joints *(A)*. Furthermore, if continued after functional surgery, this posture will stretch out tenodeses and break down joint fusions. A similar fate awaits the thumb in this patient who uses his thumb to push the "quad knobs" of the wheelchair *(B)*. Patients with these postures must be retrained to perform safer transfers and propulsion maneuvers before surgical reconstruction is considered. (*B* from Hentz V, Leclercq C: Surgical Rehabilitation of the Upper Limb in Tetraplegia. London, Harcourt Health Sciences, 2002:38-39.)

The motor examination includes an assay of residual motor groups as well as the identification of pathologic conditions, such as contracted, painful, or unstable joints. The sensory evaluation includes the measurement of two-point discrimination in the digits to assess proprioception and the identification of pathologic conditions, such as painful hypersensitivity. The currently used grip patterns are assessed (Fig. 215-4).

The patient's current functional status is assessed. Is the patient dependent or independent in bed mobility? How are transfers performed? Does the patient use a manual or electric wheelchair? What adaptive devices are used for dressing? grooming? feeding? If surgery is to be performed, is there sufficient support to get the patient through a period of greater functional dependence, or will the extra burden of care result in the attendant's quitting? For many patients, upper extremity surgery means restriction to an electric-driven chair. Can this be made available? Does the home situation permit the use of an electric wheelchair? Are the controls of the chair mounted on the nonoperated

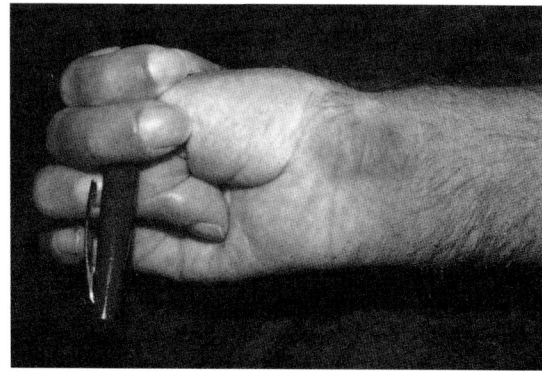

FIGURE 215-4. The manner in which the patient uses his or her hand must be evaluated. This patient uses an interweaving grip to hold utensils. (From Hentz V, Leclercq C: Surgical Rehabilitation of the Upper Limb in Tetraplegia. London, Harcourt Health Sciences, 2002:40.)

side? The patient's primary therapist plays the most important role in determining these issues.

GENERAL GUIDELINES FOR RECONSTRUCTION

Three surgical procedures are applicable for improving upper limb function in tetraplegia:

- Arthrodeses permit stabilization of joints lacking muscle stabilization.
- Tenodesis is performed either to stabilize a joint or more commonly so that another, typically more proximal movement (e.g., wrist extension) will result in the tightening of the tenodesis and movement of a more distally located joint.
- Transfer of the power of an expendable muscle-tendon unit under good volitional control compensates for the absence or ineffectiveness of function of another muscle-tendon unit.

A fourth reconstruction technique has recently been introduced. Termed functional neuromuscular stimulation, this technique uses the residual contractile properties of upper motor neuron-paralyzed muscles when they are stimulated by an extraneural source. The remainder of this chapter is devoted to a discussion of the role of surgery for improving function at the elbow, wrist, and fingers. Admittedly, it is difficult to present this in a fashion that does not bring to mind a cookbook of recipes; however, nothing could be more divorced from fact. Each patient, and indeed each upper extremity, must be evaluated and a treatment plan individualized. This cannot be stressed enough.

For cervical spinal cord injuries at the most proximal anatomic level, no expendable, and thus transferable, muscles exist. For patients injured at the more distal anatomic extreme, many potentially expendable, and thus transferable, muscles of grade 4 or grade 5 power exist. Thus, reconstructive possibilities range from procedures to merely simplify the mechanics of the hand, such as fusing a wrist joint so that this joint no longer requires external stabilizing by an orthosis, to complex multistaged procedures involving many muscle-tendon transfers. The choice of procedure depends primarily on the residual resources and, secondly, on the many intangibles, such as motivation and support. Whereas the surgical techniques are exactly those used to overcome the functional loss for patients with peripheral nerve injuries, matching the patient and the procedure requires an understanding of the real difference between the tetraplegic patient and someone with, for example, a brachial plexus injury or a combined high median and ulnar nerve palsy. A cautious approach while one gains experience pays great dividends in terms of obtaining the acceptance of team members and patients that surgery can promote greater independence for these patients. A poor outcome early in the team's experience creates a tremendous hurdle.

SURGICAL RECONSTRUCTION
Elbow Extension

Erik Moberg brought to our attention the importance of active elbow extension for the spinal cord-injured patient. The wheelchair-bound individual depends on good shoulder and elbow power and stabilization to push a wheelchair, to transfer from bed to chair, and to perform pressure releases to prevent pressure sores. For the tetraplegic patient, lack of a functional elbow extension results in a much reduced functional environment. The world of the tetraplegic patient is determined by the range of motion of his or her upper extremity. Without the ability to extend the elbow, the patient's "sphere of influence" is much reduced. The ability to extend the hand in space by an additional 12 inches results in an additional 800% of space that the hand can reach.

There are other reasons that reconstruction of active elbow extension is tremendously useful. Without active elbow extension, the tetraplegic's hands frequently fall into the face on lying supine. One cannot push a manual wheelchair up any incline without triceps function. Even as simple a task as turning on a room light switch may be impossible without active elbow extension.

DELTOID TO TRICEPS TRANSFER

There are two surgical procedures advocated for restoration of active elbow extension. In the United States, transfer of the power of the posterior half of the deltoid to the triceps tendon, as described by Moberg,[22] is preferred. This procedure is preferred when the posterior deltoid is strong and the elbow has nearly normal passive extension. The procedure, performed under general anesthesia, involves detaching the insertion of the posterior half of the deltoid from the humerus and connecting into the olecranon process of the ulna.

Surgical Technique

The surgical landmarks (Fig. 215-5A) at the level of the shoulder include the tip of the acromion superiorly, the interval between the posterior margin of the deltoid and the triceps muscle posteriorly, and the estimated point of insertion of the deltoid on the humerus. The landmark at the level of the elbow is the tip of the olecranon. The surgeon should keep in mind the neurovascular anatomy of the region, including the course of the axillary nerve and the circumflex humeral artery and the radial nerve and its relationship to the insertion of the deltoid (Fig. 215-5B).

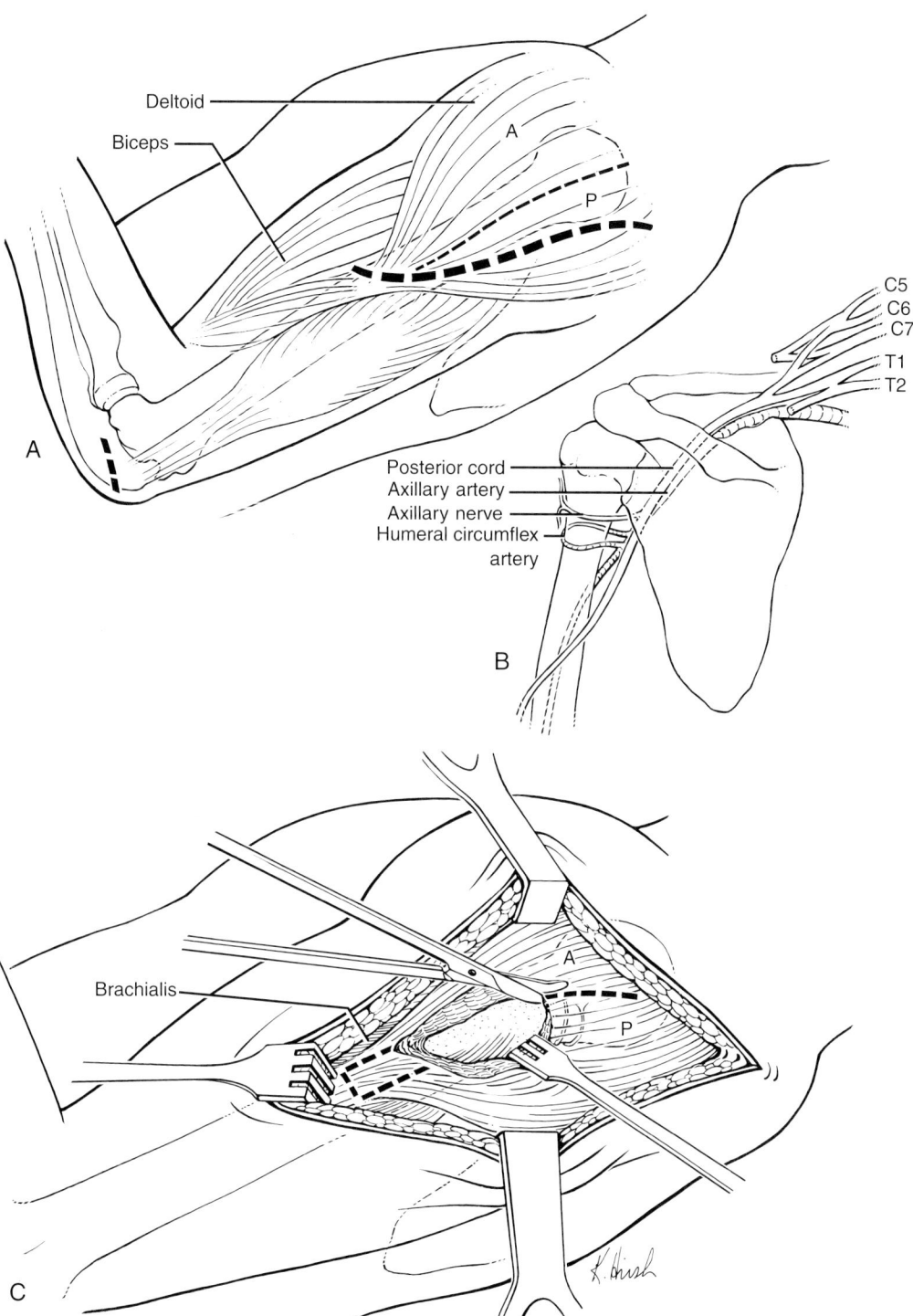

FIGURE 215-5. The authors' preferred technique for deltoid to triceps transfer is illustrated. See text for details. (From Hentz V, Leclercq C: Surgical Rehabilitation of the Upper Limb in Tetraplegia. London, Harcourt Health Sciences, 2002:100.)

Continued

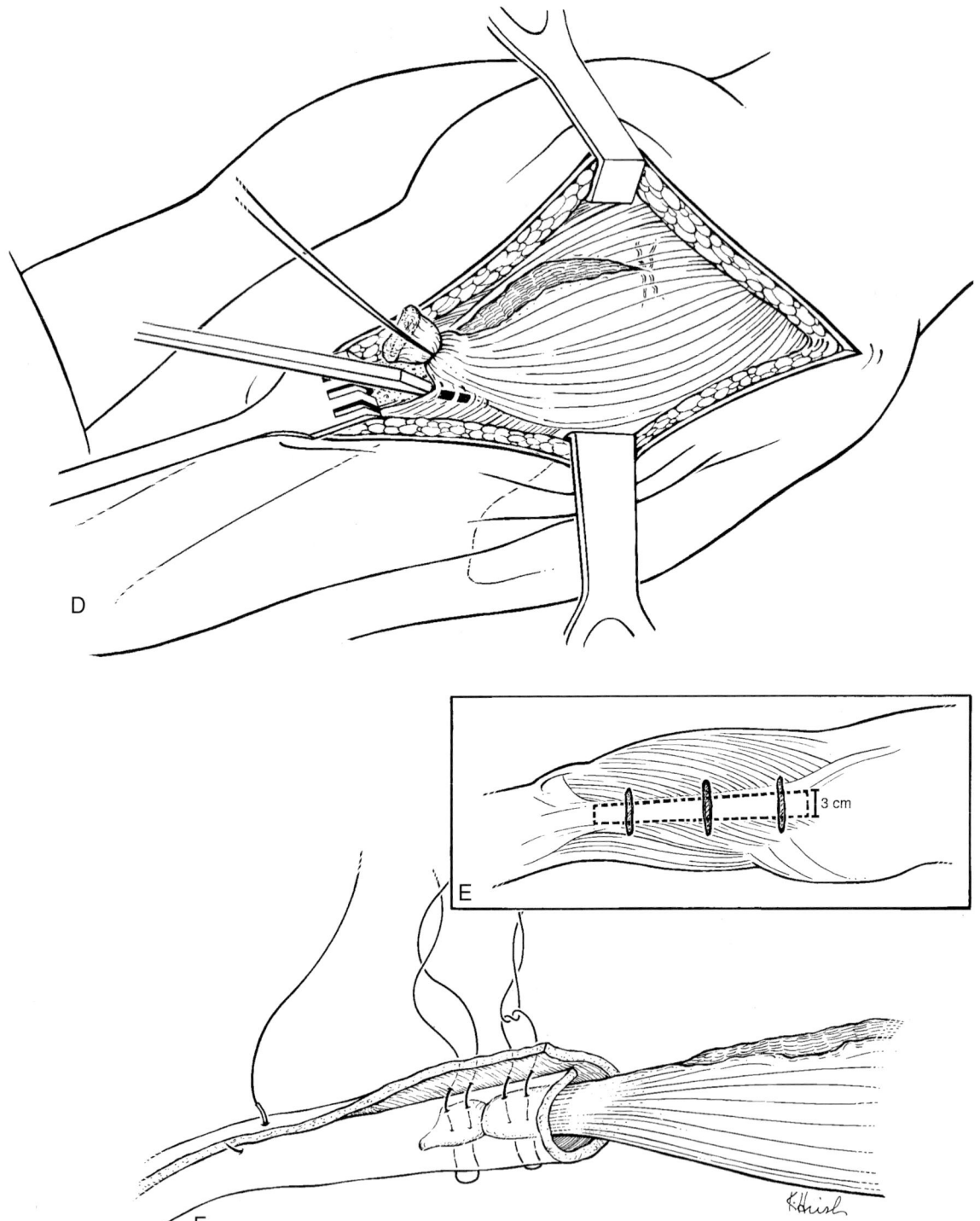

FIGURE 215-5, cont'd.

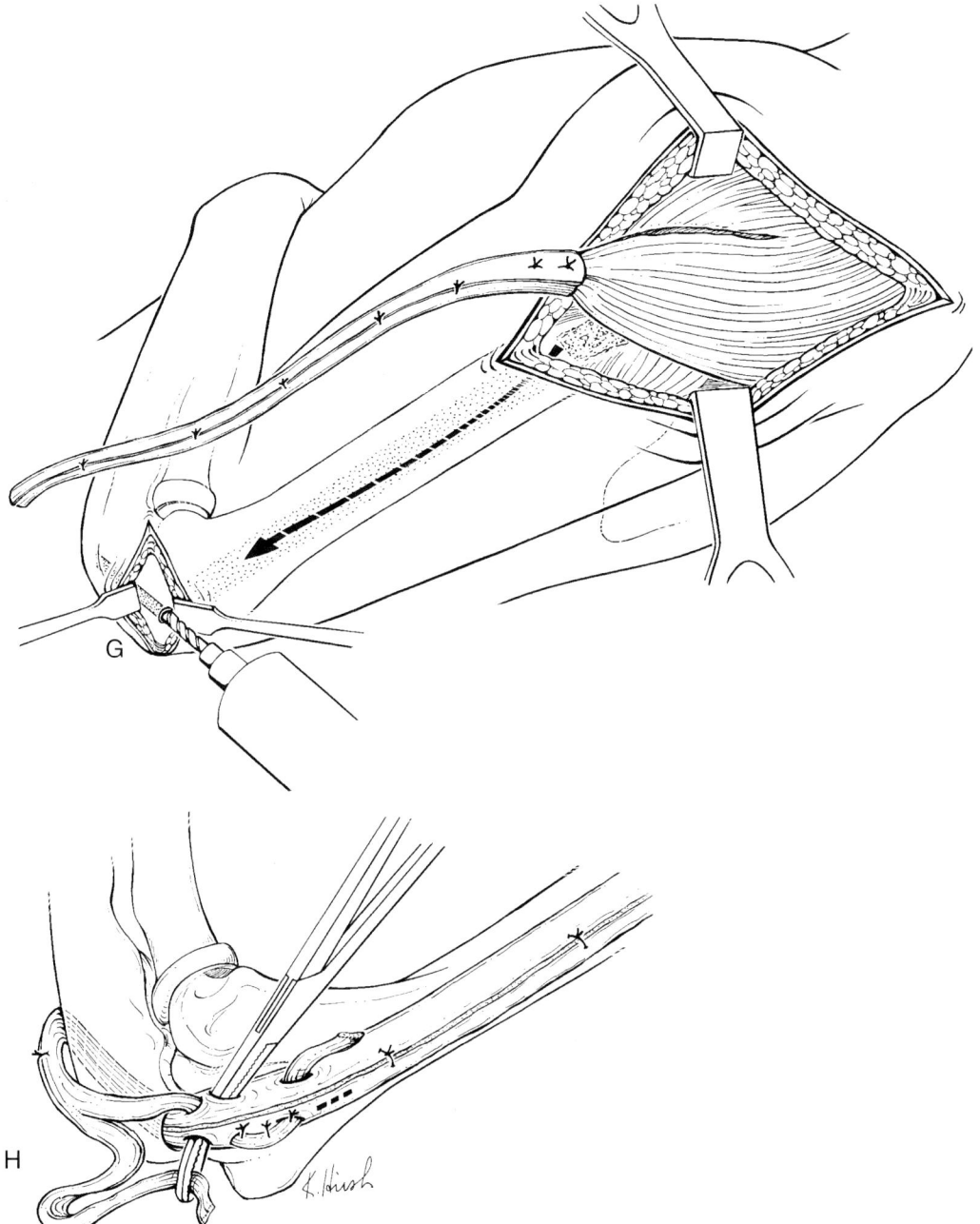

FIGURE 215-5, cont'd.

The upper incision is centered halfway between the midaxial line of the humerus and the posterior margin of the deltoid (Fig. 215-5A). The skin incision is carried to the level of the muscle fascia, and the skin and subcutaneous tissues are elevated anteriorly to just past the midaxial line of the humerus. Posteriorly, the skin flap is elevated to the confluence of deltoid and the long head of the triceps (Fig. 215-5C). The plane between these two muscles is developed by sharp or finger dissection. As the finger strikes the humerus, the fingertip can be insinuated upward through the fibers of the deltoid, separating the muscle into relatively equal anterior and posterior halves.

It is helpful to detach the insertion of the posterior half of the muscle from its point of insertion onto the humerus. This is done by sharply incising a rectangle of periosteum at the point of attachment and elevating the periosteum and the fibers of attachment off the humerus (Fig. 215-5D). Care is taken to include as much fascia and fibrous insertion as possible, including some of the fascial origin of the brachialis muscle. The radial nerve will be emerging from behind the humerus several centimeters distal to this point. Injury to this nerve has been reported as a rare but devastating complication of this procedure, so care should be exercised regarding the anatomic landmarks.

A suture is placed in the fibrous origin of the posterior half of the deltoid muscle (Fig. 215-5D), and the dissection is carried superiorly until the branches of the axillary nerve are visualized. These must not be injured, and the superior dissection should stop at this point.

The detached tendinous insertion of the hemideltoid cannot reach its proposed new point of attachment. Therefore, several methods have been proposed to attach the posterior deltoid to the triceps or olecranon, including

- autogenous tendons, such as toe extensors as initially suggested by Moberg[22]; tibialis anterior tendon, as subsequently suggested by Moberg[15]; or extensor carpi ulnaris, as proposed by Lamb[23];
- a turned-up strip of the central part of the triceps tendon,[24] with synthetic reinforcement[25];
- bone to bone attachments[26]; and
- various synthetic materials.[27]

A wide strip of the patient's own fascia lata, especially in the patient whose triceps tendon is relatively short or insubstantial, has proved useful.[11] The fascia lata strip may be obtained by a second surgical team working simultaneously.

The fascia is harvested through several transverse incisions placed over the iliotibial band (Fig. 215-5E). The ideal width is about 2.5 cm. The fascia lata is then tubed about the fibrous insertion of the deltoid with mattress sutures of nonabsorbable braided material (Fig. 215-5F). The fascia is tubed over its remaining length and will be tunneled subcutaneously to the distal incision to be made at the olecranon.

The tip of the olecranon is exposed just distal to the insertion of the triceps. The triceps tendon is split longitudinally to further expose the tip of the olecranon, and a 5-mm drill bit is used to make an oblique tunnel through the olecranon (Fig. 215-5G). A Bunnell tendon stripper is a useful instrument to "polish" this channel so that the tubed fascia lata can be passed smoothly in a proximal to distal direction (Fig. 215-5H). The fascia lata is passed into the distal exposure and separated into two tails; the tails are passed through the bone channel and woven back on themselves.

The shoulder is abducted about 30 degrees and the elbow is flexed about 30 degrees. The two fascia lata tails are then pulled to *maximally* tense the transfer, and these tails are anchored to the fascia lata tube, again

with nonabsorbable sutures. Once suturing is complete, the fascial tube should be under moderate but definite tension.

Regardless of the technique chosen, the elbow is immobilized in full extension by a light plaster or fiberglass cylinder cast for $3\frac{1}{2}$ weeks. The shoulder is kept somewhat abducted, and the patient and other caregivers are cautioned not to allow the shoulder to accidentally flop across the chest. The patient is encouraged to begin getting into his or her wheelchair on the second postoperative day. Patients are essentially totally dependent for all transfer activity while the arm is casted. An overhead, chair-mounted sling is fitted to the wheelchair. This holds the arm somewhat elevated, preventing distal edema, and helps keep the arm somewhat abducted from the body, a position that relaxes the deltoid. The overhead frame is used whenever the patient is up in the wheelchair and until the cast is removed. It is important to provide a plastic support for the wrist while the arm is immobilized within the cylinder cast. This can be removed from time to time and the wrist moved through a range of motion. We have experienced some loss of wrist extensor strength when the wrist was allowed to remain in a flexed position for too long. Another option is to include the wrist within the initial cast.

The initial cast is left undisturbed for $3\frac{1}{2}$ weeks if the elbow had essentially normal passive extension preoperatively. If the elbow had a preoperative flexion contracture between 15 and 30 degrees, the elbow is extended as much as possible at the time of surgery and casted in that position. This cast is removed between 10 and 14 days postoperatively. Great care must be taken to keep the elbow extended during this maneuver. Typically, the elbow can then be extended farther at this time by slow stretch, and the arm is recasted, now typically in nearly full or even full extension. After surgery, the elbow is immobilized in full or nearly full extension for several weeks, and the elbow is then exercised for several additional weeks by allowing progressively greater elbow flexion in a specially designed flexion stop brace (Fig. 215-6). Some months of cautious use are necessary to prevent overstretching of the transfer, and many months pass before maximal strength is obtained.

The results have been reasonably consistent. Most patients can achieve full or nearly full extension against gravity (Fig. 215-7). This allows them to position the arm in space more accurately and to control its movements. Rarely, a patient achieves sufficient power to permit independent transfer in all circumstances, but this is not a realistic goal for most patients. The majority find that they achieve more efficient transfers, pressure releases, and more efficient wheelchair mobility.

Complications are rare provided the patient follows the exercise protocol and does not overstretch the transfer by too rapidly performing full elbow flexion. In two patients, the entire deltoid muscle was transferred

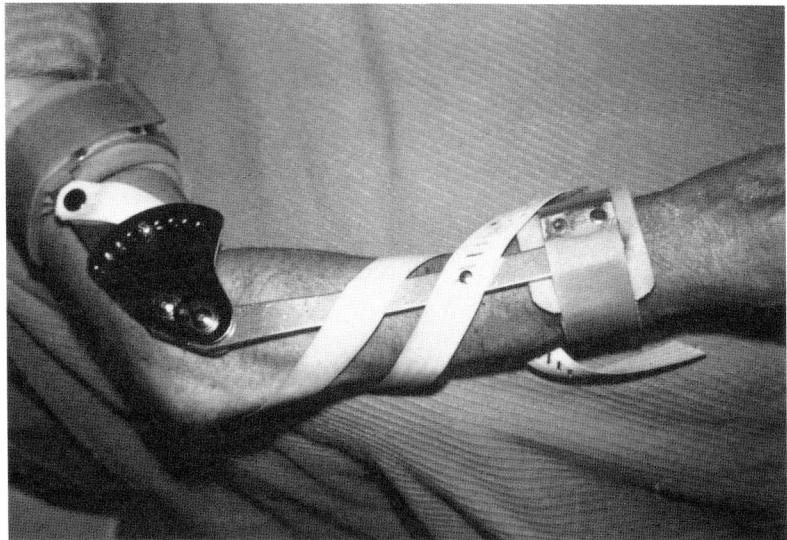

FIGURE 215-6. A type of adjustable flexion block orthosis is illustrated. This device is worn during the day for several weeks as flexion is slowly regained. (From Hentz V, Leclercq C: Surgical Rehabilitation of the Upper Limb in Tetraplegia. London, Harcourt Health Sciences, 2002:99.)

without measurably changing shoulder function. This makes sense because surgery has merely altered the point of attachment of the muscle more distally on the limb.

BICEPS TO TRICEPS TRANSFER

This transfer is indicated when there is a preexisting flexion contracture of the elbow of more than 45 degrees. In this case, the biceps is usually a deforming force, and this deforming force must be treated by tendon lengthening, tenotomy, or transfer. Although seemingly an antagonist to elbow extension, the supinator function of the biceps is used in re-education by teaching the patient to conjointly supinate the forearm and extend the elbow.

Surgical Technique

The biceps tendon can be detached from its insertion on the greater tuberosity of the radius, and the muscle-tendon unit is routed either medially[28] or laterally[29] and the tendon attached to the triceps aponeurosis. The procedure is typically performed under general anesthesia, but it can be performed under supraclavicular brachial plexus blockade. A tourniquet cannot be accommodated.

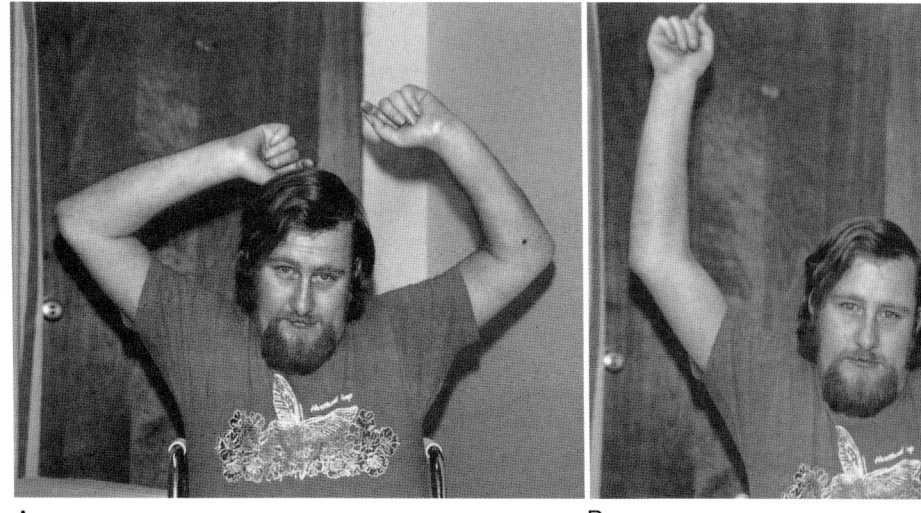

A   B

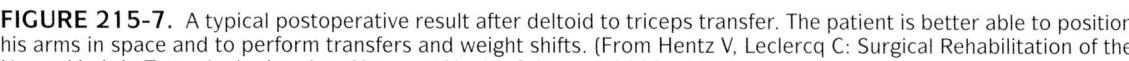

FIGURE 215-7. A typical postoperative result after deltoid to triceps transfer. The patient is better able to position his arms in space and to perform transfers and weight shifts. (From Hentz V, Leclercq C: Surgical Rehabilitation of the Upper Limb in Tetraplegia. London, Harcourt Health Sciences, 2002:108.)

The incisions that are employed depend in large measure on whether a wide exposure to the anterior aspect of the elbow joint is needed to allow adequate release of contracture (Fig. 215-8A). The distal extent of the incision should allow complete dissection of the tendon of the biceps so that it can be detached as close to its point of insertion on the bicipital tuberosity of the radius.

The incision is carried through the subcutaneous tissue, protecting the large tributaries of the basilic and cephalic veins. The soft tissues overlying the lacertus fibrosus are elevated, and the lacertus is either divided off the primary tendon or dissected distally as far as possible to provide another point of fixation to the triceps (Fig. 215-8B).

The primary tendon of the biceps is dissected to its point of insertion on the radius. Flexing the elbow and supinating the forearm assists in this exposure. The tendon is sectioned as far distally as possible (Fig. 215-8B). The biceps muscle is dissected proximally from within its dense investing fascia; the dissection proceeds proximally until the cutaneous portion of the musculocutaneous nerve is identified as it courses between the overlying biceps and the deeper brachialis muscle (Fig. 215-8C). This nerve is protected while dissection of the biceps proceeds proximally until the most distal motor branches coming from the musculocutaneous nerve are visualized.

Both medial and lateral routing of the transfer have been described. Because the ulnar nerve is typically nonfunctional in this population, we have preferred to route the biceps medially (Fig. 215-8C). It is necessary to dissect widely the arcade of Struthers and all other fascial communications about the medial intermuscular septum. There is reason to be concerned about compression of the radial nerve when the lateral route is chosen.

A second incision located posteromedially is made to expose the medial aspect of the triceps insertion. Through this incision, the medial border of the triceps is elevated and dissected to its insertion on the olecranon. The biceps muscle and tendon are then passed from the anterior to the posterior incision through the widely dissected subcutaneous tunnel. The anterior incision may be closed at this point (Fig. 215-8D).

The biceps tendon typically just reaches the tip of the olecranon, but there is infrequently sufficient tendon length to permit a strong attachment into the olecranon. Instead, the tendon of the biceps is woven into the medial border of the triceps tendon and anchored in multiple locations with stout sutures. We have judged that the proper tension is achieved when the biceps is pulled distally enough to permit the end of the tendon to touch the olecranon with the elbow in about 20 degrees of flexion. Once the tendon to tendon junctures are made, the elbow is fully extended to relax the site of approximation. The

posterior incision is closed, and the arm is placed in a cylinder cast as described before for the deltoid to triceps transfer.

The postoperative regimen is exactly like that described before except that the patient learns to trigger the transfer by extending the arm at the shoulder while trying to supinate the forearm. A flexion arrest brace similar to that described for deltoid to triceps transfer is worn, and elbow flexion is gradually increased. Electrical stimulation and biofeedback therapy have been used on occasion with improved results. Just as for deltoid to triceps transfer, one must be concerned about too rapid a remobilization of the transfer.

The results of biceps to triceps transfer are not as impressive as those of deltoid to triceps transfer. Typically, the patient cannot actively extend through a large range against the force of gravity. However, the patient does appreciate a gain in the ability to position the arm more accurately in space, and removal of a deforming force and strengthening of the antagonist decrease the chances for recurrence of the elbow contracture.

Reconstruction of elbow extension has been the single most satisfying reconstruction for our patients. Even though the overall time for rehabilitation can be relatively lengthy, the functional gain is substantial, predictable, and easily appreciated by the patient. Furthermore, the risks to residual preoperative function are practically nil. It represents an important addition to our reconstructive surgical armamentarium.

Surgical Reconstruction for the Weaker Patients: IC Groups 0, 1, and 2

For the patient assigned to International Classification (IC) group 0 with no muscles functioning at the grade 4 or higher level distal to the elbow, few reconstructive possibilities exist. For most of these patients, some type of functional orthosis must suffice. Rarely for the IC group 0 patient, fusion of the wrist might permit the patient to employ a less cumbersome functional orthosis, for example, a self-donned universal cuff rather than a long opponens splint for which the patient needs assistance in donning and doffing. Surgery may also be useful in repositioning a badly positioned part. For example, osteotomy of the radius may place the hand in a more favorable pronated position. This might permit easier manipulation of the joystick control for an electric wheelchair than can be accomplished by a hand that is perpetually supinated.

ACTIVE GRASP FOR THE IC GROUP 0 AND 1 PATIENT

Brummer[30] has proposed a clever surgical tenodesis, termed the winch procedure, that has the potential to

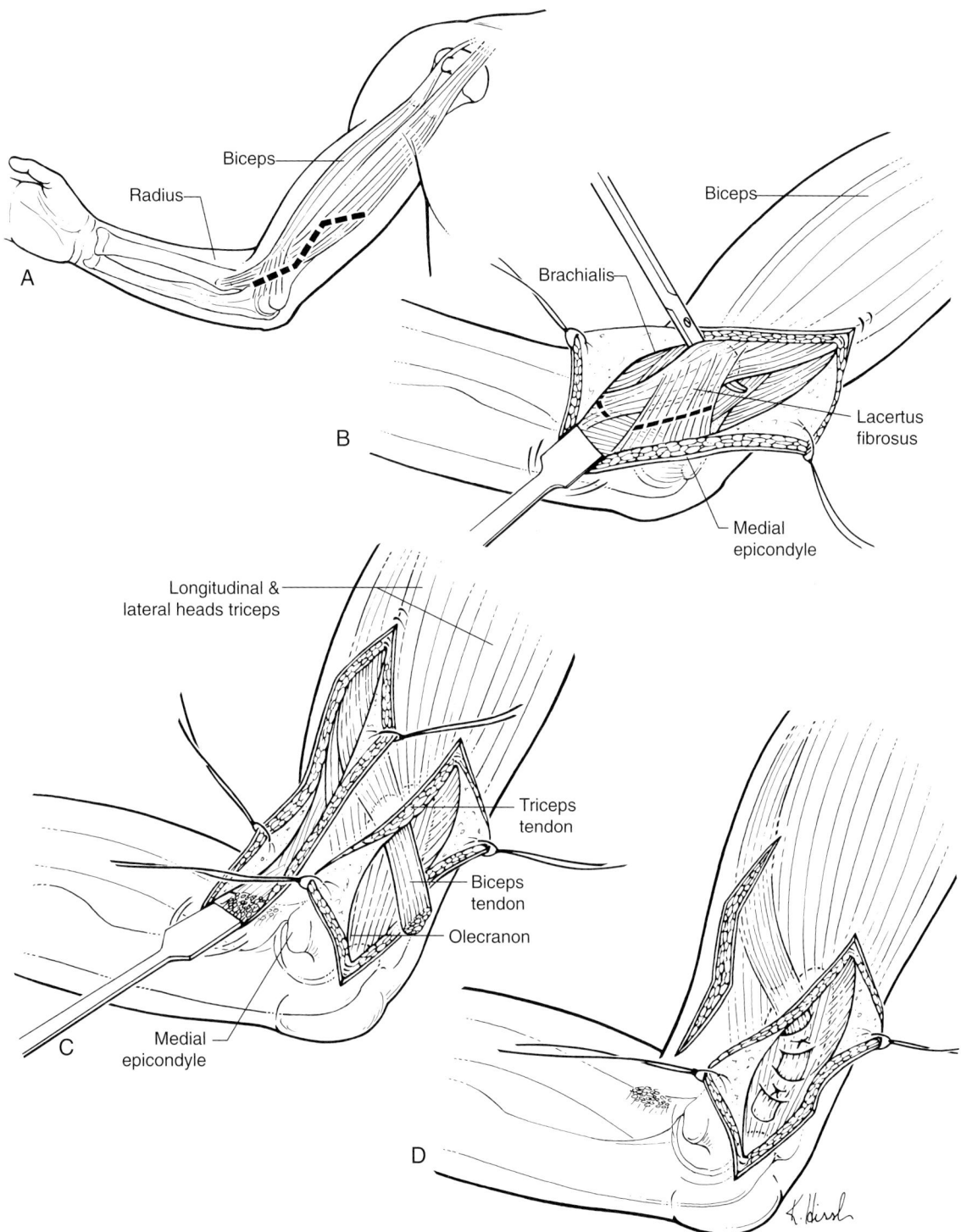

FIGURE 215-8. Biceps to triceps transfer by the medial route. See text for details. (From Hentz V, Leclercq C: Surgical Rehabilitation of the Upper Limb in Tetraplegia. London, Harcourt Health Sciences, 2002:109.)

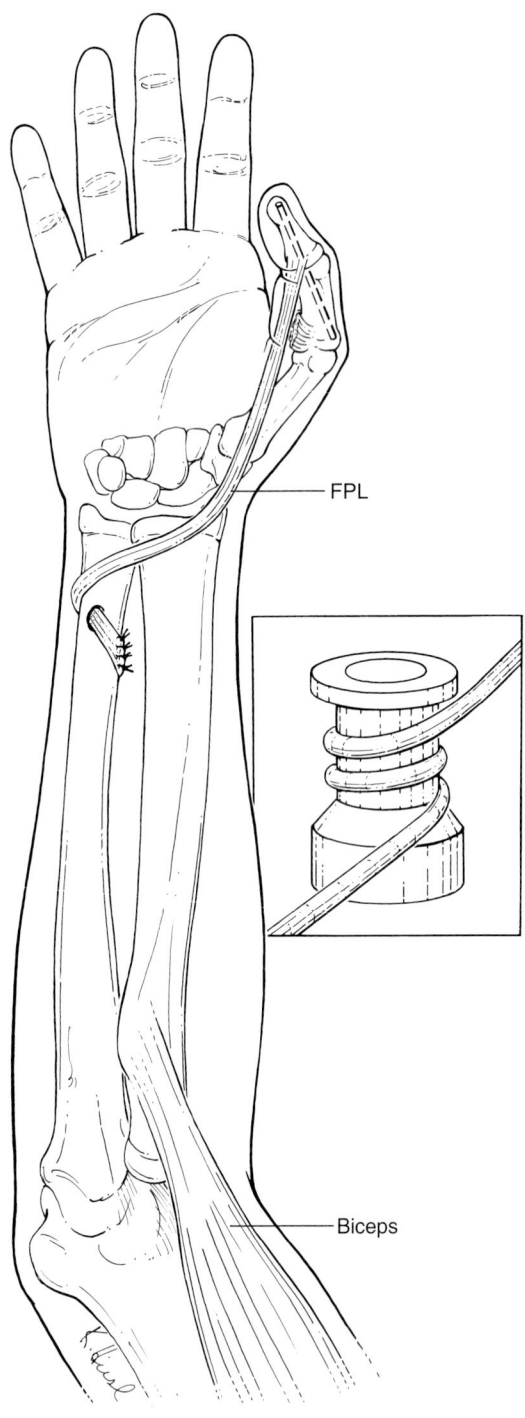

FPL

Biceps

FIGURE 215-9. The Brummer "winch" operation is illustrated. The tendon of the flexor pollicis longus (FPL) is divided at the muscle-tendon junction and is passed deep to the flexor tendons and neurovascular bundles toward the ulna. The interphalangeal joint of the thumb must be stabilized by fusion, pinning, or the split FPL to EPL procedure described in Figure 215-15. With the forearm in full supination, the tendon of the FPL is anchored to the ulna under sufficient tension to achieve key pinch between the pulp of the thumb and the radial side of the index finger with the wrist stabilized in a neutral position. Forearm pronation should allow the grip to relax. (From Hentz V, Leclercq C: Surgical Rehabilitation of the Upper Limb in Tetraplegia. London, Harcourt Health Sciences, 2002:126.)

forearm and good biceps strength. The fingers and thumb must be flexible. The wrist must be in a useful position (not contracted in excessive flexion or extension) and stabilized either by a splint (commonly) or by wrist fusion. The procedure is illustrated in Figure 215-9.

IMPROVING WRIST EXTENSION: THE IC GROUP 1 AND 2 PATIENT

In the IC group 1 patient, the brachioradialis is typically the only muscle with grade 4 function distal to the elbow. However, grade 2+ to grade 3+ radial wrist extensor function is typically present as well. The patient may be able to extend the wrist against gravity but cannot exert any force between digits and thumb through any existing natural tenodesis effect of the paralyzed finger and thumb flexors or cannot use a wrist-driven flexor hand splint unless it is equipped with a ratchet mechanism lock and release. For this patient, wrist extensor strength can be augmented by transferring the power of the brachioradialis into the more central of the radial wrist extensors, the extensor carpi radialis brevis (ECRB) tendon, which attaches to the base of the third metacarpal.[31,32] From several biomechanical studies[33,34] it has been determined that the brachioradialis becomes a more effective wrist extensor after transfer if the patient can stabilize the elbow in space. If no active elbow extension is present, the brachioradialis, because it crosses the elbow joint, may waste some of its excursion and power in flexing the elbow rather than in extending the wrist. For this reason, we prefer first to reconstruct active elbow extension and occasionally will combine deltoid to triceps and brachioradialis to ECRB transfers.

A wide dissection of the distal muscle and tendon from insertion at the radial styloid up to the very proximal forearm level is necessary to obtain the most effective potential excursion of the muscle. One can test the effect of dissection by first pulling the undis-

provide weak but perhaps useful key pinch for this very disadvantaged population. The procedure couples the active forearm supination vector of the innervated biceps with automatic flexion of the thumb to provide key pinch between the pulp of the thumb and the side of the index finger. The requirements include nearly normal passive range of motion of the elbow and

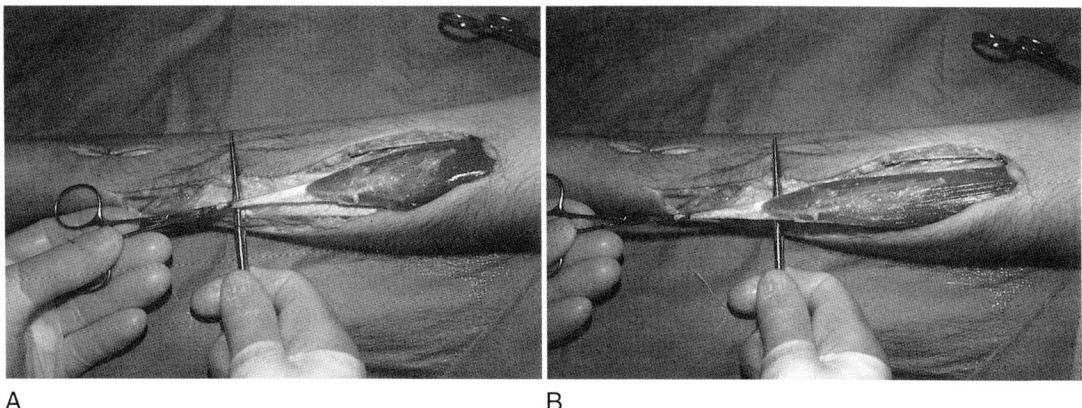

A   B

FIGURE 215-10. The brachioradialis must be dissected proximally, almost to the level of the elbow. *A* depicts the brachioradialis at its normal resting length. *B* demonstrates the amount of passive stretch (3 to 4 cm) that needs to be achieved by proximal dissection of the muscle. (From Hentz V, Leclercq C: Surgical Rehabilitation of the Upper Limb in Tetraplegia. London, Harcourt Health Sciences, 2002:134.)

sected but cut tendon end distally and measuring how much distal stretch can be achieved. After dissection, this test is repeated, and one should notice an additional 2 to 3 cm of distal stretch above that seen before dissection (Fig. 215-10). The tension on the brachioradialis should be adjusted to re-establish the normal resting length of the muscle. In adjusting the tension, it is important to place the elbow in some flexion while tension is set at the junction. Moberg[15] recommended that the elbow be set at about 40 degrees of flexion, and we have followed this guideline. This is done so that the transfer does not lose significant power at the elbow if it is flexed. The wrist is splinted in nearly full extension to relax the tendon to tendon juncture, and this position is maintained for approximately 4 weeks.

The cast is removed at the fourth week, and a removable orthosis is fitted. This can be custom-made by the hand therapist, or a suitably fitted off-the-shelf commercially made orthosis will serve equally well provided it fits properly. The orthosis is designed to maintain the wrist in some extension to further protect the tendon to tendon juncture. The orthosis is removed initially and preferably under the supervision of the therapist. The patient and attendant are instructed in the exercise protocols. The orthosis is replaced between exercise sessions. It is best worn at night for many additional weeks.

Until about postoperative week 6, the patient uses the orthosis except when exercising. Beginning about postoperative week 6, the orthosis is removed during much of the day, and the patient begins to strengthen the transferred muscle by actively contracting the brachioradialis against no resistance. The transfer is protected against resistance for an additional 3 to 4 weeks, depending on whether this procedure has been combined with additional procedures, such as a key grip

procedure or reconstruction of elbow extension by deltoid or biceps to triceps transfer.

RESTORING KEY PINCH: THE IC GROUP 1 AND 2 PATIENT

Patients functioning at the IC group 2 level, or IC group 1 patients after brachioradialis to ECRB transfer, can actively extend the wrist against gravity and against some resistance and are potential candidates for restoration of a lateral or key pinch as described by Moberg.[9] Conceptually, this is a simple operative procedure and, importantly, is essentially totally reversible should the patient decide the hand was more functional before surgery. The key pinch procedure may be combined with brachioradialis to ECRB transfer if greater wrist extensor power is deemed advantageous. It represents an automatic pinch in that the tendon of the thumb flexor, the flexor pollicis longus (FPL), is anchored to the palmar surface of the radius under such tension that with wrist extension, the thumb tip is pulled against the side of the index finger (Fig. 215-11). The other fingers are usually left supple, and the patient frequently must learn to roll these digits into some flexion to provide a platform against which the thumb can act. Gravity is needed to flex the wrist, releasing tension on the FPL tenodesis and allowing opening of the grip. Therefore, preoperative prerequisites include

- adequate passive wrist mobility
- MRC grade 4 or higher voluntary wrist extension
- supple thumb joints
- adequate flexibility in the remaining digits
- appropriate transfer and weight shift techniques so that the tenodesis is not overstretched after surgery

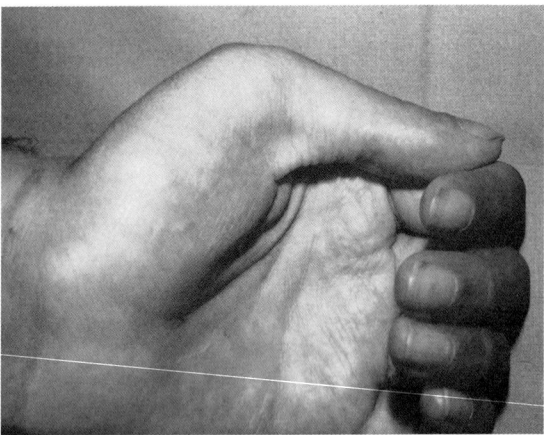

FIGURE 215-11. The preferred posture for key pinch is illustrated. The interphalangeal joint of the thumb is stabilized so that the broad pulp surface of the thumb contacts the radial border of the index finger about the level of the middle phalanx. Note the amount of FPL bow-stringing that occurs over time if the A1 pulley is released. This pulley should not be released if the thumb metacarpophalangeal joint demonstrates passive flexion of more than 45 degrees. Otherwise, the thumb flexes excessively at the metacarpophalangeal joint, and the tip of the thumb may miss contacting the index finger during pinch. (From Hentz V, Leclercq C: Surgical Rehabilitation of the Upper Limb in Tetraplegia. London, Harcourt Health Sciences, 2002:151.)

Provided that wrist extension power is adequate, the key steps of the procedure have evolved as follows:

1. The interphalangeal joint of the thumb is stabilized by pin fixation, fusion, or tenodesis of the joint effected by splitting the FPL insertion and transferring half the tendon dorsally, where it is attached to the tendon of insertion of the extensor pollicis longus (EPL).
2. The tendon of the FPL is fixed to the radius at the correct tension.
3. The thumb's metacarpophalangeal joint is stabilized against excessive flexion (necessary if this joint can be passively flexed more than 45 degrees) or against excessive extension (necessary if the joint passively hyperextends beyond 10 degrees).

The procedure is carried out preferably under regional arm block. Depending on the status of the metacarpophalangeal joint, either four or five small incisions are planned in addition to the incision on the radial aspect of the forearm for transfer of the brachioradialis to the radial wrist extensor, if this is to be done. If this transfer is indicated, it is performed as the initial operative step.

The first step is stabilization of the interphalangeal joint of the thumb. After many years of Steinmann

pin stabilization, as described by Moberg,[9] we have more recently adopted the procedure described by Mohammed and Rothwell[35] termed the split FPL transfer. This has proved to be a reliable alternative that preserves some active and even greater passive interphalangeal joint movement.

SPLIT FPL TO EPL INTERPHALANGEAL STABILIZATION. For an optimum result, the critical pulleys, including the oblique pulley of the flexor sheath of the thumb, must be preserved (Fig. 215-12A). The procedure may be carried out by the incisions outlined in Figure 215-12B or with just one incision along the radial midaxis of the thumb (Fig. 215-12A).

The zigzag incision is made, and the dissection commences by locating the neurovascular bundle on the radial side of the digit. The neurovascular bundle is included within the skin flap to protect it (Fig. 215-12C). There is frequently a small annular ligament or pulley at the level of the joint. This can be incised to visualize the FPL tendon.

A blunt probe can be used to find the small midline split in the tendon's structure. This split is lengthened both distally and proximally. When the distal dissection reaches the insertion of the tendon, the radial half of the split FPL tendon is divided at its bone insertion. The tendon end is delivered into the wound, and by pulling distally on the tendon, some additional as yet unsplit FPL is visualized. The proximal split is extended. Finally, a small window into the flexor sheath is made just proximal to the oblique pulley, and the radial half of the tendon is brought through this window (Fig. 215-12D).

If a second incision is used, it is located on the mid-dorsum of the thumb, over the course of the EPL. The radial half of the FPL is tunneled under the intervening skin, deep to the radial digital nerve, and brought out the dorsal incision (Fig. 215-12D).

The tendon slip is passed under the tendon of the EPL and then brought back over onto itself (Fig. 215-12E). The thumb interphalangeal joint is temporarily stabilized in about 20 degrees of flexion with a 0.035-inch Kirschner wire placed across the joint (Fig. 215-12E). The transferred slip of tendon is pulled distally until a slackening of the remaining tendon half is noted and then relaxed slightly so that there is equal tension on the slip of transferred tendon and on the original remaining half of the tendon (Fig. 215-12F). Pinning the interphalangeal joint before final adjustment of tension makes this step much more practical and more easily accomplished. The transferred half of the tendon is sutured to itself and to the EPL with absorbable 4-0 sutures.

FLEXOR POLLICIS LONGUS TENODESIS. The tendon of the FPL is to be anchored to the distal radius. A number of variations in the routing of the FPL have been described. Moberg's original procedure left the

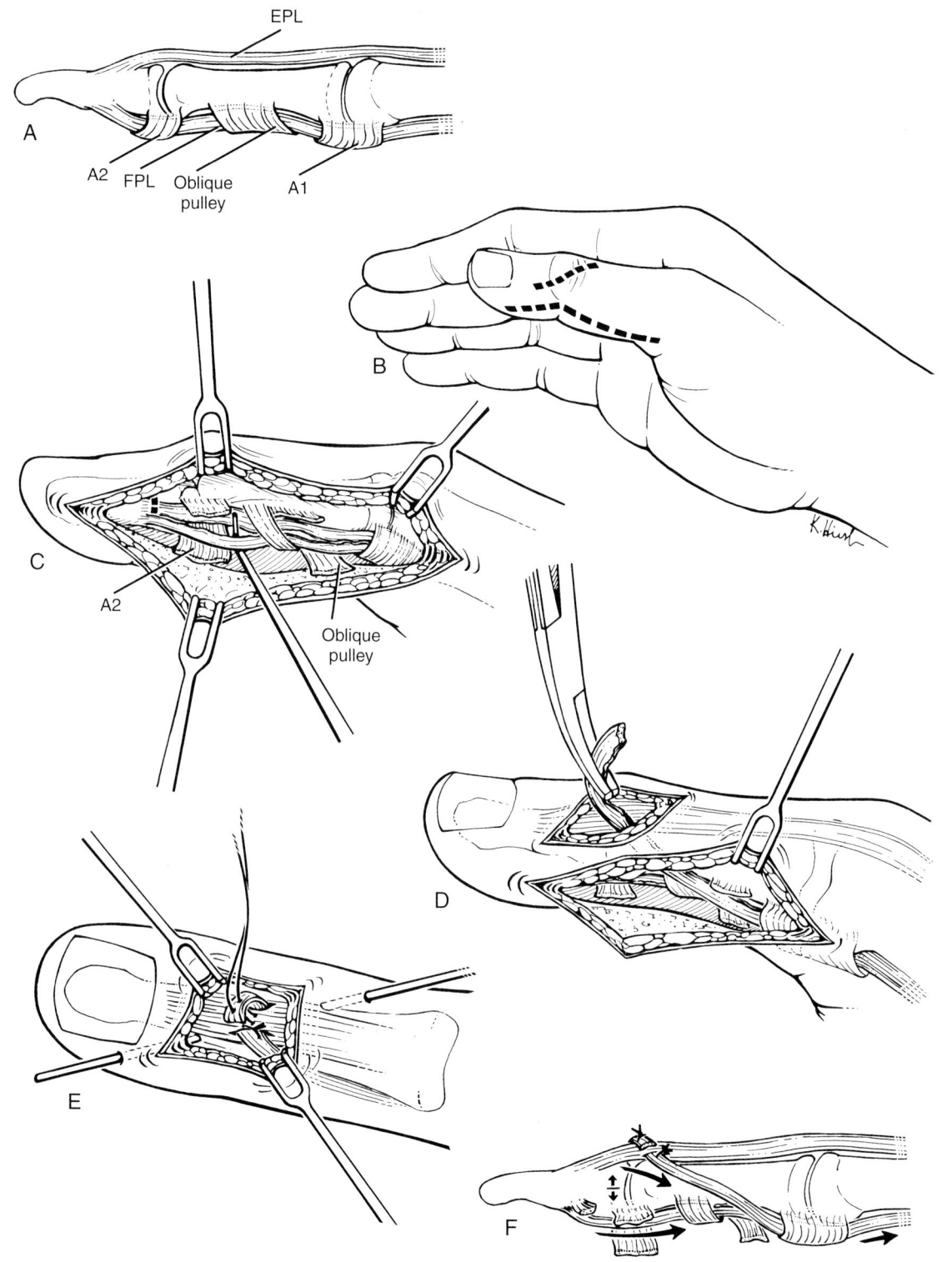

FIGURE 215-12. An effective method to stabilize the interphalangeal joint of the thumb without making it rigid is illustrated. This procedure, attributed to Rothwell and Sinclair,[35] has become universally accepted. See text for details. (From Hentz V, Leclercq C: Surgical Rehabilitation of the Upper Limb in Tetraplegia. London, Harcourt Health Sciences, 2002:141.)

FPL within its natural bursa, although he recommended releasing the A1 pulley under the thumb's metacarpophalangeal joint to increase the moment of this tendon. He and Brand later modified the technique to include withdrawal of the FPL tendon from its bursa after division of the muscle-tendon juncture in the forearm, routing it across the palm deep to the finger flexors before passing it into the forearm through Guyon canal. Moberg's original method is technically easier, but Brand's modification provides, according to his biomechanical analysis, a more favorable FPL flexor moment. We continue to use both routes of FPL transfer and frequently test each method to determine which route seems to provide a more stable thumb posture in the key pinch position when the FPL is placed under tension.

The Moberg-Brand FPL tenodesis procedure requires three incisions (Fig. 215-13A and B). The first is designed along the radial aspect of the thumb and exposes the flexor sheath of the thumb from the interphalangeal joint to the level of the A1 pulley at the metacarpophalangeal joint. The second incision is made in the palm at the level of the hook of the hamate. Through this incision, access is gained to Guyon canal. The third incision is on the volar side of the distal forearm. The landmarks to determine the location of this incision are the flexor carpi radialis and the palmaris longus tendons. The three volar incisions are illustrated in Figure 215-13A. The fourth small incision to be made last is on the dorsum of the distal aspect of the forearm (Fig. 215-13F).

After the FPL-EPL transfer is performed, the FPL tendon is identified just proximal to the A1 pulley of the thumb. This pulley should be preserved, especially if the thumb metacarpophalangeal joint can be passively flexed more than 30 degrees on preoperative testing. A small probe is placed under the FPL tendon just proximal to the A1 pulley (Fig. 215-13C).

The volar forearm incision is made and the interval between the flexor carpi radialis and the palmaris longus tendons dissected. Just deep to this interval will be the muscle-tendon junction of the FPL (Fig. 215-13C). The tendon is identified, and the muscle fibers are sharply dissected from the tendon as far proximal as possible. After the final few muscle fibers are divided, tension on the probe under the FPL at the metacarpophalangeal joint level will allow delivery of the FPL tendon into the thumb incision (Fig. 215-13C).

The third (palmar) incision is made, and the dissection is carried down through the hypothenar fat and the palmaris brevis muscle until the ulnar neurovascular bundle is located. The ulnar neurovascular bundle is retracted ulnarward to expose the flexor tendons to the little and ring fingers. A curved tendon-passing forceps is used to make a tunnel deep to these flexors and then deep (dorsal) to the adjacent flexor tendons and neurovascular structures to the ring, middle, and index fingers. The tip of the curved tendon-passing forceps is then directed toward the thumb incision. The tendon of the FPL is grasped in the jaws of the tendon-passing forceps and delivered into the hypothenar incision (Fig. 215-13D).

The same tendon-passing forceps is then introduced into the volar forearm incision, and staying deep (dorsal) to the flexor tendons and the median nerve, the forceps is gently guided across the wrist crease in an ulnar direction to exit at the hypothenar incision (Fig. 215-13E). The tendon of the FPL is grasped and withdrawn into the forearm incision.

The final part of this procedure involves the firm fixation of the FPL tendon to the radius at the proper tension. One can simplify this step by first dissecting the pronator quadratus off a small window of volar radius. The ulnar aspect of the radius is exposed so that the hole to be drilled through the radius does not interfere with the radial wrist extensor tendons. A 3- to 4-mm drill point is then used to drill a hole from volar to dorsal through the radius. The site where the drill point exits the dorsal aspect of the radius is the location for the final incision (Fig. 215-13F). A loop of 30-gauge 3-0 monofilament wire is passed through the drill hole in a dorsal to palmar direction; the tendon of the FPL is placed in the loop and then drawn through the radius and into the small dorsal incision. All the skin incisions are closed with absorbable skin sutures or subcuticularly placed sutures. The tendon of the FPL that exits the skin on the dorsum of the forearm is grasped firmly in a large clamp. By pulling on the tendon, the tension can be adjusted according to that desired by the surgeon. The proximal end of the FPL tendon is pulled so that the pulp of the thumb contacts the radial side of the index finger when the wrist is in the neutral position. When the wrist is flexed, the tension of the FPL is relaxed, and the thumb ray will extend in response to the dorsal tenodesis and viscoelastic forces. As the wrist is brought from the flexed to the neutral position, the thumb will contact the index finger. As the wrist is extended farther, the thumb exerts greater and greater force against the side of the index finger.

After satisfactory positioning of the FPL tendon, a large vascular clip is fixed across the tendon at the level of the skin, and one or two final skin sutures are placed to close the small dorsal wound (Fig. 215-13F).

The position of postoperative immobilization depends on whether the brachioradialis was transferred as part of this procedure. If this transfer has been performed, the wrist is immobilized in the neutral position and the thumb is flexed at the carpometacarpal (CMC) joint to relax tension of the FPL. If this transfer has been unnecessary, the wrist may be immobilized in 15 to 20 degrees of flexion, again to relax tension on the FPL tenodesis site.

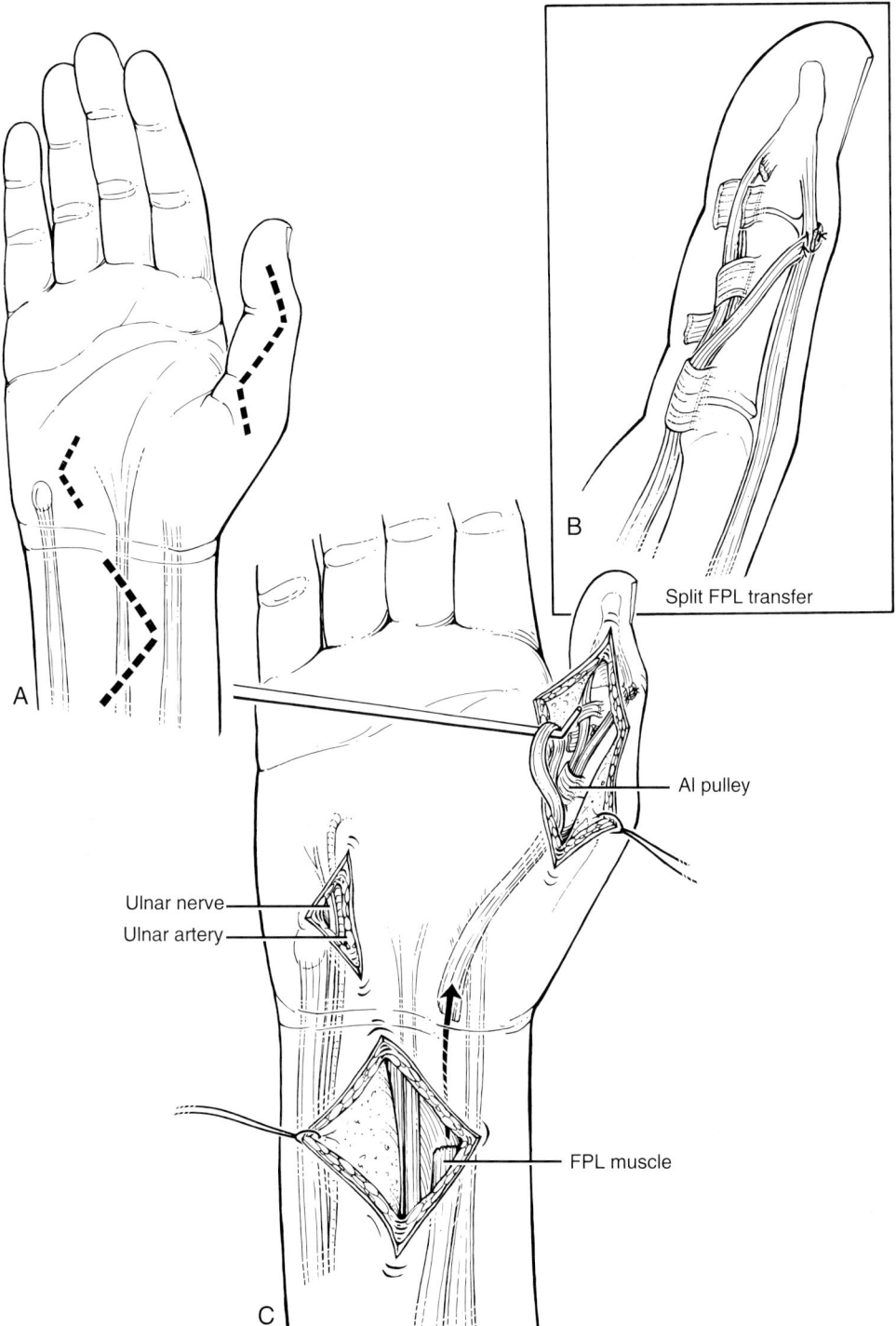

FIGURE 215-13. The Brand-Moberg modification of Moberg's original key pinch procedure is illustrated. See text for details. (From Hentz V, Leclercq C: Surgical Rehabilitation of the Upper Limb in Tetraplegia. London, Harcourt Health Sciences, 2002:142-143.)   *Continued*

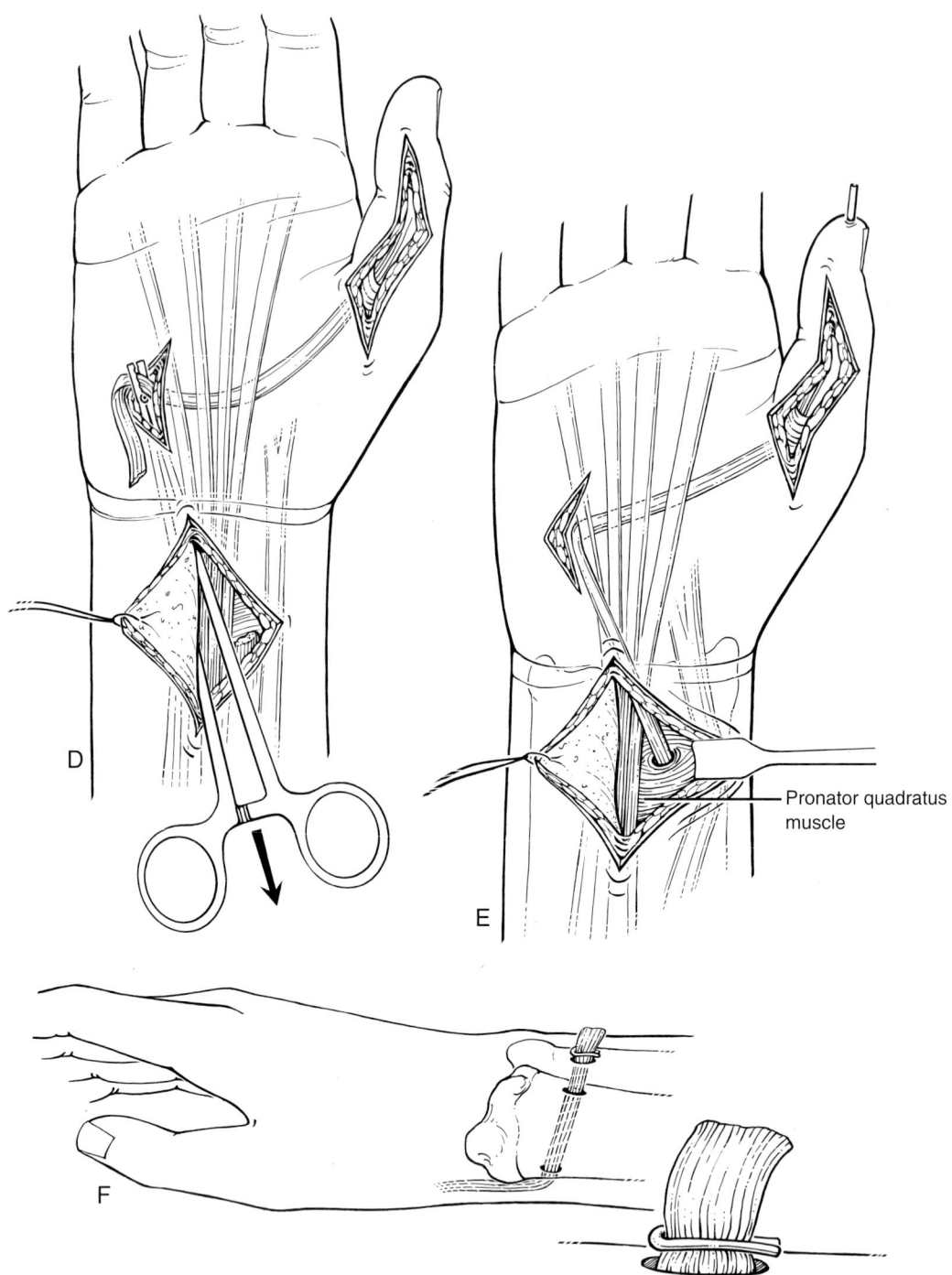

Pronator quadratus muscle

D

E

F

FIGURE 215-13, cont'd.

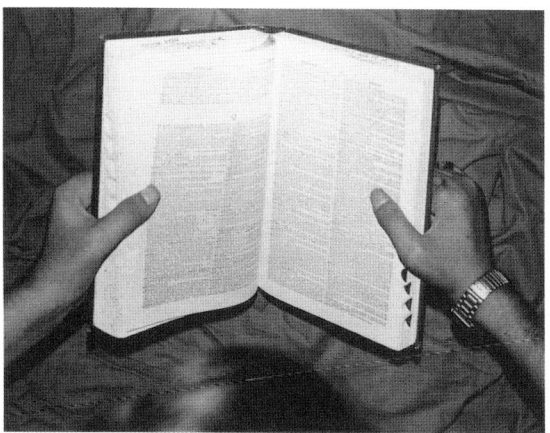

FIGURE 215-14. This IC group 2 patient has had bilateral key pinch procedures. His pinch force measures 20 newtons, and he has maintained this power for 15 years.

The hand and wrist are typically immobilized for 4 to 5 weeks, and cautious use is required for an additional 1 to 2 months to allow firm adherence of the tenodesis. We have performed this procedure on more than 50 hands, and the results have been very satisfying (Fig. 215-14). We can measure the gain in pinch strength, and it is typically proportional to the strength of the wrist extensor power but depends somewhat on the stability of the thumb and finger joints. Pinch strengths between 1 and 5 kg have been uniformly achieved. We have not had any patient ask to have the operative procedure reversed.

RESTORING ACTIVE KEY PINCH: IC GROUP 2 AND SOME IC GROUP 3 PATIENTS

After gaining experience with the key pinch procedure described by Moberg, we have chosen to modify the key pinch operation for the patient with strong wrist extension, meaning a strong IC group 2 or group 3 patient. These patients do not require augmentation of wrist extension. Instead of tenodesis of the FPL to the radius as described before, the following steps are accomplished in a single-stage procedure (Fig. 215-15):

1. The CMC joint is fused to pre-position the thumb tip to contact the index finger middle phalanx.
2. The EPL tendon is anchored to the extensor retinaculum on the dorsum of the wrist.
3. The brachioradialis muscle-tendon unit is transferred to the tendon of the FPL.
4. The split FPL to EPL transfer is performed.

Operative Procedure

The operative steps are carried out through one longer and three or four smaller incisions as illustrated in

Figure 215-15. An FPL to EPL interphalangeal joint stabilization procedure is completed as illustrated in Figure 215-12. Next, the CMC joint is exposed through an incision made along the juncture of the glabrous and hair-bearing skin over the palmar-radial aspect of the thumb's thenar eminence. The thenar muscles are reflected off the capsule of the CMC joint, and the capsule is opened. The adjacent joint surfaces are prepared for fusion by sharp excision of all cartilage and by perforation of the dense subchondral bone in several areas on the metacarpal base and the face of the trapezium. Bone is removed with a small osteotome, curette, or powered burr equally from both sides of the joint. This maintains the relative contours of metacarpal base and trapezium and good bone to bone contact between the two surfaces.

The angles of palmar and radial abduction for the CMC fusion are determined somewhat by the preoperative digital flexor tenodesis pattern and the passive range of motion at the thumb's metacarpophalangeal joint. The goal is to have the pulp of the thumb contact the radial side of the index finger over the middle phalanx as the wrist is extended. Opening of the grip is effected by wrist flexion and occurs almost exclusively at the metacarpophalangeal joint. The ideal candidate has a well-preserved digital flexor tenodesis pattern and passive metacarpophalangeal flexion that exceeds the range of CMC extension. For such a patient, the thumb ray should be positioned in only about 20 degrees of palmar abduction and almost maximum radial abduction. A thumb ray fixed by CMC fusion in great palmar abduction will interfere with transfers and pressure relief efforts and will be subject to great stress when the patient performs these maneuvers. If the patient demonstrates poor finger flexion as the wrist is extended, the CMC joint should be fused in a slightly less palmarly abducted posture. If the range of passive metacarpophalangeal flexion is small, the CMC joint should be fused in less than maximal radial abduction. If it is too radially abducted, the patient with a poorly flexible metacarpophalangeal joint will not be able to effect firm contact between pulp of thumb and index finger.

The CMC joint is temporarily pinned with a 2-mm Kirschner wire to test the preoperative hypothesis. If the position seems ideal, the joint is further stabilized. A small four-corner plate has provided sufficiently rigid bone to bone contact. Bone staples also provide excellent immobilization at the fusion site.

The third step involves firm tenodesis of the EPL to the dorsal surface of the radius. Because the CMC joint is now fused, no particular EPL rerouting is needed. Through a transverse incision made just proximal to Lister tubercle, the tendon of the EPL is located and divided at its muscle-tendon junction. The end of the tendon is brought over the extensor retinaculum and then passed under the EPL tendon just

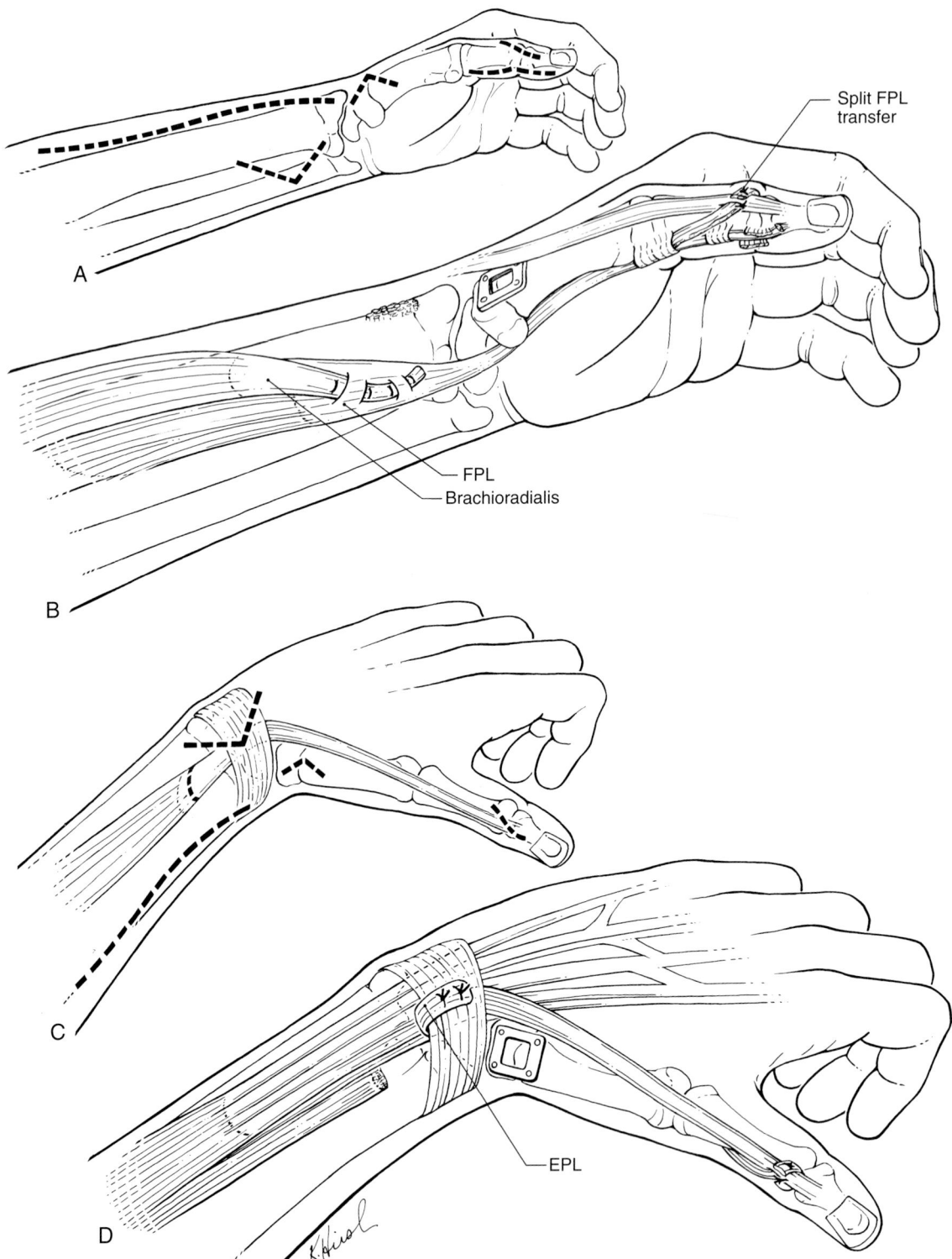

FIGURE 215-15. A procedure to restore active key pinch is illustrated. The CMC joint of the thumb is stabilized by fusion, the thumb interphalangeal joint by split FPL to EPL tenodesis; tenodesis of the EPL to the radius is performed so that the thumb extends with wrist flexion, and the brachioradialis is transferred to the FPL to provide potential voluntary pinch irrespective of wrist position. See text for details. (From Hentz V, Leclercq C: Surgical Rehabilitation of the Upper Limb in Tetraplegia. London, Harcourt Health Sciences, 2002:156.)

distal to the retinaculum. The wrist is flexed to 45 degrees, and the EPL is tensioned so that the thumb extends maximally. Several nonabsorbable sutures are used to anchor the EPL to itself and to the dense extensor retinaculum. The wrist is then passively flexed and extended and the thumb's motion observed. The thumb should reach maximum extension as the wrist reaches 45 degrees of flexion, but the pulp of the thumb should contact the radial side of the index finger as the wrist is extended to reach the neutral position.

The last procedure involves brachioradialis to FPL transfer. The FPL is identified in the volar forearm, either through the same incision used to dissect the brachioradialis or through a separate volar incision. The FPL is divided at its muscle-tendon junction, and the two tendons are directed in as straight a line as possible toward one another. The ends of both tendons are passed through one another several times, interweaving them. The ideal tension for the transfer is established as described for brachioradialis to ECRB transfer. The juncture is made with the elbow in 40 degrees of flexion, the wrist in a neutral position, and the index finger held flexed at metacarpophalangeal and proximal interphalangeal joints. The brachioradialis is pulled distally to a point midway between maximum passive stretch and fully relaxed tension (zero tension), and the FPL tendon is pulled proximally so that the pulp of the thumb just touches the radial side of the index finger. The assistant maintains this posture of both tendons while the surgeon joins the two tendons with three or four nonabsorbable sutures. Once this tendon to tendon juncture is secure, the tension of the FPL transfer and the EPL tenodesis is tested by gently moving the wrist between 45 degrees of flexion and 45 degrees of extension. It is important that the thumb still fully extend at the metacarpophalangeal joint with wrist flexion after brachioradialis transfer. The wounds are closed, and the limb is solidly immobilized in a below-elbow cast that maintains the wrist in a neutral position and the thumb metacarpophalangeal joint in some flexion. We typically place the thumb in contact with the flexed index finger.

The immobilization is continued for 4 weeks; on removal of the cast, a plastic splint is constructed that keeps the thumb and wrist in the initial position of postoperative immobilization. The splint is removed for exercises, and the initial exercises are directed at regaining the preoperative range of wrist movement. At the beginning of the fifth postoperative week, the patient is encouraged to begin practicing grasping small, light objects, and for these exercises, the therapist constructs a small hand-based splint to protect the CMC fusion. These exercises progress until the beginning of the eighth week, when greater resistance is permitted. The splint is discontinued during the daytime but is worn at night for an additional 4 weeks. The weight-bearing precautions are the same as those discussed for the FPL tenodesis procedure; no transfers are performed out of the splint until after the eighth postoperative week. The fused thumb CMC joint requires that the patient's transfer mechanics be closely monitored by the therapist.

Figure 215-16 demonstrates the postoperative result of this procedure in an IC group 3 patient.

Restoring Both Grasp and Release: IC Groups 3, 4, and 5

For our tetraplegic patients who possess additional motor resources distal to the elbow, more complicated

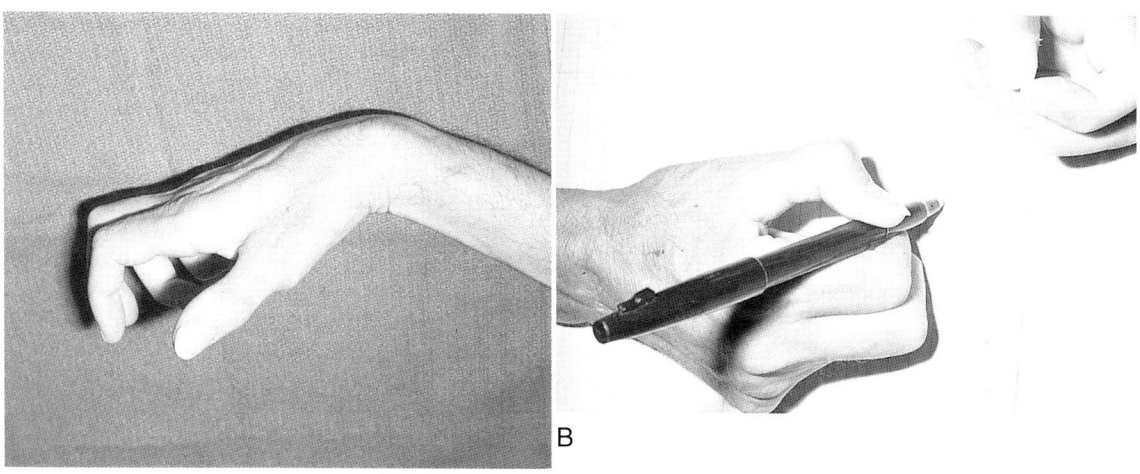

A

B

FIGURE 215-16. An IC group 3 patient after brachioradialis to FPL transfer. He has a wide opening of his first web when gravity flexes his wrist *(A)* and almost 25 newtons of force on pinch *(B)*. (From Hentz V, Leclercq C: Surgical Rehabilitation of the Upper Limb in Tetraplegia. London, Harcourt Health Sciences, 2002:157.)

reconstructions are possible but not always indicated. These patients are, of course, also candidates for either procedure described before if reversibility seems an important consideration. In the early years of our experience, only key pinch reconstruction for IC group 3, 4, and even 5 patients was offered. As we have gained confidence in being able to achieve a reliable outcome, we have extended the risk-benefit equation to include more complex procedures in these IC groups.

THE STRONG IC GROUP 3 PATIENT

Strong IC group 3 patients will have at least one of the two radial wrist extensors at MRC grade 5. The other will probably be MRC grade 4. They commonly have some function (MRC grade 2 or 3) of the pronator teres, and this assists them in pronating their wrists.

For these patients, a two-stage procedure that takes advantage of the presence of two expendable muscles for transfer, the extensor carpi radialis longus (ECRL) and the brachioradialis, may be performed. The initial procedure is directed at obtaining a reliable opening posture of the hand and is referred to as the extensor phase. Prerequisites for surgery include nearly normal passive wrist movement and reasonably flexible fingers. These patients may possess useful triceps function. If not, this function should be restored, and this can be done as part of the initial extensor phase.

The Extensor Phase

The operative steps for the initial extensor phase include

- assessing the strength of the ECRB
- identifying any accessory radial wrist extensors[36]
- passive tenodesis of the extensor tendons of the fingers (extensor digitorum communis [EDC]) and of the thumb (EPL)
- thumb CMC joint arthrodesis (described earlier)
- split FPL to EPL transfer (described earlier)

It is crucial to be certain of the true strength of the ECRB before transferring the ECRL. Robbing the patient of strong wrist extension is a grave error, and this is a risk because it is impossible to isolate the ECRB in preoperative testing. Therefore, in the strong IC group 3 patients, the ECRB tendon is exposed just distal to the extensor retinaculum under local anesthesia as the initial operative step. A probe is slipped under the tendon, and the patient is asked to forcefully extend the wrist. The surgeon then tries to displace the now tightened tendon with the probe. This is essentially impossible if the muscle is MRC grade 4 or 4+. If the ECRB is judged to be sufficiently strong, we proceed to perform the split FPL to EPL tenodesis and then fuse the CMC joint of the thumb to pre-position the thumb ray for pinch, as described before. The tendons of the EDC and EPL are fixed into a window excavated from the dorsum of the radius. Tension of this

transfer is adjusted so that the fingers and thumb begin to extend as the wrist reaches the neutral position.

The arm is casted for 4 weeks and then exercised, with avoidance of any resistance to finger and thumb extension. Now, with gravity-assisted wrist flexion, the fingers and thumb extend. This is a natural and synergistic motion and is easily learned.

The Flexor Phase

The second phase, centered on activation of the flexor tendons to the thumb (FPL) and fingers (flexor digitorum profundus [FDP]), is termed the flexor phase. It includes

- transfer of ECRL to the deep finger flexors
- transfer of brachioradialis to FPL
- intrinsic stabilization

If there is an accessory extensor carpi radialis muscle, this muscle is transferred to FPL, and the brachioradialis is used for another function, such as restoration of wrist flexion-pronation.

Through the long dorsal incision described for brachioradialis transfer, the ECRL and brachioradialis tendons are mobilized and then passed volarward, where the tendons of the brachioradialis and FPL are passed through each other and sutured. The tendons of the FDP are grouped together, and the normal finger cascade is reversed somewhat by suturing the radial two FDP tendons under slightly tighter tension than the ulnar two. The tendon of the ECRL is woven back and forth through the now combined tendons of the FDP in the manner of Pulvertaft.[37] Tension of this transfer is adjusted so that a relatively natural posture of the fingers is achieved with wrist flexion and extension. It may be preferable to tension this transfer after intrinsic stabilization is performed. The brachioradialis to FPL transfer is tensioned so that with the wrist in neutral, the thumb pulp just touches the side of the flexed index finger. If an accessory radial wrist extensor has been identified during the extensor phase, it can be transferred to the FPL, and the brachioradialis can be transferred to the flexor carpi radialis to provide better wrist flexion.

INTRINSIC STABILIZATION. For the non-tetraplegic person, the multiple functions of the intrinsic muscles are made more apparent when they no longer function. The strength of grip is considerably weakened. The fingers can no longer be widely spread apart at the metacarpophalangeal joint during finger extension. Even though the long flexors of the fingers have excursion sufficient to flex all the intervening joints, in the absence of the synchronizing effect of the intrinsic muscles, the fingertips in full flexion usually touch only to the bases of the fingers rather than fully into the center of the palm. Digital flexion begins at the distal joint under the influence of the long flexors, and the fingertip rolls into flexion rather than sweeping broadly and expansively along the spiral that the normally innervated fingertip follows. This rolling up of the fingertip will tend to push large objects out of the grasp.

The second major biomechanical function of the intrinsic muscles is also manifested in their absence. In the normal hand, the extrinsic extensors lift the proximal phalanges into extension and are assisted in extending the interphalangeal joints by the action of the intrinsic muscles. In the absence of intrinsic muscle activity, the action of the extrinsic muscles at the metacarpophalangeal joint is unopposed. In hyperextending the metacarpophalangeal joint, the extrinsic extensor forfeits the excursion that might allow it to extend the interphalangeal joint. Furthermore, this metacarpophalangeal hyperextension increases the viscoelastic tone of the long flexors and induces some flexion at the interphalangeal joints. This imbalance gives rise to a particular posture termed the claw hand characterized by metacarpophalangeal hyperextension and interphalangeal joint flexion.

In the majority of tetraplegic patients, the absence of intrinsic muscle function may also result in an imbalance between the paralyzed extrinsic flexors and extensors. The preoperative tetraplegic hand of IC groups 1 to 5 possesses only residual passive tenodesis grasp and release. For these patients, the tendency for the finger to claw as the wrist is flexed may represent only a cosmetic annoyance. However, operative procedures designed to improve digital flexion and extension in IC groups 3 and higher may accentuate the clawed posture by adding tone to both extrinsic extensors and flexors. In this circumstance, the claw deformity frequently becomes a significant functional liability in addition to further detracting from the appearance of the reconstructed hand. The deformity restricts the ability of the hand to open as widely as possible and reduces the range of objects easily grasped.

House[38] has presented convincing evidence that some type of intrinsic substitution results in a better and stronger grasp in the tetraplegic patient who is a candidate for the two-stage grasp-release procedure. Because most tetraplegic patients do not possess sufficient numbers of transferable muscles to allow intrinsic substitution by standard tendon transfer procedures, static procedures must typically suffice. One of two procedures, the first attributed to Zancolli[39] and termed the lasso procedure and the other described by House,[40] may be used for the tetraplegic patient.

ZANCOLLI "LASSO" PROCEDURE. In IC groups 3, 4, and 5, the flexor digitorum superficialis muscles are paralyzed, typically at the upper motor neuron level. As such, they retain some stretch reflexes through the intact spinal reflex arc and relatively normal viscoelastic properties. Zancolli[39] proposed use of these paralyzed muscles as an elastic tenodesis to reduce metacar-

pophalangeal joint hyperextension and lessen the clawed posture of the tetraplegic's hand. For each finger that exhibits significantly troublesome clawing, the superficialis tendon is inserted under some tension into the flexor sheath at the distal margin of the A1 pulley or even slightly more distally into the proximal part of the A2 pulley (Fig. 215-17). The superficialis tendon is redeployed from its role as the primary flexor of the proximal interphalangeal joint to become the prime flexor of the metacarpophalangeal joint. This achieves the principal goal of surgery, providing a proper balance between the flexor and extensor muscles.

The mechanical basis for this dynamic tenodesis procedure is debated. Zancolli believes that the transfer must be fixed under significant tension to still provide metacarpophalangeal flexor tone even with the wrist nearly maximally flexed. He believes that the transfer may assist in initiating some metacarpophalangeal flexion as a consequence of wrist extension's triggering some reflexive flexor digitorum superficialis contraction. He believes that this improves the sweep of the digits as they flex by resisting the tendency of the fingers to flex first at the distal interphalangeal joint.

This procedure may be performed as part of either the extensor (release) or flexor (grasp) phase of reconstruction. It is more difficult to judge the proper tension of the transfer if it is performed at the time of the extensor phase. As part of the flexor phase, the lasso procedure is preferably performed before the tension of the finger flexor transfer is adjusted.

HOUSE INTRINSIC TENODESIS. This procedure, described by House,[40] is a modification of Riordan's tenodesis procedure.[41] In the tetraplegic patient, it is frequently performed for only the index and middle fingers because these fingers are the most critical in grasp and release functions. However, the procedure (Fig. 215-18) can be performed on all four fingers as well. In this procedure, a free tendon loop is anchored at the level of the head of the metacarpal. The free ends of the tendon graft may be anchored to one of several sites on the extensor mechanism at or proximal to the proximal interphalangeal joint, depending on the finding of the preoperative examination. If the preoperative examination demonstrates that the interphalangeal joints are extended by the EDC tenodesis (with the examiner preventing metacarpophalangeal joint hyperextension), the graft may be anchored into the lateral band. If this test indicates that the extensor mechanism has become overstretched at the central slip area, the graft should be anchored into the base of the middle phalanx as demonstrated in Figure 215-18.

The Zancolli procedure may be chosen when preoperative testing demonstrates that the interphalangeal joints are extended by the EDC tenodesis

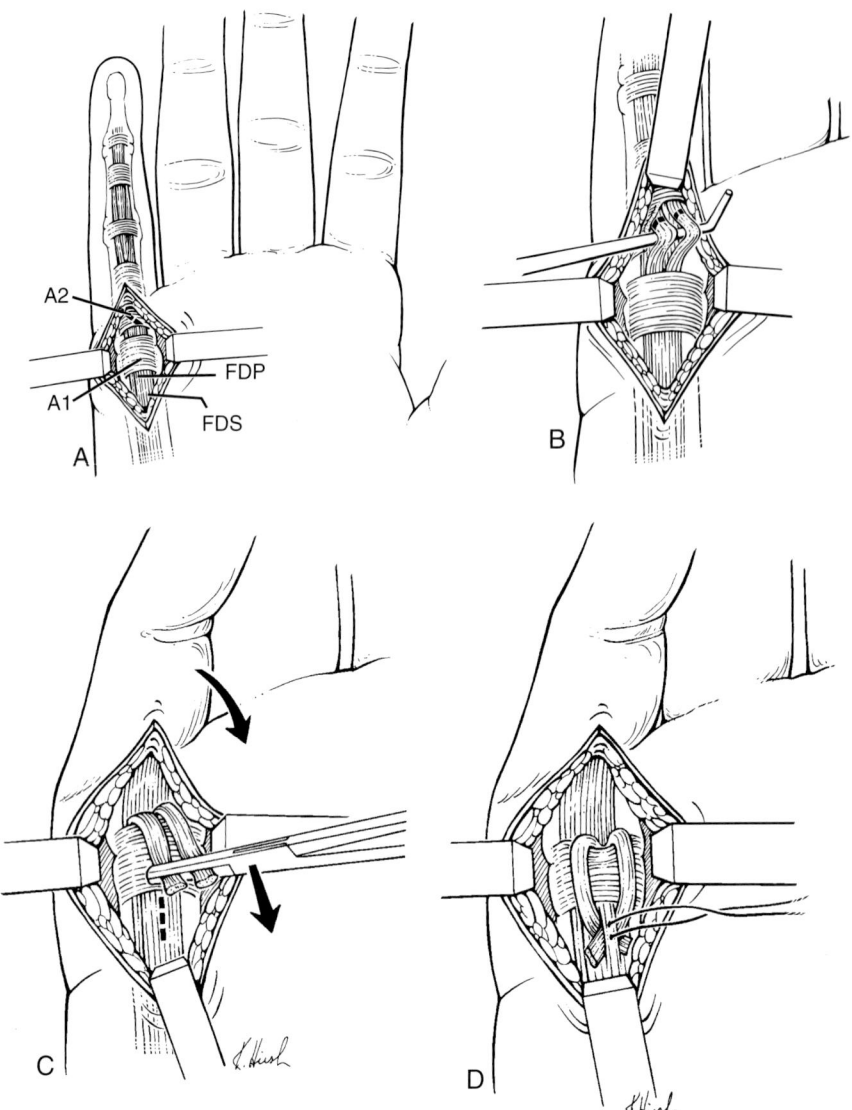

FIGURE 215-17. The Zancolli "lasso" procedure is illustrated. Either several longitudinal incisions or one longer transverse incision can be made. The flexor digitorum superficialis (FDS) is divided distal to the A1 pulley, looped about the pulley, and sutured to itself proximal to the pulley under strong tension. If the metacarpophalangeal joints remain nearly fully flexed with the wrist in neutral, proper tension has been achieved. (From Hentz V, Leclercq C: Surgical Rehabilitation of the Upper Limb in Tetraplegia. London, Harcourt Health Sciences, 2002:172.)

performed at the initial stage. If the extensor mechanism over the proximal interphalangeal joint has become overstretched, this joint will not be extended by the EDC tenodesis. In this case, the procedure described by House should be chosen.

The hand is casted with the wrist in slight flexion, the metacarpophalangeal joints in moderate flexion, and the interphalangeal joints in very slight flexion. After 4 weeks of immobilization, the cast is removed and an orthosis fitted to protect the metacarpophalangeal joints against full extension for several more weeks. No resistance is allowed for 8 weeks.

THE IC GROUP 4 AND 5 PATIENT

In IC group 4, the pronator teres is strong and available for transfer. In IC group 5, the flexor carpi radialis is strong, but experience has shown that it should not be used as a transfer. Therefore, the surgical options are similar for IC groups 4 and 5.

The pronator teres is the only functioning pronator muscle in these IC group 4 and 5 patients. However, it can be transferred and yet retain most of its pronator function if the direction of the transfer does not differ much from its original direction. In this respect, it can safely be used to activate the FPL. The brachioradialis is then available for another function. As stated before, it can be transferred to the finger extensors provided there is enough volar stabilization of the wrist. This is achieved if the flexor carpi radialis is graded MRC 3 or above. Otherwise, the results of the transfers may be unpredictable.

Alternative procedures for IC groups 4 and 5 include various combinations of procedures already described. Because patients differ, it is important to be able to plan for variations in presentation of patients

and individual functional objectives. For example, it has been our experience that patients who have had different procedures performed for each arm have been pleased with their differences. They preferentially use one hand for certain activities, such as grasping large objects, and the other for different tasks, such as manipulating smaller objects. The greatest variation in hand use has been a consequence of the management of the thumb's CMC joint. A fused CMC joint, although predictably pre-positioning the thumb, does limit the size

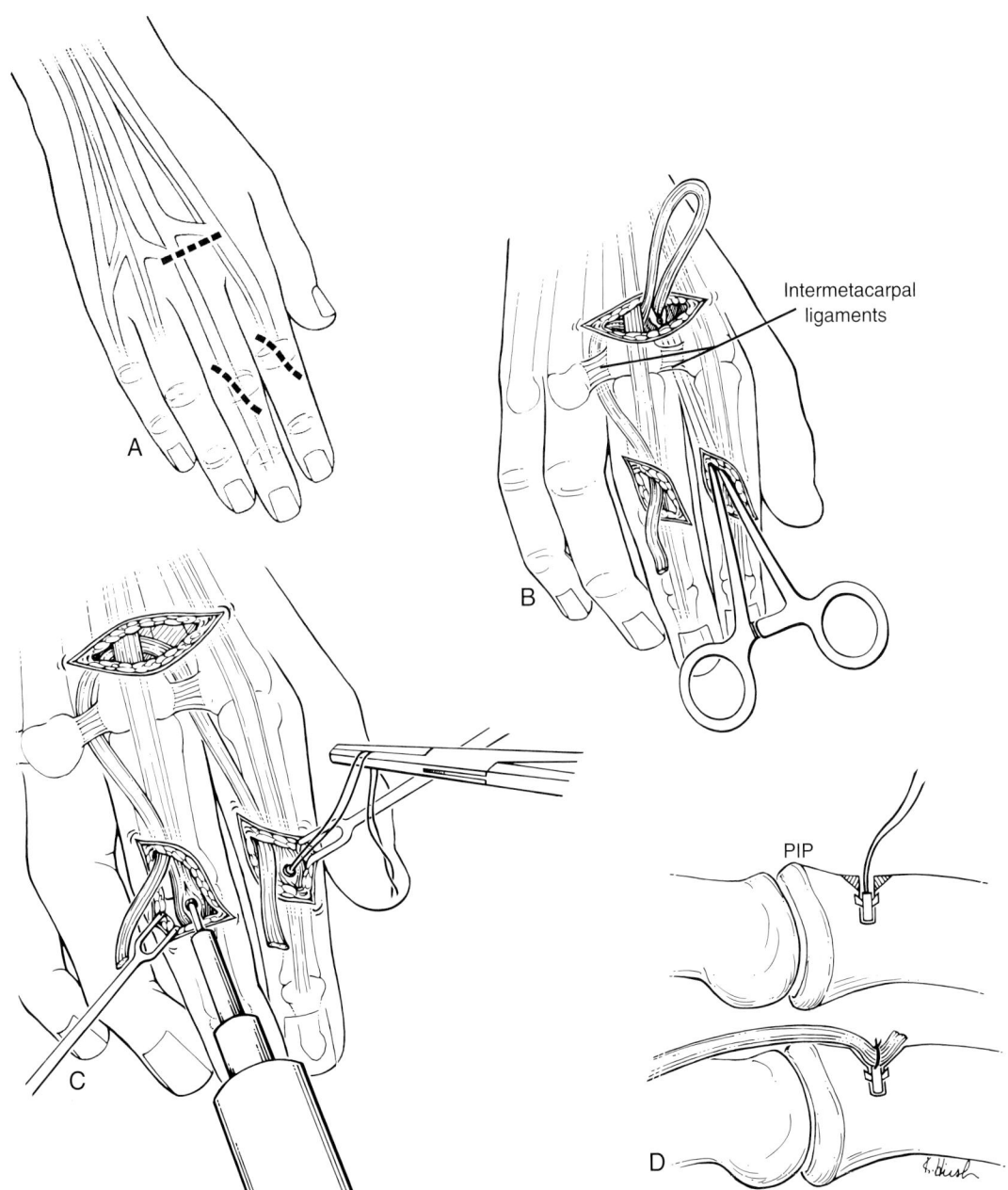

FIGURE 215-18. The House intrinsic substitution procedure is illustrated. See text for details. (From Hentz V, Leclercq C: Surgical Rehabilitation of the Upper Limb in Tetraplegia. London, Harcourt Health Sciences, 2002:173-174.)
Continued

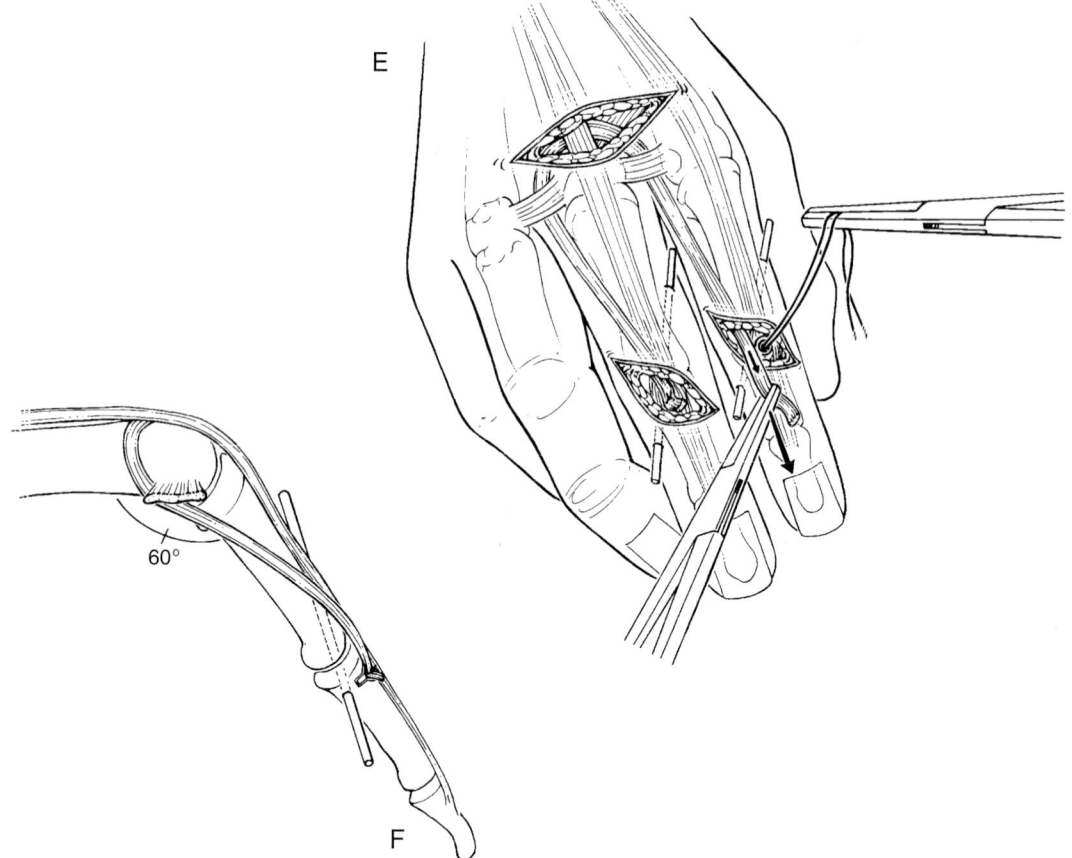

FIGURE 215-18, cont'd.

of objects easily grasped within the first web space. If the CMC joint is left mobile, the postoperative position of the thumb ray is less predictable, sometimes significantly so, but larger objects can be pushed into the first web space and held.

We have based decisions about these alternatives in large part on the preoperative presentation of the thumb's CMC joint. If the joint is completely unstable, meaning that time and poor transfer mechanics have resulted in slackening of all CMC ligaments, we prefer to fuse the CMC joint. Other options include fusing or leaving flexible the thumb's CMC joint and options regarding the number of transfers directed at strengthening thumb function, typically carried out during the flexor phase. Surgery is performed in two stages, as in IC group 3, with the extensor phase performed before the flexor phase.

The Unstable CMC Joint

EXTENSOR PHASE. If the flexor carpi radialis is weak (less than MRC grade 3, IC group 4), the extensor phase is identical to that for IC group 3:

- tenodesis of EDC and EPL to the radius
- thumb CMC joint fusion
- split FPL to EPL tenodesis

If the flexor carpi radialis is graded MRC 3 and above (typically an IC 5 arm), the fingers and thumb extensors can be activated by the brachioradialis. The procedure then includes

- transfer of brachioradialis to EDC and EPL
- thumb CMC joint fusion
- split FPL to EPL tenodesis

If brachioradialis to EDC-EPL is chosen, tension is set with the elbow in 40 degrees of flexion, the wrist in a neutral position, and the metacarpophalangeal joint in about 20 degrees of flexion. Tension should be such that during passive flexion of the wrist, the metacarpophalangeal joints start extending when the wrist reaches neutral from an extended position. The tension on the EPL tendon should be adjusted last, and its tension is typically set slightly looser than that of the EDC. The fingers should exhibit full passive flexion when the wrist is fully extended.

After 4 weeks in the cast, rehabilitation of active finger extensors is directed toward development of active extension of the metacarpophalangeal joints.

FLEXOR PHASE. The second stage is performed once the patient has been able to demonstrate active thumb and finger extension. The operative steps include

- transfer of ECRL to finger flexors (FDP)
- transfer of either brachioradialis or pronator teres to FPL
- intrinsic stabilization, if not performed at the extensor phase

Transfers of ECRL to FDP and brachioradialis to FPL have been described. An interpositional tendon graft may be needed if the pronator teres is chosen to power the FPL. The tension is adjusted so that with the wrist in neutral, the thumb rests against the lateral aspect of the index finger.

The wrist and fingers are immobilized postoperatively with the wrist in slight flexion and the fingers in 60 degrees of metacarpophalangeal and 45 degrees of proximal interphalangeal flexion. At 4 weeks, the cast is removed, and physiotherapy is conducted in the same manner as in IC group 3. The use of a manual wheelchair and shifting of the body weight onto the hands are restricted for one more month.

Stable Thumb CMC Joint

EXTENSOR PHASE. For this patient, the extensor phase typically includes the following operative steps:

- tenodesis of EDC to the radius
- tenodesis of the rerouted EPL
- split FPL to EPL thumb interphalangeal stabilization

In this case, the tendon of the EPL is divided at its muscle-tendon junction, withdrawn at the level of the metacarpophalangeal joint, and passed proximally and under the tendons of the first dorsal compartment and then toward the third compartment, where it is anchored. This provides an extensor-abductor vector when the wrist is flexed. Postoperative immobilization, rehabilitation, and precautions have been addressed before.

FLEXOR PHASE. The flexor phase can be carried out once passive mobility and muscle strength have recovered to maximum potential. The goals of this phase include transfers to provide both positional control and a powerful thumb pinch, a transfer to restore active finger flexion, and intrinsic balance. The operative steps include

- transfer of the ECRL to FDP (fingers in reversed cascade position)
- transfer of pronator teres to FPL

- brachioradialis, extended with ring flexor digitorum superficialis tendon, transferred across the palm to restore thumb flexion-abduction (Fig. 215-19)
- intrinsic substitution procedure, either lasso or House method, if not performed in extensor phase

Tension is assessed by gently passively flexing the wrist and determining that the fingers and thumb can be opened almost fully and by gently extending the wrist and judging the cascade of the fingers and the posture of the thumb. The wrist and fingers are splinted with the wrist in slight flexion; the fingers are nearly fully flexed at the metacarpophalangeal joints, and the thumb is relatively widely abducted, with the tip of the thumb touching the tip of the index finger. Immobilization is maintained for approximately 4 weeks followed by rehabilitation. The tendon junctures must be protected against great force for some additional weeks, particularly in the wheelchair-bound patient. Transfers and pressure relief activities are restricted for a full 8 weeks. Figure 215-20 illustrates the grasp and release capabilities of an IC group 5 patient after this two-stage reconstruction.

Strong Grasp and Refined Pinch: IC Groups 6, 7, and 8

Patients classified at the IC 6 level possess active digital extension but lack thumb extension. They require only addition of an extensor force for the thumb and, at the same operation, multiple tendon transfer to achieve balanced thumb pinch and strong finger grasp. Therefore, only one procedure is necessary, and their period of dependence is minimal.

Patients with an even greater number of remaining resources, such as patients in IC groups 7 and 8, can be reconstructed similar to patients with a lower peripheral nerve injury. The surgical procedures performed for these patients are directed at reconstructing some aspects of hand intrinsic muscle function and balance. There are relatively few tetraplegic patients in this category compared with the IC 2 or IC 5 categories, and we have operated on insufficient numbers to draw useful conclusions. Figure 215-21 illustrates an IC group 6 patient after reconstruction.

Other Presentations

Some injury patterns do not fit easily into the International Classification. Patients with so-called central cord injuries have hands that defy classification. These patients require prolonged studies and frequent re-examination before formulation of a surgical plan. Temporary nerve blocks have been particularly helpful in determining the procedure of choice.

FUNCTIONAL NEUROMUSCULAR STIMULATION

We have had experience implanting a system of electronics, including a programmable stimulator controlling an array of eight epimysial electrochannels. This system, developed by surgeons and engineers from the Case Western Reserve University and the Cleveland Veterans Administration Medical Center, has the capability of allowing a patient with a high spinal injury to activate and control a preprogrammed sequence of muscle contractions and thus to achieve a useful grasp for one hand.[42-45] The control mechanism is mounted externally about the opposite shoulder, allowing active and volitional shoulder movement to open and close the grip and modulate the force. Some additional movements can lock the grip in a closed position at the desired force of closure. Two

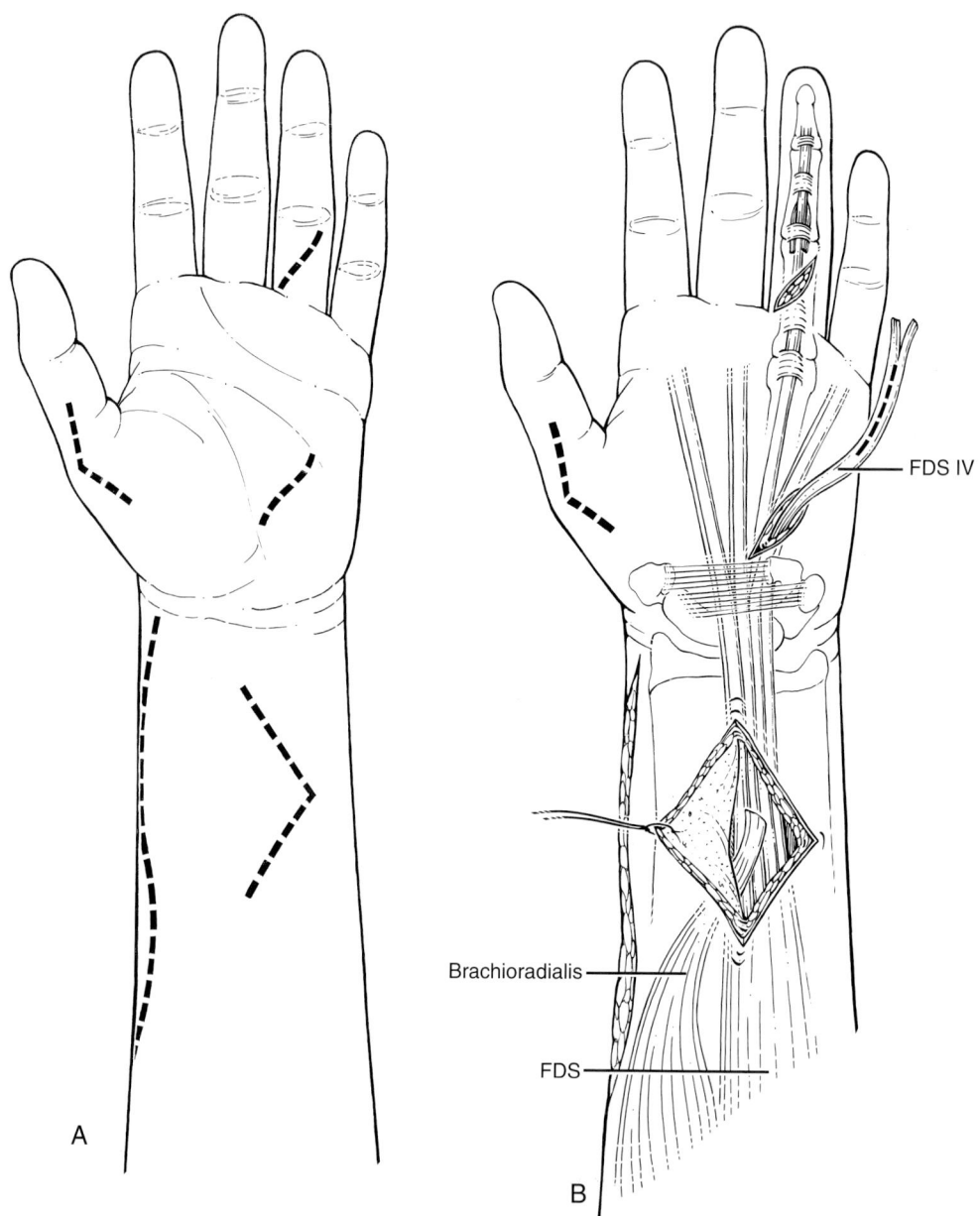

FIGURE 215-19. Transfer of the brachioradialis, extended with an interpositional tendon graft from the ring finger superficialis, passed to the thumb through a palmar fascial pulley so that the vector is one of flexion-abduction. (From Hentz V, Leclercq C: Surgical Rehabilitation of the Upper Limb in Tetraplegia. London, Harcourt Health Sciences, 2002:184-185.)

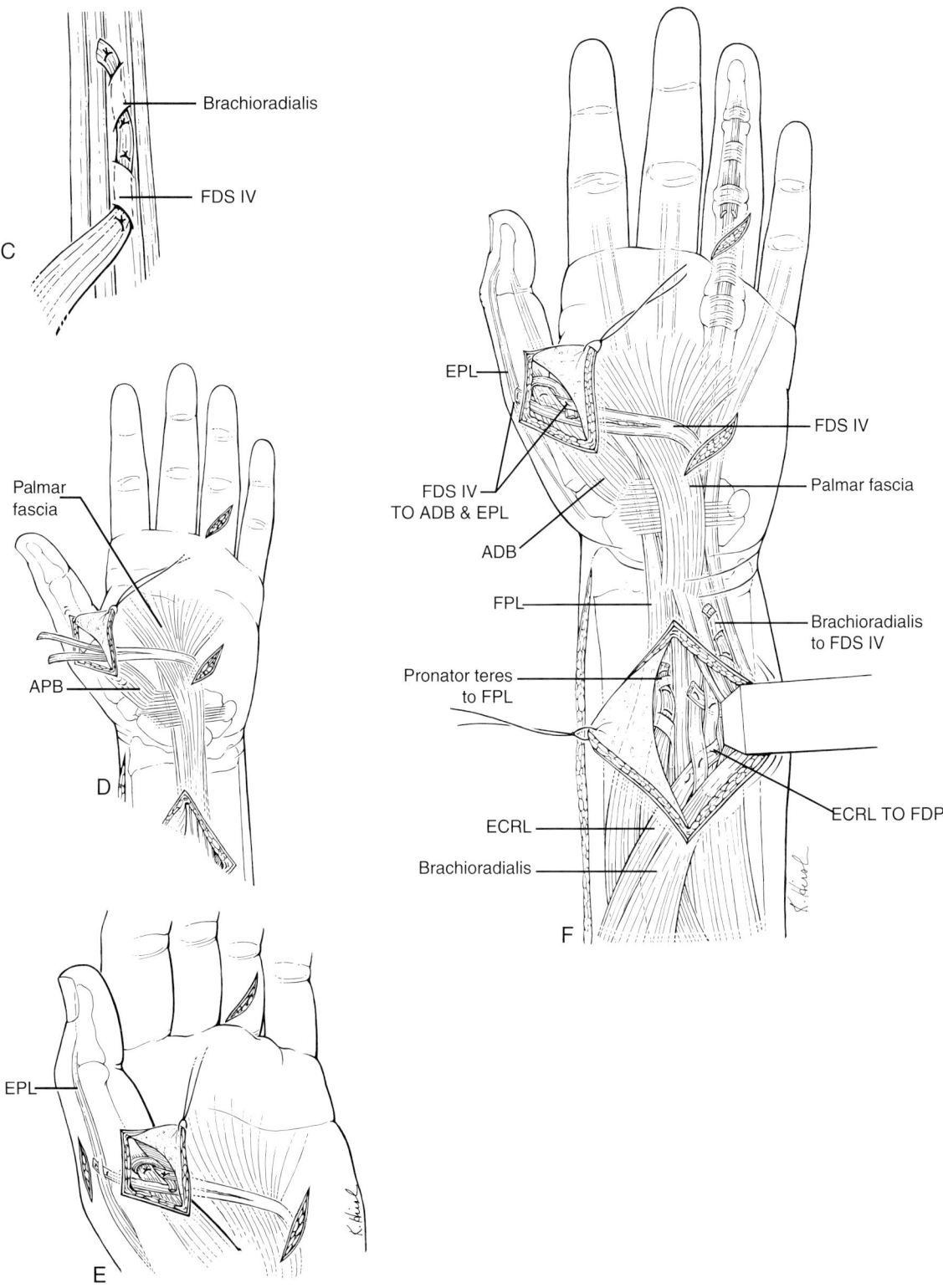

FIGURE 215-19, cont'd.

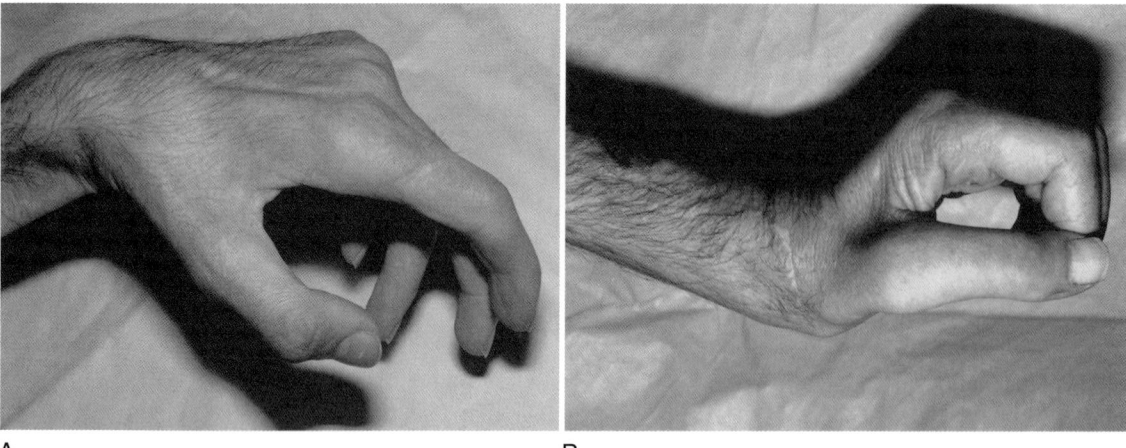

A   B

FIGURE 215-20. An IC group 5 patient has undergone the two-stage grasp and release procedure. He opens his hand by flexing his wrist *(A)* and has powerful finger and thumb flexion, augmented by wrist extension *(B)*.

different grip and release patterns can be programmed, and the patient can switch between the two patterns. These include a lateral or key pinch pattern useful for grasping smaller objects in a secure grip (Fig. 215-22*A* and *B*) and a tip-to-tip pinch or opposition pinch useful for acquiring and holding larger objects (Fig. 215-22*C* and *D*). This system of electrodes placed on predetermined upper motor neuron-paralyzed muscles has the potential to restore useful function in limbs heretofore deemed useless and unreconstructable by standard surgical techniques. Although almost 250 patients have had the system implanted at the time of this writing, the company responsible for the commercialization of this system has decided to discontinue its efforts.

RESULTS AND CONCLUSIONS

Because of the significant functional demands placed by tetraplegic patients on their upper limbs, especially the need to bear weight on their hands, the durability of operative procedures performed to enhance upper limb function in tetraplegic patients has been questioned. Perceptions about the durability of some of the earlier surgical recommendations, such as the surgically constructed wrist-driven flexor hinge hand, still influence the referral patterns to surgeons of modern-day physiatrists and spinal cord rehabilitation specialists. To provide some current perspective to this issue, we were able to locate and examine 45 patients who had been operated on at least 10 years before

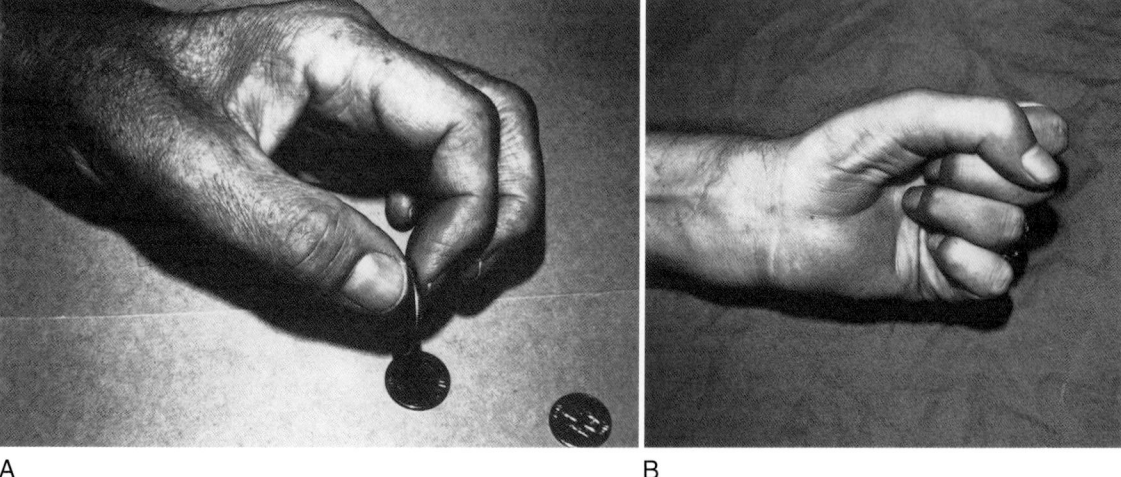

A   B

FIGURE 215-21. An IC group 6 patient has had restoration of thumb and finger flexion and intrinsic substitution in one operative step. This restored refined pinch (terminal-terminal) *(A)* and strong grip *(B)*.

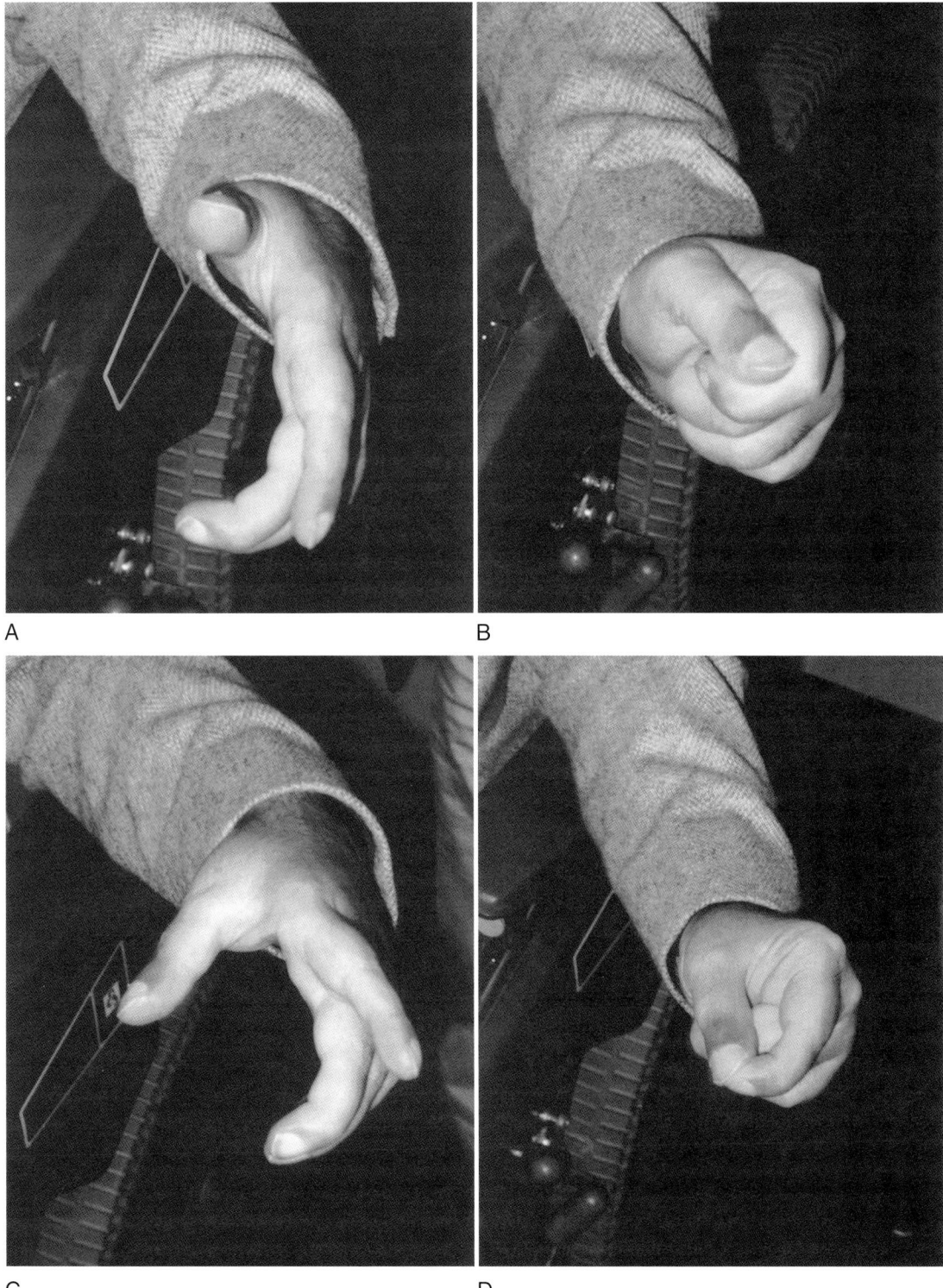

FIGURE 215-22. The two grip postures available to this patient after implantation of an eight-channel functional neuromuscular stimulator are illustrated. The patient can choose between a key grip or lateral pinch posture (*A* and *B*), useful for grasping smaller objects, and a palmar grasp (*C* and *D*), useful for grasping larger objects. The patient controls the amount of opening (*A* and *C*) by movement of the contralateral shoulder and the force of closing the grip (*B* and *D*) by movement of the opposite shoulder. (From Hentz V, Leclercq C: Surgical Rehabilitation of the Upper Limb in Tetraplegia. London, Harcourt Health Sciences, 2002:217-218.)

evaluation. We analyzed these patients according to the proposed major preoperative goals.

A primary goal was restoration of elbow extensor stabilization and active elbow extension. Two surgical procedures were employed, with relatively specific indications for each. Most commonly, transfer of posterior deltoid to triceps, as popularized by Moberg,[9] was performed. It was performed exclusively until 1985. Beginning in 1985, for patients presenting with a preoperative elbow contracture of more than 30 degrees, contracture release was combined with medial routing of biceps to triceps as popularized by Zancolli.[46]

We examined 21 patients who had undergone elbow extensor reconstruction more than 10 years earlier. Of the 15 patients who had posterior deltoid to triceps transfer, 10 had bilateral transfers. All 15 had required a motorized wheelchair as their primary means of movement before surgery. Ten years after surgery, nine now used a push chair as their standard chair and four others used a push chair at least some of the time. There were three patients who had undergone bilateral posterior deltoid to triceps transfer who were able to self-transfer in the early postoperative period. All three continued to be able to perform this monumental, for a tetraplegic, task. In the posterior deltoid to triceps group, four patients had required a preliminary release of elbow flexion contracture. One of the four examined 10 years after surgery had recurrence of contracture of more than 30 degrees.

Of the six patients who had biceps to triceps transfer (all needing contracture release), two could use a push chair but not exclusively so. None had recurrence of elbow contracture.

The second goal was the restoration of pinch for the weaker patients and pinch and grasp as well as the ability to open the hand for the stronger patients. IC group 2 patients typically had key grip fashioned by tenodesis of the FPL to the radius. Seven were evaluated longer than 10 years after reconstruction. Five had maintained pinch strength essentially equivalent to that demonstrated 6 to 12 months after surgery. Overall pinch strength in this group averaged 25 newtons.

IC group 3 patients typically had transfer of brachioradialis to FPL to restore dynamic voluntary key pinch. Six were evaluated, and all had maintained useful power that averaged 20 newtons. Thumb interphalangeal joint instability seemed to play a strong role in the diminished power seen in several of the brachioradialis-FPL patients. We now routinely employ the split FPL attachment described by Mohammed and Rothwell[35] to provide thumb interphalangeal stabilization, thus avoiding interphalangeal joint fusion.

Of the IC group 4 and 5 patients, the strong patients, 18 were re-examined. Almost all had undergone two-stage procedures, and half had elected bilateral reconstruction. Flexor power was by active transfer of ECRL, brachioradialis, or pronator teres or accessory wrist extensor, always in some combination to the thumb and digital flexors. Six had undergone some type of additional surgery in the period between their initial surgery and the date of long-term evaluation, typically adjustment of the flexor to one or another finger (usually the index) or release of a contracted proximal interphalangeal joint (usually the ring or little). Grip power had not deteriorated in these patients compared with the value measured at the 6- to 12-month evaluation after their initial surgery. Pinch force averaged 34 newtons. Typically two muscles were devoted to thumb function in these patients. We found, as did House,[38] that those patients who had some type of intrinsic stabilization, either by Zancolli[39] lasso or by House's[40] intrinsic reconstruction procedure, had, on average, more powerful grasp. This may be a product of preselection, however, the stronger patients having been selectively chosen for intrinsic substitution.

We conclude from this long-term analysis that carefully chosen upper limb reconstructive procedures in properly educated patients are both effective and durable. Systematic postoperative re-evaluation of their upper limbs should become a standard part of the more typical interval examinations of more generally studied systems, such as renal and bladder function, blood pressure, and pulmonary status. Aside from the brain, the upper limbs remain the most important residual resource for tetraplegic patients. Frequent re-evaluation of their upper limbs makes ultimate good sense.

Few of our patients perform many new activities. Typically, a good or excellent result means that the patient performs many of the same functions but with much greater efficiency. The rewards for surgeons, rehabilitation medicine specialists, and therapists are best expressed by one of our patients who replied to a question requesting his feelings on his outcome, "It's not as much as I hoped for, but it's much more than I ever had."

REFERENCES

1. Bunnell S: Surgery of the Hand. Philadelphia, JB Lippincott, 1944.
2. Bunnell S: Tendon transfer in the hand and forearm. Am Acad Orthop Surg Instruct Course Lect 1949;6:106-112.
3. Nickel V, Perry J: The flexor hinged hand. J Bone Joint Surg Am 1958;40:971.
4. Nickel VL, Perry J, Garrett AL: Development of useful function in the severely paralyzed hand. J Bone Joint Surg Am 1963;45:933.
5. Lamb DW, Landry R: The hand in quadriplegia. Hand 1971;3:31-37.
6. Zancolli E: Structural and Dynamic Basis of Hand Surgery. Philadelphia, JB Lippincott, 1968.
7. Guttmann L: Spinal Cord Injuries: Comprehensive Management and Research, 2nd ed. Oxford, Blackwell Scientific, 1976.
8. Moberg E: Upper limb surgery as a help to C5-6 tetraplegia. J Bone Joint Surg Br 1974;56:206.
9. Moberg E: Surgical treatment for absent single-hand grip and elbow extension in quadriplegia: principles and preliminary treatment. J Bone Joint Surg Am 1975;57:196-206.

10. Hentz VR, Keoshian L: Changing perspectives in surgical hand rehabilitation in quadriplegic patients. J Plast Reconstr Surg 1979;64:509-515.

11. Hentz VR, Brown M, Keoshian LA: Upper limb reconstruction in quadriplegia: functional assessment and proposed treatment modifications. J Hand Surg Am 1983;8:119-131.

12. Hentz VR: Historical background and changing perspectives in surgical reconstruction of the upper limb in quadriplegia. J Am Paraplegia Soc 1984;7:36-38.

13. Hentz VR, Hamlin C, Keoshian LA: Surgical reconstruction in tetraplegia. Hand Clin 1988;4:601-607.

14. Hentz V, Leclercq C: Management of the Upper Limb in Tetraplegia. London, Harcourt Health Sciences, 2001.

15. Moberg E: The Upper Limb in Tetraplegia. A New Approach to Surgical Rehabilitation. Stuttgart, George Thieme, 1978.

16. McDowell CL, Moberg E, Smith AG: International conference on surgical rehabilitation of the upper limb in tetraplegia. J Hand Surg 1979;4:387-390.

17. Ditunno JF, Stover S, Freed M, Ahn J: Motor recovery of the upper extremities in traumatic quadriplegia: a multicenter study. Arch Phys Med Rehabil 1992;73:431-436.

18. Curtin M: Development of a tetraplegia specific assessment and splinting protocol. Paraplegia 1994;32:159-169.

19. DiPasquale-Lehnerz P: Orthotic intervention for development of hand function with C6 quadriplegia. Am J Occup Ther 1994;48:138-144.

20. Krajnik S, Bridle M: Hand splinting in quadriplegia: current practice. Am J Occup Ther 1992;46:149-156.

21. Grover J, Gellman H, Waters R: The effect of a flexion contracture of the elbow on the ability to transfer in patients who have quadriplegia at the sixth cervical level. J Bone Joint Surg Am 1996;78:1397-1400.

22. Moberg E: Reconstructive hand surgery in tetraplegia, stroke, and cerebral palsy: some basic concepts in physiology and neurology. J Hand Surg 1976;1:29-34.

23. Lamb DW: Upper limb surgery in tetraplegia. Br J Hand Surg 1989;14:143-144.

24. Castro-Serra A, Lopez-Pita A: A new surgical technique to correct triceps paralysis. Hand 1983;15:42-46.

25. Allieu Y, Benichou M, Teissier J, et al: Restoration of the upper limb in tetraplegic patients by tendon transfers [in French]. Chirurgie 1986;112:736-743.

26. Mennen U, Boonzaier A: An improved technique of posterior deltoid to triceps transfer in tetraplegia. J Hand Surg Br 1991;16:197-201.

27. Allieu Y: Le membre superieur du tetraplegique. Conferences d'enseignment du GEM. Paris, L'expansion Scientifique, 1994.

28. Kuz J: Biceps to triceps transfer in tetraplegic patients: report of the medial routing technique and follow-up of three cases. J Hand Surg Am 1999;24:161-172.

29. Friedenberg Z: Transposition of the biceps brachii for triceps weakness. J Bone Joint Surg Am 1954;36:656.

30. Brummer H: The winch operation. The Second International Conference on Surgical Rehabilitation of the Upper Limb in Tetraplegia, Giens, France, 1984.

31. Freehafer A, Mast W: Transfer of the brachioradialis to improve wrist extension in high spinal cord injury. J Bone Joint Surg Am 1967;49:648.

32. Johnson DL, Gellman H, Waters R, Tognella M: Brachioradialis transfer for wrist extension in tetraplegic patients who have fifth-cervical-level neurological function. J Bone Joint Surg Am 1996;78:1063-1067.

33. Brys D, Waters R: Effect of triceps function on the brachioradialis transfer in quadriplegia. J Hand Surg Am 1987;12:237-239.

34. Waters RL, Stark LZ, Grubernick I, et al: Electromyographic analysis of brachioradialis to flexor pollicis longus tendon transfer in quadriplegia. J Hand Surg Am 1990;15:335-339.

35. Mohammed KD, Rothwell A, Sinclair S, et al: Upper-limb surgery for tetraplegia. J Bone Joint Surg Br 1992;74:873-879.

36. Leclercq C: Surgical rehabilitation of the upper limbs in tetraplegic patients. Chirurgie 1996;121:492-495.

37. Pulvertaft G: Repair of tendon injuries in the hand. Ann R Coll Surg 1948;3:14.

38. House J: Two stage reconstruction of the tetraplegic hand. In Strickland JW, ed: Master Techniques in Orthopaedic Surgery. Philadelphia, Lippincott-Raven, 1998.

39. Zancolli E: Correccion de la "garra" digital por paralisis intrinseca. La operacion del "lazo." Acta Ortop Latinam 1974;1:65.

40. House JH, Gwathmey FW, Lundsgaard DK: Restoration of strong grasp and lateral pinch in tetraplegia due to cervical spinal cord injury. J Hand Surg Am 1976;1:152-159.

41. Riordan D: Tendon transplantation in median-nerve and ulnar nerve paralysis. J Bone Joint Surg Am 1953;35:312-320.

42. Mulcahey MJ, Smith B, Betz R, et al: Functional neuromuscular stimulation: outcome in young people with tetraplegia. J Am Paraplegia Soc 1994;17:20-35.

43. Smith B, Mulcahey M, Betz R: Quantitative comparison of grasp and release abilities with and without functional neuromuscular stimulation in adolescents with tetraplegia. Paraplegia 1996;34:16-23.

44. Triolo R, Betz R, Mulcahey M, Gardner E: Application of functional neuromuscular stimulation to children with spinal cord injuries. Candidate selection for upper and lower extremity research. Paraplegia 1994;32:824-843.

45. Wuolle KS, Van Doren CL, Thrope G, et al: Development of a quantitative hand grasp and release test for patients with tetraplegia using a hand neuroprosthesis. J Hand Surg Am 1994;19:209-218.

46. Zancolli E: Mid-cervical tetraplegia. Sixth International Conference on Surgical Rehabilitation of the Upper Limb in Tetraplegia, Cleveland, Ohio, 1998.

Management of the Spastic Hand

ANN VAN HEEST, MD ✦ JAMES HOUSE, MD, MS

OVERVIEW OF HAND SPASTICITY

Hand spasticity is a disorder most commonly seen in association with traumatic brain injury, cerebral vascular injury, cervical spine injury, and cerebral palsy. All of these disorders have in common a central nervous system injury causing an upper motor neuron paresis or palsy. In an upper motor neuron disorder, the normal inhibitory control of tone is lost, and the resultant peripheral manifestation is spasticity. Muscle spasticity causes imbalance across joints with resultant loss of function. Cerebral palsy has the added complexity that the central nervous system injury occurs in the perinatal period, so that the effect of spasticity on the immature skeleton must be considered as well.

In the upper extremity, the typical pattern of spastic joint posturing includes shoulder internal rotation, elbow flexion, forearm pronation, wrist flexion and ulnar deviation, thumb-in-palm, and finger swan-neck or clenched fist deformities (Fig. 216-1). Although this pattern of deformity is the most common, the particular pattern and severity are individual to each patient on the basis of the extent and area of the underlying central nervous system disorder.

Spasticity in the hand does not occur as an isolated problem. Motor involvement can take the form of spasticity (increased tone), flaccidity (decreased tone), or athetosis (lack of or poor control of tone). The interplay of these various types of motor involvement is an important part of defining the problem. In evaluating a particular joint deformity, several forces often work together to exacerbate the joint deformity

(Fig. 216-2). For example, in a wrist flexion/ulnar deviation deformity, the deformity can be due primarily to spasticity of the flexor carpi ulnaris muscle. However, weakness or flaccidity of the extensor carpi radialis longus and brevis muscles can exacerbate the wrist flexion/ulnar deviation deformity because there is no active antagonist (extension/radial deviation) to the spastic flexor carpi ulnaris (flexor/ulnar deviation). The spasticity of the agonist (in this example, the flexor carpi ulnaris) as well as the strength and control of the antagonist (in this example, the extensor carpi radialis longus and brevis) must be assessed to evaluate the problem accurately.

Several disease processes that involve upper motor neuron lesions due to brain dysfunction are considered together because they have a single final common pathway: spasticity in the hand (Fig. 216-3). Traumatic brain injury is the most commonly seen in patients younger than 40 years and is typically secondary to motor vehicle accidents. Major return of function can occur up to 18 months after traumatic brain injury with cognitive improvements during many years after the injury.[1] Cerebral vascular accidents affect 1 in 1000 individuals per year; spastic hemiplegia is the most common sequela for the surviving patients. This is because the middle cerebral artery is the most commonly involved vessel, with resultant sensory and motor system dysfunction. Cerebral palsy is most commonly secondary to ischemic central nervous system injuries occurring in the perinatal period. This is most commonly associated with low birth weight with prematurity, anoxic events, or cerebral vascular bleeds or

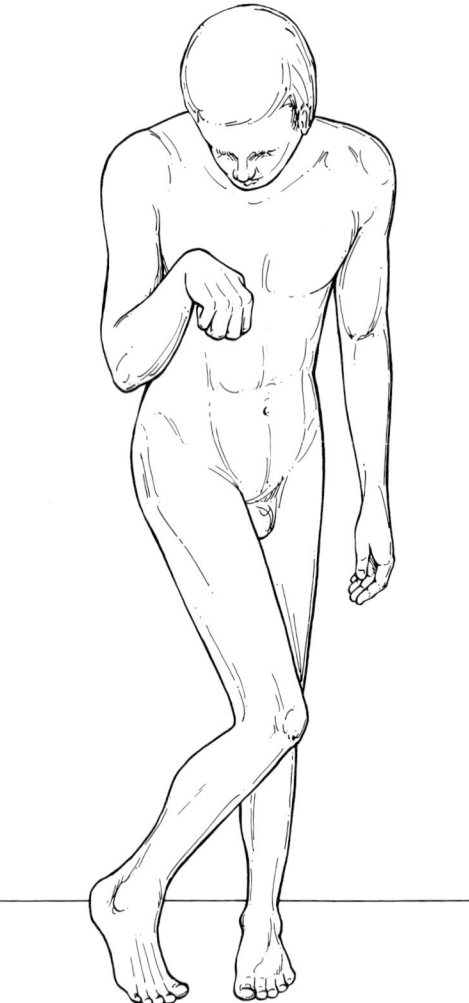

FIGURE 216-1. Typical spastic hemiplegic posturing in the upper extremity includes shoulder internal rotation, elbow flexion, forearm pronation, wrist flexion and ulnar deviation, thumb-in-palm, and clenched fist deformities.

emboli. The incidence is 0.2% (2 children per 1000 live births), increasing to 10% in the premature, low-birth-weight child.

Spasticity of the hand is not the only manifestation of these central nervous system disorders. The pattern of musculoskeletal spasticity is classified by the limb or limbs involved: monoplegia (one limb), hemiplegia (one arm and one leg), diplegia (two legs), triplegia (one arm and two legs), and quadriplegia (all four extremities).

All individuals who present with spasticity in the hand need a further evaluation of their central nervous system. If a child first presents to the hand surgeon, identification is most commonly around 1 year of age because of delayed development of normal pinch and grasp function. In this scenario, a complete neurologic evaluation is necessary, including evaluation of the lower extremities, before a diagnosis of cerebral palsy can be made. In most other scenarios, the hand surgeon is consulted for management of hand spasticity after the initial central nervous system lesion has been diagnosed. The hand surgeon must continue to work with the rehabilitation physicians and neurologists, as well as with any physicians who may be involved in lower extremity care, to maintain a multispecialty approach that appropriately coordinates services for the patient. Associated issues can include mental retardation, seizures, and speech disorders as well as lower extremity involvement that affects mobility.

In this chapter, the focus is on spastic hemiplegia secondary to cerebral palsy as the most common form of spasticity of the hand. Similar principles can be applied to other causes of hand spasticity as well.

ANALYSIS OF SPASTICITY IN THE HAND

Assessment of the patient with spastic cerebral palsy starts with the history and physical examination. Because cerebral palsy is associated with low birth weight and prematurity, associated medical problems should be noted, particularly seizures and mental retardation as indicators of more global central nervous system involvement. Developmental motor delays should be assessed. Children with spastic hemiplegia most commonly will show premature hand dominance, favoring the unaffected side even as young as 6 months. Delay of normal pinch and grasp function patterning at 1 year of age is evident. Overall use of the upper extremity should be characterized both from the history obtained from the parents and by the physician's direct observation. Overall upper extremity function in cerebral palsy is most commonly classified by a nine-level grading system (Table 216-1). General categories include the following: does not use; passive assist (poor, fair, or good); active assist (poor, fair, or good); and spontaneous use (partial or complete). Agreement with the parents on the child's present overall level of limb function lays the groundwork against which outcome of subsequent treatments can be compared.

Physical examination starts with an observation of the extent to which the individual uses the limb as well as the child's overall functional abilities. The dynamic positioning of the shoulder, elbow, forearm, wrist, fingers, and thumb is noted, particularly for grasp and release as well as for pinch function. Age-appropriate tasks or toys that require two-handed use are helpful in this assessment. The limb is then examined for passive range of motion of the shoulder, elbow, forearm, wrist, and hand, evaluating for joint contractures. Even if only the wrist and hand are to be treated, the shoulder, elbow, and forearm need to be assessed because they are

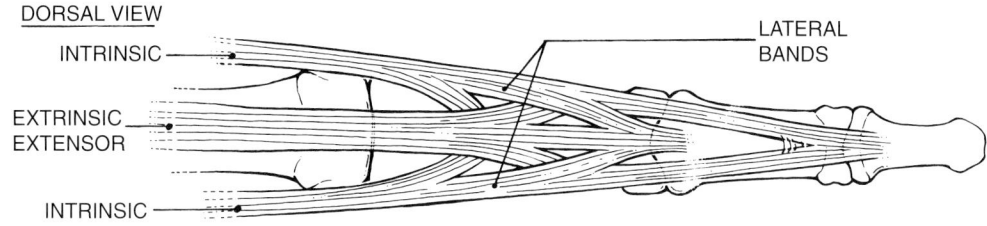

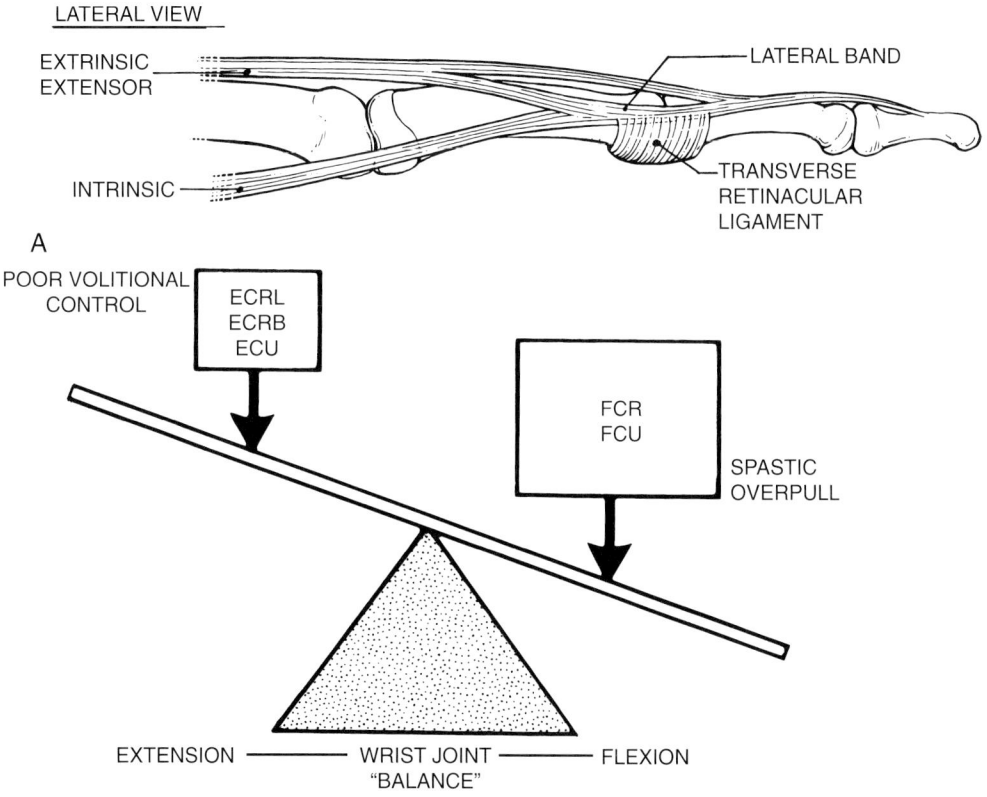

FIGURE 216-2. *A,* Normal anatomy of proximal interphalangeal joint extensors in the dorsal and lateral view. The extrinsic finger extensors (EDC, EDQ, EIP) divide over the proximal phalanx to form the central slip and two lateral bands. The finger intrinsics are the interossei and the lumbricals. The intrinsics join the extrinsic lateral band to form the conjoined lateral band, commonly referred to as the lateral band. In the normal state, dorsal subluxation of the lateral band is prevented by the volar tethering effect of the transverse retinacular ligament. *B,* Muscle imbalance causing joint deformity. Joint deformity occurs secondary to muscle imbalance. In the wrist joint, the wrist extensors are often flaccid with poor rotational control, whereas the wrist flexors are often spastic, causing wrist flexion deformity.

TABLE 216-1 ♦ UPPER EXTREMITY FUNCTIONAL USE CLASSIFICATION

Class	Designation	Activity Level
0	Does not use	Does not use
1	Poor passive assist	Uses as stabilizing weight only
2	Fair passive assist	Can hold onto object placed in hand
3	Good passive assist	Can hold onto object and stabilize it for use by other hand
4	Poor active assist	Can actively grasp object and hold it weakly
5	Fair active assist	Can actively grasp object and stabilize it well
6	Good active assist	Can actively grasp object and then manipulate it against other hand
7	Spontaneous use, partial	Can perform bimanual activities easily and occasionally uses the hand spontaneously
8	Spontaneous use, complete	Uses hand completely independently without reference to the other hand

essential for the individual to effectively position the hand in space.

Muscle tone is noted through the passive evaluation of joint mobility. Passive range of motion needs to be done slowly to overcome muscle spasticity with gentle sustained resistance. Assessment for muscle and joint contracture is performed by passive mobility of the joint and passive stretch of the muscle. If there is a loss of range of motion at both the finger and wrist joints unaffected by change in position of the wrist, both muscle and joint contractures are present. If there is full passive mobility of the joints and muscle, no contracture exists. If there is muscle contracture without joint contracture, this can be elicited by testing the effect of joint motion on a biarticular muscle such as the finger flexors. The finger flexor muscles are biarticular muscles, meaning they cross over more than one joint (the wrist joint and the finger joints). Thus, positioning of the wrist joint in flexion allows full finger extension if there is no finger joint contracture; but positioning of the wrist joint in extension will not allow full finger extension if there is finger flexor muscle contracture. This is analogous to the intrinsic tightness test. This is commonly graded as described by Zancolli (Table 216-2).[2]

Active range of motion is assessed next, including specific muscle testing for voluntary motor control of antagonist muscles. This is particularly important for muscles that are considered for tendon transfer, such as the pronator teres (for pronator teres rerouting); the flexor carpi ulnaris, extensor carpi ulnaris, or brachioradialis (for wrist extension); the extensor pollicis longus (for extensor pollicis longus rerouting); and the extensor pollicis brevis and abductor pollicis longus for control of antagonists to the thumb-in-palm deformity.

Appropriate consultation or multispecialty approach to care should be instituted before surgical intervention is considered. Several alternatives to surgical intervention exist. Consideration of the treatment pros and cons may require discussions that include the rehabilitation physicians, neurologists, and neurosurgeons to adequately explore the options of tone-reducing medications (diazepam, baclofen),

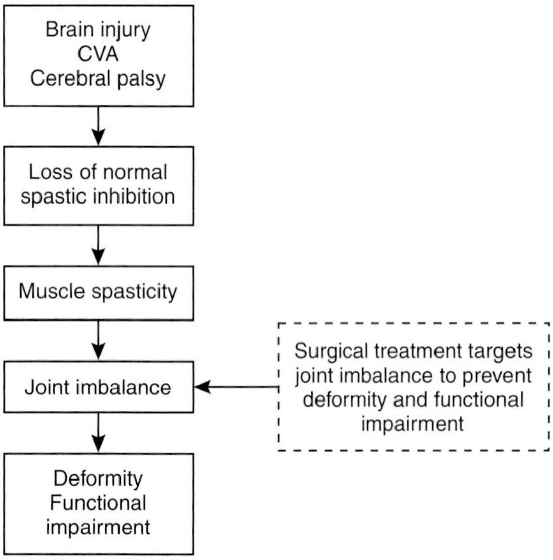

FIGURE 216-3. Sequence of events leading to limb dysfunction. Surgical treatment can address joint deformity and dysfunction at the shoulder, elbow, forearm, wrist, thumb, and fingers.

TABLE 216-2 ♦ ZANCOLLI ASSESSMENT OF WRIST FUNCTION

Group 1	Complete extension of the fingers with neutral extension of the wrist
Group 2	Finger extension with wrist flexion Subgroup a: Active extension of the wrist with the fingers flexed Subgroup b: No active extension of the wrist with the fingers flexed
Group 3	No active extension of the fingers even with maximal wrist flexion

tone-reducing injections (botulinum toxin, phenol), tone-reducing neurosurgery interventions (selective dorsal rhizotomy), and therapy interventions (splinting, stretching programs). At our institution, a spasticity management team of specialists is involved with evaluation of the patient for tone-reducing interventions and helps guide the hand surgeon to other treatment alternatives. If a patient has global problems with tone (most commonly quadriplegics), overall tone control should be obtained with tone-reducing *medications* or with *selective dorsal rhizotomy,* and control is stabilized before hand surgery intervention. Selective dorsal rhizotomy has been shown in one study[3] to have an indirect tone-reducing effect even in the upper extremity in addition to its primary direct effect in the lower extremity.

If physical examination reveals a joint or muscle contracture, particularly in a hemiplegic patient or in a patient with isolated problems to the upper extremity, initial treatment includes splinting, stretching, and therapy interventions. *Electrical stimulation* of the antagonist muscles has been advocated in the upper extremity of patients with cerebral palsy, but lasting outcomes and improved function have not been reported.[4] Electrical stimulation has been shown neither to improve digital extension nor to decrease finger flexor tightness in stroke patients.[5] If joint positioning due to spasticity significantly compromises limb function, diagnostic and possible therapeutic injections can be considered. *Phenol* has been described as a useful diagnostic adjuvant for 3 to 6 months of reduced spasticity but requires an open procedure to ensure application to the motor nerve.[6,7] It has largely been discontinued at our institution because of the risk of long-term pain in association with sensory nerve application as well as because of its unpredictable results. *Nerve blocks with local anesthetic agents* can be useful diagnostically. For example, in a stroke patient with minimal hand function but persistent skin breakdown secondary to clenched fist deformity, an ulnar nerve block at the wrist can help assess whether severe spasticity in the intrinsic muscles of the hand contributes to the deformity. Another injection modality used more recently is *botulinum toxin type A* (Botox), which works by local blockage of the release of acetylcholine at the neuromuscular junction; the reversible action lasts on average 3 to 4 months. With a reduction of tone in the specific muscles injected with botulinum toxin, a better assessment of functional control of the antagonist muscles can be performed. Therapy during the period of reduced tone has been reported to benefit functional use of the hand as well as allowing increased stretch on spastic muscles.[8,9] In the spastic mouse model, muscles have been shown to have a 15% increase in length with stretching after botulinum toxin type A injections.[10] If joint or muscle contracture exists, treatment should begin with splinting and stretching

exercises for at least 6 months, before consideration of surgical intervention.

If the patient may be a possible candidate for surgical intervention and is not a candidate for the alternative treatments or if the treatments did not resolve the patient's upper limb dysfunction, the examiner should review the history and physical examination and answer the following questions to determine the next step in treatment:

- How old is the patient?

Although some series have reported early intervention in tendon transfer surgery, results have been favorable only in surgeries involving release of severe spastic deforming muscles. A child usually needs to be at least 7 years of age to consistently cooperate with a preoperative assessment of muscle tone and control as well as with postoperative therapy protocols imperative to a successful result. Most series report tendon transfer surgeries at ages averaging 14 years (range, 4 years to adult).

- What is this patient's overall limb function as classified by House? (see Table 216-1)

Surgical intervention has been shown to improve limb function by 2.6 functional levels, particularly for children with an average baseline functional level of 2 to 3.

- What muscles are spastic and causing joint imbalance leading to limb dysfunction?

The spastic muscles may need to be released or weakened by lengthening.

- What muscles are flaccid or have poor motor control, leading to joint imbalance with resultant limb dysfunction?

The flaccid or poorly controlled muscles need to be augmented, usually through tendon transfer.

- What muscles are under good voluntary control and are available for tendon transfer?

The muscles with good voluntary control are best for good results with tendon transfer.

- Is there significant athetosis or incoordination?

In general, athetosis is associated with poor results after surgical intervention. Surgical treatment in the athetoid patient is rarely performed and usually would only involve joint stabilizations, such as fusion of the metacarpophalangeal joint of the thumb in the face of dislocation or subluxation.

TREATMENT GOALS

Treatment of the hand dysfunction centers on improving muscle balance to maximize hand function consistent with the quality of voluntary control retained. The primary lesion in the brain is not treated and remains the limiting factor to the success of the surgery. The goal is not normalization of hand use but rather improvement of joint positioning to maximize assistive hand function. Surgical treatment is indicated for patients with spastic deformity and contractures, unresponsive to nonsurgical treatment, that produce specific functional impairment and could be improved by better joint positioning.

SURGICAL PRINCIPLES

Surgical procedures to satisfy these treatment goals follow specific surgical principles (Table 216-3) to be described as they apply to wrist flexion deformity, thumb-in-palm deformity, and finger swan-neck deformity. A vast array of options exist for the surgeon treating the wrist, thumb, and fingers and a constellation of associated deformities (Table 216-4). This requires the surgeon to carefully think through the type of deformity at each joint separately and then synthesize them into a comprehensive reconstructive plan. If evaluation of the upper limb revealed significant shoulder, elbow, or forearm deformity that precludes

TABLE 216-3 ✦ SURGICAL TREATMENT PRINCIPLES

1. Release or lengthen the spastic or contracted muscles.
2. Augment the weak or flaccid muscles.
3. Stabilize the joint for severe joint instability or severe joint contractures.

appropriate positioning of the limb in space, treatment of these joint deformities should be included as part of the overall treatment plan. Because this is beyond the scope of this text, the reader is referred to other sources if this situation is present.[2,11,12]

Wrist Flexion Deformity

1. Release or lengthen the spastic muscle or muscles:
   - Fractional lengthening of the flexor carpi ulnaris or flexor carpi radialis
   - Flexor pronator slide

Most patients with hemiplegia have significant wrist flexion deformity, often accompanied by ulnar

TABLE 216-4 ✦ TREATMENT OPTIONS BY TYPE OF DEFORMITY AND TYPE OF PROCEDURE

Deformity	Elbow Flexion	Forearm Pronation	Wrist Flexion/UD	Finger Deformity	Thumb-in-Palm
Procedures*	(21)	(134)	(202)	(40)	(289)
Soft Tissue Releases	(11) Biceps lengthenings[29] (10) Brachialis lengthenings[29]	(80) P. teres releases[30] (1) P. quad release (49) Biceps aponeurosis releases	(31) FCR lengthenings[31] (15) FCU lengthenings[31] (16) Flexor pronator slides[13,14]	(14) FDS lengthenings[31]	(57) First web Z-plasties (84) Adductor and/or 1st DI releases[18] (20) FPL lengthenings
Tendon Transfers		(1) P. teres rerouting[32]	(50) BR to ECRB/L[15,16] (42) ECU to ECRB/L (28) FCU to ECRB/L[17,33] (3) FCR to ECRB/L (1) P. teres to ECRL	(8) FCU to EDC (5) BR to EDC (3) Lat. band (4) FDS tenodesis[25] (1) SORL[22]	(17) PL to APL[27] (3) PL to EPL (10) PL to EPB (25) FCR to APL (1) FCR to EPB (5) BR to APL (4) BR to EPB (1) BR to EPL (2) EPL reroutings (3) Acc. APL to EPB
Bone or Joint Stabilization		(3) Rotational osteotomies	(11) Wrist fusion with PRC (5) PRC[34]	(1) DIP fusion (2) Volar plate capsulodesis (2) PIP fusions	(48) MCP fusions[10] (4) MCP capsulodesis[20] (5) IP fusions

*Number in parentheses refers to number of times this procedure was performed in this study population; number after the procedure refers to the footnoted reference of surgical technique.

1st DI, first dorsal interosseous; Acc. APL, accessory muscle of APL; APL, abductor pollicis longus; BR, brachioradialis; DIP, distal interphalangeal joint; ECRB/L, extensor carpi radialis brevis/longus; EDC, extensor digitorum communis; EPB, extensor pollicis brevis; EPL, extensor pollicis longus; FCR, flexor carpi radialis; FCU, flexor carpi ulnaris; FDS, flexor digitorum superficialis; FPL, flexor pollicis longus; MCP, metacarpophalangeal joint; P. quad, pronator quadratus; P. teres, pronator teres; PIP, proximal interphalangeal joint; PL, palmaris longus; PRC, proximal row carpectomy; SORL, spiral oblique retinacular ligament reconstruction; UD, ulnar deviation.

deviation. If the wrist flexion deformity is mild and wrist extensor control exists, weakening the wrist flexors through fractional lengthening may be sufficient. The wrist flexors can also be effectively lengthened by moving their origin distally, a procedure termed a flexor pronator slide.[13,14] This is particularly effective if there is concomitant finger flexor and pronator tightness because the common origin of all of these muscles is released and allowed to move distally during this procedure.

2. Augment the weak or flaccid muscle (tendon transfers):
   • Brachioradialis to extensor carpi radialis brevis
   • Extensor carpi ulnaris to extensor carpi radialis brevis
   • Flexor carpi ulnaris to extensor carpi radialis brevis
   • Flexor carpi ulnaris to extensor digitorum communis (if finger extension is inadequate)

In some cases, the wrist flexion deformity is more severe, and the principal wrist extensor muscles are not functional. This may be evident on physical examination, or it may require use of a diagnostic motor nerve block or a diagnostic botulinum toxin injection to temporarily weaken the spastic wrist flexor, most commonly the flexor carpi ulnaris, to assess the patient's cortical control for wrist extension. Muscles that can be transferred to augment wrist extension include the brachioradialis, extensor carpi ulnaris, and flexor carpi ulnaris (Green transfer).[15-17] Use of the brachioradialis or extensor carpi ulnaris has the advantage of leaving both flexors intact (although they may need to be concomitantly lengthened to diminish their spastic deforming force), thus minimizing the risk of overcorrection. Use of the extensor carpi ulnaris has the advantage of diminishing the ulnar deviation forces as well for patients with concomitant ulnar deviation deformity. Use of the flexor carpi ulnaris to remove its effect as a spastic wrist flexor and to transfer its force as a wrist extensor is reserved for the most severe cases.

In all cases of transfer into the wrist extensors, the finger function must be assessed preoperatively with the wrist maintained in a neutral position. As mentioned, the finger flexor muscles are biarticular muscles so that changes in the wrist position may change finger tone and function; this needs to be evaluated preoperatively. If the finger flexors are so shortened that a clenched fist deformity ensues when the wrist is brought into extension, the finger flexors will need to be fractionally lengthened as part of the surgical procedure. If the patient does not have sufficient finger extensor control to extend the fingers (release) with the wrist in flexion, a transfer of one of these muscles into the finger extensors (extensor digitorum communis) may be indicated. If the patient does not have sufficient digital control or has too much tone with the wrist in an extended position, a tendon transfer

into the wrist extensors may result in an "extensor habitus" that will diminish, rather than help, grasp and release function. Balance of the wrist is the goal, and it is important to recognize that wrist flexion facilitates finger extension by the tenodesis effect.

3. Stabilize the joint for severe instability or contracture:
   • Proximal row carpectomy
   • Wrist fusion

If the patient has a severe wrist joint contracture limiting functional use of the hand refractory to at least 6 months of nonsurgical intervention, consideration can be given to either a proximal row carpectomy, to shorten the skeleton, or a wrist fusion, to hold the wrist in a fixed position. The proximal row carpectomy is used in combination with releases and tendon transfer surgeries if the wrist lacks sufficient mobility passively; shortening the skeleton through proximal row carpectomy can improve the wrist flexion deformity by 30 or 40 degrees of extension. This may be useful in selected cases if the wrist is fixed in 10 to 20 degrees of flexion and the surgeon wishes to preserve wrist motion to maintain the tenodesis effect. Wrist fusion has the advantage of being a predictable procedure in which the wrist is positioned and fixed intraoperatively. It is indicated only for improved cosmesis and use of the hand as a paperweight, in the skeletally mature individual, although it is possible to fuse the wrist in the skeletally immature patient if care is taken to remove only cartilaginous surfaces. The proximal carpal row may be removed as part of the wrist fusion procedure to allow some relaxation of the flexors and to facilitate positioning into slight wrist extension. The finger position must be addressed as in tendon transfer surgery (described earlier).

Thumb-in-Palm Deformity

1. Release or lengthen the spastic muscle or muscles:
   • Adductor pollicis
   • Flexor pollicis brevis
   • Flexor pollicis longus

If the primary deformity is adduction of the first metacarpal, without significant metacarpophalangeal or interphalangeal joint deformity, the primary deforming force is the adductor pollicis. Treatment includes a partial tenotomy or myotomy near its insertion (often in conjunction with a first web Z-plasty for individuals with concomitant skin contracture) or a release of its origin off the third metacarpal as described by Matev.[18]

If the primary deformity is adduction of the first metacarpal with metacarpophalangeal joint flexion deformity, without significant interphalangeal joint deformity, the primary deforming forces are the adductor pollicis and the flexor pollicis brevis. Treatment includes a surgical release of the adductor, through either a first web Z-plasty or a palmar incision as described before, with the release of the flexor pollicis brevis through the same incision.

If the primary deformity is adduction of the first metacarpal with both metacarpophalangeal and interphalangeal joint flexion deformity, the primary deforming forces are the adductor pollicis, the flexor pollicis brevis, and the flexor pollicis longus. Treatment includes a surgical release of the adductor and flexor pollicis brevis, as described before, as well as a lengthening of the flexor pollicis longus through a separate volar incision. Depending on the degree of contracture, either a fractional lengthening at the musculotendinous level (for the less severely contracted) or a Z-lengthening of the tendon (for the more severely contracted) may be performed.

2. Augment the weak or flaccid muscle (tendon transfers):
   • Donors: brachioradialis, flexor carpi radialis (if flexor carpi ulnaris is not transferred), palmaris longus, flexor digitorum superficialis
   • Recipients: abductor pollicis longus, extensor pollicis brevis (if metacarpophalangeal joint is stable), extensor pollicis longus
   • Rerouting: extensor pollicis longus

For the milder deformity *with* antagonists present, the surgical releases (adductor, flexor pollicis brevis, flexor pollicis longus) alone are sufficient. For the more severe deformity *without* antagonists present, the surgical releases need to be augmented by tendon transfers. Tendons to be transferred can be the brachioradialis, flexor carpi radialis, palmaris longus, or flexor digitorum superficialis. The choice of donor tendon is primarily based on the synthesis of the entire reconstructive plan, noting particularly that use of the flexor carpi radialis tendon is contraindicated if the flexor carpi ulnaris is used as a wrist extension tendon transfer. The recipient tendon most commonly chosen is the abductor pollicis longus because this augments first metacarpal abduction. Transfer into the extensor pollicis brevis is contraindicated if the metacarpophalangeal joint is unstable (type III thumb). Rerouting of the extensor pollicis longus tendon is used commonly, particularly if the patient has good control of the interphalangeal joint extension.[19] The extensor pollicis longus is transferred from the third dorsal compartment into the first dorsal compartment, thus changing its vector from extension/*adduction* of the thumb to extension/*abduction* of the thumb.

3. Stabilize the joint in the presence of severe instability or contracture:
   • Metacarpophalangeal joint fusion or volar capsulodesis
   • Interphalangeal joint fusion

If the primary deformity of the thumb is one of first metacarpal adduction with secondary metacarpophalangeal hyperextension deformity (subluxation or dislocation), the metacarpophalangeal joint will need to be stabilized to provide an adequate base for pinch function. The metacarpophalangeal joint can be stabilized by a volar capsulodesis as described by Filler et al[20] or by fusion.[10] In the skeletally immature individual, a fusion can be performed if the epiphysis of the proximal phalanx is significantly ossified; the distal end of the metacarpal is fused to the proximal phalanx epiphysis by use of smooth K-wires with careful technique protecting the proximal phalanx physis to preserve longitudinal growth. Another combination available, particularly for the patient with severe flexor pollicis longus spasticity and interphalangeal joint flexion deformity, includes release of the flexor pollicis longus tendon at its insertion, transfer onto the radial aspect of the thumb (palmar abduction), and fusion of the interphalangeal joint for stabilization.[21]

Finger Swan-Neck Deformity

1. Release or lengthen the spastic muscle or muscles:
   • Intrinsic slide
   • Ulnar motor neurectomy

For patients with mild swan-neck deformity secondary to intrinsic spasticity, an intrinsic slide procedure has been described to lengthen these muscles by use of two dorsal incisions to elevate and slide the interossei origins. For patients with concomitant thumb adductor spasticity, a diagnostic injection of the motor branch of the ulnar nerve with local anesthetic or phenol can be used to assess its effect on both thumb-in-palm and intrinsic spasticity disorders. If the results are favorable, an ulnar motor neurectomy can be performed just distal to Guyon canal.

2. Augment the weak or flaccid muscle (tendon transfers):
   • Lateral band rerouting

Swan-neck deformities are due to subluxation of the lateral band dorsal to the axis of rotation of the proximal interphalangeal joint.[22] This deformity can be corrected dynamically through transfer of the lateral band volar to the proximal interphalangeal joint axis, into the proximal interphalangeal volar plate by a midlateral incision as described by Tonkin.[23,24] This procedure is indicated for patients with moderate swan-neck deformities, usually 30 to 40 degrees of hyperextension, causing locking of the joint with grasp.

3. Stabilize the joint for severe instability or contracture:
   • Flexor digitorum superficialis tenodesis of the proximal interphalangeal joint

For more severe swan-neck deformity, tenodesis of the proximal interphalangeal joint can be performed through a volar incision. A distally based slip of the flexor digitorum superficialis tendon is secured into the volar aspect of the proximal phalanx as described by Swanson.[25]

Authors' Preferred Method

This example describes the authors' preferred methods of evaluation, treatment, surgical technique, and postoperative care. Note that the joints can be evaluated separately for treatment options, with a final reconstructive treatment plan synthesizing the complexities of the entire upper limb deformity.

A 10-year-old child presents with a wrist flexion/ulnar deviation and thumb-in-palm deformity interfering with her grasp-release and pinch function. She uses her hand as a poor passive assist. On passive range of motion, she has no evidence of muscle or joint contracture. On active range of motion, she demonstrates severe spasticity of the flexor carpi ulnaris with no extensor carpi radialis brevis or longus activity notable on examination. On observation of grasp and release, she can use the hand only passively by placing objects into the hand to hold because her wrist is dynamically in such a severely flexed position. She has good digital control in flexion and extension. Her thumb-in-palm posture is secondary to isolated adduction of the first metacarpal with metacarpophalangeal joint hyperextension deformity. Her thumb adducts across the palm of the hand so that the thumb sits between the index and long finger. She demonstrates good voluntary control of her extensor pollicis longus but not of her extensor pollicis brevis or abductor pollicis longus.

She was considered a possible surgical candidate for the following reasons. She is old enough to cooperate in her examination (10 years old). She has overall limb function graded as a "poor passive assist." She has spastic imbalance leading to joint deformity that limits function—the wrist flexion/ulnar deviation posturing limits her grasp and release function, and the thumb-in-palm posturing limits her pinch function.

At her thumb, the adductor is spastic, the extensor pollicis brevis and abductor pollicis longus are poorly controlled, and the metacarpophalangeal joint is unstable. By application of the surgical principles outlined before, we recommended

1. a partial adductor pollicis tenotomy (to weaken the spastic muscle);
2. a tendon transfer into the abductor pollicis longus tendon (to augment the weak muscle); note that a tendon transfer into the extensor pollicis brevis will only exacerbate the metacarpophalangeal hyperextension deformity, and so it should not be performed; and
3. a volar metacarpophalangeal joint capsulodesis (to stabilize the severely unstable joint).

Similarly at her wrist, the flexor carpi ulnaris is spastic, the extensor carpi radialis brevis/longus is poorly controlled, and the wrist joint is mobile. Diagnostic testing would be performed by injection of botulinum toxin into the flexor carpi ulnaris to better test voluntary control of the extensor carpi radialis brevis/longus as an antagonist to the flexor carpi ulnaris muscle when it is less spastic. If findings indicate that the patient has no extensor carpi radialis brevis/longus control despite diminished flexor carpi ulnaris spasticity, on application of the surgical principles outlined before we would recommend

1. fractional lengthening of the flexor carpi ulnaris (to weaken the spastic muscle);
2. a tendon transfer into the extensor carpi radialis brevis; and
3. no joint stabilizations necessary.

Available tendon transfers could include brachioradialis to the abductor pollicis longus for thumb abduction (appropriate vector and strength) and extensor carpi ulnaris to extensor carpi radialis brevis. Transfer of the extensor carpi ulnaris would help correct the ulnar deviation deformity by removing the ulnar deviation forces of the extensor carpi ulnaris, and it would help augment wrist extension by tensioning the transfer so that the wrist lay in neutral at rest.

Surgery is carried out in conjunction with the lower extremity surgeons, who removed plates placed as part of her previous lower extremity reconstruction. A tourniquet is used intraoperatively after appropriate preparation and draping.

The wrist is approached first through a curvilinear ulnar-sided incision. The extensor carpi ulnaris tendon is divided just distal to the extensor retinaculum and delivered into the proximal end of the wound by freeing its fascial attachments. Its excursion is checked; usually, approximately 3 to 4 cm indicates adequate excursion. A subcutaneous tunnel is created to a second dorsal incision made over the second dorsal compartment just proximal to the extensor retinaculum. In the interval distal to the thumb outcropper muscles (abductor pollicis longus and extensor pollicis brevis) but proximal to the extensor retinaculum, a fascial window is made, and the tendons of the extensor carpi radialis longus and brevis are identified. These tendons are usually fairly adherent because they are not under good cortical control and have not had much differential excursion. If this is found, the extensor carpi ulnaris will be transferred into both to prevent unnecessary dissection and subsequent adhesions.

Attention is now turned to the tendon transfer for the thumb. Through the radiodorsal wrist incision, the extensor pollicis brevis and abductor pollicis longus are identified. It is verified that tension on the extensor pollicis brevis tendon exacerbates the metacarpophalangeal hyperextension deformity, so this tendon is left in place. It is verified that tension on the abductor pollicis longus tendon abducts the first ray. The brachioradialis tendon is then dissected off into insertion onto the radial metaphysis, through the same incision; it is freed from its fascial insertions by extensive proximal dissection, verifying 2 to 3 cm of excursion.

Attention is now turned to release of the thumb adductor. The Matev palmar incision is made, using the distal portion of an extended carpal tunnel incision. The recurrent motor branch of the median nerve is identified and protected, as well as the palmar arch. The origin of the transverse head of the adductor pollicis muscle is then released off the third metacarpal while the deep ulnar nerve passing through the muscle near its origin is protected. Any fascial bands are released until the muscle origin is seen to "slide" radially as the thumb is brought into abduction.

Attention is now turned to the metacarpophalangeal capsulodesis. A radial midlateral incision is then made with dissection carried down onto the metacarpophalangeal joint. A radial midlateral capsulotomy is performed. The volar capsule is identified and usually found to be significantly attenuated off its volar metacarpal origin. The sesamoid bones are identified and denuded, with a corresponding area on the metacarpal neck area denuded as well. Bone suture anchors or drill holes through bone are then placed in the volar metacarpal neck with nonabsorbable suture placed through the sesamoid bones or adjacent volar plate. Tying the suture should bring the metacarpophalangeal joint into approximately 30 degrees of flexion. Slight force on the repair may allow the neutral position; assessment is made to verify that hyperlaxity or excessive flexion is not present. The metacarpophalangeal joint is pinned with a 0.045-inch K-wire to protect the repair.

Attention is now turned to sewing in and tensioning the tendon transfers, starting first with the most proximal joint. The extensor carpi ulnaris transfer is woven three times by a Pulvertaft weave through the extensor carpi radialis brevis and longus tendons. A test suture for tensioning is placed and adjusted until the wrist sits at rest in neutral. Final nonabsorbable 3-0 suture is placed. The brachioradialis tendon is then woven end-to-end into the abductor pollicis longus tendon. Because of the significant size mismatch, use of Pulvertaft weaves of the abductor pollicis longus into the brachioradialis is usually most effective. A test suture for tensioning is placed and adjusted until the thumb sits in slight abduction with the wrist at neutral, in full abduction with the wrist in flexion, and

in key pinch with the wrist in full extension. Final nonabsorbable 2-0 suture is placed. Because the brachioradialis is also biarticular, crossing both the elbow and wrist joints, the effect of elbow position is checked; it should help with thumb abduction as the elbow extends (e.g., reaching out for an object) and allow key pinch with elbow flexion.

Standard postoperative management includes long-arm cast immobilization (to protect the brachioradialis transfer) in slight wrist extension/radial deviation (to protect the extensor carpi ulnaris transfer and stretch the flexor carpi ulnaris lengthening) with the first metacarpal in extension/abduction (to protect the thumb transfer and stretch the adductor pollicis lengthening) and pinning of the metacarpophalangeal joint in approximately 20 degrees of flexion (to protect the metacarpophalangeal joint capsulodesis). For tendon transfers alone, 4 weeks of complete protection is sufficient; however, in this case, 6 weeks of complete protection is necessary to allow metacarpophalangeal joint healing. After 4 to 6 weeks of immobilization, the transfers are protected in a similar position in a forearm-based splint, with active range of motion and light activities of daily living (showers, eating) with the splint off three to five times per day. At 8 to 10 weeks after surgery, the splint is worn only at night and for protection during high-risk activities (recess, gym, play), and strengthening exercises commence.

COMPLICATIONS AND THEIR MANAGEMENT

Balance is the key, and it can be difficult to obtain. Overcorrection is due to excessively tight tendon transfers or excessive release (instead of lengthening) of spastic muscles and should be avoided through careful preoperative planning and attention to surgical technique. A key surgical principle is to leave an option to reverse the surgical correction if this is possible. Undercorrection occurs in the circumstances of release without concomitant tendon transfer, insufficient release, and undertensioned tendon transfers. If the initial procedure has resulted in undercorrection of the deformity, undercorrection is easier to manage with a subsequent additional procedure to obtain balance.

Recurrence can develop with skeletal growth,[26] but it is rare in our experience if balance is achieved at the time of surgery. Arthrodesis cannot be reversed, but "balance" or wrist position is set definitively at the time of surgery without risk of overcorrection or undercorrection. Wrist arthrodesis risks loss of function if adequate assessment of digital control is not considered as the tenodesis effect of the wrist is lost. Wrist arthrodesis should be reserved for those with the lowest level of limb function.

Lack of improved function despite better position can be due to the underlying limitations of the surgery, namely, central nervous system dysfunction and lack of selective voluntary control. These surgical corrections do not change the primary etiology (i.e., the defective central nervous system), so overall surgical results will never yield a "normal" limb. However, even better position without improved function is often a significant improvement from the patient's perspective because the limb will look more "normal" even if does not function as normal. Sensibility is also important, particularly as a predictor of spontaneous active use of the hand.

OUTCOMES OF TREATMENT

It is difficult to assess outcome as a measure of surgical results by use of functional measures such as range of motion, grip strength, or standardized testing because patients with spastic hand deformities have such varying levels of functional use, varying degrees of central nervous system involvement, and varying pictures of spasticity. By the House Upper Extremity Functional Use Classification (see Table 216-1), House et al[27] reported at least one functional grade of improvement with surgical treatment of thumb-in-palm deformities. In another review of all upper extremity surgical procedures, Van Heest and House[28] reported an average improvement of 2.6 functional levels for individuals with an average preoperative use of fair passive assist (level 2). Patients with fair to good voluntary control had the greatest functional improvement.

REFERENCES

1. Teasdale G, Skene A, Parker L, Jennett B: Age and outcome of severe head injury. Acta Neurochir Suppl Wien 1979;28:140-143.
2. Zancolli EA, Zancolli ERJ: Surgical management of the hemiplegic spastic hand in cerebral palsy. Surg Clin North Am 1981;61:395.
3. Loewen P, Steinbok P, Holsti L, MacKay M: Upper extremity performance and self-care skill changes in children with spastic cerebral palsy following selective posterior rhizotomy. Pediatr Neurosurg 1998;29:191-198.
4. Carmick J: Clinical use of neuromuscular electrical stimulation for children with cerebral palsy. Part II: upper extremity. Phys Ther 1993;73:514-527.
5. Hines AE, Crago PE, Villian C: Functional electrical stimulation for reduction of spasticity in the hemiplegic hand. Biomed Sci Instrum 1993;29:259-266.
6. Keenan MAE, Thomas E, Stone L: Percutaneous phenol block of musculocutaneous deformity in cerebral palsy. J Bone Joint Surg Am 1990;15:236.
7. Braun RM, Hoffer MM, Mooney V, et al: Phenol nerve block in the treatment of acquired spastic hemiplegia in the upper limb. J Bone Joint Surg Am 1973;55:580-585.
8. Wall SA, Chait LA, Temlett JA, et al: Botulinum A chemodenervation: a new modality in cerebral palsied hands. Br J Plast Surg 1993;46:703.
9. Van Heest AE: Applications of botulinum toxin in orthopaedics and upper extremity surgery. Techniques Hand Upper Extremity Surg 1997;1:27-34.
10. Goldner JL, Koman LA, Gelberman R, et al: Arthrodesis of the metacarpophalangeal joint of the thumb in children and adults: adjunctive treatment of thumb-in-palm deformity in cerebral palsy. Clin Orthop 1990;253:75-89.
11. Manske PR, Strecker WB: Cerebral palsy, stroke, brain injury. In Peimer CA, ed. Surgery of the Hand and Upper Extremity. New York, McGraw-Hill, 1995:1517.
12. Waters PM, Van Heest A: Spastic hemiplegia of the upper extremity in children. Hand Clin 1998;14:119-134.
13. Inglis AE, Cooper W: Release of the flexor-pronator origin for flexion deformities of the hand and wrist in spastic paralysis. J Bone Joint Surg Am 1966;48:847-857.
14. White WF: Flexor muscle slide in the spastic hand: the Max Page operation. J Bone Joint Surg Br 1972;54:453-459.
15. House JH, Gwathmey FW: Flexor carpi ulnaris and the brachioradialis as a wrist extension transfer in cerebral palsy. Minn Med 1978;61:481-484.
16. McCue FC, Honner R, Chapman WC: Transfer of the brachioradialis for hands deformed by cerebral palsy. J Bone Joint Surg Am 1970;52:1171-1180.
17. Green WT: Tendon transplantation of the flexor carpi ulnaris for pronation-flexion deformity of the wrist. Surg Gynecol Obstet 1942;75:337-342.
18. Matev I: Surgical treatment of spastic "thumb-in-palm" deformity. J Bone Joint Surg Br 1963;45:703-708.
19. Manske PR: Redirection of extensor pollicis longus in the treatment of spastic thumb-in-palm deformity. J Hand Surg Am 1985;10:553.
20. Filler BC, Stark HH, Boyes JH: Capsulodesis of the metacarpophalangeal joint of the thumb in children with cerebral palsy. J Bone Joint Surg Am 1976;58:667-670.
21. Smith RJ: Flexor pollicis longus abductor-platy for spastic thumb-in-palm deformity. J Hand Surg Am 1982;7:327.
22. Littler JW: The finger extensor mechanism. Surg Clin North Am 1967;47:415-432.
23. Van Heest A: Lateral band re-routing in the treatment of swan-neck deformities due to cerebral palsy. Techniques Hand Upper Extremity Surg 1997;1:189-194.
24. Tonkin MA, Hughes J, Smith KL: Lateral band translocation for swan-neck deformity. J Hand Surg Am 1992;17:260-267.
25. Swanson AB: Surgery of the hand in cerebral palsy and the swan neck deformity. J Bone Joint Surg Am 1960;42:951-964.
26. Thometz JG, Tachdjian MO: Long-term follow-up of the flexor carpi ulnaris transfer in spastic hemiplegic children. J Pediatr Orthop 1988;8:407.
27. House J, Gwathmey F, Fidler M: A dynamic approach to the thumb-in-palm deformity in cerebral palsy. J Bone Joint Surg Am 1981;63:216-225.
28. Van Heest AE, House JH, Cariello C: Upper extremity surgical treatment of cerebral palsy. J Hand Surgery Am 1999;24:323-330.
29. Mital MA: Lengthening of the elbow flexors in cerebral palsy. J Bone Joint Surg Am 1979;61:515-522.
30. Strecker WB, Emanuel JP, Dailey L, Manske PR: Comparison of pronator tenotomy and pronator rerouting in children with spastic cerebral palsy. J Hand Surg Am 1988;13:540-543.
31. Zancolli EA: Structural and Dynamic Bases of Hand Surgery, 2nd ed. Philadelphia, JB Lippincott, 1968.
32. Sakellarides HT, Mital MA, Lenzi WD: Treatment of pronation contractures of the forearm in cerebral palsy by changing the insertion of the pronator radii teres. J Bone Joint Surg Am 1981;63:645-652.
33. Green WT, Banks HH: Flexor carpi ulnaris transplant and its use in cerebral palsy. J Bone Joint Surg Am 1962;44:1343-4352.
34. Omer GE, Capen DA: Proximal row carpectomy with muscle transfers for spastic paralysis. J Hand Surg Am 1976;1:197-204.

Rehabilitation

Hand Therapy

CAROLYN GORDEN, OHT, CHT ✦ DONNA LASHGARI, OTR, CHT
✦ PREM LALWANI, OTR, CHT

Hand therapy is the art and science of rehabilitation of the upper extremity. Hand therapy has developed from the professions of occupational therapy and physical therapy. The hand therapist combines comprehensive knowledge of the upper extremity with specialized skills in assessment and treatment to prevent dysfunction, to restore function, or to reverse the advancement of a pathologic process in the upper extremity. The goal of hand therapy is to promote health and well-being through rehabilitation services to individuals with upper extremity dysfunction.

The specialty of hand therapy developed in response to advances in surgical techniques that enabled greater functional restoration of injured and diseased upper extremities. Specialists in hand therapy employ therapeutic techniques derived from both occupational therapy and physical therapy. Hand therapists are registered or licensed occupational therapists or physical therapists who, through advanced continuing education, clinical experience, and independent study, have become proficient in the treatment of pathologic upper extremity conditions resulting from trauma, disease, and congenital or acquired deformity. To be a certified hand therapist, one must have 5 years of experience and have passed the certified hand therapist examination. Hand therapy should be directed by an experienced therapist who has had specialized hand therapy training.

The therapist and the physician must work closely together along with the patient in a well-organized therapeutic program. Hand rehabilitation encompasses more than the hand surgery itself. It takes into account all factors that are important to the patient as well as those local factors that are amenable to the surgeon's and the therapist's skill.[1]

EVALUATION

Before treatment can begin, a baseline evaluation is necessary to determine the plan of treatment, to monitor the patient's progress, and to judge the effectiveness of treatment procedures. An evaluation can be divided into subjective and objective information.

Subjective Information

Subjective information is obtained through speaking with and listening to the patient, observation, and palpation of the hand. This type of information is important from a treatment and diagnostic standpoint (Table 217-1).

Objective Information

When objective measurements are recorded, tests that have been analyzed for validity and reliability should

TABLE 217-1 ✦ EVALUATION OF THE PATIENT: SUBJECTIVE INFORMATION

History of injury or illness
Posture of the hand: The wrist is normally in slight extension. The digits lie with increasing flexion on towels. The ulnar side of the hand and index and middle fingers are slightly supinated. The fingernails lie in the direction of the scaphoid bone. The tendon injuries or certain fractures will disrupt this posture.
Condition of the skin
Color of the skin
Edema
Sensibility: The patient is asked to describe the way the hand feels. This includes any pain, numbness, or tingling.
Any deformity
Palpation of the hand
  Any masses or nodules
  Temperature of the skin
  Texture of the skin (i.e., dry, wet, smooth, rough, scarred)
Patient's hand dominance
Patient's family, work, and avocation history

---

be used. These testing instruments must be easy to administer and produce objective measurable and reproducible data. This gives one a basis for evaluation of the patient's progress and the treatment procedures. This type of data also lays the foundation for important research and more accurate communication among professionals (Table 217-2).

Today, because of busy clinics and limited time, it is not possible to perform a number of objective tests. Therefore, to gain the types of data needed, one must choose the most appropriate and helpful tests for the particular patient. Evaluation should be repeated on an ongoing basis throughout the patient's treatment program.

HAND THERAPY PROTOCOLS FOR SPECIFIC DIAGNOSES

The following protocols treat patients with the most typical diagnoses referred by the physician for rehabilitation in hand therapy. They are adjusted for the individual patient's needs.

Tendinitis

LATERAL EPICONDYLITIS AND MEDIAL EPICONDYLITIS

CONSERVATIVE MANAGEMENT. The patient is fitted with a lateral or medial epicondylitis strap (Fig. 217-1) and occasionally a wrist immobilizer (Fig. 217-2), which places the wrist in 0 to 15 degrees of extension. The patient is instructed to wear the brace for 4 weeks. The patient is educated in ergonomics specific to the

causative factor and instructed in pain-free tendon glide exercises, icing, friction and soft tissue massage, ultrasound (with or without cortisone, depending on severity of symptoms), possible use of iontophoresis (use of cortisone driven in by electricity), and stretching. Once pain and discomfort begin to subside, progressive strengthening is initiated. This is done gradually, beginning with isometrics and advancing to isotonic and isokinetic exercises. At this point, weaning from the wrist splint is initiated. The strap is then used only as needed.

POSTOPERATIVE MANAGEMENT. At 3 to 4 weeks, therapy is started with an initial focus on edema control. A custom elbow splint fabricated from thermoplastic material may be made if pain is significant. The splint keeps the elbow in approximately 90 degrees of flexion for lateral epicondylitis and in more neutral extension for medial epicondylitis. Active range of motion (AROM) exercises are initiated, as are scar management techniques. At 6 weeks postoperatively, passive range of motion (PROM) exercise is initiated. Strengthening begins at 8 weeks postoperatively.

TABLE 217-2 ✦ EVALUATION OF THE PATIENT: OBJECTIVE INFORMATION

Joint motion	The American Society of Hand Therapy recommends certain standards in recording joint range of motion. Both active and passive motions should be recorded with a goniometer. If a discrepancy between active and passive range of motion exists, it can indicate that the problem is with tendon extension rather than in the joint itself.
Grip strength	When grip strength is recorded, notations of the spacing of the hand should be recorded on the evaluation form.
Pinch strength	The specific pinch posture (lateral or tip to tip) should be recorded.
Sensory evaluation	Monofilament testing equipment should be used for this test.
Manual muscle testing	The Medical Research Council's 0-5 scale is used.
Functional assessment tests	These might include activities of daily skills, endurance tests, and dexterity tests. Examples of these are the Jebson Hand Function Test and the Perdue Peg Board Test. These are standardized tests.
Work assessment tests	Examples include the Valpar and BTE tests.
Edema assessment	Edema assessment can be done with circumference measurements or volunteer measurements.

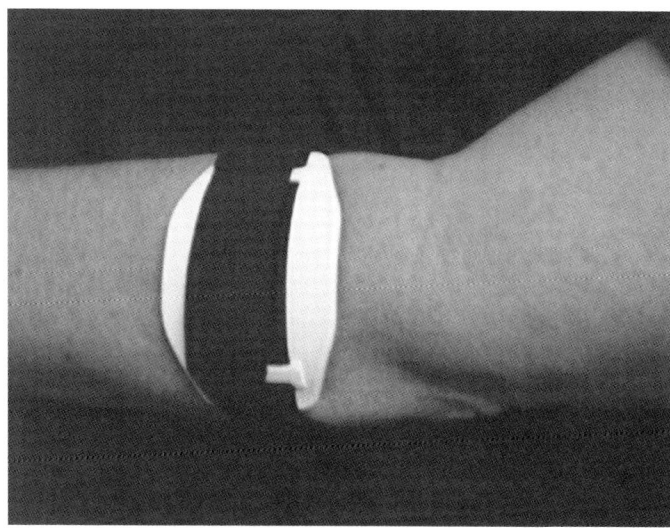

FIGURE 217-1. A forearm strap for management of lateral epicondylitis (tennis elbow).

DE QUERVAIN TENOSYNOVITIS

CONSERVATIVE MANAGEMENT. The patient is fitted with a custom thumb spica splint (Fig. 217-3); the thumb is immobilized in abduction, the interphalangeal (IP) joints are free, and the wrist is in dorsiflexion. The splint is worn for 4 to 6 weeks.

If pain has been reduced, AROM exercises and tendon gliding, soft tissue mobilization techniques, modalities (i.e., ultrasound or phonophoresis), moist heat, ice, and education of the patient are initiated. The patient is weaned from the splint as tolerated. PROM is initiated as needed, and strengthening

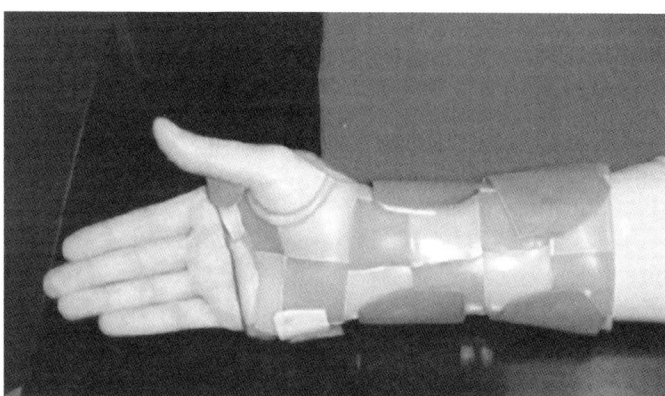

A

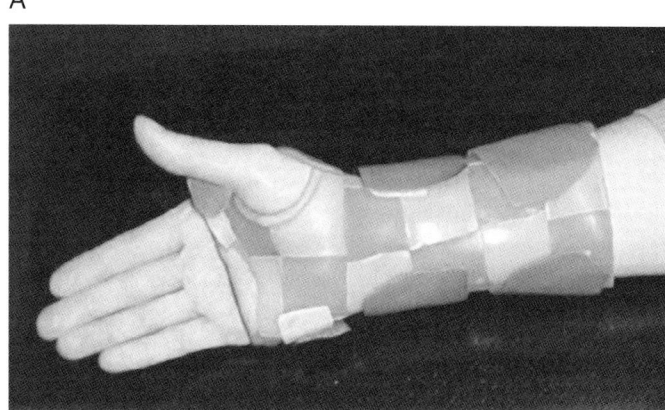

FIGURE 217-2. A and B, Standard wrist cock-up splint.

B

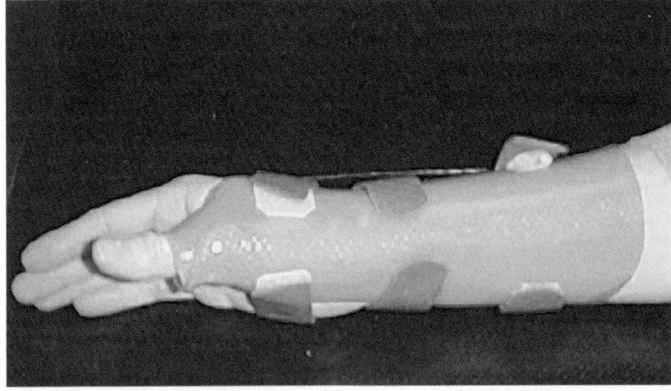

A

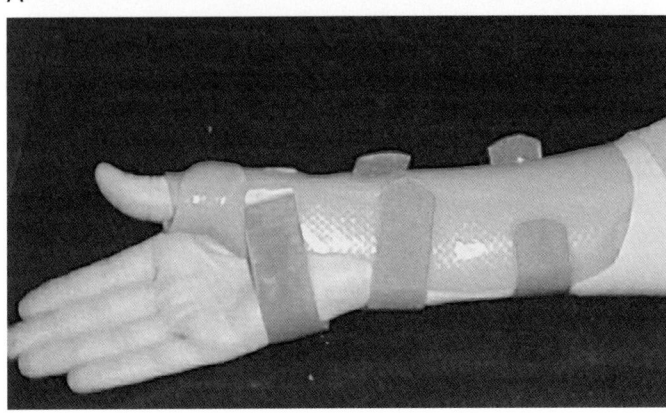

B

FIGURE 217-3. *A* and *B*, Long thumb spica splint.

follows at 6 to 8 weeks as tolerated. If pain continues at 4 to 6 weeks after full-time splint immobilization, the patient may need iontophoresis or cortisone injection.

POSTOPERATIVE MANAGEMENT. After removal of the surgical dressing, a custom thumb spica splint is fabricated (see Fig. 217-3). Edema and scar management are initiated, and AROM and tendon glide exercises are begun. Modalities as needed for pain and soft tissue mobilization are instituted. There must be a strong emphasis on education of the patient. PROM is initiated at 6 weeks postoperatively as the patient begins to be weaned from the splint, and exercises follow at 8 weeks postoperatively.

TRIGGER FINGER (STENOSING TENOSYNOVITIS)

CONSERVATIVE MANAGEMENT. The patient is fitted with a custom metacarpophalangeal (MP) joint blocking splint for 4 to 6 weeks full time (Fig. 217-4). Education of the patient is emphasized, particularly with instruction against tight and repetitive grasping; this contributes greatly to increased stress of the flexor tendon as it passes through the A1 pulley. As triggering subsides, gentle AROM and tendon glide exercises are initiated, with progression to PROM and splint weaning at 6 weeks and strengthening at 8 weeks. Should triggering and pain persist, splint immobilization may be extended, and treatment with anti-inflammatory techniques (i.e., ultrasound, phonophoresis, iontophoresis, ice massage) is initiated.

POSTOPERATIVE MANAGEMENT. After removal of the surgical dressing, the patient is fitted with a thermoplastic MP blocking splint. Education of the patient is emphasized as in conservative management; AROM and PROM exercises and edema and scar control management techniques are initiated. As pain and triggering subside, progressive strengthening is initiated.

WRIST FLEXOR-EXTENSOR TENDINITIS

CONSERVATIVE MANAGEMENT. The patient is placed in a wrist immobilization splint (see Fig. 217-2) at 0 to 15 degrees of dorsiflexion and instructed to wear the splint at night and intermittently during the day for 3 to 4 weeks. Education of the patient is important, specifically with respect to ergonomics and

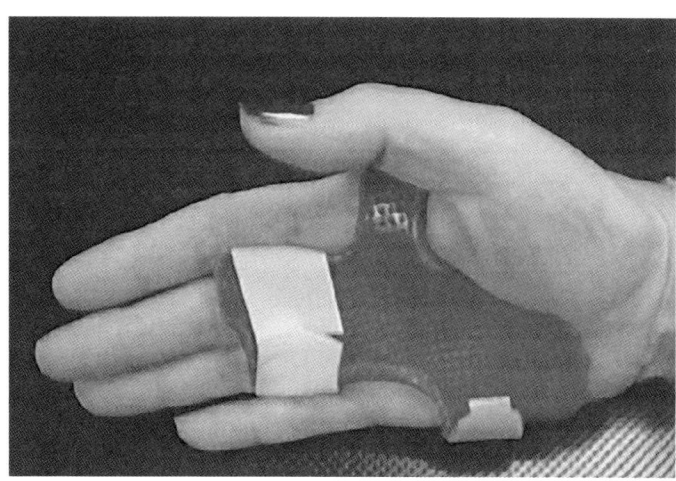

FIGURE 217-4. Night splint for trigger finger.

posture, because many of these injuries are a result of repetitive use. If the patient continues to work, the therapist may provide him or her with a semiflexible splint or possibly a rigid splint to prevent increased compensatory use, thereby preventing more proximal discomfort (particularly with individuals working on the keyboard or performing assembly work). A rigid splint is encouraged at night. Therapy starts immediately and consists of AROM and PROM exercises, tendon gliding, soft tissue mobilization, ultrasound or phonophoresis, iontophoresis (if specific tendon site is noted), moist heat, and ice. At 6 to 8 weeks, if symptoms begin to subside, weaning from the splint and progressive strengthening are initiated. If pain continues, immobilization in the splint may be extended with further reduction in overall hand use. A steroid injection may be considered. A work site evaluation may be indicated to pinpoint the cause of continued problems.

Dupuytren Contracture

POSTOPERATIVE MANAGEMENT. If the patient is seen within the first 3 to 5 days postoperatively, the surgical dressing is removed and the patient is fitted with a hand-based night extension splint. Edema control is initiated along with AROM exercises; basic wound care is taught to avoid infection. Pain and swelling will inhibit the patient from maintaining full extension, and care is taken to prevent recurrence of any flexion contractures. Once sutures are removed, whirlpool or paraffin is added; scar management, tendon gliding, and flexion splinting, if indicated, are initiated. Strengthening can begin when pain and swelling have subsided, usually around 4 to 6 weeks. Care is taken in the first few weeks postoperatively not to aggressively stretch digits into passive extension; this could compromise circulation.

Fractures

DISTAL PHALANX FRACTURES

CONSERVATIVE MANAGEMENT. The patient is frequently seen 2 weeks after initial fracture care and immobilization. A "tip" splint, immobilizing the distal interphalangeal (DIP) joint only, is fabricated; edema control and AROM exercises are initiated, provided the fracture is stable. At 3 to 4 weeks, PROM exercises are added; the patient is weaned from the splint, wearing it only at night and during high-risk activities throughout the day. By 6 to 8 weeks, resistive exercises begin, and the splint is discontinued. If a concomitant mallet deformity exists, a DIP joint immobilization splint (with the DIP joint in full extension up to 5 degrees of hyperextension) is fabricated in the same manner; however, the patient is instructed to wear this splint for 6 weeks full time while maintaining full motion at the proximal interphalangeal (PIP) joint. At 6 weeks, provided the terminal extensor tendon has tightened and is stable, AROM exercises are initiated four or five times a day; splint use continues full time between exercises. At 8 weeks, splinting can be progressed to nights only, and again, depending on stability, PROM and resistive exercises can begin with care not to overstretch the extensor tendon. Ultrasound, heat, ice, and edema control are used as indicated. If the fingertip begins to drop, full-time splinting is resumed.

POSTOPERATIVE MANAGEMENT. The patient is fitted with a DIP immobilization splint postoperatively, and gentle AROM exercises are initiated, provided the fracture is stable. Splint wear continues between exercises, and edema control and scar control (if a Kirschner pin was used) are started. At 4 weeks, PROM exercises are initiated, and splint wear can be progressed to night and high-risk activities during the day. At 8 weeks, resistive exercises are added, and the splint is discontinued.

With mallet deformities, AROM exercises, scar control, and edema control are usually started at 4 weeks postoperatively. A DIP immobilization splint is fabricated and worn between exercises and at night. This protocol continues from 6 weeks on, similar to conservative management.

PROXIMAL PHALANX FRACTURE-DISLOCATIONS

CONSERVATIVE MANAGEMENT. Therapy is initiated at 2 to 3 weeks with protective splinting, edema control, AROM exercises, ultrasound, paraffin, and ice. Provided clinical healing is present, PROM is added at 4 to 6 weeks and resistive exercises at 6 to 8 weeks. Dynamic splinting, if indicated, can be used at 6 weeks.

POSTOPERATIVE MANAGEMENT. On removal of the surgical dressing (i.e., after open reduction and internal fixation), the patient is placed in a hand-based protective thermoplastic splint. AROM exercises are initiated, as are edema and scar control techniques. At 6 weeks postoperatively, provided the fracture is healing, PROM is started and splinting is progressed to night-only and high-risk activities during the day. A dynamic PIP extension-flexion splint is considered if PIP or DIP joint contractures are present. At 8 weeks, resistive exercises proceed, and the splint is discontinued.

METACARPAL FRACTURES

CONSERVATIVE MANAGEMENT. The patient is placed in a clam-digger type splint, with MP joints flexed at 60 to 70 degrees and IP joints neutral. Provided good architectural integrity and stability are present, edema control and AROM exercises are initiated at 3 to 4 weeks after injury. PROM is initiated at 6 weeks and resistive exercises at 8 weeks. The splint is removed at 6 weeks except for high-risk activities, and it is discontinued by 8 weeks.

POSTOPERATIVE MANAGEMENT. Soon after surgery (i.e., after open reduction and internal fixation or closed reduction, depending on fracture stability), edema control, scar management, and AROM exercises are initiated. The patient is placed in either a clam-digger style splint or a rigid wrist splint, depending on the location of the fracture (i.e., proximal shaft or base or distal shaft). At 6 weeks, PROM as well as dynamic splinting is initiated to correct any joint capsule or extrinsic extensor tightness. The resting splint is usually discontinued at this point, except with high-risk activities. At 8 weeks postoperatively, resistive exercises are added.

COLLES FRACTURE

POSTOPERATIVE MANAGEMENT. Because 85% of these fractures generally require some form of reduction, protocol must vary according to the type of fracture (extra-articular or intra-articular) and the type of fracture management performed (closed versus open reduction, pins, plates, external fixation). The patient may be seen by the therapist anywhere from 1 day to 6 weeks after injury or postoperatively. If the fracture pattern and treatment allow, a rigid wrist splint is fabricated for full-time wear except during exercise (see Fig. 217-2). AROM exercises and edema and scar control techniques are initiated. The initial focus is on gaining range in all planes of wrist and forearm movement; however, the primary focus is on wrist extension and supination. At 6 weeks, PROM as well as dynamic splinting, if indicated, is initiated to prevent contracture. Progressive resistive exercises are added at 8 weeks.

Nerve Compression Injuries

CARPAL TUNNEL SYNDROME, RADIAL TUNNEL SYNDROME, CUBITAL TUNNEL SYNDROME

CONSERVATIVE MANAGEMENT. Because many nerve entrapment problems are associated with activities, job analysis is undertaken on referral if the patient is employed; ergonomic education is initiated with emphasis on job modification, workstation design, posture, and symptom management if these are thought to be factors contributing to nerve compression symptoms. For carpal tunnel and radial tunnel syndromes, the patient is given a rigid wrist splint (see Fig. 217-2) for use at night and with repetitive or heavy activities during the day. A semiflexible splint is issued for use on the keyboard or with assembly-type jobs; rigid immobilization tends to result in more proximal complications from compensatory actions. With cubital tunnel syndrome, a "heelbow" pad is issued for use during the day and night both to prevent elbow flexion and to disperse pressure off the ulnar nerve. With extreme cases, a rigid elbow extension splint is considered. AROM, tendon, and neural glide exercises as well as PROM stretch are initiated. Myofascial and soft tissue mobilization techniques are incorporated during therapy, as is heat and cold. Phonophoresis or iontophoresis is considered for treatment of nerve inflammation. As pain and paresthesias begin to subside, progressive midrange strengthening is initiated as needed. A strong home program is encouraged.

POSTOPERATIVE MANAGEMENT. After removal of the surgical dressing, scar and edema control techniques and AROM exercises are initiated. A rigid splint is provided for use between exercises (i.e., mainly for postoperative carpal tunnel release). Ultrasound can be used as well as heat or cold as needed. PROM is added at 6 weeks and progressive resistive activities at 8 weeks. Splinting is discontinued by 8 weeks. As in conservative management, a job analysis is performed for the employed patient, with the same considerations and follow-up.

Ganglion Cyst

POSTOPERATIVE MANAGEMENT. Because most ganglions do not respond to conservative management, protocol is given for postoperative ganglionectomy. The patient is typically seen 2 to 3 weeks postoperatively when edema control, scar control, and AROM exercises are initiated. The patient is fitted with a wrist splint to wear between exercises. At 4 weeks postoperatively, PROM is initiated, and the splinting is progressed to an "as needed" basis. At 8 weeks postoperatively, progressive resistive exercises are added.

Complex Regional Pain Syndromes (Reflex Sympathetic Dystrophy)

CONSERVATIVE MANAGEMENT. On referral to hand therapy, active education is initiated so patients understand this diagnosis and become active, educated participants in their treatment. When the patient is seen within the first 3 months of onset, therapy proves most beneficial. Treatment consists of range-of-motion exercises (active, active assist, and very gentle stretch, because aggressive stretch can further exacerbate the disease), transcutaneous electrical nerve stimulation, edema control, heat, splinting (if needed), tactile desensitization, and stress-loading activities. Patients are encouraged to use the extremity with functional tasks. A strong home program is initiated early in the treatment process.

Arthritis

RHEUMATOID ARTHRITIS

CONSERVATIVE MANAGEMENT. Early in the disease, the main underlying problem is synovitis as well as inflammation of the joint tissue and tendon sheaths. As the disease progresses, one sees damage to the joint structure and boutonnière and swan-neck deformities. When surgery is not yet a consideration, hand therapeutic interventions are used. The patients are initially seen for a baseline evaluation. Because the disease varies greatly from one patient to another, this evaluation is important so realistic goals can be set. Depending on whether the patient is in the acute, subacute, or chronic stage, the intensity of therapy varies, but the goals are the same. Therapy includes education about joint protection techniques, specifically in how activities of daily living are performed. Range-of-motion exercises are encouraged as appropriate to maintain muscle strength and mobility and to correct alignment of the fingers. Various modalities are

incorporated for pain and inflammation. Splinting may be used to rest the joints or to prevent or correct deformity (Figs. 217-5 and 217-6). A complete review of adaptive aids is also carried out to encourage independent function and to prevent further stress to the joints.

POSTOPERATIVE MANAGEMENT. The patients most commonly seen have had joint synovectomies, MP joint arthroplasties, correction of boutonnière and swanneck deformities, or surgery for other tendon disabilities (contracture, displacement, rupture). Because each of these varies in intensity and deformity, therapy protocols vary from one postoperative diagnosis to another; however, the principal goals of therapy remain the same. The early focus is on edema control, scar management, dynamic (as for postoperative arthroplasty patients) or static splinting, range-of-motion exercises, modalities for pain control, low-grade strengthening, and return to normal function. Again, emphasis is placed on joint protection principles, and the use of adaptive aids is encouraged, when indicated, to allow independent function while preventing mechanical stress to the joints.

OSTEOARTHRITIS

CONSERVATIVE MANAGEMENT. Osteoarthritis is far more common than rheumatoid arthritis but also varies greatly in intensity, depending on the classification (i.e., degenerative, primary generalized, or erosive). With osteoarthritis of the hand, the patients most commonly referred are those complaining of pain, loss of dexterity and strength, and stiffness and edema largely affecting the thumb carpometacarpal or the DIP joints. In therapy, a baseline evaluation is made, and realistic goals are set. The patient is introduced to various heat modalities (e.g., paraffin, moist heat packs, fluidotherapy, whirlpool) for pain control and increase in range of motion. The patient is instructed in AROM exercises, retrograde massage, joint protection techniques, and adaptive aid training. A splint may be provided to relieve stress on the affected joint or to prevent deformity. A protected strength program may be included if appropriate. Patients are prescribed a strong home program and fully educated in their disease so they can appropriately take an active role in their own care.

POSTOPERATIVE MANAGEMENT. The patients most commonly seen have undergone fusions (IP joints, wrist, thumb), carpometacarpal joint revisions, and ligament reconstruction. Goals of therapy are similar to those for rheumatoid disease. With fusions of any kind, immobilization is maintained until radiographic healing is noted. Active motion of unaffected joints is maintained early in the postoperative phase to prevent stiffness and to assist with edema control. After most

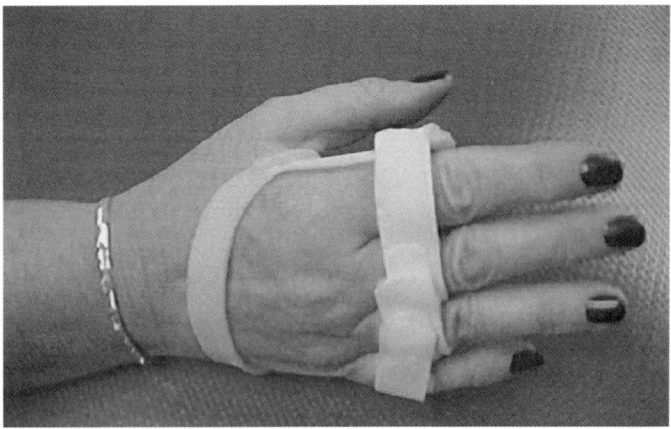

A

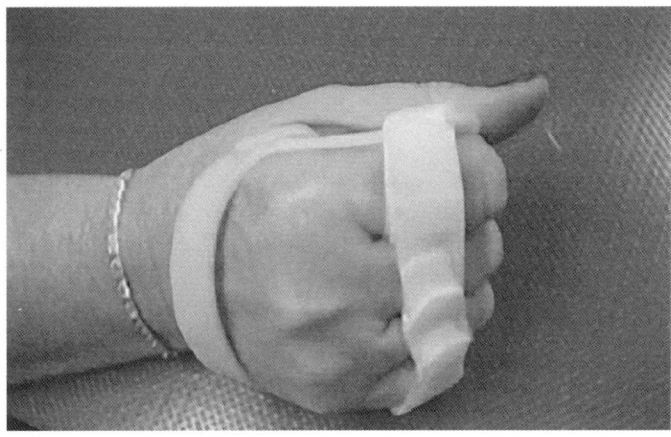

B

FIGURE 217-5. *A* and *B*, Splint to prevent ulnar drift in rheumatoid arthritis.

joint revisions or reconstructions, the postoperative joint is immobilized for 2 to 4 weeks, at which point AROM, edema control, scar management, and protective splinting are initiated. Between 6 and 8 weeks, PROM exercises are initiated, and dynamic splinting or taping may be used. Progressive resistive activities are also initiated at this time to return the patient to independent function. As in conservative management, the patient is educated in joint protection techniques, introduced to adaptive aids as needed, and given a strong home program.

Congenital Deformities

CONGENITAL LIMB DEFICIENCY

CONSERVATIVE MANAGEMENT. Provided there are no medical complications, the patient is fitted with a passive hand prosthesis as early as 3 months of age by a trained therapist. The child's parents are educated in use of the prosthesis and referred for counseling, if needed, to assist with acceptance of their child's disability. At 6 months of age, depending on the child's gross motor skills with passive use of a prosthesis, a functional hand prosthesis is considered. Because of a child's development in gross palmar prehension and hand dominance, one should not wait past 8 months of age to introduce the functional prosthesis.

CONGENITAL ADDUCTION OF THUMB (THUMB-IN-PALM)

CONSERVATIVE MANAGEMENT. The child is seen as early as possible for therapeutic intervention. The patient is fitted with a static splint worn proximal to the wrist to maintain thumb in abduction. The splint is worn nearly full time until the deformity is corrected.

CAMPTODACTYLY

CONSERVATIVE MANAGEMENT. If therapy is initiated early, before any fixed contracture, the patient is fitted with a dynamic PIP extension splint. On regaining full extension, the patient is progressed to a static night extension splint for purposes of maintaining PIP extension.

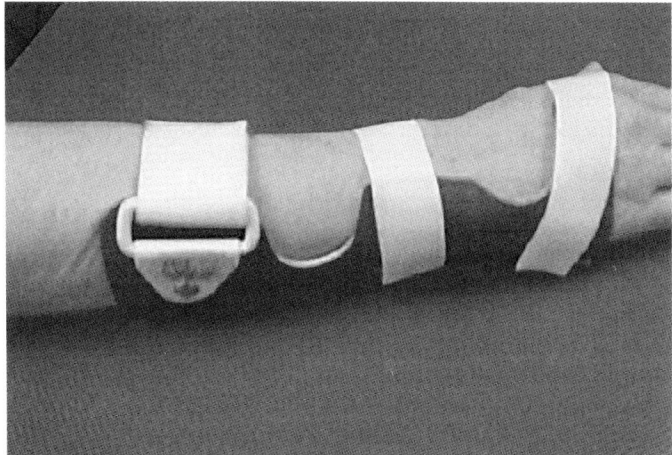

A

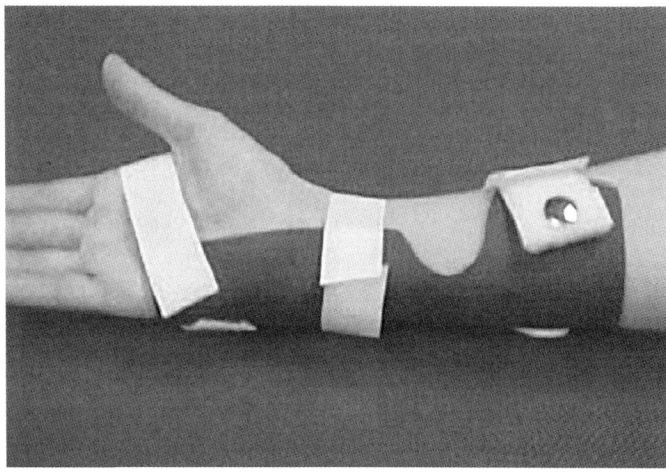

B

FIGURE 217-6. *A* and *B,* Splints for rheuma-toid arthritis that prevent radialization of the hand.

POSTOPERATIVE MANAGEMENT. At 4 weeks postoperatively, edema and scar control techniques and AROM exercises (for IP joints only) are initiated. A static splint is fabricated to place MP joints in 30 to 40 degrees of flexion (MP blocking splint). At 6 weeks postoperatively, AROM is initiated for MP joint extension, and passive flexion is begun if needed. Progressive resistive exercises are initiated at 8 weeks, and the patient is weaned from the splint.

RADIAL CLUBHAND

CONSERVATIVE MANAGEMENT. The child is generally seen shortly after birth, provided he or she has no other medical considerations. Serial casting or splinting is initiated to gently stretch soft tissue on the radial aspect of the forearm. This is maintained until further consideration is given to surgical intervention (i.e., centralization of the hand and carpus on the distal ulna or possible pollicization of the index for an absent or hypoplastic thumb).

Burns

CONSERVATIVE MANAGEMENT. On referral, the patient may be placed in a whirlpool at 98°F for cleaning and débridement of the wound. This will also help loosen eschar and adherent dressings. Sterile gauze is used to remove loose eschar. Bleeding is avoided. The wound is then covered with protective dressing, most commonly silver sulfadiazine, silver nitrate, or bacitracin. The patient is educated in dressing changes. Intensity of the wound dictates the frequency of dressing changes. Sterile techniques are used at all times. Gauze is loosely wrapped to allow as much digital range of motion as possible within restrictions of the burn. AROM exercises are encouraged. Edema is addressed immediately by elevation and active exercise. An antideformity splint is fabricated to place the wrist in neutral (if dorsal) or 30 degrees of extension (if volar). The MP joints are flexed 60 to 90 degrees, and the IP joints should be extended. The thumb is positioned in abduction and opposition. As the burn heals, scar management is initiated (i.e., lubrication, silicone gel pads, ultrasound, massage, and Jobst compression garments). For pediatric patients with palmar or circumferential burns, volar hand splints are fabricated with fingers in abduction and extension. Activities of daily living are encouraged as soon as the patient is able.

POSTOPERATIVE MANAGEMENT. The patient is generally seen 5 to 7 days after skin grafting. Most typically, the patient has been fitted with a splint in the burned hand position (wrist extension, MP flexion, IP extension) in the operating room to prevent loss of graft. Therapeutic intervention includes appropriate wound management with daily dressing changes. The skin graft site is generally not soaked because maintenance of the graft is most significant. Edema control and AROM exercises are initiated. Controlled passive motion devices may be used to restore range of motion. As the graft becomes more adherent, scar control techniques are carried out as in conservative management, and resistive exercises and activities of daily living are encouraged.

Tendon Injuries

FLEXOR TENDON REPAIR

Zones I, II, and III

POSTOPERATIVE MANAGEMENT. The patient is generally seen 3 to 4 days postoperatively, when a dorsal blocking splint is fabricated with the MP joints in 45 to 60 degrees of flexion, the wrist in 20 to 30 degrees of flexion, and the IP joints extended. The patient may follow either the Duran or Kleinert protocol. The finger is placed in rubber band flexion and allowed active extension (until the finger reaches the hood of a dorsal splint); the finger is then pulled into flexion by rubber band tension. This is done hourly. This protocol is followed to maintain full passive range of the affected digit (with special care to avoid PIP flexion contractures) and full active and passive flexion of the other digits. Edema control techniques are addressed, and when sutures are removed, scar control is incorporated. At 3 to 4 weeks after surgery, the rubber band tension is removed and the patient initiates AROM within limits of a dorsal blocking splint. At 5 weeks, the wrist is brought to neutral in the splint, and wrist tenodesis exercises can begin. Six weeks after surgery, full active extension is permitted and passive extension can be initiated. Functional electrical stimulation may be used if needed to increase tendon excursion. At 8 weeks, progressive strengthening is added, and by 10 to 12 weeks, the patient is restriction free.

Zones IV and V

With injuries in zones IV and V, the initial protocol is the same within the dorsal blocking splint; however, because of the location, controlled digital motion is not necessary except to limit finger extension to the hood of the dorsal blocking splint. At 3 to 4 weeks postoperatively, AROM of all digits is allowed within splint limits. At 5 weeks, the splint can be removed for AROM of the fingers and wrist. At 6 weeks, the splint is removed, and the protocol follows that outlined in the preceding paragraph.

EXTENSOR TENDON REPAIR

POSTOPERATIVE MANAGEMENT

Zone I (mallet deformity). The patient is seen after surgery and placed in a tip splint (Fig. 217-7) with the DIP joint in full extension to 5 degrees of hyperextension for 6 weeks. AROM exercises are initiated at that point with splint use between exercises, with progressive weaning from the splint by 8 weeks. Edema is addressed as indicated. The splint is resumed if lag recurs.

Zones II and III (extensor hood). The injured finger is maintained in a static splint that does not include the MP joint for 6 weeks, then progressed as outlined in the preceding paragraph.

Zones IV, V, and VI. Immediate static splinting occurs postoperatively with the wrist in 30 degrees of dorsiflexion, MP joints in 30 to 40 degrees of flexion, and IP joints in full extension. During the third and fourth week, gentle AROM out of the splint in protected positions is performed. The splint is shortened at 4 weeks to a more proximal level to allow flexion and extension of PIP and DIP joints. At 5 weeks, the splint is shortened to the level of the distal palmar crease to allow active flexion and extension of the MP joint as well. Active wrist motion is begun. At 6 weeks, splinting is discontinued. Dynamic extension splinting is considered if lag is noted. At 7 weeks, passive flexion of wrist and fingers is initiated, and at 8 weeks, progressive strengthening exercises are instituted. The patient may resume full activity at week 12.

Amputations

POSTOPERATIVE MANAGEMENT (SINGLE-DIGIT INJURIES, ABOVE OR BELOW ELBOW). The patient is seen 5 to 14 days postoperatively. Wound care is addressed. A protective cap splint is fabricated, and AROM exercises are initiated. Edema control is carried out by positioning and compression wraps. One can proceed with gentle passive exercises to the patient's tolerance. Transcutaneous electrical nerve stimulation or other electrical modalities can be used for pain control, and desensitization techniques are initiated. Scar gel pads can be used once sutures are removed. As pain and swelling permit, the patient is progressed to strengthening exercises. Functional use of the

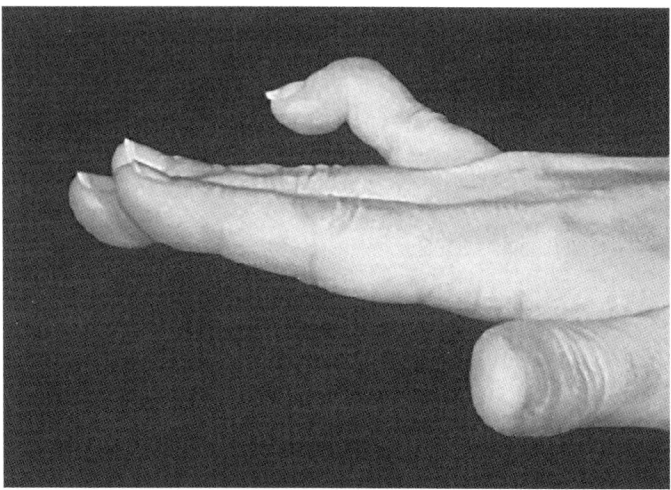

A

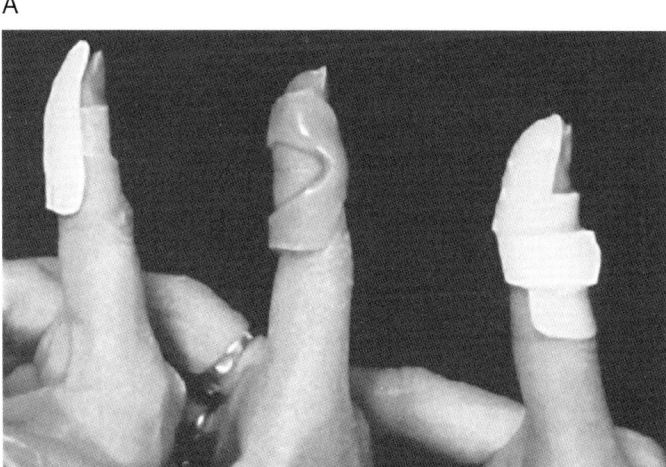

FIGURE 217-7. *A* and *B,* Mallet finger splints.   B

extremity is strongly encouraged. Because prostheses are commonly a consideration for both functional and cosmetic purposes, appropriate referrals are given to a prosthetic specialist for consultation.

Tendon Transfers

POSTOPERATIVE MANAGEMENT. The patient is typically seen 3 to 4 weeks postoperatively; AROM exercises are initiated, as are edema control and scar control techniques. Exercises are specific to the transfer performed. A protective splint is fabricated for use, generally for an additional 2 to 4 weeks, to maintain the desired position and to prevent any possible lags or undue stress on the new transfer. Electromyographic biofeedback or functional electrical stimulation may also be initiated at this time as needed. At 6 weeks postoperatively, the patient can proceed with PROM exercises, and if needed, dynamic splinting may be considered to resolve any joint or tendon tightness. At 6

to 8 weeks, the protective splint is phased out; progressive resistive exercises are initiated with the goal of returning the patient to independent functional activity.

HAND SPLINTING

Splinting of the hand can be an integral part of the final results after trauma or elective surgery.[2] Descriptions of hand splints are recorded as early as the mid-1600s. Splints must be carefully fitted, with specific goals in mind, and must be changed to meet the changing needs of the healing tissues of the hand. Most hand therapists are specifically trained to design and fit intricate hand splints, but the surgeon must understand the purposes behind good splinting (Table 217-3). Splints are also classified by type and indications (Table 217-4).

Specific principles guide the design of various splints (Table 217-5). Prefabricated splints are available in

TABLE 217-3 ✦ PURPOSES BEHIND GOOD SPLINTING

Protection
Rest
Decrease inflammation and pain
Prevent undesired motions or angles
Substitute for loss of muscle function
Resolve tendon tightness
Resolve fixed joint contractures
Increase or maintain active and passive motion

various sizes, designs, and materials. These splints can be used to save time and costs as long as the splint fits the patient properly and the desired goal is achieved (Table 217-6). When any type of splint is ordered, it is the surgeon's responsibility to provide the hand therapist with necessary information, including date of surgery or injury, diagnosis, desired function of splint or name of splint, and precautions, if any.

TABLE 217-4 ✦ SPLINT CLASSIFICATIONS

Static	A static splint prevents motion and is used to minimize or stabilize in one specific position (see Fig. 217-2).
Serial static	A serial static splint is a rigid device that maintains the hand in one position but is changed frequently to provide slow, progressive mobilization.
Dynamic	A dynamic splint (Fig. 217-8) achieves its effect by movement and force. It is a form of manipulation. In dynamic splinting, various springs, rubber bands, and coils are used to provide a constant gentle force for prolonged periods to immobilize tissue.

Indications for Each Type of Splint

Static	The static splint is indicated during the immobilization phase to allow healing, to decrease inflammation, and to provide protection. The splint can be removed for short, supervised exercise.
Serial static	A serial static splint may be used early as long as healing is not compromised. The force applied is gentle and most effective in mobilization of long-standing mature scar because prolonged positioning allows tissue to "grow" to new length. It may be initiated in the presence of edema and removed for periods of exercise.
Dynamic	A dynamic splint is most effective in the proliferation stage of scar formation when clinical response to stretch can be appreciated. The force must be of a comfortable level to allow wear for long periods.

TABLE 217-5 ✦ SPECIFIC PRINCIPLES THAT GUIDE SPLINT DESIGN

Anatomic Considerations

Maintain the transverse and longitudinal arches of the hand
Use skin creases as landmarks (i.e., digital, distal palmar crease, thenar, and wrist)
Accommodate bone prominence (i.e., radial and ulnar styloid)
Avoid compression of superficial nerves
Consider ligamentous structures
Skin and soft tissue integrity

Mechanical Principles

Use optimum rotational force of 90-degree line of pull from bone being mobilized
Increase the area of force application
Increase the mechanical advantage (first-class lever system)
Tension applied to rubber band traction should be no greater than 4 to 5 N

Precautions

Pressure areas
Poorly fitting splint
Thin skin, such as in rheumatoid arthritis
Insensitive hand
Vascular insufficiency
Vascular compromise
Partial level of understanding or cooperation level

Splint Fabrication

Custom-designed splints include those constructed of materials including
  Low-temperature plastics
  High-temperature plastics
  Plaster or fiberglass
  Wire with padding
  Component parts (Velcro, nylon cord, rubber bands, cuffs)

EDUCATION

One of the most important functions of a hand therapist is to educate the patient. Each patient is educated about the specific aspects, home care, and exercises necessary for optimum functional return after injury or surgery. In addition, education makes up a major portion of the treatment by hand therapists of patients with arthritis and repetitive stress injuries.

Joint protection education for persons with arthritis is vital to help minimize hand deformities and to lessen pain so the hands can be used more functionally and kept more mobile. Joint protection education, which usually takes three or four sessions with a patient, can be combined with night support splint

TABLE 217-6 ✦ THE USE OF PREFABRICATED SPLINTS

Commonly used prefabricated splints include
    Bunnell safety pin: three-point pressure splints, Joint-Jack
    Capner, LMB, or spring splint (extension assist splints) (Fig. 217-9)
    Futura wrist splint
    Stack splint (for mallet finger or for DIP fractures)
The principles that guide splint fabrication include
    Proper fit
    Freedom of uninvolved joints
    Comfort
    Appearance
    Education of the patient

fabrication. The trained hand therapist can assist the surgeon in educating the patient about his or her specific form of arthritis and the possible long-term effects of continuing certain joint-stressful activities. Different ways of holding implements, simple adaptive devices, education in work tasks, and task simplification techniques help reduce deforming forces on arthritic joints. Simple adaptations, such as wall-mounted jar openers, pen grips, telephone headsets, and large-handled cooking and gardening implements, can reduce ulnar deviation forces in rheumatoid arthritis and help prevent these deformities before they begin. Purchasing lighter dinner plates, using rollerball pens, and learning different ways of holding a book reduce carpometacarpal joint stresses

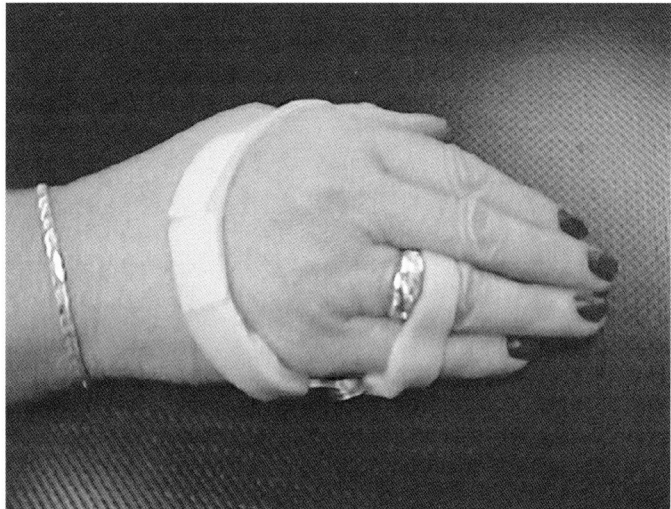

A

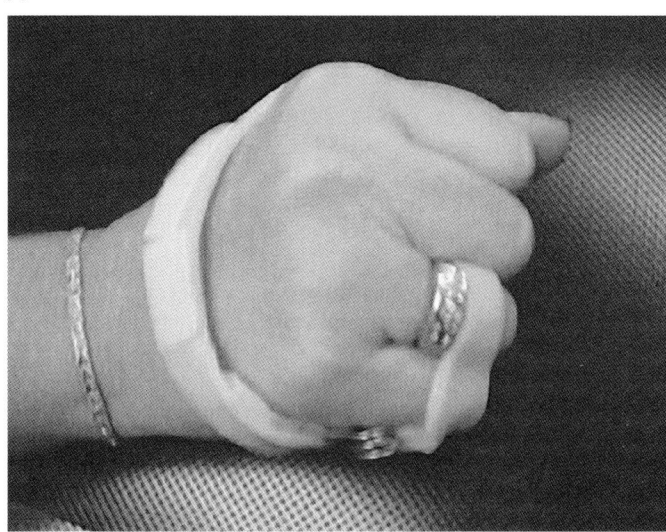

B

FIGURE 217-8. *A* and *B,* Dynamic splint for ulnar nerve palsy to prevent clawing of the fingers.

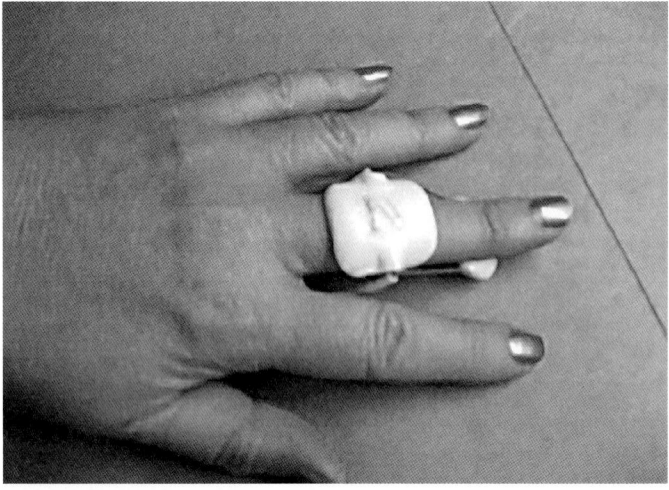

A

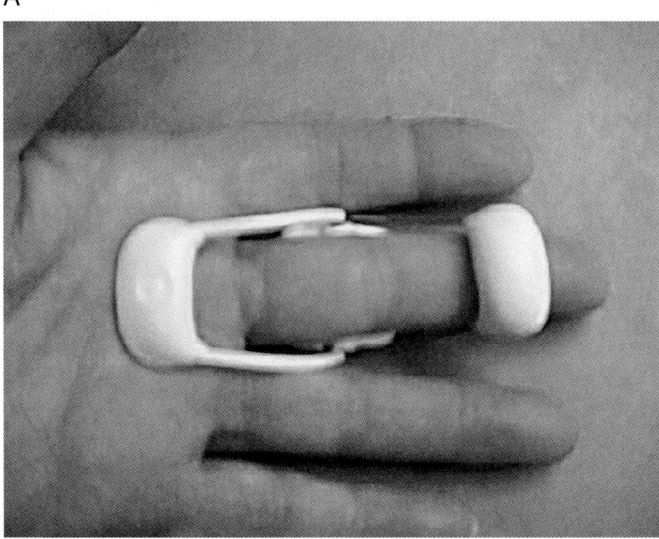

B

FIGURE 217-9. *A* and *B*, Spring-type PIP extension splint (reverse knuckle-bender).

in osteoarthritis and keep the thumbs less painful and more functional for a longer time. Because each patient is different, and an analysis of the stresses of each hand is vital to suggest ways to reduce these harmful joint stresses, it is important that a patient be referred for joint protection education when the diagnosis is first made. This is especially helpful if the patient cannot be stabilized with a medical regimen.

Repetitive stress disorders cannot heal unless the person changes what he or she is doing to cause the symptoms. An analysis of posture, positioning at the computer and arrangement of the computer components, workflow, and other workday stresses is necessary to pinpoint the cause of symptoms for suggestion of remediation. Education in postural exercises to relieve pressure on nerves, proper muscle stretches, taking breaks, and use of ergonomic adaptations

(such as split keyboards, ergonomic mice or trackballs, and telephone headsets) is a necessary component. Patients are given tips on proper exercises to begin at their gym or home to strengthen back and shoulder girdle muscles, and nutrition and rest are emphasized. Relaxation techniques, stress reduction, and deep breathing exercises may be included. The patient suffering from activity-related discomfort will not become or stay healthy unless work style changes are made.

THERAPEUTIC USE OF MODALITIES

Because many of the more common hand injury symptoms of edema, pain, and stiffness respond well to the use of modalities, modalities are often used to increase the effectiveness of the therapy regimen. In addition, a therapist may request that a home modality unit be prescribed to further speed recovery.

The modalities most frequently employed are heat, cold, ultrasound, electricity, and continuous passive motion. There are different ways to use these modalities to produce different effects on tissue. Because state licensure laws, availability of modalities, and skill levels of therapists differ from clinic to clinic, good communication between physician and therapist is essential to establish safe and effective treatment protocols.

Therapeutic Use of Heat

Heat is the most frequently employed modality in hand therapy. The main goals in the use of heat are to reduce muscle spasm and pain, to increase the extensibility of collagen scar tissue to allow more effective stretch, to increase blood flow to the area, and to reduce pain.

After injuries such as fractures that produce guarding spasms of the muscles, heat can be used to reduce ischemic pain by increasing blood flow and to change the firing rate of the muscle spindle to decrease tonic contraction. Heat is also especially effective in increasing the extensibility of collagen scar tissue to relieve joint stiffness and to increase range of motion if it is followed immediately by stretch and range-of-motion exercises or activity. Heat in itself has no lasting effect on range of motion if it is used alone.

In the clinic, three different methods are used to transfer heat into tissue: conduction, such as paraffin and hot packs, which transfer heat between two mediums; convection through a moving medium, such as fluidotherapy; and conversion, such as ultrasound, which transmits nonthermal energy (e.g., ultrasound energy) to deeper tissue, where it is converted to heat energy.

Training and experience are needed by the therapist to employ the proper surface or deep heating methods for each tissue effect and condition. For most patients, skin and sensation must be intact and edema only a minor problem.

Paraffin is commonly used with stiff hands for heating before stretch and mobilization. Elastic wraps such as Coban to stretch fingers into flexion are effective in enhancing composite flexion with use of paraffin. Paraffin is also effective as a modality to reduce the pain of arthritis and to reduce intrinsic muscle spasms. After trials and training in the clinic, home paraffin units are often recommended for regular use. Many store chains are now offering these units for around $70 for cosmetic hand treatments, and wax can be reused in home units for several months.

Well-padded hot packs are also commonly used to slowly heat forearm and hand tissues. They are especially effective in gaining range of motion after distal radius fractures; the weight of the hot pack can be used to encourage gentle supination or wrist extension while decreasing muscle spasm. Fluidotherapy, which is a modality employing whirling dry cornhusk particles, can be used both to desensitize a hypersensitive area and to introduce heat to it.

Deeper levels of heat can be obtained through certain settings of ultrasound. This use of heat is discussed in the section on ultrasound.

Therapeutic Use of Cold

The hand therapist frequently employs cold, or cryotherapy, to affect tissue. Cold causes vasoconstriction of the blood vessels and a decrease in skin temperature, which decreases the histologic evidence of inflammation in an injured area. At 10°C to 15°C, it also produces analgesia and pain relief. In persons with musculoskeletal pain, a method introduced by Travell[3] combines stretch with Fluori-Methane spray to gain range of motion with less pain. Edema is shown to be reduced best by a combination of cold and compression. However, extreme cold actually increases edema and decreases the extensibility of collagen scar.

Methods of cryotherapy employed by the hand therapist include cold packs or padded ice packs, ice massage, immersion in cold water, and Fluori-Methane evaporative spray. There are also commercially available cryotherapy units for use in the clinic. As with heat, the therapist must be experienced in the safe and effective use of cold to gain desired tissue changes.

Cold packs remain pliable, are not completely frozen, and lie easily in a conforming manner about bony structures such as the elbow and wrist. Commercial gel-filled packs can be purchased at most drug stores or made by use of zip-lock style bags filled with a mixture of 1 cup isopropyl alcohol and 3 cups water. The skin is covered with layers of moist paper towels before application of approximately 10 to 15 minutes on the hand or elbow.

Ice massage is used to treat small areas, such as for lateral epicondylitis. Small paper cups of water are frozen, the rim is torn off to expose the top half-inch of ice, and the ice is rubbed in a circular fashion over the affected area for 3 to 6 minutes. This is easily instructed for home. Cryotherapy should be avoided in persons with replants or revascularizations, healing wounds, poor sensation, Raynaud phenomenon, or diabetes with peripheral vascular disease and in those persons who react to cold with a histamine reaction such as red wheals.

Therapeutic Use of Ultrasound

Because soft tissues are composed of more than 70% water, they are an effective transmitter of sound. Ultrasound is most commonly used in the clinic to deep heat tissues to increase extensibility, to reduce inflammation, and to enhance tissue healing.

Therapeutic ultrasound is high-frequency acoustic energy generated by the application of alternating current across a piezoelectric crystal. A coupling agent, such as water-soluble gel, is applied to the skin; a treatment of ultrasound typically lasts 5 to 6 minutes for the hand and slightly longer for the arm or shoulder area, depending on the size of the area. A 1.0 MHz applicator head is commonly used for treatment of deeper tissues up to 5 cm; a 3.0 MHz applicator head is used for more shallow treatments, such as on the hand, which is bony.

Therapists are able to select from an array of applicator heads and machine settings, which vary time of treatment, area of treatment, intensity of treatment, and ultrasound frequency. Because tissue damage can result from improper use of ultrasound, therapists must understand precautions and proper technique. Ultrasound may be avoided during the acute inflammatory phase of healing, with bleeding disorders, in the early stages after tendon repairs, and over areas of impaired circulation or malignant disease. The use of ultrasound on the hand of a pregnant woman or the hand of a person with a pacemaker is generally considered safe because the treatment is focused just on the hand; however, it should never be used if there is a question of safety.

As a general rule, continuous wave ultrasound is selected for its thermal effect, and pulsed wave is selected more for enhancement of tissue healing. Ultrasound in continuous wave mode can produce deep heat before stretch to regain lost range of motion and is especially effective with stiffness after crush and fracture injuries and other scarring problems. Pulsed ultrasound is presently being used with positive results in pain reduction and edema resolution during the first few days after injury. The use of ultrasound to introduce anti-inflammatory medications through the skin, a technique referred to as ultrasound with phonophoresis, is common in the treatment of tendinitis and other conditions. Its level of effectiveness for the purpose of introducing medicine is still under study.

Therapeutic Use of Electricity

Trial uses of electricity for treatment of paralyzed limbs began experimentally in the mid-1700s, and it has been regularly used therapeutically for the past century. Current uses are facilitation of muscle contraction, pain relief, and ion induction.

Neuromuscular electrical stimulation units use pulsating alternating currents to stimulate innervated muscle tissue. These units are valuable in helping to regain range of motion by facilitating contraction of weakened muscles. Experienced therapists use this modality at approximately 2 weeks after tenolysis and approximately 6 weeks after tendon repair to assist in tendon gliding. It is used as a precursor to voluntary movement of affected weak muscle groups. Home units are easy to instruct for use by the patient on a daily basis.

Transcutaneous electrical nerve stimulation is used commonly for pain relief, and home units can provide hours of relief per day. High-voltage galvanic stimulation is used for both acute and chronic pain, for reduction of both acute and chronic edema, and for promotion of wound healing with its ability both to decrease growth of microorganisms and to increase the migration of epithelial cells. High-voltage galvanic stimulation is not used in patients with heart dysrhythmias or in attempts to stimulate denervated muscle. Home units for rental are available.

Iontophoresis is used to treat inflammatory conditions or scar by induction of topically applied ions into a small area with a low-voltage direct galvanic current. Commonly applied agents include dexamethasone for inflammatory conditions, such as lateral epicondylitis or de Quervain tenosynovitis; saline for scars, such as fully healed postsurgical Dupuytren release and laceration scars; salicylates for arthritis; and lidocaine for analgesia. Iontophoresis is contraindicated for persons with allergies to the medication being introduced, for persons with uncontrolled diabetes, around exposed metal pins or implants, and before 6 weeks after surgery. It usually causes localized redness for up to 1 hour; with steroid medication, it may cause permanent lightening of the skin under the treatment pad.

REFERENCES

1. Brand PW: Clinical Mechanics of the Hand. St. Louis, CV Mosby, 1985.
2. Cannon NM, Foltz RW: The Manual of Hand Splinting. New York, Churchill Livingstone, 1985.
3. Travell J, Simons D: Myofascial Pain and Dysfunction. Baltimore, Williams & Wilkins, 1983.

Additional Reading

Cannon N: Diagnosis and Treatment Manual for Physicians and Therapists, 3rd ed. Indianapolis, The Hand Center of Indiana, 1991.
Chai S, Dimick MP, Kasch MC: A role delineation study. J Hand Ther 1987;1(1).
Clark C, Wilgis S, Aiello G, et al: Hand Rehabilitation. New York, Churchill Livingstone, 1993.
Flatt A: Care of the Arthritic Hand, 4th ed. St. Louis, CV Mosby, 1983.
Flatt A: The Care of Congenital Hand Anomalies, 2nd ed. St. Louis, Quality Medical Publishing, 1994.
Hunter J, Schneider L, Mackin E, Callahan P: Rehabilitation of the Hand, 3rd ed. St. Louis, CV Mosby, 1990.
Malone C: Hand and Wrist Injuries and Treatment. Baltimore, Williams & Wilkins, 1989.
Puddicombe J, Nardone W: Rehabilitation of the burned hand. Hand Clin 1990;6:281-292.
Putz-Anderson C: Cumulative Trauma Disorders: A Manual for Musculoskeletal Diseases of the Upper Limbs. London, Taylor & Francis, 1988.
Wynn Parry CB: Rehabilitation of the Hand, 4th ed. London, Butterworths, 1981.

Upper Limb Functional Prosthetics

Maurice LeBlanc, MSME, CP ✦ Gerald Stark, BSME, CP, FAAOP

DESCRIPTION OF FUNCTIONAL PROSTHESES
    Body-Powered Prostheses
    Externally Powered Prostheses
    Body-Powered Versus Externally Powered
        Prostheses
    Hybrid Prostheses

BRACHIAL PLEXUS INJURY AND AMPUTATION
RATIONALE FOR FITTING CONGENITAL ARM
    AMPUTEES
    Growth
    Parents and Teachers

The functional consequences of the loss of all or part of the upper limb as a result of injury, by amputation for tumor or disease, or secondary to a congenital anomaly may be mitigated by fitting of an appropriate prosthesis (Fig. 218-1). The more proximal the loss, the more appropriate a functional prosthesis becomes (Fig. 218-2).

Aesthetic prostheses can be important to the amputee for body image and self-esteem. They can also hold objects put manually into them and hold paper for writing; in this sense, aesthetic prostheses can be functional.[1] Functional prostheses refer to those prostheses that are operational. They can be body powered with a cable and shoulder harness or externally powered with a battery and motor. Both types are described in this chapter.

It is perfectly acceptable for an amputee to choose not to wear a prosthesis. Unlike with the lower limbs, of which two are needed to walk, we can do many activities with one hand. Also, when a prosthesis is used, the residual limb is covered by a socket, and therefore the amputee loses sensation. With no prosthesis, the residual limb is free and therefore useful for sensation.

The amputee should not be forced to use a prosthesis; instead, he or she should feel like a whole person without his or her own arm and without a prosthesis. It is important for the amputee choosing not to use a prosthesis to be supported emotionally and psychologically and to receive occupational and assisted daily living training in optimal use of the residual limb.

DESCRIPTION OF FUNCTIONAL PROSTHESES

Body-Powered Prostheses

Body-powered prostheses are operated by a shoulder harness with a cable running to the prosthesis. Scapular abduction and glenohumeral flexion typically provide the force and excursion on the cable to operate the prosthesis. Major manufacturers of prosthetic components are listed in Table 218-1.

PARTIAL-HAND PROSTHESES

A partial-hand prosthesis can replace individual fingers, the thumb, and most or all of the missing digits for a person with transcarpal amputation. Prostheses can range from a simple opposition post for a missing thumb to provide prehension (Fig. 218-3) to a cable-driven prosthesis for a person missing fingers (Fig. 218-4).

CHOICE OF PREHENSORS. The prehensor is usually a prosthetic hand or a split hook (Figs. 218-5 and 218-6). There are trade-offs in the use of hands and hooks (Table 218-2).

WRIST DISARTICULATION AND TRANSRADIAL (BELOW-ELBOW) PROSTHESES

This level of prosthesis requires a wrist unit (which provides passive, manually controlled supination-pronation) and prehensor (Fig. 218-7).

TABLE 218-1 ✦ MAJOR MANUFACTURERS OF UPPER LIMB PROSTHETIC COMPONENTS

Hosmer Dorrance Corporation
PO Box 37
Campbell, CA 95008
Tel: 800-827-0070
Fax: 408-379-5263
Internet: www.hosmer.com
e-mail: hosmer@hosmer.com

Otto Bock Orthopedic Industry
3000 Xenium Lane North
Minneapolis, MN 55441
Tel: 800-328-4058
Fax: 800-962-2549
Internet: www.ottobockus.com
e-mail: info@ottobockus.com

TRS, Inc.
2450 Central Ave, Unit D
Boulder, CO 80301
Tel: 303-444-4720, 800-279-1865
Fax: 303-444-5372
Internet: www.oandp.com/commerci/trs/index.htm
e-mail: trs@oandp.com

Liberating Technologies, Inc.
(U.S. representative for Hugh Steeper, Ltd)
325 Hopping Brook Road, Suite A
Hopkinton, MA 01746
Tel: 508-893-6363
Fax: 508-893-9966
Internet: www.liberatingtech.com/
e-mail: twalley.williams@liberatingtech.com

Motion Control, Inc.
2401 South 1070 West, Suite B
Salt Lake City, UT 84119-1555
Tel: 888-MYO-ARMS, 801-978-2622
Fax: 801-978-0848
Internet: www.utaharm.com/
e-mail: info@utaharm.com

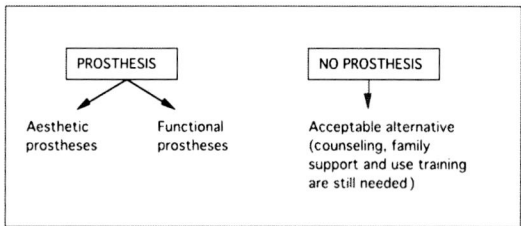

FIGURE 218-1. Algorithm of options for upper limb prostheses.

TABLE 218-2 ✦ COMPARISON OF PROSTHETIC HAND VERSUS SPLIT HOOK

Prosthetic Hand	Split Hook
Heavier in weight	Lighter in weight
More difficult to see objects being grasped	Easier to see objects being grasped
More complex mechanically	Simpler mechanically
Cannot get into pockets	Will fit into pockets
Less versatile as a tool	Versatile as a tool
More cosmetic in appearance	Not cosmetic

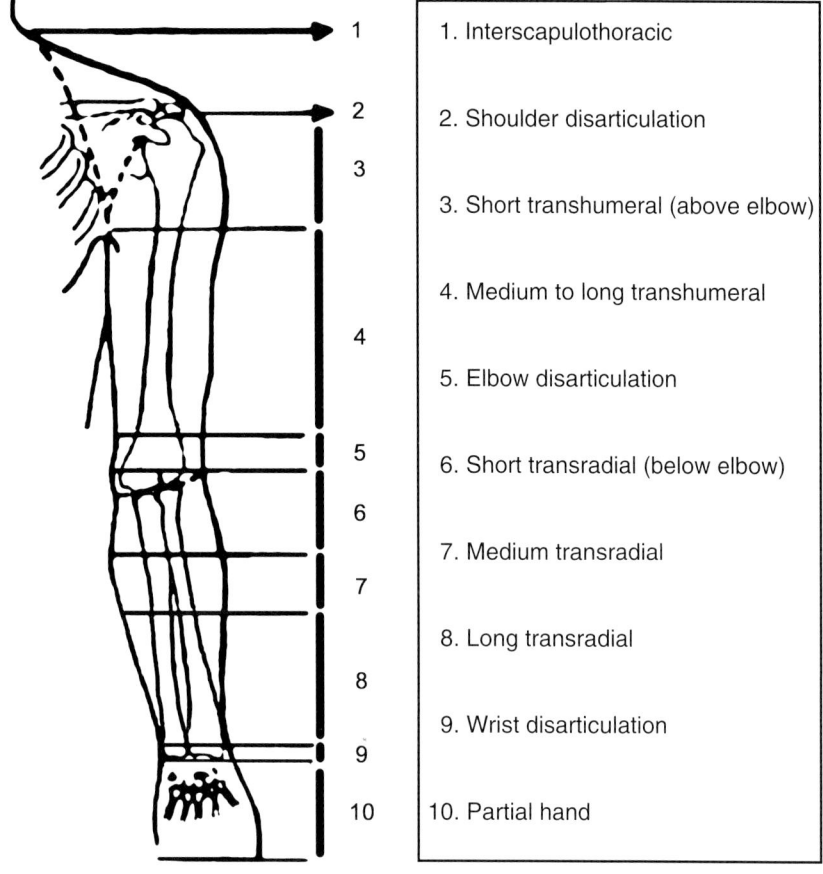

1	1. Interscapulothoracic
2	2. Shoulder disarticulation
3	3. Short transhumeral (above elbow)
4	4. Medium to long transhumeral
	5. Elbow disarticulation
5	6. Short transradial (below elbow)
6	7. Medium transradial
7	8. Long transradial
8	9. Wrist disarticulation
9	10. Partial hand
10	

FIGURE 218-2. Functional levels of amputation.[2]

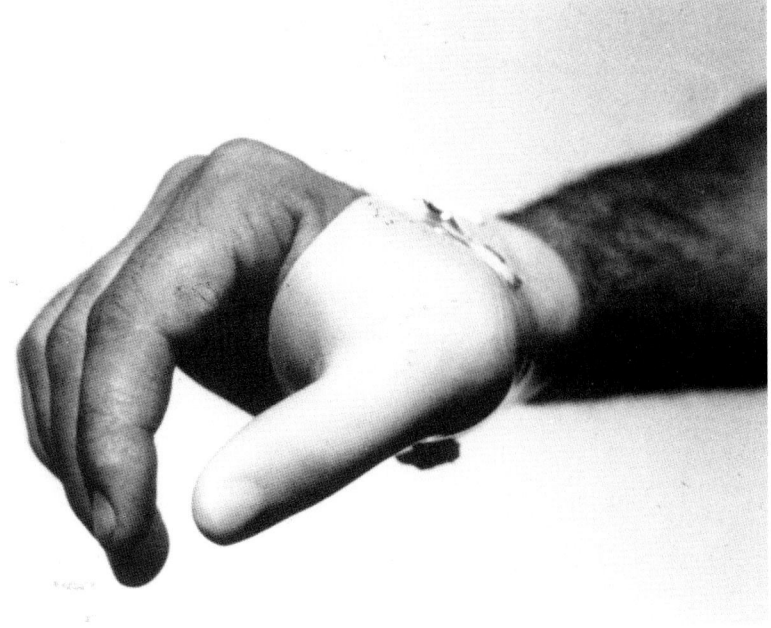

FIGURE 218-3. Opposition post. (Modified from Atkins D, Meier R: Comprehensive Management of the Upper-Limb Amputee. New York, Springer-Verlag, 1989.)

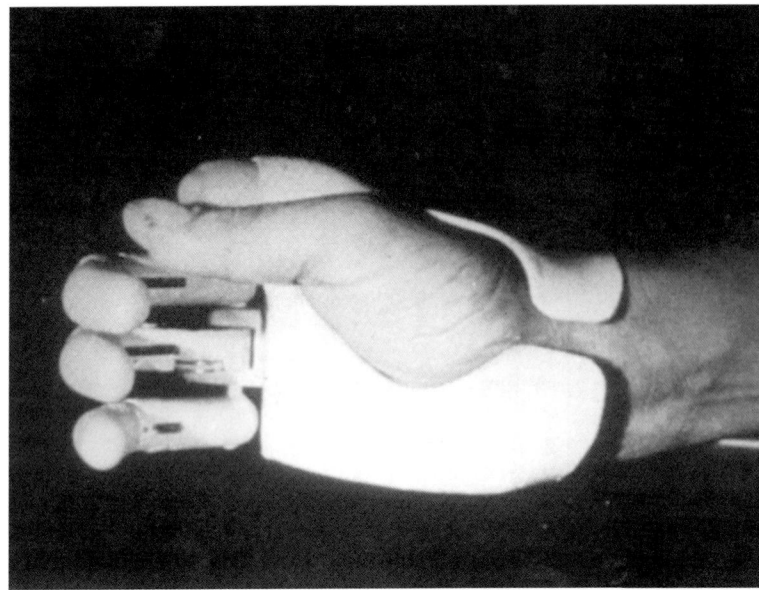

FIGURE 218-4. Cable-driven partial-hand prosthesis. (Modified from Atkins D, Meier R: Comprehensive Management of the Upper-Limb Amputee. New York, Springer-Verlag, 1989.)

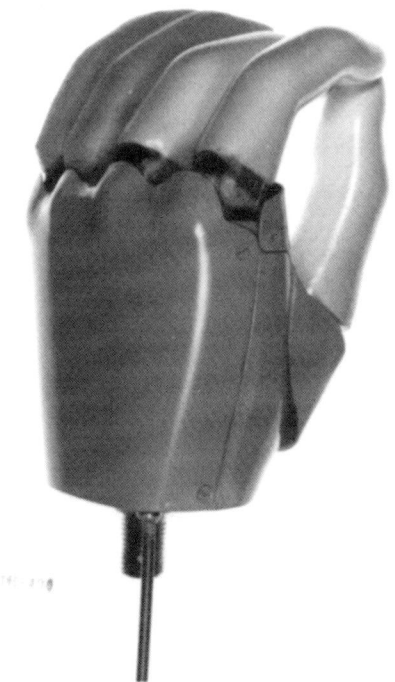

FIGURE 218-5. Hosmer Dorrance hand. (Modified from Atkins D, Meier R: Comprehensive Management of the Upper-Limb Amputee. New York, Springer-Verlag, 1989.)

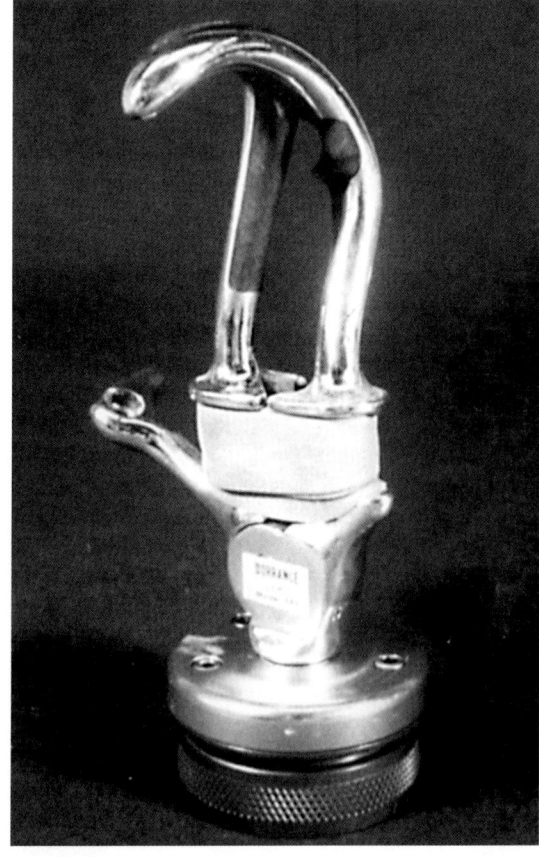

FIGURE 218-6. Hosmer Dorrance 5XA hook. (Modified from Atkins D, Meier R: Comprehensive Management of the Upper-Limb Amputee. New York, Springer-Verlag, 1989.)

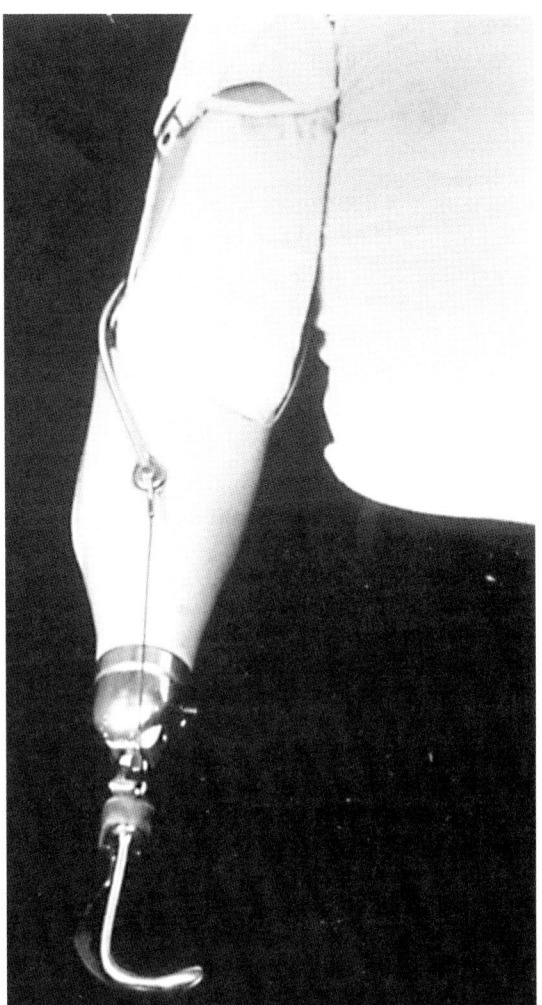

FIGURE 218-7. Medium transradial (below-elbow) prosthesis. (Modified from Atkins D, Meier R: Comprehensive Management of the Upper-Limb Amputee. New York, Springer-Verlag, 1989.)

ELBOW DISARTICULATION PROSTHESES

This level of amputation does not allow sufficient space for a prosthetic elbow, so outside hinges must be used to place the elbow joint in the proper anatomic position. With elbow function now included, the prosthetic components include the prehensor, wrist unit, and elbow hinges, which are lockable in several positions of flexion-extension (Fig. 218-8).

TRANSHUMERAL (ABOVE-ELBOW) PROSTHESES

This prosthesis is similar to the elbow disarticulation prosthesis, except that a prosthetic elbow is used instead of outside hinges (Fig. 218-9).

SHOULDER DISARTICULATION AND INTERSCAPULOTHORACIC PROSTHESES

These types of prostheses are similar in that they include a passive, manually controlled shoulder motion in addition to the prehensor, wrist, and elbow. The shoulder joint typically provides both glenohumeral flexion-extension and abduction-adduction. Only the prehensor and elbow are actively controlled by the shoulder harness and cable. The wrist and shoulder joints are manually pre-positioned for functional tasks (Fig. 218-10).

Externally Powered Prostheses

Externally powered prostheses have a battery power source and actuation of certain functions by electric motors. They are used primarily when the arm amputee

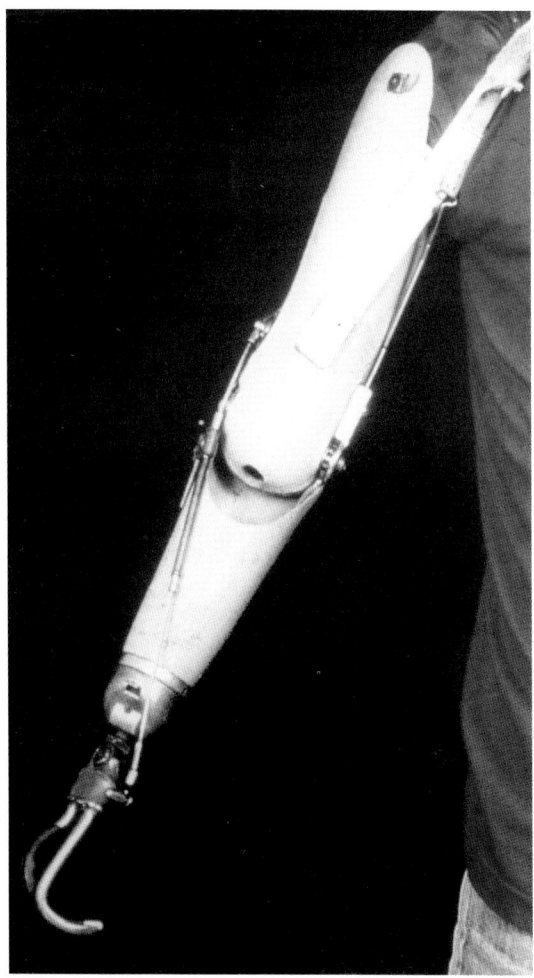

FIGURE 218-8. Elbow disarticulation prosthesis. (Modified from Atkins D, Meier R: Comprehensive Management of the Upper-Limb Amputee. New York, Springer-Verlag, 1989.)

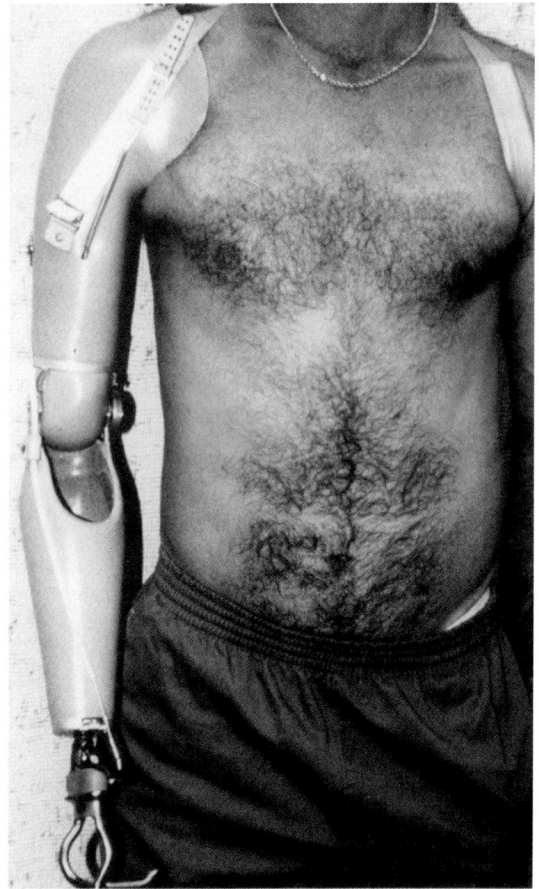

FIGURE 218-9. Transhumeral prosthesis. (Modified from Atkins D, Meier R: Comprehensive Management of the Upper-Limb Amputee. New York, Springer-Verlag, 1989.)

powered prostheses are generally heavier and require higher suspension forces, which may decrease comfort. The discomfort of body-powered prostheses comes mainly from the harness in the axilla area, which takes high forces.

APPEARANCE (EXCLUDING PASSIVE PROSTHESES)

The externally powered prosthesis generally has a better appearance because there is no external cable or hardware. The harness is simpler or eliminated, and a hand is usually chosen. It has a more modern, "high-tech" appeal.

RELIABILITY

A body-powered prosthesis generally has a simpler design and is therefore more reliable. By contrast, an externally powered prosthesis tends to have a more complex design with motors, batteries, circuits, and wires that are subject to breakage or breakdown. However, externally powered systems are becoming more modular and easier to service.

"HASSLE FACTOR"

The externally powered prosthesis requires more time and effort because of the following: charging

has limited body power to operate the prosthesis or when it is advantageous in packaging the prosthesis so that it is more self-contained than the body-powered system (Figs. 218-11 to 218-13).

Body-Powered Versus Externally Powered Prostheses

FUNCTION

A body-powered prosthesis is generally a better choice for function because there is some sensory proprioceptive feedback from the harness. A hook, which is lighter and more functional than a hand, is usually chosen.

COMFORT

An externally powered prosthesis generally requires less harness and no control force, which makes it more comfortable and less cumbersome. However, externally

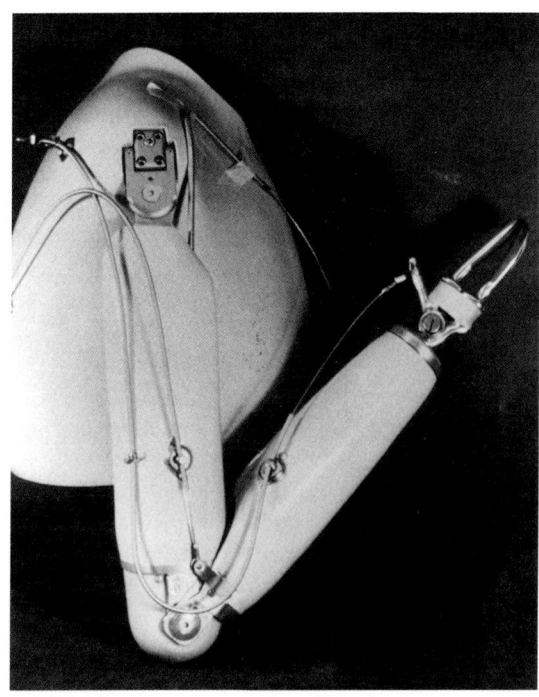

FIGURE 218-10. Shoulder prosthesis. (Modified from Atkins D, Meier R: Comprehensive Management of the Upper-Limb Amputee. New York, Springer-Verlag, 1989.)

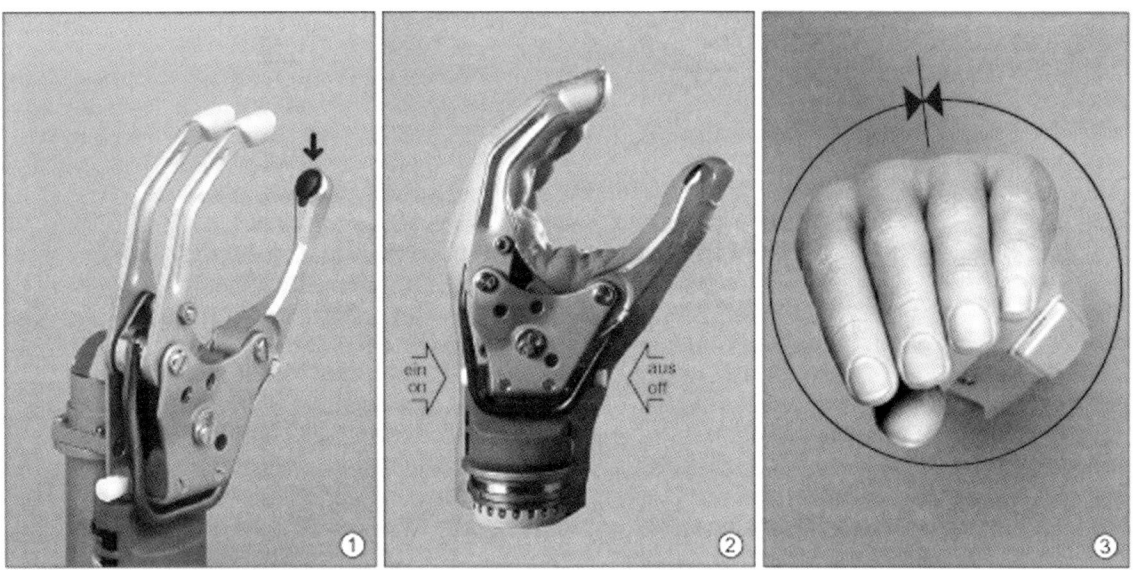

FIGURE 218-11. Otto Bock electric hand.

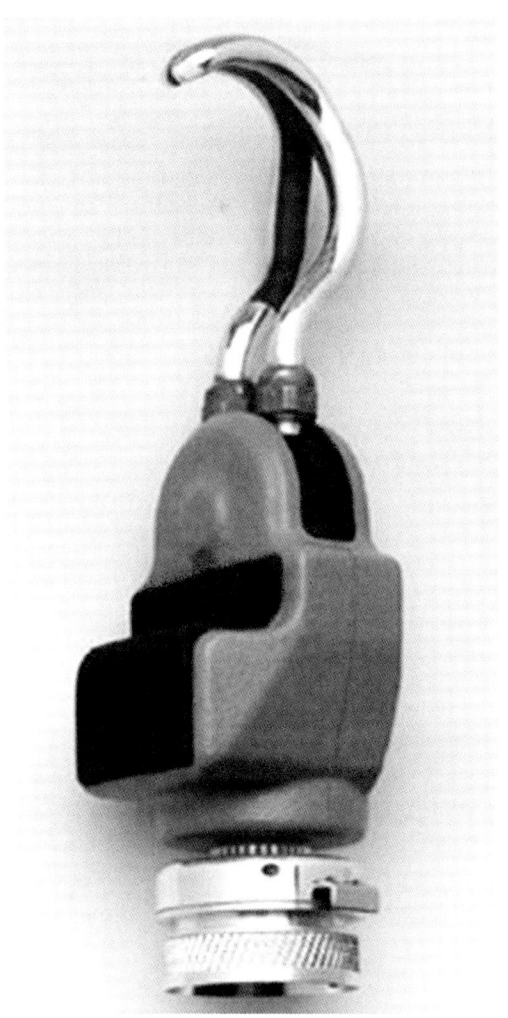

FIGURE 218-12. Hosmer electric synergetic hook.

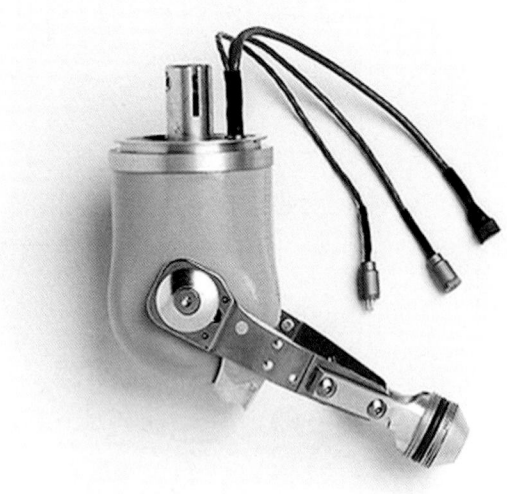

FIGURE 218-13. NYU-Hosmer electric elbow.

batteries (usually every day); care of electrodes (if used); care of cosmetic glove on hand (if used); and greater caution in activities.

Hybrid Prostheses

Hybrid prostheses can be useful to maximize function or appearance of the prosthesis in any combination: body-powered and aesthetic; body-powered and externally powered; aesthetic and externally powered. Decisions on what components to use are typically made by the amputee and the prosthetist after an analysis of needs and preferences.

BRACHIAL PLEXUS INJURY AND AMPUTATION

Brachial plexus injuries from trauma or present at birth are generally addressed in one of two ways: by making an orthosis for the flail arm or by transhumeral amputation followed by fitting of a transhumeral prosthesis. In the latter instance, the individual is provided with a prosthesis appropriate for the level of amputation (see Fig. 218-2). The primary difference is that the individual may not have active shoulder control because of avulsion of the nerve.

RATIONALE FOR FITTING CONGENITAL ARM AMPUTEES

It is recommended that congenital arm amputees be fitted with upper limb prostheses early in life so that they have the opportunity for the prosthesis to be part of their body image. In this way, they learn to use and accept the prosthesis before they become accustomed to living without it. Later in life, they can make a conscious decision whether to use prostheses.

Child amputees should be fitted with passive upper limb prostheses when they are about 6 months old so they can use the prostheses to help balance themselves when sitting and crawling. At the age when children start to walk is when they have the mental and motor ability to actively control a prosthesis. At this time, the passive prosthesis can be activated with a harness and control system, and usually a new prehensor, so the children can open and close the prehensors for eating and play activities.

Growth

When child arm amputees are between the ages of 6 months and 5 years, they usually need a new prosthesis every year because of growth. Between 6 and 10 years of age, the frequency of replacement is every 2 years because of growth. Between 11 years and the completion of growth at about 16 years, replacement is typically every 3 years. Thereafter, upper limb prosthesis replacement is dictated by wear rather than by growth. A prosthesis is usually replaced every 3 to 5 years (or more), depending on amount and type of use.

Parents and Teachers

It is important that the parents of child arm amputees accept their children and are part of the prescription and training process. Likewise, teachers must be acquainted with the prostheses so that the children can more readily be accepted, use the prostheses at school, and participate with other children in activities. A child arm amputee should be treated like a normal child with allowance for the fact that he or she has a "helper" arm.

REFERENCES

1. Fraser CM: An evaluation of the use made of cosmetic and functional prostheses by unilateral upper limb amputees. Prosthet Orthot Int 1998;22:216-223.
2. Atkins D, Meier R: Comprehensive Management of the Upper-Limb Amputee. New York, Springer-Verlag, 1989.

Additional Reading

American Academy of Orthopaedic Surgeons: Atlas of Limb Prosthetics. St. Louis, CV Mosby, 1981:95-144.
Bender LF: Prosthetics and Rehabilitation After Arm Amputation. Springfield, Ill, Charles C Thomas, 1974:70-86.
Billock JN: Upper limb prosthetic terminal devices: hands versus hooks. Clin Prosthet Orthot 1986;10:57-65.
Fletcher MJ, Leonard F: The principles of artificial-hand design. Artif Limbs 1955;2:78-94.
Klopsted PE, Wilson PD: Human Limbs and Their Substitutes. New York, Hafner, 1968.
LeBlanc MA: Patient population and other estimates of prosthetics and orthotics in the USA. Orthot Prosthet 1973;27:38-44.

Littler JW: On the adaptability of man's hand. Hand 1973;5:187-191.

Selected Articles from Artificial Limbs. Huntington, NY, Robert E. Krieger Publishing, 1970.

Setoguchi Y, Rosenfelder R, eds: The Limb Deficient Child. Springfield, Ill, Charles C Thomas, 1982.

Taylor CL, Schwarz RJ: The anatomy and mechanics of the human hand. Artif Limbs 1955;2:22-35.

Taylor C: The biomechanics of the normal and of the amputated upper extremity. In Klopsteg P, Wilson P, eds: Human Limbs and Their Substitutes. New York, McGraw-Hill, 1954:169-221.

Upper Limb Aesthetic and Functional Prosthetics

JEAN PILLET, MD ✦ ANNIE DIDIERJEAN-PILLET, MD

The hand underlies the expression of movement and gesture; mutilation of the upper limb is exposed to the eyes of others. Whatever its origin—traumatic, therapeutic, or congenital—amputation always bears social implications, and those suffering from a physical deficit find themselves torn between their desire for full social acceptance and the realities of a socially negative situation.[1] Concerning the communicative role of the hand, one cannot separate function from aesthetics, and the real disability is that a patient is unable to use his or her hand or hands because of physical reasons, psychological reasons, or physical and psychological reasons.

An individual can figuratively amputate a functional hand by not using it because it is perceived as repellent. This is what could be called, in the instance of patients with congenital amputations, acquired amputation. In fact, the demand for aesthetic prostheses does not come under the heading of luxury or improved comfort but reflects a desire to mitigate psychological injury and suffering.

A hand prosthesis can be either functional or aesthetic.[2-7] The advantages of a functional prosthesis are easy to understand. Those of an aesthetic prosthesis are less so. However, the advantages are more similar than dissimilar because the purpose of an aesthetic prosthesis is "use." If an aesthetic prosthesis can liberate an individual from the sense of abnormality by restoring the hand to its normal appearance, it will be used and therefore improve lifestyle.

Experience shows that an aesthetic prosthesis also improves function of the affected limb. To explain this twofold aesthetic and functional advantage, the prosthesis is known as a passive function aesthetic prosthesis. It may be easy to prescribe or to design a prosthesis; however, it is difficult to help the patient, and whether a prosthesis is indicated depends on the amputee's behavior more than on the amputation itself.

CHOOSING AN AESTHETIC PROSTHESIS

Patients are often demanding, even perfectionistic, and therefore difficult to please, and they have very personal prosthetic needs. First of all, it is important to establish whether the patient is affected by the hand's appearance or if he or she is responding more to external pressures from family or friends. Aesthetic "discomfort" remains, let us stress, but it is much more subjective than real and therefore does not have any direct link to the "objective" seriousness of the amputation. A patient who hides a potentially functional stump inside a pocket is just as disabled as if he or she had literally lost the hand. He or she perceives the amputation as "abnormal," and this leads the patient to avoid any "normal-looking" action that might draw attention. When the individual is with others, he or she will avoid going to the beach or to a restaurant and suffers from self-inflicted exclusion. It is also up to the clinician and prosthetist to channel expectations by warning the patient of what truly can be accomplished. Thus, when it comes to evaluating mid- and long-term results, the clinician can avoid conflicting situations.

The patient's profession is a deciding factor. It is important to know how he or she is planning to return to active life and how he or she intends to use the prosthesis. This takes into account the age and personality of the patient. In general, the younger the patient and the stronger the personality, the easier adaptation will be.

Trauma-Related Amputees

In children, domestic accidents are the major cause of amputation. Prostheses are rarely indicated in this age group, and the retention of sufficient structures to provide pinch remains the discriminating feature. If there is indeed a pinch mechanism, it is important to wait so that the prosthesis does not become more of a hindrance than a benefit. The crucial factor here is the age at which the accident has occurred. In contradistinction, a stump without a pinch mechanism must be fitted early with a prosthesis. Children who have been amputated at a very early age can be considered the same as those suffering from congenital amputation.

An adult accident victim goes through two stages: a first stage, with which surgeons are familiar, that of recent amputation; and a second stage, when amputation has occurred some time ago. The second stage is usually less well known. The behavior of recent amputees evolves throughout well-defined periods:

- an initial period that occurs immediately after the trauma and is associated with their realization of their condition;
- later, a more difficult period, that of returning to everyday life, when they realize the extent of their disability.

Whereas recent amputees are temporarily handicapped, those who have been amputees for a longer time may or may not be disabled, depending on how they have dealt with the ordeal.

Therapeutic Amputees

Acquired amputations (accidental or therapeutic) force patients to come to terms with their loss. This loss implies grieving not only for the diminishing function but also for their image, which generates an upheaval as personal as it is social and professional. In the case of therapeutic amputations, patients are faced with illness and with an extremely anguishing, serious diagnosis. The amputation is not as brutal as if it had been caused by an accident, but the unavoidable consequence of the diagnosis and treatment. Sometimes, it is refused or rejected because it is too traumatic. In cases such as these, one must stress how relative the disfigurement actually will be, thanks to the wearing of an aesthetic prosthesis. "I made up my mind after realizing that I could still go out." These words from a young woman illustrate how difficult it is to "accept" such decisions.

If, after this, other surgical procedures prove necessary because of the evolution of the patient's condition, the ensuing successive mutilations are particularly difficult to accept.

Congenital Amputees

Follow-up of patients has taught us that contrary to what we originally thought, no functional assistance is necessary. With or without a prosthesis, patients with congenital unilateral distal amputations develop their own adaptations (Fig. 219-1). Their movements might be different, but they are able to do anything without any major functional difficulty. These patients suffer from lack of normalcy in their appearance; they want to be able to go around without attracting attention. They rarely spontaneously request a functional prosthesis. In the few exceptional cases we encountered, we easily detected family pressure.

In treating congenital distal amputees, a twofold error is often made: first, by considering them mutilated; and second, by attempting to fit them with a functional prosthesis. This approach is wrong. These are not real amputations; the imperfect development is due to a congenital defect. These patients define their own perception of their body, and this view is different from ours. They see themselves as whole and normal, but different. Suggesting that a unilateral amputation patient be fitted with a functional prosthesis, of any kind, is equivalent to burdening a normal person with a third hand. This was, in fact, the reaction of one of our patients who was asked why he did not have a functional prosthesis and who said, "Doctor Pillet, what would you do with a third hand?" (Fig. 219-2). "But, when you have to carry two suitcases, you have a problem." The response: "Like you when you have three suitcases!" Therefore, patients with congenital amputations are disabled, but only from our point of view. In the 16th century, Ambroise Paré noted that "a man without arms can do almost everything another could do with his hands."[2] Contrary to traumatic amputees, patients with congenital amputations are not faced with the initial emotional impact of losing a hand or an arm. Some do suffer from the lack of normalcy in their appearance.

PROSTHETIC INDICATIONS DETERMINED BY AMPUTATION LEVEL

Unilateral Amputees

CHILDREN

The consultation is a difficult one, considering what is at stake. Between know-how and how-to, the physician's ethics and experience are challenged.

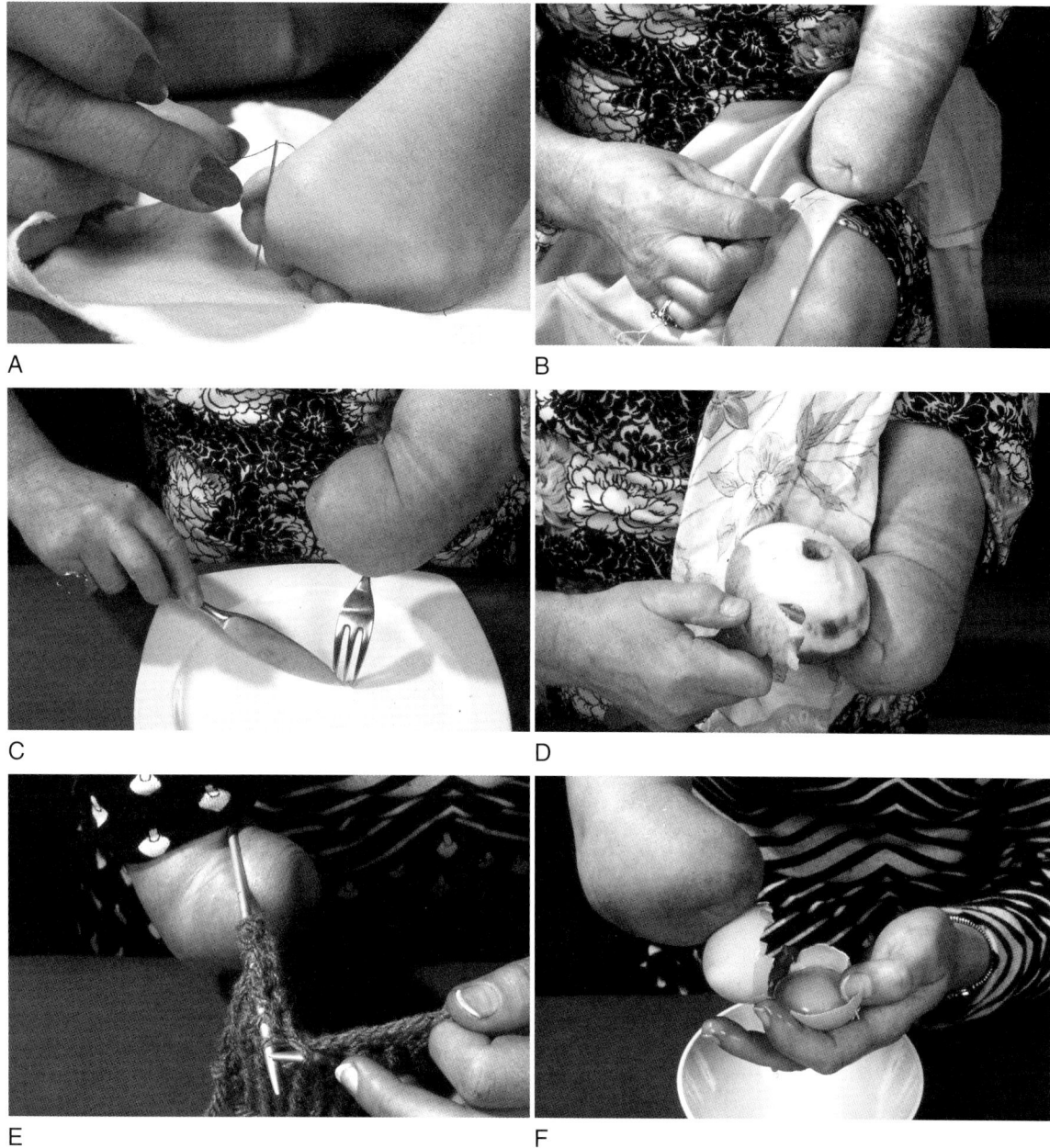

FIGURE 219-1. *A* to *F,* Adaptations of patients with congenital, unilateral distal amputations.

The psychological approach is two-tiered: parents and children. When it comes to their child's malformation, parents are addressing the functional and aesthetic aspects. They are concerned with the functional sequelae and cannot imagine how their child will develop his or her own adaptations to "do," albeit differently.

If the stump does not have a pinch mechanism (Fig. 219-3), a prosthesis can be fitted at a very young age, generally between 6 and 18 months. Being fitted at that early age ensures that the child will adjust to the presence of the prosthesis and encourages activities with use of both hands. However, before the age of 18 months, there can be cutaneous reactions.

If the stump does have a pinch mechanism, the prosthesis will be more of a nuisance than useful for everyday activities, at play or in school. In this case, it is preferable to wait until adolescence before fitting a

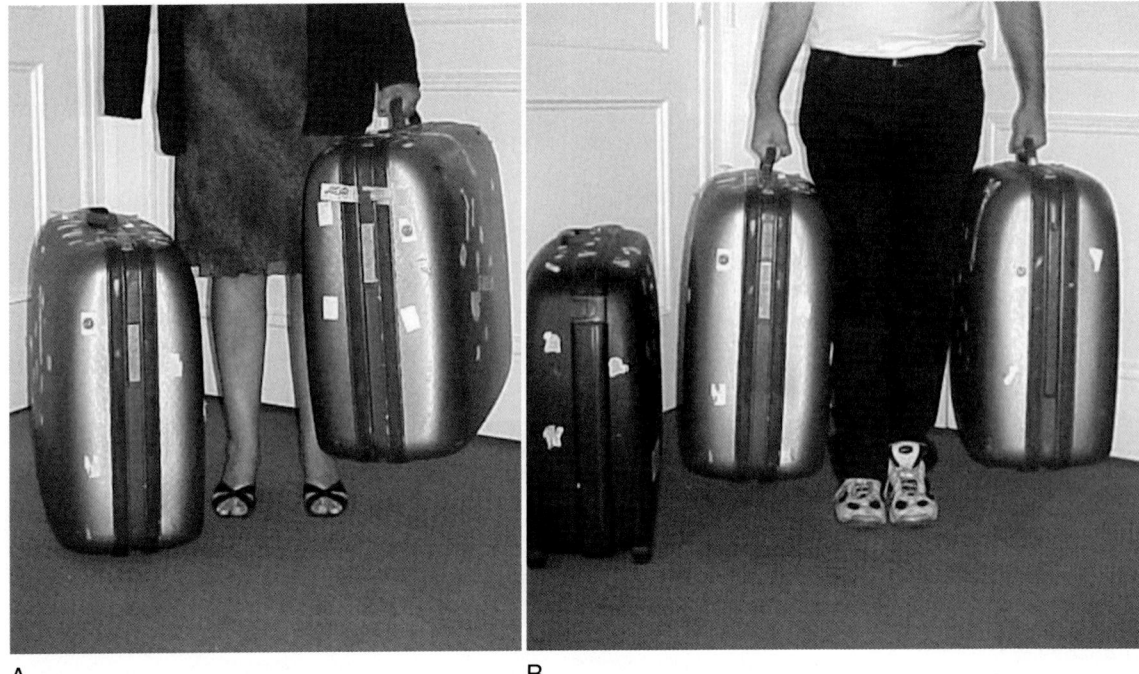

FIGURE 219-2. *A*, Patient with unilateral amputation with two suitcases. *B*, Man with two hands with three suitcases.

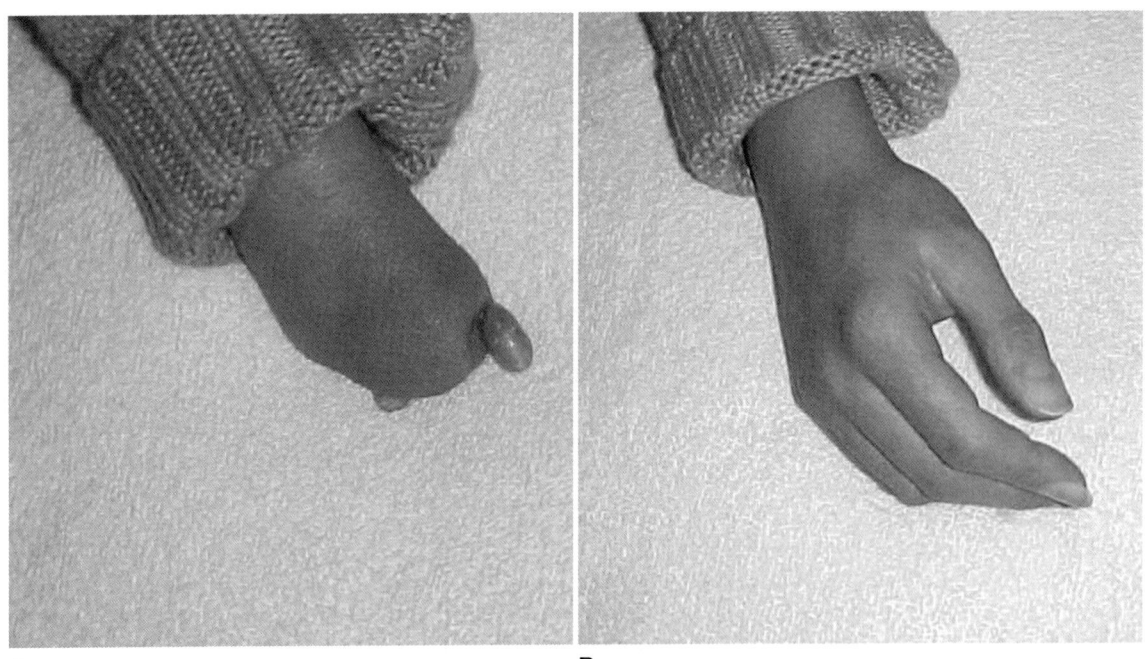

FIGURE 219-3. *A*, Stump with no pinch mechanism. *B*, Prosthesis shown in place.

prosthesis, at a time when self-image becomes all-important and the child will be more motivated to deal with the drawbacks of the prosthesis. Depending on the level of psychological distress manifested by parents, who refuse to accept the malformation, it is sometimes necessary to fit the child. In cases such as these, it is the parents we are treating, through the child (Fig. 219-4).

The first appointment is a "mirror" consultation because the parents want to know how this child will be able to live and grow up at the same time that they are asking themselves how they are going to "let" the child live and grow up. Their questions concern what their future relations with this child will be, what kind of life for the child and for them. The parents are full of anxiety and guilt. Is a malformation a disability? The question at first refers to the functional level and then moves to the level of aesthetics as soon as the child develops an astonishing dexterity and maturity, subject to their fulfilling two conditions: to let the child develop his or her own adaptations and to support the child when he or she uses intelligence to overcome difficulties.

To summarize, it is important to find out how to separate the parents' problem from the child's. They are different problems because they concern different people. It is essential to let children express themselves where their own body is concerned. However, it is so much easier to handle this among adults, bypassing the one most concerned. Consider the following scenario:

> A 6-year-old child is in tears. I ask him why.
> "I heard talk of a prosthesis . . ."
> "Do you know what it is?"

> "It's a thing you put on that looks like a hand," big sob, "I don't want one!"
> "In any case, it's up to you."
> He looks at me, hesitates, and tries to speak. "Do you find my hand ugly?"
> "What about you, what do you think?"
> "No, because I have a great time with my buddies and with my fat fingers, I'm the Boss!"

Even to make one's parents happy, how can one give up a position such as that of a boss! Unfortunately, the patient's parents, not to distress their little boy, had decided never to talk to him about his hand problem. Thus, they had no idea of their child's enviable status. This is a typical misunderstanding.

ADOLESCENTS

This is a time when joining the crowd is essential. Not only is it important to display individuality, but appearance is also of paramount importance. Physical differences are viewed as obstacles that lead to exclusion and being labeled. This is a time of fragility and of frequent relational problems. An aesthetic prosthesis can prove beneficial as long as its limitations are made explicit (Fig. 219-5).

ADULTS

The clinical approach to adults who are congenital amputees is probably one of the least well known because it is extremely specific in terms of demand and defect. These patients come to the clinician or the prosthetist to discuss, for the first time, a deformity that has bothered them for a long time. Why should this come out now? The demand corresponds to an

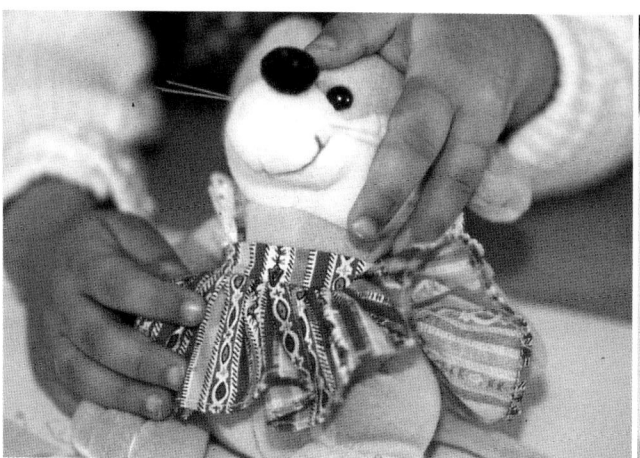
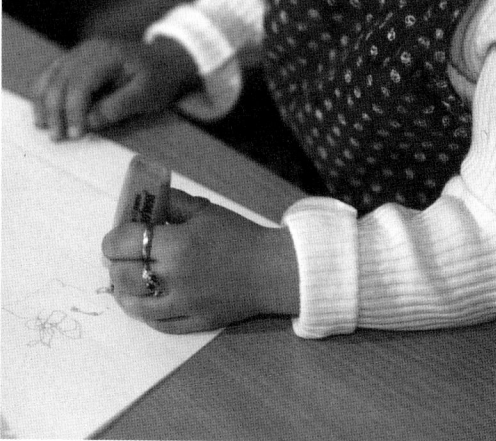

A   B

FIGURE 219-4. *A,* Stump with pinch mechanism. *B,* Prosthesis shown in place.

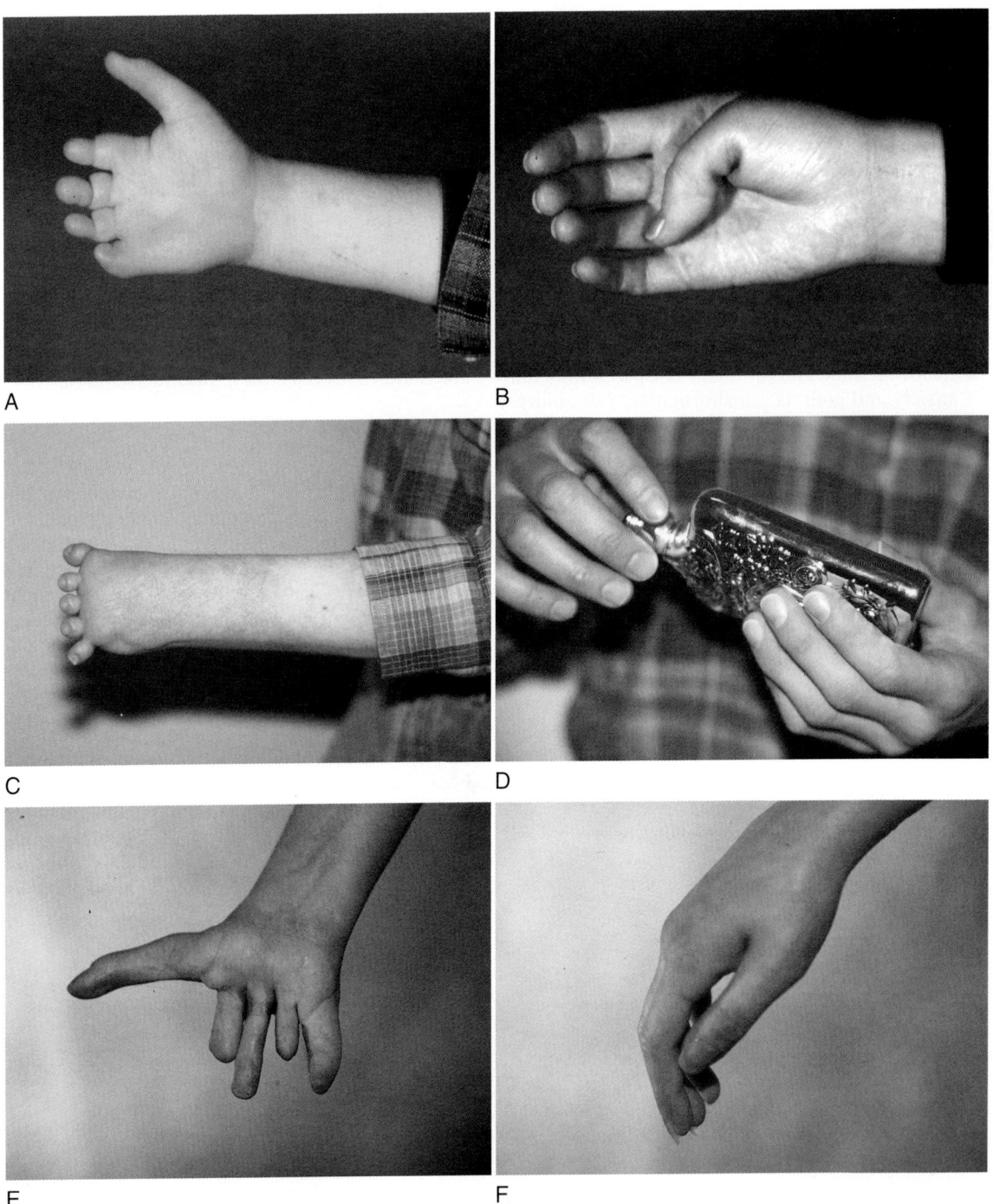

FIGURE 219-5. Patients are shown before (A, C, and E) and after (B, D, and F) fitting for a hand prosthesis.

important moment in their life that echoes their past and life experience in areas such as family and social-professional environment (a marriage, a birth, a first job, a failure), which reactivates feelings of unease concerning this deformity.

The defect is expressed as being deprived—of beauty, youth, love, and recognition. The patient does not feel complete, and this stigmatizes his or her suffering. In adulthood, the problems that were raised at the time of birth, especially the issue of transmission, re-emerge. Will they transmit their own malformation? Will they be accepted when they fall in love, not only by their partner but also by their partner's family? Will they be accepted in their social and professional environment?

In turn, they ask themselves the same questions their parents had asked themselves earlier. As an adult, an individual allows himself or herself to express the wish to hide from sight an area that generates questioning and attracts attention to, at last, feel perceived as a full human being and not seen through the malformation. Here again, it is important to explain to patients that a finger or hand aesthetic prosthesis will be, at least at first, functionally uncomfortable inasmuch as the prosthesis will give them a finger length or a hand volume they never had before, and this will require a new adaptation. If motivation is sufficient, these drawbacks will be accepted as a downside of the proposed aesthetic quality. Eventually, many patients devise their own ways of handling this.

The problem is different in the case of adult congenital amputees who have always been fitted. How do they incorporate the prosthesis? Some of them state that it is part of themselves. They use it every day, sometimes from morning to night. One cannot avoid seeing such dependency as somewhat questionable. Others wear the prosthesis in a more discriminating manner; they use it for their social and professional life and remove it at home. The difference in behavior is obvious, even in childhood.

Children who are brought up with their difference taken into account, who have enjoyed a personal life of their own, are capable of standing up for their own choices and affinities. Also, even if they are indeed aware of their difference, they do not consider it inhibiting. Children who are brought up as if they are malformed, their individuality ignored, do not have the same functional possibilities. They remain the prisoners of prejudice. It is when they become adults that the problems reappear.

SPECIFIC PROSTHESES

The presence or absence of a pinch mechanism determines whether an amputation is distal or proximal. A proximal amputation presents a stump without a functional pinch (Table 219-1).

TABLE 219-1 ◆ AMPUTATION LEVEL

Proximal (stump without functional pinch mechanism)

Above the elbow
　Shoulder
　Arm
Below the elbow
　Forearm
　Total hand

Distal (stump with functional pinch mechanism)

Partial hand
Finger

Digital Prostheses

NAILS. Nails have an aesthetic and functional role. In terms of its specific function and symbolic role, a nail that is distorted, malformed, or even partially or totally nonexistent dictates extremely precise and limited indications for prostheses in response to a demand for perfection. Physically, functional impairment is often major, and despite the fact that the lesion itself may be minor, the slightest wound affects this precise and efficient tool. It provides a very fine pinch, mainly used for picking up small objects (such as pins).

Some women will renounce this function in the name of aesthetics, preferring to wear long fingernails. A wounded nail can result in serious psychological effects. Restoring a fingernail, similar in appearance, is equivalent to treating them. However, although it is easy enough to produce a fingernail, attaching it solidly raises problems as yet not resolved. The only effective method to ensure solid attachment of a normal-looking fingernail is to cover the distal phalanx entirely with a thin thimble-type prosthesis (Fig. 219-6).

PARTIAL OR TOTAL AMPUTATION OF THE DISTAL PHALANX. Losing just one distal phalanx may cause aesthetic and functional problems for patients (Fig. 219-7). Amputations at this level require a short prosthesis (as for the nail). The prosthesis will blend perfectly with the stump in terms of shape, skin texture, and color, and it will extend over the middle phalanx, leaving the proximal interphalangeal joint free. By restoration of the finger to its original length, the pinch is improved, for example, for picking up a pencil. The prosthesis can also be used to type on a keyboard or to play a musical instrument.

PARTIAL OR TOTAL AMPUTATION OF THE MIDDLE PHALANX. Middle phalanx amputation affects lateral pinch (Fig. 219-8). In the case of multiple digital amputations, the prosthesis provides opposite support for the preserved thumb to hold light objects. If the middle

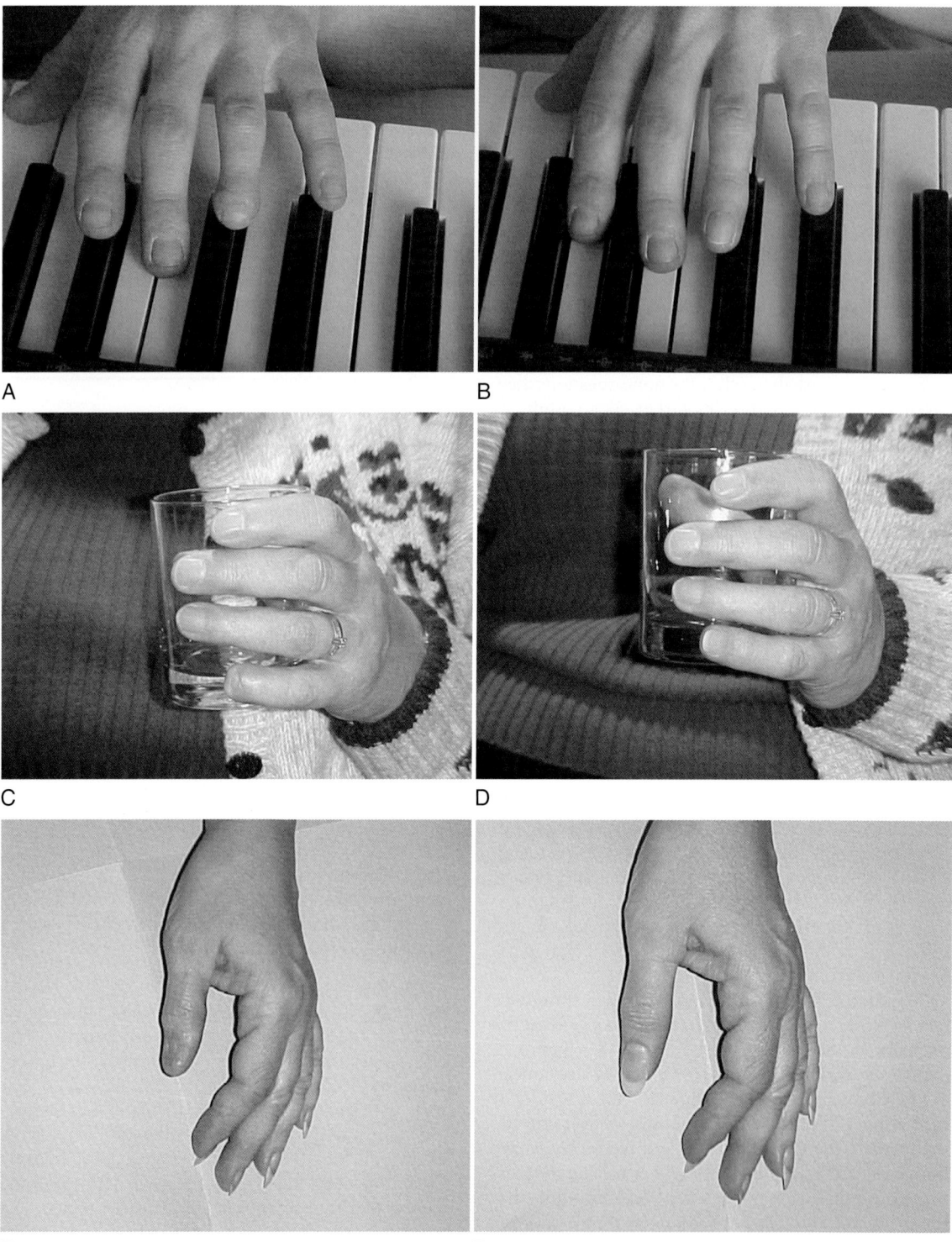

A

B

C

D

E

F

FIGURE 219-6. The only effective method to ensure solid attachment of a normal-looking fingernail is to cover the distal phalanx entirely with a thin thimble-type prosthesis. Patients are shown before (*A* and *C*) and after (*B* and *D*) fitting for a prosthesis to achieve a normal-appearing fingernail. *E* and *F,* Patient shown before and after fitting for a prosthesis to achieve a normal-appearing thumbnail.

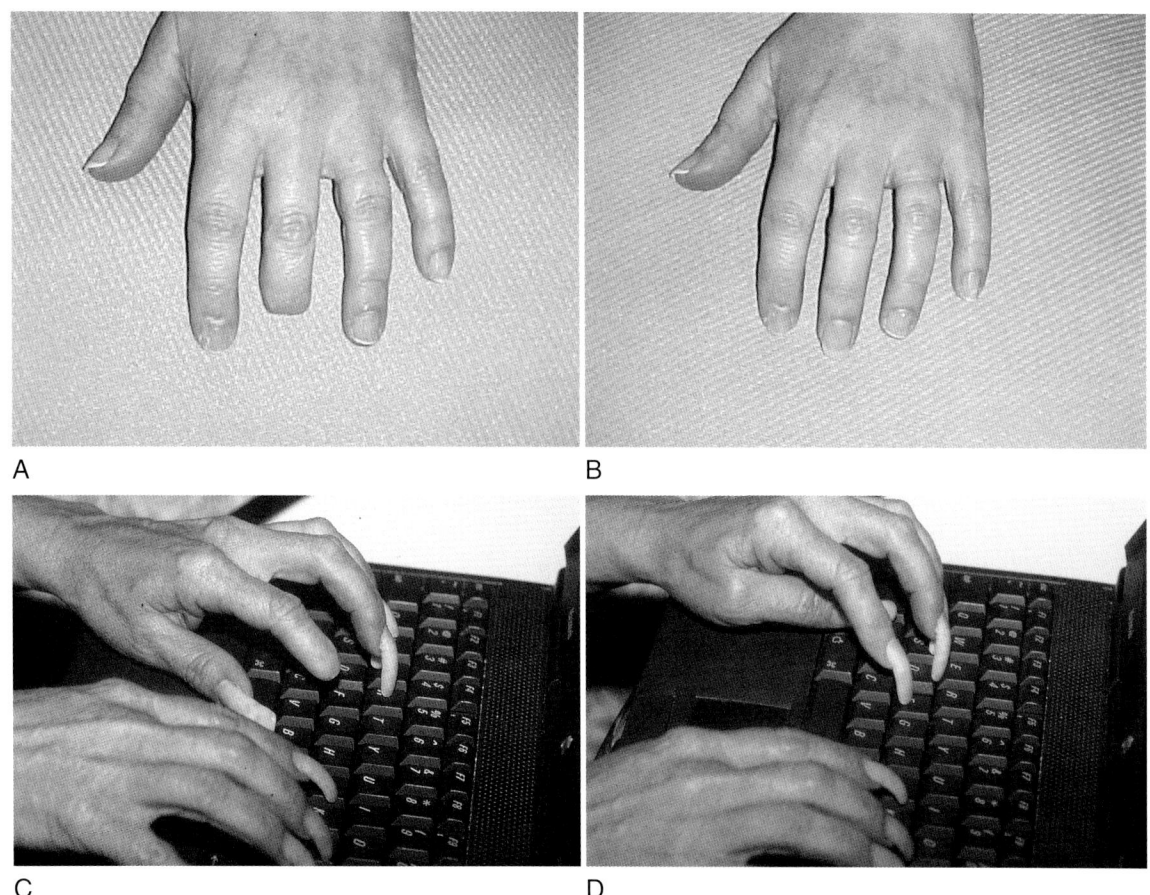

A   B

C   D

FIGURE 219-7. Amputations of a single distal phalanx require a short prosthesis (as shown in Fig. 219-6). Patients are shown before (*A* and *C*) and after (*B* and *D*) fitting for a prosthesis.

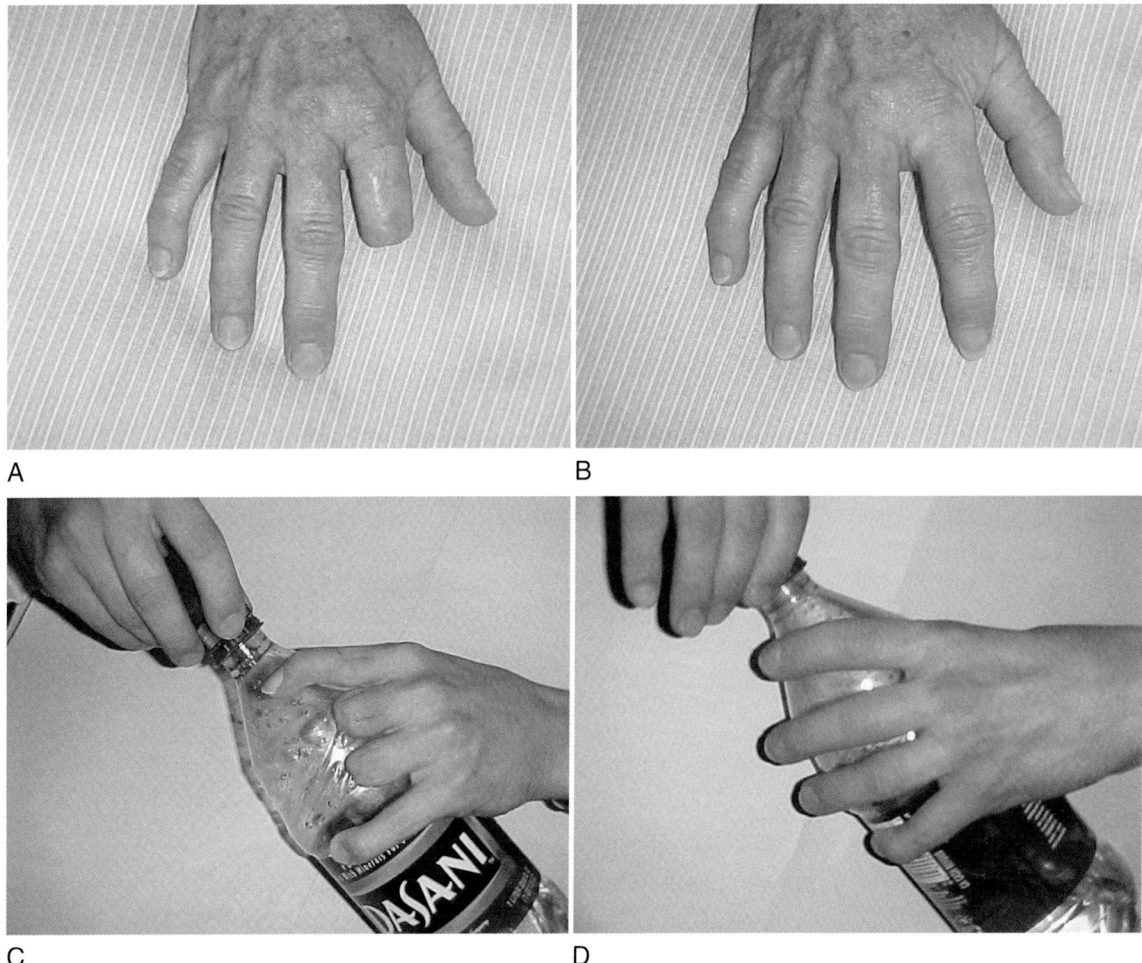

A

B

C

D

FIGURE 219-8. Amputations of the middle phalanx affect lateral pinch (*A* and *B*). Patients with multiple digit amputations require a prosthesis to stabilize fingers and to prevent dropping of small objects (*C* and *D*).

and ring fingers have been amputated, the prostheses stabilize the fingers and prevent dropping of small objects (Fig. 219-8*C* and *D*).

PARTIAL AMPUTATION OF PROXIMAL PHALANX. To ensure adequate attachment of a digital prosthesis to the proximal phalanx, a stump length of 1.5 cm is required (Fig. 219-9). With a short stump, it may be necessary to deepen the commissure (Fig. 219-10). Should the patient refuse this procedure, a special ring-based attachment can be proposed (Fig. 219-11).

PARTIAL OR TOTAL AMPUTATION OF THE THUMB. By increasing the length of the thumb, prostheses will provide adequate opposition to the fingers (Fig. 219-12). Carpal-metacarpal disarticulation of the thumb requires a hand prosthesis that will leave healthy fingers outside the prosthesis to preserve the best function possible (Fig. 219-13). Osseointegrated implants remain

a possible evolution of research. They might be indicated for situations in which a strong grasp is required. However, this technique has its drawbacks. Osseointegrated implants are still a major cause of infection because of the way they are attached, and they also result in ulcerations because of the mobility of the skin. Therefore, they should be fitted only onto a fine and immobile skin adherent to the bone. Their everyday "management" is difficult (Fig. 219-14). Experience in this area is still limited.

Partial Hand Prostheses

Metacarpal amputations can be transverse, central, or oblique. If it is a hand without the thumb, the remaining fingers are placed outside the prosthesis (Fig. 219-15). When the thumb is normal, we leave the thumb outside the prosthesis. This is the most functional solution (Fig. 219-16).

Text continued on p. 600

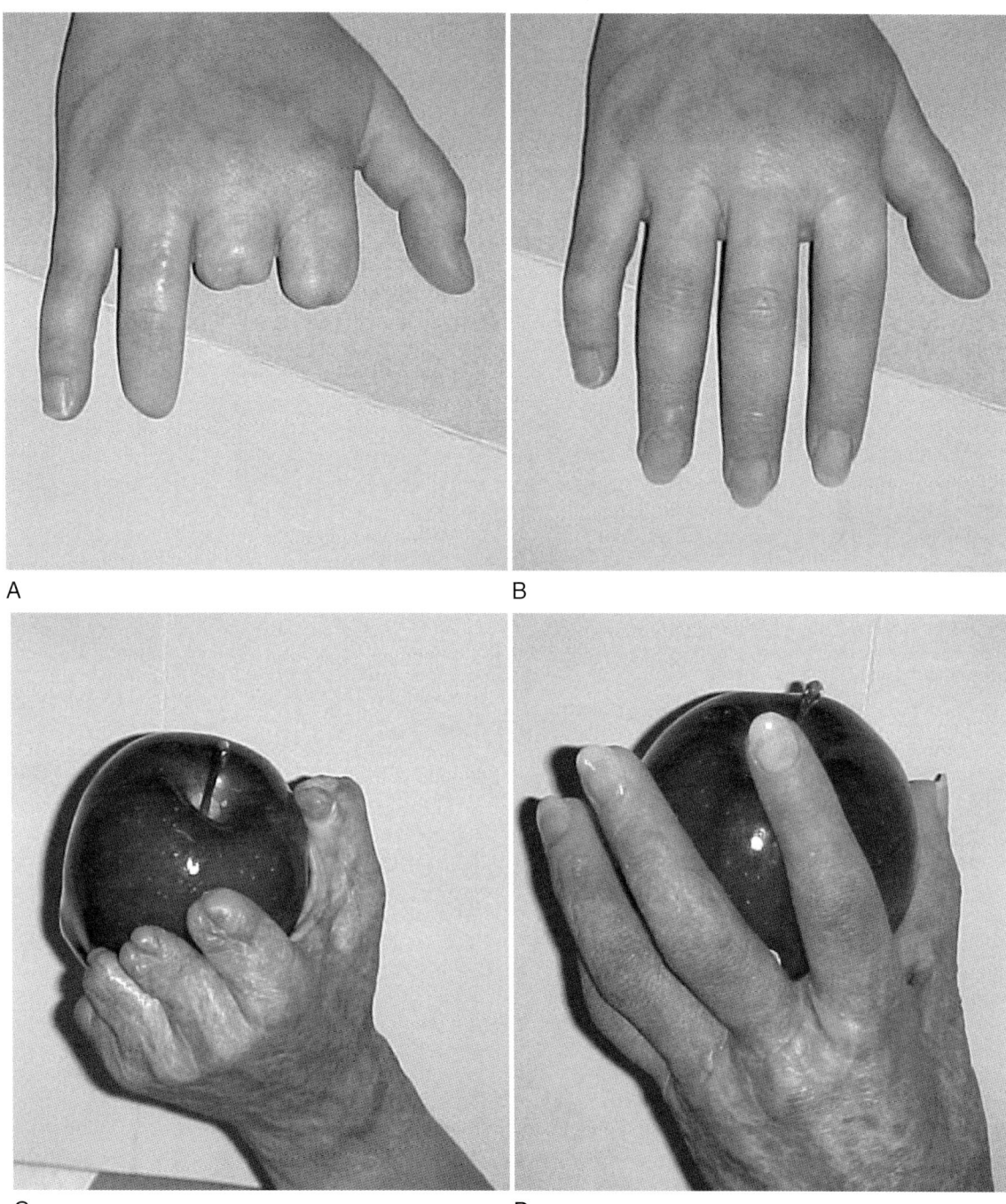

FIGURE 219-9. Patients with amputations of the proximal phalanx shown before (*A* and *C*) and after (*B* and *D*) fitting for a prosthesis.

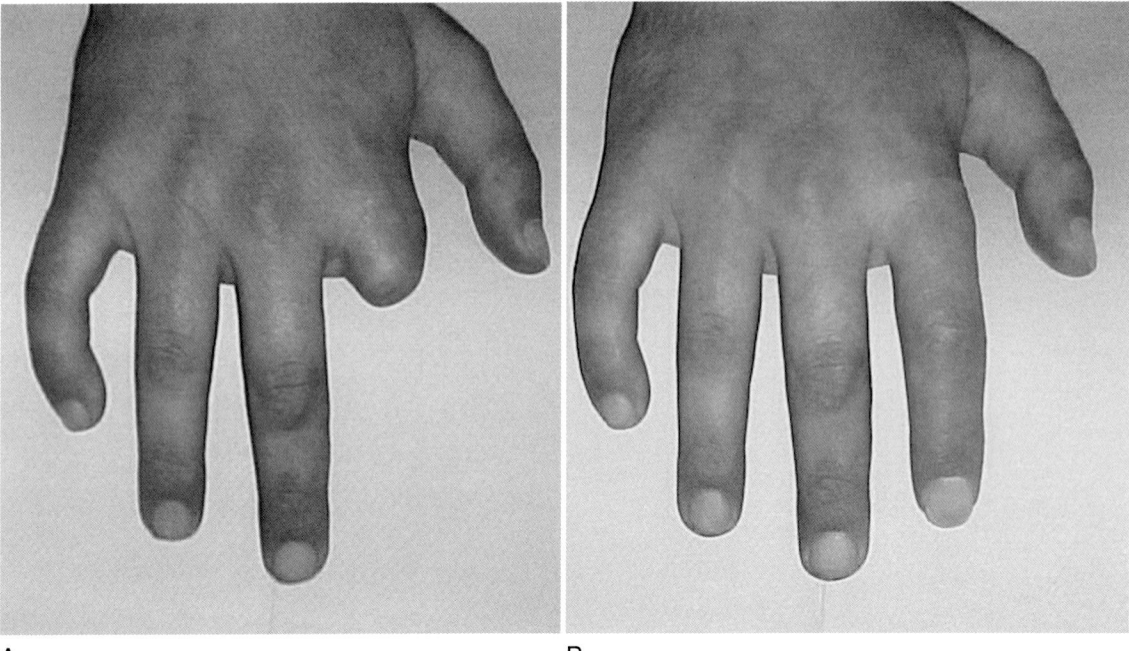

A   B

FIGURE 219-10. *A* and *B,* Patient shown before and after fitting for a prosthesis. Patients with amputations of the proximal phalanx require a stump length of 1.5 cm to ensure adequate attachment. With a short stump, it may be necessary to deepen the commissure.

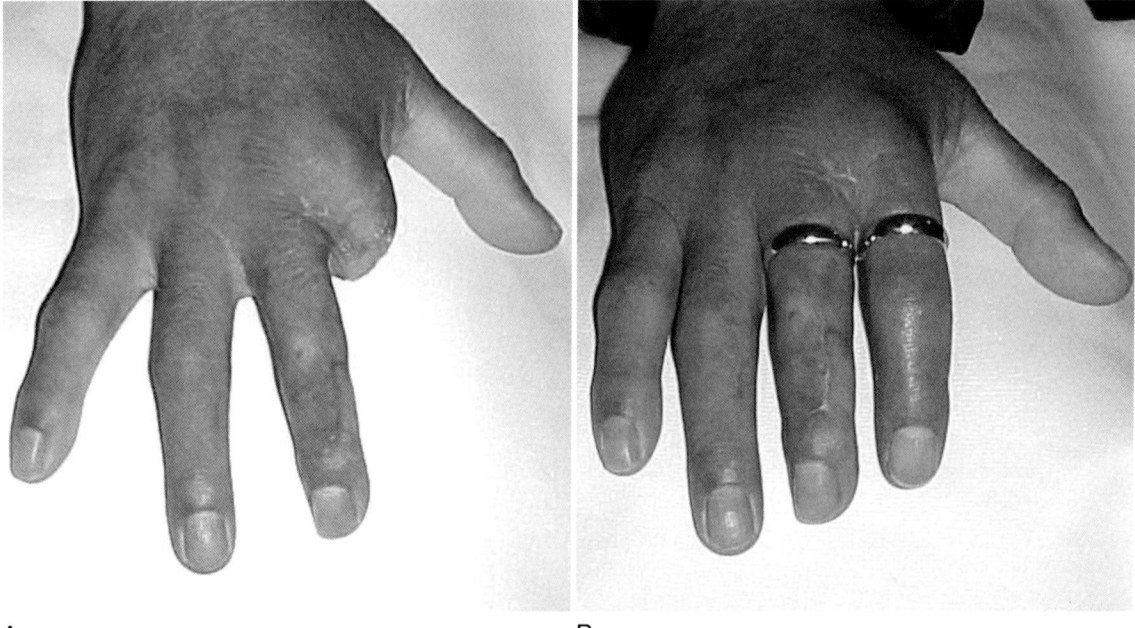

A   B

FIGURE 219-11. *A* and *B,* Patient shown before and after fitting for a prosthesis. Patients with amputations of the proximal phalanx require a stump length of 1.5 cm to ensure adequate attachment. Special ring-based attachment for the prosthesis is shown.

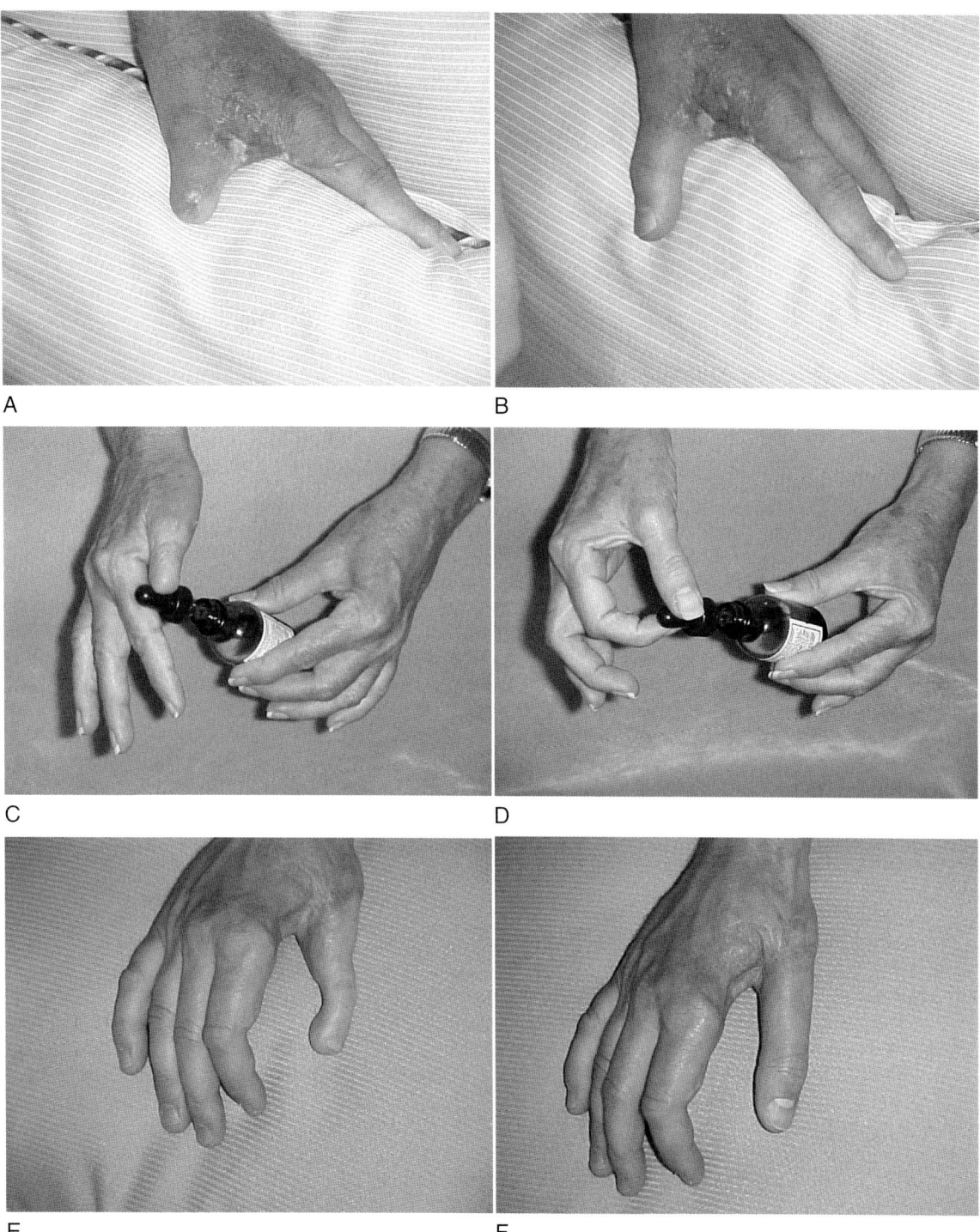

FIGURE 219-12. Patients with thumb amputations are shown before (*A, C,* and *E*) and after (*B, D,* and *F*) fitting for a prosthesis.

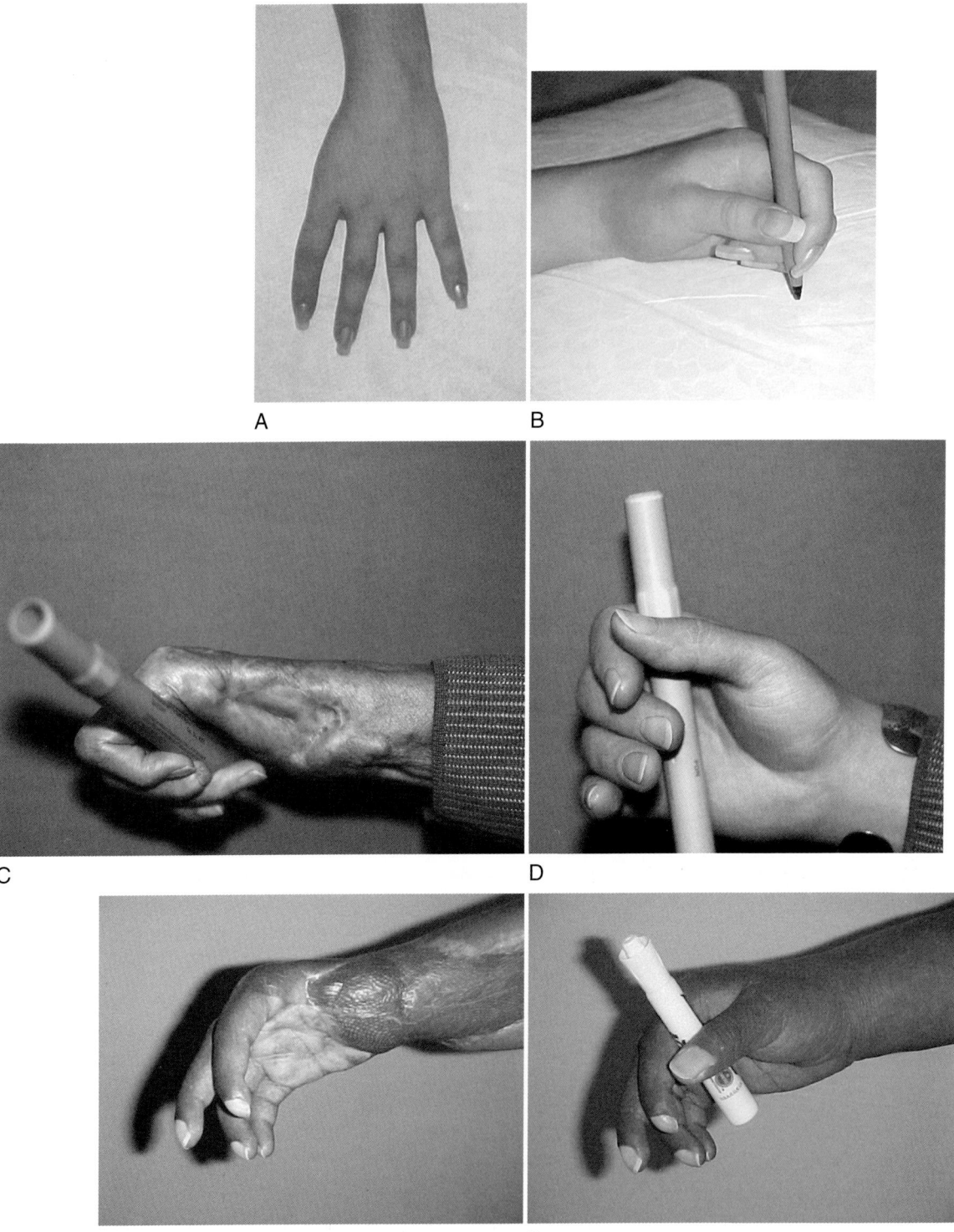

FIGURE 219-13. Carpal-metacarpal disarticulation of the thumb requires a hand prosthesis that leaves healthy fingers outside the prosthesis to preserve the best function possible. Patients are shown before (*A*, *C*, and *E*) and after (*B*, *D*, and *F*) fitting for a prosthesis.

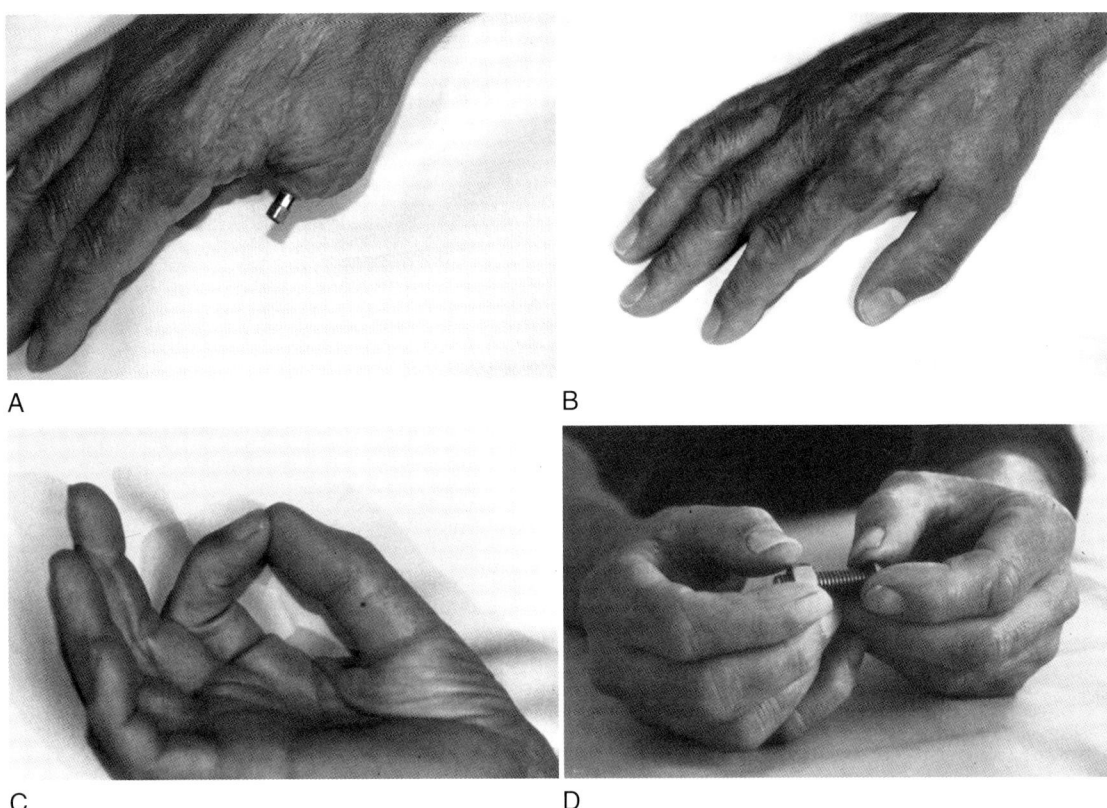

FIGURE 219-14. Patient shown before *(A)* and after *(B to D)* fitting for an osseointegrated prosthesis.

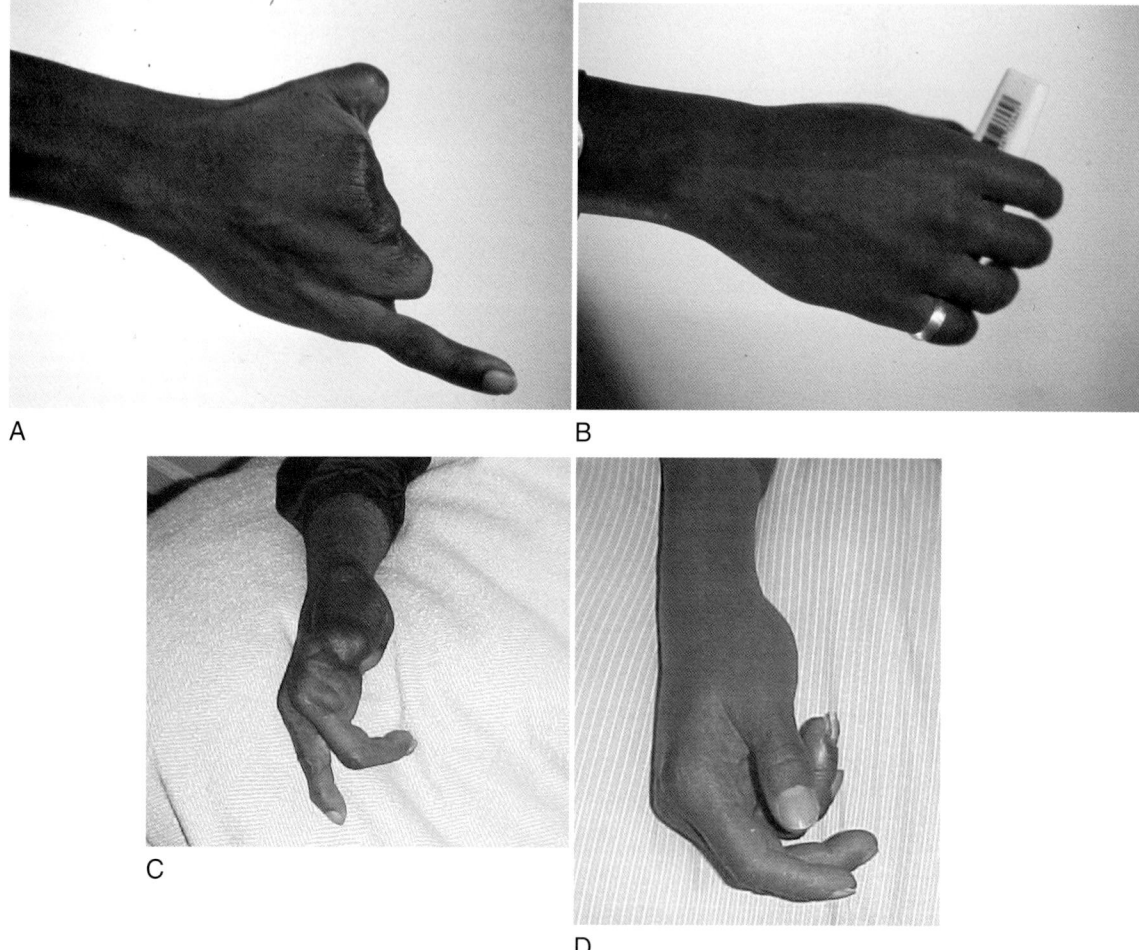

FIGURE 219-15. Patients are shown with multiple metacarpal amputations (*A* and *C*). If the patient's hand is without a thumb, the remaining fingers are placed outside the prosthesis (*B* and *D*).

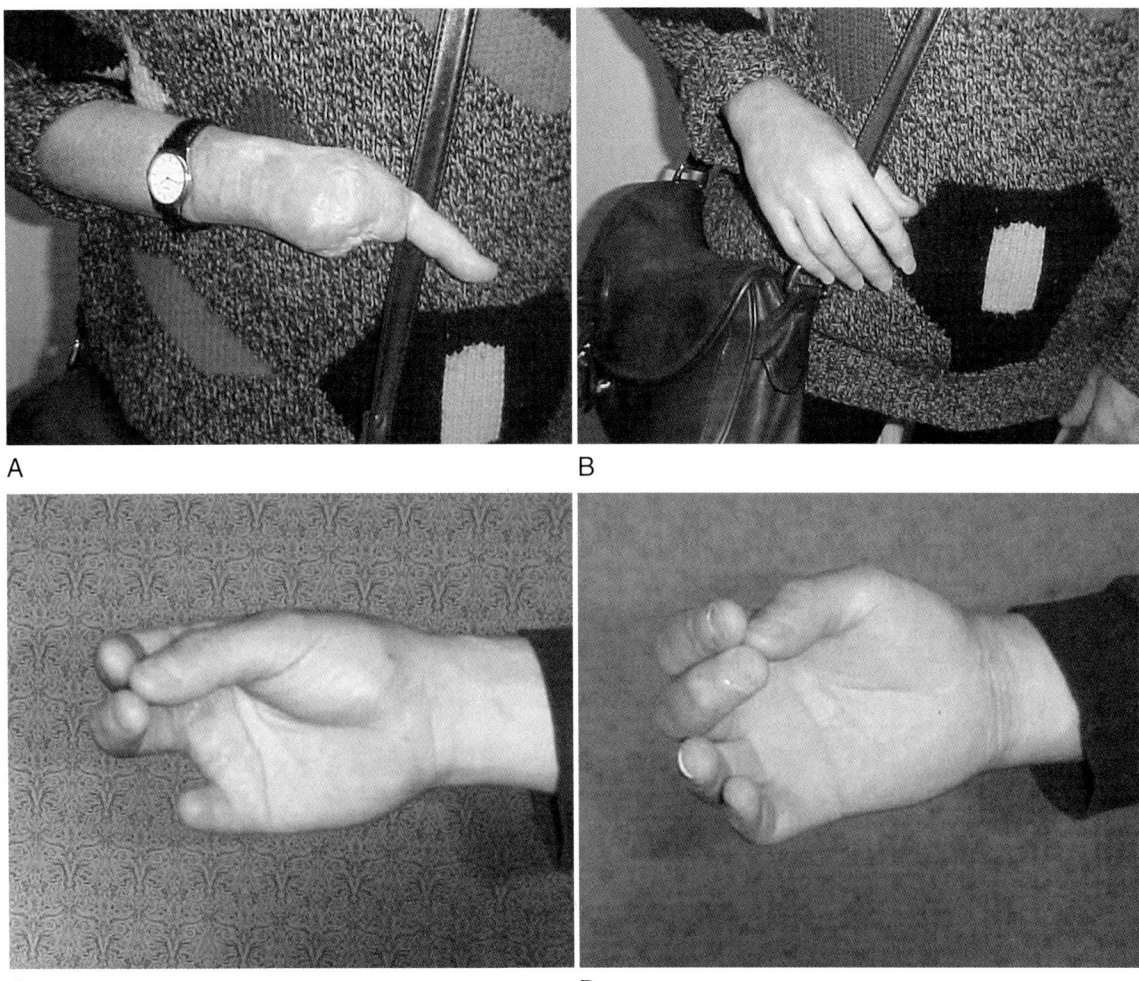

A   B

C   D

FIGURE 219-16. Patients are shown with multiple metacarpal amputations (*A* and *C*). If the patient's thumb is normal, it is left outside the prosthesis (*B* and *D*).

In partial amputations:

- If the hand has kept its anatomic shape, the remaining digital stumps are placed inside the fingers of the prosthesis.
- If the anatomic shape of the hand has been modified by surgical functional reconstructions, the prostheses are difficult to design (Fig. 219-17).

The different solutions must be carefully evaluated, taking into account the needs of the patients, which are also likely to vary.

Total Hand Prostheses

Metacarpal amputations without fingers as well as those of the wrist require a total hand prosthesis (Fig. 219-18). By restoring the hand to its initial length, the prosthesis increases the functional surface of the palm, which will enable the patient to use it as a supporting hand and for grasping objects with both hands. The prosthesis also makes it possible to hold lightweight objects placed between the fingers of the prosthesis thanks to the elastic memory of its components. In the case of carpocarpal and radiocarpal amputations, a total hand prosthesis that ends approximately 4 cm above the cubital styloid must be envisaged. A bracelet, a watch, or, in summer, a tennis band can be worn to cover the delimitation between prosthesis and skin (Fig. 219-19).

Forearm, Arm, and Shoulder Prostheses

Aesthetic prostheses concern only parts of the body that are normally exposed. Disarticulation of the shoulder results in less deformation than scapulothoracic amputation because the shape of the shoulder is preserved. Patients prefer aesthetic prostheses because they are much lighter than functional prostheses. Furthermore, because the shape of the shoulder and arm have been preserved, the aesthetics of dressing are not compromised.

Bilateral Amputees

Fortunately, bilateral amputations, except in the case of fingers, are rare (Fig. 219-20). The physical deficit is so important that it masks—at least initially—aesthetic issues. In the case of congenital amputees, aesthetic prostheses can help to not attract attention and, in some cases, enable them to re-establish more "natural" gestures. Bilateral amputees can be helped by fitting them on one side only with an aesthetic prosthesis, but the need to preserve sensitivity at least on one side means that bilateral prostheses are contraindicated. In the case of acquired amputations

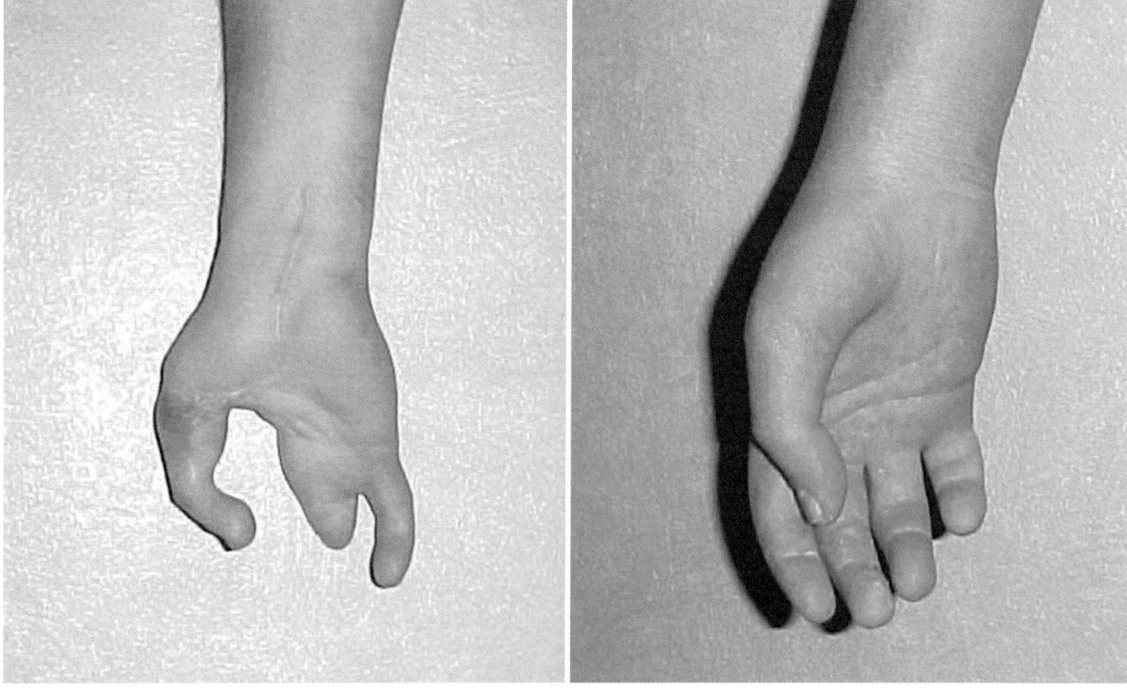

A   B

FIGURE 219-17. *A* and *B,* If the anatomic shape of a patient's hand has been modified by surgical functional reconstructions, prostheses may be difficult to design.

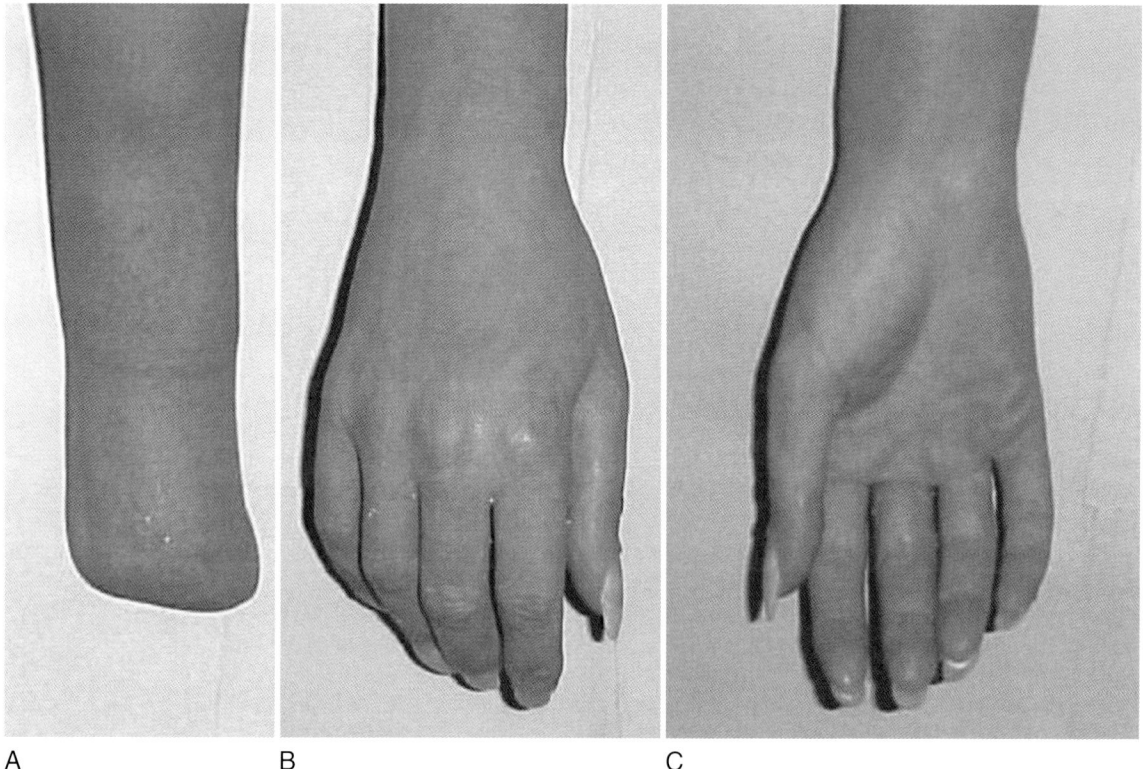

A B C

FIGURE 219-18. Metacarpal amputations without fingers as well as those of the wrist require a total hand prosthesis. Patient is shown without *(A)* and with (*B* and *C*) a total hand prosthesis.

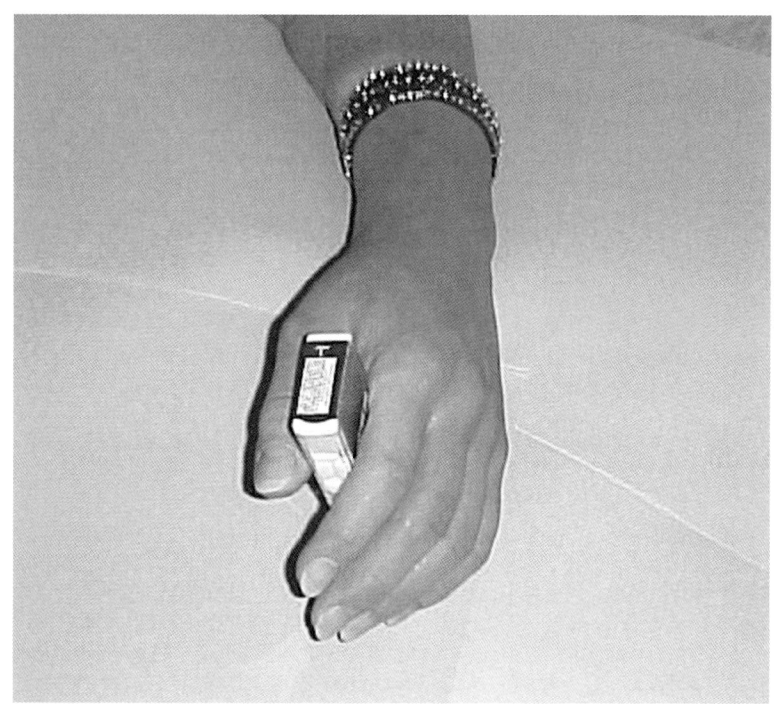

FIGURE 219-19. In the case of carpocarpal and radiocarpal amputations, a total hand prosthesis that ends approximately 4 cm above the cubital styloid is necessary. A bracelet, watch, or tennis band can be worn to cover the delimitation between prosthesis and skin.

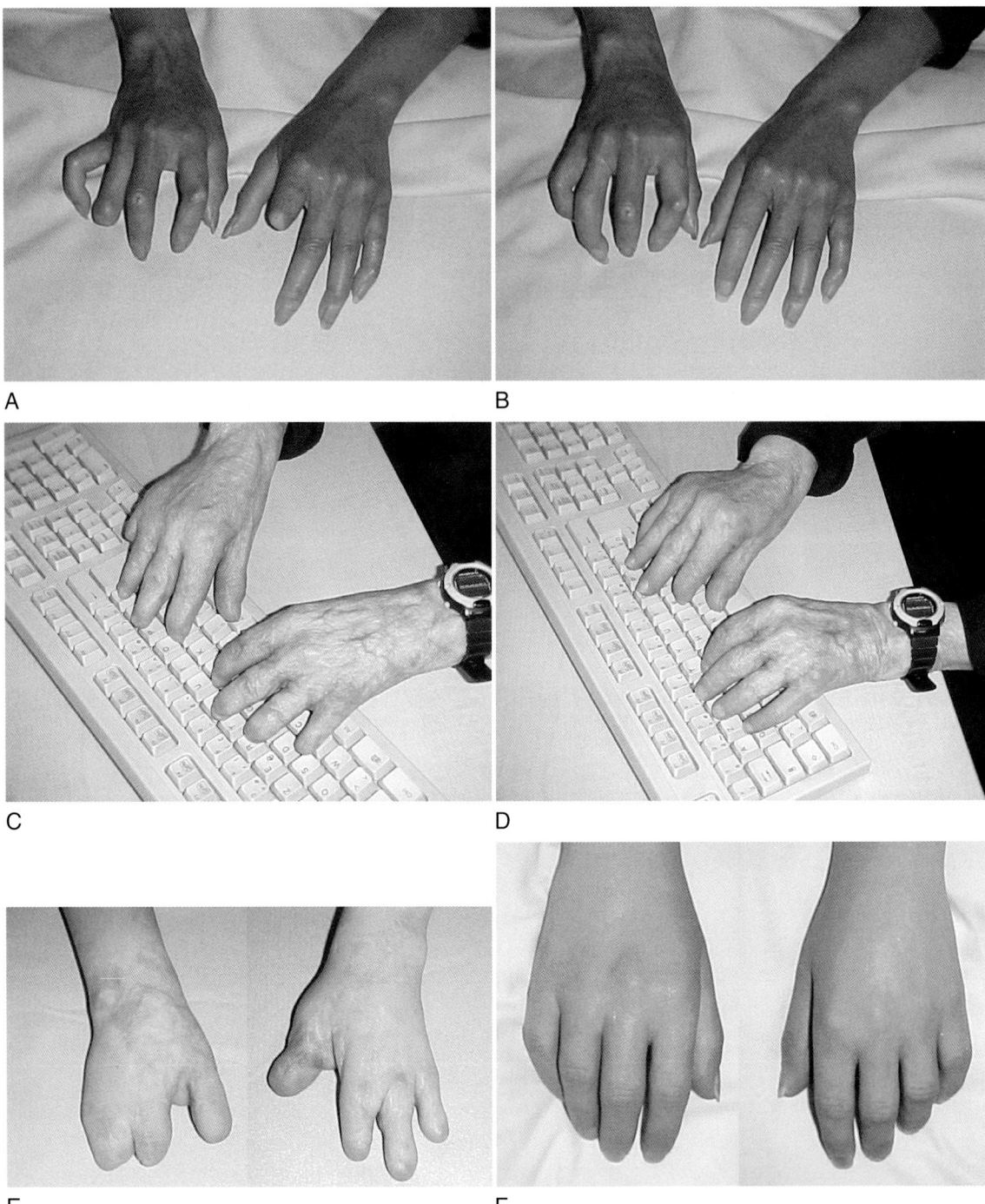

FIGURE 219-20. Patients with bilateral amputations are shown before (*A, C,* and *E*) and after (*B, D,* and *F*) fitting for prostheses.

(traumatic or therapeutic), certain patients, aware of their functional deficit, feel the need to avoid exposing their mutilation. Here, aesthetic prostheses fulfill their role, allowing these patients to re-establish social relations that would have seemed impossible without them.

A patient who had suffered burns in an explosion and had all her fingers partially amputated requested digital prostheses to return to her teaching job. When we explained to her the difficulty of wearing 10 prostheses, she answered that maybe she would not wear them all at the same time, but she would be able to choose which fingers she would wear the prostheses on, depending on her needs and activities. Since then, she uses her prostheses in an adapted manner.

Another example is that of a patient whose right hand and three fingers on the left hand had been amputated. Although she insisted on having a hand prosthesis, she prefers to leave her left hand "free" to maintain the best possible function, especially for writing.

Difficult Cases

Function, yes, but at what price? Some patients may insist on being fitted with a prosthesis, although it is obvious it will lead to discomfort and even reduced function. Loss of articulation in several fingers at metacarpal joint level means that the prosthesis must cover the entire hand, and trophic disorders will make it difficult to bear. Off-centered digital stumps almost always result in unsightly prostheses (Fig. 219-21). In these instances, patients should be advised against a prosthesis unless psychological indications prevail over

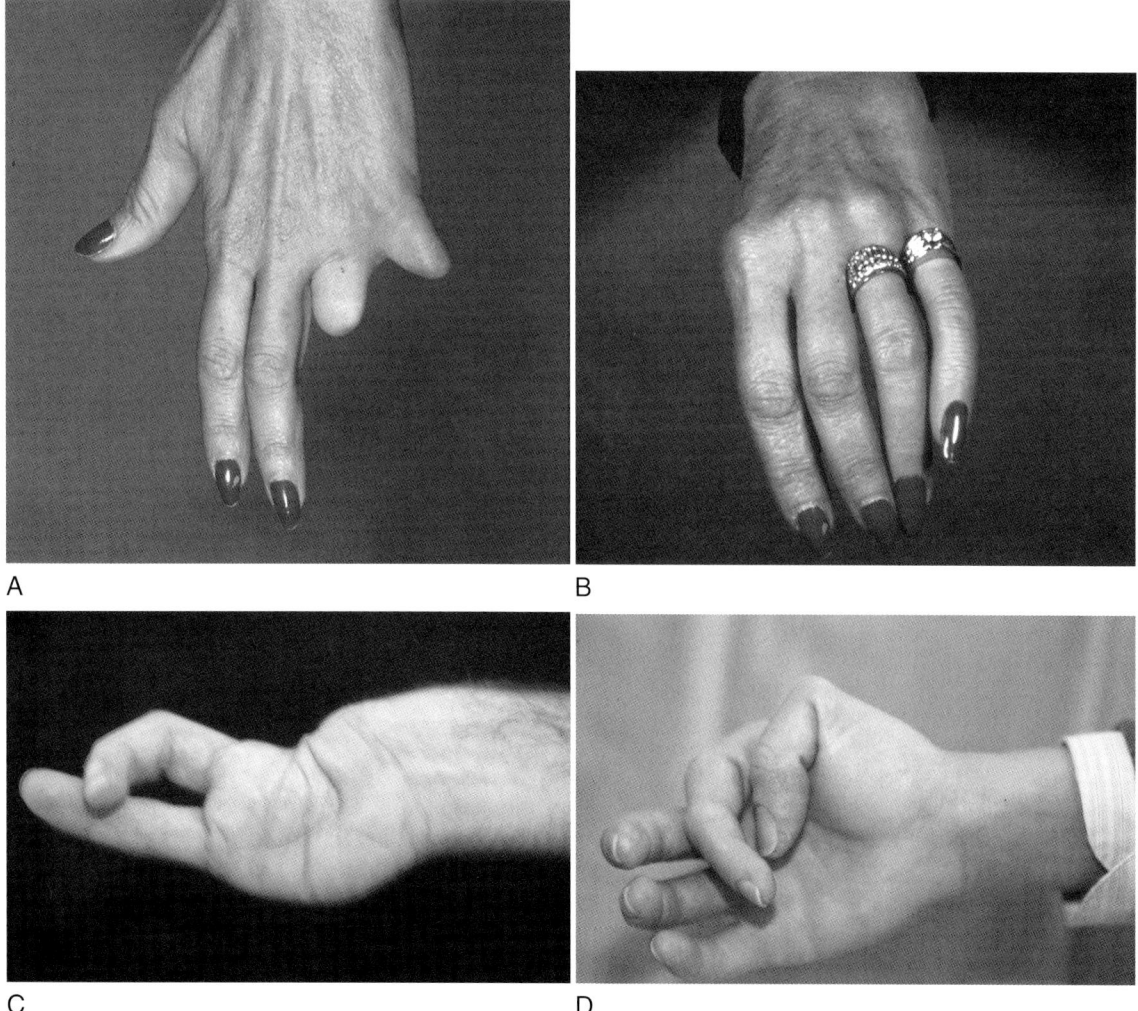

A

B

C

D

FIGURE 219-21. *A* to *D,* Off-center digital stumps almost always result in unsightly prostheses.

the drawbacks. Amputee patients must understand that a prosthesis is not a panacea.

Patients who have undergone a surgical procedure with sequelae perceived as mutilating may be difficult to fit with an adequate prosthesis. However, some patients cannot bear to see a mutilated hand or arm, or even foot (toe transplant). They will hide it, and the potential function may be underused (Figs. 219-22 to 219-24).[8]

CONTRAINDICATIONS TO AESTHETIC PROSTHESES

An absolute contraindication to wearing a prosthesis is lack of motivation or unrealistic expectations. For some patients, suitability of fitting is at the very limits of indications. Even with fairly long stumps, ensuring sound attachment, several digital prostheses on one single hand will reduce its sensitivity. When the stumps are voluminous or poorly aligned, it might prove impossible to achieve aesthetically satisfactory prostheses without the patient's undergoing a preliminary surgical alteration. Any prosthesis that does not correspond to the patient's specific needs is a contraindication because it will not fulfill expectations. This person would be dissatisfied and psychologically wounded. This trauma would be added to the trauma related to the acquired amputation or congenital malformation.

Such an experience is never without psychological repercussions. Wearing one's prosthesis all the time or putting it on selectively, even giving up wearing it altogether, is not really an issue in itself if the choice to do so is made freely. But this is very different from the case of a disappointed patient who realizes that even if the prosthesis can enable escape from the attention of others, it never can give back what was lost or offer what the patient never had.

LONG-TERM RESULTS

A review of our patients revealed a high percentage of continued use of their aesthetic prostheses in general. This may in part reflect considerable selectivity in patients fitted, those without strong motivation usually being detected and rejected at the outset. All were unilateral amputees. Most of the patients were found to fall into a well-adjusted group, which in turn could be subdivided into two subgroups. Some put on their prostheses each morning and removed them only for sleep, making the devices much a part of themselves. Others treated their prostheses much like a piece of clothing, wearing them regularly when out of the home but removing them frequently within the confines of the family circle.

A small number were found to have established peculiar attitudes toward their prostheses, but all still had a need for them. A few wore their prostheses day and night, removing them only for skin care. Others kept them available but in fact wore them only rarely— for special occasions such as holiday celebrations or family events. A very small group never wore their prostheses but refused to give them up, keeping them within reach "in case of emergency."

There seems to be little difference in use between patients with traumatic amputations and patients with congenital amputations. The highest satisfaction was in the age bracket between 15 and 40 years. The quality of the prosthesis was a major factor, as could be expected, because of its purpose being primarily aesthetic.

Finally, if the prosthesis is set aside, that may not imply that it failed but rather substantiate the excellent effect of the psychological treatment. The patient gives up the prosthesis because he or she has returned to a normal life. Having been "cured," he or she no longer requires taking the medicine and so just stops. The prosthesis has simply helped the individual come through a difficult period of life.

For the results concerning wearing of prostheses to be significant, the patient must have been fitted for at least 5 years. In reviewing 1000 of our patients fitted for at least 5 years[6] and—in the case of the patient seen for the longest time—up to 45 years, we noted the following:

- 82% of trauma-related amputees do not remove their prosthesis at work.
- Therapeutic amputees are the patients who remove their prosthesis the least. They keep it on for social activities (100%) as well as for work (93%) or at home.
- Patients with congenital anomalies wear their prosthesis for social and professional activities (95%) and remove it at home (60%).

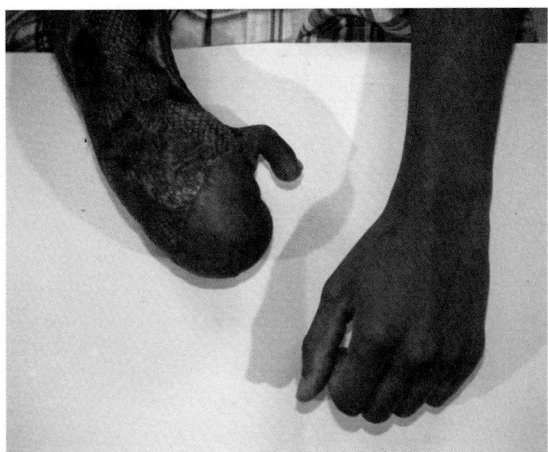

FIGURE 219-22. Patient with stump that may be difficult to fit for a functional, aesthetic prosthesis.

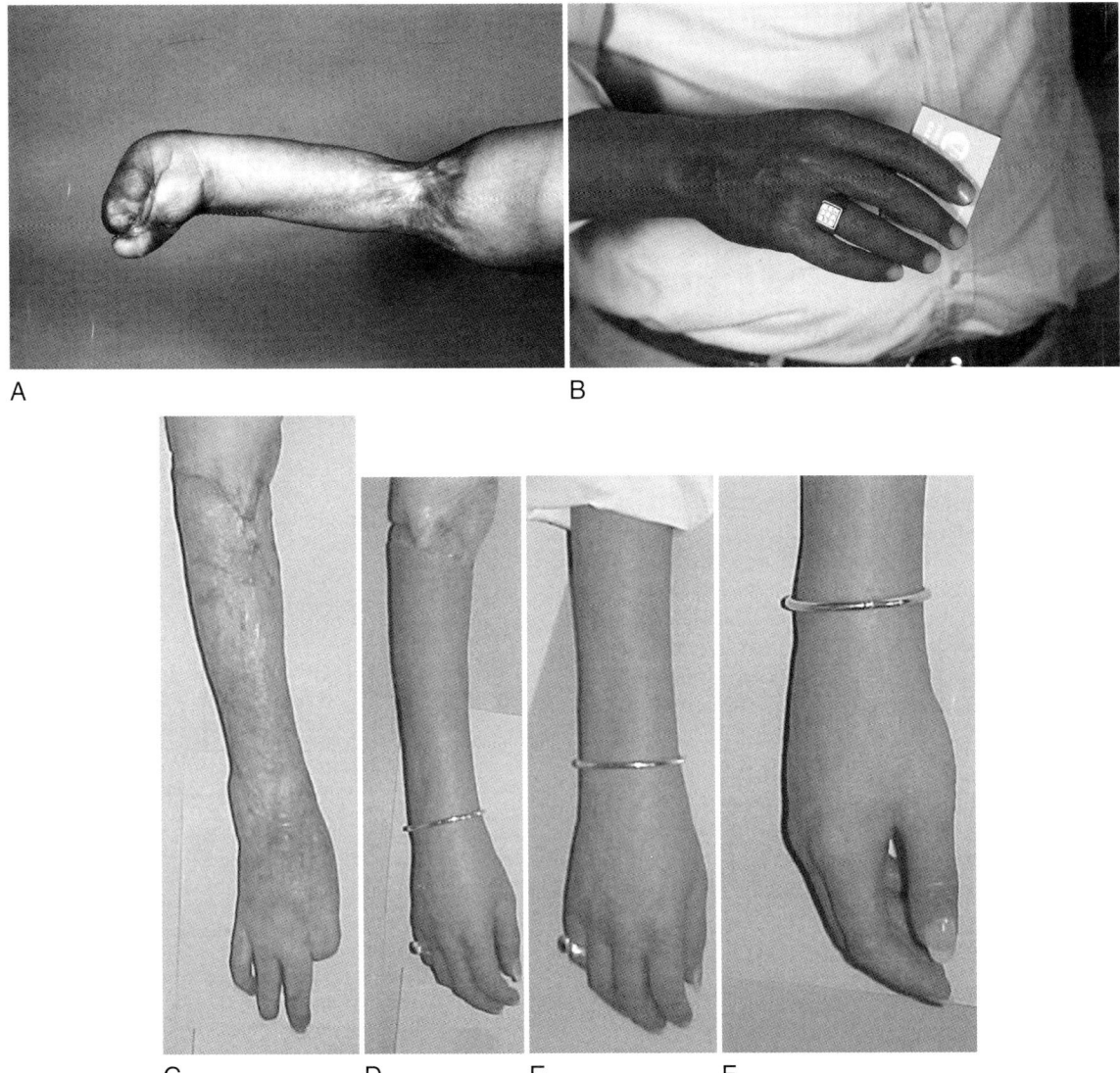

FIGURE 219-23. Two patients who presented with stumps difficult to fit with prostheses (*A, C,* and *D*). Patients with prostheses in place (*B, E,* and *F*).

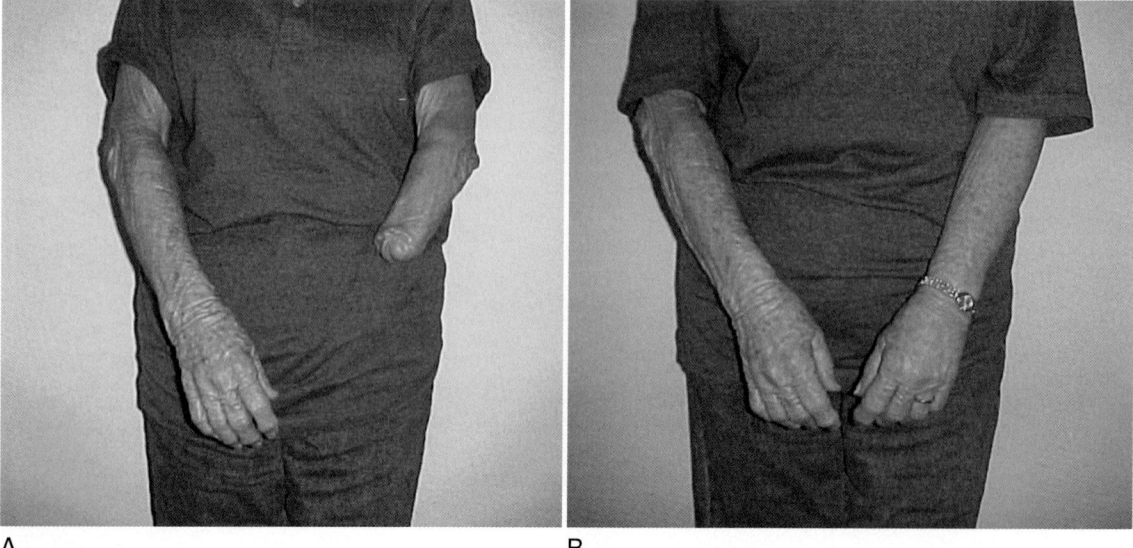

A   B

FIGURE 219-24. *A,* Elderly patients may be difficult to fit for aesthetic prostheses. *B,* Elderly patient shown with prosthesis in place.

CONCLUSION

A prosthesis cannot be reduced to a simple "covering" because each individual's demand is motivated by discomfort or even by distress. Between aesthetic prostheses and prostheses designed for life in society, we find that function and appearance cannot be dissociated. This is why the passive function of the prosthesis is so important. Gestures become, once again, more natural. Today, few would sacrifice appearance for function.

- The prosthesis is an enabler of function by treating appearance, pain, and suffering.
- It is information of first recourse. It is important for patients to be told rapidly of this possible opportunity to help them face the eyes of others and their own.
- It is a procedure of last recourse.

Physiologically and psychologically, aesthetic prosthetics cannot be an emergency response. It treats the temporary and permanent sequelae of a complex trauma. It participates in a dynamic process and thus must evolve over time, according to the physical and psychological needs of patients. The prosthesis can help overcome a difficult stage in life and be used as a temporary or long-term treatment, whether it is worn or not. This implies two qualities: aesthetic qualities, making it possible to avoid attracting attention; and the quality of comfort, making it possible to forget it.

Very demanding in terms of design and indications, an aesthetic prosthesis can contribute to alleviation of the suffering of individuals and can be conceived of only as fulfilling its social role.

REFERENCES

1. Didierjean A, Pillet J, Foucher G: L'éphémère de la beauté. Société française de chirurgie plastique reconstructrice et esthétique, Paris, Octobre 21-23, 1998.
2. Pillet J, Didierjean-Pillet A: Les prothèses unguéales. In Dumontier C: La réadaptation de la main. Paris, Elsevier, 2000. Monographie de la Société française de chirurgie de la main, 27.
3. Pillet J: Esthetic prostheses. In Gupta A, Kay SPJ, Scheker LR, eds: The Growing Hand: Diagnosis and Management of the Upper Extremity in Children. London, Mosby, 2000:1079-1090.
4. Pillet J: Aesthetic prostheses. In Buncke HJ, ed: Microsurgery: Transplantation-Replantation: An Atlas-Text. Philadelphia, Lea & Febiger, 1991:760-765.
5. Pillet J, Didierjean-Pillet A: Aesthetic hand prosthesis: gadget or therapy? Presentation of a new classification. J Hand Surg Br 2001;26:523-528.
6. Pillet J, Mackin E: Aesthetic hand prosthesis—its psychological and functional potential. In Hunter JM, Mackin EJ, Callahan AD, eds: Rehabilitation of the Hand, 5th ed. St. Louis, Mosby-Year Book, 2001:1461-1472.
7. Pillet J, Mackin E: Aesthetic restoration. In Bowker JH, Michael JW, eds: Atlas of Limb Prosthetics: Surgical, Prosthetic and Rehabilitation Principles, 2nd ed. St Louis, Mosby-Year Book, 1992:227-235.
8. Pillet J: Digital and hand prosthetic fitting. In Urbaniak J, ed: Microsurgery for Major Limb Reconstruction. St. Louis, CV Mosby, 1987;46-50.

Index

Note: **Boldface** roman numerals indicate volume. Page numbers followed by f refer to figures; page numbers followed by t refer to tables.